SECOND EDITION

Pediatric Primary Care: A Problem-Oriented Approach

Editor-in-Chief

M. William Schwartz, M.D.
Professor of Pediatrics
Department of Pediatrics
University of Pennsylvania
Senior Physician
The Children's Hospital of Philadelphia
Philadelphia, Pennsylvania

Associate Editors

Edward B. Charney, M.D.
Associate Professor of Pediatrics
University of Pennsylvania
Senior Physician
Division of Child Development and Rehabilitation
The Children's Seashore House
The Children's Hospital of Philadelphia
Philadelphia, Pennsylvania

Thomas A. Curry, M.D.
Private Practice
Schuylkill Pediatrics
Pottsville, Pennsylvania

Stephen Ludwig, M.D.
Professor of Pediatrics
University of Pennsylvania
Division Chief
General Pediatrics
The Children's Hospital of Philadelphia
Philadelphia, Pennsylvania

YEAR BOOK MEDICAL PUBLISHERS, INC.
CHICAGO • LONDON • BOCA RATON • LITTLETON, MASS.

2 3 4 5 6 7 8 9 0 CY 94 93 92 91 90

Library of Congress Cataloging-in-Publication Data

Pediatric primary care: a problem-oriented approach/M. William Schwartz . . . [et al.]—2nd ed.
p. cm.
Rev. ed. of: Principles and practice of clinical pediatrics/ editor, M. William Schwartz. c1987.
Includes bibliographical references.
ISBN 0-8151-7733-X
1. Pediatrics. 2. Family medicine. I. Schwartz, William, 1935- . II. Principles and practice of clinical pediatrics.
[DNLM: 1. Pediatrics. 2. Primary Health Care—methods. WS 100 P3653]
RJ47.P39 1990
618.92–dc20
DNLM/DLC 89-22577
for Library of Congress CIP

Sponsoring Editors: Nancy E. Chorpenning, Kevin M. Kelly
Assistant Managing Editor, Text and Reference Books: Jan Gardner
Production Project Coordinator: Karen Halm
Proofroom Supervisor: Barbara M. Kelly

Second Edition

PEDIATRIC PRIMARY CARE: A PROBLEM-ORIENTED APPROACH

To our families:

Susan, David, Charlie, Burtie, and Sloan
Linda, Laura, and Rebecca
Anne, Thomas, Brigid, and Helen
Zella, Susannah, Elisa, and Aubrey

and our mentor:

David Cornfeld, M.D.

CONTRIBUTORS

James L. Ackerman, D.D.S.
Senior Dentist
The Children's Hospital of Philadelphia
Philadelphia, Pennsylvania

David Alexander, M.D.
Assistant Professor of Pediatrics
University of Pennsylvania School of Medicine
Medical Director
The Children's Hospital of Philadelphia
Philadelphia, Pennsylvania

Herbert B. Allen, M.D.
Clinical Associate Professor of Dermatology
University of Pennsylvania
Philadelphia, Pennsylvania

Steven Altschuler, M.D.
Assistant Professor of Pediatrics
University of Pennsylvania School of Medicine
Division of Gastroenterology and Nutrition
The Children's Hospital of Philadelphia
Philadelphia, Pennsylvania

Robert Anolik, M.D.
Clinical Assistant Professor
University of Medicine and Dentistry of New Jersey
Clinical Instructor
Division of Allergy, Immunology and Bone Marrow Transplantation
The Children's Hospital of Philadelphia
Philadelphia, Pennsylvania

Balu H. Athreya, M.D.
Professor of Pediatrics
University of Pennsylvania School of Medicine
Clinical Director
The Children's Seashore House
Philadelphia, Pennsylvania

Jeffrey R. Avner, M.D.
Instructor in Pediatrics
University of Pennsylvania School of Medicine
Fellow, Pediatric Emergency Medicine
The Children's Hospital of Philadelphia
Philadelphia, Pennsylvania

Thomas Beausang, M.D.
Private Practice
Schuylkill Pediatrics
Pottsville, Pennsylvania

Louis M. Bell, M.D.
Assistant Professor of Pediatrics
University of Pennsylvania
Attending Physician
The Children's Hospital of Philadelphia
Philadelphia, Pennsylvania

Henry Berger, M.D.
Assistant Clinical Professor
University of Pennsylvania
Staff Psychiatrist
Pennsylvania Hospital
Philadelphia, Pennsylvania

Judy C. Bernbaum, M.D.
Associate Professor of Pediatrics
University of Pennsylvania School of Medicine
Director, Neonatal Follow Up Program
The Children's Hospital of Philadelphia
Philadelphia, Pennsylvania

Douglas Boenning, M.D.
Associate Director for Research
Emergency Medical Trauma Center
Children's National Medical Center
Washington, D.C.

John T. Boyle, M.D.
Associate Professor of Pediatrics
Case Western Reserve University School of Medicine
Chief, Division of Gastroenterology and Nutrition
Rainbow Babies and Childrens Hospital
Cleveland, Ohio

Karen Bringelsen, M.D.
Assistant Professor of Pediatrics
Department of Pediatrics
University of Virginia Health Sciences Center
Division of Hematology and Oncology
Children's Medical Center of the University of Virginia Health Sciences Center
Charlottesville, Virginia

Jose F. Cara, M.D.
Assistant Professor
University of Chicago
Attending Physician
Wyler Children's Hospital
Chicago, Illinois

Carol Carraccio, M.D.
Assistant Professor of Pediatrics
University of Maryland
Director, Resident Education
University of Maryland Medical Systems
Baltimore, Maryland

Rosemary Casey, M.D.
Clinical Associate Professor of Pediatrics
University of Pennsylvania School of Medicine
Associate Physician
The Children's Hospital of Philadelphia
Philadelphia, Pennsylvania

Edwin F. Castillo, M.D.
Clinical Associate
University of Pennsylvania
Clinical Associate
Philadelphia Child Guidance Clinic
The Children's Hospital of Pennsylvania
Philadelphia, Pennsylvania

Anthony C. Chang, M.D.
Instructor of Pediatrics
University of Pennsylvania School of Medicine
Instructor of Pediatrics
The Children's Hospital of Philadelphia
Philadelphia, Pennsylvania

Edward B. Charney, M.D.
Associate Professor of Pediatrics
University of Pennsylvania School of Medicine
Senior Physician
Division of Child Development and Rehabilitation
The Children's Seashore House
Philadelphia, Pennsylvania

Robert Ryan Clancy, M.D.
Associate Professor of Neurology and Pediatrics
University of Pennsylvania School of Medicine
Attending Neurologist and Director of Clinical Neurophysiology
The Children's Hospital of Philadelphia
Philadelphia, Pennsylvania

Bernard J. Clark III, M.D.
Assistant Professor of Pediatrics
Department of Pediatrics
University of Pennsylvania School of Medicine
Staff Cardiologist
The Children's Hospital of Philadelphia
Philadelphia, Pennsylvania

Mary Ellen Conley, M.D.
Professor of Pediatrics
University of Tennessee College of Medicine
St. Jude Children's Research Hospital
Memphis, Tennessee

Thomas Curry, M.D.
Private Practice
Schuylkill Pediatrics
Pottsville, Pennsylvania

Gary C. Cupit, Pharm.D.
Associate Professor and Vice Chairman for Academic Affairs
Department of Clinical Pharmacy
College of Pharmacy
University of Tennessee Center for the Health Sciences
Memphis, Tennessee

Jo Ann D'Agostino, R.N.
Nurse Coordinator
Neonatal Follow-Up Program
The Children's Hospital of Philadelphia
Philadelphia, Pennsylvania

A. Todd Davis, MD.
Professor of Pediatrics
Northwestern University Medical School
Chicago, Illinois

Margaret Delaney, M.D.
Assistant Professor of Health Care Sciences
George Washington University School of Medicine
Staff Physician
George Washington University Health Plan
Washington, D.C.

Gary R. Diamond, M.D.
Associate Professor of Ophthalmology and Pediatrics
Hahnemann University
Clinical Associate
The Children's Hospital of Philadelphia
Philadelphia, Pennsylvania

Robert Doughty, M.D., Ph.D.
Medical Director
Dupont Institute
Wilmington, Delaware

Andrew Eichenfield, M.D.
Associate Professor of Pediatrics
The Mount Sinai School of Medicine
Chief, Division of Pediatric Rheumatology
The Mount Sinai Hospital
New York, New York

Deborah L. Eunpu, M.S.
Instructor, Pediatrics
Temple University School of Medicine
Director, Genetic Counseling
Albert Einstein Medical Center
Philadelphia, Pennsylvania

Anne C. Farran, M.A.
Social Worker
Neonatal Follow-Up Program
The Children's Hospital of Philadelphia
Philadelphia, Pennsylvania

Maureen A. Fee, M.D.
Assistant Professor of Pediatrics
Temple University School of Medicine
Developmental and Behavioral Pediatrics
St. Christopher's Hospital for Children
Philadelphia, Pennsylvania

Maxine Field, Ph.D
Lecturer, Graduate School of Education
University of Pennsylvania
Philadelphia, Pennsylvania

Jonathan A. Flick, M.D.
Assistant Professor of Pediatrics
The Johns Hopkins University School of Medicine
Attending Physician
The Johns Hopkins Hospital
Baltimore, Maryland

John W. Foreman, M.D.
Associate Professor of Pediatrics
Medical College of Virginia
Medical College of Virginia Hospitals
Richmond, Virginia

Sidney Friedman, M.D.
Professor of Pediatrics
University of Pennsylvania School of Medicine
Senior Cardiologist
The Children's Hospital of Philadelphia
Philadelphia, Pennsylvania

Gertrude J. Frishmuth, M.D.
Associate Professor of Obstetrics and Gynecology
The Medical College of Pennsylvania
Assistant Surgeon (Gynecology)
The Children's Hospital of Philadelphia
Philadelphia, Pennsylvania

Ralph C. Gallo, M.D.
Assistant Physician
The Children's Hospital of Pennsylvania
Philadelphia, Pennsylvania

William Gianfagna, M.D.
Private Practice
Schuylkill Pediatrics
Pottsville, Pennsylvania

Frances M. Gill, M.D., M.P.H.
Associate Professor of Pediatrics
Department of Pediatrics
University of Pennsylvania School of Medicine
Senior Physician
The Children's Hospital of Philadelphia
Philadelphia, Pennsylvania

Linda Gordon, M.D.
Consultant in Child Psychiatry
Medical Center of Delaware
Wilmington, Delaware

Lawrence Hammer, M.D.
Assistant Professor of Pediatrics
Stanford University School of Medicine
Director, Ambulatory Care
Children's Hospital at Stanford
Palo Alto, California

Gordon R. Hodas, M.D.
Clinical Associate Professor of Psychiatry
University of Pennsylvania School of Medicine
Consultant Psychiatrist
Philadelphia Child Guidance Clinic
Philadelphia, Pennsylvania

Dee Hodge III, M.D.
Assistant Professor of Pediatrics and Emergency Medicine
University of Southern California
Director, Pediatric Emergency Room
Los Angeles County–USC Medical Center
Los Angeles, California

Marsha Hoffman-Williamson, Ph.D
Developmental Psychologist
Neonatal Follow-Up Program
The Children's Hospital of Philadelphia
Philadelphia, Pennsylvania

Paul J. Honig, M.D.
Professor of Pediatrics and Dermatology
University of Pennsylvania School of Medicine
Director of Pediatric Dermatology
The Children's Hospital of Philadelphia
Philadelphia, Pennsylvania

Helen M. Horstmann, M.D.
Associate Professor of Orthopedic Surgery
Medical College of Pennsylvania
Associate Surgeon
The Children's Hospital of Philadelphia
Philadelphia, Pennsylvania

David Jaffe, M.D.
Associate Professor of Pediatrics
Director of Emergency Department
The Hospital for Sick Children
Toronto, Ontario, Canada

Nancy L. Kashlak, R.N., P.N.P./O.
Certified Pediatric Nurse Practitioner–Oncology
Department of Pediatrics
University of Virginia Health Sciences Center
Division of Hematology–Oncology
Children's Medical Center of the University of Virginia Health Sciences Center
Charlottesville, Virginia

Richard I. Kelley, M.D., Ph.D
Assistant Professor of Pediatrics
The Johns Hopkins University School of Medicine
Staff Pediatrician
The Kennedy Institute
Baltimore, Maryland

Thomas L. Kennedy III, M.D.
Associate Professor of Clinical Pediatrics
Yale School of Medicine
Chairman, Department of Pediatrics
Bridgeport Hospital
New Haven, Connecticut

Brent King, M.D.
Instructor in Pediatrics
University of Pennsylvania School of Medicine
Fellow, Pediatric Emergency Medicine
The Children's Hospital of Philadelphia
Philadelphia, Pennsylvania

Dan F. Konkle, Ph.D.
Associate Professor of Audiology
Department of Otorhinolaryngology and Human Communications
University of Pennsylvania School of Medicine
Director, Department of Communication Disorders
The Children's Seashore House
Philadelphia, Pennsylvania

Stephen D. Kronwith, M.D., Ph.D.
Assistant Clinical Professor
Albert Einstein College of Medicine
Attending Physician
Montefiore Medical Center
New York, New York

Beverly Lange, M.D.
Associate Professor of Pediatrics
Director of Clinical Oncology
The Children's Hospital of Philadelphia
Philadelphia, Pennsylvania

Don LaRossa, M.D.
Associate Professor of Surgery (Plastic)
University of Pennsylvania School of Medicine
Director Cleft Lip and Palate Program
The Children's Hospital of Philadelphia
Philadelphia, Pennsylvania

Donna Lechner-Guskay, M.S., R.D.
Graduate Student
Hospital Administration
Yale University
New Haven, Connecticut

Mary M. Lee, M.D.
Research Fellow
Harvard Medical School
Research Fellow in Surgery and Pediatrics
Massachusetts General Hospital
Boston, Massachusetts

Susan E. Levy, M.D.
Assistant Professor of Pediatrics
University of Pennsylvania School of Medicine
Assistant Physician
The Children's Seashore House
The Children's Hospital of Philadelphia
Philadelphia, Pennsylvania

Stephen Ludwig, M.D.
Professor of Pediatrics
University of Pennsylvania School of Medicine
Division Chief, General Pediatrics
The Children's Hospital of Philadelphia
Philadelphia, Pennsylvania

Gary S. Marshall, M.D.
Assistant Professor of Pediatrics
University of Louisville School of Medicine
Attending Physician
Kosair-Children's Hospital
Louisville, Kentucky

Barry S. Marx, M.D.
Instructor in Pediatrics
Department of Pediatrics
The John Hopkins University
Baltimore, Maryland

Marie C. McCormick, M.D., Sc.D.
Associate Professor of Pediatrics
Joint Program in Neonatology
Harvard Medical School
Senior Associate in Pediatrics
Brigham and Women's Hospital
The Children's Hospital
Boston, Massachusetts

James E. McJunkin, M.D.
Chairman, Department of Pediatrics
West Virginia University at Charleston
Chairman, Department of Pediatrics
Charleston Area Medical Center
Charleston, West Virginia

Steven E. McKenzie, M.D., Ph.D.
University of Pennsylvania School of Medicine
Fellow, Division of Hematology and Oncology
The Children's Hospital of Philadelphia
Philadelphia, Pennsylvania

Marianne Mercugliano, M.D.
Clinical Fellow
Child Development and Rehabilitation
The Children's Seashore House
The Children's Hospital of Philadelphia
Department of Pediatrics
University of Pennsylvania
Philadelphia, Pennsylvania

Thomas Moshang, Jr., M.D.
Professor of Pediatrics
Department of Pediatrics
University of Pennsylvania
Senior Physician
Director of Endocrine Training Program
The Children's Hospital of Philadelphia
Philadelphia, Pennsylvania

Linda P. Nelson, D.M.D., M.ScD.
Associate Professor of Clinical Pediatric Dentistry
Department of Surgery
University of Pennsylvania School of Medicine
Director of Pediatric Dentistry
The Children's Hospital of Philadelphia
Philadelphia, Pennsylvania

Michael Norman, M.D.
Professor and Associate Chairman
Department of Pediatrics
Jefferson Medical College
Philadelphia, Pennsylvania

Jerrold S. Olshan, M.D.
Senior Fellow
Division of Pediatric Endocrinology
University of Pennsylvania School of Medicine
Senior Endocrinology Fellow
The Children's Hospital of Philadelphia
Philadelphia, Pennsylvania

Lee M. Pachter, D.O.
Assistant Professor
University of Connecticut School of Medicine
Attending Physician in Pediatrics
St. Francis Hospital and Medical Center
Hartford, Connecticut

Roger Packer, M.D.
Professor of Neurology and Pediatrics
University of Pennsylvania
Senior Physician in Neurology and Pediatrics
The Children's Hospital of Philadelphia
Philadelphia, Pennsylvania

David A. Piccoli, M.D.
Assistant Professor of Pediatrics
University of Pennsylvania
Attending Physician
Division of Gastroenterology and Nutrition
The Children's Hospital of Philadelphia
Philadelphia, Pennsylvania

Steven B. Pierdon, M.D.
Private Practice
Schuylkill Pediatrics
Pottsville, Pennsylvania

Margaret Polaneczky, M.D., M.S.
Assistant Professor of Obstetrics and Gynecology
University of Pennsylvania School of Medicine
Division of Obstetrics and Gynecology
The Hospital of the University of Pennsylvania
Philadelphia, Pennsylvania

Richard Polin, M.D.
Professor of Pediatrics
University of Pennsylvania School of Medicine
Associate Physician-in-Chief
The Children's Hospital of Philadelphia
Philadelphia, Pennsylvania

Mortimer Poncz, M.D.
Associate Professor of Pediatrics
The Children's Hospital of Philadelphia
Senior Hematologist
University of Pennsylvania School of Medicine
Philadelphia, Pennsylvania

William Potsic, M.D.
Associate Professor
University of Pennsylvania School of Medicine
Director, Division of Otolaryngology and Human Communication
The Children's Hospital of Philadelphia
Philadelphia, Pennsylvania

Graham Quinn, M.D.
Associate Professor
University of Pennsylvania School of Medicine
Surgeon, Department of Ophthalmology
The Children's Hospital of Philadelphia
Philadelphia, Pennsylvania

R. Beverly Raney, Jr., M.D.
Professor of Pediatrics
University of Virginia
Chief, Pediatric Hematology/Oncology
University of Virginia Hospital Children's Medical Center
Charlottesville, Virginia

Clyde E. Rapp, Jr., M.D.
Student Health Service
Drexel University
Adolescent Division
The Children's Hospital of Philadelphia
Philadelphia, Pennsylvania

Anthony Rostain, M.D.
Assistant Professor of Psychiatry and Pediatrics
University of Pennsylvania School of Medicine
Medical Director
Pediatric Consultation–Liaison Psychiatry Service
Philadelphia, Pennsylvania

John Sargent, M.D.
Associate Professor of Psychiatry and Pediatrics
University of Pennsylvania School of Medicine
Director, Adolescent and Psychiatry Inpatient Unit
Philadelphia Child Guidance Clinic
The Children's Hospital of Philadelphia
Philadelphia, Pennsylvania

Thomas F. Scanlin, M.D.
Associate Professor of Pediatrics
University of Pennsylvania School of Medicine
Director, Cystic Fibrosis Center
The Children's Hospital of Philadelphia
Philadelphia, Pennsylvania

David B. Schaffer, M.D.
Professor, Department of Ophthalmology
University of Pennsylvania School of Medicine
Surgeon, Department of Ophthalmology
The Children's Hospital of Philadelphia
Philadelphia, Pennsylvania

Ellen R. Schwartz, M.A., CCC/SP
Speech-Language Pathologist
Private Practice
Philadelphia, Pennsylvania

M. William Schwartz, M.D.
Professor of Pediatrics
Department of Pediatrics
University of Pennsylvania
Senior Physician
The Children's Hospital of Philadelphia
Philadelphia, Pennsylvania

Donald Schwarz, M.D., M. P.H.
Assistant Professor of Pediatrics
University of Pennsylvania School of Medicine
Attending Physician
Adolescent Medicine
The Children's Hospital of Philadelphia
Philadelphia, Pennsylvania

Steven M. Schwarz, M.D.
Associate Professor of Pediatrics
New York Medical College
Associate Director
Pediatric Gastroenterology and Nutrition
Westchester County Medical Center
Valhalla, New York

Paula Schweich, M.D.
Clinical Assistant Professor
Department of Pediatrics
University of Washington
Emergency Pediatrician
Mary Bridge Children's Hospital
Tacoma, Washington

Toni Seidl, A.C.S.W., L.S.W
Field Instructor
University of Pennsylvania School of Social Work
Bryn Mawr College School of Social Work
Coordinator for Child Abuse, Neglect and Sexual Assault
The Children's Hospital of Philadelphia
Philadelphia, Pennsylvania

Steven M. Selbst, M.D.
Associate Professor of Pediatrics
University of Pennsylvania School of Medicine
Director, Emergency Department
The Children's Hospital of Philadelphia
Philadelphia, Pennsylvania

Barbara S. Shapiro, M.D.
Assistant Professor
University of Pennsylvania
Associate Director of Pain Service
Division of General Pediatrics
Department of Anesthesiology
The Children's Hospital of Philadelphia
Philadelphia, Pennsylvania

Steven A. Shapiro, D.O.
Clinical Affiliate
Division of Oncology
Children's Hospital of Philadelphia
Chairman, Department of Pediatrics
Suburisan General Hospital
Philadelphia, Pennsylvania

William G. Sharrar, M.D.
Associate Professor of Clinical Pediatrics
University of Medicine and Dentistry of New Jersey
Robert Wood Johnson Medical School at Camden
Head, Ambulatory Pediatrics
Cooper Hospital
Camden, New Jersey

Henry H. Sherk, M.D.
Professor of Surgery
The Medical College of Pennsylvania
Chief of Orthopedics and Rehabilitation
The Medical College of Pennsylvania
Philadelphia, Pennsylvania

Gail B. Slap, M.D.
Assistant Professor of Medicine and Pediatrics
University of Pennsylvania School of Medicine
Director, Adolescent Medicine
The Children's Hospital of Philadelphia
Philadelphia, Pennsylvania

Howard Snyder III, M.D.
Associate Professor of Urology in Surgery
University of Pennsylvania School of Medicine
Associate Director
Division of Pediatric Medicine and Urology
The Children's Hospital of Philadelphia
Philadelphia, Pennsylvania

Joseph W. St. Geme III, B.S., M.D.
Pediatric Scientist Training Program Fellow
Department of Microbiology and Immunology
Stanford University School of Medicine
Stanford, California

Charles A. Stanley, M.D.
Professor of Pediatrics
University of Pennsylvania School of Medicine
Senior Endocrinologist
The Children's Hospital of Philadelphia
Philadelphia, Pennsylvania

David N. Swank, M.S.W.
Medical Social Worker
The Children's Seashore House
Atlantic City, New Jersey

Edward Sweeny, D.M.D.
Professor of Pediatric Dentistry
University of Texas Health Science Center at San Antonio
Dentist in Chief
Children's Hospital
San Antonio, Texas

William Tarry, M.D.
Associate Professor
Urology and Pediatrics
West Virginia University Health Sciences Center
Morgantown, West Virginia

Bruce Taubman, M.D.
Clinical Assistant Professor
Department of Pediatrics
Division of Gastroenterology
University of Pennsylvania
The Children's Hospital of Philadelphia
Philadelphia, Pennsylvania

Frederick Tecklenburg, M.D.
Director of Emergency Department
Medical College of South Carolina
Charleston, South Carolina

John M. Templeton, Jr., M.D.
Associate Professor of Pediatric Surgery
University of Pennsylvania School of Medicine
Associate Surgeon
The Children's Hospital of Philadelphia
Philadelphia, Pennsylvania

Andrew M. Tershakovec, M.D.
Assistant Professor
University of Pennsylvania School of Medicine
Assistant Physician
The Children's Hospital of Philadelphia
Philadelphia, Pennsylvania

Susan B. Torrey, M.D.
Assistant Professor of Pediatrics
Temple University School of Medicine
Director of Emergency Services
St. Christopher's Hospital for Children
Philadelphia, Pennsylvania

Symme W. Trachtenberg, M.S.W., ACSW
Clinical Associate of Social Work in Pediatrics
University of Pennsylvania School of Medicine
Director of Social Work
The Children's Seashore House
Philadelphia, Pennsylvania

William R. Treem, M.D.
Assistant Professor of Pediatrics
University of Connecticut School of Medicine
Associate Director
Division of Pediatric Gastroenterology and Nutrition
Hartford Hospital
Hartford, Connecticut

Jeffrey Weiss, M.D.
Clinical Professor of Pediatrics
Thomas Jefferson University
Head, Children's Health Center
Jefferson University Hospital
Philadelphia, Pennsylvania

Ralph F. Wetmore, M.D.
Assistant Professor of Otorhinolaryngology and Human Communication
University of Pennsylvania School of Medicine
Associate Surgeon
The Children's Hospital of Philadelphia
Philadelphia, Pennsylvania

English D. Willis, M.D.
Assistant Professor of Pediatrics
University of Pennsylvania
Associate Physician
The Children's Hospital of Philadelphia
Philadelphia, Pennsylvania

Robert W. Wilmott, M.D., M.R.C.P.
Associate Professor
Department of Pediatrics
University of Cincinnati
Director, Pulmonary Medicine
The Children's Hospital Medical Center
Cincinnati, Ohio

Elaine H. Zackai, M.D.
Associate Director of Pediatrics and Genetics
Director, Clinical Genetics Center
The Children's Hospital of Philadelphia
Philadelphia, Pennsylvania

Moritz M. Ziegler, M.D.
Professor of Pediatric Surgery
University of Cincinnati School of Medicine
Surgeon-in-Chief
The Children's Hospital Medical Center
Cincinnati, Ohio

Mary Beth Zitarelli, B.S., R.D.
Pediatric Nutrition Specialist
Nutrition Support Service
The Children's Hospital of Philadelphia
Philadelphia, Pennsylvania

PREFACE TO THE SECOND EDITION

In the development of the first edition of this text, I was told by a wise editor that the second edition gives the authors and editors a chance to improve on the concepts and execution of the original idea. At that point I was not sure there was enough energy remaining to modify the original effort, but did have that feeling, common to authors, that sections of the book should be rewritten or altered. The positive initial reaction and forward thinking of the planners at Year Book Medical Publishers provided an opportunity to design and produce this second edition only 3 years after the publication of the first edition. In our planning, we wanted to preserve the concept and practical spirit of the book, changing some chapters to give new staff members an opportunity to participate and to give others a chance to revise and fill in sections that readers thought were missing. We planned to rewrite one quarter of the book, update the references, and give the authors a second chance to express their thoughts. These goals were accomplished. The addition of new material such as pain management, talking to parents about child abuse and seizures, AIDS, Lyme disease, rheumatic fever, and several topics to the section on signs and symptoms filled voids in the first edition and addressed new clinical problems. The title has been changed to *Pediatric Primary Care: A Problem-Oriented Approach*. Since primary care is the focus of the book, and primary care physicians use a problem-oriented approach in practice, this new title is more accurate.

No book such as this can be assembled without extraordinary cooperation of the authors. This revision was completed 5 months ahead of schedule because of their effort. The staff at Year Book exceeded all expectations in helpfulness and positive thinking. Nancy Chorpenning, who helped with the first edition at another company and city, reappeared in her capacity in charge of pediatric texts at Year Book. Her optimistic guidance and professionalism helped make the project continue. Kevin Kelly kept us organized, kindly forgave some missed assignments, and provided the important communication liaisons. Jan Gardner and Karen Halm represented the company in a highly professional way in the production effort. To this team and their colleagues, our sincere thanks and appreciation. The assistance of Maria Rosenzweig in maintaining organization and communications with the authors and the publishers contributed to our meeting the deadline. When she carefully read the sections on the normal baby, I suspected that she had a special interest in the topic. As the book grew, so did her family. She beat us to final product by a few months. My thanks and appreciation to her and her new infant.

The associate editors carried out their assignments in a cooperative spirit, making many helpful suggestions and utilizing their increasingly professional editing skills. They receive my appreciation for their work and their kindness. Their friendship continues to be a personal treasure.

M. William Schwartz, M.D.

PREFACE TO FIRST EDITION

The opportunity to develop a textbook about primary care challenged us to organize and present information that would help those who care for children and their families in the office setting of the 1980s. Today, primary care differs from hospital-based pediatrics, where critically ill patients of intensivists, children with complicated genetic, metabolic, and congenital problems, and those requiring special surgery or diagnostic procedures dominate the hospital census. Office care has changed too. Most of the diseases that formerly called for admission to the hospital are now managed in the office, requiring new organization and problem-solving strategies. The concerns of parents today are directed more to a quality of well-being rather than survival from infections and malnutrition. Working with behavioral issues, prevention, environmental problems, and adolescence have more importance for clinical pediatrics.

In designing the book, we first defined the audience as the office-based physicians, nurses, and students who care for infants, children, and adolescents. The office was targeted as environment, and topics were selected that were managed by the primary care specialist. The scope of the chapters cover the well child, the acutely ill and injured child, problems of chronic illness, and behavioral issues. Two special chapters concerning communication with subspecialists and parents transmit information and a style that can be used to strengthen the doctor/patient relationship. In working with problems that require the skill of a subspecialist, the primary physician and nurse play an important role in continuity and communications. The section on subspecialties describes the information and management strategies that occur in the tertiary care center. The section on communication with parents is written by those who frequently are the ones who must explain an unpleasant or fatal diagnosis to parents. Since primary care physicians may also have this role, they will appreciate reading how another person has presented this information. Our theme in all sections emphasizes practicality and utility. Recognizing there are many styles and approaches to caring for children, we present our version of child care, which is reasonable and sensitive.

We achieved our personal goals of making the effort of writing this book pleasant and satisfying. In recruiting physicians from present and past staff of The Children's Hospital of Philadelphia to author the chapters, we were able to crystallize the thinking and experience of many talented faculty members, who combined a strong knowledge base with a sensitivity to children and their families. Principles of family therapy have influenced many of the writers, even though no mention of it was made in the original assignments. Working with local staff helped maintain communication to accomplish this project. Authors in other cities could have chosen to ignore a letter reminding them of deadlines, but fellow staffers had trouble avoiding the *malocchio* given them during an editor's walk through the cafeteria. We had excellent cooperation even when the editors' red pen deleted or changed cherished paragraphs. When the initial editing that emphasized reducing duplications, space budgets, and style was completed, the reviewing of galleys once again indicated the talents of coworkers with whom we are fortunate to work. The large number of writers brought various styles to this book. Although we tried to maintain a standard presentation, this diversity still remains to some degree.

Many people contributed to this work in ways other than preparing manuscripts. The project was suggested by Mimi Case and Nancy Chorpenning, who turned over the project to Diana McAninch and Stephany Scott, who continued to help and direct us to completion. The staff at Year Book was professional and kind. As the project progressed through each phase, the skills of the editorial staff were appreciated. We developed a respect for their style and expertise.

Locally, we acknowledge the abilities of Richard Wood, the former president and chairman of the board of managers of the hospital who had the foresight to build the new Children's Hospital, which helped attract the staff to work here; and Dr. Alfred Bongiovanni and Jean Cortner, who as chairmen of the department developed a plan for the staff and recruited the personnel and funding to make the program successful. On a personal level, important people in the background of setting philosophies for me include Dr. Isaac Starr, my first academic role model, who calmly faced scientific adversity by stating that "All the easy things are already done"; Lew Barness, who reminded me that "The purpose of the medical school is to teach medical students," a motto that is easily forgotten in dealing with the daily problems of academia; John Hope, a pediatrician turned radiologist, who in addition to being a premier diagnostician set a patient concern standard for all to emulate; Bill Rashkind, who combined an innovative research career with high-level patient care and was able to keep a practical perspective on any problem and, most important, to keep a sense of humor; Tom Boggs, who demonstrated how protocols could be combined with judgments made from experience; Robert Kaye, who combined medical proficiency based on a strong scientific base with extraordinary sensitivity to families' feelings; David Cornfeld, who in directing the general pediatric division and teaching program taught us about care of children and practical approach to problems. Recognition is due to the staff who helped us complete the project: Barbara Seitz, Linda Timbers, Rose Beato, Bonita Wynn, who helped prepare the manuscripts; and Pat Johnson, my assistant, who stepped in during the last phases of the book preparation and contributed a great effort to complete the project.

Finally, my appreciation to the Associate Editors, Ed Charney, Tom Curry, and Steve Ludwig. Their skills, cooperation, and hard work made this task pleasant and rewarding. During the years of this project we helped each other complete assignments, solve editorial and personal problems, and developed bonds that are treasured. My appreciation to them for their contribution and friendship. The ability to finish this project with a sense of humor and feeling of friendship is most meaningful to me.

M. William Schwartz, M.D.

CONTENTS

SECTION VI: THE PRIMARY CARE PHYSICIAN AND THE SUBSPECIALIST 797

SECTION VII: TALKING WITH PARENTS 887

section I

Well-Child Care

Well-child care (health supervision) is an integral part of the practice of medicine for those involved in the care of children and adolescents. The concept of care rendered in anticipation of problems to prevent disease serves as the foundation of primary care.

This section focuses on the content of the well-child visit. The first three chapters examine the purpose of the office visit, offer suggestions regarding the conduct of the interview, and develop a framework for examining what is to be accomplished by the visit.

Chapters 4 through 7 offer points peculiar to the physical examination of the various age groups and present topics that are frequently encountered during the evaluation of the patient and in discussion with the family.

The last seven chapters address a variety of issues that touch on the daily practice of well-child care. These include immunization practice, screening programs, obesity, accident prevention, television, day care, acquired immune deficiency syndrome (AIDS) education, the sports evaluation, and divorce.

1 EXPANDED OFFICE VISIT

Gordon R. Hodas, M.D.

Primary care physicians exert an important influence in helping children and parents to function competently. An ongoing primary care relationship becomes most significant by providing continuity that decreases parental anxiety while promoting parental competence and caretaking. The family gains a sympathetic, knowledgeable, and reliable professional who can serve as both an expert and a catalyst for parents and child during the child-rearing years.

While medical expertise is indispensable, the development of a trusting doctor-family relationship depends more on certain personal qualities of the physician that, while intangible, are also unmistakable. This skill development starts with expressing respect toward child and family and accepting them in a nonjudgmental manner. There should be empathy, whereby the physician acknowledges an appreciation of the family's goals and frustrations. The physician should display energy and enthusiasm in relating to child and family, as well as patience in response to questions and doubts. The physician should be able to rely on a sense of humor at appropriate moments, while at other times stimulating motivation in a firm yet supportive manner. Finally, the physician should maintain and convey a sense of hopefulness and a belief in family competence. The physician who believes that, despite its frustrations and uncertainties, parenting should be an essentially happy experience can convey this to the family, thereby promoting a positive family orientation from the beginning. During times of major disappointment, the physician can help the family call upon its strengths to meet the immediate crisis and eventually move ahead in an adaptive way.

This commitment to work with the family's competence and strength in all clinical situations has been called the health focus, because the ultimate task of the physician is to promote healthy functioning and effective coping in dealing with well-child care, acute minor illness, medical and psychosocial emergencies, and chronic illness.

In the following discussion, the implementation of some of the above goals will be illustrated with respect to a routine pediatric visit of a well or sick child. The same principles would also apply in acute and emergency situations.

THE ROUTINE PEDIATRIC VISIT

As shown in Table 1–1, the routine pediatric visit has three components: the interview, the physical examination, and the wrap-up. Each of these parts of the visit has medical tasks and associated interpersonal tasks; the latter are intended to promote the competence of child and parents and to strengthen the doctor-patient relationship. We will frequently refer to child and "parents." While we realize that often only the mother in a two-parent family attends routine visits for a well or sick child, it is strongly recommended that the primary care physician try to involve the other parent as often as possible, so that information and decision-making regarding the child can be more fully shared. When the physician suggests to mothers that they invite their husbands, a surprising number of fathers do come in. Even more fathers attend when invited directly by the physician, for example, during hospital contact following the birth of a newborn. The presence of both parents at least some of the time enables the physician to better understand the child's family and builds a solid foundation for future interventions during medical or psychosocial crises. With single-parent mothers, frequently another adult (mother's own mother, sister, or boy-

TABLE 1–1
Components of Routine Pediatric Visit

	MEDICAL TASK	INTERPERSONAL TASK
The interview	Chief complaint; history-taking	Connecting; establishing leadership; developing an agenda
The physical examination	Screening for illness	Creating a therapeutic experience; involving child and parents; communicating information
Wrap-up	Summarizing medical findings	Addressing the agenda; encouraging questions; formulating future goals

friend) shares caretaking responsibilities; the mother should be encouraged to bring this person at least some of the time.

THE INTERVIEW

With both initial and follow-up visits, the objectives of the pediatric interview are essentially the same. Medically, the goal is to determine the nature of any chief complaints and then to obtain data about them through history-taking. The physician has additional interpersonal psychosocial tasks; the overall goals are to promote family competence, to expand and broaden the data base, and to ensure that each office visit is goal directed and of value to the child and parents. For example, if the parents come in with recent problems, the physician should also inquire about recent successes. With parents focused on the child's ailing body, the physician should also address the child's overall physical, social, and emotional development and his family context. In this way, the physician defines his area of interest as encompassing not just the child's sick body, but the child as a whole and as part of his family.

There are two major psychosocial tasks of the physician during the pediatric interview: "connecting" with the family and establishing leadership. Listed below are the important aspects of *connecting* that involve the physician's establishing himself with child and family as a concerned, approachable helper.

1. Putting the family at ease
2. Setting the tone
3. Relating to all adults
4. Relating to the child

The physician puts the family at ease in concrete ways such as introducing himself, greeting each family member warmly, showing fondness for the child, providing chairs, and encouraging everyone to take coats off and relax. In effect, the physician connects by setting the desired tone for the visit, one of respect, collaboration, and hopefulness. This is achieved both verbally through direct comments to the child and parents, and nonverbally through the physician's manner in relating to the group. The need to relate to all adults as well as to the child constitutes the final element of successful physician connecting. In this way, everyone has a chance to contribute, more information is obtained, and the physician demonstrates that the verbal child is a person whose ideas should be respected. In addition, the physician who develops his relationship with the child at the beginning of the visit will encounter a less anxious, more cooperative child during the physical examination.

The contacting of various family members is a continuous process occurring throughout the interview, examination, and wrap-up. The physician will need to develop a comfortable style that enables him to shift his attention from one person to another in a smooth, relatively inconspicuous way. One danger is overfocusing on the mother, who is often most eager to talk, to the relative exclusion of father and child. If father is to continue to attend visits and to perceive the physician as helpful, it is essential that the physician address him regularly. Similarly, by encouraging the child to contribute, the physician paves the way for a positive relationship for many years, hopefully through adolescence. Initial contact with each family member should occur within the first several minutes of the interview, as the physician engages each person briefly in "small-talk." Each person should again be sought out as data are gathered about the child and any presenting problem.

Establishing leadership occurs almost simultaneously with connecting.

1. Relating with confidence
2. Organizing data-gathering
3. Broadening the focus
4. Developing an agenda for the visit
5. Promoting competence

The physician can establish leadership by relating confidently to the child and parents. Confidence is conveyed through firm handshakes, consistent eye contact, and a resonating voice that invites comments without being tentative. The physician's energy and enthusiasm in approaching the family also instill confidence. He or she further establishes leadership by providing the structure for organized data-gathering and helping parents to focus their concerns from the outset so that limited time can be utilized in a clearly defined manner.

Another important aspect of physician leadership involves broadening the focus. The family, especially early in the doctor-patient relationship, typically comes in with narrow expectations of their physician, as someone to give shots and treat the child when ill. While these activities are essential aspects of the physician's responsibilities, they do not incorporate other interests of a physician providing "primary care." The physician can convey his broader interests—including developmental, social, and family concerns, the importance of medical continuity, and the promotion of family competence—indirectly through questions and directly by defining his role as primary care physician.

During a particular visit, the broadening of the focus can take many forms. We recommend that the physician write down at the end of each visit the pertinent issues to be reviewed at the next visit. At that visit, the physician listens carefully to the parents' expressed concerns, then inquires about issues which the parents have not raised. On this basis, the physician can develop with the parents an agenda of specific goals for the immediate visit, which may include medical, developmental, behavioral, and family issues.

The promotion of child and family competence can occur as part of a continuing process as the physician successfully connects and establishes leadership during the office visit. Over time, the family comes to view the physician as a committed ally who also educates and challenges whenever indicated.

PHYSICAL EXAMINATION

The pediatric physical examination has a therapeutic potential which has not been fully exploited. Presenting medical concerns can be addressed by the physician in a way that promotes competence and reassurance, orienting the parents and child toward health and coping. Table 1–2 shows the role of the physical examination in promoting certain developmental psychosocial tasks of children and their parents. As these tasks are met, the likelihood of potential problems for each period is reduced. The four developmental periods considered are: (1) infancy through the second year of life; (2) the preschool period, ages 2 to 5 years; (3) the school-aged period, ages 5 to 12 years; and (4) adolescence, ages 12 to 18 years. Three major goals of the physician during the physical examination extend through each developmental period and are, therefore, not listed each time. These are the following: (1) promoting positive relationships with each parent; (2) promoting a focus on health whereby competence is highlighted under adverse as well as routine conditions; and (3) creating a therapeutic experience for child and parents while conducting the examination.

Infancy (Table 1–2) is a particularly vulnerable time for parents, yet the outcome of this period may set the tone for subsequent development. Newborns, especially first-born infants, often precipitate a crisis of anxiety and uncertainty for parents, unprepared for the demands of their new role. The infant may be seen as fragile and "not a real person." If the child should be temperamentally difficult or develop colic, the crisis intensifies.

It is in this context that the physical examination can be quite therapeutic, promoting the parents' attachment by revealing the healthy newborn to be strong, capable, and very much a person. The physician uses the examination to illustrate the child's capabilities and vulnerabilities and to show how to approach the infant, demonstrating gentleness, consistency, eye contact, expressions of affection, and an absence of punitiveness. These efforts help "hu-

TABLE 1–2
Role of Physical Examination in Promoting Psychosocial Tasks

	DEVELOPMENTAL TASKS*	POTENTIAL PROBLEMS	ROLE OF PHYSICAL EXAMINATION
Infancy (to second year of life)	Understanding infant's needs*	Lack of infant-parent attachments	Educating parents, relieving anxiety
	Promoting infant's security and trust*	Child as source of stress	"Humanizing" the infant
	Developing parental attachment*	Impaired physical or emotional development	Demonstrating gentle consistent approach to infant
	Developing mutual parental support*	Parental anxiety or depression; marital crisis Child abuse or neglect	Promoting parental competence with infant Creating a sense of adventure Promoting joint involvement in parenting Encouraging private time
Preschool period (ages 2–5 yr)	Gaining sense of initiative and separateness	Separation anxiety	Developing physician's separate relationship with child
	Developing sociability	Withdrawal and restrictive play	Promoting spontaneity and curiosity
	Pursuing eagerness to learn	Somatic symptoms	Promoting use of play
	Promoting child's curiosity and separateness while remaining vigilant*	Parental overinvolvement or parental neglect	Educating parents Promoting appropriate level of parental involvement Containing impact of acute minor illness
School-aged period (5–12 yr)	Developing sense of accomplishment	Somatic complaints	Promoting child's relationship with physician
	Strengthening sense of autonomy	School refusal	Giving child more information and responsibility
	Developing positive self-esteem	Depression	Respecting modesty Reinforcing child's cooperation
	Encouraging exploration and responsibility*	Conduct disorders	Helping child begin to develop reasonable sense of control over body Promoting parents' view of child as competent Containing impact of acute minor illness
Adolescence (12–18 yr)	Strengthening sense of independence and responsibility	Somatic complaints Substance abuse Conduct disorders	Examining adolescent alone, keeping parent informed Relating to adolescent as competent and responsible
	Developing stable body image and sense of control over body	Depression and suicide attempts Pregnancy Eating disorders	Explaining body changes Encouraging pride in body
	Dealing with sexuality	Promiscuity Pregnancy Eating disorders	Respecting modesty Explaining body changes Encouraging pride in body
	Negotiating issues of independence and closeness	Overdependency Runaway behavior Psychosis	Relating to adolescent as competent and responsible Alloting time for special concerns (sexuality, drugs, alcohol, dieting, exercise, peers, family)
	Encouraging expression of adolescent's own ideas and concerns*	Depression Conduct disorders	Alloting time for special concerns

*Denotes parental task; otherwise, psychosocial task of child.

manize" the infant for the parents; the infant is further transformed to a source of pleasure when the physician talks to him, uses humor, points out the infant's smiling and other reflexes. Because the physician's demonstration is for both parents, joint parental involvement as well as parental competence with the infant are promoted, and the potential dangers of failed attachments are rendered less likely. The physician can try to create a sense of adventure for the parents, as they both watch and help the child grow.

The preschool child (Table 1–2) is a verbal being, separate from parents and desiring to establish areas of competence. There is great interest in using speech, being sociable, and learning. The physician, therefore, now maintains an active relationship with the child as well as the parents and promotes the child's spontaneity, curiosity, and play. Participation is encouraged. The physician also utilizes the examination to assess parent-child relationships and to promote appropriate levels of parental involvement.

The tasks of the school-aged child (Table 1–2) include developing a sense of accomplishment, strengthening the sense of autonomy, and elevating self-esteem in the process. Therefore, while continuing to relate to the parents as the primary caretakers, the physician devotes further efforts toward building a relationship with the child. The child is addressed frequently, given more information and responsibility, and helped to begin to develop a reasonable sense of control over his body. The child's physical modesty is always respected through use of gowns. The parents are encouraged to see the child as competent.

During adolescence (Table 1–2), important developmental tasks include the continued development of a sense of independence and a sense of responsibility, the development of a stable body image and a sense of control over one's body, and coming to terms with one's sexuality. The physician sees the adolescent alone, keeping parents informed of major health issues. Relating to the adolescent as competent and responsible, the physician can utilize the examination to discuss such topics as physical growth, exercise, diet, weight control, acne, and menstruation.

With the adolescent the doctor encourages questions and tries to promote a positive body image and a sense of control over one's body. By offering confidentiality except in cases of attempted or threatened suicide, the physician can encourage discussion of other highly personal areas such as sexuality, birth control, drugs and alcohol, peers, and family relationships.

Summarized below are interpersonal goals and techniques, as developed by Honig and associates that promote participation and competence during a single physical examination of a verbal child.

PROMOTING RELATIONSHIP WITH CHILD
Providing transition from history to physical examination
Engaging child in conversation
Using humor
Explaining procedures
Allaying fears
Encouraging curiosity
Encouraging cooperation
Communicating information

PROMOTING RELATIONSHIP WITH PARENTS
Offering compliment(s) about child
Promoting eye contact with child
Promoting direct parental participation
Communicating information

These techniques are meaningful to a physician who has a genuine commitment to develop a doctor-family relationship based on collaboration and respect. The two major goals are promoting the relationship with the child and promoting the relationship with the parents.

With the child, the physician should strive to diminish anxiety and encourage participation as much as possible. Toward this end, the physician should announce the physical examination and allow a brief transition from history-taking to the examination so that the child is not startled. The child can be given a chance to finish undressing or to climb onto the examining table. To initiate the examination itself, the physician should explain at the child's level what will be taking place, attempting to allay fears, promote understanding, and encourage cooperation. The doctor should reassure the child that the parents are there and should ask the child to cooperate. As the examination unfolds, the physician should try to maintain an ongoing dialogue with child, at times turning to address the parents. Some of the conversation can be related to topics of interest to the child, and some should involve the physician's explaining each aspect of the examination and reassuring the child about his body. The physician can engage the child's curiosity through "tricks of examination," asking him questions, and offering a stethoscope or hammer for the child to try out.

While the physical examination is often a special time between physician and child, it is nevertheless important that the parents participate in the process. Compliments about the child serve to orient the parents positively. Promoting eye contact between parents and child is important not only for the child but for the parents as well. With younger children, a mother may participate directly when the child is examined on her lap. Parents may also participate by providing information and by helping the child to cooperate during the examination. The role of parents is especially important when shots must be given. The physician has several ways to prepare the child: simple explanations, recalling an earlier shot, using humor, and offering a toy or a familiar object. After the shot, the physician can "make peace" in several ways such as offering a kind word or a plastic strip bandage. Nevertheless, it is the parents' reassurance and comforting that matters most to the child during and after the procedure.

Finally, the physician should provide information to parents during the physical examination; this relieves anxiety and adds further legitimacy to the physician's conclusions during the wrap-up.

WRAP-UP OF THE PEDIATRIC VISIT

The wrap-up or summary of the pediatric visit affords the physician the opportunity to tie together disparate questions and findings so that the visit becomes therapeutic and important themes are reinforced. This is achieved in a variety of ways:

- Addressing agenda of visit
- Highlighting themes
- Decreasing family anxiety
- Encouraging questions
- Formulating future goals
  - Medical
  - Developmental
  - Behavioral or psychiatric
- Assigning tasks

First, the physician addresses the agenda agreed on earlier in the visit. Typically, this includes one or more medical concerns plus a behavioral or parenting question. If the physician has properly focused the interview and has utilized the physical examination strategically to promote his objectives, the wrap-up becomes the final step in a process already underway. The physician should direct his comments to both parents and to the child, allowing frequent opportunities for questions and clarification. The physician's summary should be relatively brief so that it can be easily understood. In beginning a discussion, the physician should try to use the family's own words and phrases. Physician clarity will help decrease parental and child anxieties.

Once the presenting concerns have been addressed, the physician can encourage the family to formulate future goals. These fall into three categories: medical, developmental, and behavioral or psychiatric. Medical goals may pertain to a current illness, a past illness, or the ongoing management of a chronic illness. Developmental goals may apply to the child, the parents, or both. Issues for the child include safety and anticipatory guidance, sibling and peer relationships, and development of interests and other aspects of independent functioning. Issues for the parents include the need for shared parenting and mutual support and the need for some privacy for the couple. Parents also must deal with additional planned and unplanned events that impact on child or family, such as a job change, an illness, or the birth of a baby. Behavioral and psychiatric issues that involve child or adolescent vary in severity and may include anxiety, withdrawal, disobedience, depression, suicide attempts, substance abuse, and psychosis. Issues that may involve the parents include severe marital conflict or divorce, parental depression, substance abuse, and other parental problems.

When confronted with significant developmental, behavioral, or psychiatric issues, the primary care physician must decide whether to manage them himself or initiate psychiatric referral. The task of referral is easier when parents themselves identify a problem and request help. However, the physician who has serious concerns about a child or his family must be prepared to express this directly and to recommend psychiatric consultation if indicated. In such instances, it is important for the physician to propose psychiatric consultation constructively and to reaffirm his own continuing primary care involvement.

A special challenge of the pediatric visit is for the physician to create a balance between direct problem solving and problem solving on the part of the family. Toward that goal, the physician may at times conclude many routine pediatric visits by assigning tasks to the family. These may involve a change in behavior on the part of the parents, the child, or both. The value of tasks is that they promote independent problem solving by the family while also maintaining the physician's presence as a catalyst for change during the interval between visits.

BIBLIOGRAPHY

Brazelton TB: *Doctor and Patient.* New York, Dell Publishing Co, 1970.

Carey WB, Sibinga MS: Avoiding pediatric pathogenesis in the management of acute minor illness. *Pediatrics* 1972; 49:553.

Diller LH: On giving good advice successfully. *Fam Syst Med* 1986; 4:78.

Glenn ML: Toward collaborative family-oriented health care. *Fam Syst Med* 1985; 3:466.

Glenn ML: *On Diagnosis: A Systemic Approach.* New York, Brunner/Mazel, 1984.

Hodas GR, Honig PJ: An approach to psychiatric referrals in pediatric patients: Psychosomatic complaints. *Clin Pediatrics* 1983; 22:167.

Hodas GR, Honig PJH, Montalvo B: *Interpersonal aspects of the pediatric physical examination.* William Penn Funded Grant, 1979–1982.

Honig PJ, Lieberman R, Malone C, et al: Pediatric-psychiatric liaison as a model for teaching pediatric residents. *J Med Ed* 1976; 51:929.

Klaus MH, Kennell JH: *Maternal Infant Bonding.* St Louis, CV Mosby Co, 1976.

McDaniel S, Campbell TL: Physicians and family therapists: The risk of collaboration. *Fam Syst Med* 1986; 4:4.

Rinaldi RC: Positive effects of psychosocial interventions on total health care: A review of the literature. *Fam Syst Med* 1985; 3:417.

2 INTERVIEWING

M. William Schwartz, M.D.

More than obtaining a medical history, interviewing is a challenge to gather information and develop rapport with the patient and family. If data collection were the only purpose of an interview, a computer could do an adequate job. The advocates of computer-based history neglect the other goals of history taking: developing relationships with the patient and family and establishing strategies which help increase communication and compliance. Without this rapport, a barrier develops between the two parties and important facts are withheld. If a positive relationship is present and the patient senses that the doctor cares, the chances are increased that there will be both a better history and compliance about the treatment program. This section provides hints about improving the flow of information by establishing a positive relationship with patients and eliciting information from the difficult patient.

"JOINING"

To move from a computer-type history to a more open and personal one, attention should be paid to interviewing skills and style. *"Joining,"* one of the methods which helps increase the rapport and humanism in interviewing, describes the interjection of a personalized touch to the interview. Instead of the interviewer starting with data collection, a few minutes are devoted to socialization and establishment of a relationship. Although initially awkward to the novice, this approach serves to set the atmosphere of a caring person who is seeing a patient rather than just finding out about the problem. Usually the patient makes a special effort to dress up for the visit with the doctor. If the interviewer admires a decal on the shirt, a pin, or a necklace, the patient smiles and feels more comfortable. The parents will also begin to relax and develop positive feelings toward the physician who has made an effort to put their child at ease. Likewise, if each person in the room is identified, the family feels kindly toward the busy doctor who took time to treat the people as individuals. The parents can be included in this joining process by the physician asking them questions (such as "Did you have trouble parking?") or by remarking about something that they are wearing. This technique accomplishes several goals: the patient appreciates this humanism and the doctor is signaling that he or she cares and is not rushing through the visit. Joining does not require more than a minute or two but the reward, a better history, is worth the time spent. Methods used in joining are listed below.

1. Use the patient's name
2. Ask names of all people in the room
3. Admire an object of clothing or jewelry
4. Inquire about transportation problems ("Did you have trouble parking?")
5. Talk about sports, school, interests before asking the chief complaint
6. Find similarities in preference for food, clothes, sports, etc.

TECHNIQUE

OPEN-ENDED QUESTIONS

Poor technique is another barrier to a good interview. Probably the most common problem is asking questions which will produce a "yes" or "no" answer. A different response will be given depending on the phrasing used in requesting information: "Was your pregnancy normal?" "Tell me about your pregnancy." The same is true when the physician asks: "What's happening in school?" rather than "Do you like school?" Although patients are content with brief answers, they will respond with more information if the phrasing of questions allows them the opportunity to talk. This open-ended questioning may allow a verbal patient to give an open-ended answer so that the interviewer has to maintain control of the dialogue by interrupting or refocusing the question to stay on the subject.

CLARITY

The format of the questioning is important to good interviewing. Questions should be concise. A long introduction may confuse the patient and blur the purpose of the actual question. Avoid jargon. The patient may be too shy to ask you to repeat the question or to ask a definition. The phrasing should be simple so that compound questions are not presented to the parent. "Do you take something for your headache or do you let it go untreated?" is not as good a question as "What do you do for your headache?" In the first example, a sensitive patient might feel the physician is looking for one of the options as correct and alter the response accordingly. The best questions are clear, concise, and phrased in understandable terms.

Some patients treat an interview as a courtroom session, one in which they avoid making a confession to the doctor. The television detective Columbo had a circuitous line of questioning that disarmed the suspect and facilitated the flow of information. "*What* do the kids do when you have a fight?" is a favorite Columboism. In this approach there is an assumption that there will be family quarrels; the physician is not asking if there are any disagreements but rather how the children react to them. When seeing a child with recurrent epistaxis that the physician suspects is secondary to mucosal trauma from an exploring finger, it is not wise to ask the child if he picks his nose. Since his mother told him not to do this, the physician can expect a denial from this direct line of questioning. On the other hand, the child can be disarmed if the physician assumes he does this negative behavior and asks which finger is used.

Assuming the meaning of important words can lead to communication problems. Clarification of definitions is necessary. For example, someone saying that they are "constipated" may mean that a daily bowel movement is missed, there may be straining, or the feces are hard. Certain misunderstandings can be avoided if time is taken to establish the measuring of words such as "a good baby," "poor eater," or "always has a cold." In further exploration the good baby may be one who does not cry, the poor eater may actually consume more than adequate calories but less than the parents expect, and the cold is actually a normal amount of mucus in a small airway. Errors in treatment follow poor clarification of terms.

APPROVAL

All of us like to hear we are doing a good job. Interrupting the interview with some recognition that the parent had made a good decision or exercised good judgment offers them an important approval and begins to build the desired rapport. Saying "good job" or "that was nice" creates a warm and positive inner feeling in the parent. This positive attitude should build better communication and interaction.

CLUES

In contrast to the computer history, in the personal history session, the physician can pick up visual clues and detect sensitive topics. Certain words or inflections indicate to the prepared listener that the patient is sending signals that he has material that may be ready for discussion. For example, long pauses between words may indicate that this is a sensitive topic and the speaker is seeking alternative phrases or even thinking of the problem rather than speaking. The patient should be asked why he is frowning or appears serious. He may appreciate this time to express his feelings.

PERIODIC SUMMARY

The periodic summary is a most effective technique of good communication. At the end of the history taking and again before telling the patient the diagnosis and treatment, the physician should summarize what the patient has said; this assures the patient that what he said was understood. The family will then know that what the physician is about to recommend is based on facts stated in the summary. Without this signal, the patient and family are not sure that the physician has heard what they intended to say. In addition to allowing the family to clarify any point, this summary also confirms that the physician is using the right information. A conclusion such as "Is there anything else that I should know?" indicates that the physician has time to listen and gives the patient one more chance to tell his story.

DAY HISTORY

The "day history" is an excellent technique to invoke when you desire to know more about the family interrelationships, support systems, or how judgment and interpretations are made about the children. Instead of answering direct questions, parents may be more comfortable when they talk about their daily activities. This day history is more than just a diary of events which state, for example, "Awoke at seven o'clock, ate breakfast of cereal and milk, took a nap for two hours, etc." In addition to finding out *what* happened, it should also be used to find out *why* it happened, and *who* was involved. Details about day histories reveal interesting information about support systems in the family, who helps whom, and how much organization is present in the family.

The secret of taking a good day history is to stop the person giving the daily diary at several points in the day and ask questions such as: "Why?" "How did you know?" "Who was there?"

ADDITIONAL QUESTIONS

When the physician finishes a standard interview with a patient who has presented a vague story, he may have an uneasy feeling that there is more important missing information. There may be difficulty in summarizing what has been heard. The "Who, What, Where, and When line of questions" may not always be sufficient to remove the vagueness. This may be the time to ask the five questions listed below.

1. What is wrong?
2. Why did you come *today*?
3. What do you want *me* to do?
4. What do *you* think is wrong?
5. What do *others* think is wrong?

First, the physician must obtain a clear statement of *what is wrong*. When this statement is in the family's own words, it establishes a reference point to keep the problem and concerns in focus.

Next the physician must establish *why* the patient came to see him today. When these problems are chronic or seem similar to symptoms that have been present at other times, it is important to find out reasons for this motivation. *Why today* (and not yesterday or tomorrow)? This may reveal important events or pressures such as a disease in the neighborhood or a recent change in the family, a death, or a visit by a grandparent.

"What do you want me to do?" is a blunt way of asking about the patient's agenda. The physician might not choose to use this phrase but he needs to know what the patient or the family has in mind about tests or treatment. They might think that a chest x-ray film or a "blood test" will give the answer to the problem. In these cases, the different agenda leads to dissatisfaction. Some physicians shy away from clarifying this conflict because they do not want to present an open menu for laboratory tests. This questioning should be a technique to open communications between the patient and the interviewer. Reasons for not ordering tests can be the point of discussion to resolve the communication barrier.

"What do you think is wrong?" is a question that opens up the opportunity for several responses from the patient. The patient may state that the physician's job is to determine what is wrong. In a more reasonable mode, the patient may welcome this opportunity to express concerns and questions that he may not have felt comfortable enough to discuss at the beginning of the interview. Many times, the family is concerned about leukemia and is reticent to discuss this fear. Because the chief complaint is not related to leukemia and there is nothing to suggest that diagnosis in the evaluation, the physician does not generally mention that this diagnosis was ruled out. Unless this difference is detected and discussed, the communication breakdown persists.

"What do others think is wrong?" This question helps identify who in the support system of the patient is making medical suggestions which may be different from those that are under consideration. The patient may understand the diagnostic and management issues but this is not communicated with this third party: a spouse, a neighbor, or a relative. Unless this other person is identified, the impediments to communication persist as does the unsatisfactory patient care.

While they are not required in every case, these techniques are helpful when a communication problem is detected.

3 CULTURAL CONSIDERATIONS IN PEDIATRICS

Lee M. Pachter, D.O.

The successful practice of pediatrics incorporates knowledge of normal and abnormal states of health with the talent to translate this knowledge into practice. The primary care practitioner should be sensitive to the flow of information between the patient and the practitioner and aware that this communication is not exclusively from practitioner to patient. Communication may at times be difficult due to differing perspective, experience, and background of the physician and patient. When the practitioner and patient have different cultural backgrounds, the possibility of miscommunication increases. Mistrust, unfulfilled expectations, and decreased compliance with medical therapy are some expressions of this miscommunication. In this chapter, the problem of providing health care in a transcultural setting is examined, including examples of where differences in culture may become a barrier to providing effective health care.

DISEASE VS. ILLNESS

An important distinction is the difference between disease and illness. Medical education provides a firm understanding of the disease process and its effect on the body. Disease can be defined as physical or mental impairment. Illness, on the other hand, refers to an unhealthy condition and how that condition affects the individual as both a biologic and social being. Illness may not necessarily correlate with biomedical disease categories; it can be considered a subjective experience. Patients may have a disease but not be ill, for example, those with cancer in remission or with subclinical prodromes. In contrast are patients who assume the role of being ill without biomedical disease. Illness as a concept incorporates social roles and is influenced by the patient's individual, familial, and cultural background. Harwood suggests that the concept of illness integrates the person's physiologic state with their health beliefs and behaviors.

Cultural background determines health beliefs and behaviors to a large extent, as do social class, age, and education. The primary care provider who has contact with patients and families from diverse cultural backgrounds must be sensitive to the health beliefs and behaviors of those particular cultures.

Although particular beliefs and behaviors are seen in members of a particular cultural group, it is important to point out that individuals subscribe to the standards of a group to various degrees and in varying situations. Caution should be exercised to avoid stereotyping.

Several variables may be used to assess whether a patient or family subscribes to cultural health beliefs and behaviors. These variables have been shown to correlate with an individual's or family's level of acculturation. Acculturation occurs when modification of individual or group behavior results from interaction involving intercultural exchange with a different group.

VARIABLES CORRELATED WITH ACCULTURATION

Language usage
Generational removal from migration
Age of caretaker
Amount of contact with area of cultural origin
Education (amount and location)
Community characteristics (i.e., barrio vs. suburbs)

In general, those families who have recently migrated, whose head of the household is older, whose family members keep in contact with friends and family from their initial cultural area, who have had minimal contact with health care services that provide patient education, and who live in an encapsulated cultural area with strong family and social networks may be more likely to adhere to cultural health beliefs and behaviors. Language usage has also been shown to correlate with the degree of acculturation and therefore may help to determine a family's adherence to cultural health beliefs and behaviors.

CULTURALLY DETERMINED CONCEPTS ABOUT THE BODY AND ITS FUNCTION

Many cultural groups have certain concepts with regard to the body and its function that may be at odds with standard biomedical knowledge. For example, blood and other body fluids are the focus of many health beliefs. Blood is described as high, low, bad, and thin by many traditional southern blacks; hot, cold, weak, dirty, dark, and yellow in Haitian populations, and weak, thick, and thin by many Puerto Ricans. The primary care practitioner must be aware that these terms have very specific cultural meanings in these groups. For example, in certain black populations the term high blood may refer to a folk condition described as an increase in the amount of blood in the body, possibly secondary to strong emotions or eating too much rich food, which if untreated may back up into the brain and cause a stroke. Folk treatment may consist of astringent substances, such as vinegar, that thin the blood out. If the health care practitioner who is trying to explain hypertension to a family uses the term high blood, the misunderstanding may lead to noncompliance, because the treatment of hypertension requires long-term therapy, whereas the treatment for high blood is not prolonged, because medicine taken for a long time will make the blood too thin. Harwood, in a study of Puerto Ricans in New York, demonstrated that there were differences within the sample population with regard to the definitions of low blood, weak blood, high blood pressure (alta presion), and thick blood. The practitioner must be particular in defining medical conditions and ensure that the patient and family have a similar understanding of the concepts.

CULTURE-BOUND SYNDROMES

Culture-bound syndromes are illnesses that are seen in a particular ethnic group and that do not fit into biomedically defined disease categories.

EXAMPLES OF CULTURE-BOUND SYNDROMES

Ataque de nervios, Puerto Rican syndrome (Puerto Rican)
Mal de ojo, evil eye (Mexican, Puerto Rican, other Latin cultures)
Falling out (traditional black)
Empacho, indigestion (latino)
Susto, fright (latino)
Caida de la mollera, fallen fontanelle (Mexican)

Many of these syndromes are treated by folk practitioners and do not come to medical attention, but others may be seen in the ambulatory setting because the symptoms are similar and can be attributed to biomedical entities. For example, the term empacho is used to describe a condition consisting of abdominal pain and discomfort, vomiting, diarrhea, and loss of appetite. Empacho has been described in numerous Latino communities and affects infants and children. The folk explanation is that empacho is caused by a food bolus obstructing the stomach. A mother may relate that a child can get empacho by drinking cold milk late at night. Treatment may consist of rubbing oil on the stomach and drinking orange juice mixed with olive oil, or milk of magnesia. A mother may bring her child to a curandero (a type of folk practitioner) for treatment, or she may seek medical attention from a pediatrician or family physician. In many instances, what the family considers to be empacho may be a viral gastroenteritis, and the health care provider needs to be aware of the types of treatment the child is receiving at home so as to either incorporate the folk treatments into the therapeutic plan to increase compliance or to discourage any treatments that may be potentially harmful (e.g., milk of magnesia).

LANGUAGE BARRIERS

The potential for miscommunication is greatest when the primary care provider and the patient or family do not speak the same language. In the best of all possible worlds, health care practitioners should become fluent in the languages of their patients. A realistic alternative is to have translators available when the need arises. Certain rules should be followed when choosing a translator:

1. Children should never be used to translate for adults; this may result in disruption of social roles and relations.
2. Do not ask a stranger from the waiting room to act as a translator; this would result in a breach of patient confidentiality and may strain the doctor-patient relationship.
3. It is appropriate in most cases to use an adult who the patient or parent brings to the visit for this purpose.
4. Always ask the patient or parent if the designated translator is acceptable to them.
5. Maintain eye contact with the patient or parent who is receiving the information; you may pick up important nonverbal clues.
6. Ask the translator to translate as literally as possible; make sure the translator understands the medical terms that you use.

CULTURALLY DETERMINED GENDER ROLES

Many cultures have strong rules concerning what is appropriate behavior with regard to sex roles. What can be discussed in the presence of the opposite sex is culturally determined, and the practitioner should be aware of taboos. Ac-

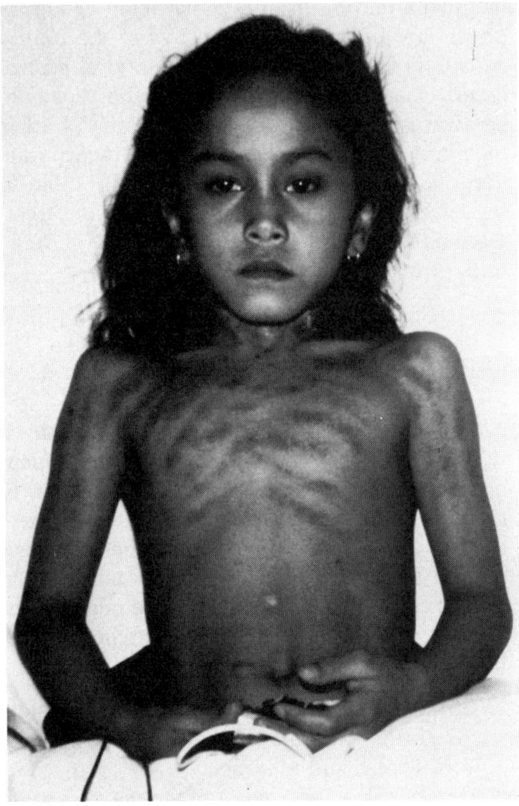

FIG 3–1
Eight-year-old Vietnamese girl with çao gio (coining) marks on chest.

cording to traditional Mexican and Puerto Rican values, a woman should not discuss sexual matters with a man. One potential problem area could be when a female adolescent comes to the office for either contraceptive planning or treatment of a gynecologic infection and the health care provider is a man, or conversely, if a male adolescent comes to the office because of a urethral discharge and the health practitioner is a woman. The patient may never actually declare the intended reason for the visit. In another example of gender role taboos, Clark relates an incident when a Mexican mother expressed concern when asked to manipulate her son's penis to release foreskin adhesions because to her that would constitute an indecent act. Awareness of these culturally determined sex roles and taboos is necessary to adequately care for all the health concerns of the patient.

CULTURALLY INFLUENCED IDEAS ABOUT CAUSATION OF ILLNESS

All cultures try to define and explain events so as to fit them into a general cognitive framework. Illness is a condition that is common to all members of a group, and therefore attempts to explain why a person gets sick is a central concept of health beliefs and behaviors. Patients often have theories of causation that may seem illogical to a person educated in the biomedical paradigm. In the patient's perspective, health beliefs and behaviors fit into a logical, cognitive framework. Some families are knowledgeable in the biomedical theories of disease and combine scientific and folk beliefs. An honest evaluation of our own beliefs may reveal this as well.

Traditional blacks may talk about natural and unnatural illness; latinos may define diseases and treatments as hot (caliente) or cold (frio); and southeast asians may refer to wind (phan) as a causative agent of illness. A culturally appropriate way of treating some illnesses caused by phan is çao gio (rubbing out the wind, or coining), which consists of applying oil to the body and rubbing the skin with the edge of a coin until actual bruising occurs (Fig 3–1). This practice should not be mistaken for child abuse, since the intention of the family is therapeutic and based on a concern for the child's well-being. The culturally sensitive clinician should discuss his or her concerns regarding the practice and alternate treatment possibilities.

A practitioner who works with a specific ethnic group needs to become aware of the basic cultural theories of causation of illness in that group. Not all people of a particular ethnic group subscribe to these beliefs; the level of acculturation is a good screening concept that the practitioner can use to assess the degree of adherence to folk beliefs and behaviors.

PHYSICIAN-PATIENT INTERACTION

All cultures have rules regarding roles and acceptable interaction between persons of different social position. Physicians are often regarded as authority figures. Some cultural groups treat authority figures with quiet respect and may not ask questions, because this would be considered inappropriate behavior. The practitioner must be supportive and should encourage questions in a nonintimidating way. Other cultures place greater emphasis on a more egalitarian exchange; the practitioner may mistake this form of interaction as being overly aggressive when in fact this is not the intent. The physician must keep in mind the cultural values of the patient and his or her family and how they are expressed when evaluating the health care encounter.

SYMPTOM PRESENTATION

Some cultural groups put emphasis on specific symptoms and may present for care more often than the practitioner may feel is necessary. The health care practitioner must be sensitive to the cultural and familial factors that enter into the decision to seek treatment for a particular symptom. For example, many in the Puerto Rican community seem to place a great deal of emphasis on symptoms of upper respiratory tract infections and may seek medical care for symptoms that others may treat at home without medical consultation. One possible explanation is that there is a high incidence of asthma in the Puerto Rican community, and families of patients with asthma are taught that a cold may bring on an episode of asthma. Some may take this to mean that colds cause asthma and therefore are overly anxious when their child displays cold symptoms. Another explanation is that during the era of rheumatic fever the Puerto Rican community was at high risk for infection. Parents remember that when they were young many died after having a sore throat. When viewed in this context, the significance of upper respiratory tract infections in this population seems more rational.

DIETARY HABITS

Diet and food preference not only are personal choices but also are culturally determined. In pediatric practice, food plays an important role. Proper nutrition is essential to the growing child; many of our treatment plans involve food as a form of therapeutic intervention; and food is used as a palatable medium to facilitate medicine taking. It is important to know what foods are appropriate and available in the community and also any general health beliefs and behaviors that may affect the diet.

Culture and ethnicity have been shown to be factors in the decision whether to breast feed. Other variables, such as socioeconomic status, level of maternal education, prenatal care, and maternal age, are also important determinants.

Every ethnic group has specific food preferences that largely determine dietary intake. The practitioner needs to be aware of the staple foods in the cultural group when making nutritional recommendations during the well-child visit. A simple but effective way of providing culturally appropriate nutritional counseling is to make up lists of foods rich in different nutrients (e.g., protein, carbohydrates, and specific vitamins) that are consumed by the particular ethnic group. This reference list can also be used when specific types of foods are used as therapy.

CONCLUSIONS

In this era of widespread media attention to biomedical topics, many people have at least a minimal knowledge of mainstream medical care. Each person fuses this knowledge with their cultural beliefs into an individual cognitive approach to illness. Caring for patients and families from different ethnic backgrounds requires knowledge of their cultural health beliefs and behaviors. Not all individuals act the same way in the same circumstances, even within an ethnic group. The job of the practitioner is to determine which patients may adhere to cultural practices and how this will affect their care.

1. Patients think in terms of illness, as opposed to disease. Think how a disease state affects the individual as a social being as well as a biologic being.
2. Factors pertaining to acculturation can provide a screening test when trying to determine if a patient subscribes to cultural health care practices.
3. Be aware that particular terms have different connotations in different cultures; be sure

that these terms have the same meaning to both you and the patient and family.

4. Encourage questions. Do not take for granted that a patient understands if he or she does not ask questions; respect for authority figures may preempt questioning.

5. When necessary, use appropriate translators.

6. Be aware of culture-bound syndromes and how they may present; try to elicit the patient's concept of causation of illness.

7. Become familiar with patients' specific food and dietary habits and incorporate them into therapeutic plans.

When dealing with conflicts arising from differing health beliefs and behaviors, patient education is both the means and the end to effective patient care. If possible, incorporate the patient's health beliefs and behaviors into the therapeutic strategy; this allows the patient and family to recognize that you respect them and their beliefs.

BIBLIOGRAPHY

Clark, M: *Health in the Mexican-American Culture.* Berkeley, University of California Press, 1970.

Guarnaccia PJ, Pelto PJ, Schensul SL: Family health culture, ethnicity, and asthma: Coping with illness. *Med Anthropol* 1985; 9:203–224.

Harwood, A: *Ethnicity and Medical Care.* Cambridge, Harvard University Press, 1981.

Harwood A: The hot-cold theory of disease: Implications for treatment of Puerto Rican patients. *JAMA* 1971; 216:1153–1158.

Harwood A: Selected issues in treating Puerto Rican patients. *Hosp Physician* 1981; Sept: 113–118.

Kleinman A, Eisenberg L, Good B: Culture, illness, and care: Clinical lessons from anthropologic and cross-cultural research. *Ann Intern Med* 1978; 88:251–258.

Scott CS: Culture, ethnicity, and medicine, in Braunstein JJ, Toister RP (eds): *Medical Applications of the Behavioral Sciences.* Chicago, Year Book Medical Publishers, 1981.

Weller SC, Dungy CI: Personal preferences and ethnic variations among Anglo and Hispanic breast and bottle feeders. *Soc Sci Med* 1986; 23:539–548.

4 THE NEWBORN INFANT

EXAMINATION

Douglas Boenning, M.D.

The initial newborn examination is important for a number of reasons. First, it establishes a baseline assessment of the child's condition at birth including measurements that will be important reference points for the rest of childhood. Second, the examination helps to identify life-threatening conditions that require immediate medical or surgical attention. Often these conditions present dramatically in the delivery room or shortly thereafter in the nursery. A third purpose is to assess or confirm the baby's gestational age based on signs of physical and neurological maturity. A fourth purpose is to screen for findings that require follow-up in the first months of life. A fifth purpose is to reassure parents that they have a healthy child, answer their questions, and establish an ongoing relationship with the family. This relationship can be promoted by conducting the physical examination in the parents' presence.

This chapter will be organized according to the components of the newborn physical examination. The salient features of the evaluation will be emphasized, recognizing that a thorough examination of the term baby can be conducted in 5 minutes. For specifics on dysmorphology or unusual findings, the reader is referred to more comprehensive texts.

HISTORY

As for a child of any age, the physical examination must be performed in conjunction with historical information. The history of the mother's medical background, pregnancy, labor, and delivery are all important elements that affect the product of her gestation. Did the mother take any prescribed medications or illicit substances during the pregnancy? Is there a history of bleeding, premature labor, or preeclampsia? Was the pregnancy complicated by any infections, illnesses, or chronic conditions such as diabetes mellitus or hypertension? Were membranes ruptured for longer than 24 hours prior to delivery, thereby putting the baby at increased risk for bacterial infections? Did the labor progress smoothly or were there abnormal decelerations in fetal heart rate? Was the baby a breech or vertex presentation? Did the mother receive local or general anesthesia for the delivery?

In the delivery room, the condition of the baby is scored using a system developed by Apgar. The baby is rated in five categories (color, cry, tone, reflex irritability, and heart rate) and a 0, 1, or 2 rating is given for each category. The maximum score is 10. Babies are rated routinely at 1 minute and 5 minutes after delivery and for every 5 minutes thereafter if the Apgar score taken at 5 minutes is less than 7. This score provides an estimation of asphyxia or some serious physiologic problem.

INITIAL INSPECTION

While a cursory inspection may have taken place in the delivery room, the formal pediatric examination generally is conducted in the newborn nursery or in the mother's room. The examiner should make sure the baby is in a warm environment. The examiner should wash his hands and instruments should be wiped clean. The baby first should be inspected for general appearance. Posture is a direct reflection of neurologic maturity and tone; arms and legs are held in flexion in the term child. Is the baby the appropriate size and weight for gestational age? The average weight for a 40-week gestation baby in the United States is 3.6 ± 0.4 kg (SD). A term baby is considered to be one with a 37 to 42 week gestation. The term child who weighs less than 2,500 g is considered small for gestational age (SGA); conversely, the term baby who weighs more than 4,000 g is considered large for gestational age (LGA). The baby born before 37 weeks' gestation is premature and often requires more careful medical management in an intensive care nursery. The baby born after 42 weeks' gestation is considered postmature and commonly has peeling skin, long fingernails, meconium staining, narrow umbilical cord, and some tissue wasting.

The order in which the examination is done is dictated by the child. If the child is asleep or quiet, the cardiorespiratory examination is best completed at this time. By convention, however, the components of the examination will be presented in the standard way in which they are organized in medical records.

VITAL SIGNS

The vital signs of the newborn include respiratory rate, heart rate, temperature, and blood pressure. The respiratory rate can be counted for 60 seconds without perturbing the baby. The rate may be irregular and normally may show pauses for up to 5 seconds. A normal respiratory rate is 30 to 50 breaths per minute. The heart rate is best assessed with a stethoscope placed at the apex. Normal heart rate for the term baby is 120 to 160 beats per minute. Temperature should be determined frequently until stable. The most accurate is the rectal temperature, with a normal newborn reading of 37° ± 0.5° C (SD). Blood pressure is best obtained with a Doppler cuff.

SKIN

Skin should be pink, warm to the touch, and have good capillary refill. In the first hours there may be some acrocyanosis of hands and feet, which often disappears with warming of the baby. Mottling is also seen with low ambient temperature and vasomotor instability. Peeling of the skin is a sign associated with postmaturity. Translucent skin with many blood vessels is associated with prematurity. Lanugo, or fine body hair, develops at 20 weeks gestation and largely disappears by birth. Lanugo may be seen on the shoulders, forehead, and lower back. Bruising and petechiae may characterize the presenting part. Birthmarks can be detected on nearly every newborn. Ninety percent of darkly pigmented children have blue birthmarks that appear like bruises on the buttocks and lower extremities. These mongolian spots represent melanocytes that did not complete the migration in the fetus from neural crest to epidermis. Other frequently seen birthmarks are the salmon patch and capillary hemangioma (Fig 4–1). A common vascular nevus usually is found on the nape of the neck, scalp, eyelids, or nasal bridge. The newborn often develops a rash or eruption in the first few days of life. The most common eruptions are milia, erythema toxicum, pustular melanosis, acne, and staphylococcal pustulosis. Skin is the organ system of the body that best shows the normal rise in bilirubin concentration during the first 4 days of the child's life. As the bilirubin level rises, jaundice progresses in a cephalad to caudal direction. The yellowness can be appreciated in natural light by putting the finger on the skin to cause blanching. Yellow pigment can also be seen in the buccal mucosa and under the tongue. Jaundice in the first 24 hours of life is serious and requires laboratory evaluation.

HEAD

The head should be assessed for size and shape. Both hands should be used in palpating fontanelles, sutures, and bones. The diamond-shaped anterior fontanelle should be open with 1 to 4 cm on each side. The posterior fontanelle is smaller and may be closed at birth. Sutures should be palpable and open. A distinct ridge at a suture line indicates an overriding bone, which requires no treatment. Prematurely fused sutures are evidence of craniosynostosis. This condition can be confirmed with skull radiographs and should be referred for neurosurgical evaluation. Molding or shaping of the head is frequently found in the baby who presented head first. A cephalohematoma is a collection of blood generally confined to one side of the head. Edema fluid or caput succedaneum extends on both sides of the suture line. Any baby who had a precipitous, traumatic, or high-forceps delivery should be examined carefully for skull fracture. Many babies will have an eschar at the site of the scalp clip inserted for monitoring during the last stages of the mother's labor. Normal head circumference is 35 cm in the term baby. If the head circumference is larger than 38 cm, the fontanelle should be

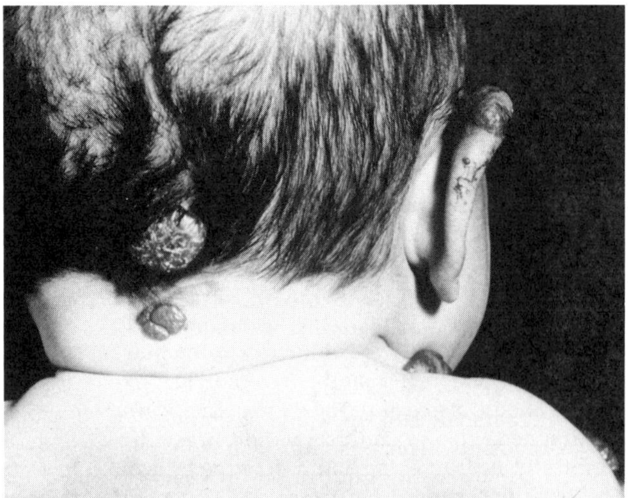

FIG 4–1
Capillary hemangioma.

carefully examined for fullness and transillumination of the head should be performed to screen for collections of fluid.

EYES

The eyes should be noted for size, shape, and slant. Their appearance should be almond-shaped with palpebral fissures that are 1.9 cm in length. Microphthalmia is associated with congenital defects and syndromes. A large epicanthal fold in an infant with a flat nasal bridge gives the appearance of crossed eyes when in fact no esotropia is present. This condition is called pseudostrabismus. An upward slant to the palpebral fissures is seen in children with Down syndrome, while the antimongoloid slant is found in such conditions as fetal alcohol syndrome. The more the examiner tries to forcibly separate the eyelids, the more difficult examining the globe can be. The preferred technique is to allow the baby to open his eyes on his own. This can be accomplished by raising the baby to an upright position and simultaneously making cooing or whistling noises. The eyes themselves often have disconjugate movements. The conjunctiva may appear injected as a result of irritation from silver nitrate drops. A chemical conjunctivitis may persist for 4 to 5 days. The conjunctiva may also reveal slight hemorrhage as a result of vessel rupture during passage through the birth canal. It is difficult to do a funduscopic examination on a newborn. The ophthalmoscope should be used to determine the presence of the red reflex bilaterally and to rule out congenital clouding of the cornea or lens. Visual acuity of the newborn is estimated to be 20/600 at birth and for the first week of life.

EARS

The size, shape, and orientation of the auricles should be observed. Malformations or malpositionings of the ear or skin tags are often associated with anomalies of the kidney or branchial pouch remnants. There is little value in performing an otoscopic examination in a healthy newborn.

NOSE

Since newborn babies are obligate nose breathers, the nares should be patent without obstruction internally. A feeding tube can be passed into each nostril to rule out choanal atresia. The baby's nose is flat with an underdeveloped nasal bridge.

MOUTH

The oral cavity should be inspected and palpated for clefts and submucous defects. On the soft palate, there may be small inclusion cysts called Ebstein pearls. Occasionally on the gums, a larger inclusion cyst or epulis is seen that appears like an erupting tooth. Any natal teeth present in the mouth usually have poor roots and should be extracted to lessen the risk of possible aspiration by the newborn. By the end of the baby's nursery stay, white curdlike material may appear on the tongue, gums, or buccal mucosa; this is oral moniliasis or thrush.

NECK

The neck should be examined for masses or lumps. Lymph nodes are usually not filled and any such finding should be considered to be related to branchial-pouch remnants or congenital malformations such as cystic hygromas. Head tilt is often a sign of wryneck or torticollis. Shortened sternocleidomastoid fibers on the affected side may be palpable as a mass in the neck. The thyroid is not palpable. Head and neck control are poor in the newborn and nuchal rigidity should not be sought as a sign of meningitis during this period.

CLAVICLES

Clavicles should be intact from manubrium to shoulders. Clavicular fractures are estimated to occur in 1% of newborns delivered vaginally. Fine clavicular fracture includes (1) a lump or irregularity of the clavicle on inspection or palpation, (2) crepitus on palpation of the clavicle, or (3) decreased or asymmetric arm movements. No treatment is needed.

CHEST

The chest of the newborn should show symmetric movement bilaterally during respiration. Asymmetric movement or hyperinflation are signs of underlying pulmonary pathologies such as pneumothorax or air trapping. Breast tissue is often enlarged bilaterally in both boys and girls. A milky secretion is present or can be expressed with slight manual palpation. This normal finding is a result of maternal estrogens. A stethoscope should be used to auscultate both sides of the chest for symmetric vesicular breath sounds. Adventitial sounds are unusual in the healthy newborn and may represent sounds transmitted from the upper airway. In the neonate with pneumonia, one of the first signs may be simply tachypnea without auscultatory findings. Decreased breath sounds in one lung field are clues to infection or lobar collapse.

HEART

The relatively rapid heart rate of the newborn in contrast to that of the adult makes it difficult to sort out heart sounds, splits, and murmurs. The physician should listen to the heart in at least five locations: the lower left sternal border at the fifth intercostal space, the apex, the aortic area, the pulmonic area, and the back. The second heart sound should be split, which is best heard at the base. Pathologic murmurs are usually accompanied by significant cyanosis in the first 24 hours. Murmurs that are heard best in the axilla or back are often due to pulmonic or peripheral pulmonary stenosis. Pulses should be felt in the femoral, brachial, and radial areas.

ABDOMEN

The abdomen of the newborn infant is protuberant with a newly cut umbilical stump. The cord should be kept clean and treated regularly with triple dye or ethyl alcohol. A defect at the base of the umbilicus or umbilical hernia is seen in approximately 20% of black babies. In the white child it is a much less common finding and should alert the examiner to question the presence of hypothyroidism. In the right upper quadrant, the liver edge is often felt 1 to 2 cm below the right costal margin. In the left upper quadrant, the spleen tip may be palpable but is usually not detected. By using deep palpation, a skilled examiner may feel masses paravertebrally that represent the kidneys. A polycystic or hydronephrotic kidney will be easily palpated as an abdominal mass. In the lower quadrant, fecal masses predominate. The complete examination of the abdomen should include a digital rectal examination, especially if there is any question about an abdominal mass. The physician should assess relative patency of the rectum and examine for anal fissures.

GENITALIA

In the girl, a white mucoid secretion or bloody discharge may be noted. This bloody discharge represents the effects of maternal estrogen withdrawal and occurs near the end of the first week of life. The labia minora often appear enlarged and a hymenal skin tag may be present at the posterior fourchette.

In the boy, the scrotum is a reflection of physical maturity. Pendulous testes with rugose scrotal skin represent a mature term newborn male. Testes are often retractile and may be palpated in the inguinal region. If no testicle is palpated, the examiner should look to see if that side of the scrotum appears underdeveloped. If so, this should raise the question of an abdominal testicle and warrants a follow-up examination for an undescended testicle. The urethral meatus should be at the end of the glands if a decision for circumcision is made. Hypospadias and chordee are contraindications to circumcision. A swelling in the inguinal area or scrotum may represent a hernia or hydrocele. Since a hydrocele is fluid-filled, its presence can be verified with transillumination.

EXTREMITIES

The upper extremities should be examined for full range of motion at all joints. Supernumerary digits occur in 0.5% of children. If only a supernumerary skin tag is present, it may be tied off at its base and allowed to necrose. If a bone is present in the supernumerary digit, re-

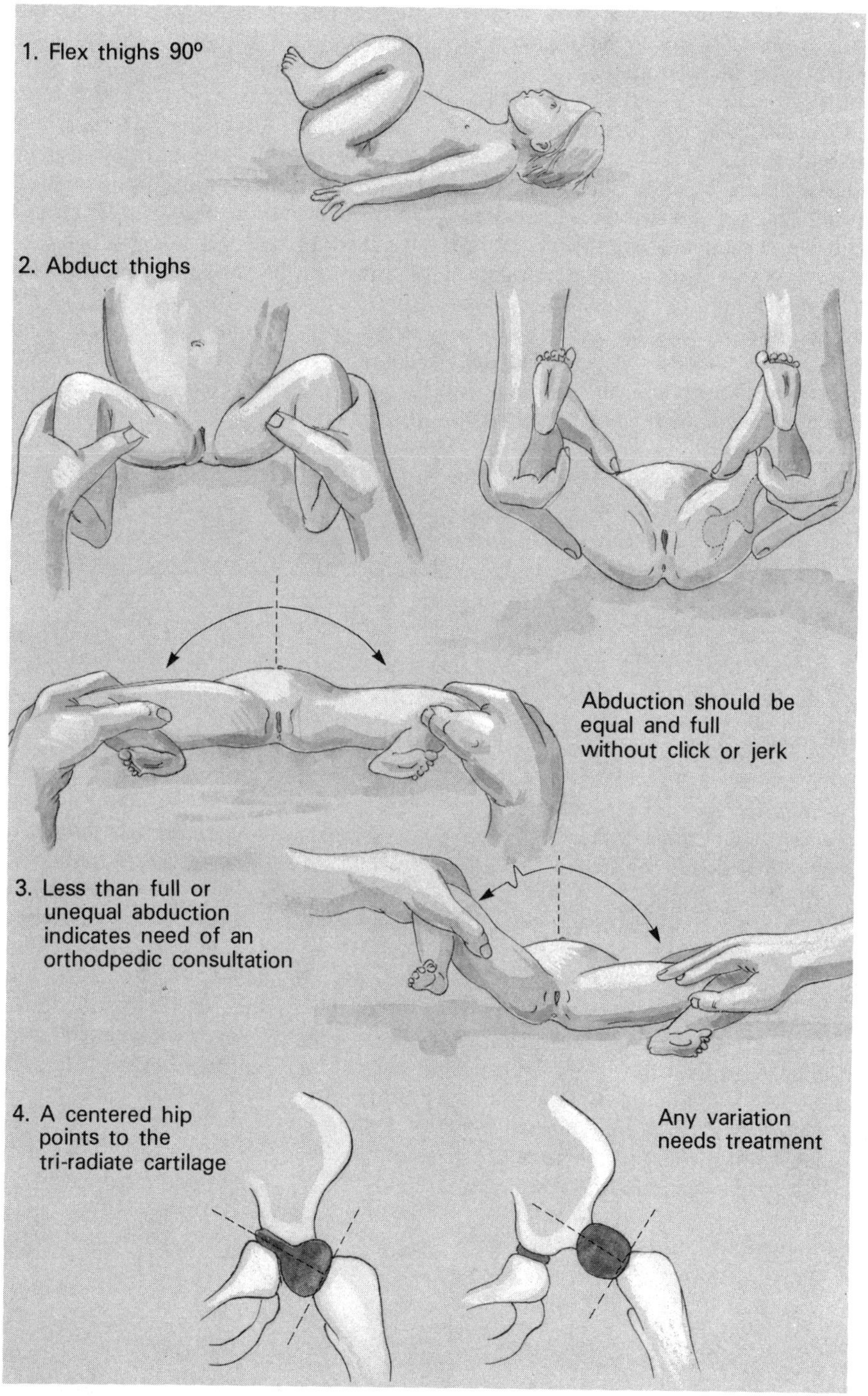

FIG 4–2

Examination of infant for congenital dislocated hip. Correct placement of thumb and finger overlying the head of femur during abduction should be noted.

ferral of the child to the appropriate surgical service is indicated. In the lower extremities, the hip merits special attention. Congenital dislocation of the hip occurs in 1 of 1,000 births. The consequences of not recognizing this defect are devastating. The examiner should be able to abduct both hips to 180° (Fig 4–2). Hands should be positioned on both thighs with thumbs in the medial position and third fingers overlying the head of the femurs. A clunking sound on abduction or adduction indicates a hip dislocation. Hip clicks are relatively common and usually disappear on their own by the time of the 1-month examination. Some authorities recommend double or triple diapering when a hip click is detected, to keep the hip and upper leg in abduction and force the head of the femur more firmly into the acetabulum. Feet are often a great concern to the parents and some anticipatory statements may save the primary care physician some grief later. Parents are often concerned about toeing-in or toeing-out. Metatarsus adductus is a medial deviation of the forefoot. All newborns will have some degree of adduction and tibial torsion which gives the impression of toeing-in. Parents can be reassured that the legs will tend to straighten as the baby becomes older and bears weight. One reassuring maneuver is to demonstrate to parents how easily the infant's legs curl into a cross-legged position. Some patience is in order to allow the lower extremities to reach a cosmetically acceptable alignment.

PROBLEMS OF NEWBORN CARE

Thomas Curry, M.D.

Health supervision of the infant less than 1 year of age requires the ability to separate specific disease entities from everyday occurrences that are variations or minor deviations from normal.

Many needless diagnostic studies and therapeutic trials have resulted from the physician's overreaction to the infant who regurgitates after feeding, has difficulty passing a bowel movement, or is awake all night crying. However, each symptom requires a thoughtful approach since it may be the harbinger of a significant medical problem. The communication of information to the family in a manner that lessens anxiety and improves parental confidence is a challenge.

The following is a discussion of problems (listed in alphabetical order) that are frequent topics of concern at the time of a health supervision visit.

CAROTENEMIA

A common concern is the infant's skin having a deep yellow coloration. On occasion, a family member associates this development with neonatal jaundice; this association produces a great deal of anxiety.

On physical examination, the skin has a distinct yellow appearance, without evidence of scleral icterus. The dietary history reveals ingestion of foods containing carotenoids over a prolonged period of time. These foods include carrots and squash.

The coloration of the skin is harmless and does not require treatment. The color lessens after a change in dietary intake is accomplished.

CRYING AND GAS

The crying, fussy, gassy infant is a frequent source of anxiety to parents, extended family, and consequently to the primary care physician.

CAUSES OF RECURRENT PAIN

Feeding problems
- Technique (too much air, nipple inappropriate)
- Volume of feeding
- Breast-feeding and technique

Problems related to gastrointestinal (GI) tract
- Reflux
- Constipation
- Allergy to milk

Head or neck
- Mental retardation
- Otitis media
- Eyes (glaucoma, abrasion)

Abdomen or extremities
- Abdomen (hernia, intussusception, torsion testicles, fissure)

Extremities (fracture, ingrown toenails, hair strangulation)

Urinary tract
- Infection

The fact that infants have fussy periods and that the symptom complex of colic develops in some has resulted in a number of folk and traditional remedies for the situation. The number of approaches in itself is testament to the inadequacy of current treatment methods.

Colic is an infant's episodic fussiness or crying (after the immediate newborn period) that is persistent over hours and days and that does not respond to simple comforting measures. During the episode, the infant will cry as if in pain and pull up his legs. Often the abdomen will be hard. Occasionally, relief is evident with passage of flatus. The attack may last for hours. Treatment of colic is discussed later in this chapter.

A detailed history is valuable in conveying to the family the physician's earnestness in dealing with the problem. Important points include: family history of colic, review of birth history, feeding history (including rate of flow from the nipple), formula changes, technique of burping, and stool pattern. Social history should focus on current family stress regarding the newborn, parents' relationship, financial problems, health problems, and expectations of the infant. This is an important time to find out if the mother is fatigued physically and emotionally, if she has free time, and how much help is available to her.

A complete physical examination should be performed. Points to be emphasized include: central nervous system (CNS), ears, eyes, mouth (dentition), abdomen (hernia, intussusception), extremities (fracture), and rectum. Announcing several times during the examination that the results of the physical examination are normal helps build the confidence of the parents.

If the history and physical examination, including review of growth to date, fail to point to any of the suggested causes of crying in infancy, little in the way of laboratory studies is required. Some physicians would insist that a urinalysis and a urine culture be obtained.

There are a number of infants who have periodic fussiness that does not fit the definition of colic. These infants do not meet the parental or extended family concept of the "good" baby. Familiarity with the literature in regard to infant temperament is very helpful in reassuring parents that the pattern of behavior they are dealing with is not a sign of disease. Reassurance that the crying or gassy infant's symptoms are not beyond the expectation of normal variation can be helpful. The family must perceive that the physician is interested and willing to take action if there is a further development of symptoms. If the physician gives the family the impression of unwillingness or reluctance to discuss the problem because of its trivial nature, little resolution of their anxiety can be expected.

CONJUNCTIVITIS

Conjunctivitis is a frequent problem during the first year of life. Symptoms that appear in the nursery immediately after the instillation of chemical drops need to be distinguished from infection that occurs during the first few days of life. Gonorrheal ophthalmia produces a profuse, purulent discharge with lid swelling. It occurs during the first week of life. Gonorrheal ophthalmia may be delayed by the use of silver nitrate or antibiotic ointments in the nursery.

Infections that occur after the infant is discharged from the nursery are frequently caused by bacteria or *Chlamydia*. The cause cannot be assumed on the basis of the time sequence alone. Patients with infection caused by *Chlamydia* may also have a cough. If the infant has had excessive tearing preceding the development of infections, evaluation for dacryostenosis may be necessary after treatment of the infection. In the older infant, conjunctivitis in the presence of an upper respiratory tract infection should suggest careful evaluation of the tympanic membranes for otitis media.

It is frequently stated that all episodes of conjunctivitis require gram staining (for intracellular diplococci), Giemsa staining (for inclusion blennorrhea), and culture (for gonococci). It should be kept in mind that this laboratory approach can be extremely expensive and may not be necessary in every circumstance if the infant is older than 1 month. The development of monoclonal antibody testing to identify *Chlamydia* may ease the problem of documenting the cause of conjunctivitis, because culturing *Chlamydia* is a difficult procedure for most community hospital laboratories.

Treatment of conjunctivitis depends on the cause. Gonococcal ophthalmia requires intense, inpatient therapy. Treatment of chlamydial conjunctivitis includes the use of oral erythromycin rather than topical agents alone. Prolonged treatment may prove to be of value in preventing chlamydial pneumonitis of the newborn.

Most cases of bacterial conjunctivitis can be treated with an ophthalmic solution of sodium sulfacetamide. Explaining to the parents the expected response time and making arrangements for a return call or visit are equally important to the institution of treatment. If the condition fails to improve after 48 hours of treatment, a culture should be obtained.

The parents of an infant with dacryostenosis should be informed of the probability of recurrence. Guidelines for appropriate surgical referral vary with geographic location. Many physicians think that surgical correction before the infant is 9 months old is rarely necessary.

CONSTIPATION

Constipation and questions related to what is perceived by parents as constipation are among the most frequent inquiries made of a primary care physician. Underlying the problem is a common misunderstanding with regard to neonatal stool patterns. The difficulty in dealing with the symptom is compounded by the occurrence of life-threatening conditions that can present as constipation during this time period (i.e., Hirschsprung disease, hypothyroidism, infant botulism).

The diagnosis and treatment of constipation must be grounded in a thorough history that includes description of stool consistency and frequency. Newborns, particularly breast-fed infants, may have a stool as infrequently as once per week. If the stool is soft, of appropriate volume, and produced with moderate effort, even though it may occur once every several days, constipation does not exist.

In reviewing family history, there can be a family predisposition to constipation or a family can be overly concerned regarding constipation. If there was delay in passage of first stool and the infant always had difficulty with stool passage, the history can be suggestive of Hirschsprung disease. Hypothyroidism is suggested by the following signs and symptoms: jaundice as a newborn, large tongue, and umbilical hernia. A history that includes difficulty with feeding such as poor suck, decreasing volume of intake, respiratory symptoms, and poor muscle tone indicates the need for further investigation to rule out infant botulism.

Physical examination includes evaluation of growth velocity and determination of the presence of the following: jaundice, large tongue, umbilical hernia, poor head control, testing of reflexes, sensory examination, particularly in lower extremities, and abnormalities of vertebral column. A rectal examination must be performed. A forward-placed anus has been associated with constipation. Partial rectal stenosis may be evident on examination. Failure to elicit an anal wink points to neurologic defect. Absence of stool in the ampulla can suggest Hirschsprung disease. If the stool is present in the rectum, a neurologic cause is less likely.

Hirschsprung disease can be confirmed with a barium enema study demonstrating a narrow segment of colon. Rectal manometry is occasionally used in diagnosis. Findings of neither test are definite and biopsy for presence of ganglion cells is necessary.

If a physician is convinced that no underlying cause of constipation exists, a variety of approaches have been used. Dietary manipulations may include a decrease in the volume of formula or decrease in amount of cereal. Additional fruit or water may be helpful. Administration of a nonabsorbable carbohydrate (malt soy extract) provides an improved stool pattern after the second day of administration. Although dietary manipulation is helpful in most cases, a rare patient may require use of a stool softener (dioctyl sodium) or glycerin suppository.

A glycerin rectal suppository for infants will frequently provide prompt relief of constipation. Unfortunately, parents will often resort to this technique with great frequency despite admonitions to the contrary.

In infants, mineral oil is not usually needed since it may lead to pneumonary aspirations and poor absorption of fat-soluble vitamins.

CRADLE CAP

Cradle cap, a crusted scaling area on the scalp, is a frequent finding at the time of physical examination of the neonate. It is important to distinguish cradle cap as an isolated physical finding rather than a more generalized condition such as seborrhea, eczema, and psoriasis. Inquiry should be made regarding a family history of such conditions. Other points to cover in the history include the treatment attempted by the family prior to the office visit. Some parents apply baby oil after the completion of shampooing. This practice temporarily improves the appearance of the scalp but after a period of time only leads to further increase in the amount of scaly material present.

On physical examination the oily scaling crust may be obvious or exposed by gentle abrasion with the fingernail. The presence of a rash behind the ears, on the neck, on the extensor surfaces, and in the diaper area should alert the physician that the condition may not solely be related to common cradle cap.

The major treatment of cradle cap is daily washing with a baby shampoo. The family should be instructed that vigorous shampooing is not precluded by the presence of a patent anterior fontanelle. Some families are hesitant regarding care of the scalp for fear of injuring the fontanelle. Frequently, this assurance is all that is needed to prevent a more extensive condition from developing.

When a diffuse process is present, the dry crusted material may be loosened with baby oil and gentle brushing. The oil treatment should be applied only prior to shampooing and only to aid in lifting the dried material from the scalp. Frequently, an antiseborrheic shampoo is necessary to complete the process. This should not be used routinely for shampooing but only in the initial stages of removal of cradle cap.

CRANIOSYNOSTOSIS

Craniosynostosis is the premature closing or fusion of one or more of the suture lines present in the skull of a neonate. Knowledge of the condition is important, for diagnosis when the infant is at an early age affords the best opportunity to avoid long-term medical complications related to increases in intracranial pressure and to prevent development of a configuration of the face and head that is aesthetically unacceptable to some families.

Craniosynostosis can occur as part of a multisystem congenital condition such as Crouzon disease or Apert syndrome or it may be an isolated finding. Diagnosis is suspected as a result of the specific configuration of the skull, palpation of a ridge along a given suture line, or abnormal head circumference. The diagnosis can be suspected at birth but may not be evident until an early well-child examination.

The myriad of terms used in describing craniosynostosis can be confusing to the practitioner who deals with the condition on an infrequent basis. The specific type of craniosynostosis is determined by the suture or suture line involved. An understanding of the condition is aided by reference to the common suture lines present in the newborn: sagittal, coronal, lambdoidal, metopic (Fig 4–3). Fusion of a specific suture results in growth in a direction parallel to the suture line that is fused. The resulting configuration of the skull is given a specific diagnosis: plagiocephaly, brachycephaly, scaphocephaly, acrocephaly, oxycephaly, and trigonocephaly (Table 4–1).

The urgency with which surgery must be performed depends on the involvement of multiple sutures. Some conditions mandate surgery when the infant is approximately 6 weeks old. Other conditions (scaphocephaly) may not have implications other than cosmetic results, and occasionally parents will refuse to have surgery performed, particularly if a parent or close relative has a skull with a similar shape. Craniosynostosis in conjunction with other anomalies may require a clinical evaluation for genetic dysmorphology.

Diagnosis can frequently be confirmed with an x-ray of the skull, although a negative finding (absence of heaped-up suture margins) does not rule out the problem. Neurosurgical consultation at an early date is recommended.

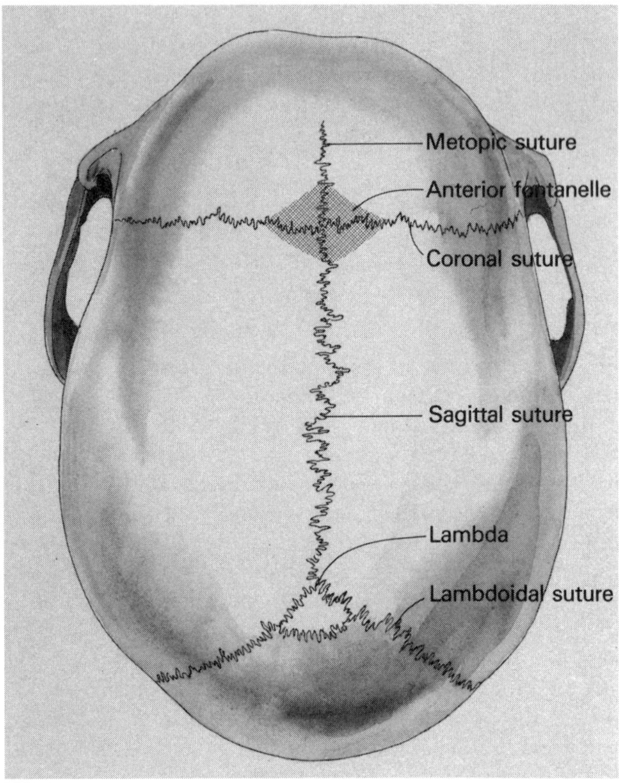

FIG 4–3
Cranial sutures present in the newborn. The specific types of craniosynostosis are determined by the suture or sutures involved in the process.

DERMOID

A lump on the skull, often first palpated by a parent, needs immediate clarification to allay anxiety and begin treatment when indicated. The lesion is not always noticed at birth or as part of the newborn examination and may not be questioned until the infant is several months old. A frequent location of palpable lesions is the occipital region; another common location is the supraorbital region, at the lateral margin of the eyebrow.

The primary differential diagnosis includes dermoid structure, lymph node, and sebaceous cyst. The location of the lesion helps to make the diagnosis. Dermoids occur at a suture line, since they are composed of embryologically derived tissue at the site where two cranial bones are joined. When a lesion is located in the occipital region, attempts should be made to define it in relation to the posterior auricular lymph nodes and the occipital nodes. A dermoid is usually midline between these anatomic markers. The dermoid has a fluid-filled

TABLE 4–1
Craniosynostosis

DIAGNOSIS	SUTURE	SHAPE
Plagiocephaly	Unilateral coronal synostosis	Facial asymmetry
Trigonocephaly	Metopic synostosis	Triangular configuration
Acrocephaly, oxycephaly	Coronal and lambdoidal	High, peaked, conical skull
Brachycephaly	Coronal and lambdoidal	Short broad cranium
Scaphocephaly	Sagittal synostosis	Long narrow cranium

consistency and is smooth surfaced; it is not fixed to the underlying structures if it is superficial to the bone. The intradeploic dermoid cannot be moved. A sebaceous cyst will frequently have a dimple present in the overlying skin.

Although many physicians will obtain x-rays of the skull to determine if there is an underlying bone defect, the absence of bone abnormalities is not conclusive evidence that there is no intracranial connection to the lesion. Midline lesions are particularly likely to be intradeploic.

Referral of a child with this lesion to an experienced surgical-anesthesia team is appropriate.

DIAPER RASH

Rash in the diaper area is a recurrent problem during the infant's first year of life. It is important to obtain a history of the rash and of the attempts made to care for it prior to instituting treatment.

The type of diaper used should be ascertained. Cloth diapers, washed at home and worn in conjunction with occlusive rubber pants, can frequently lead to maceration and inflammation of the skin. The use of antibiotics, particularly for the treatment of otitis media, can be associated with changes in bowel flora that permit overgrowth of fungus. Prior treatment with ointments and creams may have exacerbated the underlying condition; examples include the use of neomycin-containing products. Application of Vaseline can also lead to maceration and worsening of the condition.

Physical examination should not be restricted to the diaper area. The mouth should be examined for thrush. Evidence of coexisting rash behind the ears, on the scalp, intertriginous areas, face, extensor surfaces, and on the trunk may lead to a diagnosis of a more generalized skin condition that happens to be exacerbated in the diaper area. These conditions include seborrhea, eczema, and psoriasis.

Although the diaper area may have similar appearance for rashes of diverse cause, certain physical findings are helpful. A pustular eruption extending up to the umbilicus is consistent with a localized staphylococcal dermatitis. An intense red eruption with small satellite lesion or blister at the border of the rash is present with a monilial eruption (Fig 4–4).

Treatment consists of removal of the offending agents. If diapers are washed at home, particular efforts should be made regarding rinsing the diaper of residual material. Occlusive diapering that prevents evaporation of moisture from the layers of material next to the skin must also be altered.

If there is extensive inflammation and weeping, treatment with a modified Burow solution applied with a soaking diaper and followed by air drying is an important first step. If a specific cause such as staphylococcal or monilial infection is evident, an antibacterial or antifungal agent is appropriate. Use of multiple-agent creams is discouraged by many dermatologists. Contact dermatitis may be treated with a 1% hydrocortisone preparation. Potent fluorinated creams should not be used because they cause skin atrophy.

Occasionally an area of extreme skin breakdown exists particularly in the perianal region. This results in the infant crying at the time of stool passage and the contact of stool with the skin. It is appropriate to use an occlusive petrolatum only over the area of breakdown to prevent contact with stool. It must be stressed to the parent that the petrolatum is only meant to protect the area and not as a primary treatment. A perianal streptococcal infection should be considered as part of the differential diagnosis if the rash is localized to this anatomic region.

DRUG ABUSE EFFECT ON NEONATE

The infant who was exposed to drugs in utero as a result of maternal drug abuse or addiction is an infant at risk. In addition to in utero exposure an infant may have continuous drug effect if the mother is breast feeding and abusing drugs. Attributing signs and symptoms in the newborn to exposure to a specific street drug is difficult. Careful clinical observation of infants born to mothers with a single drug addiction as opposed to polydrug addiction has permitted the development of defined clinical syndromes, such as fetal alcohol syndrome.

Obtaining a history of maternal drug abuse prior to delivery may be difficult. The physi-

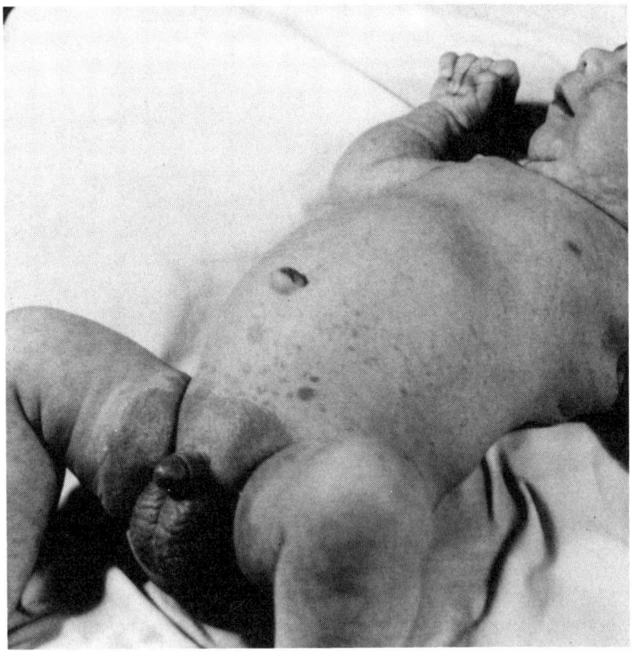

FIG 4–4
Monilial diaper rash demonstrating satellite lesions at the border of the rash.

cian need only be reminded of the pervasiveness of drug use and abuse in our society to realize the likelihood that at least some of the infants under his or her care have had drug exposure in utero. The assumption that this problem is restricted to portions of our population fails to take into account the extent to which cocaine and other drugs are viewed as recreational drugs by the age group in their reproductive years.

A physician needs to consider a diagnosis of neonatal drug withdrawal when there is a history of drug use during pregnancy and when a breast-fed infant has symptoms of drug withdrawal. The American Academy of Pediatrics Committee on Drugs has suggested the mnemonic WITHDRAWAL to aid in evaluating such symptoms.

SYMPTOMS OF NEONATAL DRUG WITHDRAWAL*

W = Wakefulness
I = Irritability
T = Tremulousness, temperature variation, tachypnea
H = Hyperactivity, high-pitched persistent cry, hyperacusia, hyperreflexia, hypertonus
D = Diarrhea, diaphoresis, disorganized suck
R = Rub marks, respiratory distress, rhinorrhea
A = Apneic attacks, autonomic dysfunction
W = Weight loss or failure to gain weight
A = Alkalosis (respiratory)
L = Lacrimation

Other symptoms of drug withdrawal include hiccups, vomiting, photophobia, and twitching.

With the widespread implementation of early discharge of newborns from the hospital, the physician needs to be mindful that although the symptoms may be present at birth or shortly afterward, definitive symptoms may not be evident until after the infant is discharged.

Treatment of a drug-addicted infant would normally take place in a hospital setting. Although pharmacologic therapy is not needed in a large percentage of infants, careful attention to caloric requirements, temperature regulation, and the changing clinical picture require initial inpatient assessment and treatment.

Hospitalization also permits the development of long-range plans for the infant at risk. Specific areas that need to be addressed include treatment of parental addiction, parental in-

*From American Academy of Pediatrics Committee on Drugs: Neonatal drug withdrawal. *Pediatrics* 1983; 72:896. Used by permission.

volvement in care of the infant, and identification of social service support in the months after discharge. An infant who has been withdrawn from drugs can have subacute symptoms that last several months.

The parent already under stress may have trouble dealing with the irritable, difficult to console baby. The infant of the mother receiving methadone is at risk for developmental delay, neurologic abnormalities in development of muscle tone, and nystagmus. Long-term medical involvement is necessary in addition to support from experienced social service professionals.

HERNIA

Hernias in the newborn usually involve questions of the location of hernia and the appropriate timing of surgery (Fig 4–5). Any lump or bulge in the inguinal region deserves consideration of a surgical consultation. Indirect inguinal hernias are common in the neonatal period. Although surgery is occasionally delayed until the infant sustains an appropriate weight gain, establishing prompt surgical contact is important. Another factor indicating surgical consultation is the occasional occurrence of an ovary or fallopian tube at the site of the inguinal hernia in the female. At times parents will report the presence of an inguinal bulge that will be gone by the time the infant is examined. This parents' observation should not be dismissed, because the hernia may slip back through the abdominal wall defect. An experienced examiner can frequently palpate a thickened spermatic cord or the tunica vaginalis rubbing on itself (silk glove sign) on the side of the previously observed bulge.

Umbilical hernias are approached differently. An umbilical hernia does not need surgical closure at an early age. Even large defects can close spontaneously, so observation and counseling are the best treatment. Many surgeons recommend waiting until the child is 4 or 5 years of age before closure is necessary. It is necessary to remind the parent that old-time therapies (such as an umbilical band or placing a coin over the hernia) are not useful and in rare cases can cause problems, particularly contact dermatitis.

Remnant umbilical structures such as a patent urachus or omphalomesenteric duct remnant may also be present. Any weeping le-

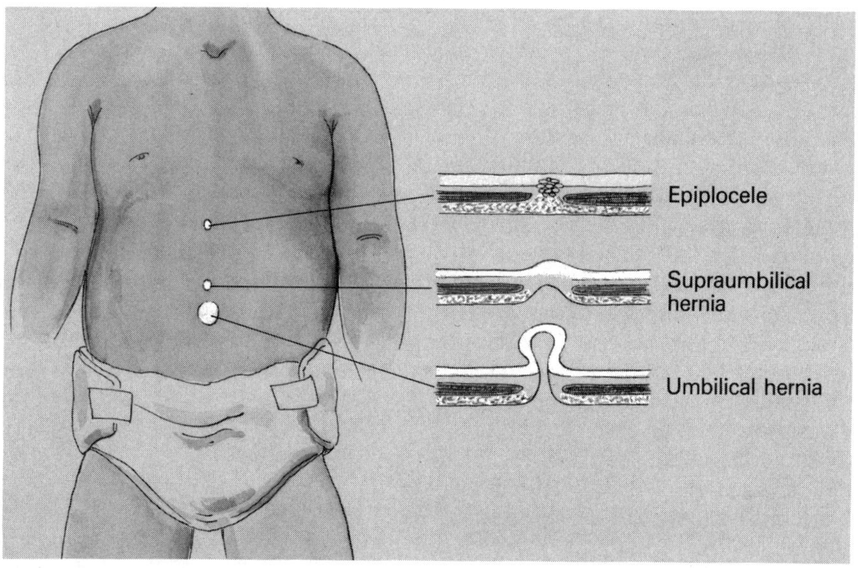

FIG 4–5
The anatomic location of midline defect in relation to umbilicus helps to determine need for surgical correction. A true umbilical hernia rarely requires early surgical intervention.

sion or structure with intermittent drainage or friable appearance should be considered a potential congenital remnant and appropriate consultation sought.

Hernias located in the midline but cephalad to the umbilicus do not close spontaneously. It is inappropriate to defer referral awaiting spontaneous closure of these supraumbilical hernias. An epiplocele is a midline defect with herniation of fatty tissue.

JAUNDICE

Jaundice persisting or developing after the infant is discharged from the newborn nursery merits an organized approach. Many primary care physicians now perform an initial in-office evaluation of a newborn 2 weeks after discharge from the hospital or birthing center. The reasons for this practice are varied, but one reason involves the frequency with which jaundice is noted at the time of this initial evaluation.

Historical points to be reviewed include prior history of jaundice in the extended family, the ethnic backgrounds of parents, and the previous neonatal history of the child's older siblings. Details of the pregnancy including symptoms of infection should be ascertained. The perinatal history must be reviewed. If the infant was not under the care of the practitioner during the newborn period, discussion with the attending physician or a review of the nursery records is helpful. If the infant had jaundice in the nursery, a review of laboratory evaluation obtained at that time is important. If the infant is breast-feeding, history should include the frequency of nursing, the use of water supplements, and the identification of the poorly feeding, poorly sleeping, dehydrated infant. Inquiry should be directed at the infant's activity level, including the level of alertness, eye contact, and response to a voice. The presence of vomiting, including the characteristics and color of emesis, should be documented. Stool and urinary patterns are also important historical points.

At the time of physical examination, documentation of weight and the change since discharge from the nursery should be noted. In addition to this, the physician should note head circumference, presence of hematoma, and results of funduscopic examination (including evaluation for cataracts and chorioretinitis). The presence of rash (including petechiae), hepatosplenomegaly, umbilical hernia, large tongue, and dry skin are all points that should be covered.

The possible conditions on which the differential diagnosis is based are numerous. If the child is breast-fed and if the findings of the historical and physical examination fail to point to a specific pathologic process, a less aggressive approach to diagnosis is warranted. A minimal laboratory diagnosis would include a bilirubin fractionation and blood type and Rh typing should be done if not performed while the infant was in the newborn nursery.

There is controversy regarding the diagnosis of breast-feeding jaundice by interruption of nursing. Gartner suggests that breast-feeding should not be interrupted simply to make the diagnosis if the serum bilirubin concentrations are less than 18 to 20 mg/dL. Maisels and Gifford suggest temporary discontinuation of breast-feeding as an appropriate therapeutic step.

Findings of laboratory tests that aid diagnosis include results of bilirubin fractionation, hemoglobin level, white blood cell (WBC) count, platelet count, reticulocyte count, blood type, results of Coombs' test, and review of the peripheral smear. Liver function tests and urine tests for reducing substances should also be performed (Table 4–2).

NASAL STUFFINESS

Nasal stuffiness, usually a benign condition, is confused with an infection or allergy. Historical information helps to assess the significance of the problem. The physician should determine the extent to which the nasal congestion interferes with the infant's sleep. Does the infant wake frequently during the night? Is there a noticeable drainage at the time of waking? Does the nasal congestion interfere with feeding? Inquiry as to whether the stuffiness bothers the infant, parent, or grandparent can sometimes place the problem in perspective. Convincing a parent that a growing infant who sleeps through the night and feeds without difficulty does not need treatment of a stuffy nose takes time but may help avoid an endless round of medication and symptomatic trials.

Nasal stuffiness that occurs in the infant during fall and winter months may be related to the heating system and breathing warm air with the resultant drying of mucus in the nose. There is no drainage associated with this problem. Use of a humidifier is frequently helpful. However, if this maneuver prompts the development of mold in the bedroom, further problems may ensue in an allergy-prone infant. On occasion, physical examination will reveal a dry mucus plug in the nares. Parental smoking, especially in a closed winter-time environment, may exacerbate the infant's nasal congestion.

If drainage has been present since birth, particularly unilaterally, consideration should be given to anatomic abnormalities such as choanal atresia. Passage of a feeding tube designed for infants will help to define the problem. Rarely is a foreign body a problem in this age group. Foreign bodies usually produce a foul-smelling discharge.

Occasionally, an infant will have persistent purulent drainage. It is appropriate to culture this material and consider antibiotic therapy for a documented bacterial rhinitis. If there is a recurrent problem, inquiry should be made regarding parental manipulation of the nares with a bulb syringe. Persistent purulent drainage should lead to consideration of an ethmoid sinus infection and x-rays of those structures.

Therapy for nasal stuffiness with decongestant or decongestant-antihistamine medication is discouraged because of frequent reactions, particularly to the antihistamine. Overuse of topical nasal decongestant results in rhinitis medicamentosus.

TABLE 4–2
Comparison of Types of Hyperbilirubinemia

DIRECT HYPERBILIRUBINEMIA	INDIRECT HYPERBILIRUBINEMIA
Hepatitis (variety of causes)	High red blood cell destruction
Inborn error (galactosemia)	Hemolysis
Cystic fibrosis	Congenital defect of red cell
Sepsis	Resolved hematoma
α-Antitrypsin deficiency	Deficiency of glucose-6-phosphate dehydrogenase, pyruvate kinase deficiency
Biliary atresia	Deficient β-glucuronyl transferase activity
Infection	Type I (Crigler-Najjar disease)
	Type II
	Breast-feeding
	Familial-transmitted neonatal hyperbilirubinemia
	Maternal diabetes
	Pyloric stenosis or other congenital obstruction
	Hypothyroidism

SEPARATION ANXIETY

As an infant approaches 6 months of age, he or she will frequently become fretful and distressed when the parent leaves. This situation is termed "separation anxiety." Variations in separation anxiety can present in the toddler. A new or inexperienced parent will be informed by friends or family that separation anxiety is a result of "spoiling" the infant. If the parents have been warned prior to the occurrence of separation anxiety (most often as part of anticipatory guidance at the 4-month visit), feelings of poor parenting or guilt can be avoided. Separation anxiety should be discussed in terms of normal development such as sitting, crawling, and other milestones.

The following suggestions can be helpful to parents. The development of a routine is important, so that the mother and father have definite time periods away from the infant. Reassurance that they are not "bad" parents to have time away from the infant must be verbalized and occasionally emphasized. The parents of an infant who experienced medical problems in the newborn nursery must particularly be encouraged to take time out from parenting.

Frequently a routine can be set up to have a reliable high-school student stay with the infant for an hour several times a week after school or for mothers to share baby-sitting duties for infants of similar ages. This program should be followed despite the fact that the infant may cry when the parents leave.

Occasionally parents will develop routines that emphasize coming and going in excess. Overstatements that "mom is leaving now" or on her return "did you miss your mom?" only serve to underline the mother's and infant's anxiety.

Reassurance that in time the intensity of the separation anxiety will abate may be helpful. Most important, the parents should be told this is a normal developmental stage that the child needs to pass through. They should be encouraged to help the child work through this separation rather than to be in constant attendance and delay the child's development.

INGROWN TOENAILS

Ingrown toenails can occur during the first year of life. Some physicians believe they are seen more often when restrictive clothing (tight socks, sleeper pajamas) is worn by the infant. The condition usually resolves if the parent is instructed to avoid tight clothing for the infant and to care for the nail properly. Proper care includes cutting the nail straight across rather than on a diagonal at the outer edges and applying gentle pressure at the nail margin after bathing the infant to eventually lift the nail plate above the adjoining skin. Rarely is nail removal necessary when the infant is this age.

TEMPERAMENT

Parents of newborn infants approach the childrearing experience with preconceived notions of the child's personality and activity level. The parents' expectations are based on prior experience or lack of experience and, occasionally, on reading information in the current popular press. Rarely do parents raise questions about the "good baby." However, they do tell their relatives, neighbors, and anyone who will listen how their child sleeps all night, feeds without a fuss, and never cries. Although such babies exist, they do not constitute the majority of infants.

During the past few decades, a considerable body of literature on child temperament has developed. It is important for the primary care physician who sees infants and their parents to recognize that infants have particular traits that characterize their behavioral style independent of their environment. Chess and associates identified nine characteristics of infant temperament that they think are primary reactive patterns that children possess:

CHARACTERISTICS OF TEMPERAMENT

Activity level
Rhythmicity
Approach-withdrawal
Adaptability
Threshold
Intensity
Mood
Distractibility

These traits may be altered by the environment but are the initial reaction that the child exhibits.

Physicians frequently encounter the "difficult child" during the first year. Because infants do not have a biologic rhythm, their sleep-awake pattern is irregular. They have an intensity of expression that is manifested by a piercing cry. They will withdraw from new environments (grandmother's house). This temperament can lead to significant stress in the family. It is this family, frequently including the extended family, that requires the physician's time for affirmation of their adequacy as parents, and reassurance as to the absence of disease or structural problems.

Specific advice is needed regarding establishment of a routine for feeding, bathing, and sleeping. A consistent approach to crying and negative reactions by all family members should be discussed. It is important to ensure that the parents of the difficult child have time away from the infant, since it is for this child that it is difficult to find a babysitter. The concepts of primary reactive pattern and infant temperament may be difficult to grasp without studying works of Carey and Chess, Thomas and Birch.

VOMITING, REGURGITATION

The difficulty for the primary care physician in assessing recurrent vomiting includes identifying those infants who have surgical causes (pyloric stenosis, intestinal obstruction); pinpointing those infants who require diagnostic evaluation for gastroesophageal reflux (GER); deciding what diagnostic tests should be performed and in what sequence; and avoiding unnecessary studies and consultation for the vast majority of infants who regurgitate small amounts after feeding without any underlying cause.

CAUSES OF RECURRENT VOMITING

- Feeding
  - Excess air
  - Overfeeding
- CNS disease
- Metabolic acidosis
- Infection
  - Sepsis
  - CNS infection
  - Urinary tract infection
- Drugs
  - Aspirin
  - Antibiotics
- Esophageal reflux
- Surgical
  - Obstruction (pyloric, intussusception)
  - Appendicitis
- Spitting of newborn

Questions to be answered in the evaluation of vomiting include: Has the vomiting been present since the infant's birth or is it a new development? When does the vomiting occur in relation to feeding? After the infant vomits, does he want to be refed? What is the color and what is the volume of vomitus? Does the infant show other signs of illness?

Physical examination must include documentation of weight, change of weight, and a plot of weight on the percentile graph. CNS examination should include head circumference, status of fontanelle, extraocular movement, and presence of appropriate reflexes. Chest examination should include evaluation for evidence of aspiration such as wheezing. Abdominal examination includes evaluation for signs of obstruction and a mass lesion, and a rectal examination should be performed.

Most obstructive lesions of the gastrointestinal tract that are congenital are diagnosed prior to the infant's discharge from the nursery (e.g., tracheoesophageal fistula, duodenal atresia). Pyloric stenosis can present in the infant from the first week until several months of age, although the usual presentation is at 3 to 6 weeks of age. With pyloric stenosis, the vomiting is forceful and projectile. The infant is frequently hungry immediately after vomiting. Despite traditional thinking, pyloric stenosis does not occur more frequently in first-born boys.

Experienced physicians can make a diagnosis of pyloric stenosis by palpation of the tumor lo-

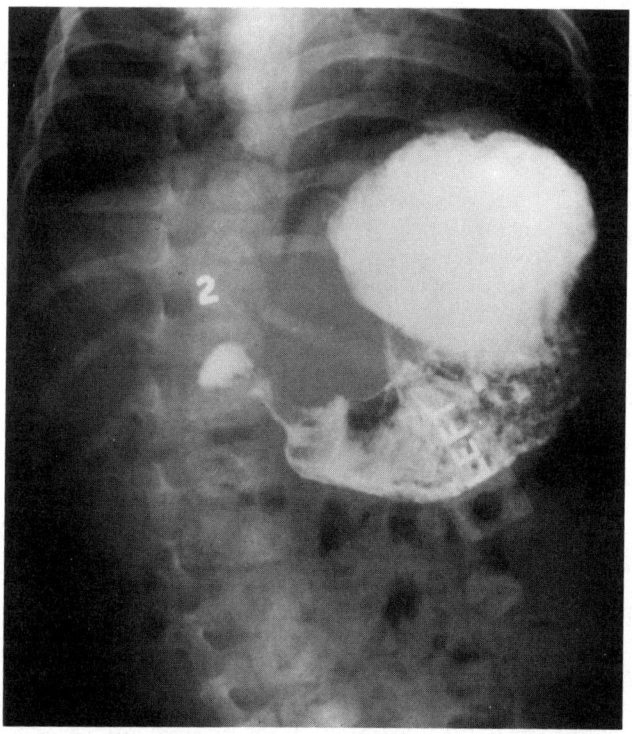

FIG 4–6
Pyloric stenosis demonstrated by barium swallow study. The procedure must be performed with care to avoid consequences of aspiration. This study has been replaced by ultrasound in many centers.

cated lateral to midline in the right upper quadrant. Ultrasound is helpful in making a diagnosis. Care must be exercised when performing a barium swallow study to avoid aspiration pneumonia (Fig 4–6).

Sepsis can present as vomiting and the physician should think of CNS and renal infection as a possible cause.

Gastroesophageal reflux occurs commonly and has been associated with a number of conditions that include asthma, anemia, and failure to thrive. The infant vomits at any time, from immediately after feeding to several hours later. The volume varies with each episode. The emesis may be preceded by crying and irritability. A variety of studies are available, with no one study currently being used universally. The traditional barium swallow study will fail to identify reflux in many cases. Overreading and overmanipulation of the abdomen may result in false-positive findings. A milk scan with technetium is slightly more sensitive but the pH probe is presently the best diagnostic test.

Once diagnosis has been confirmed, therapy should start with small, frequent, thickened feedings. A mainstay of therapy for years had been upright feeding; however, Orenstein and others have demonstrated a lack of efficacy of the upright feeding. Even though vomiting may persist, the patient may thrive. If growth velocity decreases, wheezing or other signs of pulmonary aspiration appear, or symptoms of esophagitis develop, treatment with metoclopramide is attempted. Consideration of fundoplication is necessary for the infant in whom conservative medical treatment fails to control symptoms.

BIBLIOGRAPHY

Carey WB: The difficult child. *Pediatr Rev* 1986; 8:39–45.

Fisher MC: Conjunctivitis in children. *Pediatr Clin North Am* 1987; 34:1447–1456.

Fitzgerald JF: Constipation in children. *Pediatr Rev* 1987; 8:299–302.

Gartner LM: Breast milk jaundice, in *Hyperbilirubinemia in the Newborn.* Report of the 85th Ross Conference in Pediatric Research. Columbus, Ohio, Ross Laboratories, 1983.

Hewson P, Oberklaid F, Menahem S: Infant colic, distress, and crying. *Clin Pediatr* 1987; 26:69–75.

Kokx NP, Constock JA, Facklam RR: Streptococcal perianal disease in children. *Pediatrics* 1987; 80:659–663.

Maisels MJ, Gifford K: Normal serum bilirubin levels in the newborn and the effect of breast-feeding. *Pediatrics* 1986; 78:837–843.

Marchac D, Renier D: Treatment of craniosynostosis in infancy. *Clin Plast Surg* 1987; 14:61–72.

Orenstein SR, Magile HL, Brooks P: Thickening of infant feedings for therapy of gastroesophageal reflux. *J Pediatr* 1987; 110:181–186.

Orenstein SR, Whitington PF, Orenstein DM. The infant seat as treatment for gastroesophageal reflux. *N Engl J Med* 1983; 309:760–763.

Rosen TS, Johnson HL: Children of methadone-maintained mothers: Follow-up to 18 months of age. *J Pediatr* 1982; 101:192–196.

Thomas A, Chess S, Birch HG: *Temperament and Behavior Disorders in Children.* New York, New York University Press, 1968.

Weinberger SM, Kandall SR, Doberczak TM, et al: Early weight-change patterns in neonatal abstinence. *Am J Dis Child* 1986; 140:829–832.

INFANT FEEDING

James E. McJunkin, M.D.

BREAST FEEDING

Despite the encouraging resurgence of breast feeding in the last decade, many clinicians find themselves ill-prepared to manage problems with lactation. This discussion focuses on the practical aspects of breast feeding while building on the concept that breast feeding is an appropriate and instructive standard for understanding other feeding methods.

ANATOMY AND PHYSIOLOGY

Careful inspection of the nipple reveals 15 to 25 tiny openings near the tip. Each orifice is the outlet of a lactiferous duct that drains several

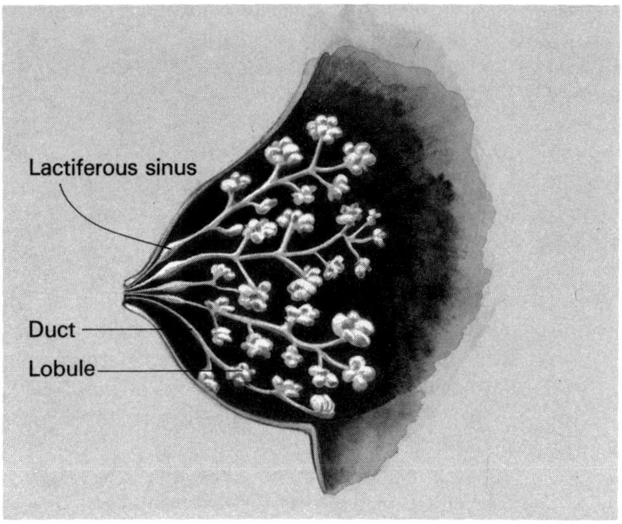

FIG 4–7
Diagram of lactiferous ducts that drain into orifice of the nipple.

branching ductules and their alveoli (Fig 4–7). The alveolar cells secrete milk into the ductules in response to prolactin, which is secreted in response to the stimulus of suckling. High estrogen levels inhibit the effect of prolactin on the alveolar cells; this explains the initial 2- to 3-day dry period and the increased production of milk on the third to fourth day when estrogen levels have fallen close to prepregnancy levels.

The alveolar cells produce milk and the myoepithelial cells, which surround the milk ductules, contract in response to oxytocin to eject milk from the ductules. This "let-down reflex" is initiated by the stimulus of suckling, but it may occasionally respond to the stimulus of the sight or sound of the infant. The milk-ejection reflex can be inhibited by maternal discomfort or anxiety.

INITIATION OF LACTATION

Natural History of the In-hospital Period

Putting the newborn to the mother's breast as soon as possible after delivery is reasonable when the baby is term, clinically stable, and warm. Nursing helps contract the mother's uterus due to oxytocin release. During the initial warm-up feedings, the mother will need instruction in technique. To start the feeding, the mother gently strokes the baby's cheek with the nipple, allowing the baby to root to the breast. The baby's mouth should engage as much of the areola as possible, allowing optimal milking of the lactiferous sinuses at the base of the areola and preventing nipple damage. Full engagement is enhanced when the mother compresses the breast between two fingers as she offers the protruded nipple (Fig 4–8).

After approximately 5 minutes of feeding at the first breast, the infant is disengaged by inserting a finger at the corner of the mouth, thus breaking suction gently. The baby is burped and then allowed to feed about 5 minutes on the second breast. The 5-minute time limit usually assures that both breasts are taken at each feeding and may prevent excessive nipple soreness. The mother alternates the breast on which the nursing is begun at each feeding, facilitating milk emptying and production at an even rate.

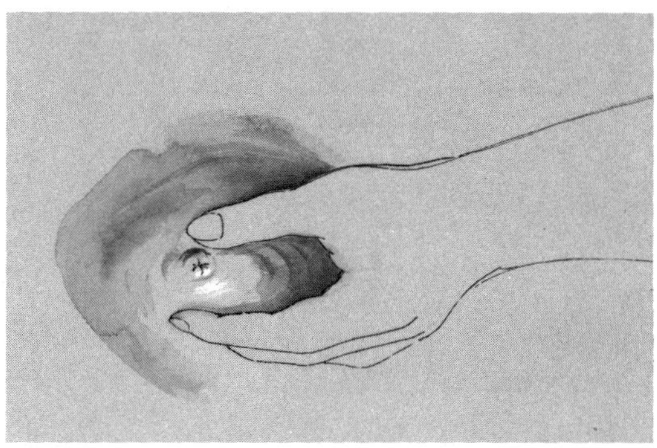

FIG 4–8
Compression of the breast between the mother's fingers can enhance engagement of the areola by the sucking infant.

The feeding frequency is dictated by the baby's demand, usually every 2 to 3 hours during the first 2 to 3 weeks. For the first 2 to 3 days, the milk supply is relatively low. The new mother needs reassurance that this period is expected and may be encouraged that although the early milk, called colostrum, is low in amount, it is high in important factors (such as IgA). By the third to fourth day, the milk begins to come in well and may even cause engorgement (see the section on engorged breasts).

PROBLEMS OF LACTATION DURING INITIATION PHASE

Inhibition of Let-down Reflex

Physical or emotional discomfort can inhibit the milk-ejection reflex; thus the most important measure to initiation is assuring maternal comfort. In practice, this means that at least one support person is available to the mother to help position the mother and baby, screen telephone calls and visitors, and help enforce a rest period for the mother at least once a day.

Nipple Tenderness or Fissuring

Nipple soreness usually occurs as a transient phenomenon that resolves as the nipples toughen over the first several days of nursing. Preparation and good technique are the best measures for preventing persistent soreness or nipple fissuring. Areolar engorgement can lead to soreness (and vice versa) and even fissuring by preventing proper engagement of the nipple.

Fair-skinned women are particularly prone to the development of fissures and should limit feeding on each breast to 5 minutes during the first few days.

Engorged Breasts

Excessive swelling of the breast is of two types, although these may occur concurrently. The first is vascular and known as *peripheral engorgement*, because it involves the body of the breast (not the areola) including the soft tissues at the periphery of the breast mass. This type of swelling usually starts on the second postpartum day and is managed with an adequately supportive bra, compresses (cold at first, warm if no relief), and oral analgesics (with codeine if necessary).

Areolar engorgement is the result of milk secretion unrelieved by proper let-down or complete emptying by the infant. This type of engorgement usually begins on the third or fourth postpartum day. In this instance the nipple becomes difficult for the baby to engage properly, with resultant nipple pain or fissuring. Treatment of areolar engorgement involves facilitating maternal comfort (and therefore the let-down reflex) and manual expression of enough milk to relieve some of the fullness before feeding the infant. Figure 4–9 illustrates the technique of manual expression. When manual expression is either too painful or provides insufficient relief, an electronic pump is an excellent supplement to gentle manual expression of the peripheral breast tissue.

Uterine Cramps

Uterine cramping occurs in response to oxytocin released during nursing. A heating pad may provide relief, but some women may require

FIG 4–9
Technique of manual expression of milk to facilitate maternal comfort when areolar engorgement occurs.

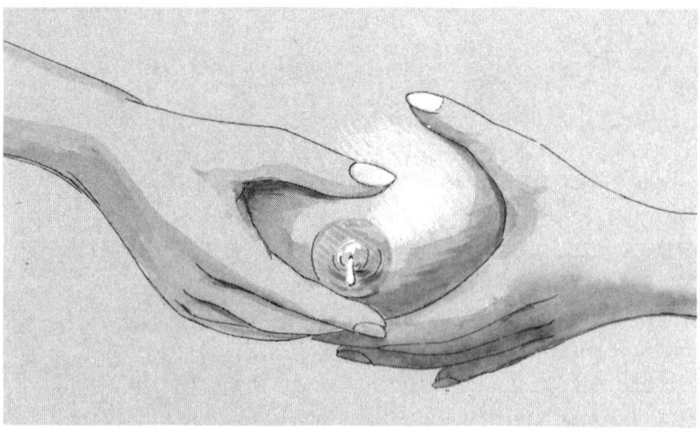

oral analgesics. The cramps will resolve spontaneously within the first few days.

Weight Loss

Ten percent weight loss during the first few days of life is reason for concern and may justifiably delay the baby's discharge until an upward trend is established. On the other hand, weight losses of 5% to 10% may well be "physiologic," especially in the primiparous mother whose milk supply may be especially slow to come in. In this instance, the mother should be reassured that this situation is likely to resolve soon and asked to bring the baby back at 7 to 14 days of age for a weight check and reexamination. This mother in particular should have adequate help at home while she is establishing the milk supply.

MANAGEMENT ISSUES AFTER DISCHARGE

HOME ENVIRONMENT

The home environment should be as supportive to the new mother as the hospital environment. Husbands, grandmothers, and others must alleviate the usual demands on the mother while she attends to a demanding newcomer who feeds every 2 to 3 hours day and night.

WEIGHT GAIN AT FIRST VISIT

While the formula-fed baby ordinarily regains birth weight by 10 days of age, the breast-fed baby may require 2 to 3 weeks to do so. When findings of the history and physical examination are otherwise normal, small deficits (a few ounces) found at the 2-week visit are best handled by observing the mother nursing the baby to determine problems of technique or nipple damage, assessing support systems at home, and by rechecking the weight during another visit 7 to 10 days later.

CONTRACEPTION

Women who breast feed experience a longer duration of postpartum amenorrhea than women who do not. This effect, related to hyperprolactinemia, cannot be considered adequate contraception; 5% to 10% of women with lactational amenorrhea become pregnant during the amenorrheic period. Therefore it is recommended that the nursing mother wishing contraception should begin to use some reasonably effective method at 4 to 5 weeks post partum.

Barrier contraceptives are the preferred method of contraception for the breast feeding mother, although oral contraceptives may be used. The bulk of evidence as reported by Lawrence and more recently by the American Academy of Pediatrics (AAP) suggests that the use of combined estrogen-progestin contraceptive pills (usually containing 30 to 50 μg of ethinyl estradiol or 50 to 100 μg of mestranol) presents no danger to the infant. There is, however, dose-related suppression of the quantity of milk produced and the duration of lactation with extended use. Therefore, if possible, it may be prudent for the breast-feeding mother to continue barrier methods until the beginning of weaning the infant.

BREAST EXPRESSION AND PUMPING

For the healthy nursing mother and infant, manual expression (Fig 4–9) or a manual breast pump will suffice to collect one or a few milk samples a day. This allows women working outside of the home to continue to provide breast milk and allows the father to provide a feeding while the mother takes a break. Some women are able to get enough milk with manual expression alone. Other women have found that a hand pump combined with manual expression will increase yield and efficiency. The best pumps provide a cyclic milking action of the breast rather than constant suction. In addition, the pump should have an adequate reservoir so that frequent decanting is not necessary.

When either the mother or the baby is sick (such as if the baby is premature), a very effective, comfortable pump is needed because lactation is only beginning to be established.

STORING BREAST MILK

Breast milk may be stored for 24 hours in the refrigerator before it is used for feeding. If the milk is to be stored for longer than 24 hours, it should be placed in the freezer directly after pumping. Frozen breast milk will keep for at least 2 weeks. The milk is stored in glass or plastic containers that have been cleaned with hot soap and water by hand or in an automatic dishwasher.

TEMPORARY BREAST REJECTION

Some infants will go through a period of rejecting one or both breasts when about 4 months of age. The cause is generally not known but suggested etiologies include teething, excessive hunger (causing a frantic eating pattern), change in the taste of the milk (perhaps occurring with ingestion of garlic or other foods), infant nasal congestion, or thrush. Return of menstruation has also been noted to be related to breast rejection. Lawrence cites rare cases in which malignancy has been diagnosed in the rejected breast, indicating that breast examination is important as well. Other than measures designed to deal with the suspected cause, breast rejection has been found to resolve with a change in position (such as the football hold) of the baby at that breast.

WEANING

The transition from breast milk to another milk should be a gradual process that optimally occurs during a period of weeks. The mother replaces one breast milk feeding at a time and allows at least a few days before replacing another feeding. The midday feedings are frequently the easiest and most sensible to initially replace, especially for the working mother who can then continue to nurse the baby morning and evening.

COMPLICATIONS OF BREAST FEEDING

LUMPS OR GALACTOCELE

Blockage of a milk duct may cause tender lumps in the breast. Therapy includes continued nursing, massaging of the area, and prefeeding application of hot packs. Tender lumps associated with fever or malaise may signal mastitis.

If blockage continues, a galactocele (milk retention cyst) manifests as a smooth swelling. Pressure on the galactocele will cause a milky or cheesy substance to be exuded from the nipple. Nursing may be continued but eventually removal of the cyst may be required.

MASTITIS

Mastitis occurs most frequently during the second or third week postpartum. A localized area of the breast becomes warm and tender with overlying redness of the skin. Systemic reactions may be severe (including fever, malaise, nausea, and vomiting) and may be noticed prior to the discovery of the inflamed area in the breast. Therefore, one must retain a high index of suspicion for mastitis in any breast feeding mother who presents with flulike symptoms.

Therapy includes continued breast feeding (starting with the infant on the unaffected side each time for the sake of comfort), warm compresses, oral analgesics, and ampicillin or erythromycin for 10 days. It is critical to start therapy as early as possible since delays of treatment are related to the development of breast abscess. Furthermore, treatment must be continued for a full 10 days, since shorter courses have been related to relapse.

MATERNAL MEDICATION AND BREAST MILK

The initial question is whether the particular medication is necessary in the first place. One also considers alternate therapies in answering this question.

If the drug is not absolutely necessary to maintain maternal health, one may still choose to give the drug if there is little or no known risk to the infant. A good question to ask in this regard is "Would direct administration of this drug in pharmacological doses be risky?" If the drug is safe for infants, it is generally fair to assume that it may be taken by the mother without subsequent harm to the baby. It must be remembered, however, that some drugs that can be taken safely during most of infancy still should not be used in the newborn period (e.g., sulfa).

If the drug is absolutely necessary for the mother's adequate functioning, then evidence contraindicating its use in breast feeding must be respected and the mother will be unable to nurse the baby. It should be remembered that

TABLE 4–3
Drugs Contraindicated During Breast Feeding*

DRUG	REPORTED SIGN OR SYMPTOM IN INFANT OR EFFECT ON LACTATION
Amethopterin†	Possible immune suppression; unknown effect on growth or association with carcinogenesis
Bromocriptine	Suppresses lactation
Cimetidine‡	May suppress gastric acidity in infant, inhibit drug metabolism, and cause CNS stimulation
Clemastine	Drowsiness, irritability, refusal to feed, high-pitched cry, neck stiffness
Cyclophosphamide†	Possible immune suppression; unknown effect on growth or association with carcinogenesis
Ergotamine	Vomiting, diarrhea, convulsions (doses used in migraine medications)
Gold salts	Rash, inflammation of kidney and liver
Methimazole	Potential for interfering with thyroid function
Phenindione	Hemorrhage
Thiouracil	Decreased thyroid function; does not apply to propylthiouracil

* From American Academy of Pediatrics Committee on Drugs: *Pediatrics* 1983; 72:375. Used by permission.
† Data not available for other cytotoxic agents.
‡ Drug is concentrated in breast milk.

the mother has the option to pump her breasts during the course of therapy if she wishes to reinstitute breast feeding when the medication is discontinued.

The AAP has developed a list of contraindicated drugs (Tables 4–3 and 4–4).

FORMULA FEEDING

METHOD AND AMOUNT OF FORMULA FEEDING

The technique of formula feeding is similar to breast feeding with the baby held close by a comfortable, unhurried parent. It is especially important that parents not develop the practice of bottle propping or putting the infant into the crib with the bottle.

Most newborns will require 5 to 6 oz/kg/day (based on caloric needs of 100 to 120 calories/kg/day and caloric density of formula of 20 calories per 30 mL). Generally this is accomplished if the parent feeds the baby on demand, usually every 2 to 3 hours in the newborn period. Infants of any age rarely require more than 32 oz of formula daily, because caloric requirements (per kilogram) decline with age and alternate food sources are available to the older infant.

TABLE 4–4
Drugs That Require Temporary Cessation of Breast Feeding*

DRUG	RECOMMENDED ALTERATION IN BREAST FEEDING PATTERN
Metronidazole	Discontinue breast-feeding 12–24 hr to allow excretion of dose
Radiopharmaceuticals	Radioactivity present in milk; consult nuclear medicine physician before performing diagnostic study so that radionuclide with shortest excretion time in breast milk can be used; prior to study the mother should pump her breast and store enough milk in freezer for feeding the infant; after study the mother should pump her breast to maintain milk production but discard all milk pumped for the required time that radioactivity is present in milk
Gallium 69	Radioactivity in milk present for 2 wk
Iodine 125	Risk of thyroid cancer; radioactivity in milk present for 12 days
Iodine 131	Radioactivity in milk present 2–14 days depending on study
Radioactive sodium	Radioactivity in milk present 96 hr
Technetium 99m ^{99m}Tc macroaggregates, $^{99m}TcO_4$	Radioactivity in milk present 15 hr to 3 days

* From American Academy of Pediatrics Committee on Drugs: *Pediatrics* 1983; 72:375. Used by permission.

COW'S MILK FORMULA

A cow's milk formula containing iron is recommended during the newborn period. Formula is available in ready-to-feed form or the less-expensive concentrate that requires dilution with an equal part of water. While vitamin and iron needs are supplied by these formulas, unless fluoridated tap water is being used to prepare the concentrate, fluoride is not and should be prescribed.

EVAPORATED COW'S MILK FORMULA

Although we would not recommend the routine use of evaporated cow's milk formulas in place of standard commercial formulas, these can be an adequate alternative if preparation is adequate and vitamin supplementation is prescribed. Preparation involves adding one can (13 oz) of the formula to 17 oz of water. While this dilution properly lowers the protein concentration, it results in too low a caloric concentration of carbohydrates. Therefore, the final step in preparation is the addition of 2 tablespoons of corn syrup (Karo), properly increasing caloric content from carbohydrates.

An infant who is fed evaporated milk will need an alternate source of iron and vitamin C. This is best provided with 1 mL daily of a multivitamin preparation with iron, which provides 35 mg of vitamin C and 10 mg of elemental iron.

Note that condensed milk has no place in infant feeding. Such milk is too high in sugar and too low in fat and protein.

WHOLE MILK

Whole cow's milk is low in iron content and the iron is less bioavailable than that of breast milk. In infants less than 5 months of age, whole milk causes occult GI bleeding more often than either formula made with cow's milk or evaporated milk. However, for infants older than 6 months who receive supplemental foods, there is no convincing evidence that whole milk is harmful. Therefore, the AAP has concluded that infants older than 6 months may be fed homogenized, vitamin D-fortified whole milk if the mother does not want to continue with breast-feeding or formula; the infant is consuming one-third of his calories as supplemental foods that provide adequate sources of iron and vitamin C; and the amount fed is limited to less than 1 L daily.

Defatted (skim) cow's milk is *not recommended* during infancy. The solute load is unacceptably high and weight gain of the infant is slowed.

SOY FORMULA

The protein component of these formulas is soy, but the carbohydrate moiety also differs from both human milk and cow's milk. Instead of lactose, corn syrup solids or sucrose is used in soy formulas. In fact, the most sensible clinical use of soy formulas at the present time is in treating secondary lactose intolerance that occurs after an episode of gastroenteritis in infants. In this case the soy formula is used for only 2 weeks.

Clear indications for long-term use of soy formula include galactosemia and primary lactase deficiency.

In families with a clear-cut history of atopic disease (particularly asthma), soy formula is considered less of an allergic risk than cow's milk and may be begun prophylactically in the newborn period. On the other hand, soy formula is *not indicated for treatment* of documented allergy to cow's milk protein. In this case, the infant gut is vulnerable to exposure to other antigens, particularly during the early months of life, and a less antigenic formula is warranted.

Soy formula is contraindicated for premature infants because the risk of developing rickets is increased. Soy formula is not recommended for the routine treatment of colic.

The practice of changing the formula for any number of other reasons as a means of doing something is to be discouraged. Continued formula changes may delay and confuse needed evaluation for true problems such as chronic diarrhea with weight loss.

FORMULAS FOR INFANTS WITH SPECIAL MEDICAL NEEDS (CASEIN HYDROLYSATES)

The casein in these formulas is prehydrolyzed and the carbohydrate source is nonlactose. Casein hydrolysate formulas are indicated for infants known to be allergic to intact cow's milk proteins. Another use of these is for the very young infant (less than 3 months of age) with prolonged gastroenteritis who needs rapid gut rehabilitation to prevent a prolonged malabsorptive state. In this situation, the gut is protected from lactose, cow's milk protein, and soy protein. In addition, at least one of these formulas provides some of the fat in the form of medium chain triglycerides, thereby easing the absorption of fats, which is often a problem for infants with special medical needs.

It is helpful to think of these formulas as medications to be started during an inpatient stay. The primary care physician faced with the decision of using these expensive formulas is usually treating an infant whose condition requires hospitalization and/or careful consultative evaluation.

VITAMIN AND MINERAL SUPPLEMENTATION

In practice, the physician needs to have a working knowledge of vitamin D, iron, and fluoride. Other texts provide more detail on other vitamin and mineral needs and deficiency states.

VITAMIN D

Rickets caused by vitamin D deficiency still occurs in the United States in some breast-fed infants. This has especially occurred in black children when exposure to sunlight is minimized and the mother is on a restricted diet. Premature infants are also at risk for rickets. We recommend prescribing vitamin D when one or more of these risk factors is present (i.e., black race, lack of sunlight exposure, restricted maternal diet, or prematurity).

The dosage of vitamin D is 400 IU/day and is available in a liquid multivitamin preparation (available with or without fluoride).

FLUORIDE

Regardless of maternal diet, fluoride is present in only trace amounts in breast milk. Therefore, all breast-fed infants should be discharged on a regimen of 0.25 mg of fluoride daily. The infant living in an area with unfluoridated water supply ($<$ 0.3 ppm) should continue to receive the 0.25 mg daily dose until the age of 2 years, when the dose is doubled to 0.5 mg daily. When the child is 3 years old, the dose is doubled again to 1 mg/day; administration continues at this level until the child is 13 years old, when it is no longer necessary.

In areas of intermediate fluoridation (0.3 to 0.7 ppm), fluoride is prescribed for infants from birth until weaning, when it is stopped temporarily until the age of 2 years. From the age of 2 to 3 years, 0.25 mg/day is given, but then is doubled to 0.5 mg/day from the age of 3 to 13 years of age.

When ready-to-feed formula is used, fluoride supplements are necessary as for the breast-fed infant. Formula concentrate prepared with fluoridated tap water obviates the need for supplementation.

IRON

Iron is low in concentration in breast milk but of relatively high bioavailability (50% absorbed). Although controversy exists over the length of time a completely breast-fed infant has a sufficient amount of iron without supplementation, it is generally agreed that iron should be added to the diet when the infant is 4 to 6 months of age. This is best done in the form of iron-fortified cereal that is usually introduced at this time. If cereal intake is a problem, then multivitamins with iron may be administered; these multivitamins contain 10 mg elemental iron per dose, of which an estimated 5% to 10% is absorbed.

It is recommended that a formula containing iron (12 mg/L) be prescribed for bottle-fed infants at birth. Studies have shown that there is no increase in GI problems such as constipation in infants receiving iron-fortified formula. Physicians therefore should avoid low-iron formulas (1.5 to 2.0 mg/L), because at least 6 mg/L is necessary for adequate absorption by the infant.

INTRODUCTION OF SOLID FOODS

Iron-fortified cereals are introduced as the first solid food when the infant is at the age of 4 to 6 months. Parents are instructed to give the baby a small amount of moistened cereal on a spoon, *not in the baby bottle.* If the baby extrudes the cereal with his tongue, he still is not ready for cereal and the parents may wait at least several days before trying again. If by the age of 6 months the baby is able to take 3 tablespoons of cereal, he will receive about 7 mg daily. Iron-fortified cereals are continued daily until the infant is 18 months of age.

After the introduction of cereal, either fruits or vegetables are begun, given in the form of commercial baby food or blenderized produce. There is no specific order in which foods must be introduced, as long as the parent waits at least several days before introducing a new food. Many pediatricians recommend that foods known to be relatively allergenic (such as citrus fruits and egg whites) be introduced later in the first year of life.

By 10 months of age, the infant may also be receiving some blenderized or mashed meat as a particularly good source of iron.

DISCONTINUING THE BOTTLE, AND BOTTLE CARIES

The use of the bottle may sometimes be avoided in the breast-fed infant who at about a year of age goes directly to the use of a cup. Formula-fed infants should begin using the cup at about 1 year of age and can generally be completely off the bottle by the age of 15 months. Discontinuance of the bottle at a later time is often met with more resistance from the child. Once the infant can drink adequate amounts from a cup or a training cup, the bottle may be rapidly and completely discontinued. The child who goes to bed with a bottle has a high risk of serious dental disease.

FAT IN THE DIET

The AAP recommends no restriction of fat in the infant diet and suggests that 30% to 40% of dietary calories come from fat during the first two decades of life, except in cases of special vulnerability. In particular, the use of low-fat milk in infants is to be generally avoided because it has contributed to failure to thrive in some cases.

BIBLIOGRAPHY

American Academy of Pediatrics Committee on Drugs: Breastfeeding and contraception. *Pediatrics* 1981; 68:138.

AAP Committee on Drugs: The transfer of drugs and other chemicals into human breastmilk. *Pediatrics* 1983; 72:375.

AAP Committee on Nutrition: The use of whole cow's milk in infancy. *Pediatrics* 1983; 72:253.

AAP Committee on Nutrition: Soy protein formulas: recommendations for use in infant feeding. *Pediatrics* 1983; 72:359.

Fomon SJ, Filer LJ, Anderson TA, et al: Recommendations for feeding normal infants. *Pediatrics* 1979; 63:252.

Kula K, Tinanoff N.: Fluoride therapy for the pediatric patient. *Pediatr Clin North Am* 1982; 29:669.

Lawrence RA: *Breastfeeding: A Guide for the Medical Profession*. St Louis, CV Mosby Co, 1980.

Olds SW, Eiger MS: *The Complete Book of Breastfeeding*. New York, Workman Publishing Co, 1972.

INFANT COLIC SYNDROME

Bruce Taubman, M.D.

Infant colic is a syndrome in which healthy infants with normal growth and development, who are usually less than 3 months old, have episodes of excessive, seemingly inconsolable crying for no apparent reason. The problem, which occurs in 10% to 20% of infants, can begin any time after birth but rarely before 1 week of age and in most cases improves significantly by 3 months of age. Behavior diaries show that these infants cry more than 2 hours a day, although parents almost always report that the crying lasts longer than 3 hours per day. The crying usually occurs at the same time of day, most often in the evening. During the crying episodes the infants are described as drawing their legs up, hardening the abdomen, turning red, and passing flatus. The infant often appears to the observer to be having abdominal pain.

The cause and treatment of the syndrome are controversial. Three major theories have been put forth. One theory assumes, because of their appearance, that these infants cry because of abdominal pain. Some believe the pain is secondary to increased abdominal gas and recommend frequent burping and simethicone for the treatment of colic. Others have looked to milk protein allergy as the cause of the abdominal pain. Jakobsson's group has published two reports showing improvement in a significant number of colicky infants given hydrolyzed casein formula and one report showing improvement in breast-fed infants when their mothers were placed on a milk-free diet. However, these reports included infants with vomiting or diarrhea, which would exclude infant colic syndrome as usually defined.

Those who assume that infant colic syndrome is caused by abdominal pain have suggested various medications for treating it. The only drug found to be effective in controlled studies is dicyclomine. The side effects of this medication include lethargy and sedation, and its effectiveness may be related more to its sedative action than to antispasmodic properties. There have been reports of apnea and death in infants given dicyclomine, and the manufacturer has warned against its use in infants.

Another popular theory of infant colic syndrome is that the immature nervous system in the infant causes them to be extremely sensitive to external stimuli; thus the crying is nonspecific and unavoidable. Attempts to quell such crying result in further stimulation of the infant and more crying. Advocates of this theory recommend putting the crying, seemingly inconsolable infant down and letting him or her cry, thereby decreasing the stimulation to the infant. To date there is only one clinical study of the effectiveness of such an approach, that by Taubman in 1984. Six parents of colicky infants were introduced to this theory and counseled to let their babies cry when they become inconsolable. There was no decrease in crying among this small group of infants. The approach was successful in helping the parents, in that five of the six thought things had improved after treatment.

The third major theory concerning infant colic syndrome states that the crying begins as an attempt by the infant to communicate wants and needs and continues, often to the point of extreme agitation, when the parents misinterpret these cries and respond incorrectly. Treatment involves counseling the parents to treat infant crying as a form of communication and teaching them how to interpret and respond to the cries correctly.

COUNSELING TECHNIQUE

Parents of infants with infant colic syndrome present many different chief complaints, including "Our infant has a lot of gas or is gassy all the time"; "Our infant cries every evening no matter what we do"; "My baby is having episodes of severe abdominal pain." In taking the history from these parents, try to determine if these babies meet the criteria for having infant colic syndrome. It is important to be sure there are no other symptoms other than excessive crying and perhaps the association of the passage of flatus. Ask specifically about vomiting, diarrhea, or constipation. Look for any preconcieved concepts of infant behavior held by the parents that may interfere with their responding appropriately to their infant's cries. Are they truly feeding on demand or are they reluctant to feed their baby freely because of concern about infant obesity? Do they have an aversion to the use of a pacifier? Are they afraid they will spoil their baby if they hold her too much? Do they believe infants should sleep a specific number of hours during certain times of the day?

After taking the history, a physical examination should be done carefully to discover any source of pain, such as otitis media, incarcerated inguinal hernia, testicular swelling, or a hair wrapped around a digit. A rectal examination should be done. A tight band in the anal canal can cause discomfort and crying with attempts at bowel movements. If found it can be easily dilated with the finger.

If after the history and physical examination you find the infant's symptoms meet the criteria for infant colic syndrome, the important concepts of infant crying and infant colic should be explained to the parents; for example, "It may appear to you that your infant is crying because of abdominal pain. This is because whenever babys cry, whether from hunger, sleepiness, or ear pain, they often look like they have abdominal pain. They draw their legs up, turn red, harden the abdomen, and pass gas. However, after taking a history and careful physical examination, I am sure your infant is not in pain. Normal infants, such as yours, rarely cry because of pain. They cry to communicate their wants and needs. You may think your infant's crying is inconsolable. This is because infant cries can be difficult to interpret. Some infants become so agitated after crying a good while that no response can calm them."

If the parents find these concepts difficult to accept, as many do, completion of a 72-hour behavior diary with precoded 12-hour diary sheets is helpful. They record the time each activity begins and ends, adding any relevant comments. The following list suggests codes to be used in recording the diary.

ACTIVITY CODE

S = Sleeping alone (not held)
SH = Sleeping held
F = Feeding
AAH = awake, alone, and happy (not held; in crib, infant seat, swing)
AAC = Awake, alone, and crying
AHH = Awake, held, and happy
AHC = Awake, held, and crying
B = Bathing

The diary allows you to quantitate the amount of crying and can be used to monitor treatment. It is difficult to get accurate information about the circumstances of the infant crying and the parental response to it by talking to the parents. The diaries give you this information. You can determine whether the parents assume all crying is pain related and only respond by walking the baby. It can be determined how much time the parents allow the infant to cry before responding. The type of responses the parents try, in what order, and how logical these responses are can also be evaluated.

After reviewing the behavior diary it is necessary to meet again with the parents and go over the information with them. For example, "Your infant is really crying a lot. Most infants cry 1 to 1½ hours a day, and your infant is crying 3 hours a day. By responding differently to the baby, we can decrease the crying significantly." The parents are instructed to assume that crying is communication and try one of five responses: feeding, offering a pacifier, putting the baby to sleep, holding the baby, or stimulating him or her. If one response does not work quickly, they are to move on to another one, trying to find the correct response before the baby becomes agitated. Never just let the baby cry. The primary care provider should review the diary, pointing out specific episodes of crying and suggesting alternate responses. Finally, the parents are given an instruction sheet on how to respond to the infant's crying (Table 4–5).

The parents should continue the behavior di-

FIG 4–10
INSTRUCTIONS TO PARENTS ON INFANT COLIC SYNDROME.

Your baby's cry is the way the infant signals you about needs. When the baby cries you respond immediately and try to determine what the infant wants. The baby's cry is a signal for one of the following:

1. The baby is hungry.
   Many babies do not feel hunger at regular intervals. There may be days when the baby wishes to feed frequently, and other times when he wants to feed less often. Feed the baby whenever appropriate. You will not overfeed the infant.
2. The baby is not hungry but wants to suck.
   There will be times when the baby does not want the bottle or full breast but does want to suck. The baby will take a pacifier readily at these times.
3. The baby wants to be held.
   If an infant cries because he wants to be held, holding will quickly stop the crying. You will not spoil the infant or make it a habit. If the baby continues to cry while being held, try something different.
4. The baby is bored and wants stimulation.
   This can be achieved by playing with the baby or putting him in an infant seat in a room where there is a lot of activity, for example, the kitchen while you are cooking.
5. The baby is tired and wants to sleep.
   Try putting the baby down in a dark quiet room. If fussing, you can leave the baby alone, but the infant should be picked up if crying loudly.

You decide in what order to try these suggestions.

NOTE

1. If after trying one of these suggestions the baby continues to cry, try another. Do not persist in any one item if the infant continues to cry.
2. Before you pick up a crying baby, be sure the baby is awake and not just crying in his sleep.
3. If you think the baby is tired, it is all right to leave the baby alone while crying, as long as the crying is off and on and does not last more than 5 minutes.

aries and have them reviewed every 2 to 3 days until improvement is observed.

If at their first visit the parents seem receptive to a discussion of crying as communication, an attempt can be made to counsel without the use of the behavior diaries.

Good anticipatory guidance can often prevent the occurrence of the infant colic syndrome. When talking to new parents, the concept of crying as communication should be explained. The importance of responding to infant cries in the development of a healthy infant-parent attachment should be discussed. Parents should be advised to feed the infant on demand, and not to be reluctant to hold their baby or use a pacifier. They should be discouraged from just letting their baby cry. When parents report that their infant is at times fussy, explain he is trying to communicate some desire that has not occurred to them. They should be encouraged to be flexible in their response at these times. They can try feeding more frequently, holding more, or offering a pacifier. Such advice should go a long way in preventing infant colic syndrome.

BIBLIOGRAPHY

Adams LM, Davidson M: Present concepts of infant colic. *Pediatr Ann* 1987; 16:817–820.

Illingworth RS: Three months colic. *Arch Dis Child* 1954; 29:165–174.

Taubman B: Clinical trial of the treatment of colic by modification of parent-infant interaction. *Pediatrics* 1984; 74:995–1003.

Taubman B: Parental counseling compared with elimination of cow's milk or soy milk protein for treatment of infant colic syndrome: A randomized trial. *Pediatrics* 1988; 81:756–761.

Wessel MA, Cobb JC, Jackson EB, et al: Paroxysmal fussing in infancy, sometimes called "colic." *Pediatrics* 1954; 14:421–424.

5 PRIMARY CARE OF THE PRETERM INFANT

Judy C. Bernbaum, M.D.
Jo Ann D'Agostino, R.N.
Marsha Hoffman-Williamson, Ph.D.
Anne C. Farran, M.A.

The survival of infants with low birth weight has been markedly improved with advances in neonatal care. The result is a significant decrease in the mortality rate among the extremely low birthweight infants—those weighing less than 1,000 g or even less than 750 g. Of 3.75 million live births annually in the United States, the number of infants who are born weighing less than 1,500 g is small (45,500), and the number weighing less than 1,000 g at birth even smaller (17,500; almost 5,000 of these infants weighed less than 500 g). This population comprises a disproportionally high percentage of children at risk for medical, neurologic, and developmental problems. As more infants with low birth weight enter the pediatric population, physicians must become expert in managing their unique medical conditions, in addition to monitoring their developmental progress and recognizing early signs of neurologic disorders. Routine physical examinations are usually not sufficient for such children; more time is needed in their assessment and in discussions with their parents than in those of the typically well child. Physicians can play a major role in the identification of problems early in their evolution. Their efforts can have a major effect on the prevention or further progression of a child's disabilities.

This chapter includes a review of conditions

frequently encountered by physicians caring for the preterm infant who has been discharged from the neonatal unit.

GROWTH

Growth rates in preterm infants vary during the first years of life and may be affected by such factors as birth weight, gestational age, severity of illness, adequacy of caloric intake during the neonatal period, ongoing or recurrent illnesses during infancy, environmental factors in the home, and heredity.

The majority of preterm infants are discharged from the hospital at 37 to 40 weeks' gestation, weighing between 4 and 5 lb. When the physician is plotting anthropometric measurements to determine growth percentiles, corrected ages should be used to adjust for the infant's premature birth. This can be done using any growth chart standardized for term infants. Corrected ages can be determined by subtracting the number of weeks the infant was born prematurely from the infant's chronologic age. Most assessments of growth are based on corrected ages until the infants are 2½ years old (corrected age) after which time chronologic ages are often used.

Growth in premature infants varies in two ways. First, differences in growth velocity among infants result in all growth parameters for some infants being between the 75th and 97th percentiles at 3 months (corrected age), whereas the parameters of other infants remain between the 3rd and 25th percentiles well beyond the first year of life. Second, individual infants demonstrate differences between the growth velocity of their head circumference, their height, and their weight. For example, the measurements for some infants are plotted between the 3rd and 25th percentiles for height and weight, while that of head circumference appears between the 75th and 97th percentile. Because of the wide range of growth that is considered within normal limits, it is necessary to assess preterm infant growth by analyzing trends in growth rather than by making assumptions based on only one set of measurements.

A common concern encountered when assessing preterm infant growth is a head circumference percentile that is significantly higher than weight and height percentiles. In preterm infants this may suggest ventricular dilation (associated with intraventricular hemorrhage, IVH) or a head that is growing while the rest of the body does not because of poor nutritional status. In most cases, this situation can be attributed to catch-up growth after a period of adequate nutrition. This is first seen as increased head growth followed by a weight and a linear growth spurt. Cranial ultrasonography is indicated in any infant who demonstrates signs of hydrocephalus, such as widely split sutures, tense fontanelle, irritability, alterations in normal behavior and activity level, or "sunsetting" (an increased amount of sclera seen above the iris caused by the eyes deviating downward). Alternately, a head circumference that is more than 3 standard deviations below the mean places the child at high risk for significant developmental disability in the future.

When the weight falls in percentiles significantly lower than length or when all growth velocity decreases, poor nutritional status or malnutrition is suggested. Special attention should be paid to growth measurements at birth and at discharge, nutritional status during hospitalization, results of cranial ultrasonography, and the status of ongoing illnesses such as bronchopulmonary dysplasia (BPD), congenital heart disease, and malabsorption syndromes associated with necrotizing enterocolitis.

NUTRITION

At the time of discharge from the hospital, most preterm infants' dietary needs are similar to those of full-term neonates. The milk source for preterm infants should be breast milk, a commercial 20 calories/oz infant formula, or other special formula (indicated because of milk intolerance, increased caloric requirements, or malabsorption resulting from bowel resection).

Increased nutritional needs are frequently encountered in preterm infants with ongoing medical problems such as BPD, congenital heart disease, malabsorption, or feeding disorders. These infants often require a 24 to 30 kcal/oz formula to maintain growth. This can be accomplished by concentrating the formula or preferably by adding caloric supplements such as vegetable oil (8.0 kcals/mL), medium-chain triglycerides (MCT oil, 7.6 kcals/mL), microlipids (4.5 kcals/mL), or glucose polymers (2 kcals/mL). Care should be taken to maintain the proper ratio of fat, carbohydrate, and protein.

Mothers of preterm infants who desire to breast feed should be strongly encouraged and supported throughout the hospitalization as well as at discharge. The breast milk of such mothers has been found to be well suited to the nutritional needs of the preterm infant, particularly during the first few weeks of life. For this reason, pooled breast milk should not be used for preterm infants.

Breast feeding a small preterm infant often requires increased support and expert guidance. Such teaching should therefore be initiated well before discharge if possible. If there is particular concern about ensuring adequate caloric intake while breast feeding is being established, a supplemental nursing system (such as Lact-Aid) may be used initially, filled with either pumped breast milk (with additional fortifier if desired) or premature formula. The use of such a system allows for adequate stimulation of milk production by the breast, which is not true with supplemental bottles. By the time of discharge, mature breast milk is generally nutritionally adequate for the healthy preterm infant.

Solid feedings should be initiated according to the guidelines of the American Academy of Pediatrics (AAP) for full-term infants. When counseling parents of preterm infants, however, dietary recommendations should be based on the infant's corrected age, not chronologic age. Solid foods should be initiated when any one of three criteria are met: the infant consistently consumes more than 32 oz of formula per day for 1 week; the infant weighs 6 to 7 kg; or the infant is 6 months old, corrected age.

Larger infants may not be satisfied with 32 oz of formula and may need to begin solid foods as early as 3 to 4 months, corrected age. Starting solid foods before 3 months is not recommended by the AAP. The premature introduction of solid foods may lead to gastrointestinal allergy, contribute to overeating, or lead to feeding problems as a result of lack of neuromuscular readiness for solid feedings. Refer to the section on infant feeding in Chapter 4 for additional dietary guidelines.

NUTRITIONAL SUPPLEMENTATION

MULTIVITAMINS

A number of factors place the preterm infant at risk for vitamin deficiencies during the first weeks of life. Low body stores of vitamins, possible defects in absorption (particularly of fat-soluble vitamins), and low intakes of formula may contribute to deficiency states. The AAP Committee on Nutrition recommends that a multivitamin supplement that provides the equivalent of the recommended dietary supplements for the term infant be supplied to preterm infants during the first weeks of life. After the infant is consuming more than 300 kcal/day or when body weight exceeds 2.5 kg, a multivitamin supplement is no longer needed, but it is a convenient method for providing the few nutrients such as vitamin D and iron that still may be required.

For infants who demonstrate poor growth because of recurrent or chronic illness or poor caloric intake, administration of multivitamin supplements should continue. These infants may benefit from special dietary counseling from a clinical nutritionist.

IRON

Low birth weight infants are especially susceptible to the development of iron deficiency anemias because their store of iron is much smaller than that of full-term infants and are insufficient to last over a prolonged period of rapid growth. Without supplemental iron, the preterm's body stores of iron will be depleted sometime after 2 months of age rather than after 4 to 6 months of age, as in normal full-term infants. The Committee on Nutrition recommends that low birth weight infants receive 2 mg of iron per kg per day starting at 2 months of age or earlier. Sufficient iron for the prevention of iron deficiency in preterm infants can be supplied through the use of iron-fortified formula or multivitamin preparations containing iron. Infants who have received multiple blood transfusions may have some protection against iron deficiency anemias because of the high iron content in packed red blood cells, 5 mg/10 mL, but because of rapid growth rates they should still receive supplementation according to the above recommendations. Preterm infants should receive iron supplements in either vitamins or formula until they have made the transition to solid foods and are consuming adequate amounts of iron-fortified cereals.

VITAMIN E

Vitamin E deficiency is rare except in premature infants in whom tocopherol requirements are unknown and in those with fat malabsorption. Vitamin E deficiency in preterm infants during the first several weeks of life can be attributed to several factors, including limited tissue stores at birth, relative dietary deficiency, intestinal malabsorption, and rapid growth. After the development of mature digestive and absorptive capacity, tocopherol absorption improves and vitamin E levels rise.

The addition of a daily multivitamin supplement that contains 5 IU of vitamin E may help correct vitamin E deficiency and achieve physiologic levels of 0.8 to 1.8 mg/dL. This may be particularly important when these infants are receiving iron-fortified formula, because iron may increase the susceptibility of infants to vitamin E deficiency.

FLUORIDE

The AAP Committee on Nutrition recommends initiating fluoride supplementation 2 weeks after birth in full-term breast-fed infants, in formula-fed infants whose community water supply is not optimally fluoridated, and in infants receiving ready-to-feed formula. Because the preterm infant is prone to enamel defects related to prolonged oral intubation, beginning fluoride supplements when preterm infants reach a postconceptual age of 40 weeks may minimize the development of caries.

ISSUES IN THE CARE OF PRETERM INFANTS

PRIMARY IMMUNIZATIONS

The AAP recommends that diphtheria and tetanus toxoids and pertussis vaccine (DTP) and poliovirus vaccine, live oral (OPV) be administered to prematurely born infants at the appropriate postnatal age. If the infant remains in the hospital, only DTP should be given, to avoid cross-infection with OPV in the nursery; the OPV can be initiated at the time of discharge, or poliovirus vaccine, inactivated (IPV) can be given at routine intervals instead.

Recent research supports these recommendations and demonstrates that preterm infants immunized with a full dose of DTP and OPV at routine intervals (8, 16, and 24 weeks after birth) are capable of producing a protective serologic response. There is no need to use a reduced dosage of DTP. Most important, a high percentage of preterm infants demonstrate *inadequate* protection (most commonly against pertussis) if given a reduced dosage of DTP at routine intervals.

Infants older than 6 months of age with chronic lung disease, such as BPD, and any of their primary caretakers should receive influenza virus vaccine in areas where this virus is known to be particularly virulent. Each year the Center for Immunization Practices Advisory Committee publishes updated immunization recommendations that should be followed.

HEARING

Preterm infants are at higher risk for hearing impairment than is the normal population. Antibiotic and diuretic therapy, exposure to incubator "noise," transient hypoxic episodes, intraventricular hemorrhage (IVH), hyperbilirubinemia, congenital infection, and prolonged intubation are examples of predisposing factors that place the preterm infant at increased risk. Routine screening for both conductive and sensorineural hearing losses should be performed early within the first year of life so that appropriate intervention can be initiated if needed. Most conductive losses are transient and should be followed up and treated as if such losses were found in a term infant. Sensorineural hearing loss, reported to occur in approximately 3% of preterm infants, is less likely to be transient. Many screening tests are now available for use in infants, but their sensitivity and reliability vary. It is important that an experienced audiologist perform the tests. Within the second year of life, it is essential that language acquisition be assessed. If there is a significant delay in language or if articulation problems are present, a formal hearing evaluation should be performed.

RETINOPATHY OF PREMATURITY

Preterm infants are at increased risk for retinopathy of prematurity (ROP). Multiple factors have been implicated in development of ROP; those most closely linked, include low birth weight, short gestation, and prolonged oxygen therapy. ROP is a disease of overgrowth of the developing retinal vessels and may lead to significant scarring and distortion of the retina. ROP has been classified into five stages, with the fifth stage the most severe.

Most ROP is reversible and may regress completely. The use of vitamin E in the prevention and treatment of ROP remains controversial. Proponents of its use generally recommend the maintenance of a physiologic serum concentration of 0.8 to 1.8 mg/dL beginning shortly after birth and continuing until full retinal maturation occurs. The use of pharmacologic levels of vitamin E (3 to 5 mg/dL) has been linked to the development of necrotizing enterocolitis and sepsis and in general is not recommended for prevention of ROP or for the treatment of less severe stages of disease.

Treatment of severe ROP with transcleral cryotherapy has resulted in a decreased incidence of retinal folds and retinal detachment. While research continues in this area, cryotherapy is recommended in the treatment of advanced active disease.

Any infant with ROP is at a 10 times greater risk for refractive errors than the same gestational age counterpart without ROP. The higher the stage of ROP, the greater the risk of more serious sequelae. For this reason, the preterm infant with previously diagnosed ROP requires close ophthalmologic follow-up.

RICKETS

Very low birth weight infants, those requiring long-term parenteral alimentation, those with gastrointestinal malabsorption, or those with cholestatic liver disease are at increased risk for rickets. Rickets has also been reported in breast-fed preterm infants.

Routine monitoring of serum calcium, phosphorus, and alkaline phosphatase levels, and if abnormal, periodic examination of bone radiographs, will allow early detection of this condition.

Treatment of rickets consists of increasing dietary calcium and vitamin D through the use of supplements of special infant formulas.

NEPHROCALCINOSIS

Renal calcification is increasingly recognized as a complication in preterm infants, especially those with extremely low birth weight and those receiving diuretic therapy with furosemide, which increases calcium excretion through the immature kidneys. Screening for nephrocalcinosis includes calculation of partial excretion of calcium (urine calcium/urine creatinine), evaluation for blood or protein in the urine, and measurements of serum creatinine or blood urea nitrogen. If any of these values are abnormal, abdominal ultrasonography to document the presence of calcifications is warranted. If confirmed, the need for diuretics should be reconsidered, and altered if current therapy includes furosemide. Follow-up ultrasound studies are suggested to document any progression or regression.

INTRAVENTRICULAR HEMORRHAGE

Intraventricular hemorrhages occur in approximately 30% to 40% of preterm infants. The degree of severity of IVH ranges from mild (grade 1) to severe (grade 4) with parenchymal damage. Infants with any degree of IVH warrant careful observation for signs of hydrocephalus. Close attention should be paid to the head circumference of infants who have sustained any IVH. Infants with grade 3 or 4 IVH should have follow-up cranial ultrasonography to document resolution of the hemorrhage or to identify any developing hydrocephalus. Follow-up ultrasound studies should be performed at 3-month intervals until complete resolution is documented. Ultrasound studies should be obtained in infants with any degree of IVH if there is a suspicion of inappropriately rapid head growth. Ultrasonography cannot be performed after the fontanelle has closed, usually at 12 to 18 months of age. In addition, infants with grade 3 or 4 IVH are at greater risk for developmental handicaps (especially in the motor areas) and warrant close screening.

PERIVENTRICULAR LEUKOMALACIA

Ischemic injury of the periventricular white matter can lead to the development of periventricular leukomalacia (PVL). The presence of a watershed area between the end zones of the cerebral arterial supply in the immature brain places the preterm infant at risk for PVL. Several studies have demonstrated an increased incidence of cerebral palsy, developmental delay, and visual impairment in infants with PVL, particularly in those infants with cysts greater than 3 mm (Fig 5–1). Infants in whom PVL is suspected should have close neurodevelopmental follow-up. Serial ultrasonography is recommended in infants in whom PVL is suspected, because cystic changes can develop several weeks to months after the initial insult.

FEEDING PROBLEMS

Although most feeding problems in the preterm infant population occur during the neonatal period, many infants exhibit long-term or recurrent problems in both sucking and swallowing. Premature infants who have transient neurologic immaturities and those who have more permanent neurologic deficits are at highest risk. Either of these infants may exhibit generalized hypotonicity or hyperactivity as well as persistence of primitive oral reflex patterns. Children with tracheostomies occasionally exhibit symptoms of swallowing dysfunction. This is probably related to limited movement of the larynx or discomfort and may be transient or persist until after decannulation. Another condition placing a preterm infant at high risk for feeding problems is deprivation of oral feeding experience for extended periods, as commonly occurs during the preterm infant's neonatal course.

Oral reflexes may be hypoactive or hyperactive. Reflexes (such as root, suck, swallow, cough, and gag) allow normal feeding and protect the airway from aspiration. Abnormal reflexes that may prevent normal feeding are the tonic bite reflex or abnormal tongue thrust. A hyperactive gag reflex is particularly troublesome because the child cannot tolerate the nipple or spoon on the tongue. This often leads to extreme oral hypersensitivity. Other causes of hypersensitivity or tactile defensiveness include intubation, suctioning, and generally noxious stimulation around the mouth. These children become resistant to any type of oral stimulation.

All of these problems are amenable to therapy if they are properly identified and appro-

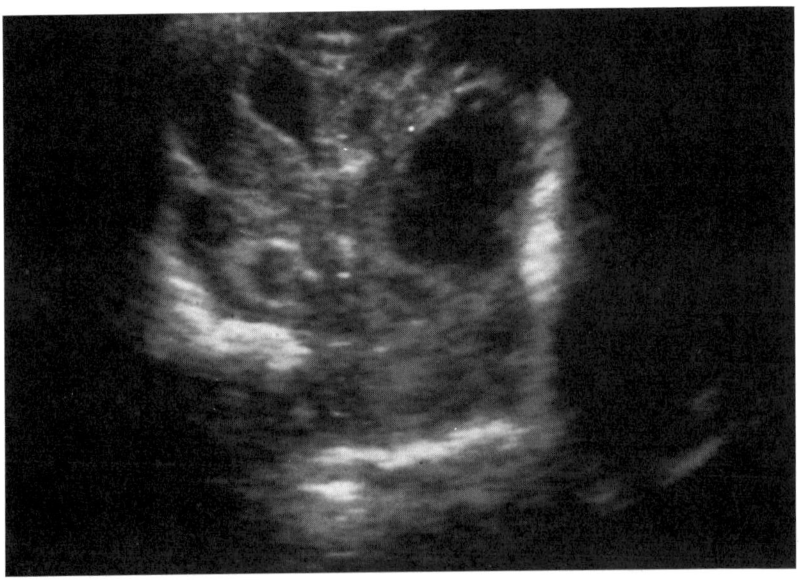

FIG 5–1
Ultrasound study of the head of an infant shows large residual cystic lesions resulting from periventricular leukomalacia. These were not evident on initial ultrasonograms obtained during the early neonatal period.

priate intervention is begun at the first sign of problems. Depending on their training, either a pediatric speech pathologist or occupational therapist can develop a feeding program that would be most appropriate once a particular feeding problem is identified.

GASTROESOPHAGEAL REFLUX

Although not unique to preterm infants, gastroesophageal reflux is common in the premature population; the presentation and therapy for preterm infants is similar to that described for full-term infants. However, it is important to remember that gastroesophageal reflux occasionally may be associated with apnea and should be considered in an apnea workup.

APNEA

Apnea in premature infants is most likely caused by the immature brain failing to trigger automatic breathing. Bradycardia often accompanies the apnea. Use of a pneumogram or thermistor, with a 12- to 24-hour recording of heart rate and respiratory rate variability, will often document the presence of apnea and bradycardia and help determine the appropriate therapeutic intervention.

Although apnea usually originates in the central nervous system, the acute onset or increase in frequency of apnea should warrant further investigation. Conditions such as infection, IVH, and anemia commonly have apnea as their initial sign. Apnea may also be associated with gastroesophageal reflux in some infants.

The mainstay of therapy for apnea and bradycardia is theophylline or caffeine, pharmacologically similar agents that are both central stimulants. Some infants may require continued therapy even after initial hospital discharge. Preterm infants, as they mature neurologically, normally "outgrow" apnea and bradycardia. Theophylline or caffeine levels should be monitored, however, and maintained at therapeutic levels only if CNS-induced apnea persists. Often an infant will require home cardiorespiratory monitoring in addition to or in lieu of drug therapy.

The need for monitoring or medication is usually determined prior to the infant's initial hospital discharge. It is the physician's task to decide when it is appropriate to withdraw either therapy. Some general principles should be followed. At least 1 month should elapse after the infant's discharge before theophylline or caffeine is withdrawn. If the infant is being monitored at home and no episodes of apnea or bradycardia occur, then the infant should be allowed to "outgrow" the medication by not increasing the dosage as the baby's weight increases. If episodes of apnea persist or increase in frequency, the theophylline or caffeine dosage can be increased after other possible causes have been evaluated. If the infant is receiving medication and is not being monitored, the theophylline or caffeine level should be maintained in the therapeutic range for 2 to 3 months and the baby rehospitalized for withdrawal of medication.

Once medication has been discontinued in the infant who is being monitored, 1 to 2 months with no monitor alarms or episodes of apnea should elapse before obtaining a pneumogram. Most often the pneumogram can be performed at home. Interpretation of results should help to determine any further monitoring needs. The majority of infants have no medication or monitoring needs beyond 6 months, adjusted age.

BRONCHOPULMONARY DYSPLASIA

Many preterm infants have BPD, a condition that develops as a sequel to respiratory distress syndrome. What role oxygen therapy, ventilatory support, or lung immaturity play in its cause is unclear. Infants with BPD often have prolonged oxygen needs or require fluid restriction or diuretic or bronchodilator therapy even after discharge from the nursery. Depending on the clinical evaluation for signs of respiratory distress, these therapies can be altered and eventually withdrawn as the child matures.

Diuretics.—Infants with BPD are often given diuretics in addition to fluid restriction, to decrease the amount of excess lung and total body water. Drugs in common use include furosemide, chlorothiazide, and spironolactone.

When diuretics are given on an outpatient basis, the infant's oral intake, estimates of output, weight gain, and serum electrolytes should be closely monitored. Because of potential electrolyte abnormalities associated with diuretics, potassium chloride supplements are usually used with all diuretics except spironolactone. Diuretics should be restricted to those patients in whom there is an apparent clinical response to the medication. Although uncommon, nephrocalcinosis has been reported in infants given furosemide. Most often these drugs do not need to be increased as the child gains weight if there are no clinical signs or symptoms of right ventricular failure or pulmonary edema. The medication can be withdrawn when the child has grown to a weight that would seem to make the drug subtherapeutic on a milligram per kilogram basis, while maintaining respiratory stability. Weaning the child from a diuretic requires frequent evaluations of body weight, fluid intake, vital signs, and auscultation of the chest.

Bronchospasm.—Many infants with mild residual BPD develop evidence of bronchospasm with viral illnesses or environmental irritants. Their airways are quite hyperactive. In many respects they have similar clinical symptoms as children with asthma. Unlike those with asthma, however, most infants "outgrow" BPD-related bronchospasm by 1 to 2 years of age. Because physicians are not accustomed to seeing bronchospasm in a child younger than 1 or 2 years, BPD-related bronchospasm in the infant is often incorrectly diagnosed as bronchitis or pneumonia, and antibiotics or cough medicine are administered. Antibiotics are usually not warranted unless a bacterial process is suspected. Cough medicines, especially those containing antihistamines, should be used with caution, because their use may lead to the development of inspissated secretions, leading in turn to worsening of pulmonary symptoms.

The use of bronchodilators such as theophylline or metaproterenol is appropriate intervention for bronchospasm related to BPD. In contrast to previous beliefs, these infants do have bronchial smooth muscle that is responsive to such medication. Theophylline is well tolerated in dosages similar to those used in children with asthma (i.e., 4 to 6 mg/kg/dose every 6 to 8 hours; therapeutic range, 10 to 20 μg/mL). Infants receiving theophylline should be closely monitored for evidence of theophylline toxicity, such as tachycardia, vomiting, and irritability. Metaproterenol, either alone or in conjunction with theophylline, is another bronchodilator in common use. The dosage for this medication is 2 mg/kg/day in three or four divided doses. These medications can be used during acute episodes either for short periods (3 to 7 days) or for several weeks until symptoms resolve. If symptoms do not resolve, readjustment of medications may be warranted or further investigation of other possible causes for the bronchospasm may be indicated.

As with asthma, maintenance doses of one or more of these medications may be needed if the infant has recurrent episodes of bronchospasm. During acute exacerbations a second bronchodilator (theophylline and then metaproteranol, for instance) can function synergistically to achieve the desired relief.

Another medication being used more commonly is cromolyn disodium. This drug acts as a mast cell membrane stabilizer and may be useful in the child with frequent episodes of bronchospasm. It is a medication given by inhalation (20 mg three times a day), and is most effective if given as routine prophylaxis.

Oxygen Requirements.—Dependence on supplemental oxygen varies with the severity of BPD. If the infant is otherwise medically stable, the need for supplemental oxygen should not necessarily preclude consideration for discharge. The supplemental oxygen required should usually be no more than 2 L/min delivered via nasal cannula. Outpatients should be followed up at frequent intervals and weaned slowly, depending on clinical stability (weight gain, good pulmonary reserve during periods of activity or feeding, and lack of significant intercurrent pulmonary illness). Ideally, if there is access to a device to measure oxygen saturation either directly (pulse oximetry) or indirectly (transcutaneous oxygen monitor), weaning can be done with more accuracy. These measurements should be done when the infant is at rest, during periods of activity and feeding, and when crying, to determine if any desaturation occurs relative to the resting state.

If the infant is medically stable based on the above criteria and not anemic, the weaning process can begin. The most important rule is to do it gradually. Studies have shown that infants with BPD who are receiving optimal oxygen show better weight gain, attain corrected

TABLE 5–1
Weaning a Patient From Supplemental Oxygen: Sample Schedule*

	AMOUNT OF OXYGEN (PER MIN)
At hospital discharge	0.5 L at all times
1 mo after discharge	0.5 L during feedings and sleep, 0.25 L when awake
2 mo	0.25 L at all times
3 mo	0.25 L during feedings and sleep, room air when awake
4 mo	Room air at all times

* Schedule assumes clinical stability, adequate weight gain, and documentation of adequate oxygen saturation. Intervals may vary depending on these criteria.

age–appropriate milestones more readily, and have fewer intercurrent respiratory illnesses than do those with borderline oxygenation. A typical weaning schedule is shown in Table 5–1. Infants should be given therapeutic doses of their previous bronchodilator or diuretic regimen until completely weaned to room air.

Rehospitalization.—Rehospitalization is common in infants with BPD, especially in the first year of life. Recurrent episodes of bronchospasm that are difficult to treat on an outpatient basis may be precipitated by outgrowing (but still requiring) medications; exposure to environmental irritants such as cigarette or fireplace smoke, paint fumes, insecticides, or kerosene heaters; and exposure to other people with respiratory viruses. In particular, infants with BPD are at higher risk for contracting debilitating respiratory symptoms secondary to respiratory syncytial virus (RSV), adenovirus, and influenza viruses. The physician should recommend that every effort be made to avoid exposure to these potential irritants.

Studies have shown a much higher rate of rehospitalization in the preterm population during the first year of life. The need arises most often from pulmonary illnesses, but poor weight gain, minor surgical procedures, or apnea and bradycardia are also potential causes. Although most episodes warrant rehospitalization, the physician should be sensitive to the effects these repeated "disruptions" have on the family unit and attempt to treat the infant as much as possible as an outpatient.

NEUROLOGIC PROBLEMS

Abnormalities of muscle tone and posture are the most common neurologic abnormalities encountered in preterm infants. Several reports in the literature describe transient muscle tone abnormalities in premature infants during the first 12 to 18 months. In general these abnormalities are evident within the first 3 months after discharge and begin to resolve by the time the child is 12 months, corrected age. In a term infant, abnormal muscle tone during the first year of life is relatively rare and is associated with an increased risk for neurologic handicaps. In the preterm infant, however, it is more common and may not carry the same prognostic importance. Misinterpretation of the significance of muscle tone abnormalities during the infant's first year of life may result in *inaccurately* describing normal premature infants as neurologically handicapped. Therefore caution should be used when labeling a condition as cerebral palsy before the infant is 18 months, corrected age. If, however, there is evidence of hemiparesis of *known* cause (e.g., porencephalic cyst or localized severe IVH), the diagnosis of cerebral palsy may be used with more certainty.

The most common abnormality of tone is increased extensor tone of the lower extremities. Figure 5–2 shows increased extensor tone seen in the lower extremities of a 6-month-old infant, corrected age. When placed in a position of support, this infant demonstrates marked knee stiffening and toe-pointing, as well as rigidity about the hip musculature. Hypertonicity that persists beyond 12 months is usually limited to a mild to moderate degree of toe-walking, which becomes evident when the child begins to walk unassisted. As expected, when lower extremity hypertonicity does not resolve by 1 year of age, these children can demonstrate a delay in walking because they are more unstable than if they were able to walk with their feet flat on the floor.

Preventive corrective measures in infancy include proper positioning so as not to reinforce and exacerbate this abnormally increased tone. It is therefore strongly recommended that these children not be placed in positions of support, such as in a walker or jumper or standing in a parent's lap. When lower extremity hypertonic-

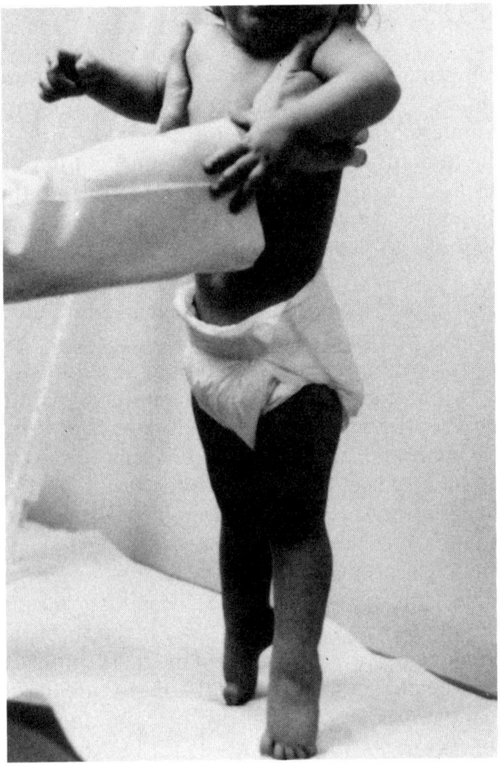

FIG 5–2
Demonstration of neurologic examination of infant with increased extension tone of lower extremities. Note stiff knees and pointed toes.

ity persists in infants older than 18 to 24 months, referral to an orthopedic surgeon may be appropriate for consideration of casting for tendon stretching or for possible release of the hamstring or Achilles tendon to ensure adequate ambulation.

Figure 5–3 shows hypertonicity of the shoulder girdle and trapezius musculature, as well as upper extremity increased flexor tone. This posture is commonly referred to as "scapular retraction." When this increased flexor tone persists until 6 to 9 months of age the infant is unable to perform the lateral-propping protective reflex and parachute reflex, respectively, because the infant is unable to extend his arms to the side or to the front. This also markedly affects independent sitting, reaching, and midline activities and can be a cause of frustration for the infant. This type of muscle tone problem is amenable to treatment with specific positions that encourage the shoulders to be brought forward, in an attempt to break up the shoulder girdle muscle hypertonicity so that reaching can be more adaptive.

Compared with the incidence of hypertonicity, decreased muscle tone is far less frequently encountered in preterm infants. Muscle hypotonicity can be evident as the persistence of an exaggerated head lag on pull-to-sit or head bobbing with the infant in a sitting position at 6 months, corrected age. Hypotonicity affecting the trunk can be evidenced as a slumped posture when the 6-month-old infant is placed in a sitting position. Hypotonicity of the trunk musculature will delay the onset of sitting until the second half of the first year. Less frequently one can see hypotonicity of either the upper or the lower extremities evidenced by a resistance or inability of the infant to bear weight on his legs in vertical suspension or on his arms in prone position; both abilities are expected in a 3- to 4-month-old term infant.

Some infants may demonstrate mixed tonic abnormalities. The most common is truncal hypotonicity coexisting with lower extremity hypertonicity.

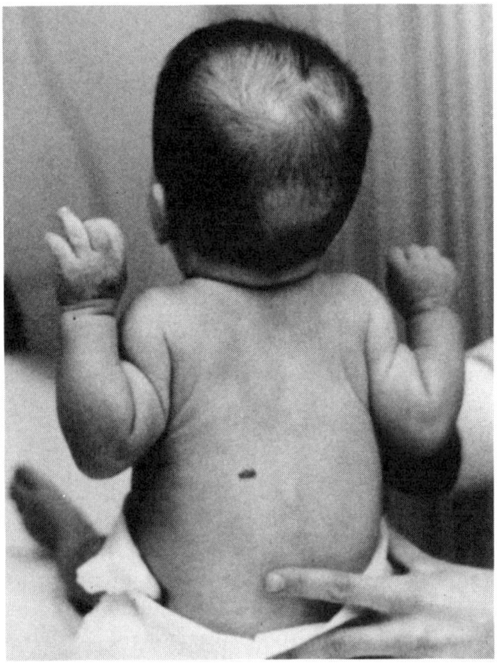

FIG 5–3
Demonstration of scapular retractions seen in hypertonicity of shoulder girdle, trapezium extremities, and upper extremities.

In isolated hypertonicity or hypotonicity or mixed tonal abnormalities, physical therapy is recommended; most of the therapy can be performed by the parent. Although it is an area of much controversy (because the natural history of these abnormalities suggests that they resolve some time within the second year of life), we do recommend formal physical therapy intervention when the tone abnormality is sufficiently involved that it affects the infant's functional status or delays the acquisition of key developmental milestones. The physical therapist can assist the child to develop adaptive measures for overcoming a functional disability.

One last neurologic problem encountered in the preterm population is the persistence of primitive reflexes. Some premature infants have reflexes such as the asymmetric tonic neck, Moro, or grasp reflexes that persist beyond the limit of 4 months of age that is thought to be normal for term infants. Although this finding is commonly encountered in full-term children with neurologic abnormalities such as cerebral palsy, persistence of primitive reflexes in the preterm infant is usually not such an ominous sign.

DEVELOPMENTAL OUTCOME

The primary care physician can play an important role in promoting the normal development of a preterm infant. The responsibilities are twofold: to screen for mental, motor, and behavioral dysfunctions for which this population is at risk and to provide emotional and educational support to parents whose task is made more difficult by the stressful neonatal period.

Screening for developmental disabilities is mandatory. Despite an improved outlook on the outcome of low birth weight infants, there remains a higher incidence of mental retardation, cerebral palsy, and learning problems in the preterm population. The majority of infants who weigh between 1,000 and 1,500 g at birth are intellectually normal after the first year of life; the remainder, approximately 10% to 13%, do have moderate or major delays in development. This represents a major improvement over the 89% incidence of handicaps in low birth weight infants born in the 1950s. The outlook for infants weighing less than 1,000 g at birth is less positive. Approximately 15% to 20% of these infants have moderate to major delays in development. Of those infants weighing less than 800 g at birth, approximately 25% are delayed developmentally.

In addition to the children who have moderate to major developmental delays, another large population of preterm children has been identified with learning problems. These are children of all birth weights who, despite normal intelligence as measured with IQ tests, have problems learning in school and often require special education. Deficits have been documented in perceptual-motor integration skills, impulse control, attention span, language skills, and integration of sensory stimuli. These learning disabilities are more difficult to identify before school age, but are serious and disabling to the affected child and family.

Screening by the community physician can be accomplished with assessment tools. The Denver Developmental Screening Test or more informal developmental interviews will provide enough information to the physician that decision for further evaluation can be made. Interpretation of the results of the developmental examination must be done in coordination with evaluation of vision and hearing abilities because any sensory impairment, even mild, can cause abnormalities in intellectual performance.

At this time, there are no norms for the development of preterm infants, so we must employ those norms standardized for a healthy term population. To correct for this difference, it is advisable to use the infant's age corrected for 40 weeks' gestation rather than the birth date. Since the developmental progress of low birth weight infants is more consistent with age from conception, using this adjusted age prevents the evaluator from being overly concerned when the infant lags behind his or her chronologic age behavior. The use of adjusted age becomes unnecessary when the infant reaches a chronologic age of 2½ years because the time span between birth and 40 weeks has become a smaller fraction of the total age. Even with correction for prematurity, these infants often demonstrate developmental lags in the first year of life. For example, most infants at the corrected age of 6 months are still not sitting upright and have only clumsy reaching skills. By the corrected age of 12 months, most infants have "caught up" to their corrected age.

Although the study of risk factors or causes of developmental handicaps has not yielded data definitive enough to predict later outcome, some factors have been identified that place a low birth weight infant at higher risk for problems: IVH (grade 3 or 4), need for transport to a tertiary care center, birth asphyxia, extended need for mechanical ventilation, and social factors.

IVH, as discussed previously, ranges from small bleeding to greater and more damaging bleeding. Developmental follow-up studies have reported that only grade 3 and 4 bleeding are associated with a risk for handicap. In particular, cerebral palsy is a frequent finding, often with no accompanying delays in intellectual skills. Periventricular leukomalacia is a relatively rare brain injury that is frequently associated with mental retardation and visual impairment. Birth asphyxia, as defined by Apgar score of less than 3 at 1 and 5 minutes, is associated with poor developmental outcome. Children requiring extended mechanical ventilation, usually an indication of BPD, generally perform in the low-average range and often demonstrate more significant delays in the preschool years while the disease is still active. The impact of social class variables such as maternal education, family income, and knowledge of child development often emerge as stronger predictors of later outcome.

Referral for further assessment and therapeutic intervention should take place when there are concerns about a specific aspect of a child's development; when there is overall delay from the child's adjusted age; when uneven or abnormal development is present; when parents seek more specific or extensive information than the physician has time or background to give.

Because problems seen in the first year of preterm infant's life are often transient, the decision to refer is often difficult; however, early referral is appropriate for this high-risk population.

Community physicians have the opportunity to affect the developmental progress of low birth weight infants by supporting the family. When these infants go home, they are quite different from term infants. Feeding and weight gain may still be a concern, sleeping and waking patterns are confused, their appearance is still disparate from that of a full-term infant, and most important, parents usually have concerns about their child's future development and may not think of the child as "normal." By showing parents the strengths and weaknesses and personality of their infant, informing them of developmental sequence, and even suggesting appropriate play and learning activities, physicians have been found to have a positive impact on parent-child relationships. Parents of low birth weight infants have experienced numerous stresses and may seek support from community physicians; by their sensitivity to the parents' concerns, physicians can help improve the family environment for the developing child.

IMPACT ON THE FAMILY

The stresses on families of preterm infants during the hospitalization are overt and dramatic. For families of preterm infants who require medically complicated home care the stresses continue to be significant after discharge. Because of these home care needs the family centers its attention on the child and normal activities become extremely difficult. The impact on these families after discharge can be described in three phases: euphoria, despair, and acceptance. Euphoria occurs during the first 6 weeks after discharge. The parents experience the thrill of having their child home. They finally feel like parents. Despair tends to set in sometime between 6 weeks and 6 months. Exhaustion may predominate. The parents may realize the child is much sicker and more developmentally delayed than they thought. During the final phase, acceptance, the parents start to integrate the child with complex medical needs into their lives. By accepting their child and the attendant life style the family is able to resume a more normal life. For the families whose preterm infants are growing, developing, and have no significant ongoing medical needs the stresses are more subtle and possibly difficult to recognize.

Many of the stresses on the families of preterm infants after discharge are described in what Green and Solnit call the "vulnerable child syndrome." Despite the infant's recovery from illness, the parents continue to experience anxiety because they perceive their infant as fragile, vulnerable, and having special needs. The behavior of the parent and child is adversely affected by this continuing belief.

The parents' perception of an infant's vulnerability persists for several reasons. Questions of the infant's survival that preoccupied the parents' emotions during the hospitalization linger after discharge. Parents also appear to lack confidence in their parenting ability. This may be due to an interruption in the normal development of parenting skills as a result of a prolonged hospitalization, or it may be related to persistent feelings that the hospital staff is more competent at caretaking. Feeling that they should be constantly happy about the infant's arrival home, parents may have difficulty admitting and expressing normal frustrations of parenting and latent anger about separation. Concerns over problems with the child's future development often lead to parental feelings that the infant remains sick, different from other infants, and warrants special status in the family.

Several parent-infant behavior problems frequently result in:

1. Feeding problems, including overfeeding and underfeeding.
2. Difficulty in separation from the mother. Mother feels that only she can do the care and wants no one else involved.
3. Overindulgence and overpermissiveness. Families have difficulty setting disciplinary limits on the child, thus interfering with normal development. The child becomes dependent, demanding, and out of control; the child, not the parent, is running the household.

What can be done to prevent the vulnerable child syndrome? First, the parents of preterm infants need more time with their physician. All the concerns that parents of full-term infants have are exaggerated in parents of preterm infants. It is important to establish rapport with the family, be sensitive to their needs, and provide support. The family needs to feel comfortable in expressing their fears and concerns to their physician. Second, families should be encouraged to normalize the caretaking of their preterm infant and their daily activities. The promotion of the normalization process is critical in the development of a healthy parent-child relationship. Third, encourage the families to be firm. Assist the parents in setting disciplinary limits and schedules. Give them permission to set limits and be in control. Fourth, educate the parents about developmental delays in preterm infants that are common and in most cases temporary.

It is important that the infant with developmental delays be enrolled in an early intervention program as soon as possible. The intervention program not only promotes developmental progress but provides an opportunity for parental involvement. As a result of direct parental involvement, the parents have a more realistic view of their child's abilities and needs.

Finally, if the parent's worries are recognized, a careful explanation and continued clarification of the infant's true health status can alleviate unnecessary concerns and promote more effective use of the primary care physician.

BIBLIOGRAPHY

Ballard RA: *Pediatric Care of the ICN Graduate*. Philadelphia, WB Saunders Co, 1988.

Bernbaum JB, Daft A, Anolik R, et al: Response of preterm infants to diphtheria-tetanus-pertussis immunizations. *J Pediatr* 1985; 107:184–188.

Feinberg E: Family stress in pediatric home care. *Caring* 1985; 38–41.

Forbes GB, Woodruff CW: *Pediatric Nutrition Handbook* ed 2. Elk Grove Village, Ill; American Academy of Pediatrics, 1985.

Green M, Solnit AJ: Reactions to the threatened loss of a child: A vulnerable child syndrome. *Pediatrics* 1964; 34:58.

Groothuis JR, Rosenberg AA: Home oxygen promotes weight gain in infants with bronchopulmonary dysplasia. *Am J Dis Child* 1987; 141:992–995.

Harrison H: *The Premature Baby Book*. New York, St Martin's Press, 1983.

Hoy EA, Bill JM, Sykes DK: Very low birthweight: A long-term developmental impairment? *Int J Behav Dev* 1988; 11:37–67.

Hurt H: Symposium on continuing care of a high-risk infant. *Clin Perinatol* 1984; 11:1.

Klein N, Hack M, Gallagher J, et al: Preschool performance of children with normal intelligence who were very low birthweight infants. *Pediatrics* 1985; 75:531–537.

Ross G: Mortality and morbidity in very low birthweight infants. *Pediatr Ann* 1983; 12:1.

Seigel LS (ed): Low birth weight. *Semin Perinatol* vol 6(special issue), Oct 1982.

Silverman WA, Flynn JT: *Contemporary Issues in Fetal and Neonatal Medicine. Retinopathy of Prematurity.* Boston, Blackwell Scientific Publications, 1985.

Vohr B, Hack M: Developmental follow-up of low-birth-weight infants. *Pediatr Clin North Am* 1982; 29:1441.

Wilson R: Risk and resilience in early mental development. *Dev Psychol* 1985; 21:795.

6 THE TODDLER AND OLDER CHILD

Watching and helping children grow gives the primary care physician special insight into human development. Variations in the physical and emotional growth of normal children make this aspect of practice both interesting and challenging. Parents who do not have the experience or knowledge of ranges of development look to the physician to determine if their child has a problem or is in the range of normal development. Therefore, the practitioner needs to keep in mind the common developmental issues that occur at various segments of the child's life and be prepared to help and advise the families.

This chapter focuses on the physical and emotional issues of the toddler. The physical examination is highlighted, rather than covered completely, as it is assumed that the reader has experience in physical examinations. Next a range of normal developmental issues is discussed in a practical manner, describing a spectrum of expected concerns of parents.

EXAMINATION

Rosemary Casey, M.D.

APPROACH TO THE EXAMINATION

The examining room should be a warm, safe environment. Children who feel cold will shiver and cry. Begin by talking to the child: ask questions, tell a story, show an instrument, help the child relax. As your examination proceeds, keep hands and equipment warm, avoid quick jerky movements, and continue to speak to the child in a calm, confident tone of voice. Use the power of suggestion to your advantage and do not ask the child's permission to perform the examination. It is usually better to say, "Show me how still you can be while I look in your ears" than to ask "May I look in your ears?"

The order of the examination must be tailored to the child's age, degree of fear, and specific complaints. Generally, it is best to postpone the objectionable parts until the end. Much of the examination can be done with a young child sitting in the parent's lap.

Although sometimes impossible to avoid, restraint should be used as little as possible. It is surprising how frequently physicians hold children down unnecessarily. A child's natural reaction is to struggle to escape, thus making the examination much more difficult to perform. A moment used to calm a child is generally time well spent.

The physician should not rush into the physical examination with frightening instruments and poking fingers. Even while taking a history, much information can be learned by observing the child and parent. The child's posture and movements and overall comfort should be noted. Degree of illness, general development, and speech skills should be determined. Some assessment of growth, nutrition, and hydration should be made. This is a particularly good time to assess respiration, to get an initial view of the skin, and to note any specific abnormal odors. The parent-child interaction and the child's personality and fearfulness can be noted at this time.

The following discussion includes common problems in physical diagnosis. For more detailed information consult the text by Barness.

BLOOD PRESSURE

Children 3 years of age and older should have their blood pressure (BP) measured annually. The rubber bladder in the cuff should cover approximately 75% of the upper arm length and should be long enough to completely encircle the arm. Cuff selection should always be based on arm size, not age. Cuffs that are too narrow will yield an artificially high BP.

The child should be relaxed and in a sitting position. Inflate the cuff to 20 to 30 mm Hg above the level at which the pulse can no longer be palpated. Next, release the pressure slowly, about 2 to 3 mm Hg per second, until a clear tapping sound is heard. This is the first Korotkoff sound and corresponds to the systolic pressure.

There is some disagreement about whether the fourth (muffling) or fifth (disappearance of all sounds) Korotkoff phase should be used as the measurement of diastolic pressure. The standard children's BP charts (Figs 6–1 and 6–2) generally use the fourth sound, but the pressure at which sounds disappear should probably also be recorded. The most common causes of error in BP determination are incorrect cuff selection, poor measurement technique, and an upset or anxious child.

Measurements of BP above the 95th percentile for age should be repeated on at least three separate occasions. Only if the BP is persistently elevated should the child be considered hypertensive. These children should undergo a careful history and physical examination to determine the extent of the further diagnostic evaluation.

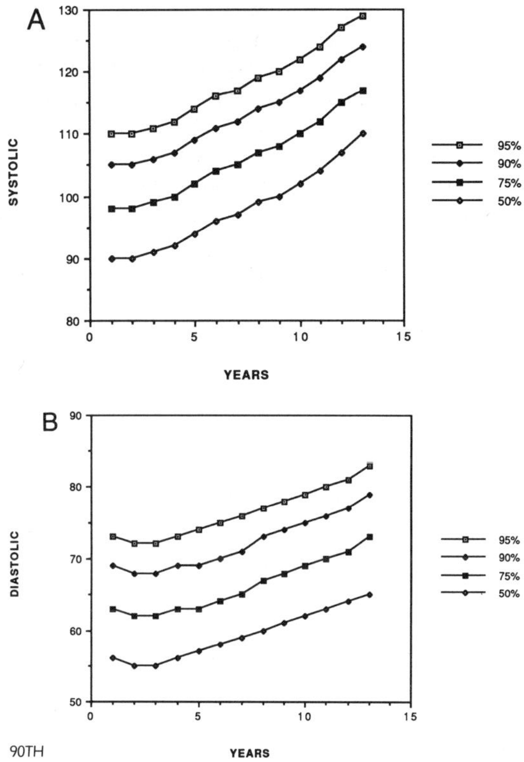

90TH PERCENTILE													
SYSTOLIC BP	105	105	106	107	109	111	112	114	115	117	119	122	124
DIASTOLIC BP	67	69	69	69	69	70	71	72	74	75	77	78	80
HEIGHT (CM)	77	89	98	107	115	122	129	135	142	148	154	160	165
WEIGHT (KG)	11	13	15	18	22	25	30	35	40	45	51	58	63

FIG 6–1

Age-specific percentiles for blood pressure measurements in boys aged 1 to 13 years; Korotkoff phase IV (K4) used for diastolic BP. (From Horan MJ, et al: Report of the Second Task Force on Blood Pressure Control in Children—1987. *Pediatrics* 1987; 79:1–25. Used by permission.)

HEIGHT, WEIGHT, HEAD CIRCUMFERENCE

The evaluation of a child's height, weight, and head circumference requires the proper use of appropriate growth charts. After the first year of life and until adolescence, a child's growth pattern is normally parallel to the percentile lines. Growth patterns that cross over percentile lines are often the first sign of some medical, emotional, or social problem. One note of caution: if a child's standing height is plotted on a chart standardized for supine length, the resultant percentiles will be falsely low.

For children whose measurements fall outside the normal ranges, tables and charts that make adjustments for parental size should be used. The method of Weaver to adjust for parental head circumference is especially helpful in the evaluation of children with large heads. With both height and head circumference, the finding of an abnormal rate of growth, known as the growth velocity, is usually more clinically important than is an abnormal measurement on a single occasion. (See also the section on growth problems, Chapter 30.)

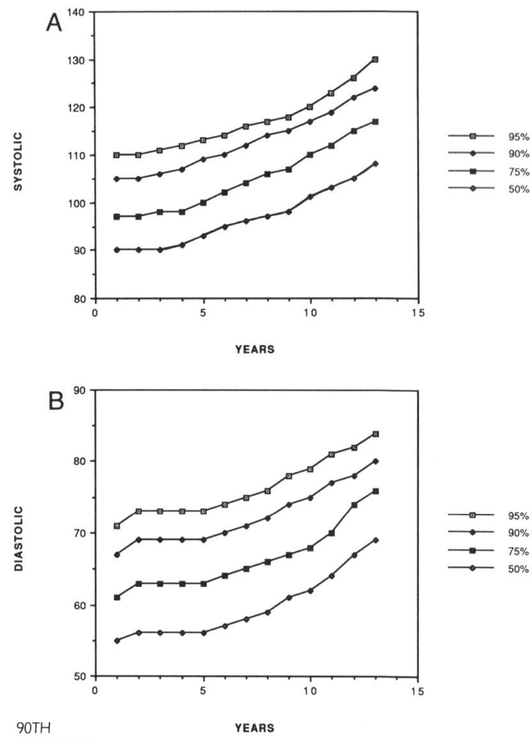

90TH PERCENTILE													
SYSTOLIC BP	105	106	107	108	109	111	112	114	115	117	119	121	124
DIASTOLIC BP	69	68	68	69	69	70	71	73	74	75	76	77	79
HEIGHT (CM)	80	91	100	108	115	122	129	135	141	147	153	159	165
WEIGHT (KG)	11	14	16	18	22	25	29	34	39	44	50	55	62

FIG 6–2

Age-specific percentiles for blood pressure measurements in girls aged 1 to 13 years; Korotkoff phase IV (K4) used for diastolic BP. (From Horan MJ, et al: Report of the Second Task Force on Blood Pressure Control in Children—1987. *Pediatrics* 1987; 79:1–25. Used by permission.)

SKIN

Bruises due to normal play activity are generally irregular in shape and are usually located on the distal extremities. In contrast, bruises from child abuse with an instrument are found on the trunk, buttocks, face, and proximal extremities and often reflect the shape of the instrument used to inflict the trauma. A bruise progresses through the following stages: 0 to 2 days, swollen, tender; 0 to 5 days, red, blue; 5 to 7 days; green; 7 to 10 days, yellow; 10 to 14 days, brown; and 2 to 4 weeks, clear.

Mongolian spots are gray or blue-black large macular lesions, usually located in the lumbosacral area and the buttocks. They are seen in 90% of black children, 80% of Oriental children, and 10% of white children. This discoloration usually fades spontaneously by adulthood and should not be confused with bruising from child abuse.

Café-au-lait spots are present in 10% to 20% of normal individuals but can also be seen in persons with neurocutaneous disorders. Six or more lesions that are 1.5 cm in diameter are presumptive evidence of neurofibromatosis in adults. In children under 6 years old, the criterion for this diagnosis is the presence of five lesions, each 0.5 cm or larger.

Acquired pigmented moles usually develop when a child is between 2 and 6 years old or during adolescence; consequently, by adulthood the average person has about 30 lesions. Fears about malignancy are unfounded unless the lesion shows rapid growth, irregular borders or nodularity, irregular darkening or bluish discoloration, an erythematous halo, spontaneous bleeding or scarring, or unless it is associated with pain or pruritus. A hypopigmented halo should not cause concern if the central nevus has benign characteristics.

The management of congenital melanocytic nevi remains controversial and depends on estimates of melanoma risks, timing of surgery, and cosmetic issues. Giant congenital melanocytic nevi have a definite premalignant potential of 1.8% to 13% before the age of 5 years. Therefore total excision of a giant congenital melanocytic nevus is recommended, as soon after birth as possible. Smaller lesions may be excised later in life (but before puberty) as long as they have a benign appearance and stable growth.

When a normally hydrated child's skin and subcutaneous tissue are pinched and then released, there is a brisk snapping back to the original position. A delay in return, called

TABLE 6–1
Chronology of Human Dentition*

	PRIMARY OR DECIDUOUS TEETH					
	CALCIFICATION		ERUPTION		SHEDDING	
TEETH	BEGINS	COMPLETE	MAXILLARY	MANDIBULAR	MAXILLARY	MANDIBULAR
Central incisors	5th fetal mo	18–24 mo	6–8 mo	5–7 mo	7–8 yr	6–7 yr
Lateral incisors	5th fetal mo	18–24 mo	8–11 mo	7–10 mo	8–9 yr	7–8 yr
Cuspids (canines)	6th fetal mo	30–36 mo	16–20 mo	16–20 mo	11–12 yr	9–11 yr
First molars	5th fetal mo	24–30 mo	10–16 mo	10–16 mo	10–11 yr	10–12 yr
Second molars	6th fetal mo	36 mo	20–30 mo	20–30 mo	10–12 yr	11–13 yr

		SECONDARY OR PERMANENT TEETH			
		CALCIFICATION		ERUPTION	
		BEGINS	COMPLETE	MAXILLARY	MANIBULAR
Central incisors		3–4 mo	9–10 yr	7–8 yr	6–7 yr
Lateral incisors	Maxillary	10–12 mo	10–11 yr	8–9 yr	7–8 yr
	Mandibular	3–4 mo			
Cuspids (canines)		4–5 mo	12–15 yr	11–12 yr	9–11 yr
First premolars (bicuspids)		18–21 mo	12–13 yr	10–11 yr	10–12 yr
Second premolars (bicuspids)		24–30 mo	12–14 yr	10–12 yr	11–13 yr
First molars		Birth	9–10 yr	6–7 yr	6–7 yr
Second molars		30–36 mo	14–16 yr	12–13 yr	12–13 yr
Third molars	Maxillary	7–9 yr	18–25 yr	17–22 yr	17–22 yr
	Mandibular	8–10 yr			

* Adapted from Losch PK: Harvard School of Dental Medicine.

"tenting," indicates poor turgor and dehydration. Hypernatremia may give the skin a "doughy" feel.

A common cause of hair loss is traction alopecia. Tight braiding can cause hair loss at the margins of the hairline or where the hair is parted.

LYMPH NODES

Lymphoid tissue grows steadily during childhood, then gets progressively smaller at puberty. Discrete, moveable, nontender nodes up to 3 mm in diameter are normally found, and can be as large as 1 cm in the cervical and inguinal regions without raising concern. Enlarged occipital and posterior scalp nodes are often seen in children with minor scalp problems such as seborrhea. Enlarged inguinal nodes are particularly common in the warm months when children run barefoot. Palpable supraclavicular nodes should never be considered normal; they are usually associated with systemic or intrathoracic disease.

TEETH

In addition to looking for obvious caries, the physician should determine the number, position, and color of the teeth. In early stages car-

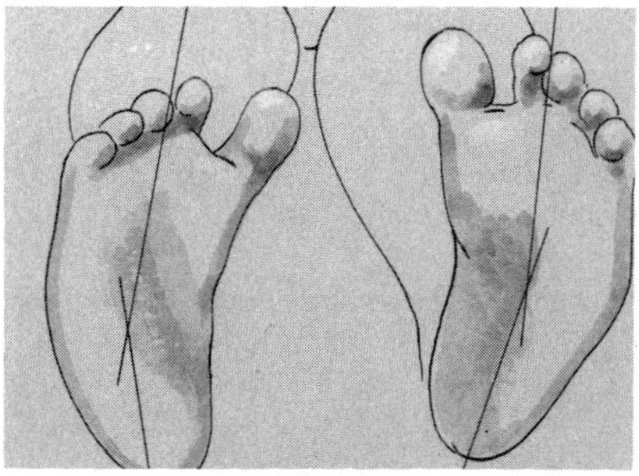

FIG 6–3
Metatarsus adductus examination demonstrates medial deviation of the forefoot.

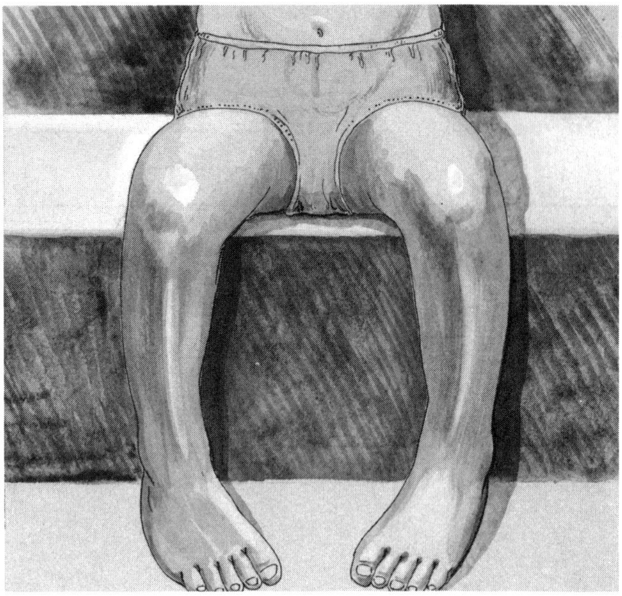

FIG 6–4
Tibial torsion with internal rotation of the foot.

ies appear as dull, opaque, whitish discolorations. The examiner should make a special effort to view the posterior aspect of the upper incisors, a common site for "baby-bottle" caries.

Table 6–1 shows the schedule for normal tooth eruption. Early or delayed tooth eruption can be seen in normal children; however, it is also associated with many specific syndromes and systemic disorders.

The deciduous (baby) teeth are normally separated by spaces. They may erupt in an irregular alignment but can realign spontaneously. The primary care physician should have the older child "open and bite" to observe for malocclusion.

Tooth discoloration that is extrinsic (superficially located on enamel surface) may be caused by poor oral hygiene, diet, or oral medications (such as iron). Unlike intrinsic discoloration, these stains can be removed with a wet gauze pad or scraped off by the dentist.

GAIT AND STANCE

Most neonates are bowlegged, but by the age of 3 to 4 years children display a knock-kneed stance (valgus angulation of about 10 degrees). By the time the child is 7 years old the knock-kneed appearance has usually spontaneously resolved.

A young child learns to walk with a wide-based gait. Foot contact with the floor is not with the heel but rather with the toe or the foot flat. Tip-toe gait should disappear by the time the child is 2 years old. The angle of toeing-out (that angle between the axis of the foot and the line of gait progression) is normally about 10 degrees; an angle of toeing-out greater than 30 degrees is considered abnormal.

In children, toeing-in is commonly due to metatarsus adductus, internal tibial torsion, or increased femoral anteversion. These conditions are evaluated by examining the sole of the foot, determining the thigh-foot angle, and measuring the limits of internal and external rotation of the hip (Fig 6–3). The normal range of thigh-foot angle is between 0 and 30 degrees of external rotation, but in children with tibial torsion some degree of internal rotation is seen (Fig 6–4). Hip rotation is best measured with the knee flexed and the child in the supine position. Internal rotation greater than 70 degrees is indicative of femoral anteversion.

BIBLIOGRAPHY

Barness LA: *Manual of Pediatric Physical Diagnosis.* Chicago, Year Book Medical Publishers, 1981.

Gundy JH: *Assessment of the Child in Primary*

Health Care. New York, McGraw-Hill Book Co, 1981.

Hoekelman R: Pediatric examination, in Bates BA (ed): *Guide to Physical Examination*. Philadelphia, JB Lippincott Co, 1979.

Horan MJ, et al: Report of the Second Task Force on Blood Pressure Control in Children—1987. *Pediatrics* 1987; 79:1–25.

Hurwitz S: *Clinical Pediatric Dermatology*. Philadelphia: WB Saunders Co, 1981.

Jacobs AH, Hurwitz S: The management of congenital nevocytic nevi. *Pediatr Dermatol* 1984; 2:143–156.

Lowrey GH: *Growth and Development of Children*. Chicago, Year Book Medical Publishers, 1973.

Staheli L: Torsional deformity. *Pediatr Clin North Am* 1977; 24:799–811.

Weaver DD, Christian JC: Familial variation of head size and adjustment for parental head circumference. *J Pediatr* 1980; 96:990–994.

PROBLEMS OF THE TODDLER AND OLDER CHILD

Rosemary Casey, M.D.

BEHAVIORAL PROBLEMS

Although the developmental tasks are the same for all children, each child approaches the challenge with his own temperament, genetic and environmental influences, and parental expectations; this results in a broad range of normal development. Thomas and Chess have demonstrated that the child's individual characteristics play an important role in the developmental process. They describe three configurations of temperament, although some children do not fit neatly into a single category. The "easy child" is characterized by regularity, positive-approach responses to stimuli, high adaptability to change, and mild or moderate intensity. The "difficult child" has irregularity, negative-withdrawal responses to new stimuli, nonadaptability to change, and intense mood expressions, which are frequently negative. The third group of children has a combination of negative responses of mild intensity to new stimuli, with slow adaptability after repeated contact; hence this group is called "slow to warm up." In discussing the clinical applications of temperament, Carey has pointed out that an awareness of a child's temperament is particularly helpful in diagnosing behavioral problems. For example, parents commonly ask for help because their child is "hyperactive." A physician who is aware of that child's behavioral style can direct the parent's attention toward the more relevant questions of attention or distractibility. Temperament alone does not predict a child's success or failure in achieving developmental goals. The same child who is considered withdrawn in one family may be praised as easygoing by another family. The physician, aware of the interaction between parental values and the child's behavioral style, can distinguish between behavioral problems that require treatment and normal behavioral differences.

There have been few studies on the incidence and prevalence of behavioral problems in preschool children. In an epidemiologic study of 3-year-old children in London, Richman and Graham found that 7% had moderate to severe problems and 15% had mild behavioral problems. The percentage of mothers worried about their child's behavior was highest when the child was 3 years old.

This section will focus on the more common behavioral problems of the toddler and older child, with particular emphasis on the normal limits and signs that intervention is necessary.

SEPARATION ANXIETY

Separation anxiety, a developmentally appropriate response for preschoolers, occurs after the child's removal from major attachment figures such as parents or from home. A child evolves from a toddler who is struggling with independence to a first-grader who is comfortable in the world of peers. Fraiberg and others have suggested that some anxiety may be crucial to the child's development of a mature ego structure. Parents who overprotect children or quickly prevent the child from feeling anxious about an unpleasant experience place these children at risk for separation anxiety disorder. This diagnosis should not be made during the preschool years or the first months of school attendance. If an older child describes persistent morbid fears or phobias of kidnapping, accidents, or dying, there is cause for concern. These children frequently have nightmares and difficulty falling asleep, particularly if they are away from home. Their anxiety can present as a physical complaint such as headache or stomachache or can manifest itself as school avoidance. In children with a separation anxiety disorder, further psychiatric evaluation and help is needed.

FEARS AND PHOBIAS

Young children have a variety of common fears, including fears of animals, darkness, and loud noises. Girls are more fearful, and the incidence peaks at 3 years of age. School-age children also fear ghosts, monsters, and certain animals, but they shift their fears to more abstract concepts such as dying. Fear can be a healthy emotion. It is often appropriate and helpful in preventing physical injury. Fear is unhealthy when it becomes excessive, spreads into other areas, and interferes with the child's normal activities. Young children who still think of their parents as endowed with special powers can usually overcome small anxieties with parental reassurance. Older children use many different approaches in overcoming their fears. Some children intellectualize their fears; others play through their terrors by acting macho or reading monster and horror stories. Most children succeed in handling their fears, and phobias are rare. Phobia is defined as persistent, excessive fear of a specific object that results in a desire to avoid that object or situation. The usual fear of insects or darkness would not be considered a phobia unless avoidance of the object was significantly stressful for the child and interfered with normal social functioning. Children with phobias know that they shouldn't be afraid, don't want to be afraid, and suffer the consequences of avoidance behaviors. The prognosis for these children is good, but treatment by experienced psychiatrists or psychologists is needed.

AGGRESSIVENESS, SHYNESS, PEER REJECTION

The 2-year-old child is still egocentric and engages mostly in parallel play with his peers. During the preschool years the child gradually learns to understand things from the perspective of others. By elementary-school age, he must be ready for rule-governed competitive and cooperative play. Each child negotiates this transition in his or her own way. Some use objects, such as teddy bears and special blankets. Others are fascinated with "superheroes" as they cope with their own vulnerability. Certain children are shy and cling more to their parents; others are more aggressive and even defy adult authority. Parental concerns about their child being "withdrawn" or "aggressive" should be dealt with in the context of a broad normal range.

It is critical that a toddler develop a healthy self-esteem and that this sense of self-worth be sustained through the school years. Chess and Thomas note that the development of self-esteem must be a social process since the child has no a priori way of assessing his achievements. The judgments of parents and others provide the initial standards. Parents need to strike a balance between being highly critical and approving to excess everything a child does.

Youngsters use aggression as a defense against imagined danger or as a way of coping with conflicting emotions (e.g., "hugging" the new baby strenuously enough to hurt). When kept in its place, aggression can be a healthy way of coping with fears. But the primary care physician must warn parents to set limits for their children. A child who loses control enough to strike a parent or be destructive is frightened and needs to have the parent step in and regain control. Extreme aggressiveness includes multiple episodes of disobedience, fighting, extreme competitiveness, and social egocentricity. This aggressiveness can lead to social isolation. Since this behavior usually will not be evident during the office visit, the physician should ask the parents or teachers to describe the duration of this behavior, the frequency of events, and specific consequences (such as injuries to other children). Unusual aggressiveness can begin during the preschool years and continue into early adulthood. The differential diagnosis of aggressive conduct disorder includes psychomotor seizures and brain damage secondary to severe trauma or infection. If these disorders are ruled out, the primary care physician can treat moderate forms of aggressiveness, but the more severe forms need to be referred for psychiatric intervention.

Children also experience shyness, daydreaming, peer rejection, and withdrawal in their socialization. The shy or isolated child tends to do well in the long run if his shyness is not accompanied by peer rejection. The daydreamer is defined by Gattman as one who is usually "off task" in the classroom, shy and anxious, neither accepted nor rejected but ignored by peers. Shyness and daydreaming must be distinguished from mental retardation, severe language delay, seizure disorders, hearing deficits, and childhood psychosis. The withdrawal seen in children with schizoid disorder is far more extreme than normal social reticence. These children are seclusive, generally unable to express strong feelings, and have few if any friends. When forced into social participation, they may become very irritable or even destructive. The primary care physician can thus distinguish these children from those with shy or sensitive temperaments.

TEMPER TANTRUMS

Temper tantrums occur commonly in children between the ages of 6 months and 6 years; they are most frequent between the ages of 1 and 3 years and should decrease over time. Tantrums reflect a child's struggle to become more autonomous. They can be caused by frustration at failing to master a developmental task, but frequently are manipulative. If a parent allows a child to get his or her way through tantrums, the child will continue to use temper tantrums as a predominant way of interacting with adults and peers. This will interfere with the child's learning appropriate social interactions such as sharing, taking turns, and making the correct verbal request. When parents ask about how to deal with temper tantrums, the physician should elicit an explicit history, looking for the frequency, specific circumstances of the tantrums, and the parents' feelings about or reactions to the child's behavior. It is normal for a parent to feel angry or frustrated, but parents who relate only negative comments (e.g., "She's always been evil") are telling you there is a significant parent-child interaction problem. In general, the parental response should help the child regain self-control (this can be done by holding the younger child or calling a "cooling-off period" in a safe place for the older child). It is important that the parent follow through to be sure that the temper tantrum has not allowed the child to get his or her own way. For example, if the child was trying to avoid something like picking up toys, the parent should physically guide him to tidying up after the child has regained control. Discipline should include praise for the desired behavior and disapproval of the undesired behavior. Temper tantrums that control the household or are constant indicate that parent and child have lost control. Barkley provides an excellent resource for pediatricians in his book, *Defiant Children: A Clinician's Manual For Parent Training*. His program is helpful in counseling parents of children between 2 and 11 years of age who display noncompliant behavior alone or in conjunction with other oppositional disorders. Children with more severe developmental psychopathologic disorders may need further help.

THUMB SUCKING

Sucking is a normal infant behavior, and nonnutritive sucking is a self-regulatory, pleasurable, consoling activity for infants. Approximately one third of infants will persist in sucking their thumbs as toddlers. If parents ignore this behavior, most children will relinquish the habit between the ages of 4 and 5 years. Parents should not intervene before the ages of 4 to 6 years. Punitive measures, bitter-tasting substances, or embarrassing comments rarely work and may have a deleterious effect by depriving the child of a positive coping mechanism. Parents raise reasonable concerns about the dental implications of thumb sucking. The primary care physician should recommend a dental evaluation for children who persist in sucking their thumbs after 4 years of age.

SEXUALITY

The healthy development of sexuality occurs well before adolescence. In her book *The Magic Years*, Fraiberg stresses that giving a child facts about sex education is not sufficient. Parents, through their example and attitudes, teach children about identification with members of their own sex. This is a very important developmental task for the preschool period. It is inevitable that infants and toddlers discover the relationship between exploring their genitals and arousal and pleasure. Masturbation probably occurs in all children of both sexes. It is a normal part of development that only becomes a problem if the child persists in masturbating in public places where it is socially unacceptable. Parents must be taught not to overreact and to help the child learn that masturbation is not an evil act but something that should be done in privacy. The older child who persists in masturbating openly or in clinging to the genitals without apparent pleasure is manifesting anxiety that requires further attention.

TOILET TRAINING

A prerequisite for successful toilet training is bowel and bladder control; that control is determined mainly by maturation and generally occurs between 1 and 3 years of age. However, toilet training is also a classic example of the toddler's struggle for autonomy. The outcome of this struggle is largely determined by the child's temperament, the parents' attitudes, and the parent-child interaction. It is usually successful when parents adopt a relaxed, nonthreatening approach once the child is ready. Brazelton refers to this as a "child-oriented approach to toilet training." In this method parents are taught to wait until the child is physically and psychologically ready (approximately at the age of 2 years). The "potty chair" is casually introduced, and gradually the child moves from sitting down on it with his clothes on to changing his soiled diapers on it, and eventually to using the potty chair correctly by himself. Whenever the child fails or resists going to the next step, parents are urged to wait and reassure the child. Some of the pressure is taken off the parents since the focus is on the child's achievement. Most children should have bowel and daytime urine control by 3 to 3½ years of age. Nocturnal bladder control should be achieved by the age of 5 to 6 years.

In general, any child older than 2½ years of age who is not toilet trained after several months of trying can be assumed to be resistant. An organic cause for toilet training resistance is rare. Urinary tract infection is probably the most common cause of daytime wetting; other causes include bubble bath urethritis, urgency incontinence, ectopic ureter, and neurogenic bladder. Children with dysuria, weak urine stream, constantly damp underwear, or wetting while running to the toilet require medical evaluation. However, most children who resist toilet training are involved in a power struggle. Schmitt has outlined a plan for treating toilet training refusal. He suggests that parents transfer all responsibility for using the toilet to the child, that major incentives be used, and that the child's progress be charted. Children should not be punished for accidents, and the babysitter or daycare center should use the same approach. Brazelton's no pressure approach to toilet training was successful in 98% of children by the age of 36 months.

BREATH HOLDING

Breath-holding spells are frightening sudden episodes in which a child cries, appears to hold his or her breath, then becomes limp and occasionally develops tonic-clonic movements. These spells occur in 5% of children between age 6 months to 6 years and are commonly categorized as either cyanotic or pallid. The cyanotic type is usually precipitated by frustration or anger; the pallid type is triggered more by painful stimuli. The cry is more obvious in the cyanotic episodes in which the child proceeds to hold his breath in expiration, becomes cyanotic, unconscious, and then sometimes twitches or develops opisthotonos. In the pallid type the breath holding or apnea is very brief before the child progresses to the same sequence of events.

The differential diagnosis must distinguish between a seizure disorder and breath holding, although cardiac disease and causes of tetany should be considered. Results of physical examination of the breath holder are normal and a careful history should rule out seizures. A precipitating factor is always present in breath holding and rarely noticed before a seizure. Cyanosis or pallor usually occurs during or after a seizure but it directly precedes the jerking movements in a breath-holding spell. The electroencephalogram (EEG), not necessary in most cases, is usually normal.

The physician should first reassure the family that the child does not have a seizure disorder and that there are no serious sequelae from breath-holding spells. All children outgrow these episodes by grade school age. Parents should be advised to treat these children normally and not spoil them in order to avoid temper tantrums. Anticonvulsants are not efficacious and should not be used for breath-holding spells.

SHOES FOR TODDLERS

Jeffrey Weiss, M.D.

Concerns about foot abnormalities are expressed and questions about shoes and corrections are asked during most well-child visits. Most of the problems can be handled without referral if a few principles and concepts are appreciated.

SHOE CONSTRUCTION

Shoe construction is divided into two major parts, the sole and the upper. The upper should be pliable and porous enough to allow for moisture evaporation. Since the ankle requires no additional support from shoes, either high-top or low-cut shoes are acceptable. A young child is less likely to step out of a high shoe; however, the leather must be flexible enough so as not to restrict ankle movement. The counter is that part of the upper that surrounds the heel and helps to maintain the shape of the rear portion of the shoe.

The sole of a shoe may have several components: the insole, outsole, filler, and welt (Fig 6–5). The upper can be stitched directly to an outsole or connected to the sole using an extra piece of leather called a welt. Welt construction is considered sturdiest and is used when wedges are applied to the shoes. In general, the sole should be flexible, bending easily at the ball of the foot.

The area of the shoe under the midportion of the arch of the foot is called the shank. Some specialists feel that a firm (steel) shank helps reinforce the arch and prevents the muscle strain that is caused by an elevated heel. Since heel elevation is really not a desirable feature for a young child's shoe, the shank is not necessary.

Shoes may have an inflare, outflare, or straight shape, depending on the angles formed by the axes of the front and rear portions of the last. The normal childhood foot is not straight but rather shows a mild forefoot inflare.

Little agreement exists among professionals concerning which shoe features are necessary for children with normal feet or helpful for children with foot deformities. Studies that compare the beliefs of pediatricians, podiatrists, orthopedic surgeons, and shoe fitters demonstrate wide differences in opinions about "proper" sole material and flexibility, shoe height, last shape, and shank stiffness. These disagreements among professionals, which confuse parents, result from a lack of objective data about the efficacy of various shoe features. Nowhere is this problem clearer than in the "great sneaker vs. shoe debate."

Questionnaire studies show that about 77% of pediatricians and 65% of podiatrists believe that sneakers are adequate as regular footwear for children, yet only 37% of parents and 28% of shoe salespeople agree that sneakers are good for the feet. There is really no evidence that wearing sneakers results in flatfoot or any foot deformity, but other questions about shoes with rubber or crepe soles have been raised. Some authors believe that rubber is actually less flexible than leather and that rubber's high coefficient of friction results in heat and moisture buildup and an increased frequency of tripping on certain types of floor surfaces. Other experts claim that the nonskid rubber sole will prevent slipping. Some argue that since sneakers come in a limited number of widths, proper fit can be a problem that may re-

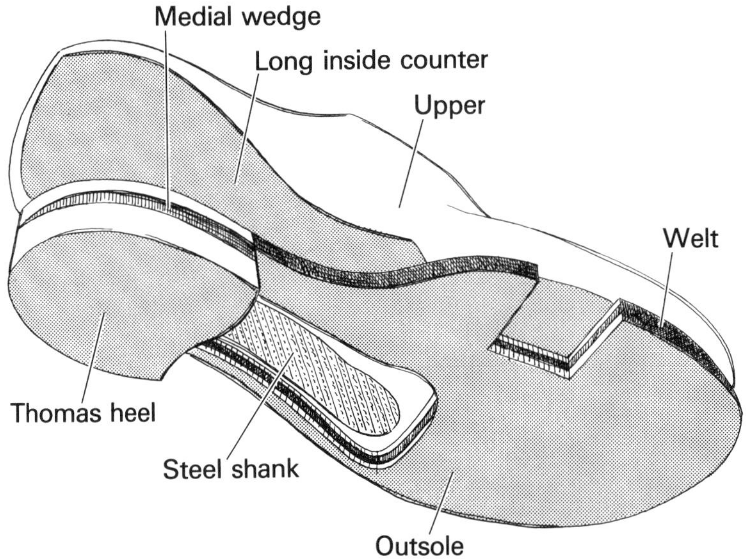

FIG 6–5
Diagrammatic representation of the components of a shoe.

sult in blisters and foot irritation. These opinions are neither supported nor refuted by any data from well-designed clinical studies.

PROBLEMS CAUSED BY SHOES

Wearing shoes can cause various irritations and inflammations of the skin of the foot. Pressures and friction due to poorly fitting shoes commonly affect the medial part of the large toe, the tips of the toes, the Achilles tendon area, the skin under the external malleolus, and the lateral aspect of the base of the fifth metatarsal. Irritation over the first metatarsophalangeal joint, known as "shoe bite," is due to leather rubbing the foot under the break (crease) of the shoe. Various substances used in the manufacture of shoes can cause shoe dermatitis, especially if excessive perspiration and moisture buildup are also present. Offending agents include rubber cements, chromates in chrome-tanned leather, nickel in lace eyelets, dyes, and antimildew preparations in shoe linings. Vesicles on the dorsum of the foot are most likely a contact dermatitis from one of these chemical agents. Patch-testing kits are available to determine the responsible agent.

Children do not develop athlete's foot, but another more serious shoe-related infection is *Pseudomonas* osteomyelitis, which can follow a puncture wound. A recent study has demonstrated that *Pseudomonas* can be cultured from the interior rubber layers of the sole in about 10% of those sneakers that have been worn.

SUMMARY

Certain points should be kept in mind by the primary care physician who counsels parents about children's shoes:

1. Shoes are worn for protection. There is no evidence to suggest that shoes are needed for support of any part of the normal foot.
2. Until a child is walking, a sock or other cloth covering is appropriate foot protection. Shoes do not help a child learn to walk better or sooner.
3. A child should be able to walk freely and naturally while in footgear. The sole must flex easily when the child walks and ankle movement should be unrestricted.
4. The bottom of the shoe should be flat. A convex surface will cause side-to-side instability and an elevated heel may stress the arch.
5. Skin irritations commonly result from new or poorly fitting shoes. In general, shoes that are a little large are better for a child than

those that are too small. Parents can be advised that shoes should be replaced before their child's toes press against the front end of the upper.

6. The upper should be made of a porous material to allow for evaporation of moisture and perspiration.

7. Shoes will not correct structural foot deformities. Flexible flatfoot, bowleg, knock-knee, and toeing-out are all seen as part of normal development. These deformities (unless severe, asymmetric, or painful) generally require no special shoes. An orthopedist may be consulted for severe foot problems.

BIBLIOGRAPHY

Barkley RA: *Defiant Children: A Clinician's Manual for Parent Training*. New York, Guilford Press, 1987.

Bleck EE: The shoeing of children: Sham or science? *Dev Med Child Neurol* 1971; 13:188–195.

Brazelton TB: A child-oriented approach to toilet training. *Pediatrics* 1962; 29:121–128.

Cowell HR: Shoes and shoe constructions. *Pediatr Clin North Am* 1977; 24:791–797.

Dyment PG, Bogan PM: Pediatrician's attitudes concerning infant's shoes. *Pediatrics* 1972; 50:655–657.

Fisher MC, Goldsmith JF, Gilligan PH, et al: Sneakers as a source of *Pseudomonas aeruginosa* in children with osteomyelitis complicating puncture wounds of the foot. Presented at Interscience Conference on Antimicrobial Agents and Chemotherapy (abstract 729), Las Vegas, Oct 1983.

Fraiberg S: *The Magic Years*. New York, Charles Scribner's Sons, 1959.

Gabel S: *Behavioral Problems in Childhood*. New York, Grune & Stratton, 1981.

Levine M, Carey W, Crocker A, et al: *Developmental Behavioral Pediatrics*. Philadelphia, WB Saunders Co, 1983.

Lombroso CT, Lerman P: Breathholding spells (cyanotic and pallid infantile syncope). *Pediatrics* 1967; 39:563–581.

Richman N, Stevenson I, Graham P: Prevalence of behavior problems in 3-year-old children: An epidemiological study in a London borough. *J Child Psychol Psychiatry* 1975; 16:277–287.

Rincover A: The parent-child connection. New York, Random House, 1988.

Schmitt BD: Toilet training refusal: Avoid the battle and win the war. *Contemp Pediatr* 1987; 32–50.

Seder JI, Dyment PG: Infant's shoes: Attitudes of podiatrists and pediatricians. *J Pod Assoc* 1980; 70:244–246.

Staheili LT, Giffin L: Corrective shoes for children: A survey of current practice. *Pediatrics* 1980; 65:7–13.

Tax HR: *Podopediatrics*. Baltimore, Williams & Wilkins Co, 1980.

Thomas A, Chess S: *Temperament and Development*. New York, Brunner Maizel, 1977.

Weiss JC, DeJong A, Packer E, et al: Purchasing infant shoes: Attitudes of parents, pediatricians and store managers. *Pediatrics* 1981; 67:718–720.

SLEEP DISORDERS

Anthony Rostain, M.D.

Sleep disorders are common during childhood and vary according to the age of the child. In infancy, most problems are related to falling asleep and nightwaking. Toddlers and preschoolers have difficulties with falling and staying asleep, night terrors, nightmares, and enuresis. For older children, nightmares, insomnia, and sleepwalking are the most common complaints related to sleep. Although estimates vary widely, a majority of children will have some type of sleep disorder during childhood.

While most sleep problems improve with minimal or no intervention, sleep disorders that are associated with organic or psychiatric illness are important to recognize and treat appropriately.

The duration of sleep changes with maturation (Table 6–2). The newborn sleeps for periods of 3 to 4 hours, with waking periods lasting 1 to 2 hours. At 1 month of age most infants sleep slightly longer at night, and by 5 months of age most sleep more than 7 hours at a time. There is a gradual decline in the length of time

TABLE 6–2
Typical Daily Sleep Time*

AGE	AVERAGE HOURS OF SLEEP (±1 HR)
Premature (29 wk gestation)	20
Newborn (full term)	18
Infant (3–9 mo)	14
1–2 yr	13
2–3 yr	12
3–4 yr	11
4–5 yr	10
6–12 yr	9.5
13–15 yr	8
16–19 yr	7.5

* From Ferber R, Rivinus M: *Med Times* 1979; 107:71. Used by permission.

spent sleeping: during the second year it averages 12 to 13 hours, with one nap during the day; from the ages of 2 to 5 years, it decreases to about 11 hours without a nap; and by adolescence it reaches the adult average of 7 to 8 hours. It is important to keep in mind that sleep patterns vary among individuals and that they are related to temperament, maturation, activity level, habits, parent-child interactions, and family characteristics. All of these factors must be assessed when evaluating a sleep disorder.

GENERAL APPROACH TO PROBLEMS OF SLEEP

Problems with sleep will be noted either as a primary complaint by the parents or as an item in the review of the child's overall behavior and development. Parents may not be aware of a problem if there are separation issues between parent and child or if there are general parenting difficulties. Management will depend on the physician's relationship with the family, the parents' ability and willingness to change, and the duration and severity of the problem.

The strategy for evaluating sleep disorders centers on differentiating three general types of problems: mild behavioral problems stemming from either parenting difficulties or "lack of fit" between the child's temperament and the family environment; stress-related sleep disturbances that are part of a significant pattern of family dysfunction or psychiatric illness; and organically based sleep disorders, which may be primary or secondary to other physical illnesses.

CHIEF COMPLAINT

The chief complaint is likely to vary according to the age of the child. Infants will have difficulty falling asleep, with waking in the middle of the night, with poorly established sleeping-waking cycles, and with fears associated with separation from parents. Toddlers tend to have problems described by parents as "can't sleep," "won't sleep," or "gets out of bed." Older children may complain of insomnia, nightmares, night terrors, sleepwalking, sleeptalking, or nocturnal enuresis. Adolescents tend to have difficulties with insomnia or hypersomnia.

DIFFERENTIAL DIAGNOSIS

Evaluation of a sleep disorder will depend on the age of the child and the nature of the complaint (Table 6–3).

HISTORY

The child's sleep milestones should be reviewed to find out at what time the child first slept through the night, stopped taking naps, and started having sleep disturbances. Current day-night sleep habits should be discussed, including naps, duration of night sleep, schedule and regularity of sleep, whether the child is a "light" or "heavy" sleeper, where the child sleeps (in relation to parents and siblings), and whether there are other people in the child's room. Prebedtime activities and bedtime rituals (e.g., story time, snacks, goodnight kisses) should also be reviewed. Special consideration should be given to details in the bedtime routine that may aid in diagnosis (e.g., scary bedtime stories or television programs, too much physical activity before bedtime, irregular habits, no fixed schedule). Some children have trouble sleeping because they are overtired.

It is important to inquire about parental responses to the sleep problem: Who is most worried? Why? How have they expressed this con-

TABLE 6–3
Common Sleep Problems by Age

AGE	PROBLEM	DIFFERENTIAL DIAGNOSIS
Infant	Nighttime waking	Normal variation
	Irregular sleep cycle	Immaturity
Toddler	Nighttime waking	Separation anxiety
	"Can't sleep"	Illness; parental disagreement (marital problems)
Preschool-aged	"Can't sleep"	Separation anxiety
	"Won't go to bed"	Fears of aggression
	"Gets out of bed"	Ineffective disciplining
	Nighttime waking	Parental anxiety; parental disagreement
School-aged	Nighttime waking	Nightmares; night terrors; sleepwalking/sleeptalking; enuresis; family stress; primary sleep disorder
School-aged and adolescent	Insomnia	Depression; anxiety; stress-related syndrome; attention deficit; delayed sleep phase syndrome
	Hypersomnia	Narcolepsy, idiopathic CNS hypersomnia, sleep-associated airway obstruction, chronic viral illness, Kleine-Levin syndrome

cern? If both parents seem to agree, what do they think is going on? If they disagree, are they communicating with each other? In this latter instance, it is very important to hear from *both* parents and to solicit their ideas in a nonjudgmental fashion. It is also helpful to inquire about the impact that the problem is having on the family. Are the parents losing sleep because of the child's problems? How are other siblings affected? What changes in family routines has the problem produced? Has it affected their parenting? Is it creating problems in the marriage? The answers to these questions will help determine the severity and complications of the problem and will aid in assessing the family's level of concern.

The presence of family stresses should be explored because sleep problems often begin in response to other family problems. Often it helps to preface such questions with a statement such as, "Kids can be sensitive to problems going on in the family, and these can cause the child to have problems sleeping. Is there anything that might be upsetting your child at home?" or "How are things at home?"

Finally, a family history of sleep disorders, neurologic diseases, or psychiatric illness must be ruled out. These must be explored carefully to ascertain any hereditary conditions or predispositions to sleep disturbances.

EVALUATION

The most important aspects of the physical examination include a careful neurologic examination, a close inspection for evidence of CNS anomalies or brain damage, and a comprehensive developmental assessment. Most organic causes for sleep disorders can be ruled out after a thorough evaluation of this type.

The child's temperament should be assessed. Is he somewhat overactive and demanding? Is he quiet and withdrawn? What kind of emotional issues is the child facing? The interaction between parents and child should be evaluated. Is there evidence of excessive manipulation? Does the child seem to obey his parents or is he generally disrespectful? Do the parents seem to have difficulty disciplining the child? Is the child perhaps being treated as older or younger than his age? Are the parents in agreement over issues of discipline? These questions are best answered by carefully observing the family in the office and by providing feedback to parents if other behavior problems are noted by the physician. Quite often sleep problems are a manifestation of behavioral rather than primary sleep disturbances.

On occasion the clinician may encounter a child with a sleep problem that is organic. If sleep apnea, narcolepsy, or seizures are strongly suspected, workup may necessitate an EEG, a tape cassette recording, or a videotape or time-lapse recording of the child's sleep. At this point most physicians would refer the patient to a sleep clinic or a psychiatrist.

TREATMENT

The treatment of sleep problems should be approached with several goals: to help the family break a repetitive cycle of interrupted sleep, reassure parents of the absence of organic disease, ameliorate symptoms, and help parents adopt an approach that they are likely to execute successfully. Although medications such as sedatives (antihistamines) or hypnotics (chloral hydrate) are not advocated for long-term use, they are helpful if given for a few nights to disrupt an acute pattern. The following is a brief outline of the most common sleep problems encountered in office practice, listed by chief complaint.

MOST COMMON SLEEP PROBLEMS

"Wakes Up"

Night waking may be due to immature diurnal rhythms or to delay in the development of "settling" in infants and to fear of separation in toddlers. In such cases parents need to be reassured that this is normal. Parents should be counseled to let the child cry for as long as necessary, to initiate bedtime rituals and positive rewards, and to avoid using hypnotics or other medications.

"Can't Sleep"

Often a child tries to go to sleep but has trouble falling asleep. This usually becomes a problem for children who are 2 years old, who grow frightened of the dark, start to hear voices, or are too excited to sleep. Treatment involves instructing parents to *reassure* the child, with a bedtime story (or similar ritual), a night-light, or letting the child take a favorite object to bed. Parents should be cautioned against getting into bed with the child, because this is a difficult habit to break. The physician should verify that parents agree with him and that they have developed a plan that suits them.

"Won't Go to Bed"

Some children resist going to sleep, either by refusing to get ready for bed or by fussing or crying excessively once in bed. This can be due to separation anxiety, to concurrent stress, or to manipulative behavior. Treatment involves teaching parents to be patient with the child. There should be adequate preparation for bedtime, including frequent reminders at 1 hour, at 30 minutes, and at 15 minutes prior to beginning the bedtime routine. The routine should be consistent and predictable, with little variation. After the parents say goodnight to the child, they must leave the room and *not* return no matter how long the child cries. Although this is initially quite anxiety provoking for parents, such patience is quickly rewarded. The child soon understands that the parents are serious and eventually goes to sleep without protesting.

"Gets Out of Bed"

This problem usually follows one of two patterns. Either the child gets out of bed shortly after bedtime and disrupts parents' evening activities or the child awakens late at night and climbs into the parents' bed. The causes of this problem are similar to those mentioned above. The difference is that parents tacitly consent to this behavior if they do not return the child directly to bed. Parents usually report ineffective attempts to reason with the child or to gently coax him back to bed.

Treatment consists of helping parents maintain *discipline*. Both parents need to agree on a consistent plan of action that they will carry out regardless of the child's protests. The specifics of such a plan will vary from family to family. Careful preparation for bedtime and predictable routines are recommended. Once the parents say goodnight, they should leave the room. The child must be monitored closely. If he is caught getting out of bed, parents must convey the seriousness of their intentions by using whatever safe and controlled measure they prefer. This must be repeated each time the child gets up. The child who climbs into the parents' bed must be taken back to his own bed immediately. Parents must be firm and unemotional in carrying out discipline of this sort, otherwise the child will find a way to persist in this behavior. It is also recommended that the parents praise the child the following morning for being so good and listening to them. "Big boys and girls sleep in their own bed," is a helpful comment that can be used to appeal to the child's wish to be more grown up.

Nightmares

Nightmares are frightening dreams that can awaken a sleeping child and cause him to cry. These dreams can be remembered and recounted by the child; when comforted by parents, the child usually returns to sleep without difficulty. Nightmares are normal occurrences. As the child gets older, he can learn to orient himself in his room and return to sleep without involving his parents.

Night Terrors

Night terrors are distinctive episodes of night waking seen primarily in preschool-aged children. The child suddenly sits up in bed and begins screaming. Parents find the child quite aroused and agitated, with sweating, rapid breathing, and "glassy-eyed" staring. In contrast to nightmares, the child is not consolable. After a few minutes he returns to sleep, with no later recall of the event. Night terrors are most frightening for parents and other family members; they need to be reassured that these are not serious or pathologic episodes. The episodes resolve spontaneously as the child grows older and do not require treatment. Use of diazepam or imipramine hydrochloride should be reserved for those children whose episodes are causing excessive family disruption or alteration of the child's behavior during the day.

Sleepwalking and Sleeptalking

Approximately 15% to 30% of all school-aged children experience one episode of sleepwalking, and 2% to 3% experience repeated episodes.

The child suddenly sits up in bed and clumsily begins to move about, occasionally arising and walking with no purpose. It is common for the child to speak in a slurred, monosyllabic, often incomprehensible manner. Repetitive finger and hand movements can also be observed. The child walks with a blank stare and seems more asleep than awake. Although capable of stumbling or bumping into furniture, the child usually avoids walking into objects. To prevent injuries, parents must use precautions such as stair guards and window bars. The episodes are otherwise harmless and usually resolve by adolescence.

The major differential diagnosis is psychomotor epilepsy, which usually produces more fatigue and confusion on awakening and is not associated with a return to bed, as with sleepwalking. If the sleepwalking or sleeptalking is thought by parents to be purposeful, a psychologic disorder should be suspected.

Insomnia in Older Children and Adolescents

Sleep problems in older children and adolescents are usually stress related. Problems include trouble falling asleep, frequent awakening, during the night, early morning awakening, daytime napping, or a chronic feeling of being tired. The physician must carefully review daily sleeping and waking habits, and must sensitively inquire into issues that may be upsetting the individual. Emotional problems in children and teenagers often present with complaints of insomnia. Depression, suicidal impulses, anxiety, drug usage, and other psychiatric disturbances must be investigated before making the diagnosis of a chronic sleep disorder. Treatment depends on the diagnosis and may necessitate referral for psychiatric care or counseling. In any case, these complaints must be taken seriously by the physician and should be handled expeditiously.

Many adolescents enjoy staying up late at night, a habit that can easily result in delayed sleep phase syndrome (DSPS). The circadian rhythm becomes readjusted, so that the adolescent has trouble falling asleep before 2:00 or 3:00 AM and cannot wake up before 10:00 or 11:00 AM the next day. School problems resulting from tardiness and absenteeism are a typical complaint. Parents report that the teenager cannot be awakened in the morning, and the adolescent complains that he or she cannot fall asleep until late at night. The primary treatment for DSPS is chronotherapy, which involves systematic advancing of the sleep-wake cycle until it is normalized. The adolescent's bedtime should be advanced by 3 hours (e.g., from 2:00 AM to 5:00 AM to 8:00 AM to 11:00 AM) over 6 days until it is normalized. Resistance to this simple technique should raise a suspicion of psychologic difficulties in the patient or family.

Hypersomnia in Older Children and Adolescents

Too much sleep or excessive daytime sleepiness is termed hypersomnia, and may be due to various disorders. Narcolepsy consists of excessive daytime sleepiness, cataplexy ("drop attacks"), hypnogogic hallucinations and sleep paralysis. It is characterized by sleep-onset REM (rapid eye movement) episodes and dissociation of the components of REM sleep. Treatment involves increasing the nocturnal sleep period and scheduling daytime naps. Occasionally low-dose pemoline or methylphenidate hydrochloride is used to control sleepiness. In idiopathic central nervous system hypersomnia, there is constant daytime sleepiness that is not associated with other symptoms or with disturbed sleep patterns. Although hypersomnia is poorly understood, there is speculation that it is associated with chronic viral illnesses such as infectious mononucleosis. Treatment with stimulants appears to be of little long-term benefit. Sleep-associated airway obstruction may result from a variety of structural abnormalities, including enlarged tonsils and adenoids, choanal atresia or stenosis, nasal septal deviation, enlarged tongue, cleft palate, and temporomandibular joint dysfunction. Associated signs include loud snoring, mouth breathing, frequent arousal during sleep, nocturnal enuresis, and a host of behavior problems such as hyperactivity and poor school performance. An evaluation of the ears, nose, and throat and treatment are necessary for these conditions. Finally, Kleine-Levin syndrome is a rare, poorly understood pattern of excessive sleep, hyperphagia, and abnormal behavior (e.g., irritability, motor unrest, excitement), which lasts for days or weeks and recurs on a regular basis from once to 12 times a year. These symptoms should result in prompt referral for psychiatric care.

BIBLIOGRAPHY

Anders T, Keener MA: Sleep-wake state development and disorders of sleep in infants, children and adolescents, in Levine MD, Carey WB, Crocker AC, et al (eds): *Developmental-Behavioral Pediatrics.* Philadelphia, WB Saunders Co, 1983.

Beltramini AU, Hertzig ME: Sleep and bedtime behavior in preschool-aged children. *Pediatrics* 1983; 71:153.

Carey WB: Night waking and temperament in infancy. *J Pediatr* 1974; 84:756.

Carskadon MA, Anders TF, Hole W: Sleep disorders in childhood and adolescence, in Fitzgerald HE, Lester BM, Yogman MW (eds): *Theory and Research in Behavioral Pediatrics,* vol 4. New York, Plenum Press, 1988.

Christopherson ER: Incorporating behavioral pediatrics in primary care. *Pediatr Clin North Am* 1982; 29:281.

DiMario FJ, Emery ES: The natural history of night terrors. *Clin Ped* 1987; 26:505.

Ferber R, Rivinus M: Practical approaches to sleep disorders of childhood. *Med Times* 1979; 107:71.

Ferber R: Behavioral "insomnia" in the child. *Psychiatr Clin North Am* 1987; 10:641.

Guilleminault C: Mononucleosis and chronic daytime sleepiness: A long-term follow-up study. *Arch Intern Med* 1986; 146:1333.

Guilleminault C: *Sleep and its Disorders in Children.* New York, Raven Press, 1987.

Hawkins DR, Taub JM, Van de Castle RL: Extended sleep (hypersomnia) in young depressed patients. *Am J Psychiatry* 1985; 142:905.

Kataria S, Swanson MS, Trevathan GE: Persistence of sleep disturbances in preschool children. *J Pediatr* 1987; 110:642.

Mark JD, Brooks JG: Sleep-associated airway problems in children. *Pediatr Clin North Am* 1984; 31:907.

Parkes JD: The parasomnias. *Lancet* 1986; 2:1021.

Richman N: Sleep problems in young children. *Arch Dis Child* 1981; 56:491.

Thorpy MJ, Glovinsky PB: Parasomnias. *Psychiatr Clin North Am* 1987; 10:623.

Zuckerman B, Stevenson J, Bailey V: Sleep problems in early childhood: Continuities, predictive factors, and behavioral correlates. *Pediatrics* 1987; 80:664.

7 THE ADOLESCENT

Primary care physicians who deal with adolescent patients must adapt their interviewing skills to address patient concerns about body image, sexuality, independence, and life roles. They must be comfortable with the developmental tasks of adolescence, family interaction, gynecology, and psychiatry. This chapter reviews the routine examination of the adolescent patient and includes topics in the areas of development, gynecology, and contraceptive counseling. Other chapters relevant to adolescent care are found in section 5 (delinquency, eating disorders, suicide, drug abuse, and family dynamics), Chapter 10 (Obesity), and Chapter 60 (section on Sexually Transmitted Diseases).

EXAMINATION

Gail B. Slap, M.D., M.S.
Clyde E. Rapp, Jr., M.D.

Examination of the adolescent patient requires an understanding of the physical, cognitive, and social changes that occur with puberty. The interview and physical examination provide a natural opportunity to discuss developmental changes with the adolescent as well as to monitor growth and screen for disease. The successful interview requires balancing the adolescent's concern about confidentiality with the parents' request for information.

HISTORY

LEGAL ISSUES

All states permit physicians to treat emancipated minors and patients older than 18 years without parental consent. The definition of emancipated minor, however, differs among the states. It usually implies (1) abdication of parental responsibilities, (2) adolescent financial independence, and (3) residence outside the parental home. In many states the age for provision of general medical care without parental consent is higher than for contraceptive care or treatment of substance abuse, pregnancy, and sexually transmitted disease. Important legal considerations in the treatment of nonemergent medical problems include maturity of the minor and assessment of the adolescent's best interests. Statutes and court precedents related to abortion change frequently and should be reviewed before proceeding in an individual case.[1, 2]

Health care providers should attempt to notify parents of an adolescent's medical care whenever possible. An adolescent who initially is reluctant to inform the parent frequently agrees to do so when the reasons for parental involvement are explained. Management usually is facilitated when the adolescent is supported by his or her parents.

APPROACH TO THE ADOLESCENT PATIENT

The interaction with the adolescent is most effective when the visit is well-structured and conducted in a relaxed, sensitive manner.

Many adolescents talk more openly when interviewed without their parents. The health provider should meet the patient and parent together, then suggest that the interview begin with the adolescent alone. If the adolescent agrees to this, a preliminary history and the physical examination should be completed while the parent remains in the waiting room. The parent then should be invited to join the adolescent in the office. This gives the provider an opportunity to review the history and physical examination with both the patient and parent, to obtain additional information from the parent, and to discuss the management plan.

Questions addressed to the adolescent should be open-ended. This encourages discus-

ADOLESCENT HEALTH QUESTIONNAIRE

This list of questions will help us to know about you and any problems you might have. It is strictly confidential. Please answer all you can *without help* from anyone else. Leave blank any you do not understand and ask your doctor or nurse clinician about them later. Circle YES or NO for each question and fill in all the blanks.

Your full name ______________________ Nickname ______________________

Birth date ____________ Age ____________ Grade in school ____________

Name of your school ______________________ How do you do in school ____________

Home phone number ______________________ Other number ______________________

1.	Do you think something is wrong with your health?	YES	NO
2.	Have you ever been in the hospital overnight?	YES	NO
3.	Are you easily upset?	YES	NO
4.	Does anything bother you about school?	YES	NO
5.	Are you having problems with your parents?	YES	NO
6.	Are you having problems with other family members?	YES	NO
7.	Do you have problems in making friends?	YES	NO
8.	Are you concerned about your sexual development?	YES	NO
9.	Do you have frequent headaches?	YES	NO
10.	Do you seem to tire easily? Are you tired a lot?	YES	NO
11.	Do you think something is wrong with your heart?	YES	NO
12.	Do you think something is wrong with your skin?	YES	NO
13.	Are you allergic to anything? What? ______________	YES	NO
14.	Do you have a cough or trouble breathing?	YES	NO
15.	Do you think you have cancer? Where? ______________	YES	NO
16.	Does it burn when you urinate (pass your water)?	YES	NO
17.	Do you have any questions about		
	Alcohol	YES	NO
	Smoking	YES	NO
	Drugs	YES	NO
	VD (venereal disease)	YES	NO
	Birth control or pregnancy	YES	NO
	Menstruation (periods)	YES	NO
18.	Do you have someone you can trust to talk to about your problems? Who? ______________	YES	NO
19.	Are there any questions or problems you would like to discuss with the doctor or nurse?	YES	NO

FIG 7–1
Adolescent Health Questionnaire.

sion rather than simple yes or no answers. A questionnaire (Fig 7–1) completed by the adolescent prior to the interview helps to identify areas of concern and may guide the interviewer's questions. Poor communication, downcast eyes, and withdrawal usually are not attributable to adolescent shyness alone. Depression is a common and often unrecognized problem in teenagers. A history of behavioral problems, poor school performance, psychosomatic complaints, or frequent medical visits points to the need for a thorough psychosocial history. This history always should include direct questioning about suicidal ideation or gestures.

Psychosomatic symptoms such as abdominal pain, headache, and chest pain are common during adolescence. If a psychosomatic disorder is suspected, several meetings with the pa-

The following is a list of conditions, problems or body parts that sometimes give young people trouble. Check each one as to whether you are troubled by it a lot, once in a while or never.

	A LOT	ONCE IN A WHILE	NEVER
Headaches			
Dizzy spells			
Eyes or trouble seeing			
Ears or trouble hearing			
Nose—stuffy or bleeding			
Colds			
Teeth or toothaches, etc			
Allergies			
Pain in back, arms or legs			
Pain when urinating (pass water)			
Stomachaches			
Bowels			
Coughing or wheezing			
Heart			
Skin trouble			
"Low blood," anemia			
Loneliness			
Anger			
Sadness			
Nervousness			
Sleep poorly			
Tired all the time			
Menstruation (periods)			

Do you have any other questions or problems? ______________________

OPTIONAL QUESTIONS:

Do you follow or believe in a particular religion? YES NO

If yes, what one? ______________________

How many people live in your home?

Brothers __________ Sisters __________ Aunts or uncles __________

Grandparents __________ Others __________

FIG 7–1 cont'd.

tient and parent(s) may help identify family dynamics that are contributing to the problem. Characteristics of the psychosomatic family include excessive parental anxiety about the adolescent's symptoms, rigidity, overprotectiveness, and lack of conflict resolution. For example, parents in the midst of marital conflict may focus their attention on the teenager's functional abdominal pain rather than on their own relationship. The adolescent's symptom draws the family together around a common issue but prevents resolution of the primary problem. An integrated, multidisciplinary approach often is needed in such situations to dispel anxiety about an organic cause and to focus attention on the psychodynamics involved.

Regardless of the presenting complaint, it may be difficult to obtain a full history until the adolescent is comfortable with the health provider. Information that is not essential for management, therefore, may be obtained more readily at a subsequent visit. The patient and parent should each leave the office with a card indicating the provider's name and telephone number. The adolescent should be encouraged to discuss all visits with the parent but also should feel free to call or schedule appointments as he or she thinks necessary.

PATIENT PROFILE, DEVELOPMENT, AND PRESENT ILLNESS

The interviewer should begin by asking why the adolescent decided to come in for the visit. The first visit should include a discussion of the adolescent's living arrangement, family members, grade and performance in school, sports or hobbies, and social milieu. Changes in the adolescent's family life (death, divorce, remarriage, new baby, change in residence or school) should be elicited. A clear notation of cigarette, alcohol, and drug use is essential.

A developmental history should be obtained from the patient and parent. This should include complications of the mother's pregnancy, labor, or delivery. The provider should note the child's length of gestation, birth weight, developmental milestones, and school history (special classes, grade repetition, peer relationships, absenteeism).

The mother should be questioned about use of diethylstilbestrol during pregnancy. Adolescent girls who were exposed to the drug in utero are at increased risk for clear cell adenocarcinoma of the vagina and cervix and should be referred for colposcopy. Adolescent boys who were exposed are at risk for benign genital lesions such as epididymal cysts and hypotrophic testes. A summary of the pediatric medical record should be included in either the history of present illness or the past medical history.

INFECTIOUS DISEASE

Adolescents must be fully immunized against diphtheria, tetanus, polio, measles, mumps, and rubella (see Chapter 8). After the primary immunization series, only diphtheria and tetanus require boosters. These are given every 10 years throughout adulthood as a combined diphtheria-tetanus injection, with the vaccine for diphtheria reduced to one-tenth the pediatric dose.

There is no need to routinely screen all adolescents with chest roentgenography. Tuberculin skin testing is indicated for adolescents who are exposed to index cases and for screening of high-risk populations.

SEXUAL HISTORY

During adolescence, 80% of boys and 70% of girls have intercourse. Only 30% of sexually active teenagers, however, report that they consistently use contraception. Consequently, teenaged girls represent 18% of sexually active females but 40% of unmarried mothers and 31% of pregnancies ending in abortion.[3] It is imperative that the health care provider discuss sexual activity and contraceptive options with the adolescent. The sexually active girl must understand that gynecologic care is an integral part of her routine medical care. When the parent is out of the room, the adolescent should be asked if he or she is sexually active. A tactful approach is to ask what kind of contraception the patient uses.

An adolescent who is considering the onset of sexual activity should receive anticipatory guidance regarding contraception and the prevention of sexually transmitted disease. All adolescents, regardless of the preferred method of contraception, should be urged to use condoms to decrease the risk of infection. The health provider should serve as a counselor and educator and should be prepared to discuss the implications of sexual activity with the adolescent. Although the number of reported cases of acquired immune deficiency syndrome (AIDS) among adolescents in the United States remains small, this is clearly a population at risk for infection. An understanding of AIDS transmission and prevention therefore is essential.[4, 5]

SUBSTANCE ABUSE

Substance abuse among adolescents is a problem of national public concern. The use of most illicit drugs increased among American high school students in the early 1970s. Peak levels of use occurred in 1978 for marijuana, 1979 for PCP (phencyclidine hydrochloride), 1980 for LSD (lysergide), and 1982 for amphetamines. It was not until 1987, however, that the cocaine epidemic among youth began to decline. It is estimated that up to 40% of persons in their late twenties have tried cocaine or crack within the past year. One in every six seniors has used cocaine, and one in 18 has used crack specifically. Consequently, although overall use is declining, this decline is beginning from a higher level than ever documented before.

There is some evidence that the use of inhalants is continuing to increase among adolescents. Furthermore, there has been no decline in alcohol or cigarette use among adolescents since 1984. In 1987 more than 90% of high school seniors had experimented with alcohol, 66% had used alcohol within the past month, and nearly 40% reported at least five drinks on one occasion within the preceding 2 weeks. Nearly one fifth of students are daily cigarette smokers when they leave high school, and most begin smoking by the age of 13 years.[6, 7]

Adolescent drug abuse usually comes to medical attention only when behavioral problems, injuries, or overdose forces the patient and family to seek help. The adolescent may admit to drug use prior to these problems if assured that the parents will not be told. It is important, however, to involve the parents in their child's problem with drugs as soon as possible. Unexplained depression, difficulty in school, behavioral change, weight loss, tachycardia, or hypertension should lead the physician to consider drug abuse. The teenager should be questioned about drug use and suicidal ideation, should understand the ramifications of drug use and driving, and should be informed of the potential for accidental overdose. Parents who abuse alcohol themselves should be informed that there is little chance that their son or daughter will stop drinking until they stop their own drinking.

NUTRITIONAL HISTORY

The growth spurt that occurs during adolescence represents one of the most rapid developmental rates experienced during the human life cycle. Most adolescent girls require at least 2,350 calories at the age of 11 years and 2,500 calories at the age of 15 years. Adolescent boys require 200 to 600 calories more than girls of the same age. The increasing popularity of fast-food chains, macrobiotic diets, and rapid-weight-loss regimens place the adolescent at high risk for inadequate nutritional intake. The health care provider should determine if caloric intake is appropriate and should educate the patient and parent of nutritional requirements. It should be remembered that adolescent girls require 18 mg of iron daily, three times the amount in the average American diet.

Eating disorders are common in the adolescent population. The obese adolescent requires close supervision and support to maximize weight reduction and nutritional adequacy. The adolescent who has signs of weight loss, secretive eating habits, distorted body image, amenorrhea, delayed menarche, and other manifestations of anorexia nervosa or bulimia should be asked directly about binge eating, self-induced vomiting, and use of laxatives or diuretics.

MENSTRUAL HISTORY

The age of menarche, the interval and duration of menses, and the presence of dysmenorrhea should always be recorded in the adolescent girl's history. The average age of menarche in the United States is 12.4 years, and 95% of girls reach menarche by the age of 14.8 years. Worldwide, the mean age of menarche is 13.5 years, and 95% of girls reach menarche by the age of 15.5 years. Menses may be irregular due to anovulation for up to 2 years following menarche. The development of dysmenorrhea during middle or late adolescence often is associated with ovulation and increasing regularity of the menstrual cycle.

Menarche can occur at any time during puberty, but is most common at Tanner stage IV.[8] Delayed puberty in girls usually is defined as no breast development by the age of 13 years or as an interval greater than 5 years between thelarche and menarche.[9] Patients who meet these criteria should undergo complete endocrine testing. Patients who have not menstruated by the age of 15.5 years should be questioned carefully for family history of delayed maternal menarche. If the patient is at Tanner stage III or IV and the mother's menarche was delayed, watchful waiting is indicated. It is important to document weight and exercise habits in young women with primary or secondary amenorrhea, because there is some evidence that a critical body weight is necessary to begin and maintain menstruation.

FAMILY AND SOCIAL HISTORY

The physician has had an opportunity by this point in the history to discuss family and social issues with the adolescent on a one-to-one basis. Time should be set aside after the physical examination to discuss family medical history, intrafamily relationships, school performance, growth and development, and social maturation with the adolescent and parent together. Parents often are concerned that the adolescent's symptoms are an early manifestation of a disease that is present in another family member. It is especially important to inquire about a family history of hypertension, diabetes mellitus, and coronary artery disease. For example, hereditary hyperlipidemia is found in 30% of teenagers whose parent(s) had myocardial infarctions before the age of 50 years. These adolescents require education about risk factors for heart disease and close surveillance of their serum lipid levels.

This part of the history taking allows the provider both to obtain information from the parent and to observe the dynamics between the patient and parent. Some conflict or disagreement is to be anticipated as the adolescent strives to achieve independence. The manner in which the parent handles these conflicts is important. Parents who repeatedly preempt authority without allowing the adolescent to discuss his or her feelings often face prolonged or exaggerated rebellion. Conversely, parents who abdicate all authority may experience less conflict but often are faced with adolescents who

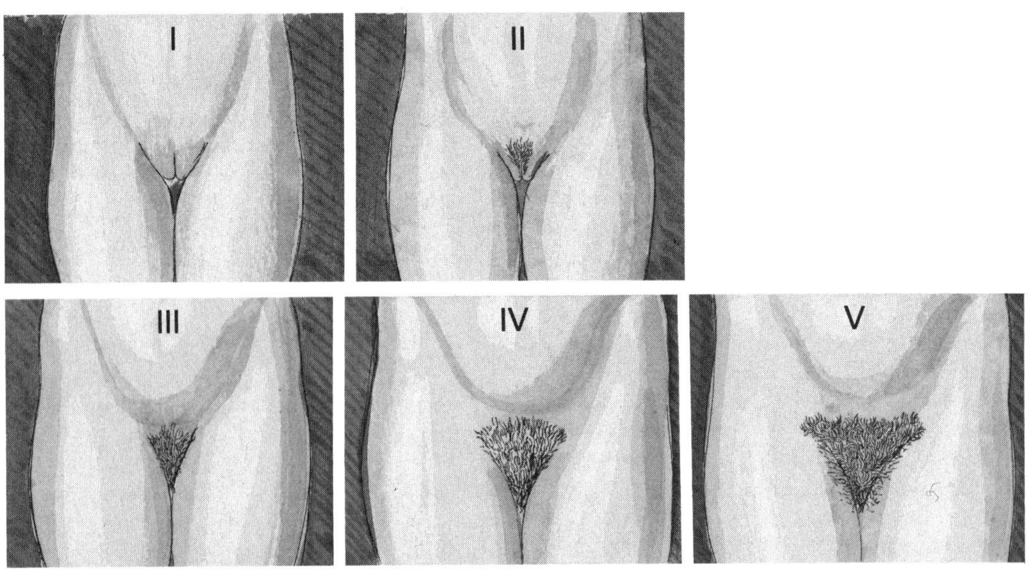

FIG 7–2

Stages of pubic hair growth in girls according to Marshall and Tanner: I, no pubic hair; II, long, pigmented hair over mons veneris or labia majora; III, dark, coarse, curled hair spread sparsely over the mons veneris; IV, abundant, adult-type sexual hair limited to the mons veneris; V, sexual hai is adult type in quantity and distribution, with spread t the medial aspect of the thighs. (Adapted from Marsha WA, Tanner JM: *Arch Dis Child* 1969; 44:291–303.)

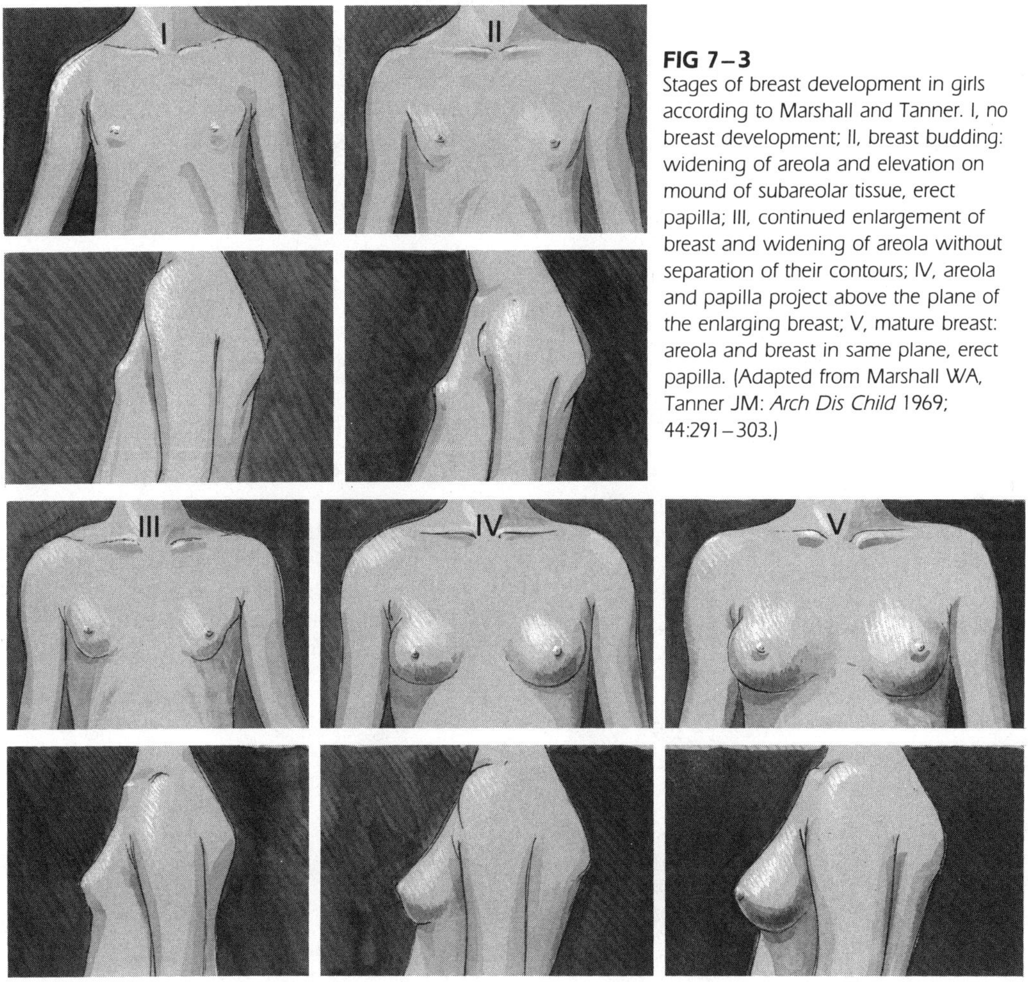

FIG 7–3
Stages of breast development in girls according to Marshall and Tanner. I, no breast development; II, breast budding: widening of areola and elevation on mound of subareolar tissue, erect papilla; III, continued enlargement of breast and widening of areola without separation of their contours; IV, areola and papilla project above the plane of the enlarging breast; V, mature breast: areola and breast in same plane, erect papilla. (Adapted from Marshall WA, Tanner JM: *Arch Dis Child* 1969; 44:291–303.)

are unable to set limits and who have difficulty achieving a smooth transition to adulthood. Both adolescent and parent may benefit from tactful suggestions for limit setting and conflict resolution.

PHYSICAL EXAMINATION

GENERAL APPROACH

The physical examination should be conducted without the parent present whenever the adolescent permits. This gives the health care provider and patient a chance to discuss normal adolescent development and sensitive issues such as sexual activity or substance abuse. Most adolescents are anxious to know if their height, weight, and sexual maturation are normal. The examiner should routinely discuss these observations both to reassure the patient and to clarify the expected changes of adolescence.

Each visit should include measurements of height, weight, blood pressure, and heart rate. Sexual development according to the method of Tanner, breast examination, genital examination in boys, pelvic examination in sexually active girls, scoliosis screening, skin examination, and visual-acuity testing should be done annually.[4]

GROWTH AND DEVELOPMENT

Height and weight should be plotted on grids to indicate the percentiles for age. However, because chronologic age correlates poorly with adolescent development, Tanner stage should also be noted. Pubic hair growth (Fig 7–2) and breast development (Fig 7–3) in girls and pubic hair growth and genital development in boys (Fig 7–4) are used to classify the sexual maturation of adolescents into one of five stages. If there are no signs of puberty by 15.2 years in a boy or 13.4 years in a girl, sexual development is considered delayed (Fig 7–5). Furthermore, if more than 5 years elapse between thelarche and menarche in the female or between initiation and completion of genital growth in the male, the progression of puberty is considered abnormal. Full medical and endocrine evaluation are indicated for delayed initiation or progression of puberty.

Increased thyroid size and activity due to growth once were considered normal findings in the adolescent patient. Thyromegaly in the adolescent now is thought to represent a pathologic process (such as chronic lymphocytic thyroiditis) and should not be attributed to normal growth.

BLOOD PRESSURE

Distribution norms for childhood and adolescent BP were established in 1977 (see Figs 6–1 and 6–2).[10] Hypertension was defined as three BP readings greater than the 95th percentile obtained over 3 months. For most adolescents, a BP reading above the 95th percentile on the initial examination will fall within the normal range on subsequent visits. A single reading above the 90th percentile probably should be repeated in 6 months and yearly thereafter.

SCOLIOSIS SCREENING

Idiopathic scoliosis affects 5% of adolescents. It usually becomes evident during the rapid growth phase (Tanner stage II to III in girls, Tanner stage III to IV in boys) and may progress very quickly during this time. Appropriate intervention requires early detection and close follow-up throughout puberty.

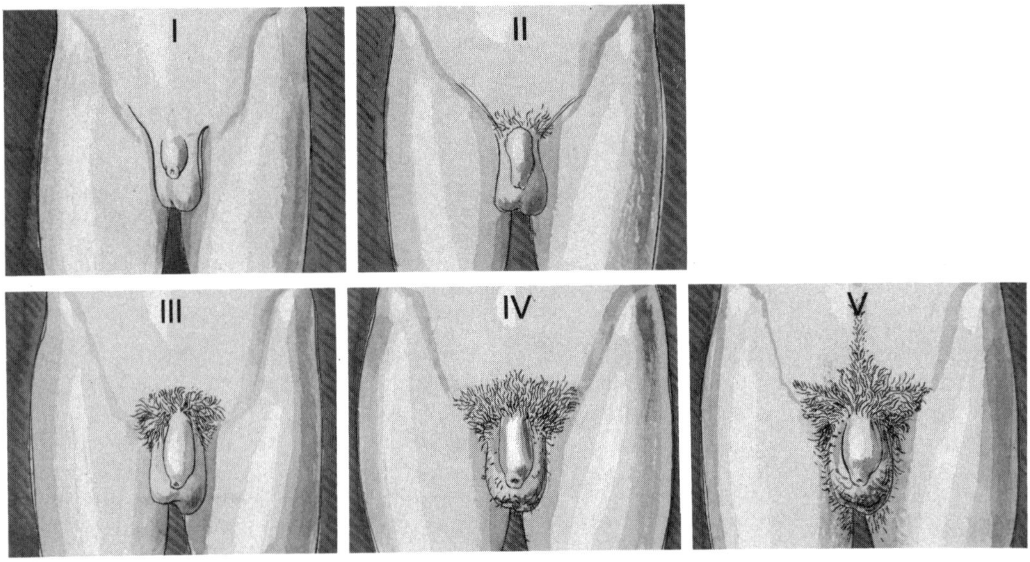

FIG 7–4

Stages of pubic hair growth and development of the external genitalia according to Tanner. Description of stages of pubic hair: I, no pubic hair; II, long downy pigmented hair at and lateral to the base of the penis; III, dark, coarse, curled hair at and lateral to the base of the penis; IV, abundant adult-type sexual hair limited to the pubic region, with no extension to the thighs; V, sexual hair is adult type in quantity and distribution, with spread to the medial aspects of the thighs. Description of genitalia stages: I, prepubertal; II, enlargement of testes and scrotum, with pigmentation and thinning of scrotum; III, lengthening of penis, further enlargement of testes and scrotum; IV, increase in width and length of penis, further enlargement of testes and scrotum, increased pigmentation of scrotum; V, adult size and shape of genitals. (Adapted from Marshall WA, Tanner JM: *Arch Dis Child* 1969; 44:291–303.)

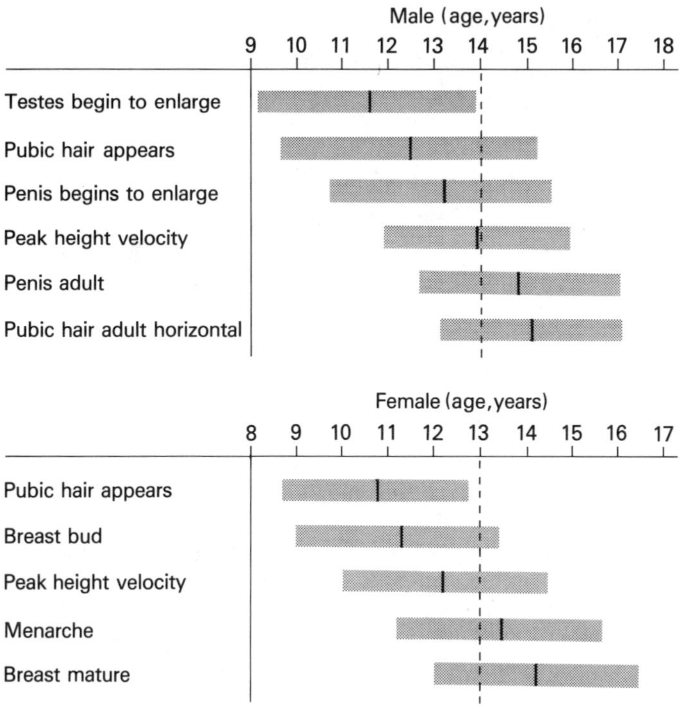

FIG 7–5

Normal timing of puberty in boys and in girls. Horizontal bars represent ±2 SD; vertical marks represent mean age of stage. (Adapted from Prader A: Constitutional delay of growth and puberty, in Chiunello G, Laron Z (eds): *Proceedings of the Serono Symposia: Recent Progress in Pediatric Endocrinology.* Orlando, Fla, Academic Press, 1977.)

The physician first should observe the patient's back for asymmetry of the shoulders, scapulae, or pelvis (Fig 7–6). The anterior chest should be examined for breast asymmetry. Next, the patient should be asked to bend forward to a 90-degree angle (Fig 7–7). This accentuates the curvature and causes protrusion of the rib cage on the convex side of the curve (Fig 7–8). The primary curve usually is to the right in idiopathic scoliosis and comprises the first part of the descriptive term (e.g., thoracolumbar). The degree of scoliosis is then de-

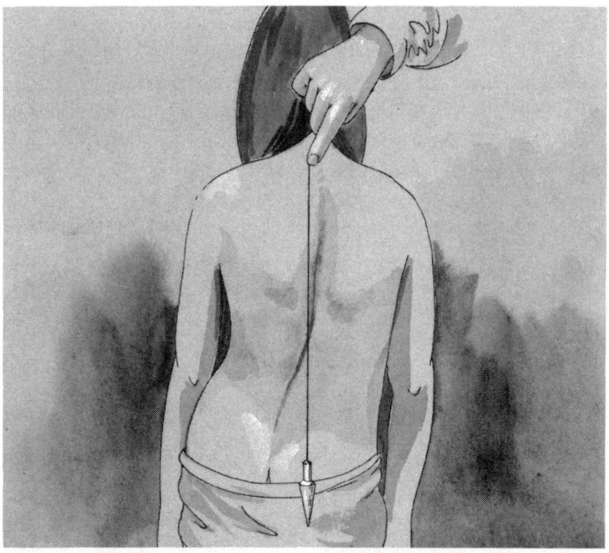

FIG 7–6

Observation of patient's back demonstrating asymmetry of the shoulders, scapula, and pelvis.

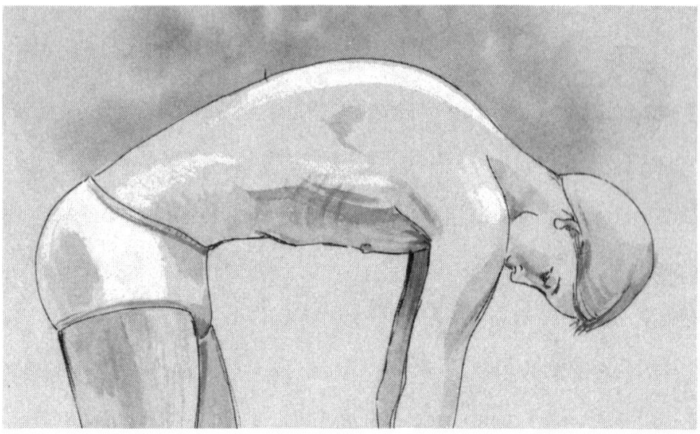

FIG 7–7
Correct forward bending position to accentuate curvature.

termined: mild scoliosis, less than 20-degree curvature; moderate, 20 to 40 degrees; severe, more than 55 degrees. A typical description might read "Scoliosis, right thoracolumbar, moderate degree." If scoliosis is detected, leg lengths should be measured, a roentgenogram of the spine should be obtained, and the adolescent should be referred for orthopedic examination.

BREAST EXAMINATION

Breast examination is important in both adolescent boys and girls. Gynecomastia occurs in 40% of adolescent boys and is most common at the age of 14 to 15 years. In 75% of the cases, it is bilateral and resolves within 2 years. Many boys with gynecomastia are too embarrassed to discuss their concerns with the health care provider; the physician should not wait until the patient asks about the gynecomastia but should reassure him that it is a normal part of development that usually resolves spontaneously. Gynecomastia that persists for more than 2 years requires medical evaluation. If no cause is found and the adolescent is troubled by the breast enlargement, surgical repair can be considered.

Breast masses are a common finding in adolescent girls and usually represent benign fibroadenomas. These lesions are persistent, freely mobile, and usually do not require surgery. Cystic lesions are less common and usually resolve with needle aspiration. Carcinoma of the breast is extremely rare in the adolescent population.

PELVIC EXAMINATION

Every sexually active adolescent girl should have a pelvic examination performed as part of the routine physical examination. It should include speculum inspection of the vagina and cervix, Papanicolaou smear, endocervical culture for gonorrhea, bimanual examination, and rectovaginal examination.

The age for the first pelvic examination of the virginal adolescent is controversial. It should always be done, regardless of age, in the adolescent with in utero exposure to diethylstilbestrol,[11] unexplained abdominal or pelvic pain, menstrual abnormality, or vaginal discharge.

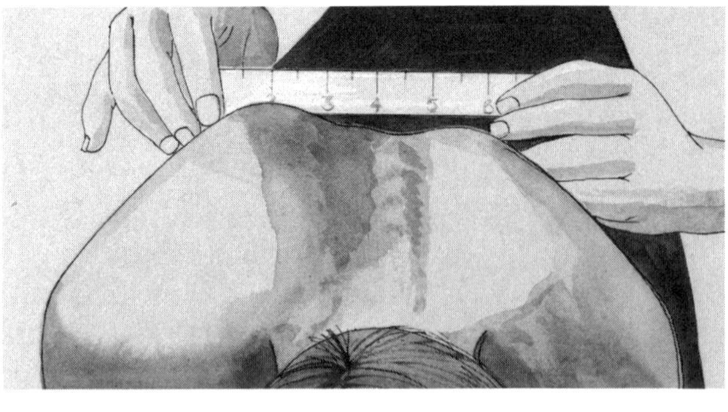

FIG 7–8
Protrusion of rib cage evident on assuming forward bending position. Protrusion occurs on the convex side of curve.

The examination should be explained thoroughly, with the aid of a pelvic model. If the adolescent refuses examination, it is best to delay it whenever possible rather than assume an aggressive approach that will interfere with subsequent follow-up and compliance. If the patient resists speculum or bimanual examination, a rectovaginal examination should be done and any discharge from the vagina should be examined microscopically and cultured.

LABORATORY EVALUATION

The laboratory tests for all adolescent patients include urinalysis, hematocrit, and cholesterol and triglyceride determinations. All sexually active girls should have a Papanicolaou smear, endocervical culture for gonorrhea, endocervical culture or antigen detection screen for *Chlamydia trachomatis,* and serologic testing for syphilis. All sexually active boys should have periodic urethral culture for gonorrhea, urethral culture or antigen detection screen for *C. trachomatis,* and serologic testing for syphilis.[4, 12, 13]

The decision to screen adolescents for antibody to human immunodeficiency virus (HIV) should be based on the patient's risk for infection. The number of reported cases of AIDS among American adolescents aged 13 to 19 years remains small relative to the total number of reported cases. However, because of the future risk confronting a young person who is newly sexually active, the physician must be prepared to answer questions pertaining to HIV infection and to counsel adolescents about protection against infection.

SUMMARY

1. Most of the history should be obtained with the adolescent alone in the office. Time should be allowed after the physical examination to interview the adolescent and parent together and to discuss the physician's impressions.
2. The physical examination should be conducted without the parent in the room. Height, weight, BP, heart rate, Tanner stage, and examination for scoliosis should be included in each visit.
3. Pelvic examination should always be performed for the sexually active girl or for the girl with in utero exposure to diethylstilbestrol, abdominal or pelvic pain, menstrual abnormality, or vaginal discharge.
4. All adolescents should have a urinalysis, hematocrit, and cholesterol and triglyceride levels. Sexually active girls should have a Papanicolaou smear, endocervical cultures for gonorrhea and *C. trachomatis,* and VDRL test. Sexually active boys should have urethral cultures for gonorrhea and *C. trachomatis* and a VDRL test.

REFERENCES

1. Legal Affairs Division, Planned Parenthood Federation of America: Litigation Update. New York, Planned Parenthood Federation of America, 1987, pp 11–22.
2. Paul EW, Klassel D: Minors' rights to confidential contraceptive services: The limits of state power. *Women Rights Law Rep* 1987; 10:45–63.
3. Dryfoos JG: *Teenage Pregnancy: The Problem That Hasn't Gone Away.* New York, Allan Guttmacher Institute, 1981.
4. Marks A, Fisher M: Health assessment and screening during adolescence. *Pediatrics* 1987; 80(suppl):135–158.
5. DiClemente RJ, Zorn J, Temoshock L: Adolescent and AIDS: A survey of knowledge, attitudes and beliefs about AIDS in San Francisco. *Am J Public Health* 1986; 76:1443–1445.
6. Johnston LD, O'Malley PM, Bachman JG: *National Trends in Drug Use and Related Factors Among American High School Students and Young Adults, 1975–1986.* Rockville, Md, National Institute on Drug Abuse, DHHS Publication No (ADM) 87–1535.
7. Johnston LD: *Summary of 1987 Drug Study Results. University of Michigan News and Information Services.* Ann Arbor, University of Michigan, 1988.
8. Marshall WA, Tanner JM: Variation in pattern of pubertal changes in girls. *Arch Dis Child* 1969; 44:291–303.
9. Prader A: Constitutional delay of growth and puberty, in Chiunello G, Laron Z (eds): *Proceedings of the Serono Symposia: Recent Progress in Pediatric Endocrinology.* Orlando, Fla, Academic Press, 1977, pp 129–138.
10. Horan MJ, et al: Report of the Second Task Force on Blood Pressure Control in Children—1987. *Pediatrics* 1987; 79:1–25.

11. Bibbo M, Gill WG: Screening of adolescents exposed to diethylstilbestrol in utero. *Pediatr Clin North Am* 1983; 28:379–388.
12. Jaffe LR, Siqueira LM, Diamond SB, et al: *Chlamydia trachomatis* detection in adolescents: A comparison of direct specimen and tissue culture methods. *J Adolesc Health Care* 1986; 7:401–404.
13. Bell TA, Grayston JT: Centers for Disease Control guidelines for prevention and control of *Chlamydia trachomatis* infections. Summary and commentary. *Ann Intern Med* 1986; 104:524–526.

PSYCHOSOCIAL DEVELOPMENT

English D. Willis, M.D.

The psychosocial development that occurs during adolescence involves the accomplishment of several developmental tasks, the most important of which are establishing independence from parents, achieving a satisfying and realistic body image, establishing a meaningful and satisfying sexual relationship, and choosing a career and achieving economic stability. Progression through each of these developmental tasks is necessary if the adolescent is to establish a sense of identity and become a healthy adult.

The psychosocial development of adolescence may be classified into three phases: early (10 to 14 years), middle (15 to 17 years), and late (17 years through mid-twenties). The adolescent's behavior is influenced by his or her phase of development. During each phase, adolescents concentrate on accomplishing a particular aspect of each developmental task. However, their psychosocial development both influences and is influenced by their ability to master each developmental task.

The assigned age range for each phase is arbitrary and varies among individuals and with different social and cultural backgrounds. Psychosocial development will also vary with differences in physical maturation. Because the range of normal pubertal development is so wide, adolescents of the same chronologic age who are at different levels of pubertal development will vary in their ability to accomplish each developmental task. In addition, adolescents at either end of the maturation spectrum, early vs. late, will behave differently from the majority.

In the care of adolescents, knowledge of normal adolescent psychosocial and cognitive development is essential. The physician is able to monitor the maturational process of the adolescent toward adulthood and counsel the parents about recent and anticipated changes in the behavior of their adolescent.

PHASES OF ADOLESCENCE

EARLY ADOLESCENCE

This phase of development usually occurs between the ages of 10 and 14 years. It is during this phase that young adolescents begin to establish independence. In their effort to develop a separate identity from their parents, they are often viewed as rebellious and difficult. The young adolescent may be quick to disagree with parents and take the opposite view on an issue to test parental values. They will often cast away hobbies or objects that link them to their childhood or demonstrate their dependence. The role of the primary care physician is to recognize these changes and to reassure the parents that this is normal separation behavior.

Emotionally, the adolescent will move away from the family toward peers of the same sex or other adults. These friends are often idolized and appear to be the center of the adolescent's "world." Adolescents within the same peer group develop similar patterns of dress, hairstyles, and speaking. It is important to the young adolescent to fit in and not appear different from his or her peers.

Coincident with psychosocial growth is pubertal development. Young adolescents must adjust to the physical changes that are occurring in their bodies. Enormous amounts of time are spent on grooming and on becoming acquainted with their new bodies. Young adolescents focus attention not only on their development but also on that of their friends, to see if their developmental changes are comparable. For the late or early maturing adolescent, this can be a particularly stressful time. It is often beneficial to acknowledge the level of development and counsel the adolescent on the maturation process.

Early adolescence is the time of sexual curiosity. Masturbation and sexual play with same-sex friends is common. Two of three boys experience their first ejaculation through masturbation. Heterosexual intercourse is also occurring at an earlier age for many; thus the discussion of sexual activity and contraceptive counseling at an earlier age is appropriate.

Cognitive maturation, the transition from concrete to abstract conceptualization, begins during adolescence. Young adolescents think concretely and are unable to relate aspects of one experience to another or relate their present actions to future consequences. They frequently respond to questions literally, not figuratively. Knowledge of the young adolescent's thinking process is important for the physician trying to obtain an accurate history or provide counseling.

MIDDLE ADOLESCENCE

During middle adolescence, ages 15 to 17 years, body awareness is heightened. Adolescents are concerned with their physical appearance and believe that others are also concerned. In an effort to become comfortable with their new bodies, greater time is invested in grooming, exercising, and experimenting with new images such as makeup and clothing styles. This is done with the purpose of developing a satisfying and realistic body image. However, their focused attention on themselves is a contributing factor to the self-centeredness of this age group.

Middle adolescents experience sexual drives and aggression and must learn to control and be comfortable with their sexuality. During this phase peer groups expand to include friends of the opposite sex. Taking risks and experimenting with sex, drugs, alcohol, and cigarettes is common. In 1983, 5% of girls and 17% of boys reported being sexually active by their fifteenth birthday; by the seventeenth birthday 27% of girls and 48% of boys were sexually active. The increase in sexual activity among adolescents makes it imperative to obtain a sexual history and provide contraceptive counseling.

Experiences of adolescents are broadened by their relationships with adults outside the family. They are exposed to new and unfamiliar situations and lifestyles. Situations in the struggle for independence are often frightening and create an ambivalence in adolescents' separation process. This ambivalence may result in increased tension with parents and other family members.

Middle adolescents have a greater ability to think abstractly. Conceptualization expands beyond past and present experiences and they are able to theorize. Their ability to understand spatial relationships and to utilize symbols improves. These new abilities are impressive to many adolescents and contribute to their already self-centered behavior.

LATE ADOLESCENCE

Late adolescence is the period from age 17 through the early twenties. During this phase one of the primary developmental tasks facing the adolescent is selecting a career and achieving economic stability. With the completion of high school, future career decisions must be made. The array of available options and the concern for economic independence contribute to the stress of this period. Those adolescents electing to continue their education prolong this growth task because of their financial dependence on family or others.

The value system of older adolescents is changing. They are often idealistic, with rigid concepts of right and wrong. Causes are embraced with conviction. Peer-group relationships are replaced by individual friendships. Older adolescents are capable of developing close, caring, and intimate relationships with a member of the opposite sex. Most have obtained a secure and realistic physical image of themselves and are capable of committing themselves to relationships with others. Relationships with parents improve because the adolescents have established a sense of identity and are no longer threatened by seeking their parents' advice or counseling. Late adolescence therefore marks the period of integration of the various developmental tasks in an effort to become an adult.

THE EFFECT OF EARLY VS. LATE PHYSICAL MATURATION

The stage of pubertal development in an adolescent appears to be a better correlate of psychosocial development than of chronologic age. Because the age range for normal pubertal development is so wide, there are great variations in behavior within any age group.

Differences in the behavioral characteristics of early- vs. late-maturing adolescents have been shown. In a previous study, early-maturing boys were judged to be more popular, self-assured, poised, and athletic; the late-maturing boys were seen as less physically attractive, less poised, more attention-seeking, and more talkative. For girls, however, there were no clear advantages in being an early maturer. Early-maturing girls, compared with late-maturing girls, exhibited less prestige, popularity, and leadership qualities. The level of self-esteem was higher in the late-maturing girls than in those who had matured early.

A correlation also exists between academic performance and timing of physical maturation. Compared with early- and mid-maturing boys, late maturing boys had less desire to complete college, were characterized less often as above average in intellectual abilities, and were less often in the upper third of their class for academic achievements. However, for girls a similar correlation between educational and intellectual achievements in early vs. late maturation did not exist. This information may be important to the health care provider when discussing behavior and school performance with the adolescent boy and his parents.

BIBLIOGRAPHY

Conger JJ: *Adolescence and Youth*. New York, Harper & Row, 1973.

Duke PM, Carlsmith JM, Jennings D, et al: Educational correlates of early and late sexual maturation in adolescence. *J Pediatr* 1982; 100:633–637.

Felice ME: Adolescence: General considerations, in Levine MD, Carey WB, Crocker AC, et al (eds): *Developmental-Behavioral Pediatrics*. Philadelphia, WB Saunders Co, 1983, pp 133–149.

Felice ME, Friedman SB: Behavioral considerations in the health care of adolescents. *Pediatr Clin North Am* 1982; 29:399–413.

Gross RT, Duke PM: Adolescence: Effects of early versus late physical maturation on adolescent behavior, in Levine MD, Carey WB, Crocker AC, et al (eds): *Developmental-Behavioral Pediatrics*. Philadelphia, WB Saunders Co, 1983, pp 149–157.

Hayes CD: *Risking the future: Adolescent sexuality, pregnancy and child bearing*, vol 1. Washington, DC, National Academy Press, 1987, pp 33–74.

Irwin CE Jr, Millstein SG: Biopsychosocial correlates of risk-taking behaviors in adolescence: Can the physician intervene? *J Adolesc Health Care* 1986; 7:825–965.

Marks A, Fisher M: Health assessment and screening during adolescence. *Pediatrics* 1987; 80(suppl): 135–158.

Neinstein LS: Adolescent health care: A practical guide. Baltimore, Urban and Schwarzenberg, 1984, pp 35–40.

Slap GB: Normal physiological and psychosocial growth in the adolescent. *J Adolesc Health Care* 1986; 7:13s–23s.

MENSTRUAL IRREGULARITIES IN ADOLESCENT GIRLS

Gertrude J. Frishmuth, M.D.

Menstruation, a cyclic physiologic discharge of blood, mucus, tissue fluids, and endometrial and vaginal cellular debris, is the result of hormonal changes produced in the endometrium by the interaction of the ovaries and the anterior pituitary gland. The flow of blood at menstruation is characteristically nonclotting, but clotting may be observed, particularly during episodes of heavy bleeding. The presence of fibrinolysin in the endometrial cavity suggests that the normal flow occurs at such a rate that clotting is prevented or there is lysis of existing clots. When there is vigorous uterine bleeding, this mechanism is rendered inoperative and clotting results. The menstrual cycle is the period extending from the onset of one normal menstrual period to the onset of the next normal period, generally 21 to 37 days. The normal menstrual blood loss is less than 80 mL (range 30 to 100 mL). The duration of the normal period is usually less than 1 week, with most of the blood loss occurring in the first 3 days. The endometrium is affected by the cyclic stimulation of estrogen and progesterone. The proliferative phase is the growth phase of the endometrium and is stimulated by estrogen. The secretory phase is the postovulatory phase of the endometrium and is stimulated by estrogen and progesterone.

PATHOPHYSIOLOGY OF ANOVULATION

In the adolescent the basic underlying defect in the physiology of menstruation is failure of ovulation. The dysfunctional uterine bleeding (DUB) that occurs is due to the hypothalamic-pituitary-ovarian axis being immature or incapable of properly releasing the necessary trophic hormones in a timely fashion to stimulate ovulation. This type of dysfunction is also frequently seen in girls during times of stress and in those who are at extremes of weight. The tonic release of follicle-stimulating hormone (FSH) is sufficient to induce some ovarian follicular development and estrogen secretion. The midcycle surge of luteinizing hormone (LH) fails to occur and anovulation results. The corpus luteum fails to develop in the ovary. Progesterone is not secreted. The loss of cyclic progesterone effect results in a continuous unopposed estrogen stimulation of the endometrium. Abnormal menstrual bleeding patterns are the end result of this chain of events.

DEFINITIONS OF MENSTRUAL IRREGULARITIES

Amenorrhea.—Amenorrhea is absence of menstruation. It is pathologic if it occurs at any time after menarche and before menopause, other than during pregnancy and lactation. It can be either primary or secondary and caused by congenital abnormalities, central nervous system lesions, sellar or subsellar lesions, systemic conditions (e.g., diabetes, malignancy, malnutrition), androgen or estrogen overproduction, thyroid and adrenal malfunction, psychiatric illness, or uterine trauma. Physiologic amenorrhea is the normal absence of menstruation before menarche, during pregnancy and lactation, and after menopause. Primary physiologic amenorrhea is the lack of the menarche in a woman at least 18 years of age. Secondary physiologic amenorrhea is the cessation of menstruation for at least 3 months in a girl or a woman after menarche has occurred.

Polymenorrhea.—Polymenorrhea designates episodes of menstrual flow occurring at an interval less than 22 days apart.

Hypomenorrhea.—Hypomenorrhea is diminution in the amount of flow while all of the characteristics of the cycle remain unaltered. This is usually seen in association with the use of oral contraceptive therapy.

Hypermenorrhea.—Hypermenorrhea is increase in the quantity of flow during a regular cycle of normal duration. This may exist without prolongation of the duration of flow (menorrhagia). In general, this is a sign of organic disease and may be accompanied by dysmenorrhea.

Menorrhagia.—Menorrhagia is excessive or prolonged menstrual bleeding. It is a sign of a disease process. The amount of blood loss can be increased, and flow duration is increased.

Metrorrhagia.—Metrorrhagia is bleeding between menstrual periods. This is the same as intermenstrual bleeding and can be of light character, even spotting. The intrauterine device (IUD) is a common cause of metrorrhagia. This pattern also suggests organic disease.

Menometrorrhagia.—Menometrorrhagia is irregular or excessive bleeding during menstruation and between menstrual periods. This is a pattern of total disturbance of the normal menstrual cycle. It is a symptom and not an acceptable diagnosis.

Oligomenorrhea.—Oligomenorrhea denotes reduction in the frequency of menstruation. An interval between the cycles of longer than 38 days but less than 3 months indicates oligomenorrhea.

Mittelschmerz.—Mittelschmerz is intermenstrual pain in the lower part of the abdomen, generally associated with ovulation. Spotty bleeding may accompany this pain.

Dysfunctional Uterine Bleeding.—This term describes all abnormal uterine bleeding with no demonstrable organic cause (genital and extragenital). This bleeding results from a disturbance in the usually finely synchronized hormonal secretory activity.

In the extremes of reproductive years, perimenarchal and perimenopausal cycles, we find that 90% of dysfunctional uterine bleeding is of the anovulatory type.

Hormonal causes of abnormal bleeding in adolescents include anovulation (approximately 90%) and ovulation (less than 10%), including failure of corpus luteum to secrete adequate progesterone and endometrial unresponsiveness to progesterone effect. The menstrual irregularity can be polymenorrhea or oligomenorrhea (with or without menorrhagia or menometrorrhagia) or amenorrhea. In adolescents it suggests disturbances of endocrine control. In the first year of menstrual life, approximately 55% of menses are anovulatory, with a steep drop to less than 7% 8 years later. It takes between 15 and 18 months to complete the first 10 menstrual cycles. The adolescent tends to have cycles of variable duration, with anovulation associated with both short and long cycles.

HISTORY

A complete history is required to be certain there is no pathologic cause for the bleeding. Associated abdominal or pelvic pain is not usually seen in patients with anovulatory bleeding. Review of the normal menstrual history should include onset, length, amount, character, and associated symptoms to establish a baseline for comparison. Age at menarche is variable but generally occurs in girls in the United States between 11 and 16 years of age (average age 12 years 4 months). The date of the last normal menstrual period (LNMP) should be recorded. Any previous pregnancy must be recorded. Previous bleeding episodes, the regularity of the menstrual cycles, and previous hormonal therapy are important considerations. One must ask about trauma, weight changes, and chronic systemic illness.

A patient with excessive and prolonged bleeding must be seen as soon as possible. It is impossible to determine accurately over the telephone the amount of the blood loss and the cause of the bleeding. The amount of blood loss can be alarming, and the number of pads required per hour must be known to estimate the amount of blood loss. A fully saturated tampon contains between 15 and 25 mL of blood; a sanitary pad can contain a somewhat larger amount. Any undue delay in the evaluation and treatment of a patient who is soaking through a pad in less than 1 hour may be hazardous.

If the patient's mother had hormone therapy during pregnancy the physician should be alert to the possibility of genital cancer. An association between clear cell adenocarcinoma of the vagina with a history of maternal ingestion of diethylstilbestrol has been shown, with the youngest child being 7 years of age. Inquiry should be made regarding the presence of episodes of nongenital abnormal bleeding or unexplained bruising to suggest the possibility of blood dyscrasia. In this age group, one should be concerned about leukemia, aplastic anemia, von Willebrand disease, and idiopathic or autoimmune thrombocytopenic purpura. The history should include a search for symptoms of hyperthyroidism or hypothyroidism. Menstrual dysfunction in hypothyroidism is more commonly menometrorrhagia than amenorrhea. Menstrual abnormalities are common in hyperthyroidism but take the form of oligomenorrhea or amenorrhea.

PHYSICAL EXAMINATION

A thorough physical examination is necessary to follow up on impressions that the physician has gathered from the history. In addition, the amount and the source of the bleeding can be better determined by physical examination. Vital signs will detect fever and orthostatic changes. The general condition of the patient is helpful in determining the acute nature of her bleeding. An abdominal examination should precede the pelvic examination. The presence of enlarged lymph nodes, liver, or spleen would suggest blood dyscrasia.

The adolescent responds to a kind, gentle physician and will be difficult to examine if the physician is brusque and hurried. An explanation and some reassuring remarks are important ingredients for obtaining a successful pelvic examination. Local pelvic causes of the bleeding are usually determined by the abdominal and pelvic examinations. Visualization of the external genitalia should allow the physician to see if the hymen is patent or not. In doing the speculum examination in the adolescent, one may first have to digitally dilate the vaginal introitus. With the use of the speculum, the physician can examine the cervix; if there are any products of conception in the cervical os, the diagnosis of an incomplete abortion can be made. Cervical neoplasia can be suspected from gross examination of the cervix. Instrumentation and discomfort should be kept to a minimum. On bimanual pelvic examination, infection should be suspected if pain in the lower part of the abdomen results from movement of the cervix either to the anterior or posterior or laterally. An enlarged uterus (e.g., pregnancy) or masses in the adnexa (e.g., ectopic pregnancy, tubo-ovarian abscess, ovarian tumor) may also be detected on bimanual pelvic examination. In some adolescents, one may not be able to do either a speculum examination or a vaginal-abdominal examination. In these cases a rectal-abdominal examination is necessary to rule out pelvic inflammatory disease and any palpable pelvic mass.

LABORATORY EVALUATION

Immediate: Complete blood count (CBC), with differential and platelet count; pregnancy test (serum, β-human chorionic gonadotropin preferred); cervical and vaginal cultures.

Delayed: Thyroid function (thyroxine and thyroid-stimulating hormone); prolactin; bleeding profile (bleeding time, clotting time, prothrombin time, partial thromboplastin time, fibrinogen and fibrin split products), FSH, LH, DHEAS, testosterone.

DIFFERENTIAL DIAGNOSIS

Organic (genital and extragenital) causes of abnormal uterine bleeding must be considered (see Tables 7–1 and 7–2).

In the adolescent, a helpful mnemonic is PIN down the diagnosis: Pregnancy and its complications will be clear by history, pelvic examination, and laboratory evaluation. Infection will be found by history, pelvic examination, and culture results (not immediately available), and by having a high index of suspicion. Acute endometritis can cause bleeding. During later stages of the disease, the bleeding can be more dysfunctional in nature. With greater chronicity, oophoritis and pelvic adhesions permit disturbances of ovarian function causing abnormal bleeding. Fever and pain point toward this diagnosis. It is interesting to note that some patients with salpingo-oophoritis–endometritis may have abnormal bleeding as a result of coexisting organic pathology. Neoplasia is rare in the genital tract of adolescents. Less than 3% of malignancy during childhood and adolescence occurs in the genital tract, and

TABLE 7–1
Genital Causes of Abnormal Uterine Bleeding

1. Pregnancy and its complications
2. Organic lesions

ORGAN	BENIGN	MALIGNANT
Vagina	Vaginitis	Epidermoid
	Postcoital	Mesonephric rest tumors
	Traumatic	Adenosis and clear cell adenocarcinoma
	Foreign body	
	Condyloma acuminata	
Cervix	Cervicitis	Squamous cell
	Polyps	Adenocarcinoma
	Endometriosis	Embryonal rhabdomyosarcoma (sarcoma botryoides)
	Tuberculosis	
	Syphilis	
Uterus	Polyps	Adenocarcinomas
	Leiomyoma	Adenoacanthoma
	Adenomyosis	Sarcoma, mixed mesodermal
	Endometriosis	
	Foreign body	
Ovary	Functional cysts	All histiogenetic classifications but especially granulosa cell (estrogen producing)
	Follicular	
	Corpus luteum	
	Polycystic ovaries	Malignant cystic teratoma
	Benign cystic teratoma	
Fallopian tube	Salpingitis	Carcinoma

the ovary is the most common site. The history and pelvic examination are of extreme importance when considering this diagnosis.

The diagnosis of DUB (predominantly anovulatory bleeding) is one of exclusion, based on history, physical examination, and pelvic examination. Less than 10% of patients with DUB will demonstrate evidence of ovulation. Abnormal bleeding in patients who are ovulating results from either the failure of the corpus lu-

TABLE 7–2
Extragenital Causes of Abnormal Uterine Bleeding

- Blood dyscrasia
  - Leukemia
  - Aplastic anemia
  - von Willebrand disease
  - Idiopathic and autoimmune thrombocytopenic purpura
  - Idiopathic bleeding-time defect
- Endocrinopathies
  - Thyroid disease
  - Adrenal disease
  - Diabetes mellitus
- Iatrogenic
- Drug therapy
  - Anticoagulants
  - Aspirin
  - Nonsteroidal anti-inflammatory agents
- Psychological
  - Stress
  - Major degrees of neurosis
  - Frank psychosis
  - Self-induced trauma

teum to secrete adequate progesterone or endometrial unresponsiveness to progesterone effect. In general, the ovulatory form of DUB tends to produce less severe bleeding patterns.

MANAGEMENT OF MENSTRUAL IRREGULARITIES

Conservative management can be considered if the hemoglobin level is over 9 g/dL and bleeding has not incapacitated the patient. A good diet, addition of iron, a menstrual record, and a periodic evaluation of the hematocrit reading are all that is needed.

Organic causes of menstrual irregularities such as pregnancy and genital lesions will require consultation with a gynecologist. Extragenital causes may require consultation with other specialists such as hematologists, endocrinologists, etc. In considering the immediate course of therapy for a bleeding patient, a physician will make a decision depending on the circumstances surrounding each patient. A patient with symptoms (weakness and light-headedness) who exhibits a slightly elevated pulse and who has marked anemia will require inpatient care; sending the patient home under these circumstances is medically risky and inadvisable.

The immediate goal in the treatment of DUB is to obtain hemostasis as soon as possible. The appropriate therapy is to supply what the patient is lacking, namely progesterone. Potent progestagenic hormones, effective when administered orally, will almost invariably stop mild-to-moderate bleeding if administered in sufficient and frequent dosage. Many preparations and regimens of progestagens have been used successfully. The most commonly used is medroxyprogesterone acetate (Provera), 10 mg daily for 5 to 10 days, to be taken orally. After cessation of medication, there will be withdrawal bleeding in 2 to 10 days (so-called medical curettage). Approximately 5 days after this bleeding episode, the patient should have her menstrual cycle regulated for 2 to 3 months by the use of oral contraceptive therapy in the usual manner. This regimen is then discontinued in anticipation that the patient's own cycle will resume.

Continuous bleeding over a long interval of time can strip the uterus of all endometrium. If no endometrial tissue is present, progesterone will be ineffective in stopping the bleeding. This is the most common presentation of adolescents with anovulatory DUB. In such cases, estrogens must also be given to stimulate endometrial growth so that tissue is available upon which the progestational agent can act. If there has been heavy blood loss, an oral contraceptive medication can be given to the patient in high doses. An oral contraceptive (containing 0.05 mg ethinyl estradiol) may be prescribed for a 21-day regimen as follows: one tablet three times a day for 3 days; one tablet twice a day for 3 days; then one tablet daily until all 21 tablets are completed. The pill is then discontinued for 7 days. The patient must be warned to anticipate a heavy flow and cramping approximately 2 to 4 days after stopping the pill. This is followed by two cycles of usual oral contraceptive therapy.

The combination pill produces both endometrial buildup by estrogenic stimulation and rapid conversion to secretory endometrium by the progestational agent. When the oral contraceptive pill is initially used, the dose is usually tapered. Regular monthly cycles with ovulation may ensue after the above regimen or the patient may continue to be anovulatory. If the patient is sexually active, oral contraceptives can be continued. To prevent a future prolonged period, it may be desirable to induce a withdrawal bleeding episode every 6 to 8 weeks with a regimen of Provera, 10 mg a day for 5 days by mouth. This is necessary only if the patient has not had a menstrual period for 6 to 8 weeks after discontinuing therapy.

CONSULTATION

Once the acute bleeding episode in an anovulatory patient is controlled, the patient must not be forgotten. If recurrent hemorrhage is a common pattern, a gynecologic consultation is recommended. If the bleeding is so severe that it warrants hospitalization for blood volume replacement and rapid hemostasis, a gynecologic consultation is recommended. Failure of oral hormone administration requires hospitalization for parenteral therapy. Rarely is dilation and curettage required to control bleeding in an adolescent. In conclusion, any referral should be made to a consulting gynecologist who is comfortable dealing with adolescents.

BIBLIOGRAPHY

Eberlein WR, Bongiovanni AM, Jones IT, et al: Ovarian tumors and cysts associated with sexual precocity. *J Pediatr* 1960; 57:484–500.

Emans SJ, Goldstein DP: *Pediatric and Adolescent Gynecology*. Boston, Little, Brown & Co, 1977.

Frisch RE: Fatness and fertility. *Sci Am* 1988; 258:88–95.

Frisch RE, Revelle R: Height and weight at menarche and a hypothesis of menarche. *Arch Dis Child* 1971; 46:695–701.

Huffman JW, Dewhurst CJ, Caparo VJ: *The Gynecology of Childhood and Adolescence*, ed 2. Philadelphia, WB Saunders Co, 1981.

Israel SL: *Diagnosis and Treatment of Menstrual Disorders and Sterility*, ed 5. New York, Harper & Row, 1967.

Kase NG, Weingold AB (eds): *Principles and Practice of Clinical Gynecology*. New York, John Wiley & Sons, 1983.

Lavery JP, Sanfilippo JS (eds): *Pediatric and Adolescent Obstetrics and Gynecology*. New York, Springer-Verlag, 1985.

Lee PA: Pubertal neuroendocrine maturation: Early differentiation and stages of development. *Adolesc Pediatr Gynecol* 1988; 1:3–12.

Speroff L, Glass RH, Kase NG: *Clinical Gynecologic Endocrinology and Infertility*, ed 4. Baltimore, Williams & Wilkins Co, 1988.

CONTRACEPTION

Margaret Polaneczky, M.D., M.S.
Gail B. Slap, M.D., M.S.

This chapter provides an overview of adolescent sexuality and contraception. The United States has the highest rates of adolescent pregnancy, live births, and abortion in the industralized world.[1] Nearly 50% of American boys and 45% of American girls aged 15 to 17 years are sexually active. Sixty percent of this sexual activity occurs without the use of contraception. One fourth of sexually active adolescents report that they never use contraception, and only one third report that they always use contraception. As a result, more than one in 10 adolescent females in the United States become pregnant, totaling more than one million pregnancies annually.[1–6] Infants born to adolescent mothers, compared with those born to adult mothers, are twice as likely to have low birth weight and twice as likely to die during the first year of life. Adolescent mothers are half as likely as older mothers to complete high school, three times as likely to separate or divorce, and seven times as likely to live below the poverty level.[2]

It is the responsibility of the primary care provider to discuss sexual activity and contraception with the adolescent patient. This chapter presents an approach to contraceptive options counseling and reviews the major contraceptive methods currently available.

COUNSELING

The primary goal of adolescent contraceptive counseling is the prevention of unintended pregnancy. To achieve this goal the health provider must educate, assess the risk for pregnancy, and help the adolescent choose an appropriate method. The adolescent seeking contraception should be ensured of confidentiality at the first visit. The possibility of parental involvement should be explored with the adolescent, but at no time should it compromise delivery of health care. Of sexually active adolescents, 25% report that they would not attend family planning clinics if their parents were informed; only 2% report that they would stop having sex.[2]

The contraceptive methods should be discussed in a factual and unbiased manner with the patient and partner. The adolescent should be shown the packet of oral contraceptives, diaphragm, condom, and spermicide. The advantages and disadvantages of each method should be described. The ineffectiveness of withdrawal, douches, plastic wrap condoms, and intermittent use of any contraceptive method should be discussed. The health provider should always explain that abstinence is an acceptable alternative and that sexual satisfaction can be achieved without intercourse.

The final choice of contraceptive method must always be the adolescent's. The adolescent who wants birth control pills but leaves the physician's office with a diaphragm is less likely to use the method effectively. Factors to be considered in helping the adolescent to select a method include the following.

TABLE 7–3
Contraindications to Adolescent Use of Oral Contraceptives

ABSOLUTE	RELATIVE
Thromboembolic disease	Severe headaches
Cerebrovascular disease	Hypertension
Coronary artery disease	Diabetes
Abnormal liver function	Gallbladder disease
Hepatic adenoma	Gilbert disease
Breast or gynecologic malignancy	Hemoglobinopathy
Pregnancy	Hyperlipidemia
Undiagnosed abnormal vaginal bleeding	Surgery within 4 wk
	Immobilization
	Lactation
	Depression
	Seizure disorder

Pattern of Sexual Activity.—A barrier method (i.e., diaphragm, condom, spermicide) is a good choice for the adolescent who has infrequent intercourse and does not wish to expose herself to the risks of the oral contraceptive or the intrauterine device (IUD). For those adolescents who have intercourse more frequently, effectiveness and spontaneity may make the pill a better choice.

Cost.—The diaphragm and oral contraceptives are less expensive methods of contraception for adolescents who have frequent intercourse than are foam and condoms.

Access to Care.—Adolescents in rural or underserved areas may benefit from methods that do not require frequent follow-up visits.

Partner Cooperation.—Methods such as the condom, diaphragm, and spermicides require partner cooperation. If this cooperation is unlikely, another method should be chosen.

Medical Contraindications.—Selection of a method must always follow a thorough medical history and physical examination (Table 7–3).

Age.—Effectiveness of use for all methods increases with the age and income of the user. Barrier methods, especially the diaphragm, are associated with high failure rates in young adolescents. The oral contraceptive has the lowest failure rate across all age groups.

Education.—The adolescent should understand the correct use of the selected method, the major and minor side effects, and the backup methods of contraception. Whenever possible, she should demonstrate correct use of the method, and should leave the office with written instructions.

Follow-up.—Method and individual needs determine the appropriate follow-up interval. All adolescents, especially the youngest, benefit from close follow-up. Telephone contact should be encouraged to alleviate concerns and answer questions.

In summary, the contraceptive method should be chosen by the adolescent and must be consistent with her life-style and resources. She should understand its proper use and should feel free to contact the health provider if questions or problems arise.[6, 7]

CONTRACEPTIVE METHODS

The question asked most frequently of health providers by women requesting contraception is "How effective is my method?"[7] The correct answer, especially for teenagers who may have difficulty with compliance, depends on both the theoretical and use effectiveness of the method. All women requesting contraception should understand that effectiveness depends on their care in using the method.

ORAL CONTRACEPTIVE

The oral contraceptive is the most popular method of contraception worldwide. The theoretical effectiveness of the pill is 99.66% (or 0.34 pregnancies per 100 women using the pill for 1 year). Its use effectiveness is 98% (2 pregnancies per 100 women using the pill for 1 year). Failure rates are much higher for teenagers, however, because 60% of adolescents who begin taking oral contraceptives discontinue them within 1 year. Of those who discontinue oral contraceptives, 27% become pregnant unintentionally within 18 months.

The health provider should be well aware of the absolute and relative contraindications to estrogen-containing birth control pills (see Table 7–3). When counseling patients about the relative risks of oral contraceptives, it is important to emphasize that the mortality rate of pregnancy-related complications (20.6 per 100,000 live births) is more than five times greater than the annual pill-related mortality (3.7 per 100,000 users). Although heart attack, cerebrovascular accident, and venous thrombosis are more common in women who use the pill, these cardiovascular risks are concentrated among women over the age of 35 years who smoke. The excess annual mortality rate among nonsmoking pill users younger than 35 years is 1 in 77,000.[7] For the adolescent who does not smoke, risk to life is virtually the same as with use of the diaphragm or condom.

Oral contraceptives carry higher rates of morbidity than the barrier methods. As many as 5% of women taking birth control pills develop hypertension. It usually is mild (10 to 20 mm Hg rise in diastolic and 20 to 40 mm Hg rise in systolic) and returns to normal within 2 to 12 weeks after discontinuation of oral contraceptives. Hypertension sharply increases the risk of cardiovascular disease among women who are taking the birth control pill. Smokers with hypertension who continue to take oral contraceptives are at 170 times the risk for myocardial infarction as are those who do not take birth control pills.

Effects of the oral contraceptive pill on the hepatobiliary system include cholestatic jaundice, pruritis, hepatic adeoma (1 per 500,000 to 1 million users), and gallbladder disease (158 per 100,000 users). The relative risk of cholelithiasis among adolescent oral contraceptive users (3.1) is higher than among older users (1.15 to 1.5). There is no evidence that the pill causes cancer of the ovary, uterus, or breast. In fact, oral contraceptive use is associated with a decreased risk for endometrial cancer, ovarian cancer, and benign breast lesions (fibroadenomas and fibrocystic changes). Other health benefits of oral contraceptive use include decreased risk for pelvic inflammatory disease, menorrhagia, dysmenorrhea, functional ovarian cysts, and premenstrual symptoms.[7–9]

Patients taking oral contraceptives should be informed of its associated risks and possible side effects. Symptoms that require immediate medical attention include severe chest or abdominal pain, dyspnea, calf or thigh pain, severe headache, and blurred vision. Minor side effects of the pill include breakthrough bleeding, breast swelling or tenderness, change in appetite, nausea, cramping, vaginitis, and depression. Although these symptoms do not impose an immediate risk and often resolve within two to three cycles, they are an important cause of discontinuation of the pill. Breakthrough bleeding is especially common with the lower potency oral contraceptives that now are used; it usually improves spontaneously within four cycles. If the bleeding continues and occurs in the first half of the cycle, the estrogen component of the pill should be increased. If it occurs during the second half of the cycle, the progestin component should be increased.

The oral contraceptive of choice contains the lowest dose of estrogen (30–35 μg) and progesterone consistent with the prevention of pregnancy. Multiphasic pills minimize the total amount of hormone delivered over the course of the cycle, thus reducing the incidence of side effects. A 28-day regimen rather than a 21-day regimen usually is preferred by adolescents because it avoids confusion about when to begin subsequent cycles. Depending on the oral contraceptive brand, the first cycle may begin on the fifth day of menses, the first Sunday after the start of menses, or the first day of menses. One pill should be taken at the same time each day until the packet is finished, and a new packet should be started the next day.

Taking the pills with meals or in the evening reduces the incidence of nausea, a common cause of noncompliance in adolescents. Although a backup method of contraception is recommended during the first cycle, it probably is necessary only if the pills are started after the fifth menstrual day. A backup method always should be used during the first few months when the progestin-only pill (minipill) is prescribed. Because the pregnancy rate for the minipill is higher than it is for combined oral contraceptives, it is best to always use a second method during midcycle. The minipill is indicated in women over the age of 35 years who want to use oral contraceptives and in women in whom use of the combination pill is contraindicated. It is used infrequently in adolescents and is not the oral contraceptive of choice.

If the patient forgets to take one pill, she should take it as soon as she remembers or with the next day's pill at the regular time. If two pills are missed, two should be taken when she remembers and two the next day. If three pills are missed, she should stop taking the pills and resume again 7 days after the last pill was taken. In all of these instances, the patient should use a backup method of contraception for at least 7 days. This is especially important if the missed pill is the first of a new cycle.

Patients who are beginning to take oral contraceptives should return for follow-up visits at intervals of 1 month, 3 months, and 6 months.

CONDOM

The high rates of sexually transmitted disease among adolescents and the emergence of AIDS as a major epidemic have prompted the use of condoms for both contraception and protection against infection. *All adolescents should be urged to use condoms during all episodes of intercourse even if other methods are used simultaneously.*

In 1987, 6.9 million women in the United States reported that they relied on condoms for contraception. The theoretical effectiveness of the condom is 98%, and it use effectiveness is 90%.[7] When a spermicide is used with the condom the effectiveness approaches that of oral contraceptives. Adolescent boys and girls should be instructed in the proper use of the condom. It should be placed on the erect penis prior to penetration, leaving a reservoir of one-half inch for semen. The condom should be held in place by the boy on withdrawal. If the condom tears or slips off, a spermicidal foam or jelly should be used immediately by the girl.

Condoms are readily available to adolescents for over-the-counter purchase. Some state medical assistance programs provide reimbursement when the condoms are purchased with physician prescriptions. Only latex condoms should be recommended, because the nonlatex brands provide less protection against HIV infection.[10] Condoms with spermicide may provide added protection against HIV infection and other sexually transmitted diseases. It remains unclear, however, whether this small amount of spermicide adds to the contraceptive effectiveness of the condom. For this reason, adolescents who rely on condoms for contraception should always use a spermicidal agent regardless of the type of condom. Noncontraceptive lubricants that can be used with the condom include K-Y Jelly and saliva. Vaseline should not be used, because it causes deterioration of the rubber.

The disadvantages of the condom include interference with sexual spontaneity or pleasure and occasional allergic reactions to rubber-containing condoms. The advantages are low costs, accessibility, medical safety, and protection against sexually transmitted disease.

VAGINAL SPERMICIDES

The vaginal spermicides include foam, suppositories, creams, and jellies. They all consist of an inert base that adheres to the cervix and a chemical that kills sperm. Theoretical effectiveness is 95% to 97%; use effectiveness is 85%. High failure rates are due to using inadequate amounts of the agent, failure to shake the foam container, failure to place the agent high in the vagina, douching within 8 hours of intercourse, and complete failure to use the agent. The spermicidal creams and jellies are less effective than foam and suppositories and are indicated for use with the diaphragm. Even the foam and suppositories, however, should be used with another method such as the condom. The major contraindication to use of vaginal spermicides is allergy to either the inert base or spermicidal agent. Noncontraceptive benefits include vaginal lubrication and decreased risk of sexually transmitted disease.

Adolescents should be instructed about proper use of these agents. The foam container should be shaken 20 times before filling the applicator. The foam then should be dispensed near the cervix within 30 minutes of intercourse. If more than 30 minutes elapses, another full applicator should be inserted. Vaginal suppositories are easy to insert but require 10 to 30 minutes for dissolution and full spermicidal effect.

CONTRACEPTIVE SPONGE

Since its introduction in the United States in 1983 the contraceptive sponge has become a popular form of birth control. It is a flattened disk of polyurethane that is impregnated with a spermicide (nonoxynol 9) and preservatives. The sponge must be moistened with tap water prior to insertion to activate the spermicide. It may be placed in the vagina up to 12 hours before intercourse, remains effective without additional spermicide for 24 hours, and must be left in place for at least 6 hours after last intercourse. Recent data suggest a use effectiveness of 86.7% (13.3 pregnancies per 100 woman-years of use). Advantages of the sponge include ease of use, availability without fitting, 24-hour effectiveness, and partial protection against sexually transmitted disease. Its cost is comparable to the combined cost of condoms and spermicide.[11]

DIAPHRAGM

The diaphragm has undergone a recent resurgence in popularity because of adverse publicity associated with the oral contraceptive and the IUD. It is a safe method of contraception, with failure rates ranging from 2 to 17 pregnancies per 100 woman-years of use.[7] College-aged women in particular are choosing the diaphragm with greater frequency and are proving to be effective users. Although the failure rate among adolescents approaches 15%, this is similar to the failure rate of oral contraceptives in this population. In both cases the rates reflect improper use and discontinuation.[12]

The diaphragm is available in three rim shapes: arcing spring, coil spring, and flat spring. The arcing spring is appropriate for most women and is the easiest of the three shapes to insert. It is available in nine different rim diameters (55 to 95 mm). The most common error in diaphragm sizing is the prescription of a size that is too small. When inserted in the vagina, the diaphragm should cover the cervix; the posterior rim should be in the posterior fornix, and the anterior rim should fit snugly behind the pubic bone. Once the diaphragm is sized, the adolescent should insert and remove the diaphragm in the office and the health provider should check its position. The patient should return to the office within 2 weeks, with the diaphragm in place, so that the provider can recheck both size and placement.

The teenager must be able to comfortably insert, check, and remove the diaphragm. If she continues to demonstrate uneasiness with this at the visit 2 weeks later, a different method should be considered. She should understand that a contraceptive cream or jelly must be used with the diaphragm and that it must remain in place for at least 6 hours after intercourse. Repeated intercourse while the diaphragm is in place requires the addition of cream or jelly with an applicator. The diaphragm should be removed after 6 hours and washed with soap and water. The only absolute contraindication to the diaphragm is an allergy to the rubber or spermicide.

CERVICAL CAP

The cervical cap was approved for use in the United States in 1988. It consists of a pliable latex dome, firm rim, and inner groove that seals the cervix when properly placed. Like the diaphragm, the cap must be fitted and the patient must be instructed in insertion and removal. The cap is available in four sizes ranging from 22 to 31 mm inside diameter. Its theoretical effectiveness (93.6%) and use effectiveness (82.6%) are comparable to the rates for the diaphragm.

The cervical cap has several advantages over the diaphragm. The cap requires less spermicide on placement, does not require additional spermicide with repeated intercourse, and remains effective twice as long as the diaphragm. Fitting and placement of the cap are more difficult, however, and fewer sizes limit its use. In addition, the effects of the cap on cervical tissue remain unclear. Consequently it is recommended only for women with a normal Papanicolaou smear who will return for a repeat test after 3 months of use. Compared with diaphragm users, cervical cap users complain more of vaginal odor, especially with prolonged use, but complain less of discomfort during intercourse.

Health providers who prescribe the cervical cap must be well-trained in its fitting, and patients need extensive instruction and practice prior to use. These factors may make the cervical cap a less popular method of contraception among younger adolescents.[13]

INTRAUTERINE DEVICE

The IUD is not recommended for adolescents. Although its theoretical and use effectiveness are 96% to 99%, users are at increased risk for pelvic inflammatory disease, infertility, ectopic pregnancy, menorrhagia, and dysmenorrhea. The IUD is indicated only in multiparous women in stable monogamous relationships. Its use requires extensive counseling, informed consent, and a physician who is well-trained in its insertion and the management of complications.

OTHER METHODS

The "morning-after pill" can be prescribed for those adolescents who have had unprotected midcycle intercourse within the past 72 hours and are not pregnant. The risk of pregnancy without the morning-after pill is 2% to 30%; the risk of pregnancy with it is 0.03% to 0.3%. Either of the following regimens are acceptable: diethylstilbestrol, 25 mg taken orally twice a day for 5 days; or Ovral (50 μg ethinyl estradiol/0.5 mg norgestrel), two tablets as soon as possible and two tablets 12 hours later. The latter regimen has a similar effectiveness, causes fewer side effects, and has not been shown to adversely affect the fetus in case of pregnancy. With either regimen nausea is common. If the patient does not menstruate within 3 weeks of its use, a pregnancy test should be done.[7]

New methods currently under investigation include the antiprogestogen RU-486 and a condom for use by women. RU-486 is not a contraceptive but an abortifactant, or means of inducing early abortion. It should not be heralded as a substitute for effective preconception birth control.

SUMMARY

1. The oral contraceptive is the most popular and effective method of contraception. The patient should understand the major and minor side effects of the pill, and should always use another method if she decides to discontinue taking oral contraceptives.

2. The simultaneous use of condoms and a spermicidal agent is a safe and effective method of contraception and also maximizes protection against sexually transmitted disease.

3. The contraceptive sponge is a popular method of contraception, with a use effectiveness between that of a condom plus spermicide and a diaphragm.

4. The diaphragm is a safe and effective method of contraception. It requires accurate sizing, careful instruction, and patient comfort with insertion and removal.

5. The cervical cap resembles the diaphragm in its use effectiveness, required fitting, and user skill in placement and removal. Because of its potential association with cervical dysplasia, it may not be appropriate for adolescents who cannot be followed up closely.

6. The IUD is not recommended for adolescents because of the increased risk of pelvic inflammatory disease, consequent infertility, ectopic pregnancy, menorrhagia, and dysmenorrhea.

7. Ovral can be used as postcoital contraception if used within 72 hours of unprotected intercourse. Because side effects are common, it should be a method of last resort.

8. Any discussion of contraception must also include counselling about sexually-transmitted disease, especially AIDS. All sexually-active adolescents, regardless of contraceptive method, should be urged to use condoms.

REFERENCES

1. Jones EF, Forest JD, Goldman N, et al: Teenage pregnancies in developed countries: Determinants and policy implications. *Fam Plann Perspect* 1985; 17:53–63.

2. Dryfoos JG: *Teenage Pregnancy: The Problem That Hasn't Gone Away*. New York, Allan Guttmacher Institute, 1981.
3. Maciak BJ, Spitz AM, Strauss LT, et al: Pregnancy and birth rates among sexually-experienced U.S. teenagers—1974, 1980, and 1983. *JAMA* 1987; 258:2069–2071.
4. Westoff CF: Contraceptive paths toward the reduction of unintended pregnancy and abortion. *Fam Plann Perspec* 1988; 20:4–13.
5. Berger DK, Perez G, Kyman W, et al: Influence of family planning counseling in an adolescent clinic on sexual activity and contraceptive use. *J Adolesc Health Care* 1987; 8:436–440.
6. Greydanus DE, McAnarney R: Contraception in the adolescent: Current concepts for the pediatrician. *Pediatrics* 1980; 65:1–12.
7. Hatcher R, Guest F, Stewart F, et al: *Contraceptive Technology, 1986–1987*, ed 13. New York, Irvington Publishers, 1986.
8. Oral contraception. *ACOG Tech Bull* 1987; 106:1–5.
9. Dickey RP: *Managing Contraceptive Pill Patients*, ed 5. Durant OK, Creative Informatics, 1987.
10. Special AIDS issue. *FDA Drug Bull* 1987; 12:17–18.
11. Edelman DA, North BB: Updated pregnancy rates for the Today contraceptive sponge. *Am J Obstet Gynecol* 1987; 157:1164–1165.
12. Fisher M, Marks A, Trieller K: Comparative analysis of the effectiveness of the diaphragm and birth control pill during the first year of use among suburban adolescents. *J Adolesc Health Care* 1987; 8:393–399.
13. The cervical cap. *Med Lett* 1988; 30:93–94.
14. Grimes DA, Mishell DR Jr, Shoupe D, et al: Early abortion with a single dose of the antiprogestin RU-486. *Am J Obstet Gynecol* 1988; 158:1307–1312.

8 IMMUNIZATION

Thomas Beausang, M.D.

Immunization, an important medical task for the primary care physician, is an attempt to prevent or modify disease. The public health goal is to confer immunity to as many as possible, with the least risk of untoward reaction, at the least cost. The decision to immunize depends on the severity of the disease, the probability of exposure, the immune status of the individual receiving the vaccine, and the effectiveness of the vaccine.

The mechanics of immunization are critical in achieving a protective response, and include dose, route of administration, technique, and the schedule for administering each vaccine. In general, it is unwise to give divided doses of a vaccine as there may be inadequate antigenic mass to stimulate an immune response. Storage of the vaccine is important, because live virus vaccines must remain able to replicate and proteins in inactive vaccines must not be allowed to denature. Schedules are devised to assure the immunization of the greatest number of susceptible individuals at a time when the protection is most likely to be durable and before exposure to natural disease. However, schedules must be adapted to an individual's particular needs and risks.

Safety of the vaccine is an important consideration. Benefits of the vaccine should outweigh the risks of natural disease. Vaccines may have side effects or adverse reactions. Side effects are frequently seen, with mild occurrences such as a sore extremity, localized redness, or moderate fever following diphtheria-tetanus-pertussis (DTP) immunization. Adverse reactions are infrequent, often severe manifestations such as seizures or cardiovascular collapse seen with DTP, paralysis following oral polio vaccine (OPV), or subacute sclerosing panencephalitis (SSPE) associated with measles immunization.

Before administering any vaccine, the physician should look for any contraindications. It is unwise to administer a vaccine during an acute febrile illness. Examples of contraindications are prior anaphylactic reactions to tetanus toxoid or a previous seizure after DTP immunization. Children who are immunocompromised should not be given live virus vaccines. If a parent or family member's immunity is compromised, live polio vaccine should be avoided and inactive polio vaccine administered. The "Red Book," the *Report of the Committee on Infectious Diseases*, should be consulted for complete details of contraindications.

CONTRAINDICATIONS FOR IMMUNIZATION

DTP
- High temperature or definite illness
- Progressive neurologic disease
- History of episode following DTP
  - Seizure
  - Encephalitis
  - Focal neurologic signs
  - Persistent screaming
  - Somnolence
  - Temperature greater than 105° F
  - Anaphylactic reaction

OPV
- Immunodeficiency or immunosuppression in patient or family member

MMR (measles-mumps-rubella)
- Pregnancy, active tuberculosis, immunodeficiency, or immunosuppression

Hypersensitivity reactions are rare. There may be allergic reactions to egg-related antigens from influenza, yellow fever, duck embryo rabies, and typhus vaccines. Chick embryo tissue culture vaccines are associated with almost no case reports of reaction involving people allergic to egg or chicken. Mercury sensitivity may occur in those receiving large amounts of gammaglobulin. There may be allergic sensitivity to antibiotics used to prevent bacterial contamination.

Records of immunizations are necessary for both physicians and parents to prevent unnecessary reimmunization and to attempt to ensure full immunization of as many susceptible persons as possible. In addition to recording the date, the National Childhood Vaccine Injury Act requires that the manufacturer, lot number, expiration date site, and the name of the person administering the vaccine be recorded. If the vaccine is refused, "informed refusal," warning of forseeable dangers of not receiving the vaccine should be documented.

In the last few years informed consent for immunization has become an issue. Despite the fact that the risk of serious reactions is low and considerable doubt exists that informed consent will prevent litigation, the signed consent of parents should be obtained for each child's immunization (just as consent forms are obtained for any surgical procedure). There should be a short general discussion with each parent about the relative risks of vaccine and the very severe disease that unprotected individuals may contract. Examples of the severe illness caused by tetanus or diphtheria may be helpful. There should also be preparation for the common, distressing, but not serious side effects, for example, the irritability, sore extremity, or mild fever seen with a DTP immunization. The measures that may be taken to relieve the child's discomfort should be discussed.

Simultaneous administration of DTP, OPV, MMR, and *Hemophilus influenzae* type b (Hib) conjugate vaccines appropriate for the child's age may be given if the individual is unlikely to return for vaccination.

IMMUNIZATION PROGRAMS

Four immunizations that should be given for everyone unless specifically contraindicated are DTP, OPV, MMR, and Hib conjugate.

DTP

DTP vaccine is composed of diphtheria and tetanus toxoids and killed pertussis organisms. Routine immunization of children should approximate the schedule outlined in this section. Diphtheria is a serious illness, with a 10% to 20% mortality rate in unimmunized children. Diphtheria does occur in adequately immunized persons but is rarely life threatening. The major contraindication is an anaphylactic reaction to a previous dose of vaccine. Local reactions are occasionally painful. Diphtheria toxoid is also available in a strength containing about one-tenth the dose of pediatric diphtheria toxoid (Td). It is administered to individuals over the age of 7 years and causes less severe reactions.

Schick testing can be done to determine immunity to diphtheria. The Schick test measures circulating antibody. The diphtheria toxin is injected and produces redness and necrosis in 2 to 5 days in patients who are susceptible to diphtheria (Schick-positive). Although Schick testing is an alternative to booster doses, it is less practical than giving a tetanus-diphtheria (Td) booster during a diphtheria outbreak. After exposure to diphtheria, a Schick test and Td booster should be administered at the same time. If the results of the Schick test are positive, a second dose should be administered in 1 month.

Tetanus has a mortality rate of about 50%. It can occur after even trivial wounds. Everyone should be immunized against tetanus. Primary immunization during infancy can be accomplished as recommended in the following schedule.

Tetanus toxoid boosters may be given as a routine booster or as an emergency booster following an injury. The decision to give an emergency booster is based on experience and past studies of antitoxin levels of individuals with known immunization histories. Routine tetanus boosters are recommended every 10 years after the child has had three primary injections and two boosters.

For clean minor wounds, no emergency booster is necessary if it has been less than 10 years since the last tetanus infection. For contaminated wounds, no booster is necessary if it has been less than 5 years since the last booster. Tetanus immune globulin (TIG) should be given if there have been less than two previous injections of toxoid or the wound has been neglected for more than 24 hours. Tetanus immune globulin is a gammaglobulin derived from hyperimmunized human volunteers. The recommended dose is 250 to 500 units intramuscularly. Tetanus toxoid should also be given at the same time as TIG but at a different site. A severe allergic reaction to a previous injection is exceedingly rare but is a contraindication to tetanus-toxoid administration.

The pertussis component of the DTP immunization has the most notoriety at the present time. Pertussis is a serious illness in infants, with a significant rate of mortality. The disease is more frequently encountered than diphtheria and tetanus. Protective immunity is probably only partially antibody mediated, and sufficient antibodies are not transmitted across the placenta to protect the infant. The killed pertussis vaccine is less effective than other vaccines in stimulating protective immunity. Children who had pertussis documented with either a culture or a positive fluorescent antibody smear need not be immunized.

Contraindications to immunization are fever, concurrent illness, and progressive neurologic disease. Symptoms of minor respiratory tract infections should not be regarded as a contraindication if the family is thought unlikely to return for immunization. Further pertussis immunizations should not be given if an acute neurologic episode (e.g., seizure, encephalitis, excessive crying, or focal neurologic signs or collapse) follows a DTP immunization. Infants who experience excessive somnolence, persistent screaming (more than 3 hours' duration), and temperature greater than 105° F should not be given further doses of pertussis vaccine. Routine immunization is recommended as listed in the schedule. Pertussis immunization should not be given after the age of 6 years. Those who have had contact with pertussis should be given a booster dose of vaccine and erythromycin because protection is not absolute. In pertussis epidemics, adolescents and adults could receive 0.25 mL of pertussis vaccine. Pertussis immune globulin has been shown to have no value for treatment or prevention of disease. The American Academy of Pediatrics Committee on Infectious Diseases makes periodic recommendations about immunizations, especially pertussis, and should be consulted for the latest opinions.

POLIO VACCINE

Polio virus infections are generally asymptomatic or undetected. Paralysis, when it occurs, is often extensive. About 5% of paralytic cases are fatal. There are two vaccines, a live attenuated vaccine given orally for types 1, 2, and 3, and an inactivated polio virus vaccine given parenterally. OPV stimulates natural immunity, producing intestinal resistance and circulating antibody. Breast feeding does not interfere with immunizations. The live virus is excreted in the stool and can infect exposed individuals. Intrafamilial spread is about 50% in some studies. Extrafamilial spread is probably 5% to 10%. Paralytic poliomyelitis secondary to vaccine occurs in 1 per 8 million individuals given the vaccine and 1 per 5 million contacts of vaccines. Although paralysis is rare, live polio vaccine is no longer routinely administered to adults. OPV should be given to infants in two or three doses at 8-week intervals, and another dose 6 to 12 months later. Multiple doses are not boosters but are given to ensure immunity to all three serotypes.

Live virus vaccine should not be administered to immunodeficient individuals including those receiving immunosuppressive therapy. Because the live vaccine is excreted and is infectious, this exclusion applies also to individuals whose family members are immunodeficient. Inactivated polio virus (IPV) is given to these individuals. Three doses of IPV are necessary for primary immunization; the first two are given at intervals of 4 to 8 weeks; the third, 6 to 12 months later. Boosters are recommended every 5 years for children and adolescents until the duration of immunity from enhanced IPV is known. Untoward reactions to IPV have not been reported. Administration of IPV does not prevent spread of wild polio virus and is impractical for large scale use in the United States. If IPV is used to immunize susceptible adults in families whose children need OPV, it is important that no strategy be used that decreases the likelihood of the children receiving their necessary immunizing dose of OPV.

MMR

Measles is often a severe illness. In outbreaks of measles, encephalitis was reported in 1 per 1,000 reported cases, with 50% having permanent sequelae. The major complication of mumps virus infection is orchitis in 15% of adult cases and, in rare cases, severe neurologic disease such as deafness. Rubella is a mild disease in childhood. However, it may have disastrous effects on a fetus whose mother is susceptible during the first trimester of pregnancy.

Children should be considered susceptible to these illnesses unless there is a history of immunization or serologic evidence of immunity. Pregnancy and concurrent immunosuppressive therapy are contraindications for MMR vaccine. Active tuberculosis is a contraindication for administration of measles vaccine. Allergy to eggs is not a contraindication. A side effect of measles vaccines produced by the attenuated strains is an illness similar to mild measles in about 10% of recipients. Patients may have fever, cough, red eyes, rhinorrhea, and rash 6 to 11 days after immunization. Severe neurologic complications occur rarely. An increased incidence of side effects has been reported in individuals receiving live measles vaccine after having had killed measles virus vaccine. These are much less severe than "atypical measles" reported with wild virus infection. Significant complications of mumps vaccine have not been reported. Occasional low-grade fever may be present for 5 to 18 days after immunization. Adverse reactions with rubella RA 27/3 vaccine are rash, fever, and lymphadenopathy. Occasional arthralgias are noted. Frank arthritis is less common and usually occurs in postpubertal girls 7 to 21 days after immunization. It is usually transient.

The MMR immunizations should be given when the infant is 15 months of age. Those immunized prior to 1 year of age should have another injection. In 1989 the Academy of Pediatrics recommended a booster at age 15 years. Vaccination of individuals with acute febrile illness should be delayed until recovery. Family members of an immunocompromised individual may be immunized with MMR vaccine because the vaccine is not transmissible. Girls of childbearing age may be immunized if there are proper precautions against pregnancy. Records of older girls should be thoroughly reviewed prior to puberty to assure they are immune.

A polysaccharide-conjugate vaccine against invasive disease caused by Hib was licensed in 1987. Hib causes serious disease, such as meningitis, cellulitis, epiglottitis, pneumonia, and septic arthritis. The vaccine should be routinely administered to all children at 18 months of age. Side effects such as fever and local reactions are generally mild. Several other conjugate vaccines are under development for infants younger than 18 months of age.

RECOMMENDED IMMUNIZATION SCHEDULE

Age 2 mo: DTP, OPV
Age 4 mo: DTP, OPV
Age 6 mo: DTP
Age 15 mo: MMR
Age 18 mo: DTP, OPV, Hib conjugate
Age 4 to 6 yr: DTP, OPV
Every 10 yr after last immunization: TD

VACCINES WITH SPECIFIC INDICATIONS

There are several other vaccines that occasionally may be used with specific indications. Rabies has the highest mortality of any infection in humans. While rabies rarely occurs in humans in the United States, knowledge of vaccine usage is important since one-half million doses are distributed each year in this country. There is a large reservoir of rabies in animals, including skunks, bats, raccoons, foxes, and in some areas dogs and cats. It is rare in small rodents and rabbits. Consultation with the local health department is important as it can provide information about risk of rabies in an area for a particular species of animal. Transmission is usually by bite. Airborne transmission has been reported in cave explorers. Local wound care is very important; the injury must be thoroughly cleaned with soap and water. Human diploid-cell vaccine (HDCV) or rabies vaccine, absorbed (RVA) are now the preferred vaccines. Passive and active immunization are recommended. Reactions to HDCV are fever, local reactions, and nausea. Serious systemic reactions, anaphylaxis, or neuroparalysis are rare. HDCV is given intramuscularly (in the deltoid) on the day of the bite and on days 3, 7, 14, and 28 following the bite. Human rabies immune globulin should be given at another site in combination with the first dose of vaccine for postexposure prophylaxis.

Influenza vaccine is recommended for children with an increased likelihood of a complication after influenza infection. These conditions include chronic cardiovascular, pulmonary, renal, metabolic, hematologic, or malignant disease. Few data are available for children less than 6 months old, but the vaccine may have value for infants with bronchopulmonary dysplasia. Because of antigenic drift, past infection is only protective to the degree that the current virus is antigenically similar to the past strains. Contraindications are anaphylactic reactions to egg protein. Inactivated influenza vaccines are formulated yearly containing antigens of several strains thought likely to be prevalent. Split virus preparations, which are more highly purified, are recommended for children since they are associated with fewer side effects. Side effects may include local induration, redness, fever, malaise, and myalgia for 1 to 2 days after immunization.

Pneumococcal infection is most severe in individuals with defective or absent splenic function. It is also the most common cause of otitis media, sinusitis, bacterial pneumonia, and occult bacteremia. A 23-valent capsular polysaccharide antigen is available. It is recommended for children with sickle cell disease, asplenia (for whatever reason), rheumatic fever, nephrotic syndrome, and immunodeficiency. It may be useful for prevention of some otitis media, although it is of limited immunogenicity in children younger than 2 years, when otitis is most prevalent. Adverse reactions include local soreness and occasional low-grade fever. Booster doses are not recommended.

A meningococcal vaccine for types A, C, Y, and W-135 is available in the United States. Most meningococcal disease in the country is caused by type b, for which there is no vaccine. Vaccines may be useful for contacts of individuals with disease due to the above serotypes. The vaccine should be administered to children aged 2 years and older with functional or anatomic asplenia.

Hepatitis B occurs in about 200,000 persons per year in the United States. Pediatric exposure occurs primarily in infants born to mothers who are chronic carriers, in family members of chronic carriers, in children subjected to frequent blood transfusions or hemodialysis, in illicit parenteral drug users, and in male homosexuals. Hepatitis B vaccine is an inactivated virus vaccine. Since infants born to HBsAg-positive mothers are at high risk for becoming carriers of HBV, they should receive hyperimmune hepatitis B serum immediately after delivery and hepatitis B vaccine in the first 24 hours of life and again at 1 month and 6 months of age.

A number of different immunizations may be

needed for foreign travel. Requirements vary with different countries. Sources of information are the U.S. Public Health Service, the *Morbidity and Mortality Weekly Report,* and the booklet *Health Information for International Travel.*

PASSIVE IMMUNITY

Passive immunity is accomplished by passive transfer of preformed immunoglobulin. The immunoglobulin may be derived from either humans or animals. Human immune serum globulin (IG) is used for replacement therapy in individuals deficient in IgG and for prophylaxis of hepatitis A, measles, and hepatitis B (if specific hepatitis B globulin is not available).

All household contacts of persons with hepatitis A should receive 0.02 mL/kg of IG as soon as possible after exposure. The use of IG more than 2 weeks after exposure or after onset of clinical illness is not indicated. Exposure of children in daycare centers has often resulted in epidemics. IG is indicated if one or more children or two or more households have hepatitis. Prophylaxis should also be given at the time of exposure to individuals in custodial care. Exposure of older children in classrooms generally does not require immunization unless there is an epidemic. Immune serum globulin is not indicated for infants whose mothers have had hepatitis A during pregnancy unless the mother has jaundice at the time of delivery. Tourists in rural villages in the tropics should receive preexposure prophylaxis.

Unimmunized individuals exposed to measles should be given 0.25 mL/kg of IG and should be actively immunized 3 months later. Susceptible immunocompromised individuals should be given 0.5 mL/kg of IG.

Immune globulin has a titer of at least 1:100 against hepatitis B surface antigen (HBsAg). Hepatitis B immune globulin (HBIG) has a titer of 1:100,000 or more. HBIG is about 75% protective in postexposure prophylaxis. A newborn infant whose mother is a carrier should be given 0.5 mL of HBIG soon after delivery and hepatitis vaccine as mentioned in the last section. Individuals exposed to blood that is positive for hepatitis B antigen should receive HBIG 0.06 mL/kg as soon as possible. The identical dose should be repeated in 1 month. Exposure to a needle stick from high-risk individuals (persons with Down syndrome, patients receiving dialysis) who have uncertain HBsAg status requires testing of serum for the HBsAg. If results are positive, HBIG should be given and repeated in 1 month. If results are negative, nothing further need be done.

After exposure to varicella, varicella-zoster immune globulin (VZIG) vaccine should be given to immunocompromised individuals including people with malignancies, immunodeficiency, and immunosuppression with medications, and newborn infants whose mothers have active varicella within a few days of delivery. Exposure should include a close contact, a playmate or sibling, or presence in the same room in a hospital. Less than 72 hours should elapse since exposure and there should be a negative disease history. The VZIG vaccine may be obtained from the regional American Red Cross office. Steroids and chemotherapy should be stopped, if possible, at the time of exposure. A live varicella vaccine is currently being used for individuals in controlled studies.

Occasionally animal-derived immunoglobulins are used for treatment of diphtheria, botulism, or venemous snake exposure. It is extremely important to test sensitivity with scratch tests followed by intradermal tests. One must be prepared to treat a severe anaphylactic reaction immediately and later be prepared to treat febrile reactions or serum sickness.

BIBLIOGRAPHY

Cherry J, Brunell P, Golden G, et al: Report on the Task Force on Pertussis and Pertussis Immunization—1988. *Pediatrics* 1988; 81:939–984.

Report of the Committee on Infectious Diseases, ed 21. Evanston, Ill, American Academy of Pediatrics, 1988.

Current trends: Rabies vaccine, adsorbed: A new rabies vaccine for use in humans. *MMWR* 1988; 37:217.

Moffet HL: *Pediatric Infectious Diseases,* vol 2. Philadelphia, JB Lippincott, 1981.

Proceedings of a Roundtable: *Haemophilus influenzae* type b: The disease and its prevention. *Pediatr Infect Dis* 1987; 6:773.

Recommendations of the Immunization Practices Advisory Committee (ACIP). Update: Preventation of *Hemophilus influenzae* type b disease. *MMWR* 1988; 37:13.

Recommendations of the Immunization Practices Advisory Committee (ACIP): Diphtheria, tetanus and pertussis: Guidelines for vaccine prophylaxis and other preventative measures. *MMWR* 1985; 34:405.

Sabin AB: Commentary: Is there a need for a change in poliomyelitis immunization policy? Opinion and analysis. *Ped Infect Dis* 1987; 6:887.

9 SCREENING

Steven B. Pierdon, M.D.

PRINCIPLES AND CAUTIONS

Screening is the evaluation of an asymptomatic population by specific means to detect the possibility of a defined condition. It is assumed that the early recognition of the condition will decrease morbidity or mortality by allowing earlier treatment. The disease or condition must be both significant and treatable to justify screening an entire asymptomatic population. In addition, the condition must occur with such frequency or be of such severity that the potential benefits to the individual and society make the screening worthwhile.

At a health supervision visit, screening procedures are part of comprehensive care that includes health maintenance, disease prevention, immunization, and anticipatory guidance. The nature of screening programs requires that the physician be prepared to go beyond the screening test to accurately diagnose and comprehensively treat identified individuals. Without follow-up, neither diagnostic studies nor treatment is assured as a result of screening. Over time, advances in technology and clinical research will mandate changes in the optimal screening procedures and schedule.

GROWTH

The monitoring of growth parameters has always been an integral part of the health supervision visit. Accurate measurements of the weight, height, and head circumference of children younger than 2 years and the plotting of these measurements on an appropriate growth curve is an important part of a child's medical record. Only by noting changes in growth chart percentiles over time can valid information be determined to allow the detection of endocrine or nutritional disorders.

Obesity is the most common growth disorder in pediatrics, found in 5% to 25% of children, depending on the definition used, and increases in frequency until adulthood. Obesity is most easily diagnosed by weight more than 120% expected for height in correlation with gross visual inspection. Stable weight for height percentiles are of less concern than changing percentiles. The majority of overweight children are mildly obese, and in many the disorder does not progress in severity. Endocrine abnormalities, eating disorders, and constitutional diseases such as inflammatory bowel disease are far less common and may be detected with other findings prior to detection with growth measurements.

The need to detect obesity and to begin counseling stems from the increasing awareness of long-term cardiovascular risks and known psychosocial, orthopedic, and respiratory problems found in the moderately and severely obese child. The plotting of growth charts during health supervision visits allows the parents to visualize their child's growth over time. These growth charts may make the parents more receptive to intervention for the obese child, and can also be reassuring to the parent concerned about appetite and nutrition.

DEVELOPMENT

Assessment of development begins with the recognition that there are subcategories and that children progress at individual rates. Accurate screening requires determination of milestones in each of the subcategories. Although global delay in attaining milestones may be seen, significant delays are often present in only one or two areas.

Development is frequently assessed by the parent's history of milestone attainment in conjunction with the physician's examination and observation in the clinical setting. This has been shown to underidentify significant numbers of children. Parental recall is frequently in error, although reporting of current milestones is apparently more accurate. There is no assurance of complete assessment of all areas without the structure of a formal testing instrument.

In spite of their general acceptance, the time requirements of formal screening tests in addition to the perceived difficulties of integrating them into office procedure have resulted in poor utilization of the tests. Formal screening devices at specific intervals should be used within the framework of health maintenance visits. The Denver Development Screening Test (DDST)* is the most widely recognized screening instrument. It is used for children aged 0 to 6 years and assesses gross and fine motor skills, language, and social development. A two-step screening procedure coordinating the Revised Prescreening Developmental Questionnaire (R-PDQ) with the DDST makes this instrument more practical in the office setting. The recommended ages for screening are quite varied; one schedule would include children who are 3, 9, 18 months, and 3, 4, 5, and 6 years old.

The DDST has been criticized for underidentifying children with speech and language disorders. Delays in the development of speech and language represent the most common type of developmental delay found with screening. Incorporating a more sensitive language screening device into the screening schedule would increase the detection rate of these problems. The Receptive-Expressive Emergent Language Scale (REEL) and the Early Language Milestone Scale (ELM) are designed specifically for children younger than 3 years old and can be administered by primary care physicians.

Surveys of current usage patterns indicate that developmental screening tests are being used as diagnostic tests or as confirmatory tests in children already thought to be developmentally delayed. This application of a screening test is inappropriate. Abnormalities of development suggested by screening should be evaluated by definitive tests or referrals, depending on the degree and type of abnormality suggested.

VISION

Visual function is a dynamic process in the infant and young child. The growth of the face, orbit, extraocular muscles, and internal structures of the eye contributes to a changing incidence of problems as well as different types of disorders, depending on the age of the child. Abnormalities found in the newborn tend to be less frequent but are often more significant. Screening for toddlers and young children usually detects several percent of the population with strabismus or amblyopia. The incidence of refractive problems found in school-aged children and adolescents varies from about 5% at preschool age to about 50% by the end of adolescence. Screening programs need to consider both the incidence and type of pathologic process most often found at the various ages.

The history given by the parents may be the first indicator of visual problems at any age. Both intermittent and fine variations of visual performance may be evident to the attentive parent. The screening process for infants includes the determination that the structure of the eye is intact and that the developing coordination of vision is age appropriate. Initial examinations of the eye should verify the normality of pupil, iris, and lens. Consideration of the size and placement of the eye may alert the examiner to congenital abnormality.

Direct ophthalmoscopic examinations should be performed in all infants for evaluation of possible cataracts. Lens opacities occur in about 1 in 250 children, and many are charac-

*DDST screening materials are available from Denver Developmental Materials, PO Box 6919, Denver, CO 80206-0919/(303-355-4729).

teristic of systemic disease, such as congenital infection or galactosemia. Cataracts may also be associated with other abnormalities of the eyes, such as microphthalmos, iris hypoplasia, and glaucoma. Discrete dots and small white plaquelike cataracts are often the remnants of the embryologic development of the eye. They may be stable and not interfere with vision. The majority of lens opacities require ophthalmologic evaluation and treatment.

The abnormal or incomplete development of binocular visual alignment with its subsequent amblyopia is one of the most common abnormalities detected by visual screening. Visual fixation usually begins within the first few weeks after birth, and by 3 months of age is present in all fields of gaze. This is demonstrated by a corneal light reflex that is symmetrically centered in the pupils of both eyes in all quadrants. Aligned corneal light reflexes distinguish the pseudostrabismus caused by a wide nasal bridge. Momentary dysconjugate movements of the eyes are common in infancy.

Amblyopia or loss of vision by disuse results from cortical suppression of the double image occurring when there is malalignment of the two visual axes. The angle of deviation between the visual axes does not correlate with the degree of amblyopia. Amblyopia is less likely to occur when the image in each eye is used alternatively than when a single image is consistently suppressed. Common compensatory behaviors such as head tilt or turning should precipitate a detailed examination for occult strabismus. The normal development of stereoscopic vision requires that strabismus and amblyopia be corrected by the age of 6 years, and preferably well before school age (see Chapters 53 and 96).

In the young infant and toddler, repeated evaluations of fixation and following should be performed to detect acquired strabismus that may have not been present in earlier examinations. Use of the cover test will demonstrate even small degrees of malalignment. Covering the dominant eye after fixation on a distant object causes movement for realignment by the nondominant eye. Uncovering allows fixation by the dominant eye and a change in alignment by the nondominant eye. Number or random-dot stereograms (Randot) show different images for monocular binocular vision (Fig 9–1).

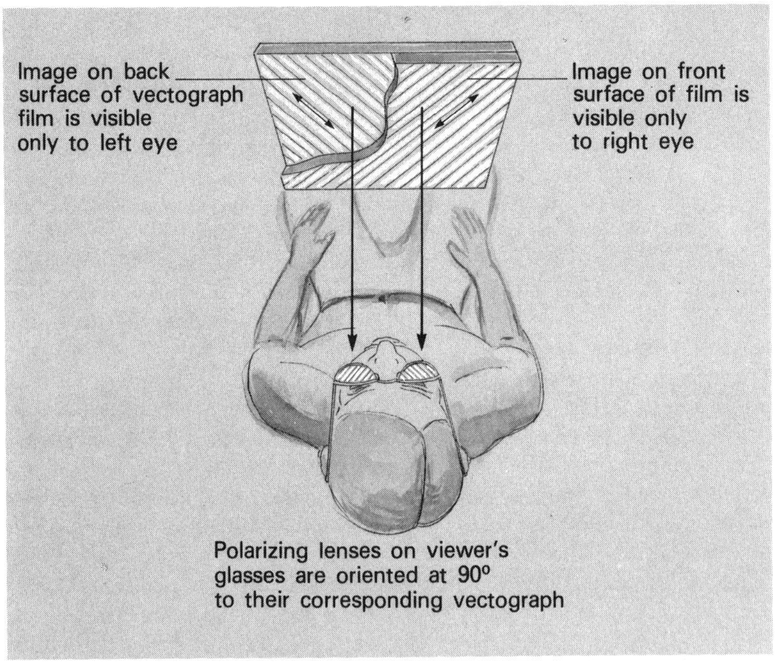

FIG 9–1

Use of stereogram permits identification of amblyopia. If vision is suppressed in one eye the child is unable to distinguish particular test items.

These represent a more standardized screening for amblyopia and can be used for children aged 3 to 5 years.

Children older than 4 years usually can undergo visual acuity screening with either picture or illiterate E charts that correlate with visual acuity. Failure to demonstrate 20/30 acuity in either eye should prompt retesting or referral for further evaluation. Screening for color blindness can be done easily with isochromatic plates at the preschool evaluation. Surprise testing for visual field is also possible in this age group. Visual acuity screening for the older school-aged child should be done every other year to aid in detection of acquired refractive errors. The local school system may provide this periodic screening.

HEARING

Delay in the diagnosis and treatment of hearing disorders can have long-term irreversible consequences for the pediatric patient. The majority of language skills are acquired during the first years of life. Even partial deficits may have significant effects on speech and language potential. Careful consideration should be given to any parental complaints about their child's hearing; this often may be the earliest indicator of difficulty. Presence of other risk factors may dictate more detailed screening even in asymptomatic patients.

Risk factors include a family history of deafness, possible congenital infections (especially rubella), and exposure to ototoxic drugs for more than 7 days. Infants discharged from the neonatal intensive care nurseries have a much higher risk of hearing loss, apparently related to prematurity, low birth weight, and associated problems of hypoxia, acidosis, and hyperbilirubinemia.

The development of speech and language is an orderly and progressive process that begins in early infancy. The receptive skills of language and the expressive skills of speech are acquired at different rates but are closely tied to each other. Receptive skills are more advanced in the young than are expressive skills. Because the disorders of speech and language are so closely tied to hearing, any recognized disorder of speech requires evaluation of hearing. Other causes of speech disorders to be considered include mental retardation, developmental abnormality, craniofacial abnormalities, and neurologic impairment.

In the infant and toddler the normal acquisition of speech is a reassuring sign that hearing is likely normal. Additional office screening includes the startle reflex in infants, which is normally present until 4 months of age. By 4 to 5 months of age the infant will recognize the primary caretaker's voice in preference to others. By 6 to 7 months of age the infant will turn to localize sounds, and more detailed screening can be done if calibrated sounds are used. Noncalibrated clickers or noisemakers should not be used. An adequate level of sound is about 50 dB for the frequencies tested. Other common milestones related to language are used to screen for age-appropriate hearing. Pure-tone testing is usually not possible in the office setting until the child is about 4 years of age. Threshold audiograms require cooperative children with cognitive development that permits them to accurately respond to minimal thresholds. The minimum screening audiogram should demonstrate hearing thresholds of 25 dB at the important speech frequencies of 500, 1,000, and 2,000 Hz. Screening audiograms should be done every 2 years in the school-aged child. This can often be coordinated with the local school system.

Otitis media, one of the most common pediatric problems, is characterized by frequent recurrence and slow resolution. The presence of middle-ear fluid is a source of conductive hearing loss that is most frequently present during the time of speech and language acquisition. Opinions differ on the seriousness and the optimal management of otitis. Certainly severe and prolonged cases are associated with high risk for significant hearing loss and need aggressive treatment. Other recommendations should be interpreted considering the potential risk of hearing loss on long-term language skills.

Further evaluation is indicated for all infants and children who have failed screening procedures or who have not responded to treatment within a reasonable time. Children who have speech and language delays should also undergo more-detailed assessment. Many neonatal units are routinely performing detailed hearing assessment for infants after discharge from intensive care units. A number of passive and active assessment instruments make detailed evaluation and diagnosis possible at all ages. Comprehensive diagnosis and treatment may require coordination of services with subspecialists, referral centers, school systems, and community organizations.

ANEMIA

Iron deficiency anemia, the most frequent abnormality of the hematologic system in the infant 9 to 24 months of age, reflects an increased rate of growth in conjunction with marginal intake of iron. Prior to the fall in hemoglobin and hematocrit values the iron stores and level of serum iron fall significantly. Associated with the fall in hemoglobin level is progressive microcytosis and hypochromasia and an increased serum level of heme precursors. Serum ferritin, free erythrocyte protoporphyrin (FEP), and mean corpuscular volume (MCV) have all been used as early indicators of iron depletion and deficiency; however, cost and technical difficulties limit their usefulness for office screening.

Screening for iron deficiency anemia is most commonly done at the 9- or 12-month health supervision visit, when fetal iron stores are normally exhausted. Results of screening performed earlier might be confused with the physiologic anemia of infancy. In cases of hemolytic disease, blood loss, or prematurity, earlier screening may be indicated. Repeated screening should be done in 2 years during the preschool evaluation and again during early adolescence.

Epidemiologic studies have shown that the frequency and severity of iron deficiency anemia in the United States have decreased significantly over the past 10 to 20 years. Treating only children with screening levels more than 2 SD below the mean would allow a significant number of those with iron depletion or iron deficiency to go untreated. An initial hemoglobin or hematocrit value less than −1 SD below the mean can be justified as the set point for a therapeutic trial of iron supplementation. Most important is assessing the response to treatment after 2 weeks. Further evaluation is indicated if the values for hemoglobin or hematocrit remain at less than 2 SD below the mean value for age or if the history and physical examination suggest other forms of anemia (Table 9–1).

Screening for anemia is a highly inefficient way to detect lead poisoning, although it may be detected in this manner. Recognition of environmental areas likely to result in lead exposure and populations likely affected will generate a high-risk population that can be more appropriately screened by checking the level of lead in the blood and FEP microtesting. In cases of microcytic anemia not responsive to a therapeutic trial of iron or of unusual or undiagnosed neurologic and behavioral problems, lead poisoning must be considered a possibility.

Recent evidence demonstrates that neuropsychologic effects can be seen with previously acceptable blood lead levels. The current definition of lead poisoning by the Centers for Disease Control has been changed from a blood lead level of 30 μg/dL to 25 μg/dL and an erythrocyte protoporphyrin level of 35 μg/dL or greater. It is possible that further studies may lower these recommended levels even farther. These changing levels for treatment could change the necessity for routine screening in the future.

CHOLESTEROL AND TRIGLYCERIDES

Elevated cholesterol and triglyceride levels are associated with increased risk for atherosclerosis and coronary artery disease in adults. Screening for elevated cholesterol and triglyc-

TABLE 9–1
Hemoglobin and Hematocrit Screening Values

	9–24 MO		5–7 YR		10–12 YR	
	HEMOGLOBIN (G/DL)	HEMATOCRIT (%)	HEMOGLOBIN (G/DL)	HEMATOCRIT (%)	HEMOGLOBIN (G/DL)	HEMATOCRIT (%)
Mean	12.5	37	13.0	38	13.5	40
−1 SD	11.5	35	12.0	36	12.5	38
−2 SD	11.0	33	11.5	35	12.9	36

eride levels in pediatric patients is based on the likelihood that atherosclerosis most likely begins in childhood. Whether this correlation can be extended to the pediatric patient has not been proved conclusively, but the evidence seems to be increasing. There has been a general trend in the United States to recommend lower-fat diets with a higher percentage of unsaturated fats as well as decreased cholesterol intake. For those children with elevated blood lipid levels, it is hoped that early dietary modifications will result in permanent dietary changes.

The recommended population for screening includes those with family histories of increased cholesterol levels, early heart attack or cerebrovascular accident, hypertension, and obesity. There is some support for universal screening, because many family histories are uncertain, and for the primary identification of index cases of hypercholesterolemia.

Screening can initially be done in children between the ages of 2 and 5 years. Random specimens are accurate if normal. One or two repeat screenings prior to adulthood would be adequate based on current information. For patients with elevated total cholesterol levels (>185 mg/dL, 90th percentile), lipid profiles including total cholesterol and high-density lipoprotein cholesterol (HDL-chol) and triglycerides after a 12-hour fast are recommended. The calculation of low-density lipoprotein cholesterol (LDL-chol) with the Friediwald formula (LDL-chol = Total chol − HDL-chol − [Triglycerides/5]) will assist in assessing cardiovascular risk. Exact treatment protocols and expectations for changes in blood levels are not well established.

URINE

The routine use of urinalysis as a screening device remains an inconsistent and unreliable method for disease prevention. It can be a more appropriate screening-diagnostic device for a high-risk population that has been identified by history and physical examination.

Hematuria is identified by screening programs in approximately 5% to 6% of children, the large majority of whom have only a transient abnormality. The incidence of proteinuria varies, depending on the study group and the age of the population, and usually is in the range of 5% to 10%. In the majority of these children reaction for protein is trace or 1+ by dipstick, and only a small percentage are found on repeated examinations to have persistent proteinuria. Hematuria in association with proteinuria requires further evaluation.

Asymptomatic bacteriuria, found in 1% of girls and 0.4% of boys, has not been proved to correlate with undiagnosed urinary tract infections and the risk of progressive renal disease. Routine screening for hematuria, proteinuria, and bacteriuria is no longer recommended by the American Academy of Pediatrics.

MASS SCREENING PROGRAMS

Screening of a large population of patients outside the framework of a health supervision visit can prove beneficial, as evidenced by the nationwide screening of newborns for phenylketonuria (PKU) and hypothyroidism. The benefit to the individual and the cost savings afforded to society by these programs have been documented by several authors. However, as pointed out in the introduction, the potential benefits to the individual and society must be considered for each screening program.

SCOLIOSIS

Scoliosis screening has become an integral part of school health programs. As the screening process has become mandatory in some states, questions arise as to the benefit of mass screening. Berwick states that scoliosis requiring further management is present in 5% of children found at screening to have positive findings. For the patient and family who require no further management, there are potential problems with being identified as having scoliosis, for example, family anxiety associated with the diagnosis and overuse of roentgenograms in the evaluation of the condition.

Screening for scoliosis as part of a health supervision evaluation is a desirable method of detection. Those patients at high risk for significant progression of the condition include girls, those with scoliosis at an early age, those with a family history of scoliosis, and those patients who have not had an adolescent growth spurt. Physical examination for scoliosis is discussed in Chapter 7.

BLOOD PRESSURE

The detection of elevated blood pressure is best accomplished as part of the physical examination performed by the primary care physician. Mass screening programs to check BP in a high school population were found by Fixler and Laird to result in an unacceptably high proportion of false positive results. The high rate of false positive findings has undesirable economic consequences, and the psychological trauma associated with identification is difficult to overstate.

The American Academy of Pediatrics Task Force on Blood Pressure Control in Children has recommended that mass screening programs not be instituted for the detection of hypertension.

METABOLIC DISEASES

The implementation of extensive metabolic screening during the newborn period has been debated for many years. Current recommendations for mass screening in the majority of states exist only for hypothyroidism and PKU. The primary care physician needs to be alert to several factors:

1. The increasing popularity of home births and alternative birth centers may result in some infants under their care who have not had appropriate screening for PKU and hypothyroidism.
2. Routine urine screening for inborn errors of metabolism performed during the first week of life does not allow time for the detection of those disorders requiring prompt treatment. The physician must be aware that the presence of unexplained vomiting, diarrhea, tachypnea, jaundice, or poor feeding requires prompt metabolic evaluation.
3. Screening for inherited errors of metabolism may be directed at the population at risk. Tay-Sachs disease is an inherited disorder of ganglioside metabolism for which there is no satisfactory treatment. The majority of affected individuals die before 4 years of age. Ashkenazic Jews have a high incidence of the disorder and may be identified as heterozygotes. Jewish couples of eastern European ancestry should be advised that tests that identify the carrier states are available.

SICKLE CELL TRAIT

Sickle cell trait is the heterozygous inheritance of hemoglobin S gene. It occurs in 1 of 12 black Americans. Screening programs for sickle cell disease are controversial because of inappropriate response to the diagnosis of the trait by members of the community, including unfair treatment at work and school by superiors who are misinformed about the carrier state and its implications.

The primary advantage of identifying sickle cell trait is its help in family planning. Any program must be voluntary and include excellent educational and counseling opportunities. Sickle cell disease is discussed further in Chapter 59.

BIBLIOGRAPHY

American Academy of Pediatrics: Vision screening and eye examination in children. *Pediatrics* 1986; 77:918–919.

American Academy of Pediatrics: Prudent life-style for children: Dietary fat and cholesterol. *Pediatrics* 1986; 78:521–524.

American Academy of Pediatrics: *School Health: A Guide for Health Professionals*. Elk Grove Village, Ill, American Academy of Pediatrics, 1987.

American Academy of Pediatrics: Statement on childhood lead poisoning. *Pediatrics* 1987; 79:457–465.

American Academy of Pediatrics: *Standards of Child Health Care*, ed 4. Elk Grove Village, Ill, American Academy of Pediatrics, 1988.

Berwick DM: Scoliosis screening. *Pediatr Rev* 1984; 5:238–247.

Borowitz KC, Glascoe FP: Sensitivity of the Denver Developmental Screening Test in speech and language screening. *Pediatrics* 1986; 78:1075–1078.

Bzoch KR, Leaque R: *Receptive-Expressive Emergent Language Scale*. Baltimore, University Park Press, 1971.

Campbell W, Camp BW: Developmental screening, in Frankeburg WK, Camp B (ed): *Pediatric Screening Tests*. Springfield, Ill, Charles C Thomas, Publisher, 1975.

Coplan J: *Early Language Milestones Scale*. Tulsa, Okla, Modern Education Corp, 1983.

Coplan J: Evaluation of the child with delayed speech or language. *Pediatr Ann* 1985; 14:203–208.
Cross AW: Health screening in schools. I. *J Pediatr* 1985; 107:487–493.
Cross AW: Health screening in schools. II. *J Pediatr* 1985; 107:653–660.
van Doorninck WJ, Liddell TN, Frankenburg WK, et al: The Denver Prescreening Developmental Questionaire (PDQ). *Pediatrics* 1976; 57:744–753.
Fixler DE, Laird WP: Validity of mass blood pressure screening in children. *Pediatrics* 1983; 72:459–463.
Frankenburg WK, Fandal AW, Sciarillo W, et al: The newly abbreviated and revised Denver Developmental Screening Test. *J Pediatr* 1981; 99:995–999.
Frankenburg WK, Fandal AW, Thornton SM: Revision of Denver Prescreening Developmental Questionnaire (R-PDQ). *J Pediatr* 1987; 110:653–657.
Friendly DS: Amblyopia: Definition, classification, diagnosis, and management considerations. *Pediatr Clin North Am* 1987; 34:1389–1401.
Grimes CT: Audiologic evaluation in infancy and childhood. *Pediatr Ann* 1985; 14:211–219.
Matkin ND: Early recognition and referral of hearing-impaired children. *Pediatr Rev* 1984; 6:151–156.
Nadler HL: Urine screening after discharge from hospital. *Pediatrics* 1981; 67:159.
Norman ME: An office approach to hematuria and proteinuria. *Pediatr Clin North Am* 1987; 34:545–559.
Reinecke RD: Ophthalmic examination of infants and children by the pediatrician. *Pediatr Clin North Am* 1983; 30:995–1003.
Prevention of Adult Atherosclerosis During Childhood. Report of the 95th Ross Conference. Columbus, Ohio, Ross Laboratories, August 1988.
Rowe LD: Hearing loss: The profound benefits of early diagnosis. *Contemp Peds* Oct 1985; 77–85.
Ruben RJ: Diagnosis of deafness in infancy. *Pediatr Rev* 1987; 9:163–166.
Simmons FB (ed): The deaf child. *Pediatr Ann* 1980; 9:12–60.
Strong WB, Dennison BA: Pediatric preventive cardiology: Atherosclerosis and coronary heart disease. *Pediatr Rev* 1988; 9:303–314.
Tongue AC: Refractive errors in children. *Pediatr Clin North Am* 1987; 34:1425–1437.

10 OBESITY

Lawrence Hammer, M.D.

Obesity is one of the most common disorders of growth and nutrition affecting children and adolescents in the United States. The medical and psychological sequelae of obesity make its prevention, early recognition, and management important. Much is currently known about the development of body fatness during childhood and the risk factors and behavioral patterns that predispose to the development of obesity in children and adolescents. Since a specific organic cause of obesity is rarely present, the primary care physician must help the family implement a program of treatment based on modifying eating and activity patterns. This chapter includes definitions of obesity, the development of adipose tissue in children and adolescents, factors that contribute to excessive body fatness, and the diagnosis and treatment of obesity.

BACKGROUND

DEFINITION AND PREVALENCE OF OBESITY

Obesity is most simply defined as excessive body fatness. A number of definitions are used for clinical and research purposes. The most accurate methods of measuring body fatness used in research are not clinically practical because they involve the use of radioisotopes or underwater weighing to estimate body fatness.

One commonly accepted definition of obesity is weight greater than 120% of ideal body weight. Ideal body weight is derived from charts giving average weight for age, sex, and height. Another popular clinical method requires growth charts that plot weight as a function of height. Though helpful when confronted with a tall, heavy child, these charts are inadequate because they assume that weight for height is constant irrespective of age. These graphs and tables tend to overestimate body fatness in adolescents and underestimate it in younger age groups.

A good indicator of body fatness is the body mass index (weight divided by height squared). Body mass index, also known as Quetelet's index, can be compared with normative data based on age, sex, and race. The body mass index does not overestimate body fatness in short individuals or underestimate it in tall individuals to the same degree as weight for height. Body mass index greater than the 95th percentile for age and sex is an acceptable definition of obesity (Table 10–1).

A clinical estimation of body fatness is obtained by measurement of skinfold thickness with standard calipers. Skinfold thickness correlates highly with other measures of body fat and is more accurate than visual assessment or weight for height in diagnosing obesity. An accepted definition of obesity uses triceps skinfold thickness greater than the 85th percentile for age, race, and sex. Normative data are available for comparison with the patient's skinfold thickness measurement (Table 10–2). The accuracy of skinfold thickness is increased by measuring multiple sites and summing or averaging these measurements; however, the single skinfold thickness measure is adequate for clinical purposes.

Obesity is seen in all parts of the world and in all ethnic groups. It is more prevalent with increasing age, and is more common in women than in men. In childhood, prevalence correlates inversely with social class for boys and girls, while in adulthood obesity is most common in lower social class women and in upper class men. Data from national health surveys indicate that the prevalence of obesity in the United States has increased 54% among 6- to 11-year-old children and 39% among 12- to 17-year-olds, to 27% and 22%, respectively, in the decade preceding the NHANES II survey (National Health and Nutrition Examination Survey) conducted in 1976 to 1980.[7]

TABLE 10–1
Body Mass Index (Reference Values)*†

AGE (YR)	MEN 50%ILE	MEN 95%ILE	WOMEN 50%ILE	WOMEN 95%ILE
2	16.3	18.4	16.0	18.5
3	15.8	17.8	15.4	17.7
4	15.6	18.1	15.3	18.0
5	15.4	18.0	15.3	19.6
6	15.3	21.1	15.3	19.3
7	15.7	19.8	15.7	19.9
8	16.2	20.8	15.9	20.3
9	16.4	21.8	16.5	25.2
10	17.3	24.4	17.0	24.1
11	17.5	26.4	18.1	26.2
12	18.0	25.0	18.8	26.3
13	18.9	24.8	19.3	28.5
14	19.6	25.1	20.4	28.8
15	20.5	26.6	19.9	26.6
16	21.6	28.0	21.0	29.1
17	21.3	28.3	21.4	31.3
18	22.1	29.9	21.6	30.7

* Adapted from Najjar MF, Rowland M: Anthropometric reference data and prevalence of overweight, United States, 1976–1980. *Vital Health Stat [11]* 1987; 238. Rockville, Md, US Department of Health and Human Services, DHHS Publication No (PHS) 87-1688.

† Calculated as weight/height^2 (kg/m^2).

DEVELOPMENT OF ADIPOSE TISSUE

The earliest stage of adipose tissue development occurs in utero. At birth the infant's body mass is 10% to 15% fat. Almost half the weight gained by the infant in the first 4 months of life is fat. By 1 year of age the child's body mass is 25% to 30% adipose tissue. The child's body fat decreases to 20% to 25% of its body mass by the age of 2 years, and begins to increase again after the adipose rebound occurs. Girls have a greater increase of body fat during adolescence than boys, so that by early adulthood, a woman's body composition includes 15% to 30% adipose tissue, whereas in men body fat remains 15% to 20% of body mass.

These changes in body composition correlate with adipocyte development. Adipose tissue development involves cellular proliferation and hypertrophy. Proliferation leads to the formation of new adipocytes by cell division and is most important in infancy and childhood. In utero, adipocyte proliferation and limited lipid filling occur. Cellular studies have demon-

TABLE 10–2
Triceps Skinfold Thickness (Reference Values)*†

AGE (YR)	MEN 50%	MEN 85%	MEN 95%	WOMEN 50%	WOMEN 85%	WOMEN 95%
1	10	13.0	15.5	10.5	13.5	16.5
2	10	13.0	15.0	10.5	13.5	16.0
3	9.5	12.5	15.0	10.0	12.5	16.5
4	9.0	12.0	15.0	10.0	13.0	15.5
5	8.0	11.5	14.5	10.5	14.0	16.0
6	8.0	12.0	17.5	10.0	14.5	18.5
7	8.5	12.0	17.5	10.5	15.0	20.0
8	9.0	16.5	22.0	11.0	16.0	21.0
9	9.0	16.0	23.0	13.0	20.0	27.0
10	11.0	20.0	26.0	13.5	21.0	24.5
11	10.5	22.0	30.0	14.0	21.5	29.5
12	11.0	18.0	26.5	13.5	21.5	27.0
13	9.0	16.5	22.5	15.0	22.0	30.0
14	9.0	15.0	23.0	17.0	25.0	32.0
15	7.5	14.5	22.0	16.5	24.5	32.1
16	8.0	18.5	28.5	18.0	27.0	33.1
17	7.0	12.5	18.0	20.0	26.5	34.5
18	9.5	17.5	22.5	18.0	27.0	35.0

* Adapted from Najjar MF, Rowland M: Anthropometric reference data and prevalence of overweight, United States, 1976–1980. *Vital Health Stat [11]* 1987; 238. Rockville, Md, US Department of Health and Human Services, DHHS Publication No (PHS) 87–1688.

† Measured in millimeters.

strated that adipocyte number remains fairly constant during the first 12 months of life, whereas filling of adipocytes with lipid continues. Adipocyte size increases during the first year of life, reaching normal adult values when the child is 9 to 12 months of age. Adipocyte number then increases steadily from the age of 1 year through puberty. A second burst of adipocyte proliferation occurs in puberty. In children who are obese, cell size and number are often increased. A proportionally greater increase in cell size than cell number characterizes individuals with adult-onset obesity. Whether development of an excessive number of fat cells during infancy and childhood contributes to the likelihood of obesity persisting into adulthood remains controversial. Factors that control adipocyte hyperplasia and hypertrophy are still incompletely understood.[8]

NATURAL HISTORY OF OBESITY

There is a growing body of evidence that obesity in infancy or childhood strongly predicts later obesity. Correlation between birth weight and weight later in life is poor; however, at each successive stage of growth the presence of obesity increases the risk for later obesity when compared with nonobese infants or children. Approximately 25% of infants who are obese remain obese after childhood. The older and fatter the obese child the more likely obesity is to persist into adulthood. Thus about 50% of obese adolescent girls remain obese as adults. Children with an earlier adipose rebound are at an increased risk for persistent obesity.[10]

Complicating the natural history of obesity in childhood and adolescence is the effect of pubertal maturation on body fatness. Data from the Ten-State Nutrition Survey demonstrate that while boys undergo a decrease in percent body fat during early adolescence and a gradual increase later in adolescence and adulthood, girls begin to increase body fat prepubertally and continue to increase their body fat into adulthood.[6]

MEDICAL AND PSYCHOLOGICAL SEQUELAE OF OBESITY

Obesity influences a variety of physiological and metabolic processes. During childhood, obesity leads to accelerated bone growth and skeletal maturation. Accelerated physical maturation with early menarche and decreased final height is often seen in obese girls. Metabolically, obesity leads to hyperinsulinemia, which increases with age in proportion to body fatness. This hyperinsulinemic state is accompanied by elevated levels of free fatty acids and glycerol. Growth hormone levels are decreased, despite accelerated growth. Decreased prolactin levels have also been reported. Levels of testosterone are decreased in some extremely obese males. Although ovarian function is intact, obese girls suffer increased rates of amenorrhea and dysfunctional uterine bleeding. In such cases polycystic ovaries should be ruled out.

There is much interest in the effect of obesity in childhood on cardiovascular risk factors such as hyperlipidemia and hypertension. Hyperlipidemia is more common among obese children and adolescents. Cholesterol and triglyceride levels increase with increased weight, and obese children have been noted to have a higher prevalence of hypercholesterolemia and hypertriglyceridemia. Hypertension is also more common among obese children and adolescents. More than 25% of hypertensive adolescents are obese. Systolic and diastolic blood pressures correlate with skinfold thickness.[5]

Other organ systems may be affected as well. Increased cholesterol turnover leads to an increased risk of cholelithiasis in obese children and adolescents. Orthopedic complications include slipped capital femoral epiphyses, Legg-Calvé-Perthes disease, and genu valgum. Intertriginous dermatitis is common. An increase in respiratory tract illness has been associated with obesity in toddlers under 2 years of age. Some patients with obesity have increased daytime sleepiness and hypoventilation (pickwickian syndrome). If hypoventilation is severe, these patients are at risk for apnea and right ventricular failure.

Perhaps the greatest consequence of obesity in childhood or adolescence is its likelihood to persist into adulthood, when obesity is associated with increased morbidity and mortality from hypertension, diabetes, cardiovascular disease, and cerebrovascular accident (CVA). It is estimated that men who are twice their ideal body weight have 12 times the expected mortality for age, and those who are only 50% above ideal body weight have 1.3 to 2.0 times the expected mortality.

Significant psychosocial sequelae have been described in obese children and adolescents. The obese child is teased, ridiculed, and rejected. The obese adolescent also has poor self-esteem, abnormal body image, and difficulty developing peer relations, leading to withdrawal and social isolation. Many obese children and adolescents experience significant depression and school failure. These psychological sequelae help perpetuate the disorder, as obese individuals often shy away from outdoor exercise and physical activity because of embarrassment over their appearance.

PATHOGENESIS AND DIFFERENTIAL DIAGNOSIS

Obesity results from an excess of caloric intake over energy expenditure. Factors that influence caloric intake include feeding patterns, composition of the diet, availability of food, and preference for certain types of food. Factors that influence energy expenditure include basal and active metabolic rate and degree of day-to-day activity. At least 95% of obesity in childhood and adolescence may be considered exogenous, or due to an imbalance of these factors. The remaining 5% of children with obesity have either a syndrome associated with obesity or an underlying endocrinologic abnormality.

Most patients with obesity have an imbalance in energy intake and expenditure. Although it is commonly believed that obese individuals have lower basal metabolism than other individuals, obese adolescents have demonstrated increased basal metabolic activity, probably secondary to increased lean mass. Though basal metabolism is not decreased, active energy utilization may be less in obese than nonobese individuals. The obese have a decreased thermogenic response to activity and carbohydrate intake, which may be a predisposing factor to the development or perpetuation of obesity. In normal individuals eating leads to a greater metabolic activity than in obese individuals. Energy utilization also decreases when obese adults are placed on hypocaloric diets. Since the obese individual does not necessarily consume more calories than the nonobese individual, this energy-conserving capability helps perpetuate the obese state.

Although overfeeding may lead to obesity, it does not appear necessary to maintain the obese state. Epidemiologic studies have not demonstrated significant differences in caloric intake or distribution of calories with respect to fat or carbohydrate in obese and nonobese children. In infancy, obesity may develop as a result of overfeeding by parents who mistake the infant's cry as an indication of hunger or who feed the infant beyond the point of satiety. Since infants less than 3 to 4 months of age do not regulate their intake as finely as older infants do, overfeeding can occur, thereby leading to excessive body fatness. Bottle feeding and earlier introduction of solid foods have been associated with more rapid doubling of birth weight; however, the efficacy of breastfeeding in protecting against obesity has not been clearly demonstrated.[1] Factors that influence intake during infancy, such as taste preference, appetite, and satiety, are still poorly understood.

Much evidence exists for a significant role of activity and exercise in moderating the effects of caloric intake on the development of obesity. Studies of infants have shown significant correlations between body weight and activity level. Among older children and adolescents, the obese appear to be less active than the nonobese. In addition, caloric energy expenditure per unit of activity is less in the obese adolescent than in the nonobese. It is not uncommon for obesity to develop after a serious illness requiring a period of bed rest and decreased physical activity. Once the obese state develops, decreased self-esteem and clumsiness often lead to further elimination of physical activity and exercise by the child or adolescent. Large periods of time spent watching television or engaged in other passive activity predispose to the development of obesity.[3]

The relative importance of familial and genetic factors cannot be underestimated. Genetic factors exert a strong influence on the development of obesity. About 40% of the offspring of one obese parent are obese, and 70% of the offspring of two obese parents are likely to be obese. Environmental modeling of dietary behavior and physical activity certainly influence the child of obese parents, yet even adopted children raised from infancy resemble their biologic parents in fatness and not their adoptive parents.[11] There may be genetic influences on metabolic rate and energy expenditure that underly this familial tendency.[9]

Although many diagnostic entities are associated with obesity, the presence of normal or increased stature, normal gonadal development, and normal intelligence rules out most of these disorders. Inherited disorders and congenital syndromes account for only 2% to 3% of cases of obesity. *Prader-Willi syndrome* is characterized by obesity, hypogonadism, mental retardation, short stature, small hands and feet, dysmorphic facies (down-turned triangular mouth, almond-shaped eyes, decreased bifrontal diameter). Infants with Prader-Willi syndrome are often hypotonic and have slow weight gain in infancy secondary to feeding problems; however, late in childhood hyperphagia and obesity develop. These children have severe behavioral problems in addition to mental retardation. Prader-Willi syndrome is the most common genetic obesity syndrome, occurring in 1 in 5,000 to 10,000 births. It is usually sporadic, but about 50% of cases are associated with deletions involving chromosome 15. The defect in Prader-Willi syndrome is probably hypothalamic. *Lawrence-Moon-Biedl syndrome* is characterized by obesity, mental retardation, short stature, polydactyly, retinitis pigmentosa, deafness, and hypogonadism. *Vasquez syndrome* is an X-linked disorder characterized by obesity, mental retardation, hypogonadism, and gynecomastia. *Alstrom syndrome* is characterized by obesity, deafness, diabetes mellitus, retinitis pigmentosa, short stature, and hypogonadism. *Cohen syndrome* is an autosomal recessive syndrome with obesity, hypotonia, and mental retardation but without hypogonadism or short stature.

Several endocrine disorders, for example, *Cushing disease* and *hypothyroidism*, may also be associated with obesity; however, their diagnosis is usually apparent from other clinical signs. In both Cushing disease and hypothyroidism the bone age is delayed, whereas most obese children have normal or advanced bone age. Patients with pseudohypoparathyroidism have short stature, hypocalcemia, and short fourth metacarpals in addition to obesity.

Children with central nervous system disease may also be at risk for obesity due to hyperphagia or hypoactivity. Meningitis, brain tumors, CVA, and head trauma have all been associated with the onset of obesity.

DATA GATHERING

Evaluation of obesity in the child or adolescent should begin with a complete history and physical examination. Since the syndromes described above account for only a small portion of childhood obesity and can generally be excluded with a good history and physical examination, few laboratory tests are needed in this evaluation. The history should include parental weight, the child's birth weight, early feeding history, age of onset of obesity, and information regarding the family's perception of the child's body habitus. It is important to obtain information regarding the feeding patterns of the household and the use of food within the family as reward or part of social functions. With older children it is important to inquire about school performance, peer relationships, relationships with members of the family, and the child's perception of his or her own body. A family history of obesity, hypertension, cardiovascular disease, diabetes, and CVA should be elicited. Any history of antecedent illness, hospitalizations, or surgery is pertinent.

A dietary history for weekday and weekend is useful, using a food diary, and an interview, with questions regarding food preferences, eating habits, snacks, where meals are eaten, and with whom. By inquiring into the family and child's eating habits, people, places, and moods commonly associated with foods are better understood. Some children binge eat, have compulsive patterns of eating, or respond to changes in emotional state with eating. Some obese children are particularly responsive to external stimuli such as the appearance, taste, or smell of food, while being unresponsive to internal cues such as a feeling of satiety. Information regarding physical activity should also be obtained, including information about daily habits such as reading and television watching. A weekday and weekend activity record is useful for this purpose.

The physical examination should include particular attention to the child's overall appearance, vital signs (especially blood pressure), distribution of fat, the presence of striae and skin irritation, the child's stage of sexual maturation, and the presence of any orthopedic abnormalities, including scoliosis, genu valgum, and slipped capital femoral epiphyses. Accurate measurement of weight and height are mandatory and the measurement of skinfold thicknesses with calipers is recommended. To rule out a congenital syndrome, observe for hypogonadism, short stature, mental retardation, dysmorphic faces, and small extremities. Signs of hypoventilation would suggest "pickwickian" syndrome. A psychological evaluation of the child and family may also be helpful, and consultation with a mental health professional can provide useful diagnostic information.

The laboratory evaluation of the obese child is not routine but directed to ruling out any disease suggested by the history and physical examination. Since less than 5% of cases have an organic basis, the testing can be very limited. If the child is short for age, a thyroid function test is needed. Chromosomal analysis can be ordered if the child has clinical signs of Prader-Willi syndrome or Turner syndrome. Urinalysis is useful as an initial screening for diabetes mellitus. A lipid profile is indicated to rule out hypercholesterolemia or hypertriglyceridemia, particularly in adolescents. If the child has a history of daytime sleepiness or apnea, pickwickian syndrome should be evaluated in a sleep laboratory with an arterial blood gas determination, pulmonary function tests, electrocardiography, and otolaryngologic consultation. Obese adolescents with amenorrhea or dysfunctional bleeding should have a pelvic ultrasound examination to look for polycystic ovaries and gonadotropin levels to evaluate hypothalamic-pituitary function.

MANAGEMENT

Obesity is a lifelong disorder. Its treatment requires patience and motivation. The importance of intervention during childhood and adolescence arises from its immediate psychological and medical effects and the tendency for obesity to persist into adulthood, when the cardiovascular effects of excess weight become more apparent. Many adolescents are concerned about their weight and body image. Many feel they are fatter than they really are. During puberty the normal increase in adipose tissue comes at a time when youth are particularly sensitive to changes in their appearance. Adolescence should therefore be an ideal time to initiate a weight-loss program, yet the combination of increasing adipose tissue and a desire to be like others with respect to diet and recreational activities leave the adolescent highly resistant to treatment. Earlier the nutritional needs of the young child for growth and development make restriction of caloric intake potentially hazardous.

The guiding principle of treatment is to change behavior so that more energy is utilized by the child for activity, growth, and metabolic processes than is consumed. Treatment can be initiated at any age as long as the nutritional needs of the child are met. The younger the child the more direct involvement parents will have to have, but family cooperation is needed for treating children and adolescents of all ages.

Management of the school-age child should be done with consideration of the nutritional requirements for growth and development. Caloric intake should be modified to provide a balanced diet without excess calories remaining for storage as fat. Reduction of caloric intake by 250 to 500 kcal/day can provide enough energy for growth without additional weight gain, particularly if restriction is focused on fatty and sweet foods. The usual goal of treatment at this age is limited reduction in weight or maintenance of weight over time while growth continues and the child's body composition normalizes. This process may take quite a while; each 20% over ideal body weight requires about a year of "catch-up" time without weight gain. If the child is severely obese periods of caloric restriction may be needed to yield actual weight loss, but this should always be done cautiously so as to allow growth to proceed.

Modifying caloric intake during childhood requires change in the eating behavior of the parent as well as the eating habits of the child. Simple dietary counseling is not adequate. Knowledge of the family's own dietary habits, with use of food for reward, pleasure, or social interaction, is important. If the family eats together, are the children given the same foods as the parents and in the same quantities? Insisting on a clean plate contributes to unnecessary caloric intake. Many children learn at an early age that their eating gives their parents a sense of pleasure and feeling of successful parenting. These children eat to please their parents rather than to satisfy their own nutritional needs or to enjoy the taste of food. The whole family may have an eating pattern that encourages excessive intake; treatment necessitates involvement of the whole family. The child should not be the target of treatment or the scapegoat in an obese family.

Treatment of obese children has generally focused on dietary modification, without sufficient emphasis on the role of exercise and increased activity in the reduction of adipose tissue and maintenance of weight. When used alone, exercise programs are often inadequate for treating obesity, but when combined with dietary change, they can be a powerful tool for initiating and maintaining weight reduction. Exercise may be particularly important in the maintenance of reduced weight. Exercise facilitates the dietary approach and decreases the inactive time during the day, when excess caloric intake occurs. Activities that encourage family participation and reduction in television viewing are especially useful in treating the whole family. Exercises, sports, and games should be selected that are appropriate for the child's age and level of fitness. As treatment proceeds, exercises that are more vigorous and demanding may be recommended. It is most important to make exercise a regular habit. Walking to school or to other activities is a good beginning. Bicycling, swimming, skating, jogging, and cross-country skiing are suitable activities for the school-aged child. The obese child is usually self-conscious about appearance and is reluctant to participate in outdoor activities, be they individual or organized group sports. It is usually best to begin with activities after school two to three times per week and increase the frequency and vigor of the activity gradually as the child begins to lose some fatness and begins to feel proud of his or her progress.

Although there are no definitive rules about who should participate in the treatment of the obese child and how often the child should be seen, a team approach with frequent visits appears to work best. The physician may coordinate visits to the office for the initial and subsequent history, examination, and follow-up. A dietitian can be called on to obtain more extensive dietary information from the child and parents and give guidance for choosing foods. Specific diets may be useful initially in treatment, but ultimately the child and parent must learn to make appropriate choices for themselves. A counselor (e.g., psychologist, psychiatrist, social worker) can be particularly helpful in establishing and maintaining the behavioral aspects of treatment, including reducing cues that stimulate eating, encouraging exercise, and reinforcing success. All of these components of treatment can be provided by the physician if desired; however, treatment may demand more time than is generally available in many practices. Visits for measurement of weight should be encouraged weekly, with positive reinforcement in the way of gold stars on a calendar or chart or other rewards (treats, privileges, money) given for achievement of reasonable goals, not only those based on weight but those for dietary modification and increased activity. Parents should also be rewarded for their achievements. Strong consideration should be given to the benefits of treating children and their parents in groups (see below).

TREATING THE ADOLESCENT

The principles that apply to treatment of the younger child also apply to the adolescent. Energy expenditure must exceed energy intake if treatment is to succeed. The components of treatment are also the same: dietary modification and increasing exercise, with emphasis on changing eating behavior and daily activity patterns. The most successful treatment programs include a combination of these components reinforced with behavior modification.

The principles of dietary modification in adolescence again require provision of adequate calories for growth and development without excessive calories for fat storage. Adolescents interested in losing weight may be eager to try the latest fad diet. This should be discouraged because these diets, though usually successful in initiating weight loss, are generally unbalanced nutritionally for the growing teen. The physician or dietitian should work with the adolescent to develop a well-balanced diet that reduces daily caloric intake by about 500 calories and provides less than 20% of calories as fat, while maintaining a level of protein intake of at least 30% to 40% of daily intake. Reliance on dietary education and counseling is rarely successful in the long run, however, unless coupled with a program designed to modify eating behavior. Teens with severe obesity (e.g., greater than 100 lbs overweight) may benefit from a protein-sparing modified fast coupled with behavior modification and group support. Such patients should be carefully monitored by a physician experienced with this approach.[2]

Exercise should be strongly encouraged in the adolescent as part of the treatment of obesity. In addition to utilizing excess calories, exercise leads to reduction in hyperinsulinemia and hypertension independent of its weight-reducing effect. After exercise, metabolic rate remains elevated for a time, appetite is temporarily reduced, and a sense of greater wellbeing is induced, which further enhances self-esteem and increases motivation for the achievement of weight loss. The greatest barrier that the obese adolescent must overcome is the initial hesitancy to exercise due to embarrassment and self-consciousness. Activities with other family members or alone rather than with peers may be more acceptable to the embarrassed teenager. Parents should be encouraged to join the adolescent in exercises such as walking, jogging, swimming, and bicycling. It is important to develop realistic goals for exercise. Periods of walking each day can be slowly increased before proceeding to jogging or bicycling. Over time the duration and strenuousness of the exercise program should be increased. Much positive reinforcement should be given for the achievement of even modest exercise goals, and a daily log of the adolescent's exercising will provide a proud reminder of progress over weeks and months.

It should be recalled that the obese adolescent often has a variety of psychological sequelae, such as anxiety, anger, and depression. The obese adolescent is at a disadvantage in developing important peer relations, particularly with members of the other sex. This is an important time for the development of confidence in dealing with social situations. These sequelae coupled with the frustration often experienced by the obese adolescent during treatment make the use of group meetings with other obese adolescents and an experienced therapist valuable. At these meetings adolescents share their frustrations, constructively discuss their eating behavior, and with the help of the therapist and support of the group, successfully begin to modify their behavior. Treatment programs in which parents attend a group separate from their obese children have been shown to be more effective than programs in which parents and children attend the same group together. Groups should meet at least once a week, particularly early in the treatment program, with an organized curriculum concerning behavior change and factors influencing behavior change. This group approach, with children and parents treated in separate groups, can be used with children or adolescents and provides group support for behavior modification.[4]

BEHAVIOR MODIFICATION IN TREATMENT OF OBESITY

Techniques of behavior modification should be employed by the physician, counselor, or dietitian as a powerful adjunct to dietary restriction and exercise in the treatment of obesity. The use of behavior modification is helpful in this setting because exogenous obesity is often maintained by excessive eating occurring as a result of endogenous and environmental cues. Each individual's eating behavior should be carefully analyzed by the therapist guiding the treatment and its immediate antecedents and consequences discovered. Treatment involves altering and limiting exposure to the antecedent stimuli (called stimulus control) and reducing the reinforcing nature of the eating behavior. A child who overeats whenever an upsetting event occurs can be given alternative suggestions for responding to discomfort. A child who eats while doing homework in the kitchen might be encouraged to do his work in another part of the house where food will not be readily available. Reducing the amount of high-calorie food available in the house also helps (environmental control). Substitution of high-calorie food with snack items such as celery and carrots should be recommended. Rewarding the child with a dessert for finishing the rest of dinner should be avoided. The child who is not hungry should not be encouraged to clean his plate. Reducing time spent watching television and encouraging activity or exercise in the evening serves the dual purposes of reducing intake and increasing energy expenditure.

Positive reinforcement can be provided in a number of ways, for example, gold stars, special outings with the family, an extra visit to a favorite place, even a rare visit to the ice cream store. Most important is that reinforcement be given for change in behavior, such as change in eating patterns and exercise, using very modest and achievable goals, rather than rewarding weight loss per se. The obese adolescent easily begins losing weight with dietary restriction, but continued loss of weight is difficult. Reinforcement for behavior change is most important to ensure continued success with treatment.

A very powerful tool for achieving behavior change is self-monitoring. Self-monitoring involves recording as accurately as possible the behavior such as eating and its immediate surrounding behaviors, with attention to timing and location. Such a record provides the therapist with a highly accurate picture of where eating occurs, in what context, with whom the adolescent usually eats, and the events that precede and follow eating that may reinforce it. Knowledge of these cues for eating and the patterns of reinforcement help the therapist and the individual in treatment understand and limit exposure to the cues and change the pattern of behavior. Self-monitoring also increases the individual's insight into his or her own behavior and independently acts to help alter that behavior. Finally, self-monitoring provides a record of achievement and success for the adolescent as treatment proceeds and weight loss continues. Combining self-monitoring with a behavior contract provides a practical approach to the problem of realistic goal setting and reinforcement. A behavior change contract might specify a daily dietary goal (e.g., the number of "red light" foods, as in Epstein's traffic light diet), a daily exercise goal, and a behavior such as keeping a daily food record. The child "contracts" with the parent for an agreed on reward for fulfillment of the contract. The reward should be age appropriate and available soon after it is earned. Young children should be able to receive a reward twice weekly; a weekly reward is appropriate for the older child. Rewards need not be expensive; an extra outing alone with the parent or to a special event may be more meaningful than material gifts.

MAINTENANCE OF WEIGHT LOSS

Many programs for treating obesity report average losses of 1 to 2 kg/wk during treatment. Most programs also report gradual regaining of weight after treatment ends. The challenge of maintaining weight loss may be greater than the challenge of initial weight loss. Most treatments, from behavioral to controlled fasting, ultimately fail unless a maintenance program is included. Maintenance requires the continuation of moderation in dietary intake coupled with a regular program of exercise. Limited self-monitoring of intake, exercise, and weight are helpful. Continuation of stimulus reduction by keeping the environment free of high-calorie foods and avoiding situations in which dietary indiscretion occurs also helps. Monthly group meetings provide further impetus and reinforcement for behavior change. During the maintenance phase, periodic intensification of treatment with further dietary restriction for several months may encourage the obese youngster to stick with the program. Any soundly conceived weight loss program for the adolescent can only succeed if he or she continues in treatment. Maintaining adherence to a program is the greatest challenge for the therapist and patient. Weight loss is difficult, requiring long periods of dedication during which success and frustration often intermingle. The treatment program should reinforce adherence, even if other goals of behavior change and weight loss are not always met. Various contingency systems using payback regimens have been very successful as adjuncts to weight loss programs. Physicians should investigate group programs available in their communities that might be suitable for children or adolescents, particularly if coupled with regular follow-up and involvement by the physician.

PREVENTION

Because the treatment of obesity requires long periods of dedication and difficult changes in eating behavior and activity, the disorder is best prevented. Knowledge of risk factors can help target efforts at prevention. Families with parental obesity have an increased risk of obesity in the children. Particular attention to overfeeding and avoidance of excessive weight gain in the first few years of life is important. Restriction of caloric intake early in childhood should be done only with careful medical supervision. The use of food as reward should be discouraged. It is wise to discourage eating in front of the television or excessive snacking between meals. Feeding should not be forced or overly encouraged if the child is not hungry. Children should not be required to clean their plates and should be encouraged to avoid junk food and high-calorie snacks. Adolescents, in particular, are prone to irregularity in their diet. It is helpful if adolescents understand that it is normal to gain weight during puberty, especially for girls, but that excessive weight gain can be avoided by regular exercise and limitation of excessive intake. The whole family should be encouraged to exercise in moderation on a regular basis. Early emphasis on healthy diet and regular exercise should be the cornerstone of the physician's approach to healthy weight management.

REFERENCES

1. Agras WS, Kraemer HC, Berkowitz RI, et al: Does a virgorous feeding style influence early development of adiposity? *J Pediatr* 1987; 110:799–804.
2. Brown MR, Klish WJ, Hollander J, et al: A high protein, low calorie liquid diet in the treatment of very obese adolescents: long-term effect on lean body mass. *Am J Clin Nutr* 1983; 38:20–31.
3. Dietz WH, Gortmaker SL: Do we fatten our children at the TV set? Television viewing and obesity in children and adolescents. *Pediatrics* 1988; 75:807–812.
4. Epstein LH, Wing RR, Valoski A. Childhood obesity. *Pediatr Clin N Am* 1985; 32:363–379.
5. Freedman DS, Burke GL, Harsha DW, et al: Relationship of changes in obesity to serum lipid and lipoprotein changes in childhood and adolescence. *JAMA* 1985; 254:515–520.
6. Garn SM: Continuities and changes in fatness from infancy through adulthood. *Curr Probl Pediatr* 1985; 15:1–47.
7. Gortmaker SL, Dietz WH, Sobol AM, et al: Increasing pediatric obesity in the United States. *Am J Dis Child* 1987; 141:535–540.
8. Poissonnet CM, LaVelle M, Burdi AR: Growth and development of adipose tissue. *J Pediatr* 1988; 113:1–9.
9. Roberts SB, Savage J, Coward WA, et al: Energy expenditure and intake in infants born to lean and overweight mothers. *N Engl J Med* 1988; 318:461–466.
10. Rolland-Cachera MF, Deheeger M, Bellisle F, et al: Adiposity rebound in children: a simple indicator for predicting obesity. *Am J Clin Nutr* 1984; 39:129–135.
11. Stunkard AJ, Sorensen TI, Hanis C, et al: An adoption study of human obesity. *N Engl J Med* 1986; 314:193–198.

BIBLIOGRAPHY

Burton BT, Foster WR, Hirsch J, et al: Health implications of obesity: An NIH consensus development conference. *Int J Obes* 1985; 9:155–169.

Epstein LH, Wing RR: Behavioral treatment of childhood obesity. *Psych Bull* 1987; 101:331–342.

Merritt RJ: Obesity. *Curr Probl Pediatr* 1982; 12:1–58.

11 ACCIDENTAL INJURY IN PRIMARY CARE PEDIATRICS

Marie C. McCormick, M.D., Sc.D.

Among children older than 1 year, injury is the most frequent cause of death and a source of substantial morbidity.[14] Mortality due to injuries ranges from 5.0 per 10,000 among infants to 4.2 per 10,000 for adolescents.[6] Death rates provide only a partial estimate of the impact of injuries as a source of morbidity, however. Injuries account for 10% to 20% of all acute conditions among children and youth reported in the National Health Interview Survey.[4]

In view of the importance of injury as a source of morbidity, many investigators have attempted to identify risk factors for injury to develop prevention strategies. This chapter reviews the results of these investigations and the implications for the primary care practitioner.

RISK FACTORS FOR CHILDHOOD INJURY

Injury during childhood is not a random event. Hence the term "accident" is increasingly being avoided by investigators, because it conveys the impression that injury may be unpredictable and unpreventable. Situations in which the risk of injury is high are understandable in terms of normal childhood activities, and can be characterized with respect to the setting in which injury occurs and the characteristics of the child and family that increase the risk for injury.

THE SETTING

Characteristics of the where and when of childhood injury suggest that most injuries are associated with play, especially unsupervised play. Most injuries occur around the home, with the kitchen the most frequent site of indoor injuries. For younger children an emerging concern is also the risk of injury in daycare settings. As children get older, however, injuries in playgrounds and in the streets are more frequent. Injury rates are higher in the spring and summer, although this seasonal pattern may vary with the type of injury.

What is not so clear is whether children who are injured are exposed to environments that can be considered more dangerous than those of children who are not injured. Careful examination of the circumstances surrounding injuries to children have led to the recognition of many specific hazards, such as improperly regulated temperature of hot water, the types of caps on containers for medications and other toxins, and the lack of child restraints in automobiles. No difference has been found in injury rates among children from environments with varying levels of specific hazards. However, the rate of injury as a function of the exposure to hazardous situations or substances remains relatively underexplored.

CHARACTERISTICS OF THE CHILD

Age.—Both the rate and type of injury vary with the age of the child. The risk is lowest in infancy (3% to 9%),[9] peaks for the toddler and preschool child (10% to 30%), and decreases to an intermediate level (5% to 20%) for older children.[17]

The risk for injury and the types of injuries experienced at different ages are related to the normal progression of developmental activities. In infancy, for example, the risk for injury remains relatively low until the child begins to attain independent mobility (e.g., walking, crawling), then accelerates markedly.[17] Associated with these activities, falls and head injuries are most frequent at this age.[17] The high rate of injuries in preschool children is consistent with their newly acquired independence in mobility and exploring behavior, especially in the home. Although falls and head injuries continue to be frequent, scalds and other burns and ingestions of toxic substances commonly found in the home are also most frequent at this age.[3] Later in childhood, both the circumstances surrounding the injury as well as the anatomic site of injury are more varied as a result of greater independence from the home and a wider range of activities. During this period, injuries sustained as a result of automobile, bicycle, and pedestrian accidents assume greater importance, as do those incurred in the course of recreational and athletic activities.[3] In adolescence, additional risks are presented by access to automobiles and use of alcohol and drugs.[5]

Developmental Progress.—The extent to which children who have injuries may vary in the way they are developing from those who do not have injuries is not clear. Compared with children without injuries, they do not differ in development as assessed by attainment of developmental milestones, social maturity, or reading readiness. In two studies children with injuries were noted to have lower IQs, but this was not true in a third study; in all cases the IQs were in the normal range. No studies have addressed areas of development that conceptually may relate more specifically to injuries, such as coordination, impulsivity, attention span, and perceptual skills. That such factors may be important is suggested by evidence of an increased risk of injuries among adults with a history of learning difficulties.

Behavior Problems.—Most investigators have focused on behavioral traits or styles of children with injuries.[14] Descriptions have varied, but a general impression emerges. Children with injuries have been noted to be more active, more aggressive, and more apt to take chances in play, more extroverted, more impulsive or less attentive, less able to cope with hazards, and more likely to be rated by teachers as having behavior problems.[2, 8, 10, 11]

CHARACTERISTICS OF THE FAMILY

Socioeconomic Status.—The most frequently examined issues concerning the relationship between childhood injuries and characteristics of the family involve the effect of socioeconomic status (SES) and stress on the family. Other factors such as injuries among other family members or level of risk-taking behavior in the family as a whole have received relatively little attention. Where differences have been noted, the role of SES in increasing the risk of injury is unclear; increased rates of injury have been observed for children from higher SES families about as often as from lower SES families. However, the frequency of certain types of injuries may vary by SES, for example kerosene-heater burns as compared with pool-related injuries.

Family Stress.—Perhaps more important than the SES is the degree to which the family may be hampered from assuring the child's safety. Stressful events in the family are thought to increase the risk of injury regardless of SES by decreasing parental attention to the child as the parents cope with the stressful event or situation. Among the stresses that have been linked to childhood injury are maternal psychiatric illness, other illness in the family, marital tensions or disruptions between the parents, parental unemployment, recent changes of residence, separations between parents and children, chronic disorganization of the family, or a combination of such events. Even relatively routine and minor stresses such as preparing the evening meal have been suggested to reduce parental supervision sufficiently to increase the risk of injury; this suggestion is consistent with the higher rates of injury in late afternoon.

The primary care practitioner is likely to encounter the injured child in a context of high use of services for other health problems and a history of previous injury. In addition to high levels of stress, maternal employment may add to the risk of injury, although whether this risk is associated with decreased supervision or daycare arrangements is not clear.[7] This pattern is consistent with descriptions of the context of the "new morbidity" generally, and suggests that such families may require additional support from their primary care practitioner in a variety of areas.

In summary, a number of factors have been associated with an increased risk of injury in children. Besides the sex of the child, the major factor appears to be exposure to hazardous situations that occurs in the course of the normal activities of development. In addition, however, the risk may be enhanced by such factors as child behavior and family stress.

PREVENTION STRATEGIES

The importance of injuries as a source of mortality and morbidity has focused attention on identifying modifiable factors leading to injury and strategies for the prevention of injuries. This attention has gradually resulted in many examples of successful prevention strategies, but these examples also illustrate the complex nature of successful strategies.

The best known successful efforts reflect legislative or regulatory activities that mandate changes in the risk of hazardous behavior. Examples include child-proof caps on bottles of medicine and poisonous substances and automobile restraint laws. Alternative successful approaches involve environmental modifications that increase safety, as in the provision of bicycle paths or changes in automobile construction. Perhaps equally well established but perhaps less well recognized is that conventional educational strategies based on nonselective approaches and reliant on passive information transfer through lectures or pamphlets have been repeatedly shown to be ineffective. What the literature suggests is that a combination of activities is more useful, for example, information on the importance of infant car seats with demonstrations of their use, or assuring access to appropriate safety devices in the context of broader community campaigns.[13, 15]

IMPLICATIONS FOR THE PRIMARY CARE PRACTITIONER

GENERAL APPROACH

The primary care practitioner should provide anticipatory guidance regarding injuries to all parents. The risk factors noted here should be used to help parents understand when injuries are likely to occur and to identify families that may require more attention. The practitioner should be aware that a number of the factors, especially family stress and child behavior problems, may also be associated with increased risk of other kinds of health problems and with inappropriate use of medical services as an expression of parental anxiety. Thus, while alert to the presence of other problems the practitioner should address approaches to the reduction of the incidence of injuries; failing that, the physician should attempt to reduce the risk of bodily harm from such injuries that do occur.

The first step is to assess parental knowledge about risks of injury and to provide information when such knowledge is lacking. Examples include the types of injuries that children incur at various ages, the dangers of household chemicals or medications, and information circulated on dangerous toys or childhood apparel. Parental awareness of the hazard presented by various factors in the environment is a basic element in the prevention of childhood injury. The provision of information is not sufficient, however, to change human behavior.

The second step is to ascertain parental attitudes concerning activities to prevent injuries. Parents may be aware of hazardous situations but may not believe that they have any power to prevent injuries; they may believe that injuries are something that happen to every child. Some parents may even believe that injuries occur as a punishment for poor behavior. In other situations, parents may encourage child risk-taking behavior as appropriate to the child's role, for example, as in the case of boys. While the primary care practitioner may have little success in changing parental attitudes, awareness of such attitudes may aid in tailoring preventive strategies appropriate to parental style.

Finally, the practitioner should assess current preventive practices. In general, the best predictor of future behavior is past behavior, and the parent who has already engaged in some preventive activities will be more successful in implementing new ones. Examples of parental behavior that are indicative of a "preventive" orientation include provision of dental care, completion of immunizations, and concern about diet and exercise.

With such information in hand, the practitioner should attempt to develop individualized strategies that will encourage preventive activities as part of the anticipatory guidance provided to every family. Insofar as possible, the strategies should be tailored so that they can be implemented as easily as possible.

One way to tailor injury prevention activities is to focus on the child's stage of development and that stage's implications for injuries. A useful adjunct to this activity is a set of questionnaires[1] that specifically link development and the risk for injury.

SPECIFIC STRATEGIES

The most efficacious way of preventing injury involves the removal of hazards from the environment of the child or protective strategies to minimize the risk of physical harm should the child be exposed to the hazard. The mechanisms by which this can be achieved have been summarized by Robertson.[3] These mechanisms involve prevention of the creation or release of hazards, modification of the hazard to reduce its potential for harm, reduction in the risk of the child encountering known hazards, and appropriate treatment for injuries that do occur, to minimize disability.

Many of the activities included in these mechanisms are beyond the scope of primary care practitioners. Examples would include the development of flame-retardant construction materials, self-extinguishing cigarettes, or safer playground equipment. However, there are a number of ways in which primary care practitioners can support injury prevention activities.

Primary care practitioners may play an important role in this regard by determining circumstances of injuries among children and identifying dangerous products. Physicians should also participate actively in campaigns to alert families to such products, for example, infant cribs with widely spaced slats through which children can push their heads, pacifiers that come apart and result in aspiration and toys with sharp points or hidden sharp parts.

When the environment cannot be made entirely hazard free, activities designed to minimize the risk of physical harm due to environmental hazards must be encouraged. Currently, as noted above, the most successful approaches to minimizing the risk of injury have involved governmental regulatory action requiring product modification or the use of protective gear, such as child-proof capping for medications and household poisons, the motorcycle helmet law, and drinking age regulations. Often such regulations are controversial, and the primary care practitioner should be prepared to answer patient questions and when appropriate provide active support of such regulations.

More difficult to implement are strategies that require behavioral change on the part of the parent or child. A major role for the primary care practitioner is the encouragement of such behavioral change. In approaching any health education activity, some basic principles may be used by the practitioner to enhance the chance of success.

A way to ease implementation of preventive activities is to emphasize those that require one-time or relatively infrequent attention. For example, reduction of risk of scald burns due to tap water can be achieved by changing the setting on the thermostat on the hot water heater. Pool injuries may be diminished by protective fencing that limits unsupervised entry to the pool. The risk of smoke or flame injury is reduced by the use of smoke detectors in the home.

Most difficult is the encouragement of strategies that require continued awareness and repetitive implementation. The classic example is the use of automobile seat belts and infant car restraints; however, other types of child-proofing activities have proved equally difficult to develop.[3] Even when preventive strategies have been successfully implemented in the home, injuries may occur when the child is in a different environment, as was the case in the trial of "Mr. Yuk" stickers in preventing poison ingestion.

In this regard, primary care practitioners should also encourage parents to be active in ensuring the safety of environments in which children spend a substantial portion of their day. This can take the form of ensuring the safety of playground equipment or the provision of appropriate protective gear for school and amateur athletics.

Finally, the practitioner should also be aware that the parents are young and at the beginning of their careers. Financial barriers may preclude the adoption of preventive activities even though the parents appreciate their importance. In this regard, measures that lower the initial

TABLE 11–1
Types of Anticipatory Guidance for Injury Prevention

AGE	INJURY	TOPICS
General	Burns	Smoke detector
Newborn	Auto injury, burns, other	Car restraints, baby furniture safety, danger of hot liquids, first aid for burns, injuries
6–18 Mo	Falls, burns, poison	Water temperature, safety gates on doors and windows, syrup of Ipecac in home, poison center telephone number, storage of toxic substances and small objects
≥2 yr	Falls, burns	Play equipment, pedestrian auto safety

costs of obtaining preventive equipment, such as programs that rent infant car seats or provide free smoke detectors, may be important adjuncts to the practitioner's anticipatory guidance.

It is unlikely that even the most conscientious parents will be able to prevent all childhood injuries. Thus the practitioner should provide adequate information on managing injuries to minimize the physical harm due to any injuries that do occur. This includes information regarding first aid at home and available emergency services.

The American Academy of Pediatrics has developed a package of materials that combines developmentally appropriate questions and educational activities for well-child care as part of their injury prevention program. The general issues dealt with in this package are summarized in Table 11–1. In addition, the primary care practitioners should be prepared to discuss appropriate babysitting and day care, the storage of firearms, the disposal of old medications, the use of child-proof caps, and the use of space heaters when needed. Special family activities such as boating or other sports may also need review.

In summary, injury remains a major source of morbidity and mortality in children. Although a variety of risk factors for injuries have been identified, these have not proved useful in selecting high-risk populations for special preventive strategies. Thus the primary care practitioner should be prepared to provide anticipatory guidance to all families on mechanisms by which the risk of incurring an injury is reduced and on measures by which any resulting physical harm from injuries that do occur is minimized.

REFERENCES

1. Bass JL, Mehta KA: Developmentally oriented safety surveys. *Clin Pediatr* 1980; 19:350–356.
2. Beautrais AL, Fergusson DM, Shannon FT: Life events and childhood morbidity: A prospective study. *Pediatrics* 1982; 70:935–940.
3. Bergman AB (ed): Preventing childhood injuries. Report of the 12th Ross Roundtable on Critical Approaches to Common Pediatric Problems. Columbus, Ohio, Ross Laboratories, 1982.
4. Current estimates from the National Health Interview Survey: United States, 1981. *Vital Health Stat [10]* 1982; 141. Rockville, Md, US Department of Health and Human Services, Publication No (PHS) 82-1569.
5. Douglass RL, Millar CW: Alcohol availability and alcohol related casualities in Michigan, 1968–1976. *Curr Alcohol* 1979; 6:303–317.
6. Health United States, 1978. Rockville, Md, US Department of Health and Human Services, Publication No (PHS) 78-1232, 1978.
7. Horwitz SM, Morgenstern H, DiPietro L, et al: Determinants of pediatric injuries. *Am J Dis Child* 1988; 142:605–611.
8. Lynch MA: Ill health and child abuse. *Lancet* 1975; 2:317–319.
9. McCormick MC, Shapiro S, Starfield BH: Injury and its correlates among 1-year-old children. *Am J Dis Child* 1981; 135:159–163.
10. Mannheimer DI, Mellinger GD: Personality characteristics of the child accident repeater. *Child Dev* 1967; 38:491–513.

11. Meyer RJ, Roelofs HA, Bluestone J, et al: Accidental injury to the preschool child. *J Pediatr* 1963; 63:95–105.
12. Newberger EH, Reed RB, Daniel JH, et al: Pediatric social illness: Toward an etiologic classification. *Pediatrics* 1977; 60:178–185.
13. Pless IB, Arsenault L: The role of health education in the prevention of injuries to children. *J Soc Issues* 1987; 43:87–103.
14. Pless IB, Stulginskas J: Accidents and violence as a cause of morbidity and mortality in childhood. *Adv Pediatr* 1982; 29:471–495.
15. Rivara FP: Traumatic deaths of children in the United States: Currently available prevention strategies. *Pediatrics* 1985; 75:456–462.
16. Shaw KN, McCormick MC, Kustra SL, et al: Correlates of reported smoke detector use in an inner-city population: Participants in a smoke detector give-away program. *Am J Public Health* 1988; 78:650–653.
17. Stallones RA, Corsa L: Epidemiology of childhood accidents in two California counties. *Public Health Rep* 1966; 76:25–36.

12 CONTEMPORARY ISSUES: DAYCARE, TELEVISION, AND AIDS EDUCATION

William Gianfagna, M.D.

DAYCARE

Multiple factors have led to the increase in the use of daycare in American society, including the loss of the extended family, greatly increased family mobility, growing economic stresses on families, and a widening acceptance of women in the workplace. More than 60% of women with children under the age of 18 years are working mothers, and fully 33% of mothers with children under 2 years of age have paid employment. This trend has been rapidly increasing since the 1960s, with little indication that it will slow down.

The *National Child Care Consumer Survey*[14] published in 1975 defined "daycare" as an arrangement by which parents delegate child care to a person outside the immediate family for more than 10 hours each week. This figure seems to distinguish casual babysitting from more formal child care. With this definition, the survey found that more than 14 million children under the age of 14 years were involved in some form of daycare. The survey revealed that maternal employment was by far the main motivator for parents to use child care. In addition, most parents believed that daycare did have benefits for the child in increasing independence and improving social skills.

Most women work because of economic need, and in the nearly 5 million households headed by women that need is most obvious and growing. For many families maternal employment helps to provide the basic necessities of life. There are, however, many other motivating factors for mothers to seek employment, including the financing of higher education for their children, relief from the constant responsibility of child rearing, and the important personal fulfillment and social rewards derived from gainful employment.

What types of daycare are sought by these families? Most children receive care in a home setting; the caregiver comes to the child's home or the child goes to the caregiver's home. The large majority of these caregivers are relatives. These small home-based arrangements account for 60% of the children in daycare. The remaining 40% of the children are involved in such diverse settings as preschool, nursery school, large group daycare centers, and parent cooperative programs.

According to Pizzo,[13] parents choose specific

child care arrangements based on the reliability of the caregiver and caregiver's responsiveness and trustworthiness. The second most important factor is cost. Larger group care of younger children is much more costly than family care. Middle- and upper-income families have wider options for child care and can benefit from child-care tax deductions; low-income groups have fewer options and tend to seek government-subsidized group care when family care is not available.

In summary, parents tend first to seek child care arrangements with relatives and in small groups of children. Cost and convenience are important considerations, as is provision of some arrangement to accommodate the care of the child when there is illness.

Despite the best efforts by working parents to provide for good alternative care for their child, most working mothers feel guilty. It is important for the practicing physician to acknowledge this common phenomenon among working parents and to be supportive of these families.

ILLNESS IN DAYCARE

Parents often remark that their child seems to have more frequent illnesses after entering daycare. Several studies comment on the incidence of respiratory tract illnesses in children in varied daycare settings in comparison with the incidence in the general population. They indicate that the incidence of minor upper respiratory tract illnesses is increased in the first 1 to 2 years of life for children in daycare compared with children remaining at home, but that there is no difference in illness frequency between the two groups after 2 years of age. Sample households in the Atlanta metropolitan area found an increased incidence of upper respiratory tract infections and ear infections in children younger than 5 years of age who attended daycare. The increased incidence of ear infections, however, was only statistically significant in full-time enrollees. Their figures estimate between 9% and 14% of upper respiratory tract infections and ear infections in children younger than 5 years of age occur as a result of attending daycare. Because most upper respiratory tract illnesses are viral, and contagious both before clinical symptoms appear and after recovery, isolation of these children is ineffective in preventing spread.

The number of acute infectious gastrointestinal illnesses is also higher in children attending daycare. This is particularly true in children younger than 3 years of age who are not yet toilet trained and have an increased propensity to oral-fecal contamination because of their personal health habits. Hand washing by both staff and children has been shown to dramatically decrease the incidence of diarrhea. Rotovirus, *Shigella*, *Campylobacter*, and *Yersinia* outbreaks have been described in daycare. Weisman et al.[15] investigated *Shigellosis* infection in daycare attendees and its spread to other family members. They found that children attending daycare are more likely to be a significant cause of intrafamiliar spread of the disease than those children who commonly are cared for at home.

Health care professionals need also to consider certain parasitic infections in children in the daycare setting. *Giardia lamblia* is a common enteric pathogen in daycare attendees, and although most of the children with positive cultures are asymptomatic, treatment may be necessary in a community outbreak. Heijbel et al.[7] recently reported chronic diarrhea in daycare attendance due to the protozoon *Cryptosporidum*. The most frequent symptoms were vomiting associated with cough and watery stools that lasted for approximately 8 days. Oöcysts can be diagnosed with special acid-fast staining of the stool.

Makintubee et al.[12] demonstrated an increased incidence of primary serious *Hemophilus influenza* type b infection among children cared for outside the home. Although not all studies agree as to the magnitude of secondary cases, prophylaxis with rifampin is presently recommended for all daycare contacts of an index case of *H. influenza* type b. This specific infection can now be considered largely preventable with the widespread availability of a conjugated *Hemophilus* vaccine, which should be given to children 18 months to 5 years of age.

Other infections are recognized because of clinical illness transmitted to the parents of children in daycare and to the caregivers of these children. Hepatitis A in infants and children is generally associated with a mild or asymptomatic illness and nearly always complete recovery. In adults, however, recovery can be prolonged and may require hospitalization. Infection and excretion of cytomegalovirus (CMV) is moderately increased in children in daycare compared with children raised at home. CMV infection is generally associated with mild symptoms, but infection in a pregnant woman poses potential serious risk to the developing fetus.

In recent years concern has escalated as to whether children with acquired immune deficiency syndrome (AIDS) should attend daycare. There now exists ample evidence to show that human immunodeficiency virus (HIV), the infectious agent of AIDS, is transmitted only by sexual contact or by innoculation with blood products. Even in intimate family settings, there continues to be no evidence that HIV is transmitted by casual contact such as hand holding, sharing utensils, or kissing. The American Academy of Pediatrics Task Force on Pediatric AIDS has published guidelines for HIV-infected children in daycare. Decisions should be made on an individual basis. Consideration should be given to the potential for other children to expose the child with AIDS to infections, the ability of the caregivers to deliver the kind of care needed to deal with such a physically and emotionally devastating illness, and whether the child could theoretically transfer the illness via open skin lesions. Even the child who bites does not represent significant risk because of the lack of evidence for transmission of HIV through saliva, which contains low concentrations of the virus. Clearly the common daycare interactions of hugging, holding hands, kissing, diaper changing, and feeding do not represent high risk activities for the transmission of HIV.

With illness, the child in daycare becomes an additional source of stress for the working mother and her family. Should the sick child be cared for at daycare or at home? Increasingly there is pressure to have the mildly ill child remain in daycare. During illness children need familiar settings and may have increasing demands for comforting. This should be taken into consideration for the ill child when deciding on where the child should stay while recuperating. The provisions of the particular daycare center for extra space for isolation and for rest as well as for the necessary staff to care adequately for sick children must be considered. Daycare centers for sick children are just now being established to care for the mildly ill child. Clearly the needs of the child and others in the group must be balanced against the stress of increased maternal absenteeism. The need for having a prearranged strategy for the care of the child with a minor illness is an important topic that should be stressed by the primary care physician when discussing child care with the mother.

CHILD DEVELOPMENT AND THE FAMILY

The psychological and emotional effects of daycare on children have always been major concerns of primary care physicians and parents alike. To date there is no evidence that well-supervised and attentive daycare has any detrimental effects on child development. Strong mother-child attachment is maintained despite prolonged care away from the home. Infants at the ages of 12 to 15 months who have spent as much as 20 hours each day with daycare providers will choose the mother over the daycare provider when approached by a stranger.

Howell[8] reviewed the effects of daycare and maternal employment on families. She concluded that when mothers are employed, both parents report that their marriages are as happy as other marriages. When both parents are pleased about the wife's employment, their marriages may even be reported to be happier. Employed mothers often spend as much or more time on a one-to-one basis with their children and report more enjoyment in the care of the child than do nonemployed mothers.

A further pressure on the family, however, may be the assumption by the mother of two full-time jobs. In many cases it is neither physically possible nor emotionally healthy for the working mother to continue to assume all of the household tasks. Most families enlist the cooperation of the husband and children to share in the household tasks to relieve the mother of this burden; this allows the working mother to have enough energy to spend unhurried and pleasurable time with her children. With proper planning and family understanding, the experience of daycare and maternal employment should neither be detrimental to the development of the child nor a source of increased stress for the family as a whole.

COUNSELING PARENTS

There are many opportunities during well-child visits for the primary care physician to offer advice and answer a family's questions on daycare. One such entry point may arise in the initial newborn office visit by questioning the mother about her plans to return to work and asking about child-care arrangements. The physician should be supportive of the parent and acknowledge the common feelings of guilt that plague working mothers. The physician can anticipate for the parents the health care needs of the child by asking if the caregiver will be able to keep the child with a minor illness or bring the child to the physician's office in case the illness requires medical care. Individual family needs including cost and convenience must also be considered when the physician is questioned about which daycare arrangements are most suitable.

Young children may benefit most by consideration of a setting with a low child-to-caregiver ratio (less than 8:1), as recommended by the American Academy of Pediatrics. Higher ratios are more acceptable for the child older than 4 years, especially if the duration of stay is short. Mothers should also be encouraged to find the time before leaving the child to tell the caregiver any early signs of illness or other special needs of the child that day. In that way caregivers can be optimally responsive and prepared.

It is hoped that an acknowledgement of the needs of the family and child regarding daycare as well as an appreciation of the importance of this issue to the community will ultimately help physicians provide improved health care for all children.

REFERENCES

1. American Academy of Pediatrics: *Health in Daycare: A Manual for Health Professionals.* Elk Grove Village, Ill, American Academy of Pediatrics, 1987.
2. American Academy of Pediatrics: *Pediatric Guidelines for Infection Control of HIV (AIDS) Virus in Hospitals, Medical Office, School and Other Settings.* Task Force on Pediatric AIDS. Elk Grove Village, Ill, American Academy of Pediatrics, 1988.
3. Aronsen S, Gilsdorg J: Prevention and management of infectious disease in daycare. *Pediatr Rev* 1986; 7:259–267.
4. Fleming DW, et al: Childhood upper respiratory tract infections: To what degree is incidence affected by daycare attendance? *Pediatrics* 1987; 79:55–60.
5. Haskins R: Daycare and public policy. *Urban Soc Change Rev* 1979; 12:3.
6. Haskins R, Kotch J: Daycare and illness: Evidence, costs and public policy. *Pediatrics* 1986; 77(Suppl):951–982.
7. Heijbel H, et al: Outbreak of diarrhea in a daycare center with spread to household members: The role of *Cryptosporidium. Pediatr Infect Dis J* 1987; 6:532–535.
8. Howell MC: Employed mothers and their families. *Pediatrics* 1973; 52:252–262.
9. Howell MC: Effects of maternal employment with child. *Pediatrics* 1973; 52:327–343.
10. Loda FA: Daycare. Pediatr Rev 1980; 1:277–281.
11. Loda FA, et al: Respiratory disease in group daycare. *Pediatrics* 1972; 49:428–437.
12. Makintubee S, Istre GR, Wand JI: Transmission of invasive *Hemophilus influenza* type b disease in daycare settings *J Pediatr* 1987; 111:180–186.
13. Pizzo PD: Counseling parents about daycare. *Pediatr Ann* 1977; 6:593–603.
14. Rodes T, Moore J: *National Childcare Consumer Survey,* vols 1–3. Washington DC, Office of Child Development, 1975.
15. Weisman JB, et al: The role of preschool children and daycare centers in the spread of Shigellosis in urban communities, *J Pediatr* 1974; 84:797–802.

TELEVISION

The impact of television on the children of our society is enormous. At least one television can be found in 98% of all American homes. During childhood, television viewing is only second to sleeping as the most time-consuming activity. Various studies trace the average weekly viewing time of television from 23 hours of television per week for our preschoolers to an incredible 54 hours per week for children during ages 4 to 5 years. By the time of high school graduation, a typical child will have viewed 15,000 hours of television, as compared with having received 11,000 hours of classroom instruction. It is hard to imagine that this quantity of television viewing would not have a powerful emotional and social impact on our children.

The primary care physician possesses a unique opportunity for anticipatory guidance regarding television viewing and its effects as well as for challenging parents to optimize their child's enormous time investment in television. The expertise of health care providers on developmental and psychological issues of child health is being increasingly demanded by parents. This expertise should include information about television.

There are nearly 2,400 scientific publications on television and human behavior. Many articles point to the negative aspects of television viewing on children. There are, however, positive potential effects of this medium on growth and development of children. A few of the general aspects noted by Devney and ten Bensil[5] include increasing the child's contact with new vocabulary, expanding his knowledge of the world around him, and exposing him to different cultures and ways of thinking. Notable positive programming for children can be found by careful parental selection. "Sesame Street" and "Mr. Roger's Neighborhood" have been extensively studied and are examples of format and pace that are specifically geared to the developmental and cognitive level of children. Public broadcasting stations present such worthwhile programs as the National Geographic Specials and NOVA, which expose children to other cultures or ways of life and encourage interest in science and nature.

VIOLENCE AND TELEVISION

Few health care providers for children need to be reminded that our children face an increasingly violent society. Somers[12] eloquently illustrates that our "culture of violence" has become a major health problem for our children and youth. The leading cause of death in individuals 15 to 24 years old is motor vehicle accidents, followed by suicide and homicide; together they account for nearly 60% of all deaths in that age group. Violent crime has been increasing at an accelerating rate, with teenagers responsible for 20% of these crimes. Most primary care physicians are all too painfully aware of the growing frequency of child abuse in our society.

Television viewing also contributes to this barrage of violence. As Rothenberg[9] states, "The average child will witness some 18,000 murders, countless bombings, beatings, robberies, and torture—an average of approximately one per minute in the standard television cartoon for children under the age of 10." Although it is true that television only shares the preponderant theme of violence with other media such as movies, magazines, and books, it must be singled out as the most accessible and influential medium for most children. As further evidence, Daven et al.[4] point to a number of reports of similar behavior by children after television viewing of daredevil and violent acts (the so-called Evel Knievel syndrome, named after the motorcycle daredevil). Wharton and Mandell[13] present case reports of imitative child abuse by parents after viewing a made-for-television film.

But is all of this exposure of children to violence on television overrated? Does television indeed just reflect our present society? Or does viewing actually encourage antisocial and violent behavior in our children?

Two of the most important studies to answer these questions were the federally funded Eisenhower Commission (1968) and the Surgeon General's Advisory Committee on Television and Social Behavior (1970). The Eisenhower Commission questioned in broad terms the influence of violence on children. The members concluded that children can and do learn aggressive behavior from what they see on a television screen, and the vast majority of experimental studies indicate that observed violence stimulates aggressive behavior. The Surgeon General's Committee focused on whether there is a casual relationship between television violence and aggressive behavior. Despite the controversy and equivocality of the federal report, the Surgeon General concluded that there was sufficient causal evidence to warrant immediate remedial action. Rothenberg has summarized the research material on television violence. He concludes that children do learn new forms of aggression while watching violence on television. Repetitive violence leads to a decreased emotional sensitivity to media violence. There is also evidence that aggression can be inhibited by reminders that the aggression is morally wrong and by awareness of the painful aftermath of that aggression.

TELEVISION COMMERCIALS AND CHILDREN

Repetitive exposure to commercials serves as another potent influence on children through television. It is estimated that the average American child will receive nearly 350,000 commercial messages by the time he is in his late teens. Most advertisers are quick to point out just how persuasive television commercials are with young viewers and will spend millions of dollars to influence target age groups to buy (or coerce their parents to buy) certain products. Each Christmas season successful marketing and selling on television create "hot items" that soon cannot be found on the toy shelves to satisfy demand. Of all Saturday morning commerical messages, 60% to 80% are for sugared breakfast cereals or snacks, many of which will be incorporated into the child's diet. Children under 5 years of age have little ability to understand the selling intent of commercials. Even the older child under 12 years of age is consistently unable to distinguish program content from commercial messages.

Commercials for drug use and health products also influence young audiences. In their study, Lewis and Lewis[7] found that 70% of fifth- and sixth-graders believed all health messages and commercials they identified. The products advertised were increasingly trusted if a parent or the child used the product. Others have shown that heavy exposure to drug advertising led children to believe that people are frequently sick and often need medication to make a quick recovery from illness.

Television viewing has other ill effects on child health. Dietz and Gortmaker[6] in the National Health Examination survey demonstrate a unidirectional causal relationship of the number of hours of television viewing with obesity in adolescents. Controlling for other variables known to be associated with obesity, each additional hour of viewing was associated with a 2% increase in the prevalence of obesity in the 12- to 17-year-old group. Only a history of prior obesity was more strongly linked than television viewing hours to later obesity in the prospectively studied adolescents.

TELEVISION AND NEW TECHNOLOGY

Cable television, electronic television games, and the videocassette recorder (VCR) exemplify double-edged technologies that have expanded traditional network television. An increased variety of positive educational and entertainment programs and films are now available to children, because 65% of households own at least one VCR. These advances also allow for increased control by children and parents over the content and duration of viewing. However, a vast repertoire of sexually explicit and violent films can now enter the home by passing conventional censorship. Health care providers should remind parents of the ever more pressing need to supervise and direct their child's exposure to these media. Overuse of electronic television games promotes physical inactivity at a time when American youth possess the lowest levels of physical fitness in years.

The American Academy of Pediatrics Committee on Communication specifically opposes the use of television-activated toys. These toys are energized by inaudible television broadcast signals. Many of these devices engage aggressive television figures in gun battles. The Committee expresses concern about the effects of these toys on the child's own creativity and imagination in play, particularly when television not only tells you what to play with but now actually plays with the toy for you as well.

COUNSELING PARENTS

What can health care providers do to improve the effects of television on their patients? The guidelines of San Francisco's Committee on Children's TV can offer some critical questions to help parents evaluate television programming. The American Academy of Pediatrics also publishes patient educational material for parents regarding television. Its handout challenges parents to limit the time children spend in front of the television and to plan their viewing schedule in advance. It further encourages parents to watch television along with their children so that they can act as interpreters of the program information and reinforce the positive experiences with a family discussion.

Physicians should be confident in informing parents of the effects of repeated television violence on the behavior and psyche of their children during the well-child visits. Physicians can emphasize the importance of parental interpretation of the value systems and commercialism espoused by modern programming.

Physicians and health care providers for children interested in affecting public policy regarding television should contact local parent-teacher associations and regional television action groups. These coordinated action groups are working with parents and physicians toward the healthful and effective use of this most formidable teacher of our children—television.

REFERENCES

1. Action for Children's Television. Newtonville, Mass.
2. American Academy of Pediatric's Committee on Communications: The commercialization of children's television and its effects on imaginative play. *Pediatrics* 1988; 81:900–901.
3. Comstock G, Fisher M: *Television and Human Behavior: A Guide to the Pertinent Scientific Literature*. Santa Monica, Calif, Rand Corp, 1975.
4. Daven J, O'Conner FJ, Briggs R: The consequences of imitative behavior in children "Evel Knievel syndrome." *Pediatrics* 1976; 57:418–419.
5. Devney R, ten Bensil R: Television and children: A physician's guide. *Minn Med* 1979; 67:822–837.
6. Dietz WH Jr, Gortmaker SL: Do we father our children at the television set? Obesity and television viewing in children and adolescents. *Pediatrics* 1985; 75:807–812.
7. Lewis CE, Lewis MA: The impact of television commercials on health related beliefs and behavior of children. *Pediatrics* 1974; 53:431.
8. Rothenberg M: Effects of television violence on childhood and youth. *JAMA* 1975; 234:1043–1046.
9. Rothenberg M: Television and children. *Pediatr Rev* 1980; 1:329–332.
10. Rubinstein EA: Television and the young viewer. *Am Sci* 1978; 66:685–693.
11. Somers A: Violence, television and the health of American youth. *N Engl J Med* 1976; 294:811–817.
12. Wharton R, Mandell F: Violence on television and imitative behavior impact on parenting practices. *Pediatrics* 1985; 75:1120–1123.
13. Zuckerman, DM, Zuckerman BS: Television's impact on children. *Pediatrics* 1985; 75:233–239.

AIDS EDUCATION

Since the discovery of human immunodeficiency virus (HIV) as the cause of acquired immune deficiency syndrome (AIDS), public health officials and others concerned with child health have been developing strategies to prevent the spread of AIDS. Because there is no cure for AIDS once symptoms develop, one strategy is the education of school-aged children and adolescents to reduce the chance that they will become infected. The school-age pediatric and adolescent populations represent target groups likely to respond to educational efforts. The pediatric health care professional is in a position to be a positive force for appropriate AIDS education. A background in child development enables him or her to make recommendations on what is appropriate material to present on AIDS. Because of other health-related issues, the preexisting relationships with school nurses, administrators, and parents may be exploited to influence and guide decisions and policy on the AIDS curriculum and general health education in the schools, where most of the formal dissemination of information will take place. In addition, the primary physician has the opportunity to directly discuss and answer questions about AIDS with both the child and family at the time of health supervision visits.

Primary health care professionals as well as school nurses and school health teachers need to be informed on an ongoing basis about AIDS research. They should know the natural history of AIDS, which groups are at high risk, and associated high-risk behaviors, in addition to understanding the prevention of transmission of HIV, so that age-appropriate formal instruction can be added to the school health curriculum. Ideally all teachers and parents should possess basic knowledge about AIDS so that answers can be given to children at the time of inquiry rather than defer the answers to a professional later; children are most receptive when answers are given immediately. There now exists a wealth of educational information available to both parents and educators for this purpose. Most formal educational recommendations on AIDS engage those attending school but do not address the issue of the adolescent or young adult not attending school who may be at even higher risk of becoming infected. The U.S. Public Health Service, along with the media, promotes educational campaigns designed to discourage drug abuse; to encourage seeking of professional help for drug abuse, and more controversial, to promote safer sex with the use of condoms.

EARLY ELEMENTARY SCHOOL

The primary purpose of AIDS education in the young school-aged child is to relieve anxiety about the AIDS epidemic. Because transmission occurs via sexual activity and from contact with infected blood, as in sharing needles for intravenous drug abuse, young school-age children are not commonly affected. These children should be told that AIDS is very hard to catch. Early school-aged children may in the future be increasingly exposed to others in school who have acquired AIDS in the perinatal period. It is important for them to know that touching someone or being in the same classroom with a child with AIDS will not cause them to get the disease. This presents an additional opportunity to discuss and develop compassionate and accepting attitudes toward children with other handicaps in the classroom. Young children should be taught that medical scientists and physicians all over the world are working to find a cure for AIDS.

MIDDLE SCHOOL

The educational objectives in middle school consist of further discussion of the basic principles of transmission of HIV and presentation of the high-risk behaviors to be avoided. Children in this age group can begin to understand some of the basic principles of infectious disease and become acquainted with the concept of HIV as a microorganism, a living thing too small to be seen with the unaided eye. Middle school–aged children should be taught that the infection can be spread by the use of a needle contaminated with the blood of an AIDS patient, from an infected mother to her baby during pregnancy, or from sexual contact either between a man and a woman or between two men. Most sources do not define the term sexual contact in their recommendations, but teachers and parents will need to be comfortable with some direct discussion of what the term means based on the age and experience of the group and the prevailing moral standards of the community. For these purposes, sexual contact can be explained to this age group as a special way that adults touch each other. Such a discussion should include definition of the words homosexual, heterosexual, and gay.

Children should be aware that people of all races and in all parts of the United States can become infected, and although most patients are adults, teenagers can acquire the disease as well. Those who are infected can be without symptoms for a long while and still pass the disease to another person. The children should be told that they will not be able to look at a person and see anything that will tell them that he or she has AIDS. Reinforcement must be given to the idea that casual contact, such as sitting next to someone or being in the same classroom with a person with AIDS, is not dangerous. These children should be told that the way to avoid AIDS is to not have sexual contact with another person and to not use intravenous drugs.

JUNIOR AND SENIOR HIGH SCHOOL

The adolescent and young adult not only need explicit information regarding the facts about AIDS but the material must be presented in such a way that the adolescent believes that he or she should and can change personal behavior to prevent being infected with HIV. Adolescents not only represent a high-risk pediatric group, but some experts think they are the next potential population segment to have a dramatic increase in the incidence of AIDS. Belying this statement is the tendency for adolescents to possess a sense of invulnerability and immortality and to engage in multiple behaviors that may place them at high risk of contracting HIV. These behaviors are well known to health professionals working with adolescents. By the age of 16 years, depending on the racial and ethnic groups examined, 30% to 50% of girls and 45% to 60% of boys report having had sexual intercourse. Fewer than 20% of all sexually active teenagers use any type of contraception, and each year in the United States more than one million teenaged girls become pregnant. Sexually transmitted disease infects more than two million adolescents each year. Illegal drug use is prevalent among adolescents and young adults, although the percentage of intravenous drug users remains small. AIDS is but one crisis area among many calling for a comprehensive approach to adolescent health education.

Adolescents should be taught that HIV is the cause of AIDS and that the initial illness may be a flulike syndrome, which will then disappear. The patient can remain asymptomatic for months or years; however, the disease can still be transmitted during this period. Additional information should be given about secondary infections, including pneumonia and meningitis, that the lymph glands throughout the body can become enlarged and that a rare type of cancer known as Karposi's sarcoma may develop. Specific details of how the virus can be transmitted should be stressed, including all types of vaginal, anal, and oral intercourse, both homosexual and heterosexual; transmission by use of infected drug injecting equipment; and transmission by a mother with AIDS infecting the unborn baby. It is important to discuss the theoretical possibility of transmission from deep mouth kissing if there is direct mucous membrane exposure to infected blood or saliva. Increased risk comes from unprotected intercourse between men and with multiple partners of either sex, such as men or women who are prostitutes. Adolescents should be informed that once infection occurs and symptoms appear, there is no cure and the patient will eventually die. Children and adolescents should feel optimistic, however, that worldwide research for a future vaccine offers the hope of protecting those not yet infected by the virus. Perhaps the most important message for adolescents is that the most effective way to eliminate the chance of infection with HIV and other sexually transmitted diseases is by not engaging in sexual contact and by not using illegal intravenous drugs. Parents, educators, and professionals should not be fearful of supporting sexual abstinence or letting the teenagers under their care know why they make this recommendation. Abstinence offers the teenager freedom from worry about pregnancy and other sexually transmitted diseases, freedom from overcommitment to one relationship, and the ability to maximize future plans and options. Educators can discuss the healthy ways to have romantic relationships during adolescence without sex. It is unrealistic, however, to believe that all adolescents will adopt this behavior strategy. Therefore, those adolescents who continue to be sexually active should be instructed to use latex condoms, carefully applied, during every act of sexual intercourse. The use of spermicides offers additional protection, although no method provides 100% coverage.

The adolescent should be told where to obtain necessary medical services if he or she believes they may be already infected with HIV or any other sexually transmitted disease. It is important to encourage patients to be tested so that further spread can be eliminated, and to inform the patient that although there is no cure, drugs can be used and appropriate medical care given.

Is there any evidence that education has any real impact in altering behavior in high risk groups or in adolescents at risk for AIDS? Brown and Fritz have reviewed the medical literature and give mixed results. There is evidence that educational efforts are successful in changing behavior in homosexual and bisexual men and in intravenous drug abusers in San Francisco. However, the review of the success of sex education programs reveals that sex education does increase knowledge and dispel myths but that this knowledge does not necessarily lead to a change in behavior, such as the use of birth control or of condoms with each sexual contact. Which approaches will optimize AIDS education in adolescents and children? Behavior modification appears to be most successful if the program gives the adolescent decision-making skills and enables participants to practice coping with the pressures of how to say no to drugs or sexual intercourse. Children and adolescents conform to peer pressure as peers help move the adolescent away from the family toward independence. Programs with peers as role models or individuals whose opinion the peer group values may lead to successful transfer of information about AIDS into alteration of high risk behaviors.

SUMMARY

The AIDS crisis may act as a focal point for the development of comprehensive health education for children and adolescents. Primary health care professionals can play an important advisory and direct teaching role for school-aged children in the prevention of AIDS. The anxiety about AIDS in the early school-aged child can be reduced by simple and direct explanation. Middle school–aged children should be taught about basic infectious disease spread and should understand who is at risk for AIDS. Further, they can be taught to avoid certain behaviors associated with contracting AIDS. Adolescents and young adults need full, explicit, current information on how the virus is spread, and should be given strategies for decreasing the risk for infection. The material should be offered in such a way as to maximize self-determination and decision-making skills and in settings in which peer groups can rehearse effective ways of avoiding high-risk behavior.

BIBLIOGRAPHY

American Academy of Pediatrics: Acquired immunodeficiency syndrome education in schools. Committee on School Health Policy Statement, June 1988. *Pediatrics* 1988; 82:278–280.

Asch-Goodkin J: AIDS: What shall we teach the children? *Contemp Pediatr* 1988; 5:50–84.

Asch-Goodkin J: AIDS on the home front: Schooling and foster care. *Contemp Pediatrics* 1988; 5:76–90.

Barbour SD: Acquired immunodeficiency syndrome of childhood. *Pediatr Clin North Am* 1988; 34:247–268.

Brown LK, Fritz GK: AIDS education in the schools: A literature review as a guide to curriculum planning. *Clin Pediatr* 1988; 27:311–316.

Centers for Disease Control: Guidelines for effective school health education to protect the spread of AIDS. *MMWR* 1988; 37(Suppl S–2):1–9.

Centers for Disease Control: Human immunodeficiency virus infection in the United States: A review of current knowledge. *MMWR* 1987; 36(Suppl S–6):1–48.

ADDITIONAL INFORMATION

AIDS, Sex and You; Facts about AIDS and drug abuse, AIDS Suite 700, 1555 Wilson Blvd., Rosslyn VA 22209.

National AIDS Information Line: 1-800-342-AIDS.

Understanding AIDS. Publication No HHS-88-8404, US Department of Health and Human Services, Public Health Service, Centers for Disease Control, PO Box 6003, Rockville, MD 20850.

13 ROLE OF THE PRIMARY CARE PHYSICIAN IN ATHLETIC PROGRAMS

Ralph C. Gallo, M.D.

Owing to an increase in the number of young people involved in sports programs and the renewed awareness of fitness in our society, the primary care physician is faced with questions related to the participation of children and adolescents in sports and recreational programs. The level of sophistication in sports physiology, psychology, nutrition, and medicine today makes it imperative that the primary care physician become more aware of the advances in the field. Proper screening, examination, counseling, guidance, and supervision can help prevent personal injury, foster good health practices, and put youth sports in the right perspective psychologically and developmentally. There is also a role for the primary care physician as a team physician. This position requires a person who is both competent and willing to work with coaches and athletes in achieving maximum physical and psychological benefit for the participant.

EXAMINATION FOR SPORTS COMPETITION

Preparticipation examination of children and adolescents should be approached as an important screening step, not just as a brief review of a previous physical examination or signing a school form.

History taking should include eliciting carefully any history of head injury and unconsciousness, allergy and symptoms suggestive of exercise-induced asthma, musculoskeletal injury, and previous treatment. Inquiry about sudden unexplained death in a relative under the age of 50 years may detect hypertrophic cardiomyopathy or other cardiac causes. Additionally it is useful to ask about nutritional practices, conditioning, training programs, and sources of psychological stress. Problems in these areas can often predispose to injury.

The permission form is signed by the young athlete if old enough and also by either parent or primary care physician as a verification and review of the athlete's responses. A questionnaire (such as the one in Fig 13–1) together with the results of the examination is presented to the officials responsible for the youth sports program. The team physician can review the evaluation and incorporate it into the athlete's program if needed.

The physical assessment should be divided into key areas that will produce data useful for

Medical History (to be completed by student athlete with help of parent or physician)

1.	Are you physically healthy and able to participate in sports?	Yes	No
2.	Have you been told not to participate in a sport before?	Yes	No
3.	Have you ever been unconscious or lost your memory from a blow on your head?	Yes	No
4.	Have you ever had a fracture or dislocation?	Yes	No
5.	Have you had a knee or ankle injury?	Yes	No
6.	Have you had other injuries (other than the usual minor ones)?	Yes	No
7.	Are you under a doctor's care now for any medical condition?	Yes	No
8.	Do you take medicine on a regular basis for any condition?	Yes	No
9.	Do you have allergies (hay fever, hives, asthma, or to medicine)?	Yes	No
10.	Have you had surgery or been hospitalized in the past 5 years?	Yes	No
11.	Are you on a diet or are you concerned about weight or nutrition?	Yes	No
12.	Are you under any stress that might affect sports performance?	Yes	No
13.	Do you have any concerns about your health or other questions you would like to discuss with a physician?	Yes	No
14.	Are you presently in a conditioning or weight training program (Nautilus, Universal, weights, running, swimming, etc.)?	Yes	No
15.	Has anyone died suddenly in your family under age 50?	Yes	No

Date of last tetanus booster ______________ Polio vaccine ______________________

EXPLAIN ANY QUESTIONS ANSWERED WITH "YES" BELOW.

_______________________________ _______________________________

Signature of student athlete *Signature of parent or physician (family)*

FIG 13–1
History questionnaire for sports participation.

Physical Assessment

1. Body composition/growth/maturation Weight ______ Height ______
   Tanner stage: Prepubertal Early pubertal Midpubertal Late pubertal
   Body fat vs. lean mass: Too much Adequate Too little
2. Cardiopulmonary examination:
   Heart rate (resting) ____________
   Heart rate (after exercise) ____________
   BP (resting) ____________
   BP (after exercise) ____________
   Murmur or arryhthmia of significance ____________
   Previous cardiac condition affecting endurance or sports play ____________
   Exercise-induced bronchospasm/asthma ____________
3. Musculoskeletal examination: Adequate ______ Injury prone ______
   Flexibility: Adequate for sports ______ Too much ______ Too little ______
   Strength: Adequate for size and age ______ Not adequate ______
4. Other medical condition or finding affecting participation Yes No
   (e.g., dental, eyes and vision, abdominal, paired organs, skin, acute infection)
5. Urinalysis: Normal ______ Protein ______ Blood ______
6. Recommendations/limitations/conditioning or training program?

FIG 13–2
Physical examination for sports participation (yearly).

general participation and for selection or possible elimination of a specific sport. The profile might be used to direct a child to a different, more appropriate sport or perhaps to open areas that were otherwise formerly closed to a child. The key areas of the physical assessment are highlighted in Figure 13–2.

Important points to be covered during the general examination include assessment of eye and vision function, paired organs, abdominal palpation for enlarged liver and spleen, and urinalysis to detect renal dysfunction.

The important functional areas of a sports-oriented examination are analysis of body composition and growth that includes sexual and physical maturation staging, functional cardiopulmonary examination, and musculoskeletal assessment including strength and flexibility.

By plotting height and weight on a standard growth chart, one can estimate body growth velocity. An estimation of ideal weight has implications for aerobic fitness and appropriate matching of athletes for certain contact or collision sports. In an office setting, measurement of subcutaneous fat folds with calipers in several locations (triceps, subscapula, abdominal, suprailiac) is the most practical, quickest, and least expensive way to estimate lean body mass and fat content. This measurement is performed by isolating a fold of skin and subcutaneous fat between the thumb and forefinger. After applying tension, the thickness of the double fold of skin with underlying fat (not muscle) is read from the caliper and the percent of body fat is found by referring to standardized, age-appropriate tables.

It is useful to note the general physique and body type of the young athlete being examined. A tall, thin, lanky boy with a relatively small thickness of neck muscle mass would not be suited to be a lineman in football as neck injury is a real concern.

In the final aspect of growth analysis, the youth's stage of sexual and related physical development should be determined using the Tanner staging of sexual maturation (see Chapter 7). The patient can be placed in sports with peers of similar physique, particularly from early adolescence onward. Differences in maturation may mean great differences in physical strength, and this can predispose to injury, particularly in contact and collision sports. It is especially disturbing to see a 14-year-old boy (ninth grade, Tanner stage II) wrestling a 17-year-old boy (twelfth grade, Tanner stage V) because they are the same weight and the coach does not have a more competitive wrestler to use and does not want to forfeit the match.

The cardiovascular and pulmonary examinations specifically address the question of whether the patient can safely and effectively play sports. The examination should include detection of murmurs and arrhythmias and measurement of the blood pressure (BP), both at rest and after an exercise test. If an abnormality is more pronounced during and after exercise, further evaluation of the condition is needed before sports participation should take place. Referral to a cardiologist is appropriate at this point. The primary care physician usually has the advantage of knowing the child's history prior to the time of sports participation and thus most congenital heart disease will be detected prior to sports participation. For the child with congenital heart disease, decisions have to be made as to the advisability and limits, if any, of sports participation. The child with a high percentage of body fat and poor cardiovascular fitness will fatigue easily, be at risk for injury, and be at risk for health problems as an adult. The issue of sports participation should be a springboard for counseling such a patient on improving his fitness and health.

During the primary care office visit, the most basic method used to stress the young athlete's cardiovascular system is exercise (steps, running, push-ups) until the system is adequately challenged (maximal heart rate). Then the physician should measure BP and recovery heart rate as well as listen for murmur and arrhythmias. One can use a graded method such as a bicycle ergometer to provide increments in workload in a more structured manner, while measuring heart rate response and BP. These methods are more than adequate in an office setting.

Evaluation of the musculoskeletal system in the athlete consists of examining for any obvious structural abnormalities, injuries, and disability. Assessment of strength and flexibility with recommendations for conditioning are appropriate. Young athletes stress their bodies through intense physical activity, contact, collision, weight lifting, running, and other activities. The result is repeated microtrauma to the growing musculoskeletal system (stress fractures, overuse syndromes) or perhaps an episode of macrotrauma (a dislocation or head injury).

Adolescents begin to lose flexibility in the movement around their joints. Assessment of flexibility becomes important for participants in a physical activity with high demands on muscles and joints, such as a collision sport or one with sudden changes in direction. If a certain joint is not flexible enough, musculoskeletal injury (e.g., strains, pulls, tears) will occur when there is stress of sudden movement changes and when excessive force is applied, especially at the velocity with which high school and college sports are played. Likewise, if the joint is too lax, one is subject to injury due to the inadequacy of the supporting structures around bone and muscle. Each major joint should be examined for degree of tightness and range of motion. Stretching, muscle strengthening exercises, or both should be prescribed to counteract or improve the particular situation encountered. Avoidance of certain activities, refinement of others, or use of supportive equipment (taping) might be indicated. Referral to an athletic trainer or sports medicine center for troublesome cases might be appropriate.

As flexibility often decreases, muscular strength increases with adolescence and young adulthood. Relative deficiency in strength can be attributable to genetic endowment, lack of weight training, and lack of proper rehabilitation of an injured muscle. Methods of testing muscle strength are basically restricted to performance tests such as pull-ups and push-ups and to estimates of resistance generated against a force applied by the examiner. As an example, one might ask the patient to flex the biceps and resist extension or to forcibly extend the knee against resistance. Use of aids such as hand grips to gauge relative strength is also possible. Attention should be paid to any area of relative weakness specific to the sport (weak neck in a football lineman or wrestler or weak quadriceps in a swimmer). Equipment such as the Cybex, which is an isokinetic instrument used to test specific muscle groups, is most accurate but beyond the scope of a primary care office.

DISQUALIFYING CONDITIONS FOR SPORTS PARTICIPATION

There are different categories of youth sports. The categories are collision sports (football, rugby, lacrosse, hockey), contact sports (wrestling, basketball, soccer, baseball, volleyball), noncontact sports (crew, swimming, gymnastics, tennis, track, cross-country), and leisure sports (bowling, golf, archery, field events). A child might not qualify for one category because of a medical problem and the inability to safely meet the demands of the sport. The American Medical Association Committee on the Medical Aspects of Sports as well as other medical organizations have published guidelines for qualification or disqualification in sports activity. One must individualize even when using these guidelines. Acute, systemic, uncontrolled or severe illness is the major reason why a child might be restricted from all competitive sports. The period of disqualification is only for the period that the above condition exists. A child with uncontrolled major motor convulsions is quite different from one who is under good control. Acute infections, such as mononucleosis, do not allow for competition until adequate recovery has occurred. There are specific cautions for specific sports. An adolescent with splenomegaly should avoid a collision or contact sport. A sport requiring great endurance might be fine for a child with a history of multiple concussions but a collision sport might be contraindicated. Individualize! Find an appropriate activity if possible. Try not to exclude a child from something that might be of physical and emotional benefit.

Two issues of great concern and which are getting much media attention are acquired immune deficiency syndrome (AIDS) and drugs. In future years primary care physicians will have to address one or both of these issues when dealing with young athletes. The question of whether a child with AIDS can participate in school sports (particularly contact and collision sports) is bound to be controversial, with legal ramifications. Medically, the question is whether there is a significant risk of transmission of the virus during close contact (assuming blood mixing from injury) in athletic competition. The question will have to be adequately dealt with by physicians and schools. Evidence is lacking that transmission occurs through such secretions as saliva, but one can only imagine the public concern should it occur. The decisions will be complex and not purely medical.

WEIGHT CONTROL IN SPORTS

Sometimes there is great pressure from coaches or peers for adolescents to gain or lose weight to be more successful at a given sport. Wrestlers are notorious for being pressured to lose so that they can compete at a lower weight category and have an advantage over a smaller opponent. The adolescent must be counseled that the purpose of youth sports is not to win at all costs, including that of potentially harming the body. Weight loss or weight gain should be managed by the primary care physician. Determine ideal weight based on percentage of body fat. Set realistic goals: 2 pounds per week is enough. Balance calories between appropriate amounts of protein, carbohydrate, and fat. Include exercise. Watch out for fad diets and inappropriate dietary supplements. Avoid unnatural states such as use of anorectic agents, diuretics, and rubber sweat suits in steam rooms. Replace body fluids during intense activity to prevent dehydration. This seems reasonable enough but it is precisely what thousands of young people are not doing as they try to be successful athletes.

CONDITIONING AND TRAINING

The primary care physician is in a good position to advise on the basics of conditioning. Different sports have different training needs. Some require aerobic training to develop capacities to compete in that sport (long-distance running). Aerobics require sustained moderate exercise (running) on a regular basis to improve cardiovascular fitness and muscle function. Anaerobic training is achieved by increased work or intensity or speed over shorter distances. Short intense sprints followed by active rest (jogging), which is known as interval training, is the basis for a conditioning program to build strength, endurance, power, and speed. Specific muscular strength is achieved through weight training and one must caution all against doing this to excess and preadolescent patients against doing it all for fear of injury to the growing musculoskeletal system. The importance of a flexibility program was previously mentioned.

ATTENDANCE AT GAMES

Many physicians are requested to leave the office and be present at the field or arena of competition. One must be prepared to take on the responsibility of being a team physician in attendance at games. Adequate medical supplies for injury treatment, emergency medical services, an ambulance at contact sporting events, establishment of procedures for handling injuries, delegation of responsibilities, communication with coaches and officials, and provision for transporting and referring injured players are just some of the items that should be worked out *before* the game begins. The physician should know the laws and be familiar with medical liability and the specific insurance provisions at the school district or league.

SPORTS FOR SPECIAL GROUPS

Participation sports and other physical activity can and often do have psychological benefits in the development of children and adolescents. Learning to work toward constructive goals, achieving competence, developing physical abilities to potential, and relating to peers as teammates and competitors are all part of the growth experience of sports participation. For the child or adolescent with a handicap or chronic illness, these factors become even more important. Many youngsters have not had opportunities because they have a disability and are excluded from sports programs. There is a growing awareness of this need, and more programs are becoming available. Success is defined in youth sports as trying, participating, and feeling good about the effort. Children who are retarded can participate in the Special Olympics. Blind athletes can compete in many sports, including track and field, swimming, and wrestling. Hearing-impaired youth have a relatively full schedule of sports, including football and cheerleading. Amputees have wheelchair sports and also compete with nondisabled youths in sports such as wrestling. The primary care physician is in a position to encourage patients with handicaps to participate in athletics.

SPORTS ACTIVITY AND THE CHILD TAKING MEDICATION

The adolescent with essential hypertension can play most sports if the condition is under control. Mildly elevated BP does not preclude most participation. Certain activities such as isometric exercise and intense weight lifting can be aggravating factors and should be cautioned against in those with moderate hypertension. For those playing high school and grade school sports, antihypertensive medication is not usually illegal.

Wheezing, shortness of breath, and symptoms of upper respiratory tract disorders are often exacerbated during exercise. Exercise-induced bronchospasm in a child who is otherwise asymptomatic is fairly common and can be diagnosed by history and observation of the symptoms during vigorous or sustained physical activity. Other cardiac or pulmonary causes should be ruled out by history and physical examination. The inhaled β-adrenergics such as albuterol are useful both diagnostically and therapeutically. The athlete is told to inhale the medication 15 minutes before competing. Advantages of inhaled medication are the avoidance of some of the systemic side effects of oral medication, which would be undesirable during competition. Oral bronchodilators and other medications still have their place for the asthmatic needing them for maintenance. Swimming and interval sports are tolerated better than running or continuous activity sports. Cromyln sodium (Intal) is another useful drug for the patient with asthma and is legal at all levels of athletic competition. Many youth with exercise-induced asthma respond to use of cromyln sodium before practice and competition.

Children with well-controlled diabetes need not be restricted from competition, but careful monitoring of the level of blood glucose and adjustment of insulin dose is needed. Hypoglycemia can be a problem, and insulin requirements may have to be reduced during training. Nontraumatic epilepsy that is controlled should not exclude a child from sports, whether taking anticonvulsants or not.

Common in college, Olympic, and professional sports is the use of anabolic steroids to achieve greater levels of performance. With these athletes as role models and with the availability of these drugs to high school students, a serious potential problem is created. The extent of use among young athletes, school policy on drug testing, education of youth as to the multisystem dangers of anabolic steroids, and decisions on strategies for dealing with users are areas that physicians may be involved with.

BIBLIOGRAPHY

Birrer R, Brecher D: *Common Sports Injuries in Youngsters.* Boston, Med Deck Inc, 1987.

Eisenstadt W, et al: Allergic reactions to exercise. *Physician Sports Med* 1984; 12.

Galioto F Jr: Identification and assessment of the child for sports participation: A cardiovascular approach. *Clin Sports Med* 1982; 1:383–396.

Harvey J: The participation examination of the child athlete. *Clin Sports Med* 1982; 1:353–370.

Hulse E, Strong WB: Pre-participation evaluation for athletes. *Pediatr Rev* 1987; 9:173–182.

Smilkstein G: Health evaluation of high school athletes. *Physician Sports Med* 1981; 9:73–83.

Smith NJ (ed): Sports medicine. *Pediatr Clin North Am* 1982; 29:1305–1320, 1383–1399.

Strong W, Steed WB: Cardiovascular evaluation of the young athlete. *Pediatr Clin North Am* 1982; 29:1325.

The uniqueness of the young athlete: Schering Symposium on Sports Medicine. *Am J Sports Med* 1980; 8:372–376.

14 DIVORCE

Anthony Rostain, M.D.

Divorce is not a single event, but a long and complicated process involving a series of transitions or stages, including predivorce, separation, adjustment, reorganization, and remarriage. These stages present different challenges to family members and occur over variable lengths of time.

STAGES OF DIVORCE

Predivorce.—The predivorce stage is filled with emotional tension and marital conflict. As the marital crisis intensifies, children are often brought into the marital conflict and may develop behavioral changes or "moodiness."

Separation.—This stage begins on the day that one spouse departs from the home. Profound disruption of daily routines takes place as negotiations begin over the terms of the divorce. Irrational and immature behavior is often demonstrated by both spouses. Financial problems, dependence on grandparents, and disruption of well-established social support networks all contribute to the regressive behavior commonly observed in the children.

The uncertainty, disorder, and confusion contribute to the children's sense of insecurity, and they may show signs of profound sadness, marked hostility, or apparent withdrawal. Emotional outbursts at home or at school and poor academic performance are common. Doctor visits for minor problems may suddenly increase, as if both parents and children are looking for reassurance from the trusted physician.

Adjustment.—After a time the family's changed circumstances require new coping mechanisms. Schedules are rearranged and living habits altered. The formerly unemployed housewife may take an outside job. New social supports for parents *and* children are enlisted with greater ease and frequency. After a fair amount of experimentation with different rules and routines in both the custodial and noncustodial households, the turmoil of earlier phases begins to subside. If antagonisms and resentments between parents develop into a recurrent pattern of challenges over parenting, mutual disrespect, and constant conflict, children will continue to be dragged into the parents' fights.

Reorganization.—After new equilibrium is reached and life seems to be reorganized, the divorce appears to be an accepted fact of life. Routine parent-child issues reemerge with both custodial and noncustodial parents. Children's views and expectations of parents grow more balanced and secure. The child's sense of self, although altered, is more integrated.

Remarriage.—Most divorced parents remarry. Initially this may precipitate strong emotional reactions from the children: stepparents can be challenged, angry or acting-out behavior may be directed at biological parents, and a new "readjustment" phase is initiated. In most cases, once it becomes clear to the children that they have not lost the remarried parent, family relationships eventually restabilize.

CHILD'S RESPONSE TO DIVORCE

The child's response to divorce varies according to a number of factors. Individual temperament, developmental level, predivorce adjustment, previous emotional difficulties, the role of the child in the parents' antagonisms prior to the split, the immediate circumstances of the divorce and parental behavior in its aftermath all interact to determine the child's responses to the situation. For the most part, divorce is an extremely painful experience that initiates a grieving process in children. The characteristic features of this grief and mourning are similar to those of reactive depression. John Bowlby has identified four stages of grief following the death of a loved person: numbness or shock; yearning, searching for the lost figure; disorganization and despair; and reorganization. Children seem to go through a similar process after divorce. Unlike death, however, the more "voluntary" loss of one parent, who goes away but is not gone forever, can add confusion to the grieving process. Children ask, "How can I belong to two people who don't love each other?"

Many children remain torn between two warring parents who use them to fight their battles. Love expressed to one parent is interpreted as rejection by the other one. The child may be made to feel guilty for his anger at the parents for divorcing. This guilt is complicated by an initial sense of helplessness that the child experiences when his efforts to help the parents stay together have failed.

The child's feelings of vulnerability and insecurity are intensified by the new life circumstances: fluctuating parental attention (due to parental grief and upset), unstable family routines, weakened family ties, high mobility, decreased economic resources, less available social support structures, and unpredictable parental behavior. The specific reactions will vary according to the child's age and level of cognitive and emotional functioning.

Infants may react with increased fretfulness, poor sleep, poor appetite, or decreased activity. Toddlers may react with regression in toilet habits, greater irritability, and more dependence on their mother. Preschoolers may become more aggressive, throw tantrums, have problems sleeping, become possessive of objects and people, and show signs of autoerotic activity. Older preschool children may become frightened, confused, and sad. Although their play, as well as their fantasies, may reflect denial of the divorce, children at this age tend to blame themselves for the breakup and often display a general bewilderment and helplessness.

Young school-aged children have a better cognitive understanding of the changes resulting from parental divorce. They can express sadness, longing, and the wish for reconciliation more directly, although they tend to become restless, whiny, moody, anxious, and aggressive. Many children can successfully deny some of these painful feelings, and can find gratification outside the home. By contrast, grade-school children (7- to 8-year-olds) seem more affected by the divorce. They show pervasive sadness and grief, fear about the future, feelings of deprivation, and a strong sense of loss. They are often preoccupied with wishes for reconciliation and may experience conflicts in loyalty. Preadolescents react similarly but with more direct expressions of anger and shame. They appear more self-controlled and engage in a multitude of activities to cope with underlying feelings of loss and rejection. Some increase their participation in school-sponsored programs or attempt to master new skills. Others attempt to take on the role of the departed parent at home. A few may act out by lying or stealing in situations in which they are likely to get caught. The majority experience identity confusion, loneliness, powerlessness, and conflicts in loyalty. There may be somatic complaints (e.g., headaches, cramps, abdominal pain) and a decline in both school performance and peer relationships. Occasionally these children may demonstrate precocious sexuality or assume the role of "parental child," both of which are responses marked by "pseudomaturity."

Adolescents are particularly vulnerable to parental divorce because of the primacy of their developmental task: separation and individuation. The teenager's "search for identity" can be disrupted and accelerated by divorce. Although they don't often feel responsible for the breakup, most express concerns about future personal and marital plans. They may become moralistic and self-righteous, especially in their attitudes toward the parent they believe to be "wrong." A majority will use distancing as a coping mechanism: general aloofness, self-involvement, increased social activity, rebelliousness, and staying away from home. Parents often complain that the adolescent doesn't seem to care about the family. This may be an adaptive response insofar as it prevents the teenager from getting enmeshed with either parent, and is consistent with the tasks of separation and individuation.

Most children survive their parents' divorce without major psychologic or emotional sequelae. With time and understanding from the primary adults responsible for their care, children eventually work through their grief and attain a stage of readjustment. Several risk factors for poor resolution of grief must be kept in mind, including continued parental conflict, depression or psychiatric illness in the custodial parent, continued family instability (nonresolution of divorce), overinvolvement of the custodial parent with the child, and previous emotional disorder in the child. Evidence of any of these conditions should alert the physician to the need for psychiatric referral.

INDICATIONS FOR REFERRAL

Child
- Depression
- Withdrawal from peer relationships
- Severe or persistent school problems
- Behavior problems
- Other sign of emotional maladjustment

Family
- Parental conflict
- Parental depression
- Continued family instability
- Parental overinvolvement
- Other sign of family dysfunction

PEDIATRIC MANAGEMENT OF DIVORCE

The sensitive pediatrician or family physician can play an important child advocacy role for children when parents divorce. The physician is in a unique position to provide emotional support to the children, to help parents fulfill their responsibilities as parents, and to offer neutral, objective advice to parents who request it. The primary care physician's role is to offer immediate emotional first aid, to monitor the child's and the family's progress in coping with the divorce, to provide anticipatory guidance, and to offer referral to psychiatric or counseling services when these seem indicated. To do this, the physician must feel comfortable with his own feelings, must be familiar with the predictable responses of parents and children to the divorce process, and should know about the variety of community resources available to help families of divorce.

Although the practitioner usually hears of the divorce from one parent, it is important to speak with the other parent to be able to take a position of impartiality and respect for both spouses. The informant should be reassured that the physician is interested in providing support to the family during this difficult process. A subsequent appointment should be made to discuss issues related to the children's reactions to the divorce. It is preferable to meet with both parents together to emphasize that despite their divorce both will remain parents to the children. If the antagonism between them is too great, it will be necessary to meet separately. In either case, the physician should establish his expertise as a child advocate, primarily interested in preventing emotional problems in the children.

IMMEDIATE STEPS

In the early stages of the divorce the physician should focus the counseling on communication and other issues that may be upsetting the children. When possible, both parents should inform the children of the divorce and explain the changes that the children can anticipate. Children will worry more if they are not informed in advance of the plans that will affect them. Stress the importance of extended family ties, of continuity of place and routine, and of parental acceptance of children's questions and expressions of sadness and anger. In these early stages children fear the loss of emotional support from *both* parents, who may be preoccupied with their own reactions to the breakup. It will be necessary for the physician to emphasize repeatedly the children's need to maintain contact with both parents.

The predictable responses of children of different ages should also be explained in a calm and objective manner. Since parents are filled with guilt about the emotional trauma their children are experiencing, they need to be reassured that although their children will undergo strong emotional reactions in the ensuing months, most children adjust to divorce without severe psychological disturbances. Parental guilt is itself an obstacle to the children's coping with divorce.

The physician should maintain contact with the noncustodial parent, usually the father. The father should understand his importance to the child, his current and future role in raising the child, and the need to maintain an open line of communication. By meeting with the father, the primary care physician is practicing preventive psychiatry and helping to promote an easier adjustment process for the children. By knowing the concerns, feelings, and attitudes of the noncustodial parent, the physician is better able to monitor the divorce process in an objective manner. Both sides of the story will become available and a fuller picture will emerge.

PLAN OF ACTION

As a first step of the plan of action, the resources of each parent and of each child should be assessed. On the basis of their strengths and abilities, parents can be advised about rational allocations of responsibility in situations they must negotiate between themselves, such as visitation schedules, special events, discipline, school performance, purchase of clothing and other necessities, and transportation. Their obligations as parents must be clarified and met or their children will suffer the consequences.

Potential problem areas should also be assessed. Over what issues are the parents in conflict? Are the parents responding appropriately to the children? Are they emotionally available to them? Are the children having a particularly hard time, and if so, why? Based on these concerns, the physician may decide to schedule several meetings to discuss problems that seem to be developing or to refer the family for counseling. The children should be met alone to assess their coping abilities and to provide reassurance and emotional support.

The physician's plan must include methods for maintaining open communication among members of the family as well as between family and physician. Children should be encouraged to express their feelings directly to their parents. Parents should be counseled about the evolution of feelings over time and about the process by which children and parents eventually achieve a new balance. The need for parents to talk to each other about child-rearing issues should be emphasized. All family members should be reassured that their physician is interested.

CUSTODY

Custody battles are painful, ugly, and costly for everyone. If it appears that a custody fight is imminent, every effort should be made to refer the parents to a divorce counselor or mediator, a professional who specializes in helping parents to resolve custody disputes *outside* the courtroom. Since neither parent forfeits his or her right to pursue a legal judgment should this step fail to produce a mutually acceptable outcome, this alternative should be seriously considered by both parents.

If the physician is called into the courtroom to offer expert testimony, a few guiding principles should be kept in mind: (1) Use reason and sensitivity, and above all be honest. (2) Comment only on direct observations from interviews with the children and parents. (3) Try to offer an opinion regarding the preference of the child, the capacities of each parent, the strength of the parent-child bond, and the best chances for providing continuity of place, routine, and parental contact for the child. (4) Avoid having the child choose the custodial parent unless he or she is willing and is capable (adolescent-aged). (5) Avoid commenting on criticisms or accusations raised by either parent unless they are established as being true and are potentially harmful to the child. As child advocate, the physician should emphasize the child's right to visitation with the noncustodial parent, to maintenance of current lifestyle if possible, and to representation by an attorney if it appears that neither parent has the child's best interests in mind.

The choice of joint custody should always be considered when the possibility exists for both parents to work out their disagreements. For certain families joint legal custody has proved to be the best solution. It avoids a "winner-takes-all" situation and provides each parent with a sense of continued involvement in raising the children. Studies have shown that in cases in which the parents make the effort to cooperate, children adjust well.

THE TWO-FAMILY CHILD

The concept of the "two-family child" is helpful in that it emphasizes the importance of *both* parents in the life of the child and serves to remind parents that any rivalry between them only harms the child. The child lives in two families, and these families should be as consistent as possible. It is natural for some differences to exist; but parents must try to maintain similar approaches to discipline, homework, housework, and daily routine. If they are unable to agree with each other, parents will soon notice their children begin to manipulate them, using arguments such as "At Mommy's house we do this" or "Daddy lets us stay up later than you do." As with nondivorced families in which parents fail to be consistent, children will play each parent against the other, making the task of discipline extremely difficult and frustrating.

The custodial parent should be encouraged to resume a normal life pattern as quickly as possible. Frequent contact with the noncustodial parent may be necessary in the early stages to reassure the children that they are still effective together as parents. The custodial parent should avoid confiding in the children and involving them in the emotional, financial, and social concerns of an adult. Commonly, the oldest child assumes a "parental" role in the home, but that child must avoid becoming a substitute for the departed spouse.

The noncustodial parent must not play "camp counselor" but should establish a home environment for the children that includes a stable living area, assigned tasks around the house, and regular bedtime and other routines. These are important insofar as they provide the children with a sense of belonging in the new home of the noncustodial parent. Visitation time should not be shared with other adults except on special occasions. The parent should wait for several months before introducing new lovers or friends to the children, and this should be planned well in advance.

SINGLE-PARENT FAMILIES

When the noncustodial parent has departed from the family and lost regular contact with the children, a single-parent family evolves. These families require special consideration from the physician. The first step is providing support to the parent and the children, who likely feel abandoned. Available resources from the extended family and the community need to be assessed and utilized.

Single parents need reassurance that they can manage the tasks of child rearing albeit under different circumstances. The goal is to help the parent achieve a sense of authority, confidence, and competence in parenting. This may mean that the parent will need help from the oldest child or a grandparent. The partnership that results must be under the parent's control; otherwise his or her authority will be undermined and a sense of helplessness will result.

As the family adjusts to its new situation, the physician will need to monitor the emotional development of the children to identify problems requiring psychiatric referral. The physician can anticipate having to spend extra time with single parents during times of crisis, developmental transition points, and whenever the family undergoes structural change.

Infrequent and irregular contact with the noncustodial parent presents a problem for the children. If possible, this parent should be contacted directly by the physician and encouraged to make regular visits and phone calls to the children. Usually the custodial parent is resentful and finds it difficult to hide this from the child. A sensitive pediatrician can create an opportunity for the child to discuss feelings about the missing parent. The child must be reminded that there is a caring adult who can accept him nonjudgmentally.

DAILY CRISIS AREAS

Predictable problems of daily living can become crisis areas for families of divorce. The practitioner who employs foresight, sensitivity, and common sense can help divorcing parents avoid crises. The adults should understand that they need to work together as parents when the need arises, while also maintaining their "separateness" as divorced individuals. Consistency between parents does not imply they do everything exactly the same way but that they respect each other's individuality and avoid undermining the other's parental authority.

School.—In the early stages of divorce the child may have problems with school performance and peer relationships. Both parents should be encouraged to inform the child's teacher about the divorce and to request that each of them be notified of any difficulties with the child's behavior or performance in school. Each parent should maintain interest in and knowledge of the child's academic development. Instead of parents blaming each other for the child's difficulties, school problems must be approached calmly and rationally. Parents should try to meet together with teachers to learn directly about the nature of the child's problems. Parents who are incapable of working together may need to be referred for therapy. In these cases the physician must make use of his own relationship with the parents to convince both to accept the referral. Therapy is for the divorced family, not just the distressed child.

Special Events.—Birthdays, holidays, school plays, recitals, athletic events, and graduations all require special consideration from parents. Despite negative feelings that the parents may continue to harbor toward each other, each parent must make an effort to attend events that hold special significance for the child. This does not require that they attend *every* event, nor that they go to these together. However, children have a right to expect that their parents will show an appreciation for the special activities in which they are involved. In addition, parents must learn to explain directly to their children their reasons for choosing not to attend a particular occasion. It is not acceptable for parents to use the excuse that they do not want to encounter each other there; this will only make the child feel guilty and ashamed.

Ideally, parents should negotiate holiday and birthday plans well ahead of time. Differences must be worked out without involving the child in the dispute; otherwise these special occasions will become unhappy events marred by conflict and turmoil. Each parent should be warned against becoming competitive and using these events to prove they love the child most. This forces the child into loyalty conflicts. Finally, parents can expect the child to express sadness or anger or to voice reconciliation wishes during these moments. Parents may need to be reassured that these are natural feelings for the child and that eventually the parents will learn to take these feelings in stride.

Discipline.—Divorced parents often need help concerning issues of discipline. During the early stages of the divorce, children may exhibit regressive or challenging behavior. Parents should not be alarmed to find increased testing of limits or acting out. If the parents are overwhelmed with guilt or are too self-absorbed with their own emotional turmoil, they will find it difficult to enforce limits in the home. The physician can be of most value by listening to the parent's concerns, providing another perspective on the child's (or the parent's) behavior, and helping parents anticipate conflict situations or devise strategies for carrying out disciplinary measures. The physician should emphasize the competence and responsibility of both parents for enforcing discipline. Often these problems resolve as the family reorganizes itself. Most problems can best be handled when there is consistency of approach between the custodial and noncustodial parents.

On occasion these problems become chronic. This may signal continuing parental conflict despite the divorce or may reflect the child's efforts to manipulate the parents and play them against each other. By misbehaving, the child may also be seeking attention, trying to rescue a depressed parent, or attempting to reunite the parents. It is important that the physician make a careful assessment of the entire family before glibly offering advice about discipline. The physician should not perpetuate the problem by siding with either parent or by giving repeated suggestions to a "helpless" parent who has been wronged by the ex-spouse.

Illness.—When children get sick there is a danger that illness episodes will be used by parents to accuse each other of neglect. Parental guilt, already high, is quickly intensified when children are ill. The physician can confront this directly by clarifying that the child's sickness is *not* a reflection of poor parenting, by gently cautioning against parental overreaction, and by making certain that the separated parent knows about the illness and that his or her concerns are addressed.

Physicians can expect an increase in office visits for minor illnesses and physical complaints during the early stages of divorce. The child or parents may be looking for emotional reassurance from the physician, who must handle such situations sensitively and use them as opportunities to monitor the divorce process. If these visits become chronic, it is important to look for a pattern of parent-child interaction whereby parental anxiety causes the child to express his emotions through physical symptoms, which in turn causes parental overprotectiveness and enmeshment with the child. Skillful intervention is required to break this cycle. The physician may suggest that even though the child does not appear to be too ill, it would be a good idea to schedule a return visit to see how things are going. Gradually the focus of such visits can shift from the physical complaints to the emotional issues that are troubling the child and the parent.

Remarriage.—The remarriage of one or both parents signals the beginning of a new phase of family development. Of special concern to the pediatrician is the restructuring of roles in the new family. The success of this new family arrangement depends on a number of factors. First, the child needs to know that he still has access to the parent who has remarried and that this change does not mean abandonment or rejection. Second, the child needs to understand that the stepparent is *not* a replacement for the biological parent and that he is not being asked to choose one over the other. Third, the child has the right to express feelings about the stepparent and to develop a relationship with him or her independent of the remarried parent. Fourth, the stepparent has the right to provide both nurturance and discipline to the child in collaboration with the biological parent. This must be done within a framework that is mutually acceptable to biological parent, stepparent, and child. Finally, the new marriage partners must create a satisfying relationship independent of the child. The creation of a new "distance" between parent and child can be a painful process if the divorce has created parent-child bonds that are either very tight or very loose. The remarriage can also increase anxiety and competition between the biological parent and the stepparent of the same sex. The astute clinician will be aware of these different dimensions and will be able to help locate the problem should difficulties arise. Efforts should be made to meet the stepparent and to offer the family ongoing support.

CONCLUSION

Divorce has become a common experience for millions of children. It is a painful and complicated process involving a fundamental restructuring of family relationships, patterns of daily living, and definitions of personal identity. Primary health care practitioners who work with children are in a unique position to provide support, continuity, and guidance to families and to play an advocacy role for children affected by divorce. To do this successfully the practitioner must feel comfortable with his or her own feelings; must demonstrate concern, sincerity, and patience; must be knowledgeable about children's reactions to the divorce process; and must have a good understanding of the particular child and family, their strengths, weaknesses, needs, and resources. Effective intervention can minimize the emotional complications, provide direct support to the individuals involved, and give the practitioner a tremendous sense of personal as well as professional satisfaction.

BIBLIOGRAPHY

Anthony EJ: Children at risk from divorce: A review, in Anthony EJ, Kovpernic C (eds): *The Child and His Family—Children at Psychiatric Risk.* New York, John Wiley & Sons, 1974.

Bowlby J: *Attachment and Loss,* vol 3, *Sadness and Depression.* New York, Basic Books, 1980, p 180.

Brun G: Conflicted parents: High and low vulnerability of children to divorce, in Anthony EJ, Kovpernic C, Chiland C (eds): *The Child and His Family—Vulnerable Children.* New York, John Wiley & Sons, 1978.

Caplan G: Preventing psychological disorders in children of divorce: General practitioner's role. *Br Med J* 1986; 292:1431.

Caplan G: Preventing psychological disorders in children of divorce: Guidelines for the general practitioner. *Br Med J* 1986; 292:1563.

Child Custody Consultation: Report of the Task Force on Clinical Assessment in Child Custody. Chicago, American Psychiatric Association, July 1982.

Derdyn AP: Children in divorce: Intervention in the phase of separation. *Pediatrics* 1977; 60:20.

Despert JL: *Children of Divorce.* Garden City, NY, Dolphin Books, 1962.

Francke LB: *Growing Up Divorced.* New York, Simon & Schuster, 1983.

Galper M: *Co-parenting.* Philadelphia, Running Press Book Publishers, 1978.

Gardner R: *The Boys and Girls Book About Divorce.* New York, Bantam Books, 1971.

Goldstein S, Solnit A: *Divorce and Your Child: Practical Suggestions for Parents.* New Haven, Conn, Yale University Press, 1984.

Grollman E (ed): *Explaining Divorce to Children.* Boston, Beacon Press, 1969.

Guidubaldi J, Perry JD: Divorce and mental health sequelae for children: A two-year follow-up of a nationwide sample. *J Am Acad Child Psychiatry* 1985; 24:531.

Hancock E: The dimensions of meaning and belonging in the process of divorce. *Am J Orthopsychiatry* 1980; 50:18.

Hazen BS: *Two Homes to Live In: A Child's Eye View of Divorce.* New York, Human Sciences Press, 1983.

Hetherington EM: Divorce: A child's perspective. *Am Psychol* 1979; 34:851.

Hetherington EM, Cox M, Cox R: Long-term effects of divorce and remarriage on the adjustment of children. *J Am Acad Child Psychiatry* 1985; 24:518.

Jellinek MS, Slovik LS: Divorce: Impact on children. *N Engl J Med* 1981; 304:557.

Kalter N, Pickar J, Lesowitz M: School-based developmental facilitation groups for children of divorce: A preventive intervention. *Am J Orthopsychiatry* 1984; 54:613.

Kalter N: Long-term effects of divorce on children: A developmental vulnerability model. *Am J Orthopsychiatry* 1987; 57:587.

Kappelman MM, Black J: Children of divorce: The pediatrician's responsibility. *Pediatr Ann* 1980; 9:343.

Krementz J: *How It Feels When Parents Divorce.* New York, Alfred A Knopf, 1988.

Luepnitz D: *Child Custody.* Lexington, Mass, Lexington Books, 1982.

McDermott JF: Divorce and its psychiatric sequelae in children. *Arch Gen Psychiatry* 1970; 23:421.

Ricci I: *Mom's House, Dad's House.* New York, Macmillan Publishing Co, 1980.

Rofes EE: *The Kids' Book of Divorce: By, For and About Kids.* Lexington, Mass, Lewis Publishing Co, 1981.

Roman H, Haddad W: *The Disposable Parent.* New York: Holt Rinehart & Winston, 1978.

Shamsie J: Family breakdown and its effects on emotional disorders in children. *Can J Psychiatry* 1985; 30:281.

Sinberg J: *Divorce is a Grown Up Problem: A Book About Divorce for Young Children and Their Parents.* New York, Avon Books, 1978.

Sugar M: Children of Divorce. *Pediatrics* 1970; 46:588.

Visher E, Visher J: *How to Win as a Stepfamily.* New York, Dembner Books, 1982.

Wallerstein J, Kelly J: *Surviving the Break-up.* New York, Basic Books, 1980.

Wallerstein JS: Children of divorce: The psychological tasks of the child. *Am J Orthopsychiatry* 1983; 53:230.

Wallerstein JS: Children of divorce: Preliminary report of a ten-year follow-up of older children and adolescents. *J Am Acad Child Psychiatry* 1985; 24:545.

Wallerstein JS: Children of divorce: Emerging trends. *Psychiatr Clin North Am* 1985; 8:837.

Weiss RS: *Going It Alone.* New York, Basic Books, 1979.

Weiss RS: *Marital Separation.* New York, Basic Books, 1975.

part II

Assessing Signs and Symptoms

Assessing a patient's problems and organizing an evaluation challenges the primary care physician to be both complete and economic. This section highlights the major concerns for parents of sick children. After the common etiologies of the problem are listed, the major items are discussed in more detail. The discussion of the data-gathering process, history, physical examination, and laboratory testing includes hints and approaches for an office-based evaluation. Some problems that require the help of consultants are mentioned; the methods described should not be used as a prescription but should be modified in the light of the resources available in local practice.

Likewise, the flow sheets offer an approach to working through the problem. As in any such attempt to simplify the diagnostic process, there are other attractive options that work well so the approach suggested in the diagrams needs to be modified with common sense and practicality.

15 ABDOMINAL MASSES

M. William Schwartz, M.D.

Many abdominal masses are discovered by a parent while bathing or dressing the child or by the physician during routine physical examination. Rarely is the mass associated with other signs or symptoms such as pain or fever. The problem requires immediate attention, and the primary care physician should have an organized approach to expedite the evaluation and management of the abdominal mass.

DIFFERENTIAL DIAGNOSIS

CAUSES OF ABDOMINAL MASSES

Trauma

Pseudocyst of the pancreas

Infection

Abscess
- Appendix
- Other

Allergic/immunologic

Large bladder
- Transverse myelitis

Endocrine-metabolic

Liver
- Glycogen storage disease
- Nutritional deficiency
  - Kwashiorkor
- Hyperalimentation

Spleen
- Gaucher disease
- Histiocytosis X

Uterus
- Pregnancy
- Hematometria

Tumor

Liver
- Metastatic disease
  - Neuroblastoma
  - Wilms tumor
  - Gonadal tumor
- Infiltrative disease
  - Leukemia
  - Histiocytosis
  - Granuloma: tuberculosis, sarcoidosis

Spleen
- Leukemia

Kidney
- Wilms tumor

Adrenal gland
- Neuroblastoma

Lymphoid tissue
- Lymphoma

Connective tissue
- Rhabdomyosarcoma

Congenital

Liver
- Cysts
- Congenital hepatic fibrosis

Spleen
- Congenital anemia
  - Spherocytosis

Kidney
- Ureteropelvic obstruction
- Cystic disease: multicystic, polycystic

Dilated ureters

Bladder
- Urethral valves

Intestine
- Duplication
- Omental cysts

Ovary
- Dermoid
- Follicular cyst

Multiple etiologic

Ascites

Constipation

DISCUSSION

An effective organization of the differential diagnosis combines the age of onset with the location of the mass. Young children commonly have congenital causes, mainly genitourinary malformations or tumors such as Wilms tumor and neuroblastoma. Older children have infectious and oncologic masses. In adolescent girls, tumors, cysts, or teratomas may develop in the reproductive organs.

Newborns with masses may have either multicystic dysplasia or polycystic kidneys. Multicystic kidneys contain cysts of various sizes that may have surrounding islands of functional glomeruli that sustain life for a period of time or they may have no functional tissue. This malformation may occur with urethral valves or pulmonary malformations or it may be an isolated problem.

Polycystic kidneys may be "infantile" or "adult." These terms are somewhat misleading since both occur in infants and children. Infantile polycystic kidneys, an autosomal recessive disorder, consist of many dilated tubules that form sacules. Relatively few of the nephrons are functional, so the prognosis is poor. Some forms of polycystic kidneys are associated with liver cysts and fibrosis that typically cause portal hypertension in the third decade. The adult form has small cysts that remain functional and do not cause any clinical problems until adulthood when hypertension is the major problem. Within each group are many variations of anatomic changes and functional disability.

Ureteropelvic obstruction, the other frequent anomaly that presents as an abdominal mass in the newborn, is caused by narrowing at the juncture of the renal pelvis with the ureter. The stricture will cause hydronephrosis that, if severe, will be discovered as an abdominal mass. In less severe cases, mild hydronephrosis may present as hematuria after mild trauma.

Patients with urethral valves may have lethargy or failure to thrive and an enlarged firm bladder. Often there is ureteral reflux and dilated tortuous ureters. A voiding cystourethrogram will outline the urethral valve and reflux, if present. Renal ultrasonography will demonstrate any associated hydronephrosis.

Wilms tumor and neuroblastoma are two main abdominal tumors of childhood. Few patients have any associated signs, although some have either hematuria or hypertension. Imaging of the mass with ultrasound (US) or computed tomography (CT) will help differentiate the two masses. In the first year of life, a special form of neuroblastoma, stage IVs, may regress without any specific treatment.

Dermoid cysts or cystic teratomas in adolescent girls are the most common ovarian tumor in children or adolescents. These tumors contain tissue from all three germ layers, including skin, hair, and sebaceous glands; 10% to 20% are bilateral. Usually detected on a rectal examination or coincidentally on an abdominal x-ray film, the tumors may enlarge to present as an abdominal mass. The major complication of dermoid cysts are torsion and peritonitis although most cause no symptoms.

Pseudocyst of the pancreas is seen in patients after trauma, usually in cases of child abuse. After it is damaged, the pancreas undergoes autodigestion and forms a pseudocyst. This mass, not easily palpable, is demonstrated with ultrasound studies. If the history does not reveal any major trauma, then an investigation for child abuse should be undertaken.

A mass in the lower mid-abdomen frequently is shown to be an enlarged bladder, usually a neurogenic bladder. Neurologic problems, such as transverse myelitis or spinal trauma, may produce contraction of the bladder sphincter and urinary retention. Since the second to fourth sacral nerves innervate both the anal and bladder sphincters, stimulating the skin on the buttocks and looking for contraction of the anus serves as a test for the integrity of these spinal nerves.

DATA GATHERING

HISTORY

For most problems of abdominal masses, the history offers limited information. Age will help in some cases, since many congenital problems appear in infancy, such as infantile polycystic kidney and multicystic kidney. Most cases of Wilms tumor occur in 3- to 5-year-old children. Masses associated with reproductive organs usually appear during early adolescence.

Constipation is a common cause of masses in the left lower quadrant; therefore, a series of questions about constipation should be asked, including diet, frequency of bowel movements, medications, and left-sided pain. A history of blunt abdominal trauma should make one suspect a pseudocyst of the pancreas and child abuse. Growth charts should be completed to see if there is a growth problem that might suggest the possibility of urethral valves. Patients with urethral valves have a weak urinary stream.

Polycystic disease of the kidney is familial, so a family history may lead to the diagnosis.

PHYSICAL EXAMINATION

The physical examination will be more helpful in establishing the diagnosis. A description of a mass should include the location, degree of firmness, tenderness, and sharpness of the border. The location of the mass is usually related to the underlying structure. For example, a right upper quadrant mass is related to the liver; a left lower abdominal mass is associated with a feces-filled intestine or an ovary. Renal masses are in the flanks. Some masses, such as an omental cyst, are not in a fixed location but move as the patient's position changes.

The other characteristics of the mass (firmness, tenderness, and sharpness of the border) also aid in the focusing of the diagnostic possibilities. A hard liver should make one suspect a metastatic process, while a soft, full, and tender liver is congested, as seen in patients with heart failure or hypoalbuminemia. Likewise, the hard spleen may be infiltrated with cells from Gaucher disease, while the soft spleen is more likely from a hemolytic anemia. A large hard bladder is secondary to an obstruction, while a soft bladder is from a neurologic process such as a spinal cord injury or transverse

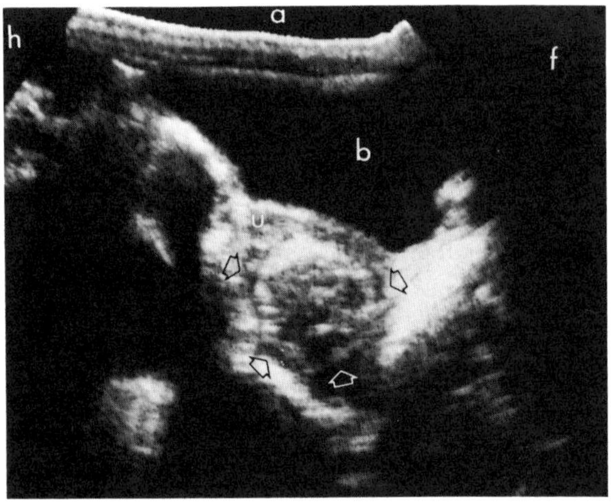

FIG 15–1
Nine-year-old child with chronic abdominal pain. US was helpful in outlining the mass with a calcification in the center *(arrows)*. At surgery, the diagnosis of a teratoma was confirmed. *a* = anterior; *b* = bladder; *f* = caudad; *h* = cephalad. (From Haffer JO, Slovis TL: *Introduction to Radiology in Clinical Pediatrics*. Chicago, Year Book Medical Publishers, 1984, p 110. Used by permission.)

myelitis. Most tumors are hard. Tenderness usually comes from a stretched capsule or impingement of the mass on other organs or nerves. Ill-defined borders may indicate a spreading tumor or a deep organ, in which case palpation is difficult because of overlying normal structures.

Common errors in physical diagnosis include not being able to recognize the spleen from the left kidney and not appreciating how far to the left of the midline the left lobe of the liver can appear. Often, this left lobe may be confused with the spleen.

LABORATORY EVALUATION

Ultrasonography (US) has simplified the evaluation of abdominal masses (Fig 15–1). Although it has taken some of the challenge from the bedside clinician who had impressive physical diagnostic skills, this test helps speed up the identification of the mass. In most cases, the organ can be identified, cysts located, and either a diagnosis can be made or direction can be given to the next step in the diagnostic process: biopsy, CT, or magnetic resonance (MR) imaging. US has helped decrease the number of contrast radiologic studies, laparoscopies, and diagnostic biopsies. Cysts of any organ are easily outlined. Ureteropelvic obstruction, renal cysts, tumors, and thick-walled bladders are identified with US. The origin of a large mass may be traced to the pelvis and calcifications identified that suggest the diagnosis of a pelvic teratoma.

Other helpful screening tests include the complete blood cell count (CBC), especially if anemia, malignancy, or infection is suspected. If there is anemia, further testing with reticulocyte counts and Coombs test will complete the screening (see Chapter 59 for anemia evaluation.) Renal function tests, urine cultures, and serum chemical analyses are important when a mass from the genitourinary system is being considered.

Special testing is indicated by the specifics of

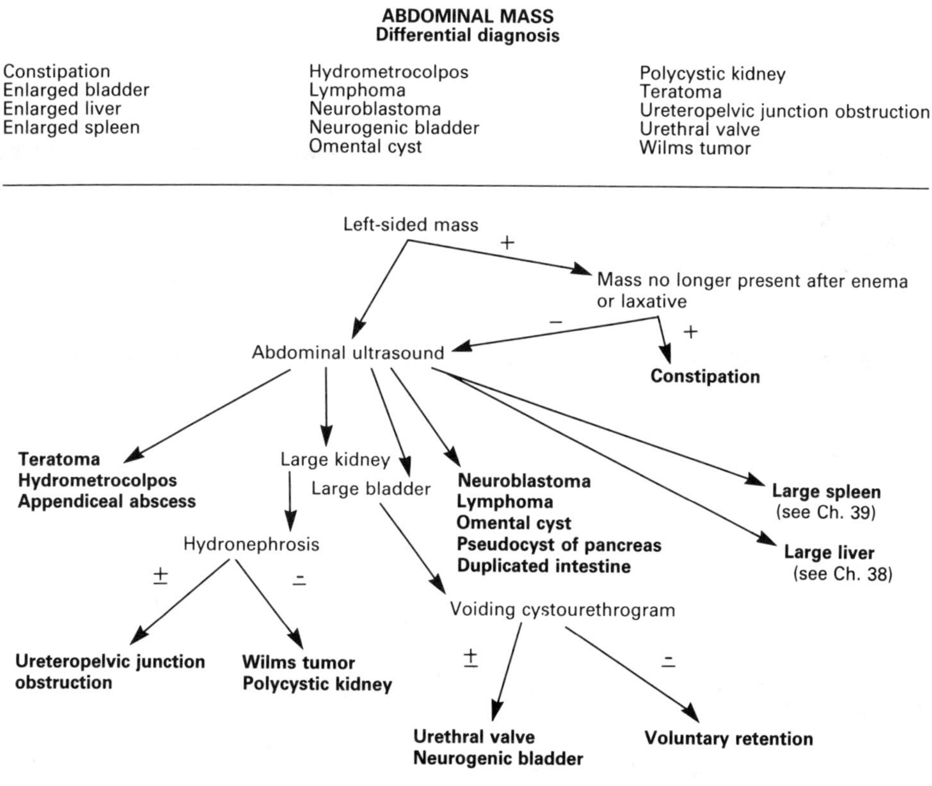

FIG 15–2
"Decision tree" for differential diagnosis of abdominal masses.

the case. Tests such as abdominal CT may help the surgeon or oncologist better outline the mass. Barium studies can better define a mass secondary to intestinal duplication. Screening for vanillylmandelic acid (VMA) or quantitative analysis of VMA will help confirm a neuroblastoma.

INDICATIONS FOR CONSULTATION OR REFERRAL

With the exception of the mass secondary to constipation, most patients with abdominal masses need consultation with appropriate specialists. If the left lower quadrant mass is thought to be secondary to constipation, an enema may relieve the primary problem, but further attention should be directed to the causes of this problem.

DISCUSSION OF ALGORITHM

Since many masses located on the left side are secondary to constipation, this must be ruled out first. After that step, the masses must be evaluated expeditiously, since they may be malignant, infectious, or if benign, cause pressure on other organs or torsion and progress to acute abdomen (Fig 15–2). Other problems of pregnancy, trauma, and malnutrition should be considered as well as anemia and hepatomegaly secondary to heart failure or liver disease.

Abdominal US plays a pivotal role in the evaluation, since it demonstrates the characteristics of the mass and often suggests the correct diagnosis. The remainder of the evaluation will be determined from the results of US.

BIBLIOGRAPHY

Bloom DA, Brosman J: Multicystic kidney. *J Urol* 1978; 120:211–15.

Coldman AJ, Fryer CJH, Elwood JM, et al: Neuroblastoma: Influence of age at diagnosis, stage, tumor site, and sex in prognosis. *Cancer* 1980; 46:1896.

Edelmann CM Jr (ed): *Pediatric Kidney Disease.* Boston, Little, Brown & Co, 1978.

Ein SH, Darte JMM, Stevenson CT: Cystic and solid ovarian tumors in children—44 year review. *J Pediatr Surg* 1970; 5:148.

16 ACUTE ABDOMINAL PAIN

Brent King, M.D.

In the majority of children acute abdominal pain is caused by a self-limiting condition. The physician must distinguish these children from the few whose illness is more serious. In making this distinction, the clinician should be aware of the child's age and developmental level, because these influence the history, physical examination, and differential diagnosis. Whereas the older child and adolescent may be able to give a concise history of abdominal pain and to cooperate with the physical examination, the signs and symptoms in the younger child are more often nonspecific and results of the physical examination can be misleading. Furthermore, many common childhood illnesses have features that may be confused with acute abdomen.

DIFFERENTIAL DIAGNOSIS

COMMON CAUSES OF ACUTE ABDOMINAL PAIN

Trauma

Child abuse

Infection
Viral or bacterial gastroenteritis
Infections that may be confused with acute abdominal pain
- Pneumonia
- Urinary tract infection
- Otitis media
- Streptococcal pharyngitis
- Meningitis
- Mononucleosis

Mesenteric lymphadenitis
Sexually transmitted disease
Mechanical
Intussusception
Volvulus
Malrotation
Testicular tortion
Tortion of testicular appendage
Ovarian tortion
Toxin
Food poisoning
Accidental ingestion
Metabolic
Renal stone
Diabetes
Inflammation
Anaphylactoid purpura
Inflammatory bowel disease
Other
Hemolytic uremic syndrome
Dietary indiscretion
Constipation
Appendicitis
Appendiceal abscess
Functional abdominal pain
Peptic ulcer
Mittelschmirtz
Sickle cell anemia

DISCUSSION

Trauma.—Trauma is a rare cause of abdominal pain throughout childhood, and significant abdominal pain does not occur as a result of minor trauma. Any child with significant abdominal pain reported to result from incidental trauma such as a fall from bed should be considered an abused child until proved otherwise. Adolescents often participate in dangerous activities that may result in abdominal trauma, but because these activities may have been proscribed by their parents, they may be unwilling to explain the circumstances.

Trauma severe enough to cause significant intra-abdominal injury should be managed with the assistance of an experienced surgeon.

Gastroenteritis.—Gastroenteritis is the most common cause of acute abdominal pain at any age. The infant usually has diarrhea, with or without vomiting, often preceded by symptoms of an upper respiratory tract infection. Fever may also be present. Stools will be passed more frequently and will be watery. The pain associated with gastroenteritis is colicky and diffuse. The examination may reveal hyperactive bowel sounds. Tenderness, if present, is most often diffuse. Viruses, especially rotovirus, commonly cause gastroenteritis in infants and young children. Bacterial pathogens include *Salmonella* and *Shigella,* and less commonly certain strains of *Escherichia coli* and *Campylobacter.* Diarrhea that is bloody or contains large numbers of white blood cells on microscopic examination is likely bacterial and should be sent for stool culture. Treatment is conservative and aimed at maintaining adequate hydration. Antibiotics should be withheld until stool culture results are available. Exhaustive evaluation is best reserved for those cases that do not resolve spontaneously.

Constipation.—Constipation may cause abdominal pain, usually left-sided. The stools are usually hard, and their volume may be either large or small. Abdominal distention is often present. The physician may be able to palpate doughy stools in the bowel. The possible causes of constipation are numerous, varying from functional to serious diseases such as Hirschprung disease.

Intussusception.—Intussusception, the process in which a segment of bowel telescopes into a more distal segment, is the leading cause of acute bowel obstruction in infants, and is most common during the second 6 months of life. Most intussusception is ileocolic, although ileoileal intussusception does occur. The classic features of intussusception are colicky abdominal pain, vomiting, a sausagelike right upper quadrant mass, and bloody "currant jelly" stools. There may be a paucity of abdominal contents on palpation of the right lower quadrant (Dance sign). Some of these symptoms, including abdominal pain, may be absent, and therefore a high index of suspicion must be maintained. Diagnosis (and often reduction) may be accomplished with a barium enema study (air contrast enema has a lower success rate). In those cases in which the intussusception cannot be reduced or recurs, surgery is usually indicated, and a surgeon should be involved when the diagnosis is suspected. When intussusception is diagnosed in an older child, a search for an underlying disease is warranted.

Malrotation.—Malrotation is a congenital condition in which the mesentery is abnormally attached to the bowel, allowing the bowel to twist. The patient usually has constant, severe, abdominal pain and bile-stained vomitus. The onset may be acute or may be preceded by minor gastrointestinal symptoms, such as "feeding difficulty." Volvulus can cause extensive ischemic injury to the bowel in a short time, and emergency surgery is necessary. In the patient with suspected malrotation, plain flat and upright abdominal radiographs may demonstrate loops of small intestine overriding the liver. If volvulus has occurred, plain films often show air-fluid levels and dilated bowel loops proximal to the obstruction and a paucity of bowel gas distally. A barium esophagogram is usually diagnostic.

Colic.—Colic syndrome occurs most frequently in infants younger than 3 months of age. The cause of colic is unknown, but the symptom complex consists of paroxysms of extreme irritability accompanied by apparent abdominal pain, with "drawing up" of the legs and a distended, tense abdomen. These episodes may persist for hours, and tend to recur, usually in the late afternoon (see Chapter 6 for discussion of colic).

Appendicitis.—Of all causes of acute abdominal pain in childhood, appendicitis causes the greatest concern. It can be difficult to diagnose, especially in children younger than 6 years. Appendicitis is most common during late childhood and early adolescence, with 12 years being the average age of occurrence. The pain begins as colicky, sometimes vague, periumbilical pain that increases in intensity and migrates to the right lower quadrant over 12 to 24 hours. However, only a third to half of affected children have these classic symptoms. In many children the pain begins in the right lower quadrant, and in others the pain does not migrate. Anorexia is present in the majority of children. Vomiting is also common, occurring after the onset of abdominal pain. The physical examination is often more helpful than the history. The patient usually appears ill and objects to any movement. Signs of peritoneal irritation are frequently present.

The diagnosis of appendicitis is made on clinical grounds. The laboratory data are often equivocal. Most patients have mild leukocytosis. Urinalysis is negative for white blood cells unless the inflamed appendix lies near the ureter, in which case a few leukocytes may be seen. Occasionally a fecalith will be seen on plain radiographs, but films are usually normal (Fig 16–1).

The patient with suspected appendicitis

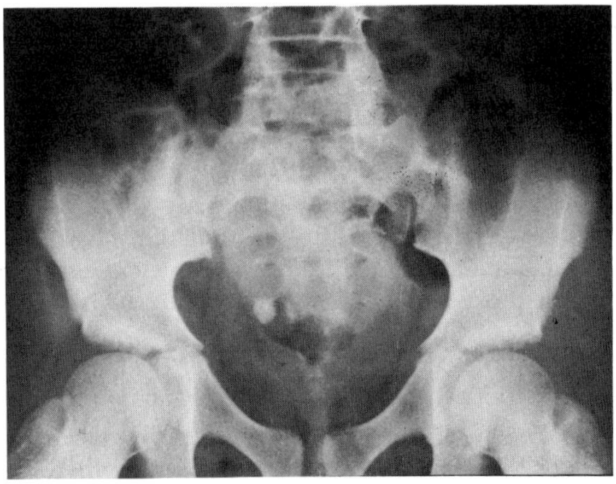

FIG 16–1
Nine-year-old child with abdominal pain. Calcification in the right lower quadrant was part of a teratoma. (From Haller JO, Slovis TL. *Introduction to Radiology in Clinical Pediatrics.* Chicago, Year Book Medical Publishers, 1984, p 110. Used by permission.)

should be seen by a surgeon without delay, because most appendixes rupture within 48 hours of the onset of symptoms. Those children in whom results of physical examination are equivocal but in whom the diagnosis is being considered should be admitted to the hospital for serial abdominal examinations.

A child with a history that includes symptoms of appendicitis, with sudden relief of pain followed by gradual return of pain and fever, probably has a ruptured appendix or an appendiceal abscess. Immediate surgical consultation is mandatory.

Mesenteric Lymphadenitis.—Mesenteric lymphadenitis is a poorly understood disorder that can mimic appendicitis so closely that it may be difficult to differentiate the two. Mesenteric lymphadenitis sometimes occurs concurrent with or shortly after a viral infection. Adenovirus may play a role in this disease. Symptoms that help to differentiate mesenteric lymphadenitis include generalized lymphadenopathy, pain that is diffuse rather than localized, and lymphocytosis. In most cases the diagnosis is made either when a normal appendix is found at laparotomy or on clinical grounds when the symptoms fail to progress during a period of observation.

Sickle Cell Crisis.—The patient with sickle cell anemia will sometimes present with a painful crisis localized to the abdomen, often mimicking acute abdomen. The history of sickle cell disease and previous similar crisis is reassuring but should not lull the physician into a false sense of security. Observation in the hospital allows for both intravenous hydration and serial abdominal examinations.

Torsion of Testis.—Torsion of the testis, usually occurring in prepubertal boys, is a result of inadequate attachment of the testis to the intrascrotal subcutaneous tissue. This gives the testis the potential to rotate, which may result in infarction of the testis. The patient most often has acute onset of scrotal pain, but the pain often is referred to the abdomen and that abdominal pain may be the chief complaint. In addition, nausea and vomiting are frequently associated with torsion, which may direct attention to the abdomen rather than to the scrotum. The scrotal examination is diagnostic. The involved testicle is swollen and lies higher in the scrotum than its mate. Torsion of the testis is a surgical emergency; when torsion is suspected, consultation should be sought without delay.

Food Poisoning and Dietary Indiscretion.—A careful history will help determine whether the child has overeaten or eaten too much of an unfamiliar food. Nausea and vomiting may be present, along with mild, diffuse abdominal pain. Signs of acute abdomen are absent. In the majority of cases laboratory evaluation is not warranted. Treatment consists of support and dietary modification.

Food poisoning can be more difficult to diagnose. The patient may have a history that suggests the diagnosis; for example, consumption of a salad made with mayonnaise or cream points to staphylococcal food intoxication, whereas eating stuffed poultry suggests salmonellosis. More often, however, the dietary history is equivocal. Vomiting, usually the prominent feature of food poisoning, occurs before the onset of maximal abdominal pain. Fever may also be present. The pain is crampy, and signs of acute abdomen are usually not seen, although in occasional patients the pain may be severe enough to require observation in the hospital to rule out significant intra-abdominal disease. Hospitalization may also be required if supportive measures fail to prevent dehydration.

Cholecystitis.—Cholecystitis is rare in childhood. It is most often diagnosed in patients who have hemolytic anemia (sickle cell anemia, its variants, or hereditary spherocytosis), but may occasionally be seen in an otherwise normal adolescent. The symptoms of childhood cholecystitis are similar to those in adults: colicky abdominal pain in the right upper quadrant that is exacerbated by intake of fatty foods. Pain may also be referred to the right scapular region. Nausea and vomiting are frequently reported. Evaluation should proceed with the aid of a surgeon.

Renal Calculus.—A renal stone may appear in childhood, but more likely in adolescence. The expected symptom is unilateral flank pain that radiates to the lower abdomen and is colicky and severe. Frank hematuria occurs frequently. Management is aimed at making the patient comfortable until the stone passes and at identifying an underlying cause. Common causes of urolithiasis are urinary tract infection and hypercalcuria; the remainder of stones are idiopathic except for the few caused by rare metabolic diseases.

Pelvic Inflammatory Disease.—Pelvic inflammatory disease (PID, acute salpingitis), a disease of sexually active females, causes much diagnostic uncertainty. It may be difficult for the physician to differentiate PID from acute appendicitis. There is usually a history of previous sexually transmitted disease; however, many patients deny sexual activity and deny or are unaware of having a sexually transmitted disease. Other risk factors include multiple sexual partners and use of an intrauterine device. The usual patient is a young woman with abdominal pain that began shortly after the onset of her menstrual period and is associated with vaginal discharge. In severe cases the patient may also have right upper quadrant pain, which suggests FitzHugh-Curtis syndrome, a gonococcal perihepatic abscess. The physical examination yields variable findings; signs of peritoneal irritation may be present, but the patient may instead have diffuse abdominal tenderness. On pelvic examination the examiner will often find cervical discharge and adnexal tenderness. In addition to the history and physical examination, a more protracted course of pain may help to differentiate PID from acute appendicitis. Admission to the hospital should be considered for those patients who have fever, severe pain, or recurrent disease and for those in whom the diagnosis of acute abdomen cannot be ruled out.

Ectopic Pregnancy.—Any postpubertal female patient with severe acute abdominal pain should have a urine pregnancy test performed, because ectopic pregnancy may cause acute abdomen and is a disease with high mortality if untreated. Ectopic pregnancy is rare, occurring in fewer than 1% of all pregnancies. The history may include symptoms of early pregnancy such as missed or scanty menstrual period, morning sickness, and breast tenderness. Uterine enlargement is a frequent finding. Examination will demonstrate an adnexal mass in about half of these patients. Cervical motion tenderness also occurs, and may lead to the mistaken diagnosis of PID.

DATA GATHERING

HISTORY

Important early clues to serious disease that are useful at all ages include pain that interrupts the child's usual activities, pain that worsens over time, and an ill-appearing patient either lying still or vomiting.

Among the most important signs of abdominal pain or a significant intra-abdominal process in infants are vomiting, diarrhea, anorexia, irritability (particularly paradoxical irritability), and drawing up of the legs.

Vomiting occurs with many childhood illnesses. A careful history of the course of the illness and the quality of the vomitus may help in identification of the cause. The vomiting of acute abdomen usually occurs later in the course of the illness, often after a period of increasing irritability and crying that is pain related. In contrast, vomiting occurs early in the course of infectious gastroenteritis. Vomiting is particularly worrisome if it is bile stained, indicating bowel obstruction, or projectile, indicating obstruction at or near the pylorus.

Diarrhea, that is, increased stool quantity, frequency, water content, or any combination of these features, is most often associated with acute infectious gastroenteritis, but may be associated with more serious conditions. Particularly significant is passage of bloody mucus, the "currant jelly" stool of intussusception.

The family will sometimes report that the child's fretfulness seems to increase with rocking or cuddling. This paradoxical irritability usually represents serious disease. Paradoxical irritability occurs in acute abdomen because rocking and cuddling serve to disturb the intra-abdominal contents much as an examiner does when attempting to elicit rebound tenderness. Most infants with serious intra-abdominal disease prefer to lie still in the supine position with the legs flexed to relieve abdominal pressure.

PHYSICAL EXAMINATION

The physical examination of the infant with symptoms of intra-abdominal disease should not be limited to the abdomen. Most infants have a group of nonspecific symptoms that may suggest an abdominal cause.

The physician should first observe the child and his or her interactions with the caretaker. The active and playful infant is unlikely to have serious disease. Children with significant intra-abdominal disease usually display one of two behaviors: (1) They may lie quietly, and become irritable with the slightest movement, which suggests acute abdomen, or (2) they may have periods of near normal activity punctuated by irritability and writhing, which should lead to consideration of colicky pain such as caused by intussusception.

Infants will be most comfortable if examined in the parent's arms or lap. The examination should proceed slowly, with the invasive or painful portions of the examination deferred to the end. The abdomen should be inspected for distention and for bruises or other signs of trauma. If found, an explanation should be sought from the family and child abuse should be considered. With a warmed stethoscope the examiner first listens for bowel sounds; the child may prefer to have the parent hold the stethoscope. Absent bowel sounds is suggestive of bowel obstruction. After auscultation, the examiner proceeds with very gentle palpation and percussion, focusing on one small area at a time. The physician may discover point tenderness or guarding that seems related more to one area than to others. Depending on location and quality, masses may represent stool in the bowel, appendiceal abscess, the olive of pyloric stenosis, intussusception, or a true tumor. Paucity of bowel contents in the right lower quadrant (dance sign) suggests intussusception. A child who cries at the physician's slightest touch may be more cooperative if palpation is performed at least partially by a parent or caretaker. The usual test for rebound tenderness can be just as effectively performed by gentle side to side rocking or percussion; this method saves the child undue discomfort. With a well-lubricated small finger, rectal examination can be performed without trauma, and may yield valuable information.

Examination of the older child and adolescent should be guided by the child's own behavior and desires. Many children and adolescents are more comfortable if a parent or caretaker remains close by during the examination. The child's modesty should be respected insofar as possible without sacrificing a complete examination. The traditional abdominal examination can be performed, although the more gentle tests for peritoneal irritation should be used in place of the rebound tenderness test. Absent bowel sounds, exquisite point tenderness, the presence of peritoneal irritation, abdominal rigidity, involuntary guarding, and abdominal mass are the most significant findings on abdominal examination.

Pain in the right lower quadrant produced by palpation or by rocking or percussion is indicative of appendicitis. Clues to the diagnosis of generalized peritonitis are absent bowel sounds and a rigid abdomen. Voluntary guarding may sometimes be differentiated from involuntary guarding by distracting the child. Colicky abdominal pain associated with right upper quadrant mass suggests cholecystitis. Similar pain in a young girl with a mass in a lower quadrant is likely related to ovarian torsion, tubo-ovarian abscess, or rarely ectopic pregnancy.

Since pneumonia, streptococcal pharyngitis, and urinary tract infection may all cause abdominal symptoms, a complete physical examination is required. The evaluation of abdominal pain in the sexually active adolescent girl should include a pelvic examination. The external genitalia and introitus are first examined for signs of trauma such as tears and bruising. Young women may be unwilling to admit to forcible rape or sexual abuse, but these may cause intra-abdominal injury. Purulent cervical discharge, cervical motion tenderness, and adnexal mass are signs of PID. Bloody discharge most likely represents normal menstrual bleeding, but may also be seen in ectopic pregnancy or threatened abortion.

LABORATORY EVALUATION

After a complete history and physical examination the physician will often have to rely on laboratory studies and imaging techniques for a certain diagnosis. Diarrheal stools may be easily evaluated by microscopic examination after staining with methylene blue or Wright stain. Stools that are bloody or contain large numbers of white blood cells should be sent for culture.

The urinalysis is a useful screening device in the patient with somewhat nonspecific symptoms. The physician can quickly identify pyuria and glycosuria, which may be indicative of urinary tract infection and diabetes mellitus, respectively. Hematuria often represents cystitis or renal stone, but may indicate more serious renal disease. In the adolescent a urine pregnancy test can be obtained. Finally, the degree to which the urine is concentrated allows the clinician to estimate the patient's state of hydration.

In patients with concomitant pharyngitis and those who have been exposed to streptococcal pharyngitis a throat culture or a rapid antigen test should be obtained. Abdominal pain can be present prior to the onset of pharyngitis in these patients.

Chest x-ray examination may be helpful in the patient with fever and cough, because lower lobe pneumonias may cause abdominal pain.

Plain radiographs of the abdomen are rarely helpful. Occasionally air-fluid levels or a fecalith may be seen, but unless these studies are immediately available to the physician, obtaining plain films will only serve to delay appropriate referral of the child with suspected acute abdomen.

Serum electrolytes and glucose levels may prove helpful in evaluation of excessive vomiting or diarrhea, but are not routine. More extensive metabolic profiles should be reserved for specific indications.

INDICATIONS FOR CONSULTATION OR REFERRAL

Most acute abdominal pain is related to self-limiting conditions that can be managed easily by the physician in an outpatient setting. A small number of children will benefit from hospitalization. Patients with suspected appendicitis, malrotation, intussusception, ectopic pregnancy, or peritonitis and those who appear to have sustained significant intra-abdominal trauma should be seen by a surgeon early in the course of diagnostic evaluation, because delay in treatment may result in significant morbidity or even death. Likewise, diabetes, sickle cell disease, inflammatory bowel disease, and other such disorders are best managed with the assistance of appropriate subspecialists.

DISCUSSION OF ALGORITHM (FIG 16–2)

The physician should first ask about trauma and look for evidence of abdominal trauma such as bruising. Inasmuch as significant abdominal trauma is rare in young children, child abuse should be considered unless the history of the event given by the caretakers is plausible and fits with the pattern of injury. When trauma appears to be the cause of abdominal pain, perforated viscus, splenic rupture, bowel wall hematoma, and contusion of the abdominal muscles must be considered in the evaluation. Surgical consultation should be sought early.

In the absence of trauma, the physician should try to fit the symptom complex with a known syndrome. A 1-year-old infant with paroxysms of crying and drawing up of the legs who also has bloody stools may well have intussusception.

When a recognizable pattern cannot be found in a febrile infant, the child should be examined for infections that cause abdominal pain. In the older infant streptococcal pharyngitis can cause abdominal pain, and a throat culture should be considered. Urinalysis, complete blood cell count, chest x-ray, Mono-Spot test, and stool cultures may be diagnostic. When results of these laboratory tests are negative or the child is afebrile, imaging techniques such as abdominal ultrasound may lead to a diagnosis. Surgical consultation should be sought when the diagnosis is unclear.

A dietary history should be included in the evaluation to help identify dietary indiscretion and perhaps to point to common causes of foodborne disease, such as *Salmonella* and *Staphylococcus*.

Some consideration should also be given to the possibility of sexually transmitted diseases, acquired from sexual abuse or early sexual experimentation.

If no syndrome is recognized, the physician must attempt to differentiate surgical from non-

ACUTE ABDOMEN
Differential Diagnosis

Accidental Injury
Accidental Ingestion
Anaphylactoid Purpura
Appendicitis
Child Abuse
Constipation
Ectopic Pregnancy
Food Intolerance
Gastroenteritis
Hemolytic Uremic Syndrome
Mechanical Obstruction
Mononucleosis
Pneumonia
Renal Stones
Sickle Cell Anemia
Tortion of Ovary or Testicle
Trauma
Urinary Tract Infection
Viral Syndrome

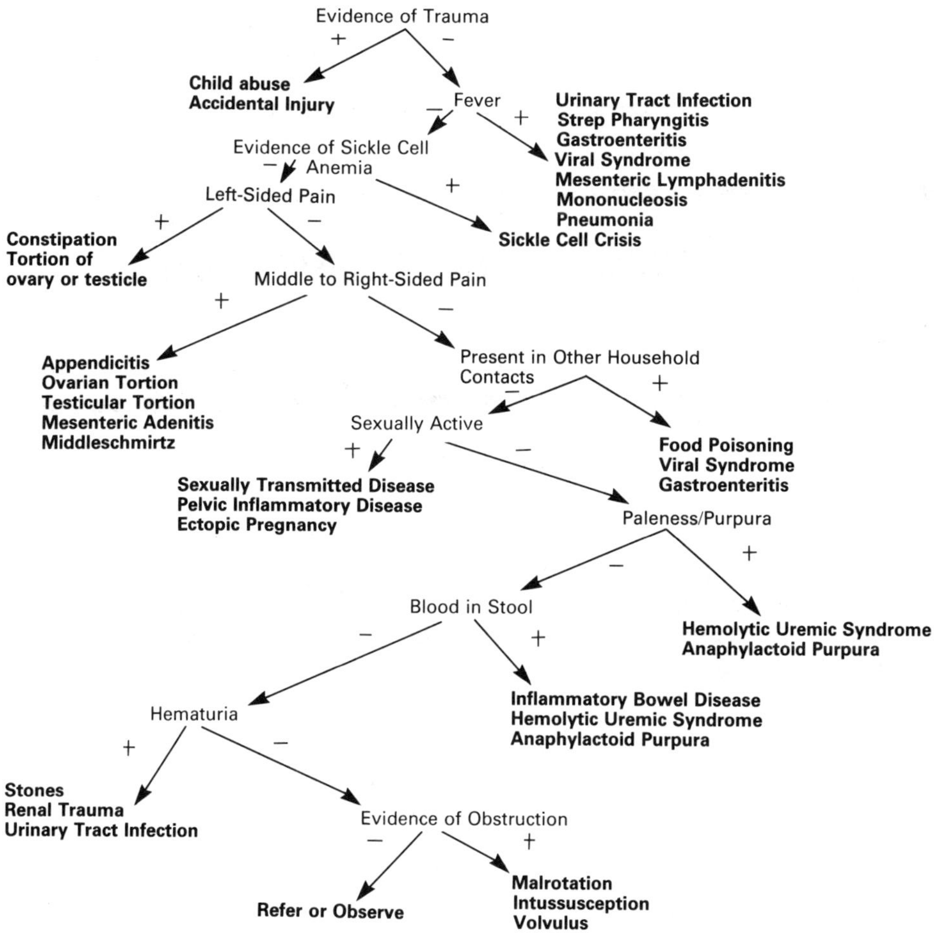

FIG 16–2
"Decision tree" for differential diagnosis of acute abdominal pain.

surgical abdomen. Although not infallible, the presence of such signs as rebound or motion tenderness, involuntary guarding, and other signs of peritoneal irritation should lead to prompt surgical consultation.

Urinalysis is useful in the evaluation of pain in those patients who are not thought to have acute abdomen and in whom there is no ready explanation for the symptom. This test is easy to obtain and can quickly rule out diabetic ketoacidosis, urinary tract infection, and renal stone. Hematuria plus abdominal pain may be the result of anaphylactoid purpura or hemolytic uremic syndrome. When urinalysis is also normal, the physician should consider gastrointestinal disorders such as inflammatory bowel disease or constipation.

When the abdominal pain persists without

positive physical or laboratory findings, it is wise to enlist the aid of a surgeon before further evaluation.

Adolescents differ from younger children in that they are more independent of their families and are more often involved in sexual exploration and in experimentation with alcohol and other drugs.

Sexually active teenage girls who have abdominal pain should undergo a pelvic examination, because it can be difficult to differentiate PID from other causes of acute abdominal pain in this age group. A urine pregnancy test should be performed in all postmenarcheal girls who have significant abdominal pain, because ectopic pregnancy can mimic appendicitis and other causes of acute abdomen.

Those patients who have acute abdominal pain that persists, have surgical abdomen, or do not have an apparent self-limiting disorder will benefit from consultation with a surgeon. Collaboration with a subspecialist may be necessary to manage sickle cell crisis, hemolytic uremic syndrome, or inflammatory bowel disease. Most other problems related to abdominal pain may be managed by the primary care physician.

17 CHRONIC ABDOMINAL PAIN

M. William Schwartz, M.D.

Chronic abdominal pain presents a special challenge to the primary care physician since there are few classic symptom complexes and many of the entities that cause pain share many common signs and symptoms. The problem requires use of a logical approach and a battery of questions that helps to direct the evaluation.

DIFFERENTIAL DIAGNOSIS

Most diseases causing abdominal pain do not present in classic and predictable ways. Children with ulcer disease do not have the same symptoms seen in adults. Likewise, urinary tract infections rarely cause flank pain. One way to view this complex problem is to consider each of the abdominal structures as the possible source of pain. For children this list includes the liver, spleen, kidney, bladder, lymphatic system, intestines, and blood vessels. In older patients, the uterus and fallopian tubes also contribute to the causes of pain. Since the pain in about 90% of the patients is psychophysiologic, this diagnosis should be considered in parallel with the less frequent organic causes and not brought into consideration when the diagnostic list is exhausted. The major causes of chronic abdominal pain are summarized below.

CAUSES OF CHRONIC ABDOMINAL PAIN

Trauma
Pseudocyst of pancreas
Hematoma
Infection
Giardiasis
Urinary tract infection
Tubo-ovarian abscess
Toxins (partial list)
Aspirin
Lead poisoning
Hydralazine
Corticosteroids
  Pancreatitis
  Peptic ulcer
Inflammatory/allergic/immunologic
Inflammatory bowel disease
  Ulcerative colitis
  Regional enteritis

Metabolic/genetic
Lactase deficiency
Lactose malabsorption
Sickle cell anemia
Hemolytic anemia
Gallstones
Kidney stones
Diabetes mellitus
Hyperlipidemia
Porphyria
Tumor
Lymphoma
Leukemia
Brain tumor
Rhabdomyosarcoma
Congenital/structural
Intermittent volvulus
Pancreatitis
Stricture of pancreatic duct
Ovarian cyst
Multiple etiologic
Behavioral
  School avoidance
  Family tension
  Identity problem
Constipation
Abdominal epilepsy
Periodic syndrome (Apley)
Irritable bowel
Aerophagia

DISCUSSION

Apley reports approximately 90% of chronic abdominal pain is nonorganic. The pain in these patients is usually periumbilical, does not interfere with sleep, and is not related to meals. The pain may occur at specific times of day such as at bedtime or during school or stressful experiences. Although severe, the pain does not usually radiate. Apley also writes about the periodic syndrome that includes headache, vomiting, fever, joint pains, and abdominal pain. In working with these children, the physician should keep in mind that the pain is real and is symbolic of a communication dysfunction—the pain is trying to say something that words cannot.

Pancreatic disease is frequently overlooked in children with chronic abdominal pain. Pancreatitis, although more frequently associated with alcoholic adults, may be secondary to trauma, congenital strictures of the pancreatic duct, or biliary stones that migrate and block the pancreatic duct. Pseudocysts are commonly associated with child abuse. Both are detected with abdominal ultrasonography (US).

Abdominal epilepsy, a controversial topic because it is not accepted by all, may be a seizure equivalent. Patients with this problem have severe intermittent pains that are followed by lethargy or sleep. Patients may have paroxysmal EEG abnormalities and may be relieved of pain coincident with phenytoin (Dilantin) therapy.

There are no specific clues to detecting tumors that cause abdominal pain. Usually the pain is persistent and does not fit into any more obvious category. Abdominal US is an efficient screening technique to identify the problem.

One third of the patients with ureteropelvic obstruction have abdominal pain and vomiting. Careful history may indicate that the pain is worse after meals or ingestion of large amounts of fluids. The pain can be either periumbilical or upper abdominal. This can be documented with intravenous pyelography (IVP) or renal scan and a diuretic that will increase the formation of urine producing swelling of the renal pelvis and pain.

DATA GATHERING

HISTORY

The goal of the workup is the development of a series of questions that will point to a few diagnoses as well as exclude others. First, try to determine if the evidence leads to an organic or psychologic etiology (Table 17–1).

Though not infallible, the answers to these questions help to rearrange these differential diagnoses into a list of likely causes for the pain and direct the laboratory investigation into a more efficient process (Fig 17–1). Additional information comes from observing the affect of the patient as the pain is described. The patient may be vague about the details of the pain, may relate the problem with a flat affect, or make extra efforts to assure the physician that the pain is present with a facial grimace and an occasional flexion of the trunk. The patient then looks around the room to see who observed these actions.

TABLE 17–1
Important Considerations in Diagnosing Chronic Abdominal Pain

Considerations	Meaning
Related to meals (postprandial)	Cholecystitis, pancreatitis, ureteropelvic obstruction
Associated with milk ingestion	Lactase deficiency
Related to fatty foods	Cholecystitis
Pain awakens patient at night	Organic causes
Location of pain	Central pain (behavioral), peripheral pain (organic), left-sided (constipation)
School absences	If excessive, school avoidance
Family history of anemia	Hemolytic anemia causing gallstones
Associated with diarrhea	Inflammatory bowel disease, irritable bowel syndrome, giardiasis
Family changes or tension	Irritable bowel, functional abdominal pain

PHYSICAL EXAMINATION

In addition to the general physical examination, special attention should be directed to finding: (1) bowel gas, (2) hard stools, (3) masses, and (4) localized pain. It is more common for those who can point to one spot for the pain to have an organic cause. Periumbilical pain is usually from a psychological etiology, whereas pain in the flanks or in the upper or lower part of the abdomen is more likely from an organic problem. It is important to examine the abdomen for gas pockets since this may be the only clue to the cause of pain. Likewise the left lower quadrant should be checked for the hard stool associated with pain from chronic constipation. Careful attention should be paid to deep palpation for masses and organomegaly. Not having the patient relax is the most common error in the physical examination of the abdomen. A tense abdominal wall if a patient is resistant will have the same consistency as an enlarged liver or spleen. A few extra moments of reassurance or a bottle given to an infant will make the findings of this part of the examination more reliable.

LABORATORY EVALUATION

Sometimes the physician strongly considers a psychological basis for the problem and may be tempted not to order any tests. This may not be consistent with the parents' agenda, which may include laboratory tests to confirm the clinical impression. On the other hand, the numerous laboratory aids available cause the concerned physician to make important choices to control the costs and discomfort to the patient. The advantages of some of the important tests are listed in Table 17-2.

The approach to the patient requires some assumptions from the physician. If the evidence leads to a psychological cause, the laboratory work can be either minimal (complete blood cell count or urinalysis) or nothing. However, if the parents indicate that they need more laboratory documentation, then the minimal workup may include sedimentation rate, abdominal US, or a plain roentgenogram of the abdomen. The abdominal US image will demonstrate the gallbladder, pancreas, and kidneys and, if present, it will reveal a tubo-ovarian abscess, a mass such as a lymphoma, or a cystic ovary.

The lactose breath test is used to document a lactase deficiency but there is controversy about the relationship of lactose malabsorption

TABLE 17–2
Important Laboratory Tests

Tests	Information
Sedimentation rate	If high, inflammatory bowel disease
Urine culture	Urinary tract infection
Abdominal ultrasound	Pancreatitis, cholecystitis pseudocyst, abscess, ovarian cyst, tumor
Lactose breath test	Lactase deficiency
Stool ova and parasite *Giardia*	Giardiasis
Diuretic IVP or radionuclide study	Ureteropelvic obstruction
Endoscopy	Inflammatory bowel disease
Barium enema	Inflammatory bowel disease
CBC	Hemolytic anemia, sickle cell anemia, lead poisoning

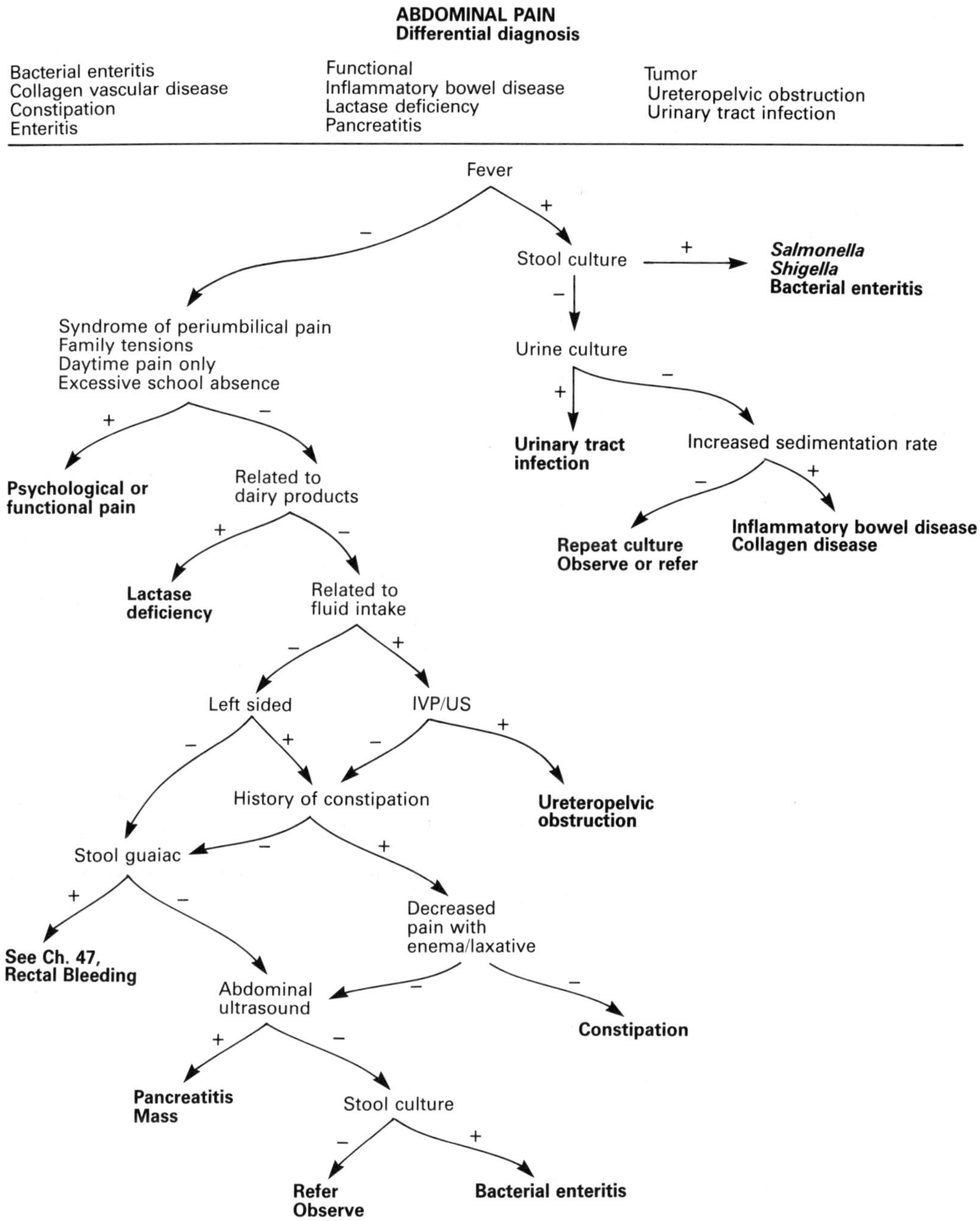

FIG 17–1
Decision tree for differential diagnosis of chronic abdominal pain.

and recurrent abdominal pain. This test measures the amount of hydrogen released by lactose that is not absorbed because of deficiency of the lactase enzyme. Some gastroenterologists use a positive lactose breath test as evidence for lactase deficiency causing pain. Wald et al. believe that previous studies that presented evidence for the relationship between lactose malabsorption and recurrent abdominal pain were not well controlled. They conclude that there is no relationship between lactose malabsorption and abdominal pain.

INDICATIONS FOR CONSULTATION OR REFERRAL

The best therapy is an interested physician who listens to the family tell the history and does not jump into an open-ended evaluation. There are times that the child and the family need another opinion. This does not necessarily mean that the referral should be to a gastroenterologist, surgeon, or a psychiatrist, but rather to a person who understands the problem and has time to collect information and explore psychosocial areas.

DISCUSSION OF ALGORITHM

The thrust of the evaluation is to make a positive search for a psychological cause of the pain, because this will be the final diagnosis in the majority of the cases. The physician should keep in mind a model of this pattern of history, physical examination, and family dynamics. If the patient's condition fits the description of chronic abdominal pain, a modest laboratory examination is necessary. If there are features of the pain that do not fit the description of chronic abdominal pain, then a more detailed evaluation is warranted. Abdominal US has changed the approach to the workup since it allows for rapid return of information about the abdominal organs that may be the cause of the pain.

BIBLIOGRAPHY

Apley J: *Child With Abdominal Pain*, ed 2. Oxford, England, Blackwell Scientific Publications, 1975.

Apley J, MacKeith R, Meadow R: *The Child and His Symptoms*, ed 3. New York, Blackwell Scientific Publications, 1978.

Barr RC, Levine MD, Watkins JB: Recurrent abdominal pain of childhood due to lactose intolerance. *N Engl J Med* 1979; 300:1449.

Douglas EG, White PT: Abdominal epilepsy: A reappraisal. *J Pediatr* 1967; 78:59.

Ein SH, Darte JM, Stephens CA: Cystic and solid ovarian tumors in children: A 44-year review. *J Pediatr Surg* 1970; 5:148-156.

Jordan SC, Ament ME: Pancreatitis in children and adolescents. *J Pediatr* 1977; 91:211.

Kelalis P, Culp OS, Stickler GB, et al: Ureteropelvic obstruction in children: Experience with 109 cases. *J Urol* 1971; 106:418.

Pena SD, Medovy H: Child abuse and traumatic pseudocyst of the pancreas. *J Pediatr* 1973; 83:1026.

Stone RT, Barbero GJ: Recurrent abdominal pain in childhood. *Pediatrics* 1970; 45:732.

Wald A, Chandra R, Fisher SE, et al: Lactose malabsorption in recurrent abdominal pain. *J Pediatr* 1982; 100:65.

18 BREAST ENLARGEMENT

Jerrold S. Olshan, M.D.
Thomas Moshang, Jr., M.D.

The differential diagnosis of breast enlargement ranges from normal changes, as those seen during puberty or in the newborn, to manifestations of serious systemic illnesses. The purpose of this chapter is to act as a guide for differentiating between common pathologic and physiologic conditions resulting in breast enlargement (Fig 18–1).

DIFFERENTIAL DIAGNOSIS

CAUSES OF BREAST ENLARGEMENT

Nonglandular breast enlargement

Trauma
Infection, abscess
Hematoma, lipoma, neurofibroma, lymphangioma
Neoplasm (sarcoma, carcinoma)
Obesity

Glandular breast enlargement

Boys and girls
- Neonatal physiologic breast buds
- Toxin
- Feminizing tumor (gonadal, adrenal, hepatic)

Prepubertal girls
- Premature thelarche
- Precocious puberty

Pubertal boys
- Adolescent gynecomastia
- Hypogonadal states (Klinefelter syndrome, Kallman syndrome, congenital or acquired testicular failure)
- Androgen resistance syndromes

DISCUSSION

Overweight children commonly appear to have increased breast tissue without any real increase in actual glandular tissue, which can be easily mistaken for true glandular hyperplasia. Trauma with subsequent hemorrhage or fat necrosis, inflammation, infection, or other benign masses are common causes of nonglandular breast enlargement that may be mistaken for true increased breast tissue, and usually can be differentiated on thorough physical examination. Malignant neoplasms of the breast in children are exceedingly rare.

Breast enlargement is considered to be part of normal development in newborns and adolescents. Sixty percent to 100% of neonates of both sexes have some degree of physiologic breast hyperplasia. Although this hyperplasia usually lasts only 1 to 3 weeks, it may persist into the second year of life. The rich hormonal milieu in utero responsible for neonatal breast hyperplasia may also result in galactorrhea.

During puberty in girls, elevated levels of estrogens result in normal breast budding, which may begin unilaterally or bilaterally. Adolescent gynecomastia or breast budding seen during puberty is the most common cause for breast enlargement in boys. More than 50% of boys aged 14 to 15 years have some degree of gynecomastia. This usually consists of bilateral, although frequently asymmetric, subareolar enlargement that is somewhat tender. In 90% of these adolescent boys, the breast tissue recedes within 2 years without therapy. Obesity may exaggerate the gynecomastia seen in pubertal boys from increased peripheral conversion of androgens to estrogens by excessive adipose tissue.

Enlargement of the glandular breast tissue, in either sex, can result from increased circulating levels of estrogens or estrogen-like compounds from either endogenous or exogenous sources. Endogenous hormones may be responsible in uncommon or rare conditions, such as feminiz-

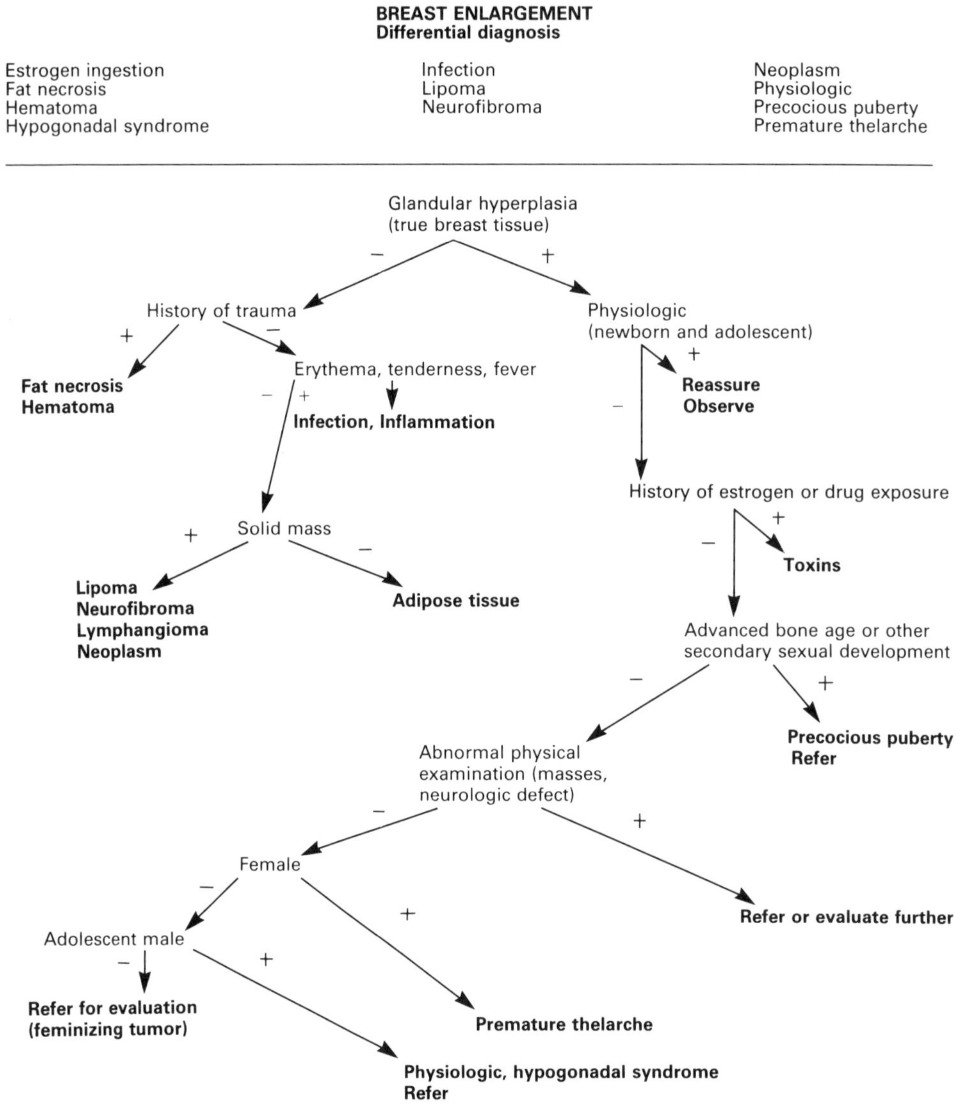

FIG 18–1

Decision tree for differential diagnosis of breast enlargement.

ing tumors of the adrenal gland, liver, or gonads, whereas exogenous hormones can be found in a variety of estrogen-containing products (Table 18–1). Digitalis is thought to be an estrogen precursor and, as such, has effects similar to other estrogen-containing medications. In pubertal boys, drugs that decrease androgen activity, such as ketoconazole and spironolactone, which inhibit testosterone synthesis, or cimetidine, which inhibits androgen binding, can result in breast enlargement. Marijuana use has been linked with breast enlargement as well as galactorrhea. It is possible, although not documented, that other abused street drugs can result in breast enlargement.

In girls, isolated breast development with no other pubertal changes before the age of 8 years is referred to as premature thelarche (Fig 18–2). This benign condition of prepubertal girls is not a result of elevated circulating estrogens but is thought to represent increased end-organ sensitivity to normal circulating estrogen levels. These girls are otherwise normal and have normal bone age. It is important to recog-

TABLE 18–1
Toxins Associated with Breast Enlargement

Estrogens
Estrogen contaminated food products
Oral contraceptive pills
Diethylstilbestrol
Topical estrogen creams
Digitalis
Anti-androgens,
Ketoconazole
Spironolactone
Cimetidine
Hydroxyzine
Unknown mechanism
Isoniazid
Tricyclic antidepressants
Diazepam
Penicillamine
Cannabinoids (Marijuana)

nize premature breast budding from other breast masses, because surgical removal of breast buds will prevent breast development.

Breast enlargement that occurs prior to the age of 8 years in girls and is accompanied by other pubertal changes such as growth spurt, maturation of the gonadal-pituitary axis, and advancement of bone age is considered precocious puberty (see Chapter 93). The varied etiology of precocious puberty is shown below. Idiopathic precocious puberty is the diagnosis in the vast majority of cases.

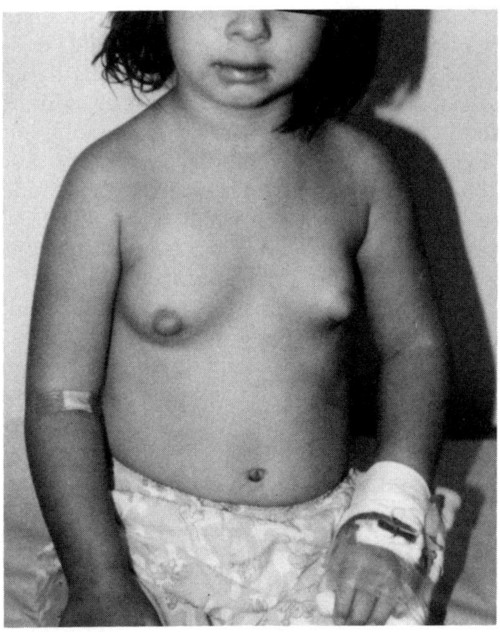

FIG 18–2
Isolated bilateral breast development of unknown cause. This patient has no other secondary sexual development.

PRECOCIOUS PUBERTY SYNDROME
Idiopathic
Central nervous system (neoplasms, infection, hydrocephalus)
Neurofibromatosis
McCune-Albright syndrome
Hypothyroidism
Gonadal tumor congenital adrenal hyperplasia

In pubertal boys, aberrations from the normal ratios of androgens to estrogens may result from decreased testosterone production, decreased end-organ responsiveness to androgens (testicular feminization), increased conversion of androgens to estrogens, or increased estrogen production. Decreased testosterone production can be seen in any of the forms of hypogonadism. With a frequency of roughly one in 600 live births, Klinefelter syndrome (XXY) is one of the most common chromosomal abnormalities and is probably the most common cause of hypogonadism in men. In children with Klinefelter syndrome often no abnormalities are noted until puberty, when there is evidence of testicular failure, with small testes and poor virilization. Approximately one third of these patients will develop gynecomastia, from both decreased levels of testosterone and increased levels of estradiol.

In some boys there is no discernible cause for the breast enlargement and biochemical evaluation yields normal results. The diagnosis is idiopathic gynecomastia in these children, unless there is a family history, in which case the diagnosis is familial gynecomastia.

DATA GATHERING

HISTORY

Important information includes a detailed history of the duration of the breast enlargement, any associated signs or symptoms suggesting the onset of puberty, or findings suggestive of nonendocrine systemic illnesses. A careful history of possible trauma or drug ingestion is also important.

PHYSICAL EXAMINATION

The initial goal of the physical examination is to discern whether there is true glandular hyperplasia. The presence of true breast development is suggested by other findings of estrogenization, such as darkening of the areolar region, protrusion of the areola and nipple above the plane of the breast, or thickening of the vaginal mucosa. Attention should be paid to height, weight, blood pressure, and presence of accompanying secondary sexual characteristics. In boys, determination of testicular volume is essential in assessing pubertal status.

LABORATORY EVALUATION

A careful history and physical examination often preclude the need for any further evaluation. Bone age, however, may aid in differentiation of premature thelarche from other disease entities: Bone age is normal in premature thelarche and advanced in most cases of true estrogenization.

INDICATIONS FOR REFERRAL OR CONSULTATION

The vast majority of cases of breast enlargement can be dealt with appropriately at the primary care level. The following findings in children after the newborn period would raise concern: gynecomastia in a prepubertal boy; precocious puberty; significantly advanced bone age; or evidence of systemic or central nervous system disease. These children deserve a more complete evaluation, with further laboratory testing or referral.

A more complete endocrinologic evaluation would include determination of circulating levels of estradiol, testosterone, androstenedione, dehydroepiandrosterone, follicle-stimulating hormone, and luteinizing hormone. Assessment of the hypothalamic-pituitary axis with a gonadotropin-releasing hormone stimulation test would further clarify the pubertal status. Chromosomal analysis is necessary to exclude the diagnosis of Klinefelter syndrome in the hypogonadal boy with elevated gonadotropin levels.

Pelvic US can show cystic changes or enlargement of the ovaries that can be present during puberty and can be useful in assessing the developmental status of the ovary.

THERAPY

For the adolescent boy, in whom there is rarely pathologic breast enlargement, the psychologic and emotional concerns of the patient are of primary importance and require a dedicated physician to provide the reassurance necessary to support the patient over the usual several years needed for spontaneous regression of gynecomastia.

In other situations of breast enlargement, treatment is usually in the hands of an experienced pediatric endocrinologist and is initially directed toward treating the underlying condition to stop the progression of glandular hyperplasia. In the case of precocious puberty, for example, long-acting gonadotropin releasing hormone analogues often are used. In other cases of recent-onset gynecomastia, a variety of antiestrogens and weak androgens have been tried, with varied success. Among these, testolactone is one of the more promising agents.

In long-standing breast enlargement, regardless of cause, the initial glandular hyperplasia is replaced by fibrosis and is unresponsive to any medical therapy. If there is enough enlargement to cause serious psychologic or cosmetic concern that cannot be dealt with by appropriate counseling, surgery is the only alternative.

19 CHEST PAIN

Steven M. Selbst, M.D.

Chest pain, a fairly common complaint in pediatric practice, occurs in about 1 in every 200 children who see a doctor because of illness. The pain, often chronic and recurrent, may resemble the syndrome of chronic abdominal pain. Chest pain affects children of all ages, with the highest incidence occurring at age 12 to 13 years. In general, chest pain probably affects boys as often as girls. This chief complaint has considerable importance because it often causes great concern in the patient and family, who fear that the chest pain is a symptom of serious cardiac disease.

DIFFERENTIAL DIAGNOSIS

COMMON CAUSES OF CHEST PAIN

Trauma
Hemothorax
Pneumothorax
Fracture
Infection
Pneumonia
Upper respiratory tract infection
Pericarditis
Myocarditis
Toxin/environmental
Caustic ingestion
Foreign body
Drugs of abuse (cocaine)
Allergy/inflammatory
Pleurisy
Costochondritis
Tietze syndrome
Asthma
Lupus erythematosus
Tumor
Metastatic disease
Congenital
Mitral valve prolapse
Anomalous coronary arteries
Sickle cell disease
Multiple etiologic
Esophagitis
Pulmonary embolus
Anxiety
Hyperventilation
Arrhythmia
Acute chest syndrome (sickle cell disease)

The differential diagnosis of childhood chest pain is extensive. In addition to thinking of the problems classified by cause, another approach is to look at each organ system that may be involved in producing pain.

ORGAN SYSTEM INVOLVEMENT IN CHEST PAIN

Musculoskeletal
Chest wall pain
- Trauma
  - Hemothorax
  - Pneumothorax
- Rib fractures
- Costochondritis
- Tietze syndrome

Gastrointestinal
Esophagitis
Caustic ingestions
Foreign bodies
Respiratory
Asthma
Pneumonia
Upper respiratory tract infection
Pneumothorax
Pleurisy (e.g., secondary to systemic lupus erythematosus)
Pulmonary embolus
Cardiac
Dysrhythmia

Mitral valve prolapse
Myocardial infarction
Idiopathic hypertrophic subaortic stenosis
Pericarditis
Myocarditis
Pneumopericardium
Ischemia (congenital heart disease)
Anomalous coronary arteries
Drugs of abuse (cocaine)
Psychogenic
Anxiety
Hyperventilation
Miscellaneous
Breast tumor
Sickle cell disease
Vaso-occlusive crisis
Metastatic disease

DISCUSSION

Studies have shown that young children (younger than 12 years) with chest pain are more likely to have cardiorespiratory problems and that older children (more than 12 years old) are more likely to have psychogenic pain. The broad category of musculoskeletal problems is the most common cause of chest pain in pediatric practice. Usually due to overuse (strain) of chest wall muscles, this pain may occur following extensive exercise or minor trauma (as with wrestling or football) or from, direct trauma to the chest, i.e., from automobile accidents that may result in hemothorax or pneumothorax. Less severe injuries can still cause rib fractures that will produce marked chest pain. In addition, costochondritis is a common cause of chest pain. The cause of this entity is not known, but it is believed that inflammation of the costochondral junctions produces chest pain.

GI problems have been known to cause chest pain since the esophagus is more pain-sensitive in its proximal portion. Esophagitis, or indigestion, often presents as chest pain and should be the presumed cause if there seems to be a definite relationship between the onset of pain and the consumption of certain foods. This pain may be worse when the individual is in the recumbent position.

Respiratory disease also produces chest pain. Children with an exacerbation of asthma, pneumonia, or other upper respiratory tract infection may complain of intermittent chest pain. These are usually associated with coughing or fever, and, in fact, may be due again to overuse of chest wall muscles. Moreover, pneumothorax can cause sudden severe chest pain that is often associated with dyspnea and cyanosis. Such pneumothoraces may occur spontaneously (uncommon) or in association with cystic fibrosis, asthma, or trauma.

Parents and physicians are most concerned about cardiac disease when a child complains of chest pain even though it is an uncommon cause. Supraventricular tachycardia in an older child may cause sudden or intermittent chest pain. Mitral valve prolapse has been found to cause chest pain in children.

Cardiac problems are found in fewer than 5% of children with chest pain; however, mitral valve prolapse is no more common in children with chest pain than it is in the general population (see Chapter 92).

A myocardial infarction is an exceedingly rare cause of chest pain in children. However, this may occur when anomalous coronary vessels exist. Adolescents who use cocaine may be at risk for myocardial infarction. Cocaine causes tachycardia, increased oxygen demand, hypertension, and coronary artery vasospasm. Children who have had Kawasaki disease may be at risk for future myocardial infarctions.

Idiopathic hypertrophic subaortic stenosis, an uncommon congenital problem that may cause angina-like pain, is often exacerbated by the Valsalva maneuver, which causes decreased venous return to the heart.

Finally, infections of the cardiac structures may cause chest pain. Of these, pericarditis is the most common and usually precipitates chest pain that may be characterized as dull pressure or sharp pleuritic type pain or even referred to as angina-like pain. Pericarditis may be caused by a bacterial infection (*Staphylococcus aureus, Hemophilus influenzae, Neisseria meningitidis, Streptococcus pneumoniae*), viral infection (coxsackievirus and echovirus), tuberculosis, acute rheumatic fever, or trauma. Concomitant fever, malaise, and diffuse myalgias are seen with pericarditis that is viral in origin. Pericarditis is often associated with a pericardial effusion. Similarly, myocarditis is caused by a virus, usually coxsackievirus B or echovirus. It is also seen secondary to mumps or infectious mononucleosis. With this infection, there is intermittent, substernal, dull chest pain. Pleuritic type chest pain may be present if there is accompanying pericarditis.

Psychogenic factors or anxiety are among the most common causes of chest pain in the pediatric age group. While there is some controversy about the role of stress in causing or resulting from chest pain, at least one study found that many children with chest pain had school phobias, separation anxiety, or fear of illness in association with the symptom of chest pain. With such chest pain, hyperventilation may be obvious or signs of anxiety may be more subtle. Girls and boys are both susceptible to anxiety-induced chest pain, which accounts for about 20% of episodes of chest pain in children.

There are other miscellaneous causes of chest pain. For instance, a primary or metastatic intrathoracic tumor is a rare possibility. Also, some adolescent boys will complain of chest pain that is the result of physiologic breast hypertrophy and girls may complain about painful breast cysts. In addition, children with sickle cell disease may have a vaso-occlusive crisis that causes chest pain and usually, pain in other extremities. Of further interest is the finding that chest pain may be associated with cigarette smoking. One study of adults and adolescents indicated that chest pain was significantly more common in smokers than nonsmokers. This was true for all types of chest pain, regardless of coffee and alcohol consumption. More data are needed to assess the role of smoking as a factor in the development of chest pain. Finally, studies found that in a large number of children (2% to 45%) a specific cause for chest pain could not be found despite a thorough evaluation.

DATA GATHERING

HISTORY

In evaluating the specific complaint of chest pain, one must first establish the *severity* of the pain. The primary care physician needs to know if the pain is severe enough to cause limitation of activity or, most notably, school absence. Information about the *frequency* and *duration* of the chest pain is also important. For instance, a child with constant or frequently occurring intermittent chest pain probably has a more serious problem (not necessarily organic in etiology) than the child with one brief, mild episode of pain. Next, one needs to ascertain the *type* and *location* of the chest pain. This is sometimes difficult to assess since young children often cannot well describe or localize the pain sensation. However, a classic description of sharp, pleuritic chest pain that occurs intermittently and may be relieved by sitting up and leaning forward should lead one to consider pericarditis. Likewise, a "burning" sensation in the sternal area may suggest esophagitis. Furthermore, one needs to learn the *onset* of the chest pain. Chest pain that is temporally related to eating meals or particular foods should lead one to consider esophagitis (reflux) as a cause of chest pain. Likewise, one should question the patient and family about any recent choking episodes, since foreign body ingestions may have been forgotten soon after the event. Similarly, it is extremely important to ask about possible trauma to the chest. While major trauma or direct chest trauma is easily recalled, a history of recent strenuous exercise is often overlooked. Such activity could easily cause chest wall pain as well as rib fractures or more serious injuries such as pneumothorax. Other *precipitating factors* such as anxiety must be questioned. Since chest pain in children is often a manifestation of unrelated stress, it is important to uncover the presence of school phobias, sleep disturbances, and other somatic complaints or the presence of family turmoil that may be temporally related to the onset of chest pain. Teenage girls need to be specifically questioned about the likelihood that they are pregnant, since this may occasionally be the stressful situation that is manifesting itself as chest pain. An adolescent girl should also be asked about the use of birth control pills, which are rarely linked to pulmonary embolism. Any adolescent with sudden onset of pain should be questioned about the possible use of drugs such as cocaine.

Although chest pain in children does not have the same ominous prognosis as in adults, the complaint must be taken seriously. One study has found that almost half the children with "psychogenic chest pain" had a positive family history for chest pain. Also, since some congenital problems may be inherited, it is important to find out about heart disease in the patient's family. A previous history of known heart disease in the patient may suggest that the chest pain reflects exacerbation of the long-standing problem. History of smoking in the patient and family may be important.

Finally, a review of systems is needed to see if there are *associated complaints* that may imply that the patient's chest pain is part of a systemic illness, for example, infection, collagen vascular disease, acute rheumatic fever, Kawasaki disease, and sickle cell disease. Fever, malaise, and myalgia may indicate that an infection such as pericarditis or myocarditis is responsible for the chest pain. Similarly, an associated cough would lead one to consider pneumonia, asthma, or an upper respiratory tract infection. In addition, chest pain that is associated with palpitations, syncope, or lightheadedness is more often due to anxiety or mitral valve prolapse. One needs to know what treatment has been tried previously and which medicines, positions, or therapeutic regimens seem to relieve the child's chest pain. For example, chest pain that resolves regularly when the child is allowed to sleep with his parents suggests an emotional problem.

PHYSICAL EXAMINATION

It is important to distinguish hyperventilation from true dyspnea so that proper referral and treatment can be instituted. Such hyperventilation is often accompanied by carpopedal spasm, acral paresthesias, headache, and lightheadedness. A general examination may be quite helpful in detecting the cause of the chest pain. For instance, poor growth or cyanosis may suggest serious underlying disease. Also, a rash or joint swelling may indicate the existence of a collagen vascular disease with secondary chest pain. Likewise, the abdominal examination is important, and, at least in one series of chest pain, examination of a teenager's abdomen revealed a large mass that was determined to be an unsuspected uterine pregnancy. Similarly, skin bruising elsewhere on the patient may give a clue to previously inapparent chest trauma. In addition, one should concentrate on additional signs of anxiety during the examination (e.g., excessive hand wringing, muscle tightness, tics). While these may reflect only the fear of examination, at times they may indicate an underlying stressful situation at home.

Finally, it is necessary to concentrate on examination of the chest itself. Inspection may reveal evidence of trauma or asymmetry due to underlying heart disease or scoliosis. Auscultation may reveal significant cardiac murmurs, tachycardia, or dysrhythmias, or perhaps an apical nonejection systolic click indicating mitral valve prolapse. Also, a friction rub at the left sternal border may suggest pericarditis and muffled heart sounds may suggest an effusion. Moreover, asymmetric breath sounds may indicate a pleural effusion, pneumonia, or, rarely, an intrathoracic tumor. Rales or wheezing implies lower airway disease. Palpation of the chest is useful since musculoskeletal chest pain is frequently reproducible by palpation or movement. For instance, pain induced by palpation of the costochondral junctions is characteristic of costochondritis. This should be distinguished from the extremely rare condition known as Tietze syndrome in which there is actual swelling and tenderness of the costochondral junction. Also, if a pneumothorax is present, subcutaneous emphysema may be palpable at the upper chest or neck.

LABORATORY EVALUATION

For most children with chest pain, laboratory tests rarely provide positive information to make a diagnosis. However, a chest x-ray film is indicated if fever is present or if significant trauma has occurred. A chest x-ray film is also useful if signs or symptoms suggest cardiac disease or pulmonary pathology, but this is not a useful procedure in diagnosing muscle overuse syndromes or costochondritis.

An electrocardiogram (ECG) may be quite helpful if the results of the history or physical examination suggest a dysarrhythmia. It may also provide confirming evidence of pericarditis if marked elevation of the ST segment is noted or of effusion if there is decreased voltage present. Moreover, an ECG that shows T wave inversion in the inferior leads may suggest mitral valve prolapse, especially if the results of the history and physical examination are consistent with this. An ECG will indicate the rarely occurring myocardial infarction or strain.

Additional laboratory tests are rarely needed and should only be ordered if specifically indicated.

A drug screen should be considered in any adolescent with acute severe pain. The value of an ECG in most children with chest pain has not been established, but this test is probably not indicated if the results of the history or physical examination do not suggest cardiac disease.

A complete blood count (CBC) and sedimentation rate may be useful if an infection is suspected but are not of value with common conditions like costochondritis or asthma. Finally, most chest pain from esophagitis does not require documentation with roentgenograms.

INDICATIONS FOR CONSULTATION OR REFERRAL

Once the cause of chest pain has been established, treatment can be appropriately begun. For the most part, this includes only therapy aimed at relieving symptoms. Heat, analgesics, and rest will suffice for the very common musculoskeletal problems discussed earlier. Likewise, antacids are usually effective for GI inflammation with referred chest pain. Antibiotics or bronchodilators may be required if lower airway disease is determined. A pleural effusion should be aspirated while the patient is in the office (or by a consultant) for diagnosis and relief of symptoms.

The rare child in acute severe distress with dyspnea or cyanosis or evidence of major trauma should be immediately referred to an emergency department. Supplemental oxygen may be useful enroute. Also, one should arrange for a hospital admission and rapid referral if a pericardial infection or effusion is suspected. Such an effusion should be aspirated for diagnostic purposes during echocardiography. Likewise, if any evidence of cardiac disease is found at the time of initial evaluation, elective further workup by a pediatric cardiologist would be appropriate. Finally, children found to have significant stress can usually be treated by the primary care physician. However, occasionally chest pain is only a minor symptom of major underlying psychopathology and referral to an appropriate specialist for counseling would be indicated in these cases.

The child with "idiopathic chest pain" requires additional consideration. There is no evidence that a chest x-ray film would be useful for such a patient if the results of the history and physical examination are not revealing. Extensive laboratory tests do not seem to be worthwhile or justified, although an ECG may provide some useful information or reassurance. Certainly, such patients require follow-up care and reevaluation as many have persistent chest pain for several months or years.

Most children and their parents can be reassured that chest pain does not have an ominous prognosis. While long-term follow-up data are not available, there is little reason to believe that serious cardiac or pulmonary disease will be eventually found if not immediately apparent. However, persistent chest pain may indicate underlying stress or organic disease (such as asthma). Thus the complaint should never be dismissed lightly.

DISCUSSION OF ALGORITHM

A "decision tree" for differential diagnosis of chest pain is presented in Figure 19–1. First, determine if the patient is experiencing acute distress; if so the patient needs emergency care. If there are no major airway problems, the patient should be screened for cardiac problems, pulmonary infection, gastric reflux, or systemic disease. Many patients who have chest pain are under emotional stress, and a careful history of psychosocial concerns may help to make this diagnosis. Still, in one third of patients the evaluations may not yield a diagnosis; these patients need to have close follow-up and be treated symptomatically.

BIBLIOGRAPHY

Asnes R, Santulli R, Bemporad J: Psychogenic chest pain in children. *Clin Pediatr* 1981; 20:788–791.

Driscoll DJ, Glicklich LP, Gallen WJ: Chest pain in children: A prospective study. *Pediatrics* 1976; 57:648–651.

Freidman G, Sieglaub A, Dales L: Cigarette smoking and chest pain. *Ann Intern Med* 1975; 83:1–7.

CHEST PAIN
Differential diagnosis

Anxiety
Asthma
Cardiac disease
Costochondritis
Foreign body
Gastroesophageal reflux
Muscle strain
Myocarditis
Pericarditis
Pleural effusion
Pleurisy
Pneumonia
Pneumothorax
Rib fracture
Sickle cell disease
Tumor

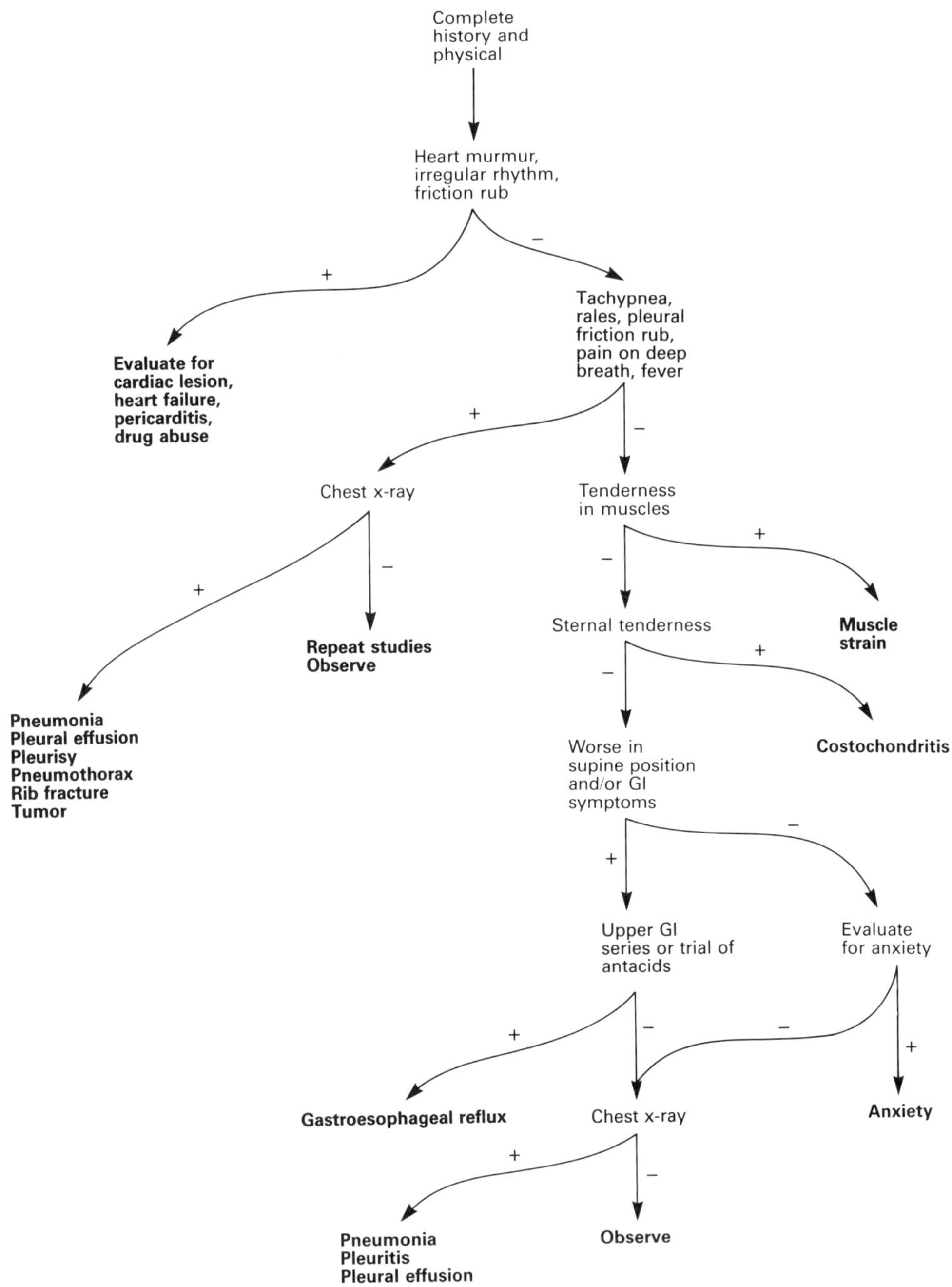

FIG 19–1
Decision tree for differential diagnosis of chest pain.

Pantell RH, Goodman BW Jr: Adolescent chest pain. *Pediatrics* 1983; 71:881–887.
Rowland TW, Richards MM: the natural history of idiopathic chest pain. *Clin Pediatr* 1986; 25:612–614.
Selbst SM: Chest pain in children. *Pediatrics* 1985; 75:1068–1070.
Selbst SM: Evaluation of chest pain in children. *Pediatr Rev* 1986; 8:56–62.
Selbst SM, Ruddy RM, Clark BJ, et al: Pediatric chest pain: A prospective study. *Pediatrics* 1988; 82:319–323.
Woodward GA, Selbst SM: Chest pain secondary to cocaine use. *Pediatr Emerg Care* 1987; 3:153–154.

20 CONSTIPATION

Steven Altschuler, M.D.

Constipation occurs in 5% to 10% of children. Normal defecatory patterns may range from several bowel movements each day to one movement every few days. The diagnosis of constipation is dependent on a history of difficulty passing stools, pain on defecation, or a decrease in frequency of passing stools.

DIFFERENTIAL DIAGNOSIS

COMMON CAUSES OF CONSTIPATION

Functional/acquired
Local anatomic abnormalities
Ectopic anus
Rectoperineal fistula
Proctitis or colitis
Extrinsic lesion causing rectal compression
  Abscess
  Neoplasm
Intrinsic colonic motor disorder
Hirschsprung disease
Metabolic and endocrine disorders
Pharmacologic agents
  Opiates
  Phenothiazines
Myelomeningocele
Spinal injury or tumor

DISCUSSION

In the majority of cases, the cause of constipation is functional or acquired. Functional constipation frequently occurs in infancy after dietary manipulations, such as early introduction of solid food, excessive intake of cow's milk, or a switch from breast-feeding to formula-feeding. A history of fussiness, colic, or excessive gas is frequently elicited in addition to the usual symptoms of difficulty passing stool, pain on defecation, or decreased frequency of passing stools. Constipation with the resultant passage of large, hard stool may also lead to fissure formation and result in blood streaking on the outside of the formed stool. The pain from the fissures then can contribute to additional constipation.

During the period of toilet training, constipation may become chronic and lead to impaction and secondary encopresis (fecal soiling). Fecal soiling in a previously toilet-trained child may be the first symptom of severe long-standing constipation. The presence of secondary encopresis also implies there is fecal impaction and abnormal colonic function from chronic constipation and distention. Parents may interpret encopresis as chronic intermittent diarrhea or as a child's weapon in a psychological conflict.

Important historical information includes urinary frequency, abdominal pain and distention, anorexia, and irritability. The physical examination will frequently reveal abdominal distention, a tubular mass arising in the left pelvis and following the anatomical course of the colon, and normal anal sphincter tone and a dilated rectal vault with a large soft fecal impaction on digital examination. Treatment of encopresis requires long-term therapy to reverse the chronic distention and return to normal function.

Besides a functional cause, the differential diagnosis of constipation includes a number of organic and anatomic abnormalities. These far less common disorders are conveniently divided into local and anatomic abnormalities, intrinsic colonic motor disorders, and extrinsic neurologic disorders.

Local anatomic abnormalities that may present with constipation include an ectopically placed anus, congenital anal stenosis, rectoperitoneal fistula, external rectal compression from an abscess or neoplasm, and proctitis or colitis. The intrinsic anal rectal abnormalities usually present in early infancy. In fact, they may be evident in the immediate newborn period. These abnormalities may be subtle, thus they can be overlooked unless specifically sought.

Constipation as a result of extrinsic lesions and inflammatory conditions usually occurs in the older child and adolescent. Usually acute in onset, there is frequently a change in stool caliber. When colitis or proctitis is the underlying cause, there may be rectal bleeding without an external anal fissure.

The classic intrinsic colonic motor disorder is Hirschsprung disease, a congenital aganglionosis. The colon in Hirschsprung disease is characterized by an area of transition from normal bowel containing ganglia to aganglionic bowel. The child with Hirschsprung disease usually has a history of constipation from birth. In most patients the disease is diagnosed within the first month of life. Clinical findings in these patients include abdominal distention, bilious vomiting, and failure to pass meconium in the first 24 hours of life. Radiologic evaluation will frequently reveal evidence of intestinal obstruction.

The infant or child with Hirschsprung disease will have a history of intermittent abdominal distention, failure to have a bowel movement without the aid of an enema or laxative, and no history of stool withholding. Encopresis does not occur because the aganglionic segment is at a state of tonic detraction, thus preventing leakage. At the time of the physical examination, the infant or child has abdominal distention and an empty rectum and tight internal sphincter on rectal examination. Thus the history and physical examination are very helpful in distinguishing Hirschsprung disease from functional constipation.

Extrinsic neurologic disorders such as myelomeningocele, spinal injury, or tumors cause constipation by interfering with extrinsic intestinal innervation. The onset of constipation may occur prior to the occurrence of more classical neurologic symptoms. Physical examination may reveal changes in anal sphincter tone, evidence of neurogenic bladder, and subtle changes in lower extremity strength and reflexes.

INDICATIONS FOR CONSULTATION OR REFERRAL

Since most cases of constipation occur as a functional disorder, very few patients require referral to subspecialists or admission to an inpatient facility. Functional constipation (unless complicated by fecal impaction, encopresis, or long-standing duration) can be handled in the outpatient setting. Therapy for constipation includes (1) enemas, (2) bowel training, (3) high fiber diet, and (4) laxatives.

Enemas.—Enemas are included in the treatment protocol to relieve fecal impactions within the rectum. The patient should receive enemas daily for 3 days. On the first day, an adult-size mineral oil enema is given. The next 2 days, adult-size Fleet enemas are given. Parents should be instructed to have children retain enemas for 15 to 20 minutes. Removal of the fecal impactions will immediately end episodes of encopresis.

Bowel Training.—This part of the program emphasizes bowel retraining. Parents should be instructed to have the child sit on the toilet twice a day for 15 to 20 minutes. Care should be taken to ensure that the child is comfortable and can place his or her feet flat on the floor.

CONSTIPATION
Differential diagnosis

Anticholinergic drugs	Functional	Myelomeningocele
Botulism	Hirschsprung disease	Sacral mass
Constipation	Hypothyroidism	Tethered cord
Dietary imbalance	Mental retardation	Transverse myelitis

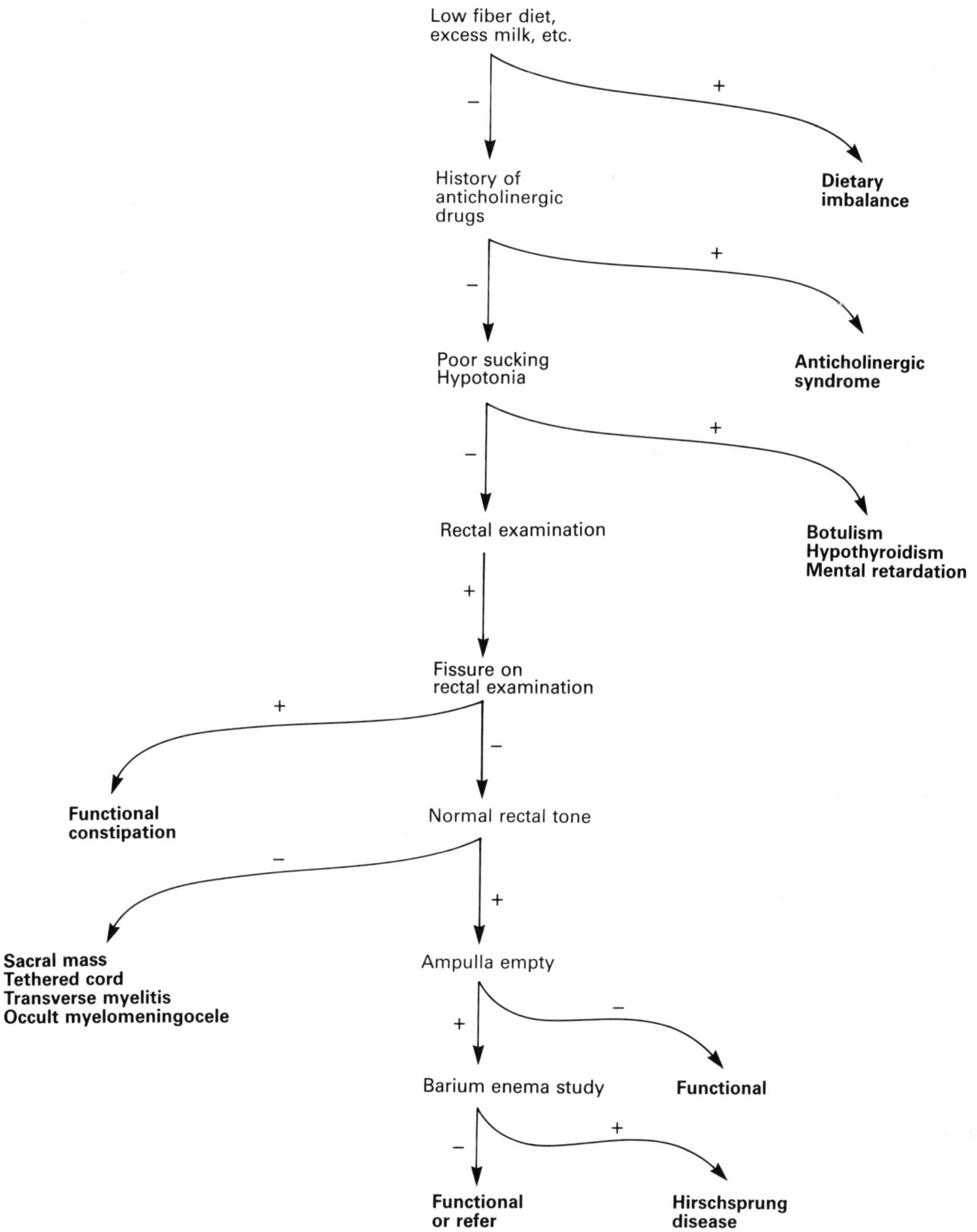

FIG 20–1
Decision tree for differential diagnosis of constipation.

Optimal times for toilet sitting are usually in the morning and evening after meals. After the child has had a bowel movement or after 20 minutes, toilet sitting time should be considered over. Over time, daily toilet sitting will develop as a routine.

High Fiber Diet.—A high fiber diet is instituted to add bulk to the daily diet and thus increase bowel peristalsis. Episodes of bowel spasm and the accompanying pain will also decrease in frequency. In general, fluids should be encouraged in the diets, but milk, apple juice, and tea should be limited to about two 8 oz glasses each day.

Laxative.—A nonstimulating laxative is generally used in constipated children. Kondremul, a mixture of mineral oil and Irish moss, acts as a lubricant and bulk-forming agent. This medication softens stools and prevents stool withholding. The initial dose should be 1 to 3 tbsp/day. If there is no response within 4 days, the dose should be increased to effect a response. This dose should be maintained until a leakage of oil occurs or regular bowel movements have occurred for 1 month. Kondremul may decrease the absorption of fat-soluble vitamins, therefore, a multivitamin should be taken while the medication is being received.

Failure of this regimen generally occurs when the initial "cleanout" with enemas has been ineffective. Occasionally, a constipated child will have to be admitted to the hospital for a closely supervised initial cleanout.

DISCUSSION OF ALGORITHM

An algorithm for the differential diagnosis of constipation is presented in Figure 20–1. The major problems underlying constipation include functional constipation, neurologic defect, Hirschsprung disease, and local problems. First, the rectal area is examined for fissures, fistulae, or abscesses. Next, a rectal examination will detect decreased tone that indicates a problem in the S2–4 innervation. If present, a comprehensive neurologic examination is needed. Otherwise, Hirschsprung disease should be considered. These patients have abdominal distention, poor weight gain, and empty ampulla on rectal examination. For those remaining patients who do not have bleeding, are taking no medication that contains atropine, and may have had decreased bulk or fiber in their diet, a diagnosis of functional constipation can be made.

BIBLIOGRAPHY

Abrahamian FP, Lloyd-Still JD: Chronic constipation in children: Longitudinal study of 186 patients. *J Pediatr Gastroenterol* 1984; 3:460–467.

Arhan P, Devroede G, Jehannin B, et al: Idiopathic disorders of fecal continence in children. *Pediatrics* 1983; 71:774–779.

Caresky JM, Weber TR, Grosfeld JL: Total colonic aganglionosis: Analysis of 16 cases. *Am J Surg* 1982; 143:160–168.

Davidson M, Kugler MM, Bauer CH: Diagnosis and management in children with severe and protracted constipation and obstipation. *J Pediatr* 1963; 62:261–275.

Fitzgerald JF: Constipation in children. *Pediatr Rev* 1987; 8:299.

Levin MD: Children with encopresis: A descriptive analysis. *Pediatrics* 1975; 56:412–416.

Schnaufer L, Kumar APM, White JJ: Differentiation and management of incontinence and constipation problems in children. *Surg Clin North Am* 1970; 50:895–905.

21 COUGH

Robert W. Wilmott, M.D., M.R.C.P.

Cough, one of the most common symptoms in pediatrics, has many causes. Recurrent or chronic cough should always be evaluated for underlying conditions such as asthma, sinus disease, or cystic fibrosis, because most normal children do not cough except when they have a respiratory tract infection. Persistent cough is always abnormal in *infants* and should lead to a search for underlying causes such as cystic fibrosis, gastroesophageal reflux, congestive heart failure, or chlamydial infection.[1,2] A chronic cough can be defined as one that has lasted for more than 8 weeks, although it may be appropriate to be concerned about a cough that has lasted 3 weeks or more, especially in an infant.[3]

COMMON CAUSES OF COUGH

Trauma
Foreign body in tracheobronchial tree
Infection
Pneumonia
Pharyngitis
Laryngitis
Sinusitis
Pertussis
Parapertussis
Influenza
Tuberculosis
Toxin
Hydrocarbon ingestion
Tobacco
Woodburning stove
Inflammatory
Asthma
Allergy
Metabolic/genetic
Cystic fibrosis
Circulatory
Congestive heart failure
Multiple etiologic
Psychogenic
Gastroesophageal reflux
Bronchopulmonary dysplasia

UNCOMMON CAUSES OF COUGH

Trauma
Foreign body in ear or esophagus
Infection
Tuberculosis
Pneumocystis
Cytomegalovirus
Visceral larva migrans
Schistosomiasis
Psittacosis
Mycosis
Humidifier fever (protozoa)
Rickettsiae
Hydatid cyst
Immunologic
AIDS
Congenital immune deficiency
Vasculitis
Sarcoidosis
Wegener granulomatosis
Tumor
T cell leukemia
Teratoma
Lymphoma
Congenital
Tracheoesophageal fistula
Vascular ring
Laryngomalacia
Bronchogenic cyst
Pulmonary sequestration
Pulmonary lymphangiectasia
Immotile cilia syndrome
Multiple Etiologic
Bronchiectasis

DIFFERENTIAL DIAGNOSIS

Asthma is the most common cause of chronic cough in children, and symptoms of wheezing may be unrecognized by parents. The term "cough variant asthma" is used to describe asthma in which coughing is the main complaint.[4, 5] Asthma is relatively common; 8% to 10% of schoolchildren have recurrent coughing and wheezing consistent with this diagnosis (see Chapter 51). Other symptoms of asthma include nocturnal coughing and coughing or wheezing after exercise, after laughing, or when exposed to cold. Physical examination may reveal that the patient has a barrel deformity of the chest from gas trapping or a Harrison sulcus (depression) around the lower chest. The diagnosis of asthma is supported if the chest radiograph shows gas trapping or peribronchial thickening.

Inhalation of a foreign body is a common cause of persistent coughing in children. For example, a young child may choke on a small toy or food such as a peanut or candy, and older children sometimes inhale objects that have been held in the mouth, such as a pen top. A foreign body lodged in the airway usually causes persistent coughing, but there may be no symptoms unless secondary infection develops. Fixed, localized wheezing suggests the diagnosis of an inhaled foreign body, which may require evaluation with bronchoscopy or fluoroscopy of the chest. A retained foreign body or impacted cerumen in the ear may also cause reflex coughing because of stimulation of Arnold's nerve.[6]

Infection of the respiratory tract at any level may cause coughing. Pharyngitis is also associated with fever, sore throat, and local erythema. It is usually caused by a viral infection such as parainfluenza, influenza, or adenovirus, although it may be caused by bacteria such as β-hemolytic *Streptococcus* or occasionally by *Staphylococcus aureus*.

Laryngitis is similar in many ways to pharyngitis, except the cough is more noticeable and harsher and the child may lose his or her voice. Supraglottic infection with *Hemophilus influenzae* can produce acute epiglottitis. Coughing is not a major symptom of this disease, in which rapid onset of toxicity, severe inspiratory stridor, drooling, and sore throat are typical. Inspiratory stridor and coughing are also features of acute laryngotracheobronchitis (croup). Croup is usually caused by parainfluenza, influenza, or respiratory syncytial virus. There is a prodromal upper respiratory tract infection and a harsh, barking cough. The inspiratory stridor and respiratory distress of this disease may not become apparent for 1 or 2 days, usually during the night. Laryngitis does not require specific evaluation unless it persists. Croup may be difficult to distinguish from acute epiglottitis. Lateral x-ray examination of the neck is indicated in children with persistent stridor of acute onset to rule out epiglottitis, which causes a characteristic "thumb sign" due to swelling of the epiglottis and aryepiglottic folds. Patients with severe obstruction should be transferred to a pediatric center for evaluation and consideration of intubation or tracheostomy. In such cases, it is usually best to avoid delaying the referral to obtain studies such as a lateral neck x-ray film, and to arrange an attended transport as quickly as possible.

Pneumonia produces consolidation of the alveolar spaces and infiltration of the alveolar septae. Fever, respiratory distress, and symptoms of systemic toxicity are found in association with coughing, which is more noticeable in the early stages. Viral pneumonia is more common than bacterial pneumonia in young children. Infants are especially prone to infection with cytomegalovirus and adenovirus. Viruses still account for the majority of cases in school-aged children, but pneumonia due to pneumococcus or *Mycoplasma pneumoniae* is more common in infants. Other causes of pneumonia include *Chlamydia* in infants and pertussis in unimmunized children. The clinical diagnosis of pneumonia is confirmed by the demonstration of consolidation on the chest radiograph, and the specific cause may be sought with appropriate cultures, counterimmunoelectrophoresis, or demonstration of the antigen with latex agglutination methods.

Cystic fibrosis is an important cause of persistent coughing. Typical symptoms are recurrent respiratory infection, poor weight gain, wheezing, coughing, and large foul-smelling bowel movements containing oil and grease. The diagnosis should also be considered in any child who develops nasal polyps or rectal prolapse. Physical examination in untreated cases may reveal finger clubbing, barrel-shaped deformity of the chest, and signs of poor nutrition. Children with such symptoms should undergo a sweat test.

Bronchopulmonary dysplasia is a chronic lung disease that develops in premature infants who have had mechanical ventilation. The characteristic symptoms are tachypnea, coughing, wheezing, and blue spells from either severe bronchospasm or collapse of the large airways due to an acquired weakness of the airway wall.[7] Physical examination may reveal intercostal retractions and persistent respiratory distress, barrel-shaped deformity of the chest, expiratory wheezes, inspiratory crackles, and poor physical growth. The chest radiograph characteristically shows emphysema, with areas of consolidation, atelectasis, and focal hyperaeration. The diagnosis of bronchopulmonary dysplasia is usually readily apparent from the typical history; however, sometimes the presence of blue spells can lead to the consideration of other causes, such as gastroesophageal reflux, seizures, and idiopathic apnea.

Chronic sinusitis is difficult to define in children. Typical symptoms are chronic nasal obstruction, persistent nasal discharge, facial pain (or tenderness), and a trickle of infected mucus from the nasopharynx down the posterior pharyngeal wall, associated with a recurrent cough that is especially bad at night. Examination of the throat may reveal mucopurulent secretions or granular mucosa on the posterior pharyngeal wall. Children with chronic sinusitis demonstrate mucosal thickening, air-fluid levels, or opacification on radiographs of the sinuses and appear to have chronic low-grade sinus infection. Many such children also have allergies, which predispose them to infection. Chronic sinusitis is therefore sometimes difficult to distinguish from asthma, with which it may be associated.[8]

Cigarette smoking should always be considered in the older child with respiratory symptoms. It is uncommon for smoking to be the sole cause of symptoms in children, but it may trigger latent airway reactivity. Careful physical examination may reveal yellow staining of the fingers, teeth, or tongue. Passively inhaled cigarette smoke probably affects all age groups, especially young children, and it has been reported that infants exposed to such smoke in their homes are significantly more likely to have lower respiratory tract infections. Irritating vapors and odors from paints or insecticide sprays cause coughing and wheezing, particularly in children with asthma.

Psychological illness may produce a chronic cough without any apparent physical signs or abnormalities on the chest radiograph. Typically these children have a dry trumpet-sounding cough. The cough usually disappears when the child is asleep and is much worse when attention is drawn to it (for example, during a consultation with a physician). If the cough does not resolve with simple reassurance, the child should be evaluated by a pediatric pulmonlogist, and if psychogenic cough is suspected, referral to a psychiatrist is recommended.

LESS COMMON CAUSES OF PERSISTENT COUGH

Immune deficiency is a serious but uncommon cause of chronic cough. Increased susceptibility to bacterial infections is a feature of immune deficiency syndromes that affect humoral antibody production, bacterial phagocytosis, or bacterial killing. Bronchiectasis or chronic pulmonary infection often develops in patients with these disorders and causes chronic cough with expectoration of infected sputum. Acquired immune deficiency syndrome is increasing in frequency in children and may present with persistent coughing and an abnormal chest radiograph due to an opportunistic infection with pneumocystis, cytomegalovirus, mycobacterium, or legionella.

Congenital malformations of the esophagus, larynx, or trachea are a rare cause of persistent cough. Diagnoses to be considered include cleft larynx, tracheoesophageal fistula (Fig 21–1), and a vascular ring (Fig 21–2). Other associated symptoms such as coughing after swallowing, poor feeding, or stridor may suggest the correct diagnosis.

Mediastinal tumors may produce airway obstruction associated with stridor and dry cough. Benign tumors include teratomas and cystic hygroma. Malignant tumors such as lymphoma, T cell leukemia, and thymic neoplasia are rarer and usually lead to additional symptoms. Primary tumors of the lung are extremely uncommon in children.

Bronchiectasis (Fig 21–3) and immotile cilia syndrome produce recurrent respiratory infections and persistent cough. The clinical fea-

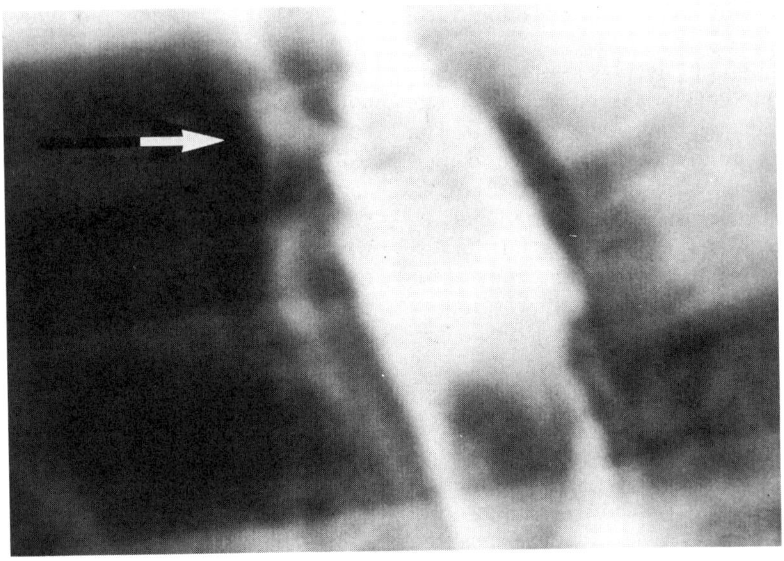

FIG 21–1
The barium swallow study of a child with an H-type tracheoesophageal fistula demonstrating the fistula *(arrow)* and aspiration of contrast material into the trachea.

tures of a chronic productive cough, finger clubbing, and intercurrent exacerbations are similar to those seen in cystic fibrosis and immune deficiency. In addition, children with immotile cilia syndrome usually have recurrent otitis media and chronic sinusitis. Approximately 50% of those with the dynein arm defect also have situs inversus (Kartagener's syndrome).

Tuberculosis, although relatively uncommon,

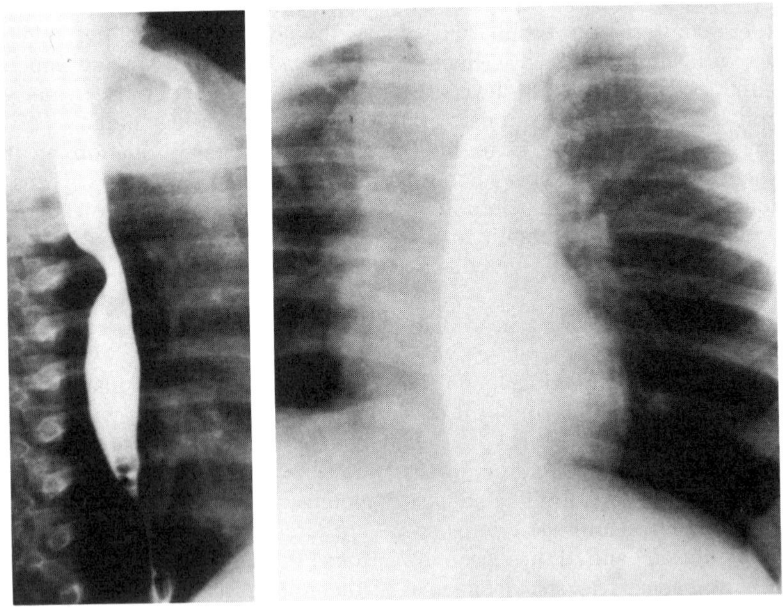

FIG 21–2
The barium swallow study of an infant with stridor demonstrating a vascular ring that makes a bilateral impression on the esophagus in the anteroposterior projection. At surgery, she had a double aortic arch.

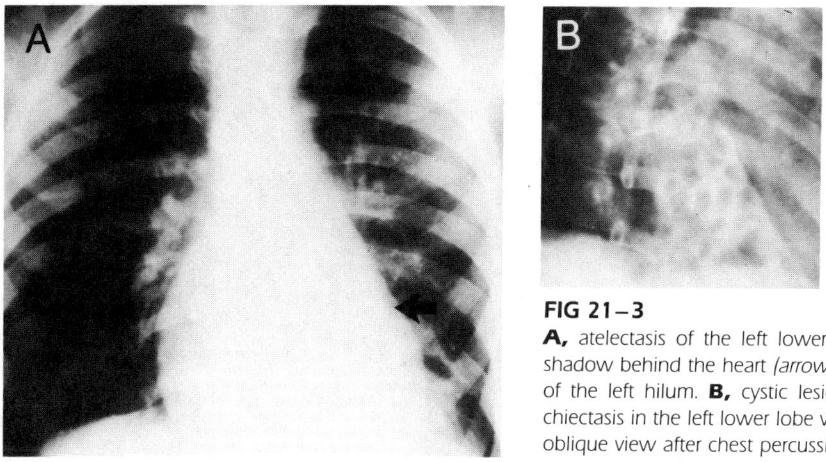

FIG 21–3
A, *atelectasis of the left lower lobe with a dense linear shadow behind the heart (arrow) and inferior displacement of the left hilum.* ***B,*** *cystic lesions due to saccular bronchiectasis in the left lower lobe were demonstrated with an oblique view after chest percussion and postural drainage.*

is still a problem affecting economically disadvantaged people such as North American Indians and recent immigrants from Southeast Asia. Patients with an undiagnosed persistent cough should therefore undergo a skin test for tuberculosis. The intradermal tuberculin test is more reliable than the tine test, and the latter should be reserved for routine screening in low-risk groups. The chest radiograph may show a primary complex (Fig 21–4), tuberculous pneumonia (Fig 21–5), or progressive lesions.

LABORATORY EVALUATION

The chest radiograph is the single most useful tool in the diagnosis of respiratory disorders in general, and is abnormal in many of the conditions described. Two views of the chest should be requested, with evaluation for gas trapping, increased bronchial line shadowing, alveolar infiltrates, reticulonodular shadowing, and localized emphysema. Localized emphysema or a persistent infiltrate should lead to a search for an inhaled foreign body (Fig 21–6). Right and left lateral decubitus films may help with this diagnosis. If the foreign body is in a main bronchus, there is often gas trapping in the affected lung, which never deflates even if placed in a dependent position. Older children may cooperate with inspiratory and expiratory radiographs, which also can be used to assess localized emphysema. Fluoroscopy of the chest by a pediatric radiologist is the best noninvasive way to identify a foreign body. The radiograph should also be evaluated for hilar and mediastinal adenopathy, because these may be the only clues to rarer conditions such as tuberculosis and sarcoidosis (Fig 21–5).

The complete blood count and differential may show eosinophilia in an allergic child with asthma. In young children with cystic fibrosis it may reveal hypochromic anemia or neutrophilia. The white blood cell count is often abnormal in children with pneumonia, and is usually increased in bacterial pneumonia, with band forms and toxic granulation. In viral pneumonia there may be lymphocytosis or in severe cases lymphopenia. The most extreme

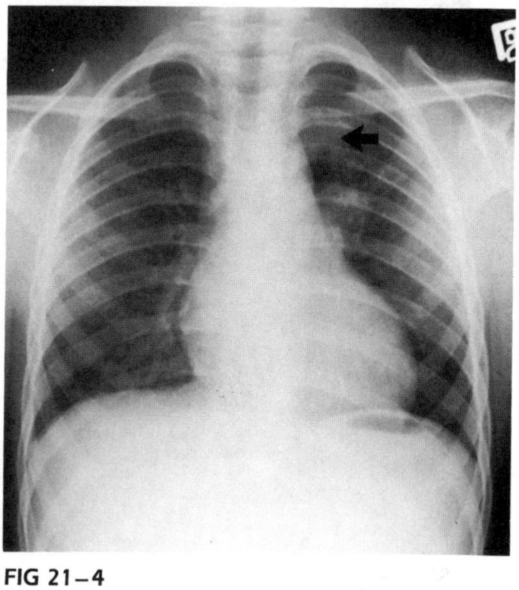

FIG 21–4
A primary tuberculous complex with left hilar adenopathy and a pneumonic infiltrate in the left upper lobe (arrow).

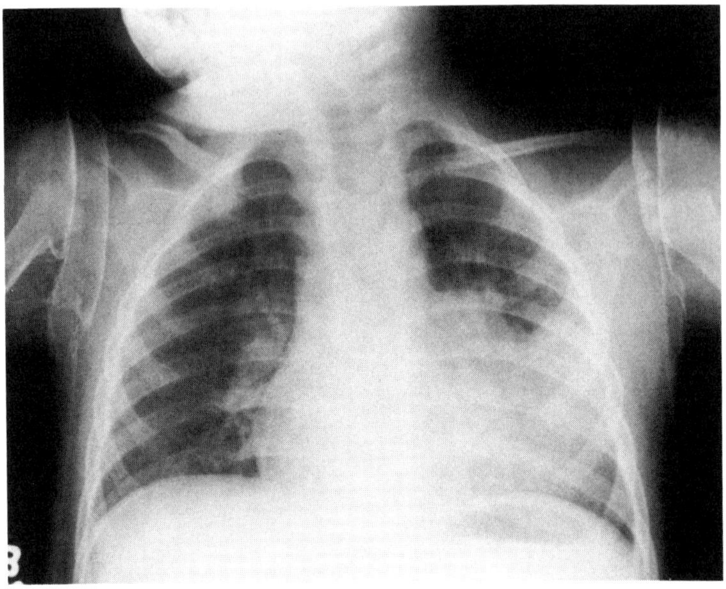

FIG 21–5
Primary tuberculosis with an extensive lingular infiltrate.

form of lymphocytosis is seen in children with pertussis, although this finding may be absent in the early stages.

Pulmonary function tests before and after administration of bronchodilators often help in the diagnosis of chronic cough. They are most valuable in diagnosing asthma by showing airflow obstruction. If the diagnosis is difficult to establish, most asthmatic children will show exercise-induced bronchospasm if tested before and after a standardized treadmill running test.[4]

A sweat test should be performed in any child who has symptoms that suggest cystic fibrosis. The test should be performed with the pilocarpine iontophoresis method of Gibson and Cooke[9] at a hospital with an accredited cystic fibrosis center. The chloride electrode

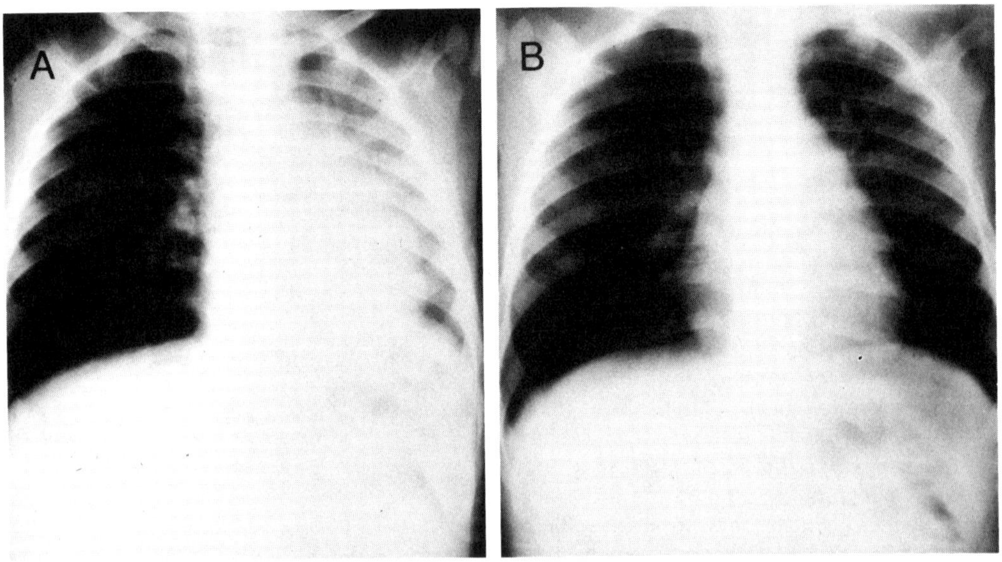

FIG 21–6
A, atelectasis of the left lung from a peanut in the left main bronchus. **B,** same patient after bronchoscopy.

COUGH
Differential diagnosis

Allergy	Cystic fibrosis	Reflex cough
Asthma	Epiglottitis	Sequestered lobe
Bronchiectasis	Foreign body	Sinusitis
Bronchiolitis	Immune deficiency	Tuberculosis
Cough variant asthma	Pneumonia	Tumor
Croup	Psychogenic	Upper respiratory tract infection (URI)

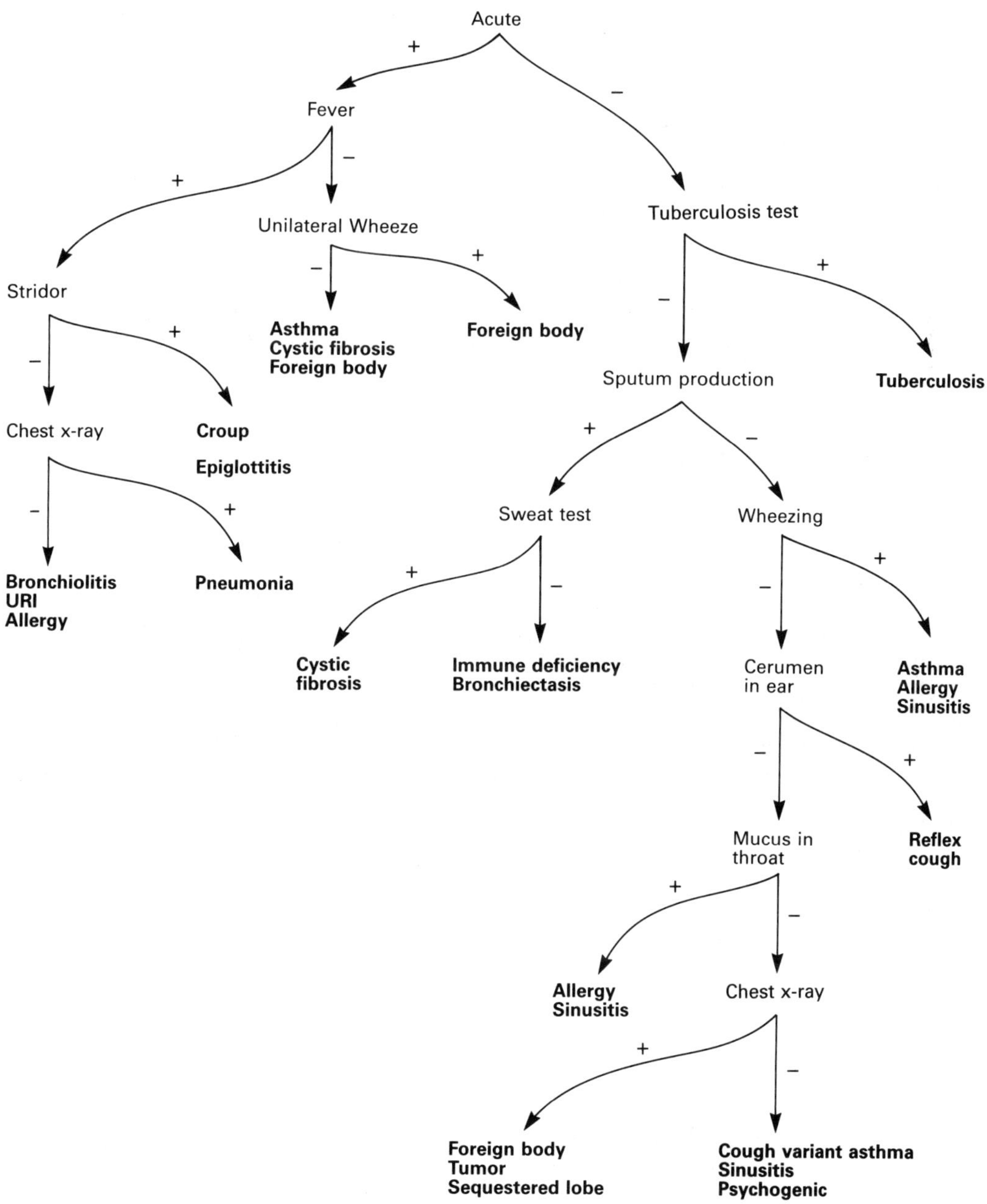

FIG 21–7
Decision tree for differential diagnosis of cough.

method is unreliable, and is not recommended. A screening system with encapsulated reagents and a solid-state device for iontophoresis has recently been marketed.

INDICATIONS FOR CONSULTATION OR REFERRAL

The child with severe symptoms, cyanosis, respiratory distress, or stridor, should be evaluated for inpatient care. Cyanosis may indicate incipient respiratory failure, and arterial blood gas measurements are indicated. If the blood gases are abnormal, the child may require specialized care. Children should also be referred for evaluation if the cough is persistent or if the diagnosis is unclear, particularly if there is a possibility of a serious underlying cause, as may be indicated by weight loss, poor general health, or reduced activity.

DISCUSSION OF ALGORITHM

An algorithm for the differential diagnosis of cough is presented in Figure 21–7. In evaluating cough, the first task is to differentiate between acute and chronic disease. Acute cough probably has an infectious cause. Foreign bodies should also be considered, especially if there are unilateral signs or findings on the radiograph.

Patients with chronic cough should be examined for signs of a systemic disease such a wasting, pallor, fever, sputum production, digital clubbing, and wheezing. These findings may help to lead to the specific tests to make the diagnosis. Coughing may be a sign of asthma, so a careful history of allergic symptoms is important. As cystic fibrosis may be present even in healthy looking children, a sweat test should be considered in children with persistent cough. Chest radiographs are helpful, both in establishing a diagnosis and in ruling out organic disease. A psychological cough is usually "seal-like," increases at times of stress, and disappears during sleep.

REFERENCES

1. Eigen H: The clinical evaluation of chronic cough. *Pediatr Clin North Am* 1982; 29:67–78.
2. Cloutier M: Finding the cause of chronic cough in children. *J Resp Dis* 1980; 1:20–28.
3. Schuller DE: Persistent cough in childhood. *Immunol Allergy Pract* 1986; 8:378–384.
4. Cloutier M, Loughlin GM: Chronic cough in children: A manifestation of airway hyperreactivity. *Pediatrics* 1981; 67:6–12.
5. Konig P: Hidden asthma in children. *Am J Dis Child* 1981; 135:1053–1055.
6. Wolf AP, May M, Nuelle O: The tympanic membrane: A source of the cough reflex. *JAMA* 1973; 223:1269.
7. Sotomayor JL, Godinez RI, Borden S, et al: Large airway collapse due to acquired tracheobronchomalacia in infancy. *Am J Dis Child* 1986; 140:367–371.
8. Rachelefsky GS, Katz RM, Siegel SC: Chronic sinus disease with associated reactive airway disease in children. *Pediatrics* 1984; 73:526–529.
9. Gibson LE, Cooke RE: A test for concentration of electrolytes in sweat in cystic fibrosis of the pancreas using pilocarpine by iontophoresis. *Pediatrics* 1959; 23:545–549.

22 ACUTE DIARRHEA

Jonathan A. Flick, M.D.

Acute diarrhea, one of the most frequent presenting complaints during childhood, is usually a self-limited illness, but the impact of the disease on society as well as the individual should not be underestimated. Worldwide, acute diarrheas are the major cause of death during childhood. In the United States, diarrhea and consequent dehydration account for a significant percentage of pediatric hospital admissions.

In adults, diarrhea is usually defined as greater than 200 mL of stool output each day. In children, it is defined as an increase in the frequency, water content, or volume of the stools compared to the child's normal pattern. It is important to remember that there is wide variability in "normal" from child to child. Breast-fed infants will typically pass a loose or seedy stool with each nursing. In the older infant or child, the frequency of bowel movements may vary from several times a day to once every several days.

The signs and symptoms accompanying acute diarrhea may include fever, vomiting, abdominal pain, and the passage of blood or mucus in the bowel movement. In cases of persistent or severe diarrhea, the clinical picture becomes dominated by signs of dehydration and acidosis, with decreased urine output and lethargy often noted. Infants are at particular risk for these complications, owing to their relatively large intravascular volume and surface area, as compared to older individuals. Fortunately, in the majority of instances the disease is short-lived.

DIFFERENTIAL DIAGNOSIS

COMMON CAUSES OF DIARRHEA

Infection

Viral
- Rotavirus
- Norwalk agent
- Adenovirus
- Coxsackie

Bacterial
- *Salmonella*
- *Shigella*
- *Campylobacter*
- *Yersinia*
- Pathogenic *Escherichia coli*
- *Aeromonas hydrophila*

Parasitic
- *Cryptosporidium*
- *Giardia lamblia*
- *Entamoeba histolytica*
- *Strongyloides stercoralis*
- *Trichuris trichiura*

Extraintestinal
- Urinary tract infection
- Otitis media
- Hepatitis

Toxin

Food poisoning
- *Clostridium perfringens*
- *Staphylococcus aureus*

Antibiotic-associated
- *Clostridium difficile*

Laxatives

Thyroxine

Allergic/Immunologic

Food allergy

Milk protein

Soy protein

Hemolytic uremic syndrome

Henoch-Schönlein purpura

Other
Intussusception
Neonatal drug withdrawal

DISCUSSION

Most episodes of acute diarrhea are infectious in origin. In the United States, viral agents predominate. In contrast, bacterial and parasitic pathogens are of major etiologic significance in less developed countries.

Acute diarrhea may also accompany infection elsewhere in the body (so-called parenteral diarrhea). Thus, urinary tract and upper respiratory tract infections may be associated with increased bowel movements or stool water. The mechanism of this change is unclear but may involve alterations in bowel motility, changes in diet, or effects of antibiotic treatment.

A number of systemic illnesses affect the gastrointestinal tract and may be associated with diarrhea, sometimes bloody in nature. Examples include the hemolytic uremic syndrome and Henoch-Schönlein purpura.

Rotaviruses are the most common cause of nonbacterial gastroenteritis in infancy and childhood. Infection occurs in both sporadic and epidemic patterns, with a peak incidence during the cooler months of the year. The virus is spread person to person by the fecal-oral route. The incubation period extends from 48 to 72 hours with the illness usually having a 5- to 8-day duration. Fever and vomiting are characteristic and may precede the diarrhea. Respiratory symptoms are also common.

Another group of viruses, the Norwalk-like agents, has been estimated to cause one third of epidemic viral gastroenteritis in the United States. Typically acute in onset, it predominantly affects older children and adults. Nausea, vomiting, abdominal pain, fever, headaches, and myalgias accompany the diarrhea. The illness seldom lasts for more than 3 days.

Of the bacterial pathogens listed earlier, *Salmonella* and *Shigella* account for the majority of infections seen. Both organisms invade the intestinal mucosa and, therefore, blood, mucus, and white blood cells may be found in the stool. In contrast to the winter predominance of viral diarrhea, bacterial diarrheas are more common during the summer and fall. Fever and respiratory symptoms are common in *Shigella* infections but are usually not seen in nontyphoidal salmonellosis.

With the advent of selective culture media and conditions, *Campylobacter* and *Yersinia* organisms have emerged as common agents of acute diarrhea. The peak incidence of *Campylobacter* infections is in the age group of 1 to 5 years though infection has been noted in neonates and occurs in all age groups. In temperate climates there is an increased incidence in the warmer months. The most common symptoms are fever occurring in 80% of patients, bloody diarrhea in 50%, abdominal pain, and vomiting. Diarrhea develops 1 to 3 days after the onset of abdominal pain. It is initially watery, profuse, and foul-smelling and characteristically becomes bloody after several days. The duration of the acute illness is from 3 to 5 days but a recurrent or relapsing course has been reported.

Yersinia enterocolitica affects primarily children under 3 years. While most cases are mild, it can cause a mesenteric lymphadenitis or appendicitis-like picture that may mimic an "acute" abdomen. The diarrhea may last from 1 to 2 weeks and is sometimes bloody. An associated reactive arthritis has been noted. Unlike most other enteric bacterial infections, *Y. enterocolitica* occurs more frequently during the winter.

Aeromonas has recently been recognized as a frequent cause of acute diarrhea in children as well as adults. The severity of infection is variable, ranging from an asymptomatic carrier state to severe watery and sometimes bloody diarrhea. Fever and vomiting are present in one third of patients. Infection has been associated with drinking untreated well water or spring water. Specialized techniques are required for identification of the organisms in stool culture specimens.

Far from being unusual, *Giardia lamblia* is the most common intestinal parasite in the United States. There is a high incidence of giardiasis in children attending daycare centers and in residents of institutions for the handicapped and mentally retarded. The clinical picture is variable, ranging from an acute, self-limited enteritis to chronic diarrhea with malabsorption and failure to thrive. Nausea, abdominal cramping, and bloating are common. An asymptomatic carrier state also occurs.

Cryptosporidia are parasitic protozoans that may produce a self-limited diarrheal illness in normal individuals. Upper abdominal cramping, anorexia, nausea, and vomiting are frequent accompanying symptoms. A more chronic, severe, and sometimes fatal infection may occur in immunocompromised individuals.

Amebiasis is endemic in certain areas of the world, including Central and South America and Asia. Recent travelers to and immigrants from such areas who develop bloody diarrhea should have stool examinations for ameba. Serologic testing is also available.

Food poisoning results from the consumption of food contaminated with bacterial toxins. The three most common organisms responsible for the illness are *C. perfringens, S. aureus,* and *Vibrio parahaemolyticus.* Typically there is severe crampy abdominal pain, profuse watery diarrhea, and vomiting. Recovery is prompt, usually within 24 to 48 hours. Antibiotic therapy is not indicated.

There are also noninfectious causes of diarrhea to be considered. The hemolytic-uremic syndrome frequently presents with a gastroenteritis-like prodrome. Abdominal pain, bloody diarrhea, and colitis may precede the development of renal disease by several days to weeks. A decrease in urine output plus paleness, petechiae, or prolonged bleeding at a venipuncture site should alert the physician that the case is more than a case of infectious diarrhea. Most patients (but not all) will have anemia, increased reticulocyte count, and azotemia. Bloody diarrhea and abdominal pain are also common features of Henoch-Schönlein purpura.

DATA GATHERING

HISTORY

As the majority of acute diarrheas are infectious in origin, a history of contact with a similarly affected individual should be sought. Inquiries should be made about not only the health of family members but about that of daycare and school contacts as well. Information about recent travel, family pets, and the source and quality of the family drinking water may help establish the source of infection. Often, however, a source cannot be identified.

Accompanying symptoms of fever or vomiting should be established. A history of abrupt onset of fever, more than four stools per day, absence of vomiting, and the presence of blood or mucus in the stool suggests a bacterial pathogen and a stool culture is indicated. In contrast, bloody diarrhea does not often occur in rotavirus infection.

A history of recent antibiotic exposure will alert one to the possibility of antibiotic-associated colitis. This is a diarrheal disorder produced by a toxin elaborated by *C. difficile,* an anerobic organism whose proliferation in the intestinal tract is favored by antibiotic-induced alterations in the normal gut flora. *Clostridium difficile* may be identified by culture or assay for its cytotoxin.

As the state of hydration is a function of the difference between intake and output, it is important to obtain information about thirst, fluids consumed, frequency of urination, and stool output. Increased thirst may reflect hypovolemia, although vomiting often precludes significant oral intake. Diminished urinary frequency and volume can be difficult to assess in the infant and toddler still in diapers because of mixing of urine and feces.

PHYSICAL EXAMINATION

The physical examination of the infant or child with acute diarrhea has two main objectives: determination of the state of hydration and assessment for evidence of chronic disease. Rarely will a specific pathogen be diagnosed by physical examination alone. An erythematous maculopapular rash is seen not only in patients with typhoid fever but may be present in those with *Shigella* and viral infections as well. Similarly, arthritis is nonspecific, having been reported with enteritis caused by *Shigella, Yersinia,* and *Campylobacter* organisms.

An estimation of the degree of dehydration must be made from the clinical signs and symptoms. In addition to serving as a baseline to follow during the course of the illness, the patient's weight, when plotted on a growth chart, may serve as the first clue to an underlying chronic disease process. Diarrhea with failure to thrive leads to the consideration of a malabsorption syndrome (see Chapter 23). If a recent preillness weight is available, comparison with the current weight will provide an accurate assessment of the loss in body water. When a recent weight is not known, determination of vital signs, examination of skin turgor, mucous membranes, anterior fontanelle, and the peripheral circulation will allow one to classify the dehydration as mild, moderate, or severe. When possible, blood pressure with the patient in the supine and upright positions should be recorded. Features of the physical examination important in estimating the magnitude of dehydration are listed in Table 22–1.

The abdominal examination may be revealing. While hyperactive bowel sounds are sometimes heard, high-pitched rushes are unusual in acute gastroenteritis and suggest an intestinal obstruction. In the infant or young child who passes a bloody diarrheal stool, an intussusception must be considered. A sausage-shaped mass may be palpated, most often in the right upper quadrant. An emergency barium enema study with attempted hydrostatic reduction is indicated. Rebound abdominal tenderness indicates peritoneal inflammation and may be seen with bacterial or ulcerative colitis.

LABORATORY EVALUATION

Several simple laboratory tests can be helpful in defining the nature of the diarrhea and its impact on the child. A history of bloody diarrhea should be confirmed by Hematest or Hemoccult testing, as the appearance of blood may be mimicked by a number of agents. Food colorings used in juices or gelatin can impart a red color to the stool; black or tar-colored stools can result from licorice, iron, or bismuth compounds that are present in certain over-the-counter antidiarrheal medications.

The finding of fecal leukocytes, particularly in the presence of fever, vomiting, or blood or mucus in the stool, increases the likelihood of a bacterial infection. Fecal leukocytes may be detected by adding five drops of methylene blue to a fecal smear. Specimens with greater than five leukocytes per high-powered microscopic field are considered positive.

A stool culture should be obtained when blood is present, when a bacterial pathogen is suspected, or when hospitalization is planned. Ideally, the laboratory will handle the specimen so as to identify not only *Salmonella* and *Shigella* but *Campylobacter, Yersinia, Aeromonas* and *C. difficile* organisms as well. Several enzyme immunoassays are available for the diagnosis of rotavirus infections (i.e., Rotazyme). While not indicated routinely, these tests may be useful in prolonged illnesses, in hospitalized patients, and in investigations of nursery, school, or community outbreaks of diarrhea. When a parasitic infection is suspected, a fresh or preserved stool specimen should be obtained for ova and parasite examination.

A routine urinalysis and determination of levels of serum electrolytes should be performed when dehydration is clinically apparent. The urinary specific gravity provides information on the child's avidity for fluid, while examination of the sediment may suggest the presence of an underlying urinary tract infection as the cause of the diarrhea. In patients re-

TABLE 22–1
Clinical Assessment of Dehydration

	Dehydration*		
	Mild (5%)	Moderate (10%)	Severe (15%)
General appearance	Alert, thirsty	Thirsty, irritable, or lethargic	Drowsy or unresponsive
Heart rate	Postural increase	Resting tachycardia	Marked increase
Blood pressure	Normal or postural decrease	Mild decrease	Frank hypotension
Respirations	Normal	Rapid	Deep and rapid
Skin	Dry, normal turgor	Tenting	Poor turgor and perfusion
Peripheral pulses	Normal	Rapid, thready	Weak or unattainable
Eyes	Tears may or may not be present	Dry	Sunken
Mucous membranes	Tacky	Dry	Very dry

*Percentages (5%, 10%, and 15%) refer to the fluid deficit in infants (i.e., 0.05 L/kg). In older children, the approximate deficits are 3%, 6%, and 9%.

quiring hospitalization, measurement of levels of electrolytes (sodium, chloride, potassium, carbon dioxide), BUN, and creatinine are necessary to provide proper fluid management (see Chapter 55, Dehydration).

MANAGEMENT

Most episodes of acute diarrhea can be managed expectantly, while observing the child closely for signs of developing dehydration. Management has traditionally included a period with the patient fasting or taking clear liquids, though support for this approach is based more on theoretical concerns than on controlled studies. Rarely should such a diet be maintained for more than 24 to 48 hours, as nutritional deficits may develop along with "starvation stools." A period of transient lactose intolerance is relatively frequent, particularly in infantile rotaviral gastroenteritis. Refeeding such infants with a soy-based, lactose-free diet is often recommended.

Antidiarrheal drugs (such as kaolin, paregoric, loperamide, or diphenoxylate) are rarely indicated and may mask ongoing fluid loss into the intestinal lumen. In addition, in the case of bacterial infections, there is a risk of promoting bacterial proliferation and delaying toxin elimination.

Antibiotics are not indicated in most episodes of acute diarrhea, including viral gastroenteritis and food poisoning. In *Campylobacter* and *Yersinia* infections, antibiotics may eliminate the organisms from the stool but there is no substantial evidence that the clinical course of the disease is altered. Fecal excretion of *Salmonella* is not reduced by antibiotics, though treatment is indicated in infants less than 3 months of age and in immunocompromised individuals because they are at increased risk for systemic spread of the infection. In normal hosts, *Cryptosporidium* infections are self-limited and therapy is not required. Symptomatic *Aeromonas* infections respond promptly to oral antibiotic therapy, with most strains being susceptible to trimethoprim-sulfamethoxazole.

Antimicrobial therapy is also indicated in documented cases of shigellosis, salmonellosis, and amebiasis and when diarrhea is associated with an extraintestinal infection such as otitis media or cystitis. Antibiotic-associated diarrhea often responds to discontinuation of the offending agent, though oral vancomycin or metronidazole therapy is sometimes required.

INDICATIONS FOR CONSULTATION OR REFERRAL

Most cases can be managed in the outpatient setting. Rarely do patients with acute diarrhea need referral.

The decision to hospitalize the infant or child with acute diarrhea is based on several factors. If significant dehydration is present, intravenous therapy may be required to correct fluid deficits and acid-base status. Hospitalization may also be indicated in cases of mild dehydration, if it could be expected to progress because of the child's inability to tolerate oral fluids. The young infant is at greatest risk of having this complication develop. Inhospital observation is also warranted when peritoneal signs are present, indicating a possible "surgical abdomen."

DISCUSSION OF ALGORITHM

An algorithm for differential diagnosis of acute diarrhea is presented in Figure 22–1. The assessment of acute diarrhea includes the identification of patients who have blood in the stool; this identification then leads to the diagnosis of either a bacterial or parasitic infection or the hemolytic uremic syndrome. Another branch helps identify extraintestinal infections such as otitis media or urinary tract infection. If there is no history of antibiotic exposure or contact with family and friends who have diarrhea stemming from food poisoning, a presumed diagnosis of viral enteritis can be made.

BIBLIOGRAPHY

Brown KH, Gastanaduy AS, Saavedra JM, et al: Effect of continued oral feeding on clinical and nutritional outcomes of acute diarrhea in children. *J Pediatr* 1988; 112:191–200.

Fischer MC, Agger WA: Cryptosporidiosis. *Am Fam Physician* 1987; 36:201–204.

Gorbach SL: Bacterial diarrhea and its treatment. *Lancet* 1987; 2:1378–1382.

ACUTE DIARRHEA
Differential diagnosis

Antibiotic-induced diarrhea
Enteritis
Food dyes
Food poisoning
Hemolytic uremic syndrome
Intussusception
Otitis media
Urinary tract infection

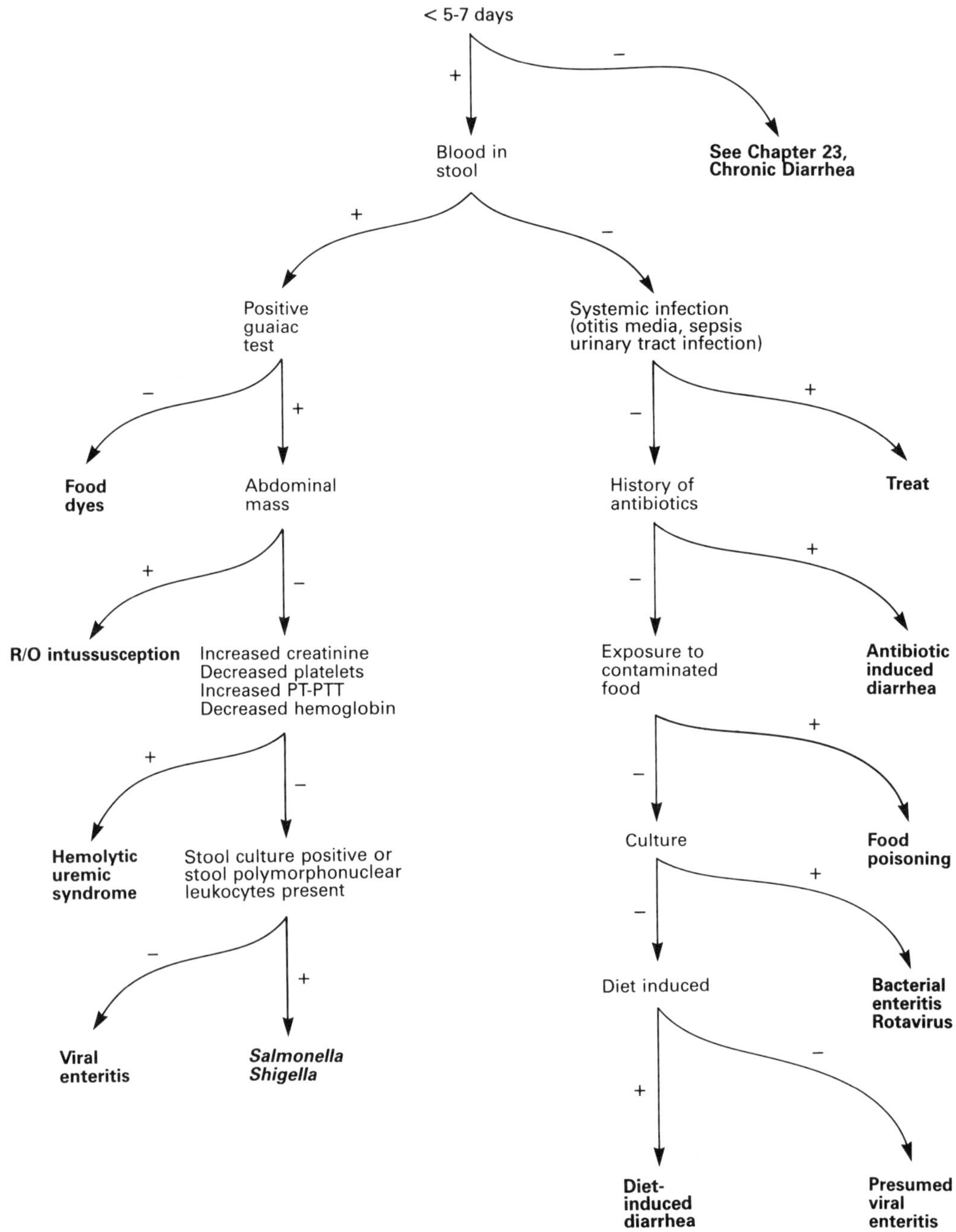

FIG 22–1
Decision tree for differential diagnosis of acute diarrhea.

Pickering LK, Englekirk PG: Giardia lamblia. *Pediatr Clin N Am* 1988; 35:565–577.

San Joaquin VH, Pickett DA: *Aeromonas*-associated gastroenteritis in children. *Pediatr Infect Dis J* 1988; 7:53–57.

Simmonds SD, Noble MA, Freeman HJ: Gastrointestinal features of culture-positive Yersinia enterocolitica infection. *Gastroenterology* 1987; 92:112–117.

Uhnoo I, Olding-Stenkvist E, Kreuger A: Clinical features of acute gastroenteritis associated with rotavirus, enteric adenoviruses, and bacteria. *Arch Dis Child* 1986; 61:732–738.

23 CHRONIC DIARRHEA

Steven M. Schwarz, M.D.

By definition, diarrhea may be considered chronic if it persists beyond 2 weeks and is characterized by stools of loose to watery consistency. While persistent diarrhea may be responsible for significant morbidity (particularly in infants under 3 months of age) characterized by poor growth and weight gain, it may also present as a relatively benign condition associated with normal growth over a period of months to years. Assessment of the nature of any underlying etiology includes attention to any protracted effects of diarrhea, including dehydration and malabsorption leading to malnutrition and growth failure. To fully understand the syndrome and approach it with a rational diagnostic scheme, it is important to consider the major mechanisms responsible for the diarrheal state.

CAUSES OF CHRONIC DIARRHEA

Infection
Viral
Bacterial
Parasitic
Urinary tract
Drugs, toxins
Antibiotic-related diarrhea
Allergic-Inflammatory
Crohn disease
Ulcerative colitits
Protein intolerance
Immune deficiency
Endocrine/metabolic
Carbohydrate malabsorption
- Sucrase-isomaltase deficiency
- Glucose-galactose malabsorption
- Lactase deficiency (late onset)
- Postinfectious lactase deficiency

Diet related
- Overfeeding
- Dietetic sweets, fruit juices (sorbitol)
- Chronic nonspecific diarrhea

Pancreatic insufficiency
- Cystic fibrosis
- Schwachman syndrome
- Enterokinase deficiency

Hyperthyroidism
Malnutrition
Tumor
Ganglioneuroma
Malignancy related
Chemotherapy related
Radiation enteritis
Graft vs. host disease
Congenital anatomic
Blind loop
Partial obstruction
Fistulas (Crohn disease)
Malrotation
Hirschsprung disease
Celiac disease
Lymphangiectasia
Multiple etiologic
Toddler's diarrhea

Secretory diarrhea
- Enterotoxigenic
- Tumor related
- Congenital chloridorrhea
- Bile salt malabsorption

Irritable bowel syndrome
Motility disorders
- Collagen vascular disease
- Pseudo-obstruction
- Diabetes mellitus

Constipation-paradoxical diarrhea

DIFFERENTIAL DIAGNOSIS

Chronic diarrhea presents as a perplexing problem because of the long differential diagnosis and the considerable uncertainty regarding the appropriate diagnostic evaluation. Nevertheless, a careful history and physical examination and the use of relatively few readily available diagnostic tests will allow the primary care physician to reach a diagnosis in over 95% of cases. This chapter will suggest an initial course of evaluation that may obviate the need for subspecialist intervention in the majority of patients.

CARBOHYDRATE MALABSORPTION

Certain acute disorders that involve damage to the brush border membrane, such as viral gastroenteritis, result in reduction of hydrolytic activity and malabsorption of carbohydrate. It is now well recognized that this secondary carbohydrate intolerance (most prominently for lactose) may persist for weeks or months after recovery. Diarrhea occurring as a consequence of carbohydrate loss is of two types, osmotic and fermentative. The latter results from malabsorbed sugars broken down by colonic bacteria into lactic and acetic acids, accompanied by H_2 formation. The diarrhea that follows is often explosive, watery, and vinegar-smelling.

IMPAIRED INTESTINAL TRANSPORT OF NUTRIENT, WATER, AND ELECTROLYTE SECONDARY TO MUCOSAL DAMAGE

The apical plasma membrane of the small intestinal epithelial cell, or brush border membrane, is the final common pathway for nutrient and electrolyte transport across the mucosal surface. Disruption of the structural and functional integrity of this membrane leads to impaired hydrolysis of nutrients and distorted water and electrolyte fluxes. In more severe states of loss of mucosal integrity (such as the celiac syndrome), reduced intestinal surface area and damage to the brush border membrane affects absorption of all nutrient classes and may be associated with luminal excretion of water and electrolytes. Various other insults to mucosal epithelial cells (e.g., viral infection) lead to increased cellular turnover and population of the surface epithelium with immature crypt cells containing reduced levels of brush border enzymes. Malabsorption of unhydrolyzed and unabsorbed nutrient molecules, particularly monosaccharides and disaccharides, exert an osmotic effect intraluminally resulting in increased water excretion.

ACTIVE WATER AND ELECTROLYTE SECRETION

Secretory diarrheas are characterized by continuance of the diarrheal state under conditions of absence of oral feedings; these syndromes manifest fecal sodium losses in excess of 70 mEq/L/day. Certain bacteria may release toxins that affect intestinal transport systems, resulting in active secretion of water and electrolytes. These effects are typically mediated by cyclic adenosine monophosphate (cAMP) that stimulates sodium secretion by inhibiting the coupled absorptive process for sodium chloride. Various tumors release vasoactive substances (e.g., catecholamine-producing ganglioneuromas, pancreatic tumors secreting vasoactive intestinal polypeptide) that stimulate an intestinal secretory state. Rarely, intestinal hypersecretion occurs as a congenital phenomenon (familial chloridorrhea).

BILE SALT, FAT MALABSORPTION

Any disorder that damages the terminal ileum may result in bile salt malabsorption. Subsequent bacterial deconjugation of bile salts in the colon leads to fluid and electrolyte secretion induced by bile acid. Fat malabsorption, either consequent to ileal dysfunction and bile salt loss, or secondary to disease of the upper small bowel (e.g., celiac) or pancreas (e.g., cystic fibrosis) may present with bulky, foul-smelling stools (steatorrhea) or as watery diarrhea induced by bacterial production of hydroxyl-fatty acids in the colon.

OTHER MECHANISMS

Hypermotility states may result from the presence of vasoactive substances (prostaglandins, serotonin). These syndromes are often associated with active secretion (as well as malabsorption) of water and electrolytes. Conversely, decreased motility, often noted in collagen-vascular disorders, and diabetes mellitus lead to secretory and malabsorptive diarrhea secondary to bacterial overgrowth. Dietary-related diarrheal syndromes are less well understood. In recent years, there have been increasing reports of the relationship between chronic diarrhea and ingestion of large quantities of sorbitol. Sorbitol is found in high concentrations in certain fruit juices (apple, pear) and some sugarless candies. The association of the chronic nonspecific diarrhea syndrome (toddler's diarrhea) with excessive carbohydrate or fluid intake raises intriguing questions concerning intestinal "thresholds" for fluid and nutrient absorption, particularly in young children, and it additionally suggests altered developmental patterns of colonic motility.

DISCUSSION

For the purposes of evaluation in pediatrics, it is useful to consider the etiologic possibilities in terms of age at presentation rather than diagnostic category. Thus evaluation is divided into cases occurring in three age groups: newborn to 3 months, 3 months to 3 years, and greater than 3 years.

Children in the Age Group of Newborn to 3 Months

MAJOR CAUSES OF CHRONIC DIARRHEA

Postinfections
Protein intolerance
Cystic fibrosis
Short bowel syndrome
Transport, enzyme defects
Malnutrition
"Intractable diarrhea"

Here, protracted diarrhea often heralds severe absorptive-secretory defects and is complicated by the development of malnutrition-associated diarrhea. Culmination in the syndrome of intractable diarrhea of infancy, a well-described but poorly understood entity, necessitates an extensive diagnostic workup and often requires central venous alimentation. Office management of chronic diarrhea in this age group includes a careful clinical assessment to ascertain requirement for hospitalization and an initial workup aimed at confirming or ruling out common diagnostic entities.

The infancy period is most likely one to be complicated by significant morbidity from protracted diarrhea. In the infant who appears to be thriving, however, overfeeding and the passage of normal "breast-milk stools" often present with an associated complaint of diarrhea. In the breast-fed infant, it is not unusual to observe as many as ten liquid stools per day. This is probably related both to the particular colonic bacterial flora in the infants and the high lactose content of breast milk. Clearly, any newborn who is fed excessive quantities of formula may develop diarrhea secondary to increased fluid intake and demonstrate osmotic effects from malabsorption of nutrients that may exceed normal absorptive capacity.

Postinfections.—In a previously well infant, the sudden onset of diarrhea suggests an infectious etiology. When diarrhea is accompanied by heme-positive stools, bacterial pathogens such as *Salmonella*, *Shigella*, and *Campylobacter* species are suspected. These agents as well as viral pathogens (particularly rotavirus) are often associated with a protracted course secondary to mucosal injury resulting in disaccharide intolerance, confirmed by the presence of Clinitest-positive stools (liquid part) with pH less than 6.0. Use of a formula free of disaccharides, particularly lactose (e.g., Prosobee, disaccharide-free Isomil) in a clinically stable baby may avoid the need for hospitalization secondary to dehydration from an osmotic diarrhea.

Protein Intolerance.—When diarrhea develops after the introduction of formula feedings at birth or after weaning from the breast, infants may be manifesting cow's milk or soy protein intolerance. Diarrhea is often marked by heme-positive or even grossly bloody stools and the clinical syndrome ranges from a thriving, well baby with some occult gastrointestinal (GI) blood loss to a severely toxic infant with frank enterocolitis. Vomiting may be an associated symptom in more morbid cases. Although the precise mechanism has not been elucidated, absorption of intact macromolecules in the newborn may lead to specific protein sensitization, with subsequent injury to GI mucosa. Recent evidence, in fact, suggests that this sensitization takes place even in breast-fed infants whose mothers ingest cow's milk protein. In the clinically stable child, appearance in the stool of neutrophils or eosinophils (with or without peripheral eosinophilia) suggests the diagnosis after infectious causes have been ruled out. It is important to emphasize that a high percentage of protein-sensitive infants will react to soy and goat's milk as well as cow's milk protein. Therefore, a hydrolyzed protein formula (Nutramigen) should be used in an infant suspected of protein intolerance. In more severe cases, hospitalization for initial parenteral therapy may be required followed by the institution of an elemental formula (Pregestimil), necessitated by mucosal injury affecting absorption of all nutrient classes. After mucosal recovery, documented by renewed carbohydrate tolerance, gradual reintroduction of the suspected formula (initially in very small amounts) is undertaken as a rechallenge. Recrudescence of symptoms, usually heralded by early carbohydrate malabsorption, confirms the diagnosis.

Cystic Fibrosis.—When clinically apparent in the first 3 months of life, cystic fibrosis is often complicated by malabsorptive stools secondary to pancreatic insufficiency; the syndrome thus presents with chronic diarrhea and failure to thrive. The physician should suspect cystic fibrosis in any infant with such a clinical course, particularly one with associated pulmonary disease or a positive family history. Although the finding of elevated sweat chloride levels are diagnostic, this test is difficult to perform in small babies, because of the inability to obtain adequate quantities of sweat. Until the infant is old enough to be diagnosed specifically, finding a reduced or absent stool trypsin content can be considered presumptive evidence for cystic fibrosis. Under these conditions, a therapeutic trial of pancreatic enzyme replacement is indicated until an adequate sweat test can be performed (see Chapter 54).

Short Bowel Syndrome.—With the development of refined surgical techniques and the advent of parenteral nutrition, infants are now surviving catastrophic small-intestinal illnesses resulting in extensive resections. These resections include those for congenital omphalocele and gastroschisis, following resections for small bowel atresias, and the surgical treatment of necrotizing enterocolitis. The primary care provider should be aware of the long-term consequences of these problems, since obviously initial management involves prolonged hospitalization involving both surgeons and gastroenterologists. Thus, despite the intestine's ability to adapt effectively following resections (e.g., ileum assuming functions of resected jejunum), loss of the terminal ileum invariably leads to bile salt loss with secondary secretory diarrhea and steatorrhea. Therefore, infants will require a formula containing medium-chain triglycerides (Portagen), which does not require micellar solubilization for absorption. The use of cholestyramine, an anion exchange resin, may be required to treat diarrhea induced by bile acid loss. If the infant with jejunal resection survives the initial postoperative and long recovery period, ileal adaptation will often obviate the need for an elemental diet.

Transport and Enzyme Defects.—Transport and enzyme defects often present with severe, protracted diarrhea leading to inanition. Congenital glucose-galactose malabsorption is manifest by watery, acidic stools after the initial glucose-water feeding at birth; it may be differentiated from mucosal injury-related malabsorption by normal tolerance to fructose. The most common congenital disaccharidase abnormality is sucrase-isomaltase deficiency, which presents with diarrhea after the introduction of sucrose-containing foods (fruits, juices), usually at 3 to 4 months. Congenital lactase deficiency is an extremely rare disorder.

Children in the Age Group of 3 Months to 3 Years

MAJOR CAUSES OF CHRONIC DIARRHEA

Postinfections
Chronic nonspecific diarrhea
Giardiasis
Celiac disease
Protein intolerance
Sucrase-isomaltase deficiency
Hirschsprung disease

Diagnoses associated with the development of chronic diarrhea in this age group overlap somewhat with those diagnoses for the age group of birth to 3 months. Although chronic bacterial infections are uncommon, an important disease is protracted diarrhea associated with *Clostridium difficile*. Postinfection carbohydrate intolerance occurs commonly in children up to 1 year of age. Similarly, the onset of protein intolerance often occurs after 3 months (although it rarely persists beyond 2 years), particularly in previously breast-fed infants. A brief comment should be made concerning Hirschsprung disease (intestinal aganglionosis). Although the disorder classically presents with chronic (from birth) constipation, a life-threatening enterocolitis may develop in certain cases; and this may be confused with infections or idiopathic inflammatory bowel disease. In general, however, the majority of children with persistent diarrhea in this age group fall into two broad categories: those with chronic nonspecific diarrhea, who manifest no nutritional deficits, and those with specific malabsorption syndromes associated with steatorrhea.

Chronic Nonspecific Diarrhea.—In the child who presents with a prolonged history of diarrheal stools while continuing to thrive and grow normally, the most likely diagnosis is chronic nonspecific diarrhea (CNSD), or "toddler's diarrhea." These children will have one to as many as 12 loose to watery stools per day, which often appear to contain "undigested" food particles (actually nondigestible cellulose matter that has not undergone disintegration by colonic action), but they are rarely troubled by nighttime diarrhea. In children in whom weight loss or poor weight gain is evident, the cause is invariably caloric deprivation secondary to dietary restrictions. Once caloric intake has been documented and normalized and infection ruled out by adequate cultures, the presence of diarrhea in a well, growing child invariably reflects CNSD. Although the precise mechanisms responsible are not known, some children may benefit from an increase in the fat: carbohydrate ratio in the diet or by a reduction in fluid intake (when excessive). Antidiarrheal agents are of no value in CNSD, and the syndrome will resolve by the age of 3 to 4 years in almost all children.

Giardiasis.—Infection with this protozoal organism represents the most common cause of chronic malabsorption in North America. Although *Giardia lamblia* infestation may present as an acute diarrheal syndrome, the more common course is that of a chronic illness marked by steatorrhea and poor weight gain. Suspicion is particularly high in patients with immunoglobulin deficiency, in whom the infection may be a recurring problem. Although many authors suggest the technique of duodenal aspiration to recover the organism (which resides in the upper small bowel), we have found the culturing of a *fresh* stool specimen or one preserved for only a short time in formalinized transport medium will lead to a positive diagnosis in well over 90% of cases. At present, the treatment of choice is either Furoxone, 7 mg/kg/day, or metronidazole, 20 mg/kg/day, for a 7-day course.

Celiac Disease.—Although a common cause of malabsorption in individuals in Europe, the diagnosis of celiac disease is made less frequently in North America. Nevertheless, it is important to consider this diagnosis in appropriate clinical situations, since specific therapy with dietary gluten restriction may be necessary to reduce the occurrence of intestinal lymphoma observed in untreated adult patients. The syndrome occurs as a result of a sensitivity to gliadin, the protein fraction of gluten present in wheat, barley, rye, oats, and malt. The likely etiology of celiac disease is genetic, manifested by a dominant gene of low penetrance, resulting in incidence figures of roughly 1:3,000. Most cases are evident within 1 year of the introduction of gluten-containing products to the diet. The usual clinical course is marked by a falloff in percentile levels from standard growth curves, with the falloff in weight preceding that of height; and it is associated with the presence of foul, bulky stools resulting from steatorrhea. The physical findings of a protuberant abdomen with wasted buttocks and extremities always raises the possibility of cystic fibrosis and giardiasis as the major differential diagnoses to be considered. The presentation may be considerably more subtle, particularly in older children, and there have been recent reports of cases manifested solely by growth failure without diarrhea. Once the diagnosis is suspected and appropriate laboratory studies suggest malabsorption, the patient is referred for peroral small intestinal biopsy; a flat villus lesion that responds to gluten withdrawal is diagnostic.

Children in the Age Group of 3 to 18 Years

MAJOR CAUSES OF CHRONIC DIARRHEA

Giardiasis
Celiac disease
Late-onset lactose intolerance
Inflammatory bowel disease
Crohn disease
Ulcerative colitis

Chronic diarrhea is a less frequent complaint after 3 years of age. Because CNSD invariably resolves by this time, this major nonpathologic cause of diarrhea observed in younger children no longer presents a problem. In fact, the only significant causes of chronic diarrhea after the age of 3 years that do not represent an underlying disease process are chronic constipation resulting in overflow stools and late-onset lactose intolerance. Giardiasis and even celiac disease may become manifest at any age and must be considered in any patient whose course suggests a malabsorptive state.

Late-Onset Lactose Intolerance.—With the exception of white persons of Northern European extraction, lactose intolerance is a common, developmentally-related phenomenon in older children and adults, with over 95% in some ethnic groups being affected. Clinical manifestations result from absent intestinal lactase leading to malabsorption of lactose and an osmotic, fermentative diarrhea. Excessive gas production may cause crampy abdominal pain. When noted by positive breath H_2 testing in a patient under 5 years of age, lactose malabsorption usually reflects underlying small bowel mucosal dysfunction. In older children, however, lactase deficiency usually is a genetically mediated phenomenon without associated gastrointestinal pathologic findings. This diagnosis should be considered in the older patient presenting with diarrhea, abdominal pain, and flatulence, particularly when the child appears otherwise clinically well. A trial of a lactose-free diet is both diagnostic and therapeutic. Long-term management, especially in younger children, may involve treatment of milk with Lact-Aid, a yeast-derived lactase that predigests the offending sugar.

Crohn Disease.—Crohn disease, or regional enteritis, represents an idiopathic, inflammatory condition that may involve any portion of the digestive tract; however, the terminal ileum and colon are the most frequently affected areas. Malabsorption is an infrequent complication, except in cases in which severe jejunal and ileal involvement results in nutrient and bile salt loss. The most common presenting symptoms include diarrhea (with or without blood), fevers, abdominal pain, and growth failure, with poor growth and weight gain most commonly occurring as a consequence of reduced caloric intake. In fact, Crohn disease, like celiac disease, should be considered in any child manifesting inadequate growth and development, even if the patient is otherwise relatively asymptomatic. Laboratory aids to diagnosis include findings of anemia, thrombocytosis, an elevated erythrocyte sedimentation rate, and hypoproteinemia. Barium studies will often reveal characteristic mucosal abnormalities, but definitive diagnosis requires colonoscopic-biopsy evidence of chronic inflammation with granulomas and giant cells (see Chapter 61).

Ulcerative Colitis.—Evaluation of ulcerative colitis parallels that of Crohn disease, since the presenting signs and symptoms are similar. However, ulcerative colitis may appear in much younger children (with some reported cases in children under 1 year of age) and bloody diarrhea is a more common presentation. Because this disease only affects colonic mucosa ("backwash" ileitis is a relatively uncommon condition in pediatrics), malabsorption is not a problem. Proctosigmoidoscopy with cultures and biopsies should always be performed, since bacterial colitis and amebiasis must be ruled out. Medical treatment, including the use of salicylazosulfapyridine and corticosteroids, is similar to that employed in Crohn disease.

DATA GATHERING

HISTORY

Obviously, an attempt to rule out every cause of chronic diarrhea in each patient is a futile and costly exercise. In infants, the most common cause of protracted diarrhea is postinfectious lactose-intolerance. In this group of patients, requirements for inpatient evaluation and treatment are clearly dependent on the infant's state of hydration. Failure to improve while not taking anything by mouth and receiving intravenous (IV) therapy suggests the possibility of a secretory process. In the older infant and child, after a complete dietary and travel history is obtained, the course of diagnostic workup depends largely on the clinical state of the patient. Several screening studies may then direct further workup.

LABORATORY EVALUATION

Stool Examination.—Stool examination is important not only to confirm the diarrheal state but also to give some clues as to the cause. Thus, watery, acidic, explosive stools suggest carbohydrate malabsorption, while foul bulky ones indicate steatorrhea. Similarly, mucoid stools with or without diarrhea with occult blood (Hemoccult-positive) indicates the possibility of protein intolerance in infants, inflammatory bowel disease in older children and adolescents, and infection in all age groups. Specific tests on fecal material should include:

1. pH, reducing substances (to rule out carbohydrate malabsorption)
2. Wright's stain for polymorphonuclear neutrophils, eosinophils (infection, allergy)
3. Hemoccult test for occult blood
4. Cultures for ova and parasites
5. Sudan stain for fat

Growth Curve.—The growth curve is the most important single piece of information required to establish the likely nature and chronicity of the problem, and it should include weight, height, and weight-for-height assessments. Thus, a sudden weight falloff while maintaining height percentile suggests a relatively acute process. On the other hand, reduction of both weight and height percentile levels from previous growth points indicates chronic illness and may reflect chronic caloric deprivation (e.g., in inflammatory bowel disease) or malabsorption.

Hematologic Studies.—Results of hematologic studies will provide evidence for nutritional deficits (levels of albumin, total protein, folate, vitamin B_{12}) and suggest an infectious or other inflammatory etiology (values for complete blood cell [CBC] count and erythrocyte sedimentation rate).

Malabsorption Studies.—In a case in which chronic malabsorption is suspected, certain screening studies will aid in assessing absorptive function.

Lactose Breath H_2.—This noninvasive study measures H_2 levels in expired air, formed by colonic bacterial fermentation of unabsorbed lactose. If results are abnormal (i.e., $H_2 > 10$ ppm above baseline) in patients less than 5 years of age, small bowel disease should be suspected.

Carotene and 1 Hour Blood D-xylose Absorption.—These are additional screening studies of small intestinal function. Carotene levels are only useful if dietary carotene intake is adequate; a value of > 100 mg/dL is normal. A serum carotene < 50 mg/dL suggests malabsorption.

72-Hour Fecal Fat.—When properly carried out, this test is the most definitive test for steatorrhea. On a diet containing 100 g of fat, fat excretion should not exceed 7 g/day.

When the workup suggests a malabsorption syndrome, and cystic fibrosis and giardiasis have been ruled out, patients should be referred for peroral small intestinal biopsy.

INDICATIONS FOR CONSULTATION OR REFERRAL

Decisions to hospitalize patients with chronic diarrhea and refer them for subspecialist care are dependent on both the clinical severity and complexity of the problem. The dehydrated infant will obviously require IV hydration. Similarly, the condition of the infant (or even older child in some cases) who presents with inanition and severe failure to thrive may be evaluated more rapidly in an inhospital setting, and this patient often requires IV nutrition (central or peripheral) while his condition is being evaluated. Figure 23–1 illustrates the basic guidelines for the outpatient evaluation of chronic diarrhea. Obviously, diagnosis of specific entities requiring invasive intervention (e.g., celiac

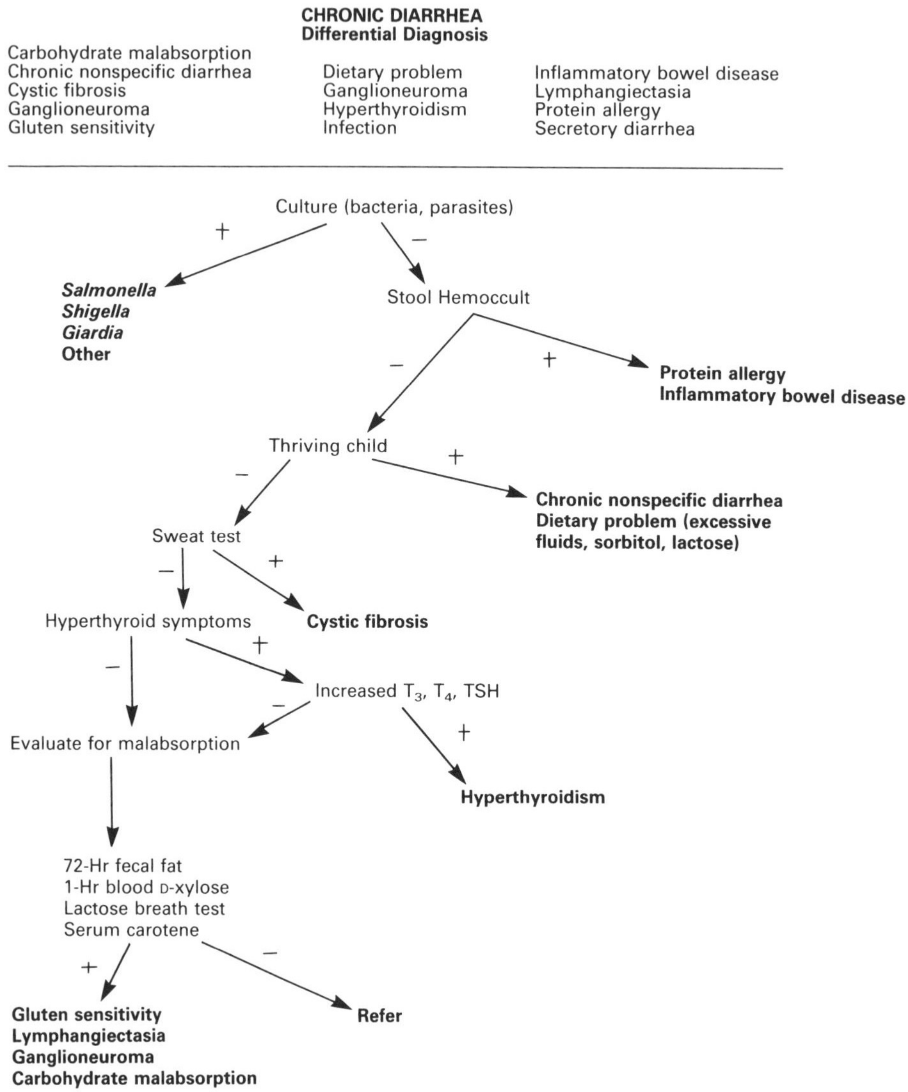

FIG 23–1
Decision tree for differential diagnosis of chronic diarrhea.

disease, inflammatory bowel disease) will require consultation by a pediatric gastroenterologist. However, in the majority of cases, workup can be completed by the primary care physician.

DISCUSSION OF ALGORITHM

The first major branch in the "decision tree" in evaluation of chronic diarrhea includes a careful dietary history, stool culture, and testing of the stool for pH, Clinitest, Wright stain for white blood cells, and stool hemoccult testing. At this point, those with infections or food intolerance can be identified and treated. For those who still have diarrhea and are not thriving, an investigation should be carried out for inflammatory bowel disease or malabsorption. A diagnosis of CNSD is reserved for those children with normal laboratory tests who continue to grow despite failure to respond to dietary manipulations.

BIBLIOGRAPHY

Ament ME, Barclay GN: Chronic diarrhea. *Pediatr Ann* 1982; 11:124.

Anderson CM: Malabsorption in children. *Clin Gastroenterol* 1977; 6:355.

Barr RG, Perman JA, Schoeller DA, et al: Breath tests in pediatric gastrointestinal disorders. *Pediatrics* 1978; 62:393.

Calvin RT, Klish WJ, Nichols BL: Disaccharidase activities, jejunal morphology, and carbohydrate tolerance in children with chronic diarrhea. *J Pediatr Gastroenterol Nutr* 1985; 4:949.

Cohen SA, Hendricks KM, Mathis RK, et al: Chronic nonspecific diarrhea: dietary relationships. *Pediatrics* 1979; 64:402.

Davidson M, Wasserman R: The irritable colon of childhood. *J Pediatr* 1966; 69:1027.

Greene HL, Ghishan FK: Excessive fluid intake as a cause of chronic diarrhea in young children. *J Pediatr* 1983; 102:836.

Hyams JS, Leichtner AM: Apple juice. An unappreciated cause of chronic diarrhea. *Am J Dis Child* 1985; 139:503.

Lo CW, Walker WA: Chronic protracted diarrhea of infancy, a nutritional disease. *Pediatrics* 1983; 72:786.

Phillips SF: Diarrhea: a current view of the pathophysiology. *Gastroenterology* 1972; 63:495.

Sunshine P, Sinatra FR, Mitchell CH: Intractable diarrhea of infancy. *Clin Gastroenterol* 1977; 6:445.

Sutphen JL, Grand RJ, Flores A, et al: Chronic diarrhea associated with *Clostridium difficile* in children. *Am J Dis Child* 1983; 137:275.

24 DIZZINESS

Roger J. Packer, M.D.

Dizziness is a nonspecific term used to describe diverse symptoms including light-headedness, weakness, unsteadiness, or the illusion of rotational movement. The significance and proper evaluation of the condition of the dizzy child is dependent on a better understanding of what the patient is actually experiencing when dizziness occurs. If the child complains of feeling a sense of whirling or rotation of himself or the environment, then he is suffering from vertigo, which implies dysfunction of the vestibular system.

In this chapter discussion is limited to vertiginous dizziness.

DIFFERENTIAL DIAGNOSIS

COMMON CAUSES OF VERTIGINOUS DIZZINESS

Infection
Otitis media
Mastoiditis
Labyrinthitis

Toxins
Aminoglycosides
Ethycrynic acid
Salicylates
Quinine

Trauma
Immediate or delayed

Tumor
Brain stem glioma
Acoustic neuroma

Multiple etiologic
Cholesteatoma
Migraine
Epilepsy
- Complex partial
- Simple partial

Benign paroxysmal vertigo
Benign recurrent vertigo
Multiple sclerosis
Ménière disease

DISCUSSION

Vertigo may be conceptualized as occurring either on a peripheral basis, secondary to dysfunction of the vestibular apparatus, or on a central basis, following impairment of the vestibular nuclei or their brain-stem connections.

In childhood, peripheral vertigo is more common than central vertigo and may rarely occur as a complication of acute and chronic otitis media. Mastoiditis and associated suppurative labyrinthitis with vertigo, fever, and pain, are rare in the antibiotic era but, when present, cause redness and warmth behind the ear. Variation of the mastoid pneumatization may make diagnosis somewhat difficult. Cholesteatomas, masses of desquamated epithelial cells occurring primarily or associated with chronic otitis media, invade bone and may result in labyrinthitis and vertigo. Small bits of whitish debris in the middle ear are seen extruding from the perforated tympanic membrane. Radiologic studies disclose destruction of the temporal bone.

Vestibular neuronitis (viral labyrinthitis) usually occurs in children over 10 years old but may occur at any age. It is often associated with intercurrent upper respiratory tract infection or middle ear infection. Viral labyrinthitis is most symptomatic during the first 2 weeks of illness, slowly improving during the following 2 weeks. Results of vestibular function tests are abnormal during the disease, and spontaneous nystagmus is common. Findings of audiologic tests are normal. Two entities frequently confused with vestibular neuronitis, Ménière disease and benign positional vertigo, are rare in childhood. Ménière disease results in recurrent paroxysmal vertigo, tinnitus, and hearing loss. Benign positional vertigo is manifest by intermittent vertiginous episodes associated with rapid changes of head position. Toxic labyrinthitis may occur following the administration of various drugs (most noteworthy, the aminoglycosides). The onset of this illness is usually insidious, and the diagnosis may be missed if a careful history of drug intake is not performed. Other drugs that may rarely cause a similar toxic labyrinthitis include ethacrynic acid, salicylates, and quinine.

Vertigo may occur secondary to trauma. Sudden vestibular damage, occurring immediately after trauma, with resultant vertigo, nausea, vomiting, and spontaneous nystagmus, poses little difficulty in the differential diagnosis. Posttraumatic vertigo occurs days and sometimes weeks following head trauma and is manifest with sudden changes of head position. This is associated with abnormal vestibular function as demonstrated by testing. In contrast, dizziness, as a component of the postconcussion syndrome, is rarely associated with vertigo or abnormal vestibular testing.

Benign paroxysmal vertigo, which occurs between the ages of 1 and 3 years, is heralded by acute episodes of imbalance. During the attack, which may occur in clusters, the child seems frightened, becomes pale, and, if standing, either reaches for support or falls but does not lose consciousness. Subjective symptoms are difficult to ascertain. Infrequently, these are associated with upper respiratory tract infection or middle ear infection. The cause of these attacks is unknown, although some believe it to be the equivalent of a migraine attack. Results of radiologic, audiographic, and electroencephalogram (EEG) studies are normal. Findings of tests of vestibular function are usually consistent with peripheral vestibular dysfunction.

Vertigo on a central basis is uncommon in childhood, although it may occur as a component of epilepsy or migraine. Vertiginous symptoms may uncommonly be the sole clinical manifestation of partial complex (temporal lobe) seizures and during these attacks vestibular function is said to be normal. However, usually the vertiginous symptoms are associated with other symptoms referrable to the temporal lobe and abnormalities are noted on EEG. Vertigo may also occur prior to onset of a seizure, and thus be the "aura" of a more complex event. Vertiginous migraine may mimic temporal lobe epilepsy, but the history of associated headaches makes clinical differentiation possible. Similarly, vertigo may occur during a migraine attack.

When vertigo occurs secondary to tumors of the posterior fossa such as brain-stem gliomas, it tends to be overshadowed by associated neurologic deficits. Acoustic neuromas and other tumors of the cerebellopontine angle do present with vertigo but are rare until adulthood. Other rare reported causes of central vertigo are encephalitis, increased intracranial pressure, and syringobulbia. Multiple sclerosis can, in rare cases, present as vertigo in the adolescent.

DATA GATHERING

HISTORY

The key to the proper diagnosis and management of the child's complaint is determining what the child or parent means by dizziness. If the patient's symptoms are that of true vertigo, differentiation between peripheral and central etiologies is of major importance and is often possible. Complaints of tinnitus, hearing loss, pain, or a sensation of fullness in the ear, as well as nausea and vomiting are much more frequent with peripheral lesions. The history of intermittent episodes of severe vertigo is much more consistent with peripheral disease, as central vertigo tends to be persistent and somewhat milder.

PHYSICAL EXAMINATION

Important features on the physical examination include evidence of redness or warmth behind the ear, suggesting mastoiditis, serous labyrinthitis, or bacterial labyrinthitis. Careful cranial nerve examination is mandatory for diagnosis, since involvement of the fifth or seventh cranial nerve implies central vertigo. The fifth cranial nerve supplies sensation to the face and motor innervation to the muscles of mastication. Mass lesions in the pontocerebellar angle may result in paraesthesias of the face with abnormalities of pain, cold, and touch sensation and, less often, in deviation of the jaw to the side of the lesions. The seventh cranial nerve innervates the muscles of the face, and disruption of its fibers causes weakness of the upper and lower portions of the face. The corneal reflex tests for the integrity of both the fifth and seventh cranial nerves; its loss may suggest subtle asymmetries of cranial nerve function. A neural-sensory hearing loss, indicating eighth cranial nerve dysfunction, may be of cochlear or primary eighth nerve origin. Differentiation is often impossible at bedside and requires further audiologic evaluation. Spontaneous nystagmus may result from either central or peripheral vertigo. Nystagmus due to vestibular dysfunction is commonly a jerk nystagmus with a fast and slow component, the fast component being toward the side of the impairment and increasing as one looks toward the lesion. It is primarily horizontal and decreased by fixation. A central basis for the nystagmus is likely if there are vertical or purely rotatory components to the nystagmus and if nystagmus changes direction when the direction of gaze is altered.

Extremely helpful in the diagnosis of vertigo are the inclusions of special tests that simulate the symptom. Not only should the patient's objective responses be evaluated during these procedures, but the child should be asked if these tests reproduce the subjective complaint. If they do not, the importance of any abnormality observed is questionable. The Nylen-Barany maneuver is performed after seating the child on the edge of the examining table. The subject is then asked to quickly lie back and his head is tilted 45° backward and 45° to one side and maintained in this position for 60 seconds. The eyes are observed for the onset, duration, and direction of nystagmus. The child is then returned to the sitting position and the maneuver is repeated, with the head turned to the opposite side. If nystagmus occurs, there is evidence for vestibular abnormality that can often be separated into central or peripheral categories (Table 24–1).

LABORATORY EVALUATION

Performance of additional tests after the initial evaluation is dependent on the clinical impression. These tests should not be done routinely and are included only to help understand what

TABLE 24–1
Nylen-Barany Maneuver

Test	Central Vertigo	Peripheral Vertigo
Nystagmus	Yes	Yes
Latency	Immediate onset	Few sec delay
Adaption	No	Yes
Fatigue	No	Yes (disappears on repetition)
Subjective vertigo	Usually absent	Present

DIZZINESS
Differential diagnosis

Anemia
Anxiety
Arrhythmia
Benign paroxysmal vertigo
Brain tumor
Collagen vascular disease
Depression
Heat exhaustion
Hyperventilation
Hypoglycemia
Hypotension
Labyrinthitis
Mastoiditis
Ménière syndrome
Meningitis
Myositis
Otitis media
Paroxysmal atrial tachycardia
Posttraumatic vertigo

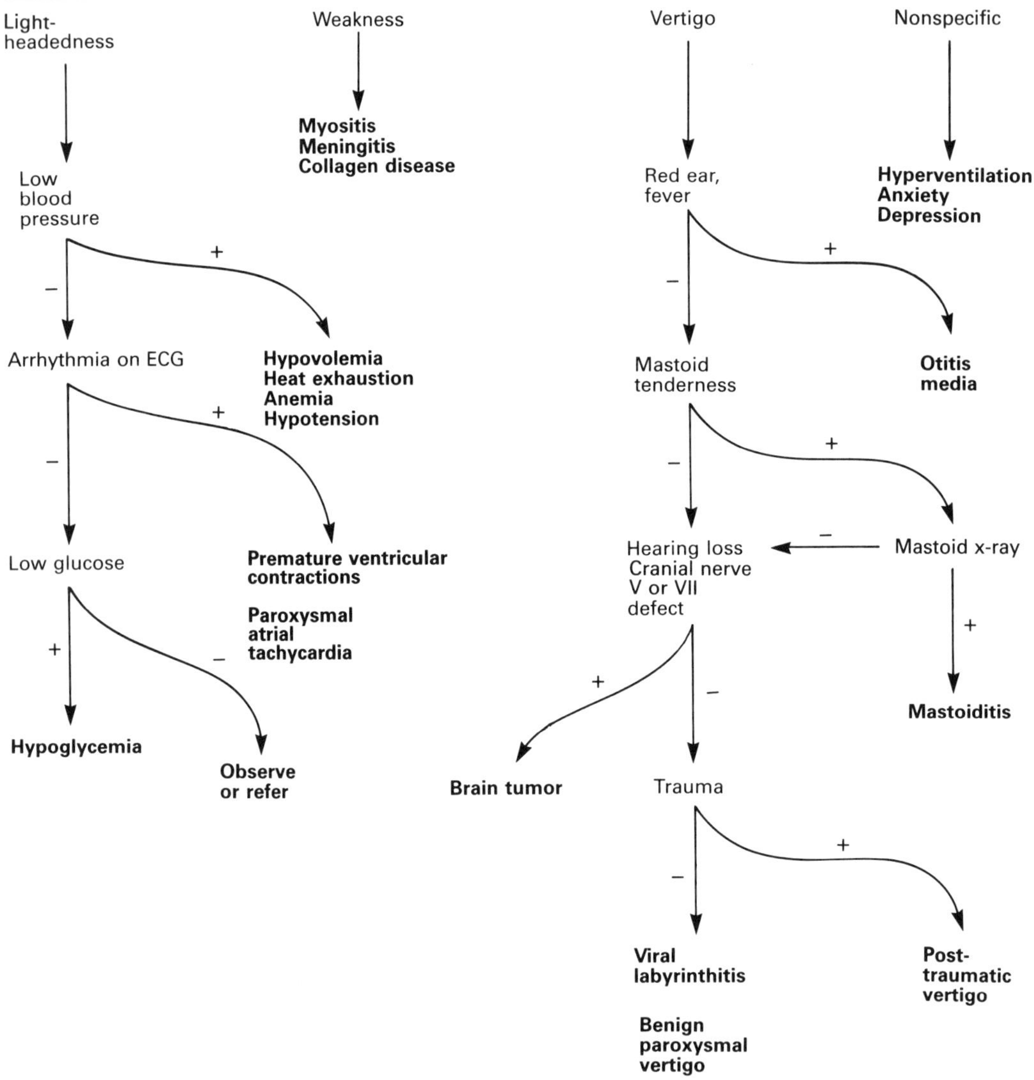

FIG 24–1
Decision tree for differential diagnosis of dizziness.

the neurologist or otolaryngologist may do in the evaluation. Caloric testing, which is irrigation of the ear canals with both warm and cold water, may be used to confirm vestibular dysfunction. Electronystagmography is a more sophisticated means of monitoring caloric responses and involves electrorecording the rate, direction, and amplitude of the nystagmus quantitatively with the eye open and closed. Audiometry should be performed if there is a suspicion of hearing loss. Other tests of auditory function, such as auditory recruitment, are useful in differentiating cochlear from eighth nerve dysfunction in the older child.

Roentgenographic studies are mandatory if one suspects central vestibular disease or labyrinth destruction. Roentgenograms of the skull and mastoid area, including tomography of the auditory canal, are useful in the detection of infectious or destructive lesions. Computed tomography with contrast enhancement or magnetic resonance imaging are procedures of choice if there is evidence of fifth or seventh nerve involvement. An EEG should be obtained only if there is a high index of suspicion that the vertigo is a seizure equivalent.

INDICATIONS FOR CONSULTATION OR REFERRAL

The majority of causes of vertigo are benign, self-limited illnesses, and reassurance is the major aspect of therapy. In most cases, if the etiology is not readily apparent and there is no evidence of associated neurologic dysfunction or labyrinth destruction, the child may be treated symptomatically and the condition reevaluated before proceeding with more specific laboratory studies. In acute labyrinthitis, meclizine (12.5 mg twice a day to 25 mg twice a day for children over 12 years of age) results in symptomatic improvement of nausea and unsteadiness. Treatment of benign paroxysmal vertigo is hard to evaluate since the clinical course is unpredictable. There may be improvement with the use of diphenhydramine (5 mg/kg/day).

DISCUSSION OF ALGORITHM

A careful history will help develop the further evaluation of dizziness (Fig 24–1). These symptoms include: lightheadedness, dysequilibrium, weakness, and vertigo. Lightheadedness is usually associated with other systemic problems such as hypertension, hypoglycemia, and drug ingestion. Dysequilibrium and weakness tend to be secondary to neurologic problems. Vertigo should make one consider mastoiditis, deficits of the fifth, seventh, or eighth cranial nerves, or trauma.

BIBLIOGRAPHY

Britton BH: Vertigo in the pediatric and adolescent age group. *Laryngoscope* 1988; 98:139–146.

Deonna T, Zeigler AL, Despland P, et al: Partial epilepsy in neurologically normal children: Clinical syndromes and prognosis. *Epilepsia* 1986; 27:241–247.

Dix MR: Vertigo. *Practitioner* 1973; 211:295.

Drachman DA, Hart CW: An approach to the dizzy patient. *Neurology* 1972; 22:323–334.

Eviatar L, Eviatar A: Vertigo in children: Comments on pathogenesis and management. *Clin Pediatr* 1974; 13:940.

Fenichel GM: Migraine as a cause of benign paroxysmal vertigo of childhood. *J Pediatr* 1967; 71:114.

Koenigsberger MR, Chutorian AM, Gold AP, et al: Benign paroxysmal vertigo of childhood. *Neurology* 1970; 20:1108–1113.

25 EARACHE

William Potsic, M.D.

Because earache is one of the most common complaints of pediatric patients, it is important to develop a plan for diagnosis and management. Although the great majority of patients will have an otologic cause for the earache, the diagnosis of earache can be a challenge because pain may be referred to the ear and surrounding structures from multiple areas of the head and neck. These areas are any structures innervated by the cranial nerves (V, VII, IX, X, and XI) and cervical nerves C2-3. They include a number of structures that may or may not be visible at the time of direct examination in the office.

Otologic causes of ear pain usually produce severe, constant earache and are associated with fever. Nonotologic pain is usually intermittent, less severe, and not accompanied by fever. In our experience, we found 85% of cases with ear pain are from infection; 7% from referred pain; 5% from eustachian tube dysfunction and serous otitis media; and 3% from miscellaneous causes.

DIFFERENTIAL DIAGNOSIS

COMMON CAUSES OF EARACHE

Trauma
Barotrauma
Blunt trauma
Sharp trauma
Thermal injury

Infection
External otitis
Acute supportive otitis media
Mastoiditis
Infected preauricular sinus
Perichondritis
Lymphadenitis
Sinusitis
Aphthous ulcer

Allergic-immunologic
Neuralgia

Tumor mass
Cholesteatoma
Rhabdomyosarcoma
Facial neuroma
Cystic hygroma
Arteriovenous malformation

Multiple etiologic
Eustachian tube dysfunction, effusion
Referred pain, dental
Temporomandibular
Psychogenic pain
Tic
Migraine
Myofacial pain
Parotiditis
Parotid duct stone

DISCUSSION

The diagnosis of earache involves careful history and examination of the ear by inspection and pneumatic otoscopy. Otologic causes of earache are usually infections but may be from trauma or tumors.

Otologic causes of earache are the most common and present with severe, steady pain. External otitis causes pain with chewing or manipulating the pinna. A foul discharge is present in the inflamed, edematous external canal.

Acute suppurative otitis media causes deep, steady, and severe pain that is not aggravated by chewing. Very young children may just be fussy or lethargic but older children either pull at their ear or specifically state that their ears hurt. Otoscopy reveals an inflamed and bulging eardrum. (A normal eardrum is shown in Fig 25–1).

The earache associated with eustachian tube dysfunction is mild and associated with a steady sensation of fullness. Intermittent acute exacerbations may be present for 30 minutes to 1 hour as the negative pressure fluctuates. Barotrauma usually causes severe sudden pain that resolves spontaneously in 1 hour.

Nonotologic causes of ear pain consist of problems in the head and neck that refer pain to the ear. These include dental and temporomandibular joint pain (trigeminal nerve), Bell palsy, and aphthous ulcers (facial nerve), tonsillitis and adenoiditis (glossopharyngeal nerve), and esophageal foreign body and thyroiditis (vagus nerves). Referred pain from the cervical nerve $C_{2\text{-}3}$ include: lymphadenitis, infected cysts, cystic hygroma, hemangioma, and arteriovenous malformation. Cervical spine injury and neuralgia also cause ear pain.

DATA GATHERING

HISTORY

Since most ear pain is secondary to infection, a careful history should include information about fever and symptoms of upper respiratory tract infection. Traumatic causes should also be excluded. Other important information includes evidence of dental problems, pain on chewing (temporomandibular joint) or after eating food, especially some foods that stimulate saliva flow (parotid pain).

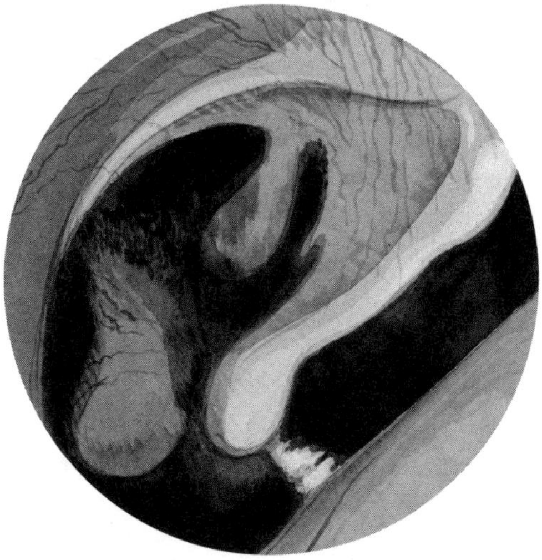

FIG 25–1
Normal eardrum showing translucent tympanic membrane and middle ear structure: malleus in center and incus and stapes above it.

PHYSICAL EXAMINATION

When the otologic examination is normal, the source of the problem must be searched for by examining the oral cavity, pharynx, and neck region. The signs and symptoms of the primary problem are often overshadowed by ear pain but they usually cause some difficulty that is detectable to the patient if he is asked while the history is taken. The most common reason for referred ear pain in children is dental problems or aphthous ulcerations of the oral cavity. Erupting teeth, caries, or gingivitis may also cause referred pain. The pharynx and nose should be examined carefully to search for pharyngitis, tonsillitis, or evidence of sinusitis. The neck must be palpated for cervical adenitis, thyroiditis, or cysts.

LABORATORY EVALUATION

When the cause of the referred pain is not apparent, a roentgenographic sinus series may be helpful to demonstrate the presence of sinusitis. In addition, the complete evaluation of otalgia may need to include a dental examination with dental x-rays and an otolaryngology consultation for a complete head and neck examination including nasopharyngoscopy, hypopharyngoscopy, and laryngoscopy.

Children with severe debilitating pain or severe ear infection may need admission for intravenous antimicrobial therapy and narcotic medication for pain control.

INDICATIONS FOR CONSULTATION OR REFERRAL

Earache of otologic origin usually resolves in 4 to 8 hours after antibiotic therapy is started. If the pain persists after 24 hours, other reasons for the pain should be investigated. The help of an otolaryngologist or neurologist may be needed. If no cause for the pain is apparent by history, physical examination, or laboratory tests, a tension-pain syndrome may be present.

EARACHE
Differential diagnosis

Barotrauma
Dental caries
Otitis externa
Otitis media
Serous otitis media
Temporomandibular joint (TMJ) pain
Tension
Trauma
Tumor

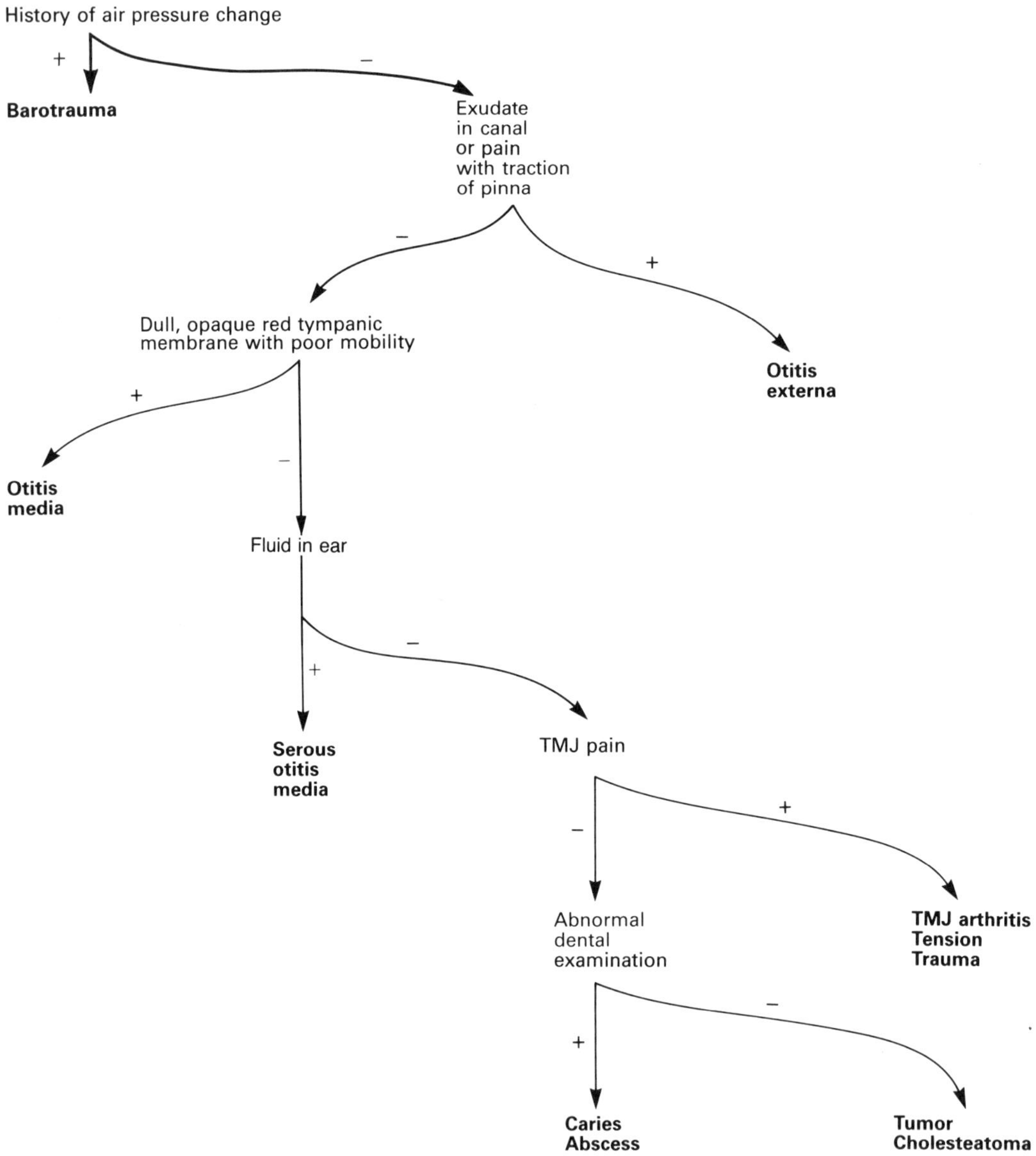

FIG 25–2
Decision tree for differential diagnosis of earache.

DISCUSSION OF ALGORITHM

An algorithm for differential diagnosis of earache is presented in Figure 25-2. A careful physical examination will detect either external otitis or otitis media, secretory otitis, or cholesteatoma. Neck trauma and dental problems should be excluded. If no diagnosis is made, causes of referred pain from surrounding structures should be considered.

BIBLIOGRAPHY

Bluestone CD, Shurin PA: Middle ear disease in children: Pathogenesis, diagnosis, and management. *Pediatr Clin North Am* 1970; 3:15.

Bluestone CD, Klein JO, Paradise JL, et al: Workshop on effects of otitis media on the child. *Pediatrics* 1983; 71:639–652.

Chasin WO: Otalgia (the ear), in Bluestone CD, Stool SF, (eds): *Pediatric Otolaryngology*. Philadelphia, WB Saunders Co, 1983.

Potsic WP: Management of trauma of the external ear, in English M, (ed): *Otolaryngology*. New York, Harper & Row, 1979.

Potsic WP: Pediatric otorhinolaryngology (the ear), in Rudolph AM, et al (eds): *Pediatrics*, ed 18. New York, Appleton-Century-Crofts, 1982, p 885.

Potsic WP, Handler SD: *Primary Care Pediatric Otolaryngology*. New York, Macmillan Publishing Co, 1986.

Tremble GE: Referred pain in the ear. *Arch Otolaryngol* 1965; 81:57–63.

26 EDEMA

Michael E. Norman, M.D.

Edema is the accumulation of excessive salt and water in the extravascular (e.g., interstitial) spaces. Digital pressure may or may not produce an indentation, and often there is a "doughy" feel to the subcutaneous tissue. Edema may be generalized or localized, but is usually confined to the dependent extremities and the distensible soft tissues, such as the periorbital region, scrotum, and labia majora. Trauma or infection often produces edema at the site of injury. Pathophysiologic causes of edema include decreased plasma oncotic pressure, increased venous or lymphatic hydrostatic pressure, and increased vascular permeability due either to the release of inflammatory mediators, as in an allergic reaction, or to vasculitis, as in collagen vascular disease.

DIFFERENTIAL DIAGNOSIS

The etiology of edema may be divided according to whether the edema is localized, especially if asymmetric, or generalized.

CAUSES OF EDEMA

Localized
Trauma
Infection
Lymphatic obstruction
  Lymphedema praecox
Allergic reaction
Immediate-type hypersensitivity

Generalized
Toxins
Drugs
Contraceptives

Metabolic/genetic
Malnutrition
Protein-losing enteropathy
Premenstrual swelling
Inappropriate level of antidiuretic hormone (ADH)
Congenital
Biliary atresia
Lymphedema praecox
Multiple etiologic
Cardiac
- Congestive heart failure
- Pericardial tamponade
- Constrictive pericarditis

Hepatic-biliary
- Hepatitis
- Cirrhosis

Renal disease
- Nephrotic syndrome
- Glomerulonephritis
- Renal failure

Gastrointestinal
- Protein-losing enteropathy
- Cirrhosis

Endocrine
- Hypothyroidism
- Mineralocorticoid excess

DATA GATHERING

HISTORY

Indolent localized edema such as "puffy eyes" on awakening is usually due to an infection such as periorbital cellulitis, an allergic reaction, or nephrotic syndrome. Traumatic edema is usually apparent from the history. Allergic reactions may or may not be evident, either on the basis of past medical or family history or exposure to a known allergen. In such cases the presence of pruritus, urticaria, laryngeal obstruction, or abdominal pain suggests the diagnosis. Lymphatic obstruction is almost always unilateral and provides a "woody" feeling to the affected extremity.

PHYSICAL EXAMINATION

Generalized edema may be insidious, with only progressive weight gain offering a clue to the diagnosis. This is particularly true in lean, muscular individuals. Careful attention must be paid to sudden changes in shoe or belt size. Pitting edema may become apparent only after firm direct pressure with the fingertips; the forehead and shin are favored places to perform this examination. Ascites should be looked for with palpation and percussion. In edema secondary to particular organ system involvement, the symptoms and physical signs are referable to that particular system and are usually obvious; they are not discussed here. Bloating and cyclical symptoms point to premenstrual edema in the menstruating girl. Occasionally a severe allergic reaction will cause generalized edema.

LABORATORY EVALUATION

The presence of localized edema other than bilateral periorbital edema rarely requires any investigation other than bacterial cultures for suspected primary infection (e.g., cellulitis) or urticaria secondary to infection (e.g., strep throat). Bilateral periorbital edema or generalized edema always necessitates a complete urinalysis, unless there are obvious symptoms and signs of congestive heart failure, constrictive pericarditis, or pericardial tamponade. Proteinuria indicates the need for further investigations to differentiate idiopathic nephrotic syndrome (levels of serum albumin and cholesterol, 24-hour urine sample for measurement of total protein excretion) from glomerulonephritis (determination of antistreptolysin O, C3 complement, antinuclear antibody [ANA] titer). The absence of proteinuria is compatible with hepatobiliary disease or vasculitis. A low level of serum albumin without proteinuria indicates protein-losing enteropathy, cirrhosis, or malnutrition. Determinations of erythrocyte sedimentation rate, ANA titer, and anti-DNA antibodies are often helpful in vasculitis. Edema with associated hyponatremia but inappropriately concentrated urine suggests ADH excess.

INDICATIONS FOR CONSULTATION OR REFERRAL

Patients who should be considered for referral or consultation include those with suspected anaphylaxis with laryngeal edema or edema of

EDEMA
Differential diagnosis

Allergy	Hepatic disease	Pregnancy
Cellulitis, infection	Lymphatic obstruction	Premenstrual swelling
Collagen disease	Lymphedema praecox	Renal failure
Glomerulonephritis	Nephrotic syndrome	Trauma
Heart failure	Pericardial effusion	Vasculitis

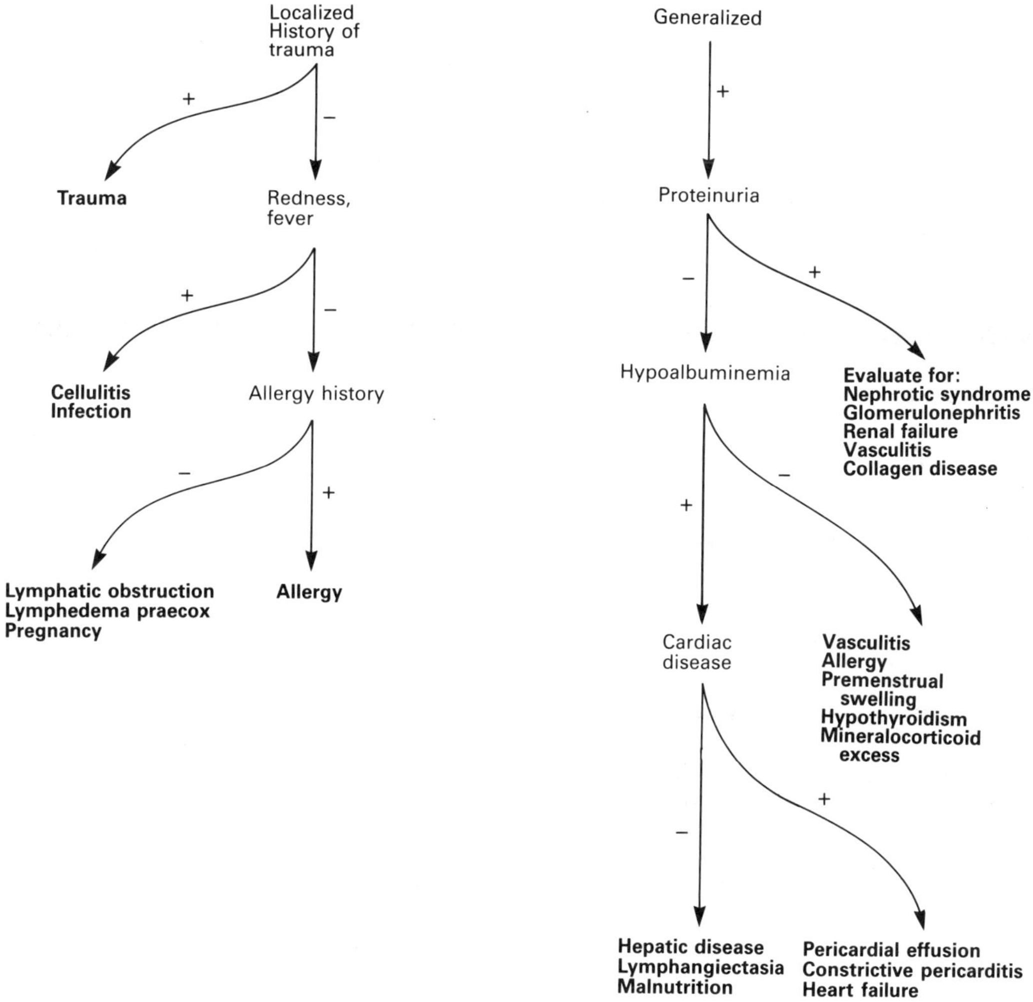

FIG 26–1
Decision tree for differential diagnosis of edema.

the abdominal viscera; unexplained generalized edema; and specific disease such as protein-losing enteropathy or cirrhosis.

DISCUSSION OF ALGORITHM

A decision tree for differential diagnosis of edema is presented in Figure 26–1. The first task is to determine if the edema is localized or generalized to more than one area of the body. Localized edema is likely secondary to trauma, infection, allergy, or lymphatic obstruction (lymphangiectasia or tumor). Generalized edema is usually secondary to heart failure, increased protein loss, or decreased protein production. The patient should be examined for heart failure, the urine tested for protein, and the serum albumin level measured. If the diagnosis cannot be confirmed by these investigations, the patient may have vasculitis, serum sickness or allergy, premenstrual swelling, or generalized lymphangiectasia.

BIBLIOGRAPHY

Baglia R, Levy JE: Pathogenesis and treatment of edema. *Pediatr Clin North Am* 1987; 34:639.

Schwartz MW: Edema, in Fleisher G, Ludwig S: *Textbook of Pediatric Emergency Medicine*, ed 2. Baltimore, Williams & Wilkins Co, 1988, pp 156–158.

Gauthier B: Edema, in Gauthier B, Edelman CM (eds): *Nephrology and Urology for the Pediatrician*. Boston, Little Brown & Co, 1982.

Lewis JM, Wald ER: Lymphedema praecox. *J Pediatr* 1984; 104:641.

27 ENURESIS

Jeffrey Weiss, M.D.

Enuresis, the involuntary passage of urine, is a poorly understood symptom with several possible causes and corresponding treatments. To evaluate and treat this common and annoying problem, the primary care physician should follow a logical stepwise approach of first defining the problem, screening for infection, and developing a reasonable treatment plan.

The term *primary nocturnal enuresis* means that the child has never kept a bed dry for a continuous period of several months. In contrast, secondary enuresis implies that nighttime bladder control was achieved for at least a 3-month period before the wetting resumed. About 85% of all cases of enuresis fall into the primary class. Both primary and secondary enuresis can be caused by maturational, organic, or psychosocial problems but many authorities think that secondary enuresis is less likely to be due to a simple maturational factor.

DIFFERENTIAL DIAGNOSIS

COMMON CAUSES OF NOCTURNAL ENURESIS

Maturational

Small bladder capacity
Immature sleep arousal pattern

Organic

Urinary tract infection
Urinary tract structural abnormality
Bladder innervation disorder
Myelomeningocele
Diabetes mellitus
Diabetes insipidus
Hyposthenuria (inability to concentrate urine)

Sickle cell anemia and trait
Sensitivity to certain foods (milk, eggs, orange juice)

Emotional

Temporary stress
Regressive behavior (birth of a sibling)
Severe emotional disturbance

DISCUSSION

Most nocturnal enuresis is due to maturational factors. Boys are affected twice as often as girls, and nearly 75% of patients have a positive family history. The underlying pathogenesis may be an immature sleep pattern or small urinary bladder capacity. Studies correlating the electroencephalogram with enuresis indicate that these children are actually asleep when wetting occurs, usually shortly after bedtime. Children with maturational enuresis show little evidence of emotional maladjustment. Organic causes of bedwetting account for less than 5% of all cases. Most of those are due to a urinary tract infection. An organic cause should be considered likely if the child had previously been dry at night for a prolonged period or if daytime wetting accompanies the nocturnal enuresis. Temporary stress and regressive behavior commonly cause bedwetting, especially in preschool children. However, in rare cases enuresis is a symptom of severe emotional disturbance. These children tend to be older than most enuretics, and wetting may occur just prior to morning awakening; symptoms of neurosis are often obvious.

DATA COLLECTION

HISTORY

When asking about the wetting pattern, determine if the enuresis is primary or secondary, whether it is associated with diurnal enuresis, whether the wetting is constant or sporadic, and at what time of the night wetting usually occurs. Daytime frequency can be due to the small bladder capacity found in maturational enuresis; however, the presence of dysuria or an abnormal urinary stream suggests urinary tract infection.

The physician must know which treatments have already been attempted, how successful these were, and whether a punitive approach had been tried. This information will be particularly important in planning the future management.

The family history should focus on enuresis in other family members. Questioning about sickle-cell disease, food allergy, and diabetes is only occasionally helpful. Although a review of systems is part of any thorough evaluation, significant information is rarely obtained in cases of nocturnal enuresis. Since enuresis is probably not related to coercive toilet training, lengthy discussions of this topic may serve only to generate parental guilt.

The child's behavior patterns should be discussed in detail. Specific attention should be paid to how he feels about the enuresis and whether this problem is affecting self-image and limiting the child's social activities. Asking about family dynamics and stresses is necessary to uncover hidden psychological factors. Even with maturational or organic enuresis, an understanding of how the family is responding to the problem is important. Parents should be asked why they are seeking help at this particular time and what bothers them the most about their child's problem.

PHYSICAL EXAMINATION

Since organic problems rarely are the cause of enuresis, the physical examination is not usually diagnostic. However, the external genitalia should be examined carefully, especially for abnormalities of the urethral meatus. To detect urinary tract problems, the physician should observe the urinary stream and examine the child for costovertebral-angle tenderness and bladder distention. If a child has the urge to void, an estimation of bladder capacity can be made by measuring the urine volume. A neurologic examination (to look for bladder innervation disorders) should include an evaluation of lower extremity muscle strength, deep tendon reflexes, and sensory functioning. In addition, rectal sphincter tone and the anal wink reflex should be assessed since both the bladder and the rectal area are innervated by sacral nerves II to IV.

LABORATORY EVALUATION

In most cases of nocturnal enuresis, a urinalysis with a screening test for infection (such as the nitrite-reaction or Uricult) is the only test needed. Even this test rarely adds much information to a carefully obtained history and physical examination. Routine sickle-cell testing in black children with enuresis is often recommended. Urine culture, pyelography, cystourethrography, and renal ultrasonography should be reserved for children whose symptoms suggest organic disorders.

TREATMENT

At present there is no treatment modality that is 100% successful for eliminating enuresis. As summarized below, the methods most commonly used include counseling, medication, and behavior modification with buzzer alarms.

SUMMARY OF TREATMENT

- Counseling
  - Child and parent education
  - Active role for child
  - Motivation: physician interest, star charts, rewards
- Bladder exercises
  - Stretching bladder
  - Urine stream interruption
- Elimination diet
  - Avoid milk, eggs, citrus fruits, and corn
- Hypnosis
- Medication (for special circumstances)
  - Imipramine (Tofranil)
- Buzzer-alarm conditioning

Before any successful treatment can begin, the family must understand that enuresis is a problem that is out of the child's conscious control. It is important that the child's enuresis is not perceived as bad behavior. Parents should realize that not only is enuresis a very common problem, but that it usually resolves spontaneously. Because scolding, restricting fluids, and waking the child generally do not help (and may actually delay the eventual cure), these methods should be discouraged.

The child must take an active role in the treatment process, taking responsibility for the symptoms himself. Therefore, the physician should communicate directly with the child during office visits and phone contacts. The enuretic child must understand that he will be responsible for all aspects of his problem, including changing and washing the pajamas and sheets.

With motivational counseling, positive reinforcement should be given when the child stays dry. Keeping a calendar with stars and using small rewards can be quite helpful. Interest from a strongly optimistic physician can be a strong reinforcement factor to keep the child's motivation high. While the cure rate with motivational counseling itself is not well known, many authorities feel that this safe approach is quite useful as an adjunct to other forms of treatment.

Many children with nocturnal enuresis have been found to have a small functional bladder capacity (less than 4 oz in children who are 6 years old). Starfield has described a method to stretch the bladder, in which the child is told to postpone voiding as long as possible and the urge to urinate is gone. When sensing an uncomfortable feeling, the child is instructed to void into a measuring cup. The goal is to increase the bladder capacity steadily so that the child can get through the night without wetting. A second exercise, known as stream interruption, is designed to increase the child's ability to withstand bladder spasms. Here, the child starts to void and then stops the urine flow for a 10-second count before emptying his bladder. In Starfield's studies, about 35% of the children were successfully treated when bladder stretching exercises were used for 6 months. The successful treatment occurred in children with the greatest increases in bladder capacity.

Some children stopped wetting the bed when certain foods were eliminated from their diet. One study showed that milk, eggs, citrus fruits, and corn were most frequently found to be associated with enuresis. A 2-week trial of dietary therapy places little burden on the child or the family and may occasionally be worthwhile.

Imipramine is the medication most commonly used in the treatment of enuresis. It may work by anticholinergic action on the bladder or by altering the sleep cycle so as to improve arousal. Cure may occur rapidly, but there are frequent relapses. This medication may be a common cause of serious accidental ingestion or may even produce pulse rate and blood pressure changes when appropriate amounts are given. The dose ranges between 25 mg and 75 mg, depending on the child's age. Some children do better when the medication is given at supper rather than at bedtime. Imipramine should not be given to children younger than 5 or 6 years of age.

In recent years, enuresis alarms have been shown to be the most effective treatment for bedwetting. The old bell-and-pad systems (that woke the family, were difficult to use, and occasionally caused skin ulcers) have been replaced by inexpensive (about $35) alarms that work on hearing-aid batteries. Small sensitive electrodes attach to the child's underwear and generally do not cause skin irritation. The two most popular models are the Wet Stop and Nytone buzzers. The physician will find it helpful to have a demonstration model, with detailed instruction sheets, in the office.

The buzzer-alarm conditioning method works slowly, but about 75% of enuretics are dry within 4 months after the initiation of therapy. By the end of the first month, the "puddles" in the bed are smaller each night. Some dry nights occur in the second month, and cure is seen by the third or fourth month. The alarm is used until there are no nights with wetting for 3 weeks. Some children get up to go to the bathroom at night; others learn to inhibit their micturition reflex until bladder contractions subside. About 10% to 15% of children have relapses, but reconditioning is usually easy. Symptom substitution (the appearance of new emotional symptoms that replace the enuresis) has not been a problem with buzzer conditioning techniques. The motivation and cooperation needed to utilize the buzzer-alarm system

NOCTURNAL ENURESIS
Differential diagnosis

Maturational	Organic	Emotional
Small bladder capacity	Urinary tract infection	Temporary stress
Immature sleep pattern	Urinary tract structural abnormality	Regressive behavior
	Bladder innervation disorder	Severe emotional problem
	Diabetes mellitus or diabetes insipidus	
	Sickle cell anemia or trait	

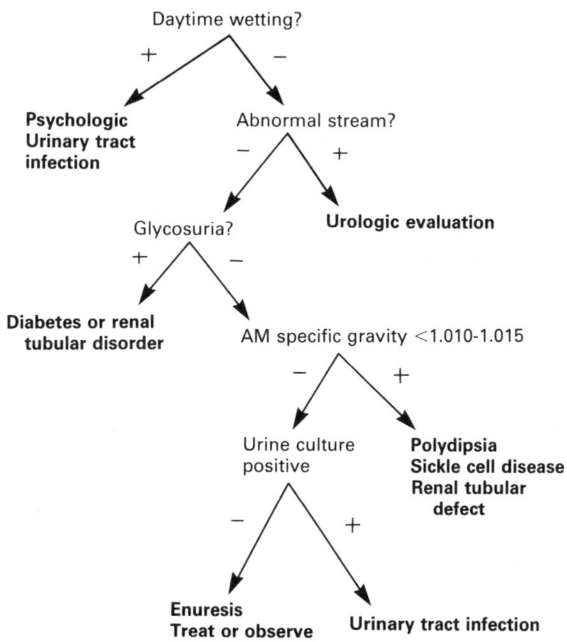

FIG 27–1
Decision tree for differential diagnosis of nocturnal enuresis.

usually requires that the child be at least 8 years old. If the child is older than this, failure is most often associated with either family difficulties or behavior problems.

INDICATIONS FOR CONSULTATION OR REFERRAL

Most cases of nocturnal enuresis can be managed by the primary care physician. At the time of the initial evaluation, a combination of motivational counseling, bladder stretching exercise, and elimination diet can be tried. If significant improvement has not occurred within 2 weeks, and the child is at least 8 years old, a buzzer-alarm system is the next step. Use of medications depends on the physician, who must be aware of the potential side effects and relapse rates.

Referral to a urologist is indicated if the child has repeated urinary tract infections, urethral reflux, constant daytime dribbling, or an abnormal urinary stream. Children with severe family or behavioral problems require psychiatric consultation.

DISCUSSION OF ALGORITHM

An algorithm for the differential diagnosis of nocturnal enuresis is presented in Figure 27–1. In the vast majority of children only a careful history, physical examination, and urinalysis are required. Some experts recommend a urine culture for all enuretic children, but the yield is extremely low. It is probably more cost efficient to reserve urine culture and sensitivity for patients in whom the problem likely is organic, such as secondary or diurnal enuresis. Ultrasound and radiologic studies are very rarely necessary. All black children should be tested for sickle cell anemia and trait.

BIBLIOGRAPHY

Cohen MD: Enuresis. *Pediatr Clin North Am* 1975; 22:545–560.

Dische S, Yule W, Corbett J, et al: Childhood nocturnal enuresis: Factors associated with outcome of treatment with enuresis alarm. *Dev Med Child Neurol* 1983; 25:67–80.

Olness K: The use of self-hypnosis in the treatment of childhood nocturnal enuresis. *Clin Pediatr* 1975; 14:273–279.

Ritvo ER, Ornitz EM, Gottlieb F, et al: Arousal and nonarousal types of enuretic events. *Amer J Psychiat* 1969; 126:1.

Schmitt BD: Nocturnal enuresis: An update on treatment. *Pediatr Clin North Am* 1982; 29:21–36.

Shelov SP, Gundy J, Weiss JC, et al: Enuresis: A contrast of attitudes of parents and physicians. *Pediatrics* 1981; 67:707–710.

Starfield B, Mellits ED: Increase in functional bladder capacity and improvements in enuresis. *J Pediatr* 1968; 72:483–487.

SUGGESTED READING FOR PARENTS

Scharf M: *Waking Up Dry: How to End Bedwetting Forever*. Cincinnati, Writer's Digest Books, 1986.

Schmitt BD: Nocturnal enuresis: An update on treatment - Parent instruction sheets. *Pediatr Clin N Am* 1982; 29:21–36.

28 FACIAL WEAKNESS

Roger Packer, M.D.

Acute facial paralysis is usually marked by either weakness in eyelids and/or facial expression, including furrowing of the brow and upward or downward movement of the corner of the lips. There may also be decreased lacrimal and salivary gland secretions as well as diminished taste sensation on the anterior two-thirds of the tongue. Weakness in only the lower portion of the face (central) results from contralateral upper motor neuron damage, whereas weakness in the upper and lower portion of the face (peripheral) results from lower motor neuron damage of the seventh cranial nerve.

DIFFERENTIAL DIAGNOSIS

COMMON CAUSES OF FACIAL WEAKNESS

Congenital
Möbius syndrome
Hypoplasia angulus oris
Trauma
Infection
Meningitis
Encephalitis
Lyme disease
Mastoiditis
Otitis (acute and chronic)
Herpes reactivation (Ramsey Hunt syndrome)
Sarcoid
Neoplastic
Intrinsic brain tumor
Posterior fossa tumor
Leptomeningeal dissemination
Bone (mastoid) tumor
Cholesteatoma
Rhabdomyosarcoma
Autoimmune
Gullain-Barré syndrome
Myasthenia gravis
Miscellaneous
Bell palsy (possibly viral)
Myotonic dystrophy
Muscular dystrophy
Congenital myopathy
Melkersson-Rosenthal syndrome

DISCUSSION

Facial weakness recognized immediately after birth is most likely traumatic in origin. This is usually secondary to intrauterine sacral pressure on the peripheral portion of the seventh nerve, although it may occur in traumatic deliveries with or without the application of forceps. These traumatic etiologies are clinically distinguishable from the Möbius syndrome, which is usually bilateral and involves other cranial nerves (especially the sixth cranial nerve nuclei, bilaterally). An often misdiagnosed condition is congenital hypoplasia of the depressor angulus oris muscle, resulting in an inability to depress the lower lip. Children with this condition are often referred for evaluation of facial weakness of the other side of the face, as parents note that the child's mouth pulls to the opposite side when crying (which is in reality an inability to depress the lip on the aplastic side). The importance of the recognition of this condition is not only its distinction from a more extensive cranial nerve involvement but the association of hypoplasia of the angulus oris with other congenital anomalies, especially cardiac anomalies.

The next major distinction in the diagnostic process is whether the acquired facial weakness is secondary to interruption of cortical input to the facial nerve nucleus or from direct nuclear nerve damage. Although interruption of cortical control of the facial nerve is relatively uncommon, its recognition is mandatory. Etiologies of so-called central facial weakness are similar to those of acute hemiplegia of childhood, including cerebrovascular accidents, primary central nervous system and metastatic tumors, traumatic injury, and a postseizure state.

Peripheral or lower motor neuron weakness is the common cause of facial weakness and the most common etiology is Bell palsy, which is a unilateral process.

Idiopathic or Bell palsy was initially believed to be secondary to primary or secondary ischemia of the facial nerve as it exits through the facial canal. There is now increasing evidence that Bell palsy is not a result of ischemia but rather is an acute cranial polyneuritis secondary to reactivation of herpes simplex virus.

Other causes of seventh nerve dysfunction are more frequent in children than they are in adults. Conditions that may mimic Bell palsy include lesions within the brain stem such as infiltrating tumors and demyelinating disease. Meningitis of bacterial, fungal, or neoplastic origin may selectively cause facial nerve dysfunction.

Isolated facial nerve palsy has recently been associated with central nervous system Lyme disease.

A rare variant (the Fisher variant) of acute postinfectious polyradiculitis (Guillain-Barré syndrome) may initially present with facial weakness. Rarely a child may have idiopathic cranial nerve neuropathies. Infections or neoplastic lesions (cholesteatomas, rhabdomyosarcomas) may compress the facial nerve outside of the brain stem. Acute and chronic otitis media may result in facial nerve dysfunction, although this complication is much less frequent in the antibiotic era. Herpetic involvement of the geniculate ganglion (Ramsay Hunt syndrome) may selectively cause facial weakness. Traumatic injury, especially to the base of the brain or the side of the face, may result in disruption of the facial nerve. Muscular causes of facial weakness are bilateral and slower in evolution. Rarely, a child may suffer from the Melkersson-Rosenthal syndrome, which is a triad of recurrent facial paralysis, facial edema, and furrowing of the tongue of unknown etiology.

DATA GATHERING

HISTORY

The basis of appropriate management of acute acquired facial palsy is careful clinical evaluation. Patients with idiopathic (Bell) palsy usually suffer a paralysis of one side of the face that has evolved over a few hours. The child's face may have suddenly pulled to one side or the child could not close one of his eyes while sleeping. Another presentation is difficulty in eating or drinking, as substances in the mouth fall out of the involved side. If the child is old enough, however, there is frequently the complaint of a dull ache or sharp pain behind the ear for 1 to 2 days prior to the onset of the weakness. Information concerning recent headaches, fever, or rashes should be obtained at the initial evaluation. In addition, the child should be questioned about recent tick bites or tick exposure, which might suggest Lyme disease.

PHYSICAL EXAMINATION

A careful neurologic examination for the extent of weakness and associated neurologic deficits is mandatory in all cases of acquired facial palsy. The presence of greater involvement of the lower face suggests a supranuclear lesion and is usually associated with evidence of hemiparesis on the involved side. More extensive brain stem dysfunction is suggested by the presence of associated cranial nerve deficits, such as the inability to completely abduct the eye on the side of weakness (abduction of the eye controlled by the sixth cranial nerve), sensory loss in the face or the absence of the corneal reflex (sensation conveyed by the sensory component of the fifth cranial nerve), jaw muscle weakness (innervated by the motor portion of the fifth cranial nerve), abnormal palatal movements (innervated by the ninth and tenth cranial nerves), or abnormal tongue movement (innervated by the twelfth cranial nerve). It should be remembered that in idiopathic Bell palsy there are frequently mild sensory alterations to touch and pin sensation that often may confuse the diagnosis. The presence of bilateral facial weakness, ataxia, or systemic illness suggests meningeal involvement or the Gullain-Barré syndrome.

Obviously, it is also necessary to complete a careful otolaryngolic examination for signs of inner ear or mastoid bone involvement. The presence of a vesicular eruption in the outer ear suggests herpetic involvement of the geniculate ganglion.

If after careful clinical evaluation there is no other evidence for other sites of neurologic or otolaryngolic involvement, a diagnosis of Bell palsy is likely. The yield from additional tests such as complete blood cell count or glucose is quite low in children and probably need not be obtained in an otherwise well child. In a child with a history of recent tick exposure, especially in areas where Lyme disease is endemic, blood should be drawn at the time of presentation for determination of Lyme titers. If these titers are consistent with recent infection, a spinal tap should be performed. At present there is no evidence to support the routine need for cerebrospinal fluid evaluation in children with facial palsy who are otherwise well. Similarly, computed tomography or magnetic resonance imaging is not indicated in children with isolated, unilateral facial weakness. Skull x-ray films with special views of the internal auditory meatus and formal audiologic evaluation are often recommended for all patients with acquired facial palsy, but in the otherwise asymptomatic patient for whom follow-up can be assured, this can probably be delayed. Electrodiagnostic tests such as measurements of nerve conduction velocity and muscular denervation are unreliable in the first 72 hours of illness. These evaluations can be carried out later in the course of illness, if necessary, to confirm the diagnosis and supply prognostic information.

INDICATIONS FOR CONSULTATION OR REFERRAL

The management of acute facial nerve paresis of any specific cause is appropriate neurologic, neurosurgical, or otolaryngologic referral. Neurologic consultation should be immediately obtained if there is evidence of disruption of cortical control of seventh nerve function or associated cranial nerve deficits. Otolaryngologic consultation should be immediately obtained in children with signs of inner ear or mastoid bone involvement. If there is any evidence of meningitis of whatever cause, the patient should be immediately hospitalized and appropriately treated. Facial weakness secondary to trauma usually requires careful radiologic evaluation and appropriate neurosurgical or otolaryngologic consultation. We recommend that any patient without any recovery between 5 and 7 days of the active onset of paresis be referred for neurologic evaluation and electrodiagnostic studies. It is also reasonable to obtain otolaryngologic consultation in such patients for consideration of decompression of the facial nerve within the facial canal.

Most children with idiopathic (Bell) palsy can be treated by their primary physician, and we presently recommend a 10-day course of oral prednisone (60 $mg/m^2/day$) in divided doses for 7 days, tapered over the next 3 days. The effects of such therapy are hard to document, because the natural history of idiopathic Bell palsy is improvement in most cases. This is especially true in children with only partial paralysis at diagnosis. However, since there does seem to be some benefit for early steroid therapy in patients with severe involvement and the potential side effects of a short course of treatment are minimal, we recommend treatment for all children with acute Bell palsy. If a child is seen after the first few days of illness (arbitrarily 4 days), there is little evidence that steroids are beneficial. In such patients, we do not recommend the use of prednisone. The role of surgical decompression for acute Bell palsy is controversial and, by and large, we do not refer patients for surgical decompression.

During the period of facial weakness, if the patient cannot close his eyes, artificial tears (three times daily and at night) should be applied to the eye. Eye patches can be used to protect the cornea but are usually unnecessary except during sleep.

The prognosis for the vast majority of patients is excellent as most patients recover fully. In children, the muscle weakness is usually partial at onset and these patients uniformly do well. In those patients with complete paralysis at onset, some recovery can also be expected, but it is within this group of patients that partial or delayed recovery occurs.

All patients with idiopathic (Bell) palsy should be seen within 5 days following the ini-

FACIAL WEAKNESS
Differential diagnosis

Bell palsy
Birth trauma
Brain tumor
Cerebrovascular accident
Cholesteatoma
Hypoplasia angulus oris
Lyme disease
Meningitis
Otitis media
Mastoiditis
Möbius syndrome
Rhabdomyosarcoma
Trauma

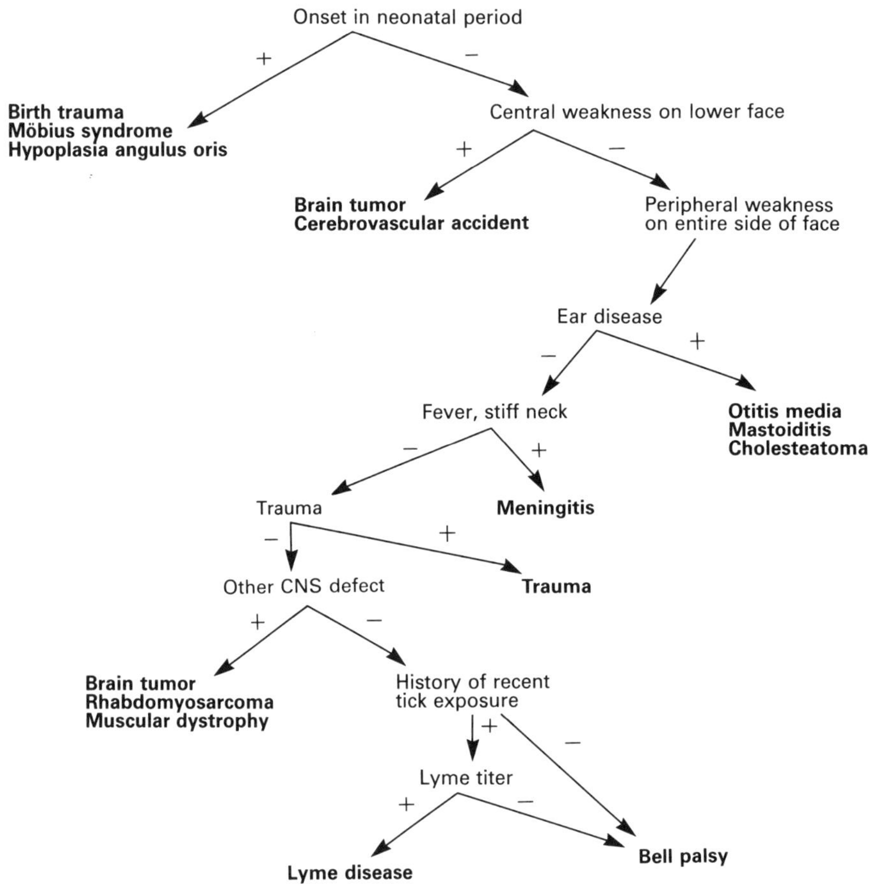

FIG 28–1
Decision tree for differential diagnosis of facial weakness.

tial diagnosis. If at this point there is evidence for some facial movement, chances for full recovery are excellent within the next 2 to 3 weeks. In those patients with no evidence of facial movement at this point, the chances of residual weakness is greater, and nerve conduction velocity measurements are prognostically helpful.

DISCUSSION OF ALGORITHM

An algorithm for the differential diagnosis of facial weakness is presented in Figure 28–1. If the condition is not congenital, a differentiation should be made between central or peripheral weakness. Those with a central cause most likely have a brain tumor or a cerebral vascular accident. Next, systemic problems such as brain tumor, meningitis, rhabdomyosarcoma, encephalitis, or ear abnormalities should be considered. Those who have none of these problems most likely have Bell palsy.

BIBLIOGRAPHY

Adour KK: Diagnosis and management of facial paralysis. *N Engl J Med* 1982; 307:348–351.

Adour KK, Wingerd J, Bell DN, et al: Prednisone treatment for idiopathic facial paralysis (Bell's palsy). *N Engl J Med* 1972; 287:1268.

Kansu T, Us O, Sarpel A, et al: Recurrent multiple cranial nerve palsies. *J Clin Neuro Opthalmol* 1983; 3:263–268.

Manning JJ, Adour KK: Facial paralysis in children. *Pediatrics* 1972; 49:102.

Nelson KB, Eng GD: Congenital hypoplasia of the depressor anguli oris muscle: Differentiation from congential facial palsy. *J Pediatr* 1972; 81:16.

Paine RS: Facial paralysis in children. *Pediatrics* 1957; 19:303.

Pachner AR, Steere AC: Neurological manifestations of Lyme disease: Meningitis, cranial neuritis and radiculoneuritis. *Neurology* 1985; 35:47–53.

29 FAINTING

Edward B. Charney, M.D.

A child with a history of an episode of brief, sudden loss of consciousness and muscle tone should be examined. During this fainting or syncopal event, the child is often limp, unresponsive, and diaphoretic, with decreased blood pressure, diminished deep tendon reflexes, slow pulse, and dilated pupils. The period of unconsciousness usually lasts for only a few seconds, and there is generally mental alertness immediately on awakening. Tonic-clonic movements of the extremities should only be present if there has been a prolonged period of unconsciousness.

DIFFERENTIAL DIAGNOSIS

COMMON CAUSES OF FAINTING

Congenital

Structural heart lesions

Arrhythmias

Metabolic

Anemia

Hypoglycemia

Allergic

Tussive (coughing) episodes with asthma

Infection

Tussive episodes, particularly with pertussis

Multiple etiologic
Vasovagal
Orthostatic
Hyperventilation
Breath holding
Hysterical

DISCUSSION

Congenital heart disease, particularly severe aortic or pulmonic stenosis and tetralogy of Fallot, may result in fainting episodes, particularly during or just after the child has been involved in strenuous physical activity. Cardiac arrhythmias such as congenital complete atrioventricular block with episodes of loss of consciousness (e.g., Adams-Stokes disease) or a prolonged QT interval are unusual causes of fainting in childhood. The presence of prolonged QT interval is associated with either autosomal recessive deafness or an autosomal dominant trait in families with normal hearing.

Metabolic causes of fainting include anemia and hypoglycemia. Allergic causes of fainting are those conditions (e.g., asthma) associated with severe coughing spells. This form of fainting, referred to as tussive syncope, probably results from the hypoxia and reduced cardiac return from the Valsalva maneuver or respiratory spasm experienced after completion or strenuous coughing. Tussive syncope may also be seen in any respiratory tract infection process (e.g., pertussis) that produces this excessive or strenuous coughing.

The majority of cases of fainting in children are caused by those conditions listed as multiple etiologic. Vasovagal syncope, the most common form of fainting, results from a sudden loss of resistance in the peripheral circulation. These attacks are usually precipitated by emotional upsets. Orthostatic hypotensive fainting, infrequently encountered in children or adolescents, is associated with an excessive and prolonged fall in blood pressure on assuming the erect position from a recumbent position. Hyperventilation fainting, particularly seen in adolescents, and breath-holding spells, particularly seen in the infant or toddler, are usually associated with stress or sudden emotional upset or fear. Hysterical fainting spells tend to be more common in adolescents.

DATA GATHERING

HISTORY

Determination of whether a period of loss of consciousness was a fainting episode or a seizure can often be accomplished by a detailed history. Questions in the history should first focus on whether there were associated tonic-clonic movements, incontinence, confusion on awakening, and most important, what was the duration of unconsciousness. These distinguishing characteristics of a seizure and fainting are outlined in Table 29–1.

Additional history, with particular attention to the events preceding the fainting attack, may often be diagnostic. Vasovagal syncope or fainting is often precipitated by emotional upsets such as feelings of fear, pain, anger, apprehension, and fatigue. Often the emotional trauma of procedures such as venipuncture or dental treatment may precede these attacks. Another common historical note is that the fainting spell occurred during a formal religious service marked by prolonged erect posture of the child, in a warm and poorly ventilated environment. Orthostatic fainting is characteristically associated with a history of loss of consciousness occurring soon after suddenly assuming an upright position. Fainting attacks from anemia are usually preceded by light-headedness or giddiness, whereas those attacks associated with hypoglycemia are frequently preceded by pallor

TABLE 29–1
Distinguishing Characteristics for Fainting and Seizure

Characteristic	Fainting	Seizure
Duration of unconsciousness	Usually seconds	Often 5 min or longer
Tonic-clonic movements	May be present only if unconsciousness is long	Frequently present
Incontinence	Absent	May be present
Confusion on awakening	Generally absent	Marked

FAINTING
Differential diagnosis

Anemia
Anxiety
Arrhythmia
Breath holding
Cardiac lesion
Hyperventilation
Hypoglycemia
Hysteria
Orthostatic fainting
Seizure
Tussive syncope
Vasovagal syncope

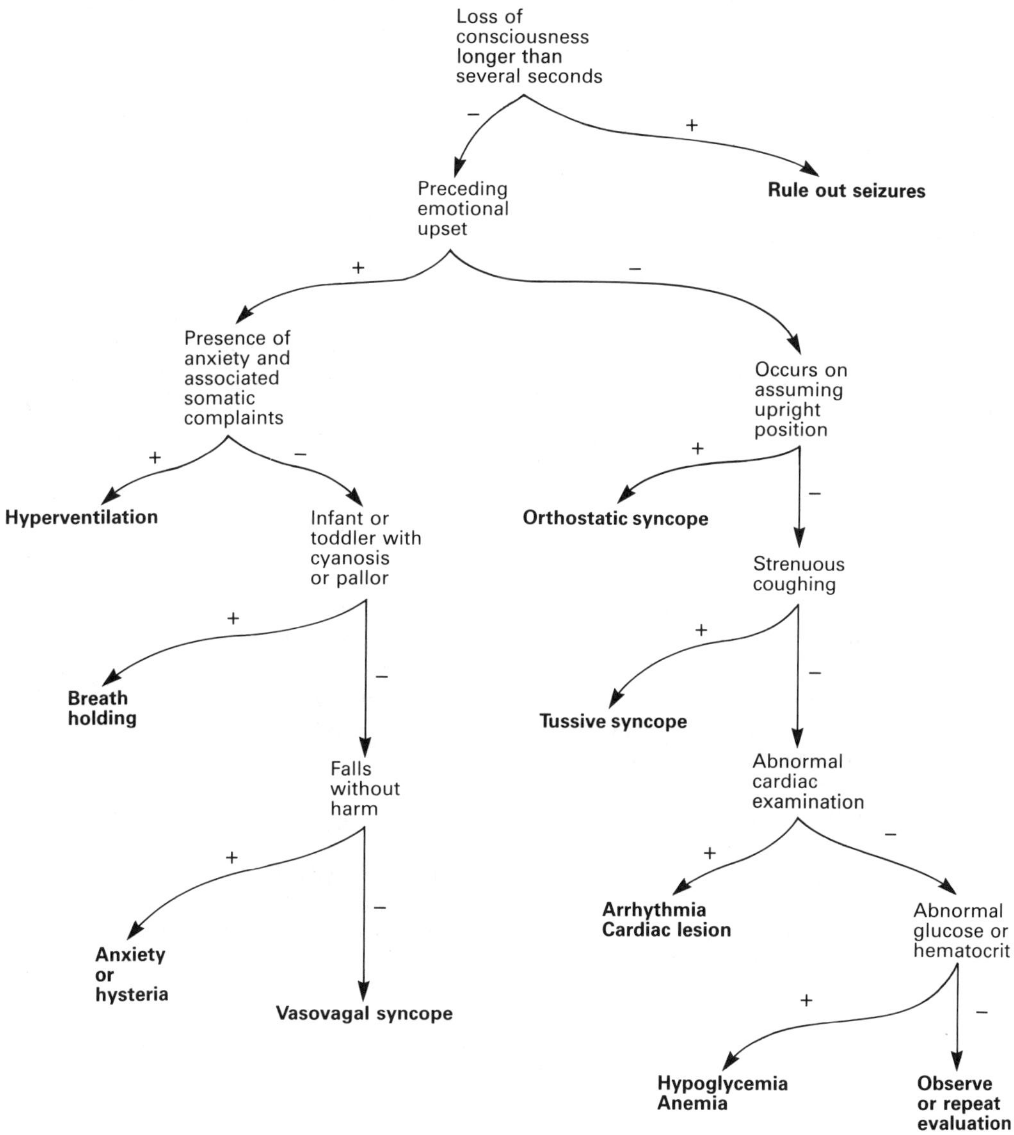

FIG 29–1
Decision tree for differential diagnosis of fainting.

and sweating. Tussive fainting is caused by strenuous coughing.

Hyperventilation with fainting is often precipitated by anxiety and may be associated with complaints of chest pain, palpitations, numbness, and particularly breathlessness prior to loss of consciousness. Fainting may also be induced consciously when hyperventilation is coupled with a Valsalva maneuver by children "at play." Breath-holding spells are frequently precipitated in an infant or toddler by emotional upset and are either of the cyanotic or pallid nature. Cyanotic spells are usually precipitated by the cry of anger after being restrained or punished or after a playmate has grabbed a toy. Pallid spells are often preceded by a sudden pain or fright such as from hitting the head after a minor fall. Hysterical fainting is often the diagnosis for children who fall repeatedly before an audience and do not hurt themselves, and the attack may be preceded or accompanied by dramatic moaning. Further history may reveal significant psychosocial stress in the child's home, family, and school.

PHYSICAL EXAMINATION

The physical examination is generally normal in children who have experienced a fainting episode. Particular attention should be directed to cardiac auscultation to determine the presence of the systolic murmurs of aortic or pulmonic stenosis or arrhythmias. Clinical cyanosis may be suggestive of heart disease, and paleness may represent anemia.

LABORATORY EVALUATION

An electrocardiogram rhythm strip and values for serum glucose and hematocrit should be obtained in all children with their initial complaint of fainting. If seizures are a consideration, then an electroencephalogram may be requested.

INDICATIONS FOR CONSULTATION OR REFERRAL

Children with recognized or suspected cardiac lesions should be referred to a cardiologist for further evaluation and initial management. Hyperventilation or hysterical fainting may require referral for professional counseling.

DISCUSSION OF ALGORITHM

An algorithm for differential diagnosis of fainting is presented in Figure 29–1. The two major tasks of evaluation of fainting are ruling out major organic causes, heart disease, and seizures and working through the history to rule out hypoglycemia and tussive syncope. After this process, the less well-defined entities such as vasovagal, orthostatic, and stress should be explored. Many times the cause of fainting cannot be determined. These patients should be followed up for recurrence. If the problem persists, either the evaluation should be repeated or the patient should be referred.

BIBLIOGRAPHY

Lockman LA: Nonepileptic paroxysmal disorders, in Swaiman KF: *Pediatric Neurology: Principles and Practices*, ed 2. St. Louis, CV Mosby, 1989, p 443.

30 GROWTH PROBLEMS

M. William Schwartz, M.D.

Problems with growth, either poor weight gain or short stature, present an opportunity for an interesting diagnostic evaluation. Many solutions become apparent after the initial assessment; others require special laboratory tests. In some situations, observation and the proper setting will help make the diagnosis. The designation failure to thrive serves as a convenient diagnosis in those children who do not gain weight or grow linearly. It is not a final diagnosis but a label for a problem that needs further definition.[1]

DIFFERENTIAL DIAGNOSIS

The majority of patients with growth problems will be found to have inadequate nutrition, social interaction problems, gastrointestinal disease, or neurologic disorders. A number of studies have outlined what diagnoses are made after evaluation.[2–6] Table 30–1 shows the cause of failure to thrive in a series of patients from one center. The following list includes the major problems that affect growth. Many unusual problems are not included because of rarity or because the children usually have symptoms other than growth problems.

TABLE 30–1
Etiology of Failure to Thrive in a Series of Patients*

Constitutional short stature, 56%
Isolated human growth hormone deficiency, 7%
Intrauterine growth retardation, 6%
Maternal deprivation syndrome, 3%
Chromosomal anomalies, 3%
Hypothyroidism, 3%
CNS disease, 6%
Skeletal disease, 4%
Congenital heart disease, 2%
Respiratory disease, 2%
GI disease, 2%
Renal disease, 1%
Immune deficiency, 1%
Other metabolic disease, 3%

*From Horner JM, Thorsson A, Hintz R: Growth deceleration patterns in children with constitutional short stature: An aid to diagnosis. *Pediatrics* 1978; 62:59. Used by permission.

COMMON CAUSES OF GROWTH PROBLEMS

Infection
AIDS
Urinary tract infection
Tuberculosis

Congenital/anatomic
Congenital heart disease
Gastroesophageal reflux
Pyloric stenosis
- Posterior urethral valves
- Sequestrated lobe of lung
- Diaphragmatic hernia
- Aspiration pneumonia

Metabolic/nutritional
Malabsorbtion
Malnutrition
Diabetes mellitus
Diabetes insipidus
Growth hormone deficiency
Hypothyroidism
Renal tubular acidosis
Short bowel syndrome

Genetic
Cystic fibrosis
Chromosomal anomaly (e.g., Turner syndrome)
Genetic short stature
Sickle cell anemia

Immunologic
Inflamatory bowel disease
Immune deficiency

Miscellaneous
Constitutional growth delay
Cerebral palsy
Cocaine abuse by mother
Fetal alcohol syndrome
Genetic short stature
Liver disease
Placental insufficiency
Renal failure

DISCUSSION

Most of the problems listed above are discussed throughout this text (see index). A few of the more common problems are presented here.

Insufficient Nutrition.—Usually detected with a careful history, most cases of poor growth result from inadequate caloric intake. The families may give an initial history that lacks sufficient detail or contains unreliable information. Infants require at least 80–125 kcal/kg for growth in the first year, then 70 to 115 kcal/kg for the next 3 years. Sometimes asking the parent to complete a diary of food intake will document that the child's actual caloric intake is insufficient for good growth.

Family Dysfunction.—Often family dysfunction and social problems contribute to poor caloric intake. The families expend most of their energy coping with daily problems and conflicts, with the result that child does not get sufficient feeding. Observations made through a one-way mirror in a family therapy unit showed the variance between the history and what actually transpired at feeding time. This is not a conscious effort to decieve the physician but another symptom of the distracted, disorganized caretaker saying what they believe rather than what happened.

Constitutional Short Stature.—Constitutional short stature describes a growth pattern where there is normal size at birth followed by delayed growth velocity for 1 to 2 years. After the third year the child is small but has normal growth velocity; thus although the linear size is small, eventual height will be within the normal range. The clues to this diagnosis are the growth record, growth velocity calculations, and bone age radiographs. The bone age is less than the chronologic age and equal to the height age (Fig 30–1). Delayed bone age indicates more potential for growth.

Genetic Short Stature.—The child with the familial trait of short stature differs from one with constitutional short stature by having a family history of short adult stature and a bone age equal to chronologic age. These patients will be short adults, whereas those with constitutional short stature will be taller.

DATA GATHERING

HISTORY

Obtaining a record of previous growth patterns will help establish the onset of the problem and allow calculation of growth velocity or the amount of growth in a year (see Chapter 93). Some children whose parents are concerned about short stature are really at the 3rd or 10th percentile and have normal growth velocity. The family history may also reveal information about other members who had growth delay suggestive of genetic short stature or constitutional short stature.

Because family problems are often the basis for growth problems, obtaining a reliable history requires skill and time. Often the patient will give answers to questions to satisfy the interviewer rather than accurately describe what is going on at home. More time and concentration are required to allow the patient to feel comfortable and give details to a nonjudgmental listener so that the child can be helped. A day history (see Chapter 2) in which the parent gives a detailed account of a typical day provides information about the details of feeding plus an indication of the family interactions and support systems. After hearing that the underweight patient eats "a good balance of meat, vegetables, and fruit," press for details of favorite foods or foods that are disliked to document the caloric intake. If it seems as if the intake is good, inquire about stool problems, which are seen in malabsorption or cystic fibrosis. Other symptoms, such as cough (cystic fibrosis), developmental delay, change in stool pattern, or weak urinary stream (posterior urethral valves), will lead to possible diagnoses.

Decreased intake or increased losses are com-

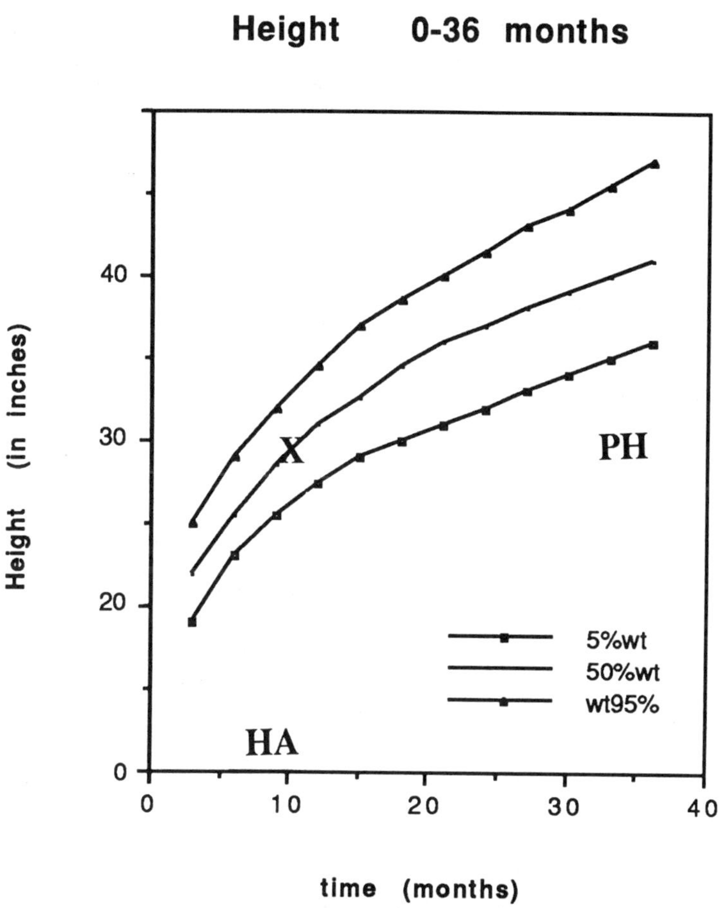

FIG 30–1
Calculation of height age. Intersect patient height *(PH)* with 50% line *(X)* on growth chart. Look down age marks to determine the age that corresponds with this height *(HA)*.

mon causes of poor growth. A complete dietary history can detect a problem with inadequate caloric intake or suggest a malabsorption problem when the patient has not grown despite a large intake. For those with a good nutritional and social history, look for the problem of increased losses, either gastrointestinal or urinary. An increased number of loose stools leads to consideration of cystic fibrosis, steatorrhea, short bowel syndrome, and food intolerance. Urinary losses, characterized by polyuria, lead to consideration of diabetes mellitus, diabetes insipidus, renal tubular disorders, or chronic glomerulonephritis. Vomiting suggests gastroesophageal reflux, pyloric stenosis, or metabolic diseases.

The birth history, including duration of gestation and birth weight, may yield clues to the diagnosis. A full-term infant with a low birth weight suggests placental insufficiency, or cocaine or alcohol abuse by the mother. Patients with placental insufficiency may have persistent small size; those small infants exposed to cocaine usually grow normally if the family provides adequate calories.[7]

PHYSICAL EXAMINATION

The physical examination should emphasize careful assessment of the chest, because conditions such as aspiration pneumonia or pulmonary anomalies such as diaphragmatic hernia may escape early detection. Heart murmurs are sometimes undetected prior to evaluation because of growth problems. A protuberant abdomen and wasted buttocks suggests malabsorption, such as with gluten sensitivity or cystic fibrosis. In a short teenaged girl with an increased carrying angle and webbed neck, Turner syndrome may explain the growth problem.

LABORATORY EVALUATION

In the majority of cases, the laboratory tests are limited. Since the two major causes of poor growth, poor intake and social problems, are detected with the history, laboratory tests should be reserved for confirming specific diseases suggested by the history or physical examination or for screening those patients in whom the initial assessment does not suggest a specific problem. Screening tests that are most helpful include bone age, urinalysis, thyroid function tests, and chemistry panel. The somatomedin level, a screening test for growth hormone function (Chapter 93), is helpful in specific patients who are older than 5 years without chronic illness, thyroid disease, or malnutrition.

INDICATIONS FOR CONSULTATION OR REFERRAL

Usually a careful history with special attention for nutrition and family interaction problems, documentation of growth velocity, and bone age will suffice to make a diagnosis. If after working through the flow sheet the diagnosis is unclear, or if results of a laboratory test conflict with the history, consultation may help to detect a rare cause of growth failure.

DISCUSSION OF ALGORITHM

The first phase follows the scheme of determining the major causes of growth problems in infants, which are poor nutrition and dysfunctional parenting (Fig 30–2). If these problems are detected, counseling and support followed by observation are sufficient treatment in the majority of the children.

For those with a good nutritional and social history, look for increased losses, either gastrointestinal or urinary. Increased or loose stools lead to consideration of cystic fibrosis and other diseases in which malabsorption is the major feature. Urinary losses, characterized by polyuria, lead to consideration of diabetes

GROWTH FAILURE
Differential Diagnosis

AIDS
Aspiration pneumonia
Celiac disease
Cocaine abuse
Congenital heart disease
Constitutional short stature
Cystic fibrosis
Cerebral palsy
Chromosomal anomaly
Diabetes mellitus
Diabetes insipidus
Gastroesophageal reflux
Genetic short stature
Growth hormone deficiency
Fetal alcohol syndrome
Hypothyroidism
Immune deficiency
Inflammatory bowel disease
Liver disease
Malabsorption
Malnutrition
Metabolic disease
Neurogenic bladder
Placental Insufficiency
Posterior urethral valve
Pyloric stenosis
Pulmonary problems
  Sequestration
  Diaphragmatic hernia
Renal failure
Renal tubular acidosis
Sickle cell anemia
Social problems
Tuberculosis
Turner syndrome
Urinary tract infection

A. Poor growth

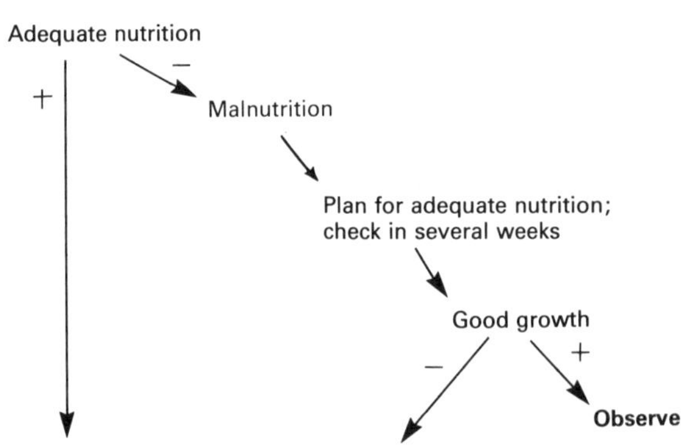

Continued.

FIG 30–2
Decision tree for differential diagnosis of growth failure.

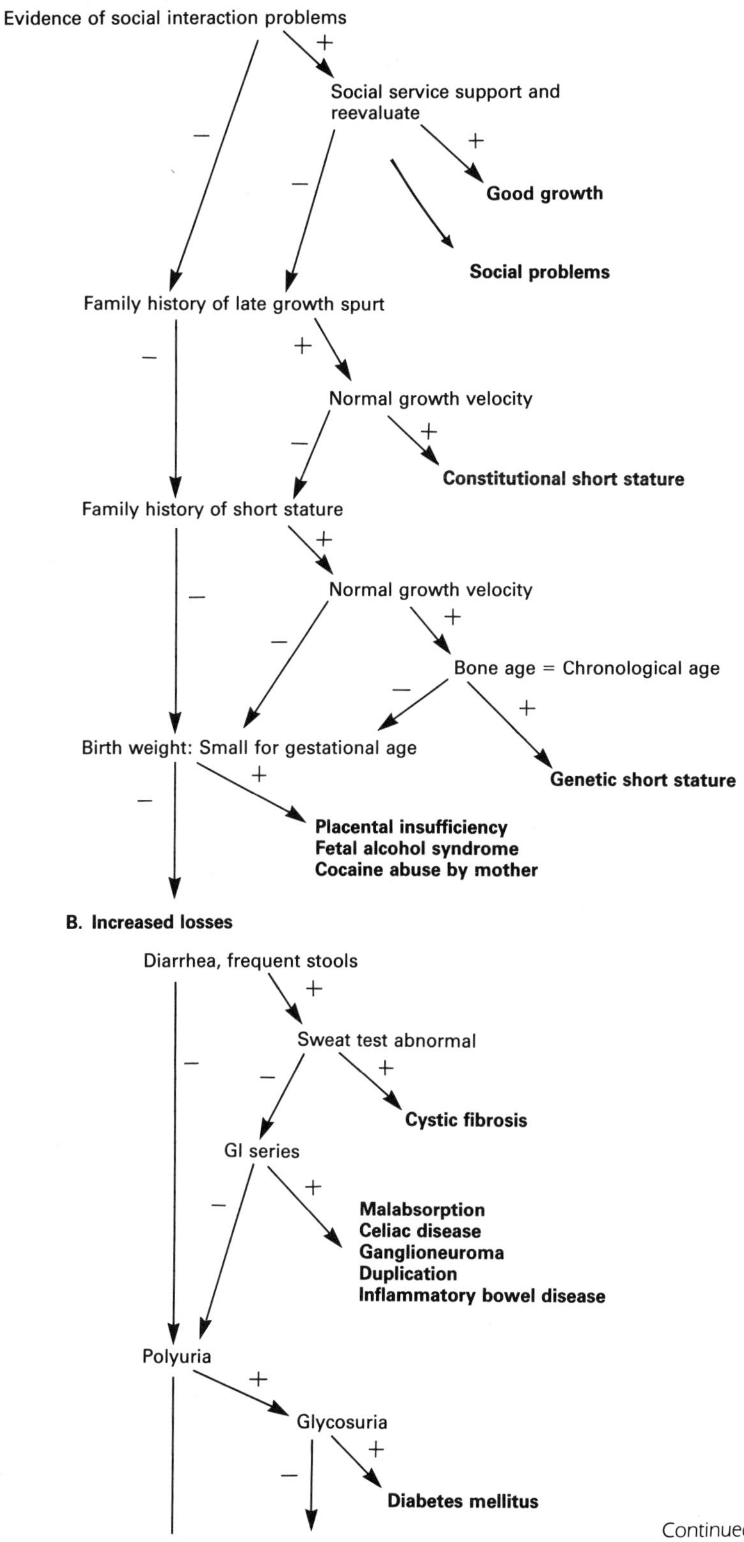
Evidence of social interaction problems
+
−
Social service support and reevaluate
+
−
Good growth
Social problems
Family history of late growth spurt
−
+
Normal growth velocity
−
+
Constitutional short stature
Family history of short stature
+
−
Normal growth velocity
−
+
Bone age = Chronological age
−
+
Birth weight: Small for gestational age
+
−
Genetic short stature
Placental insufficiency
Fetal alcohol syndrome
Cocaine abuse by mother
B. Increased losses
Diarrhea, frequent stools
+
Sweat test abnormal
−
−
+
Cystic fibrosis
GI series
+
−
Malabsorption
Celiac disease
Ganglioneuroma
Duplication
Inflammatory bowel disease
Polyuria
+
Glycosuria
+
−
Diabetes mellitus

Continued.

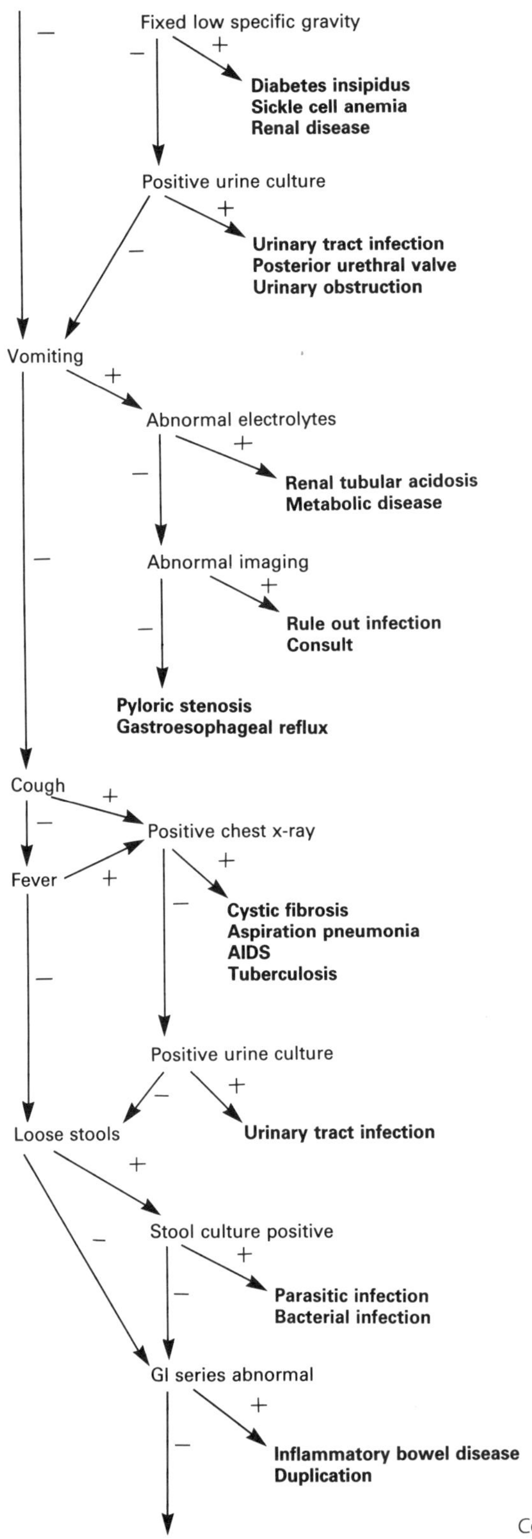
Fixed low specific gravity
+
–
–
Diabetes insipidus
Sickle cell anemia
Renal disease
Positive urine culture
+
–
Urinary tract infection
Posterior urethral valve
Urinary obstruction
Vomiting
+
Abnormal electrolytes
+
–
Renal tubular acidosis
Metabolic disease
–
Abnormal imaging
+
–
Rule out infection
Consult
Pyloric stenosis
Gastroesophageal reflux
Cough
+
–
Positive chest x-ray
Fever
+
+
–
Cystic fibrosis
Aspiration pneumonia
AIDS
Tuberculosis
–
Positive urine culture
–
+
Loose stools
Urinary tract infection
+
Stool culture positive
–
+
–
Parasitic infection
Bacterial infection
GI series abnormal
+
–
Inflammatory bowel disease
Duplication

Continued.

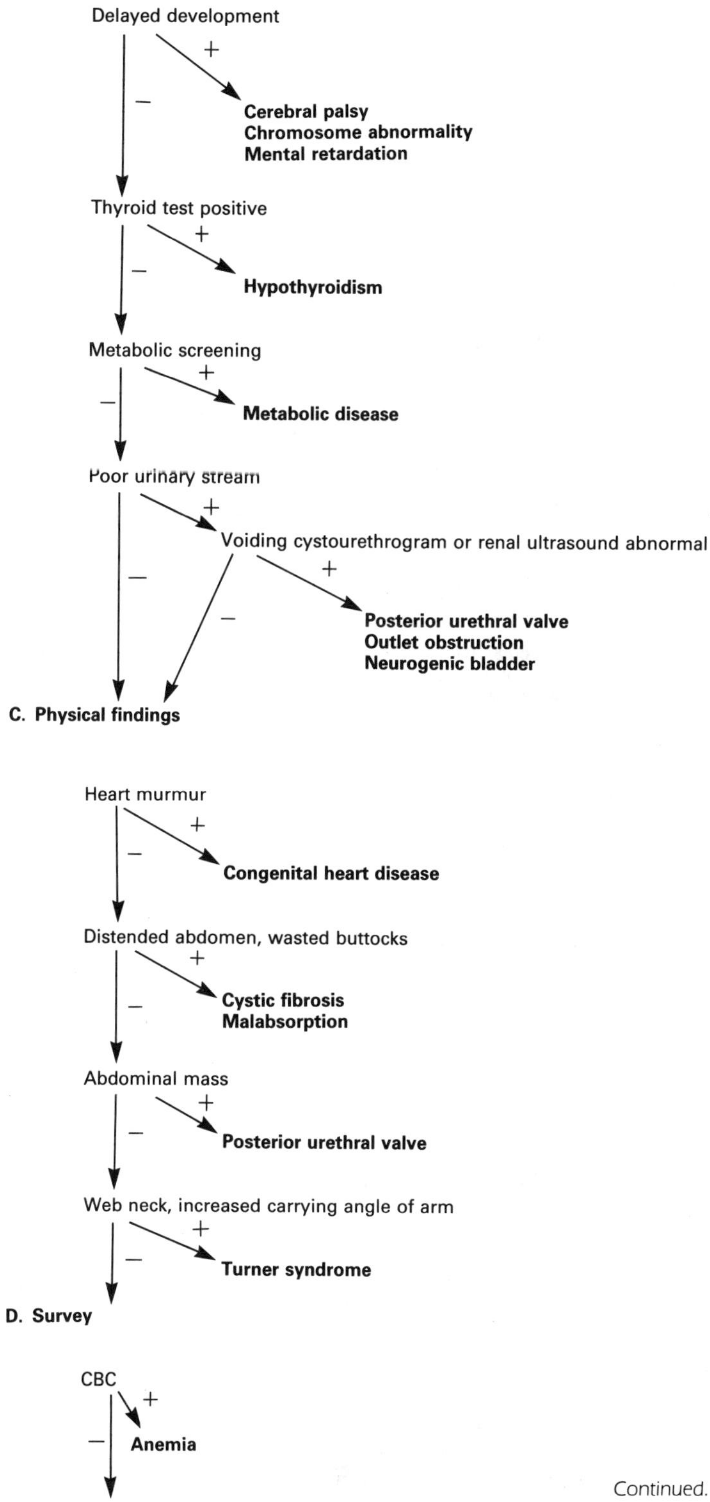
Delayed development
+
−
Cerebral palsy
Chromosome abnormality
Mental retardation
Thyroid test positive
+
−
Hypothyroidism
Metabolic screening
+
−
Metabolic disease
Poor urinary stream
+
−
Voiding cystourethrogram or renal ultrasound abnormal
+
−
Posterior urethral valve
Outlet obstruction
Neurogenic bladder
C. Physical findings
Heart murmur
+
−
Congenital heart disease
Distended abdomen, wasted buttocks
+
−
Cystic fibrosis
Malabsorption
Abdominal mass
+
−
Posterior urethral valve
Web neck, increased carrying angle of arm
+
−
Turner syndrome
D. Survey
CBC
+
−
Anemia

Continued.

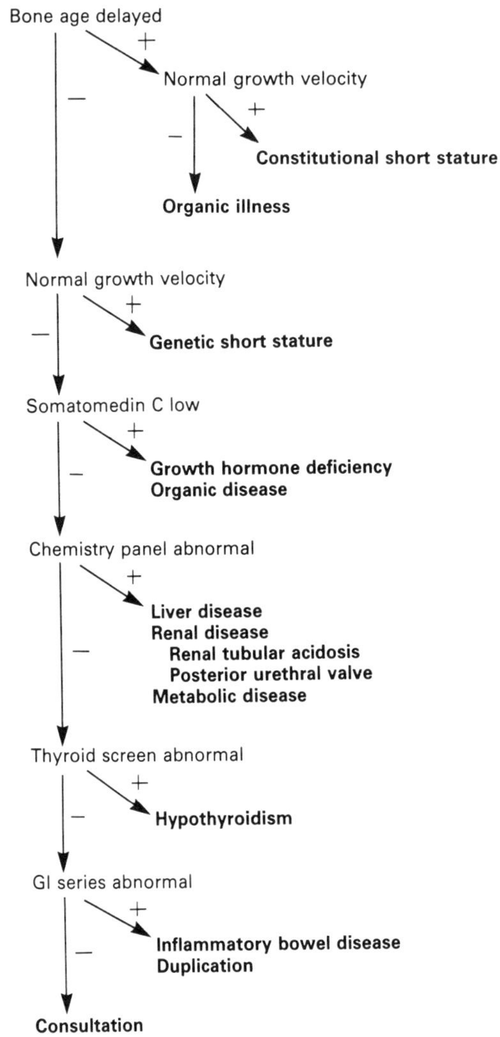

mellitus if there is glycosuria or renal disease or diabetes insipidus if there is low specific gravity or osmolarity. Vomiting suggests gastroesophageal reflux, pyloric stenosis, sepsis, or metabolic disease.

Next, ask a series of questions about symptoms that may lead you to consider specific diseases, for example, cough (cystic fibrosis or other pulmonary problems), diarrhea (malabsorption, fever, delayed development), and poor urinary stream (posterior urethral valves).

Physical findings may detect such problems as congenital heart disease (murmur), cerebral palsy (neurologic deficit), abdominal mass (posterior urethral valves), and increased carrying angle of the arm, and webbed neck (Turner syndrome).

Family history may detect the normal growth velocity seen in constitutional short stature or genetic short stature. Neonatal history may reveal that the infant was small for gestational age or had neonatal complications resulting in short bowel syndrome. The latter should be known from a general history.

If this general screen does not help suggest a diagnosis, a general survey may. Laboratory tests include bone age determination, chemistry panel, thyroid function tests, and somatomedin levels. Since this system helps detect the cause of the growth problem in the majority of cases, any that remain undiagnosed require either another pass through the system or referral to a consultant.

REFERENCES

1. Stickler GB: "Failure to thrive" or the failure to define. *Pediatrics* 1984; 74:559.
2. Horner JM, Thorsson A, Hintz R: Growth deceleration patterns in children with constitutional short stature: An aid to diagnosis. *Pediatrics* 1978; 62:59.
3. Goldbloom R: Growth failure in infancy. *Pediatr Rev* 1987; 9:57.
4. Sills RH: Failure to thrive: the role of clinical and laboratory evaluations. *Am J Dis Child* 1978; 132:75–967.
5. Barbero GJ, Shaheen E: Environmental failure to thrive: A clinical view. *J Pediatr* 1967; 71:639–44.
6. Berwick DM, Levy JC, Leinerman R: Failure to thrive: Diagnostic yield of hospitalization. *Arch Dis Child* 1982; 57:347–51.
7. Glaser MH, Heagarty MC, Bullard DM, et al: Physical and psychological development of children with early failure to thrive. *J Pediatr* 1968; 73:690–698.

31 HAIR LOSS

David Alexander, M.D.

Hair loss, a common diagnostic problem, has an extensive list of differential diagnoses, but only a small number of disorders account for the etiology in the vast majority of children. These common causes of alopecia can be easily identified and treated by the primary care provider.

DIFFERENTIAL DIAGNOSIS

COMMON CAUSES OF HAIR LOSS

Trauma
Trichotillomania
Traction alopecia
Hot-comb alopecia
Chemical trauma secondary to permanent-wave or hair-straightening solutions
Infection
Tinea capitis
Pyoderma
Varicella
Drugs and toxins
Heavy metals, including thallium, lead, and arsenic
Antimetabolites
Antithyroid drugs (methimazole)
Carbamazepine
Immunologic
Alopecia areata
Systemic lupus erythematosus
Endocrine metabolic
Hypothyroidism
Hypoparathyroidism
Hypopituitarism
Homocystinuria
Argininosuccinic aciduria
Congenital
Trichorrhexis nodosa
Menkes syndrome
Monilethrix
Trichorrhexis invaginata
Ectodermal dysplasia
Cartilage-hair hypoplasia
Incontinentia pigmenti
Multiple etiologic
Telogen effluvium
Myotonic dystrophy

DISCUSSION

Trauma.—Trauma is responsible for two of the most common causes of childhood alopecia. Trichotillomania, the compulsive pulling of one's hair results in irregular patches of incomplete hair loss. These areas are most frequently on the scalp, but the eyebrows and eyelashes may also be involved. The hairs within these patches are short and broken off at varying lengths. The scalp underlying these patches is usually normal.

Almost all cases of trichotillomania resolve spontaneously. Since this disorder frequently represents a habit analogous to nail biting, most parents should be reassured that this should disappear with time. In some children, however, and more frequently in adolescents, trichotillomania may be indicative of a more serious psychological problem that requires psychiatric evaluation.

Hair styles that cause excessive tension on the hair shafts for a prolonged period of time such as ponytails and cornrows may lead to traction alopecia. The reversibility of alopecia is related to the duration of the traction. Most cases in children are reversible, but prolonged traction may lead to fibrosis of the hair root and resulting irreversible alopecia. Treatment of these patients consists of advising them to avoid hair styles that cause traction.

Other hair care routines may lead to traumatic alopecia. The use of a hot comb may lead to alopecia at the periphery of the scalp. Hair-straightening or permanent-wave solutions may also lead to hair damage and resulting alopecia.

Infection.—Probably the most common cause of childhood alopecia is fungal infection of the scalp and hair. *Trichophyton tonsurans* has replaced *Microsporum* species as the most common causative organism. The clinical appearance of fungal infections varies widely with the organism involved and with the severity of infection. The mildest form consists of small patches of alopecia with broken hairs and mild scalp scaling. More extensive involvement may lead to severe inflammation and kerion formation involving larger portions of the scalp. In *T. tonsurans* infection, the patient's initial complaint may be only of dandruff without any associated alopecia.

Once the diagnosis of fungal infection is made, treatment should begin with griseofulvin at a dose of 10 mg/kg/day. A pediatric suspension containing griseofulvin 125 mg/5 mL is available. Bone marrow suppression has occasionally been seen in patients receiving griseofulvin. Hepatotoxicity has also been reported and the drug is contraindicated in patients with known liver disease. Selenium sulfide shampoo used twice weekly has also been shown to be sporicidal and useful as additional therapy in the treatment of fungal infections. Once a case of fungal infection is diagnosed, other family members should be examined for evidence of infection and treated as necessary.

Immunologic.—Alopecia areata is a condition characterized by the sudden appearance of round, nonscaling, noninflammatory patches of hair loss on the scalp or any other hair-bearing area of the body. The disorder, most frequently seen in children and young adults, has a variable course and prognosis. Although the etiology of this disorder is not understood, the increased incidence of Hashimoto thyroiditis and other rheumatic or autoimmune disease in patients with alopecia areata and their families point to an immunological basis. Extensive hair loss may precede total scalp balding (alopecia totalis) or loss of all body hair (alopecia universalis). In general, more extensive hair loss is associated with worse prognosis for eventual hair regrowth. Many different regimens have been used in an attempt to treat this condition, but none has been definitively shown to be of any real benefit. Injection of corticosteroids into the lesion is the most widely used therapy. Probably most important of all in the management of patients with this disorder is psychological and emotional support.

Toxins.—Many drugs have been reported to cause hair loss, as listed earlier in the chapter. Toxicity with thallium and lead may also lead to alopecia. Hair loss associated with drugs and toxins is usually reversible after the discontinuation of the causative agent.

Nutritional.—Severe malnutrition can lead to hair loss. Isolated deficiencies of vitamin A and zinc can also produce alopecia. It is also important to realize that excessive dosages of vitamin A may lead to hair loss.

Endocrine.—Alopecia may be seen in patients with several endocrine disorders including hypothyroidism, hypopituitarism, and hypoparathyroidism. These children will have other signs and symptoms suggesting these diagnoses.

Congenital.—A host of congenital disorders is associated with alopecia, as listed under differential diagnosis. In most of these disorders, alopecia will be only one component of a larger symptom complex.

Multiple Etiologic.—Several different stressful circumstances including febrile illnesses, surgery, anesthesia, and crash dieting have been associated with premature cessation of growth of otherwise normal hairs. Once the hairs stop growing, they enter a resting phase during which they may be shed. This disorder is known as telogen effluvium. Hair loss usually occurs within 2 to 4 months after the stressful event, followed by regrowth of normal hair.

DATA GATHERING

HISTORY

Although the differential diagnosis of alopecia is long, a screening history and physical examination can rule out most of the less common causes. A history that the child has had otherwise normal growth and development and has had no other serious medical problems can rule out most of the uncommon etiologies for alopecia. Once these are ruled out, history taking should be directed toward identifying either infectious or traumatic causes of alopecia. Important questions to ask while taking the history include: Have the parents seen the child pulling on or playing with his hair? Is there a family history of childhood baldness? Is there a family history of autoimmune disease? Has the child been taking any medications? Is there a history of high fever, surgery, or rapid weight loss during the past 6 months?

PHYSICAL EXAMINATION

A general physical examination should be performed for all children with alopecia. Once the results of the general examination are found to be normal, attention should obviously be paid to the hair and scalp. Diffuse alopecia might suggest telogen effluvium. Patchy alopecia, especially if seen with scalp scaling is suggestive of fungal infection. Trichotillomania should be considered if there are irregular patches of hair loss with the hairs within these patches broken off at varying lengths. Wood's lamp examination findings, if positive, may be useful in the diagnosis of fungal infection. It is important to realize, however, that fluorescence is not a characteristic of *T. tonsurans*.

LABORATORY EVALUATION

Because of the frequency and variability in the clinical presentation of fungal infection, culture should be performed for all children presenting with alopecia. A new dermatophyte test medium (DTM) has made routine office cultures for superficial fungal infection easy and inexpensive. Samples of scalp scrapings or hairs should be pressed gently directly onto the surface of the medium, and cultures kept at room temperature. If positive, growth should be visible on the medium in 3 to 4 days. If the growing fungus is a pathogenic dermatophyte, a color change from yellow to red should be seen in the medium around the fungus. If no growth is noted within 14 days, the culture is interpreted as negative.

INDICATIONS FOR CONSULTATION OR REFERRAL

The etiology of the alopecia will give an indication about which patients can be managed by the primary physician. Alopecia caused by traction, toxins, and infection can be corrected with relatively simple treatment. Usually the alopecia areata, a chronic problem, is best shared with an interested dermatologist.

DISCUSSION OF ALGORITHM

The first step includes a complete history and physical examination to rule out those metabolic, immunologic, and neurologic problems (Fig 31–1). Then causes such as traction, drugs, chemicals, and fungal infection should be ruled

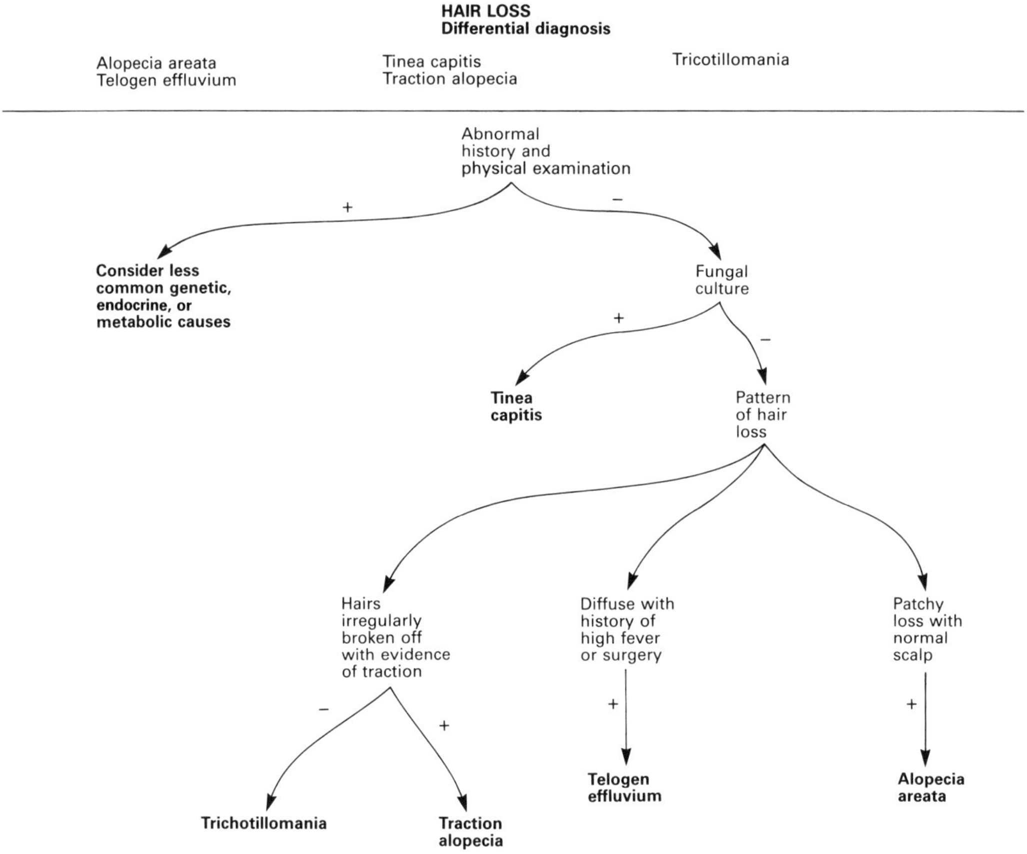

FIG 31–1

Decision tree for differential diagnosis of hair loss.

out. If there is a history of high fever, surgery, or stress, a diagnosis of telogen effluvium can be considered. At this point, alopecia areata is likely and the patient can be referred.

BIBLIOGRAPHY

Krowchuk DP, Lucky AW, Primmer SI, et al: Recurrent status of the identification and management of tinea capitis. *Pediatrics* 1983; 72:625–631.

Price V: Disorders of the hair in children. *Pediatr Clin North Am* 1978; 25:305–320.

Stroud JD: Hair loss in children. *Pediatr Clin North Am* 1983; 30:641–657.

Weston WL: *Practical Pediatric Dermatology*. Boston, Little, Brown & Co, 1979.

32 HEADACHE

Edward B. Charney, M.D.

The primary care physician is frequently called on to assess the condition of a child complaining of a headache. Although in the vast majority of these children headaches are benign, parents are often fearful of a more serious medical problem. Assessment of the child within the office setting can often help establish the cause of the headache and provide guidance for therapeutic management.

DIFFERENTIAL DIAGNOSIS

COMMON CAUSES OF HEADACHE

Infection
Meningitis
Encephalomyelitis
Brain abscess
Sinusitis
Dental abscess
Viral syndrome

Tumor
Brain neoplasm

Congenital
Brain vascular anomaly
Hydrocephalus

Trauma
Result of trauma of the head

Multiple etiologic
Migraine
Hypertension
Pseudotumor cerebri
Tension
Psychogenic
Ocular
Seizure

DISCUSSION

Fever associated with any infection process (e.g., viral syndrome, pharyngitis) is the most common cause of headache in children. Headache associated with fever frequently occurs over the frontal and bitemporal regions from increased intracranial vasodilation. Infections of the central nervous system including purulent bacterial meningitis and viral encephalomyelitis can produce headache by inflammation of pain-sensitive structures at the base of the brain and over the convexity. There are often, however, associated changes in mental status (e.g., seizures, confusion) and nuchal rigidity or neck stiffness. Headaches from a brain abscess may result from the increased intracranial pressure and traction on neighboring pain-sensitive vessels and dura. There are frequently focal defects (e.g., cranial nerve palsies, gross motor weakness) present on neurologic examination in these children. Dental abnormalities such as caries or gingivitis may result in a dental abscess that can have referred pain to distant points with either frontal, temporal, retroauricular, or global headaches. Inflammation and swelling of the sinusoidal ostia, the most pain-sensitive areas of nasal and paranasal structures, are commonly the cause of sinus headaches. Usually there is also localized pain and/or tenderness over the sinuses. Although ethmoid and maxillary sinuses are present at birth, frontal sinuses usually are not sufficiently developed until the child is 6 to 10 years of age and, therefore, frontal headaches should not be attributed to sinus infection in the preschool child.

Tumors of the brain, although a relatively uncommon cause of headaches in children, are often the major fear of parents bringing their child in for office assessment of a headache complaint. Brain tumor headaches resulting from the increased intracranial pressure and traction on neighboring pain-sensitive vessels and dura are often accompanied by neurologic abnormalities (e.g., ataxia, head tilt) and/or ocular abnormalities (e.g., papilledema, diplopia, squint, decreased visual acuity) within 2 months after the onset of headache complaints. These headaches may also be associated with vomiting, exacerbation with positional changes, and awakening the child from sleep.

Trauma-related headaches are generally uncommon, are associated with loss of consciousness, and probably result from irritation of extracranial and intracranial pain-sensitive structures by small hemorrhages, edema, or vascular changes. They usually occur soon after return of consciousness and their prolonged persistence (several weeks to months) may be associated with a history of numerous psychogenic somatic complaints.

Major causes of headaches in children that are caused by either multiple or unknown causes include: migraine, hypertension, muscle contractions of head and neck, pseudotumor cerebri, and psychogenic. Migraine is a common cause of recurrent headaches in childhood. Family history is usually positive for similar migraine headaches. There are three well-recognized stages in these headaches including vasoconstriction of cerebral arteries, vasodilation, and edema that are correlated with specific clinical manifestations. During the vasoconstrictive phase there may be transient visual disturbances (e.g., photophobia, scintillating scotoma), other sensory disturbances (e.g., paresthesias, nausea) and motor deficits (e.g., speech difficulties, hemiparesis) that occur. The vasodilation phase is marked by pain that is usually unilateral at the onset, often becomes generalized after 1 to 2 hours, and may last up to 1 or 2 days. During this painful period, the child often tries to avoid noises and bright lights and may find relief through prolonged sleep. There may be episodes of complicated migraine during the vasoconstrictive phase as ischemia results in transient hemiplegia or ophthalmoplegia. The edema, or final stage, often may be marked by a steady and dull headache accompanied by nausea.

Systemic hypertension, an unusual cause of headaches in children, is often associated with diastolic pressures of greater than 100 to 110 mm Hg and frequently is a clinical sign of acute glomerulonephritis or other renal disease (e.g., systemic lupus erythematosus, membranoproliferative nephritis). Pseudotumor cerebri (a syndrome of headache with elevated intracranial pressure and papilledema without clinical, laboratory, or radiologic evidence for focal lesions or hydrocephalus) has no known specific cause. Although more commonly encountered in young adult girls, it may be seen in children. Often the headache is aggravated by factors that affect the cerebrospinal fluid pressure, such as straining, coughing, and positional changes.

Tension headaches result primarily from sustained contraction of the skeletal musculature of the head and neck. Emotional stress or fatigue can frequently precipitate the pain that is usually in the back of the head and neck or, on occasion, is generalized. These headaches tend to be much more common in the adolescent than in the younger child. Psychogenic headaches, not uncommon in children, although frequently precipitated by stress in the environment, are not thought of as having musculature contraction as causing the headache. Rather, psychogenic headaches may represent depressed or hypochondriacal state or function for secondary gain, as in school avoidance.

Ocular abnormalities such as refractive errors, astigmatism, strabismus, and impaired convergence may cause headaches. Although controversy still exists as to this cause-and-effect relationship, ocular headaches should be relieved with proper corrective lenses. Headaches associated with a seizure disorder may occur either as aura of a major motor seizure during the postictal stage or as the only manifestation of the seizure. (If no observable seizure activity is noted, then a significantly epileptiform electroencephalogram (EEG) is necessary to establish this diagnosis.)

DATA GATHERING

HISTORY

The history should include characteristics of the headache (e.g., frequency, time of day, prodrome, associated nausea, vomiting, or motor disturbances), family history of headaches, environmental stress, head trauma history, and school attendance record. Although findings of the neurologic and ophthalmologic examination may often remain normal up to 2 months after the onset of brain tumor headaches, there frequently is a history of vomiting, exacerbation by positional changes, awakening from sleep, or increased severity and frequency of the headache during this time period. Children with this history should be followed up regularly (once or twice a month) for evaluation of any changes in the physical examination. A positive family history of headaches, associated prodrome with motor or sensory disturbances, and relief through prolonged sleep or darkened room is suggestive of migraine headaches. If none of the aforementioned historical details are present, additional information must be acquired regarding stresses at home or school that may result in tension or psychogenic headaches. School avoidance headaches are commonly characterized by prolonged school absenteeism and occurrence on weekday mornings with relief during other periods of the day and weekends.

PHYSICAL EXAMINATION

The absence or presence of fever in a child complaining of a headache is often the critical information that helps direct the physician's initial office assessment. In the febrile child, particular attention must be directed to identifying any abnormalities on the neurologic examination that suggest an infectious process of the central nervous system. Nuchal rigidity, changes in sensorium, and Kernig's or Brudzinski's signs are characteristic of purulent bacterial meningitis or viral encephalomyelitis, whereas cranial nerve palsies or focal weakness may be signs of a brain abscess. For the febrile child with headaches and normal results on a neurologic examination, attention should be directed at examination of the sinuses and dentition. Sinus headaches are suggested with findings of localized tenderness and pain to gentle finger tapping over the sinuses in a child with nasal mucosa congestion. Abnormalities of the dentition with localized tenderness and pain over the teeth or gums may suggest a dental abscess. If the neurologic, sinuses, and dental portion of the examination are unremarkable, physical evidence for other infectious processes (e.g., pharyngitis) should be looked for. In the majority of cases, results of the entire physical examination will be normal and the headache is part of a viral syndrome.

Although a detailed history is often the most important part of assessing the afebrile child complaining of headache, particular attention must also be directed toward obtaining an accurate blood pressure, neurologic and ophthalmologic examinations, and linear growth measurements. Children with acute glomerulonephritis may present with headache complaints secondary to their hypertension; however, there are usually other objective complaints (e.g., hematuria, edema) that bring the child to the attention of the physician. Abnormalities of the neurologic or ophthalmologic examination may be better understood by obtaining a history of whether or not they are persistent or transient in nature. Persistent abnormalities such as ataxia, hemiparesis, or squint are highly suggestive of an underlying brain tumor, whereas transient motor disturbances may be compatible with migraine headaches. A sudden onset of severe headache with a stiff neck and a decrease in the level of consciousness may be characteristic of an intracranial hemorrhage secondary to a congenital vascular anomaly.

Headaches in a child with evidence of deceleration in linear growth over a period of several months, a history of polydipsia, polyuria, and normal findings of a neurologic examination are suggestive of the slow-growing brain tumor, craniopharyngioma.

LABORATORY EVALUATION

Laboratory investigations in the primary care physician's office setting may be limited to lumbar puncture and analysis of cerebrospinal fluid for suspected meningitis or encephalomyelitis, requests for roentgenograms of the sinuses or dentition for suspected sinusitis or dental abscess, requests for an EEG for suspected seizures, and urinalysis with a measurement of specific gravity for suspected nephritis or craniopharyngioma-associated diabetes insipidus. Additional laboratory diagnostic workups may be ordered by consultants.

INDICATIONS FOR CONSULTATION OR REFERRAL

Any child with persistent neurologic abnormalities should be referred to a neurologist or neurosurgeon for further diagnostic workup with computed tomography or magnetic resonance imaging. The child with suspected abnormalities on ophthalmologic examination should be referred to an ophthalmologist for formal consultative examination. Children with suspected migraines may benefit from a referral to a neurologist for both definitive diagnosis and management. For the child with psychogenic head-

HEADACHE
Differential diagnosis

Brain abscess
Brain tumor
Dental disease
Encephalitis
Hypertension
Intracranial hemorrhage
Meningitis/encephalitis
Migraine
Post-trauma headache
Pseudotumor cerebri
Sinusitis
"Strep" throat
Tension
Viral syndrome

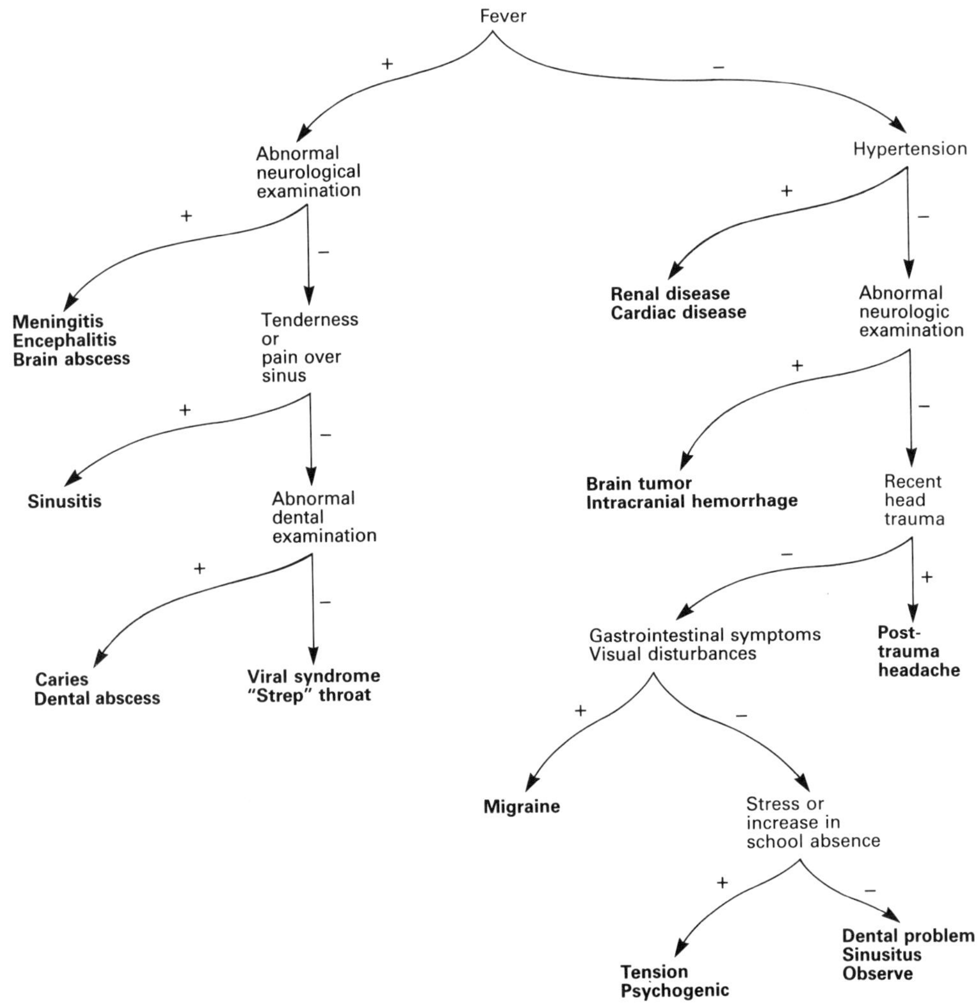

FIG 32–1
Decision tree for differential diagnosis of headache.

aches, referral of both the child and family for professional counseling may be necessary and beneficial.

DISCUSSION OF ALGORITHM

An algorithm for differential diagnosis of headaches is presented in Figure 32-1. The first step in the evaluation is to diagnose or rule out meningitis, hypertension, or brain tumor. Next, dental and vision problems are considered. A careful history will help diagnose migraine headaches. If these pathways are not productive, then tension or stress are the likely cause of headaches.

BIBLIOGRAPHY

Honig P, Charney E: Children with brain tumor headaches. *Am J Dis Child* 1982; 136:121.

Rothner AD: Headache, in Swaiman KW: *Pediatric Neurology: Principles and Practice*. St Louis, CV Mosby, 1989, p 185.

33 HEMATURIA

Michael Norman, M.D.

Hematuria in children presents in two ways: the accidental discovery of asymptomatic microhematuria on routine urinalysis or a complaint of abnormal color of the urine (red, brown, or Coke-colored). In considering the differential diagnosis and the indication for a workup, an operational definition of significant hematuria is required: 10 or more red blood cells (RBCs) in a freshly voided urine specimen is convenient, though arbitrary. Confirmation may then be obtained by documenting hematuria in several first morning urine specimens examined over several days. Hematuria should be differentiated from hemoglobinuria or myoglobinuria, which presents with a dipstick-positive finding for blood but few if any RBCs in the corresponding urine sediment. Conditions that rule out lysis of RBCs include a freshly voided urine specimen that is suitably acid (pH <7.0) and concentrated (specific gravity >1.015). Early morning urine specimens yield the best results.

Prevalence figures suggest that 4% to 6% of children will have at least one episode of hematuria sometime during childhood. Persistent or recurrent asymptomatic microhematuria is found in 0.1% to 0.5% of school-aged children.

DIFFERENTIAL DIAGNOSIS

COMMON CAUSES OF HEMATURIA

Trauma

Infection

Pyelonephritis
Cystitis
Sepsis

Toxin

Penicillin and derivatives
Cyclophosphamide
Phenacetin

Inflammatory

Glomerulonephritis
Collagen disease
Subacute bacterial endocarditis
Anaphylactoid purpura (vasculitis)
Hemolytic uremic syndrome
IgA nephropathy

Metabolic-endocrine

Cystinuria

Kidney stone
Idiopathic hypercalciuria
Bleeding disorders
Hemophilia
von Willebrand disease
Tumor
Wilms tumor
Leukemia
Congenital
Obstruction
  Ureteropelvic
  Stricture
Medullary sponge kidney
Multiple etiologic
Renal vein thrombosis
Benign recurrent hematuria: familial or nonfamilial

DISCUSSION

Although the differential diagnosis of hematuria is extensive, relatively few causes are seen in clinical practice. These are listed below in decreasing order of frequency:

1. Urinary tract infection
   a. Bacterial
   b. Viral (e.g., cystitis)
2. Trauma
   a. Kidney
   b. Bladder
   c. Local (e.g., urethral, meatal)
3. Benign recurrent hematuria
4. Glomerulonephritis
   a. Poststreptococcal infection
   b. Berger disease
   c. Henoch-Schönlein purpura

Perhaps 5% of children will have nephrolithiasis or hypercalciuria, sickle cell trait or anemia, tumor, a bleeding diathesis, or postexercise hematuria. It is useful when commencing an evaluation of hematuria to determine whether the bleeding is coming from the upper or lower urinary tract. This is likely to reduce the number of diagnostic investigations required.

DIFFERENTIATING BETWEEN LOWER AND UPPER TRACT HEMATURIA

Upper urinary tract
No terminal hematuria
No clots
Red, brown, Coke-colored
Proteinuria (>2+)*
RBC casts
Lower urinary tract
Terminal hematuria
Clots
Red
Proteinuria (<2+)*
No RBC casts

Benign Recurrent Hematuria.—Benign recurrent hematuria is an idiopathic disorder, more common in boys than in girls, and the most frequent cause of referral to a nephrologist. It typically occurs in an asymptomatic child with normal findings on physical examination. The hematuria is usually microscopic and may be persistent or intermittent. Episodes of gross bleeding may occur but are not a prominent part of the history. Family history may be positive for similar findings. The hematuria may subside over time. Prognosis for preservation of renal function is excellent.

Immunoglobulin A Nephropathy (Berger disease).—IgA nephropathy may produce either persistent or intermittent hematuria. The characteristic feature, proved with renal biopsy results, shows deposition of IgA in the mesangium of all glomeruli. These glomeruli may be otherwise normal or show focal nephritis. In many cases, gross hematuria and RBC casts occur. Those patients with IgA nephropathy plus proteinuria have a less favorable prognosis than those without proteinuria. About 10% to 20% of patients with IgA deposition may develop renal failure. These patients have marked glomerular disease compared with the majority of patients who maintain good renal function.

Hypercalciuria.—Many patients who have hematuria may have hypercalciuria, defined as the excretion of more than 4 mg of calcium per kilogram of body weight per day. This problem commonly seen in adults with kidney stones is being recognized more frequently in children, reaching 40% to 60% in some series. The characteristics include greater than 4 mg/kg of calcium in a 24-hour urine collection or a spot

*With dipsticks, the maximum readable protein concentration in grossly bloody urine that is due to RBCs and plasma proteins is 2+.

urine calcium/creatinine ratio greater than 0.2; family history of kidney or gallbladder stones; absence of other signs of renal disease, such as proteinuria or azotemia; and calcium oxalate crystals. The condition is rare in blacks. Many patients will develop renal stones in adulthood. The hypercalciuria may develop from either increased absorption of calcium in the intestine or increased excretion in the renal tubules. Good hydration to maintain high urine volume plus dietary restriction of sodium seem to decrease the hematuria. Reduction of calcium intake and use of hydrochlorothiazide are helpful in some patients.

Poststreptococcal glomerulonephritis or the nephritis of Henoch-Schönlein purpura is more likely to present with a history of upper respiratory tract infection, strep throat or pyodermia, hypertension, edema, and oliguria. Children with severe abdominal pain, vomiting, pallor, and diaphoresis should be suspected of having renal colic. Black children should undergo sickle cell screening tests. Children with hematuria due to hydronephrosis or a kidney tumor may have a palpable flank mass. Hematuria due to a clotting defect is virtually always associated with a positive finding of a medical or family history of bleeding or hemorrhage elsewhere in the body.

DATA GATHERING

HISTORY

Children with urinary tract infections usually have other signs and symptoms, such as fever; abdominal, flank, or suprapubic pain; and urinary urgency, frequency, or dysuria. It should be noted, however, that the passage of gross blood is irritating to the bladder and urethra and may mimic the symptoms of urinary tract infection. Some patients may have local irritation of the urethra from trauma, masturbation, or chemicals such as a bubble bath. A family history of stones may be the initial clue to the detection of hypercalciuria.

PHYSICAL EXAMINATION

The external genitalia should be examined for signs of trauma. A careful abdominal examination can help detect flank masses consistent with Wilms tumor, renal vein thrombosis, or obstruction. Blood pressure measurements are also important.

LABORATORY EVALUATION

Since certain dyes, hemoglobin, myoglobin, and beets can cause the urine to appear bloody, the urine should be examined microscopically to find RBCs. Tests to determine the presence of myoglobin and hemoglobin will also give false positive results for blood with the dipstick method. Relatively few laboratory or radiologic investigations are required to diagnose the cause of hematuria in children. In 70% to 80% of children with gross hematuria a specific cause is usually found. The urine sediment is the key to initiating a workup. Heavy pyuria and positive gram staining suggest bacterial infection; urine culture is then mandatory, whether the results of gram staining are positive or negative. Patients with glomerular bleeding are likely to have proteinuria (>2+), and those with RBC casts have some form of glomerulonephritis until proved otherwise. Sometimes several urine sediments must be carefully scanned to find casts. After urinalysis, two approaches can be taken.

(1) For suspected trauma, obstruction with or without kidney stones, or tumor, a renal ultrasound (US) is useful and noninvasive. Intravenous pyelography (IVP) will demonstrate structural details by documenting the site of obstruction, confirming extravasation of blood or urine outside the kidney, and demonstrating compromised or absent renal perfusion. If trauma to the lower urinary tract is suspected, voiding cystourethrography should be performed.

(2) If glomerulonephritis is suspected, a test to measure the serum creatinine level to estimate glomerular filtration rate (GFR) and determination of antistreptolysin O and C3 to document poststreptococcal glomerulonephritis should be performed. Occasionally the history of vague musculoskeletal complaints is elicited, suggesting the need to screen for lupus nephritis with an antinuclear antibody titer. A family history of nephritis should prompt a search for visual abnormalities and sensorineural hearing loss.

HEMATURIA
Differential diagnosis

Benign hematuria	Hemoglobinuria	Stones
Bleeding disorder	Hypercalciuria	Trauma
Drugs	Infection	Tumor
Glomerulonephritis	Myoglobinuria	Ureteropelvic junction (UPJ) obstruction
Hematoma	Sickle cell anemia	

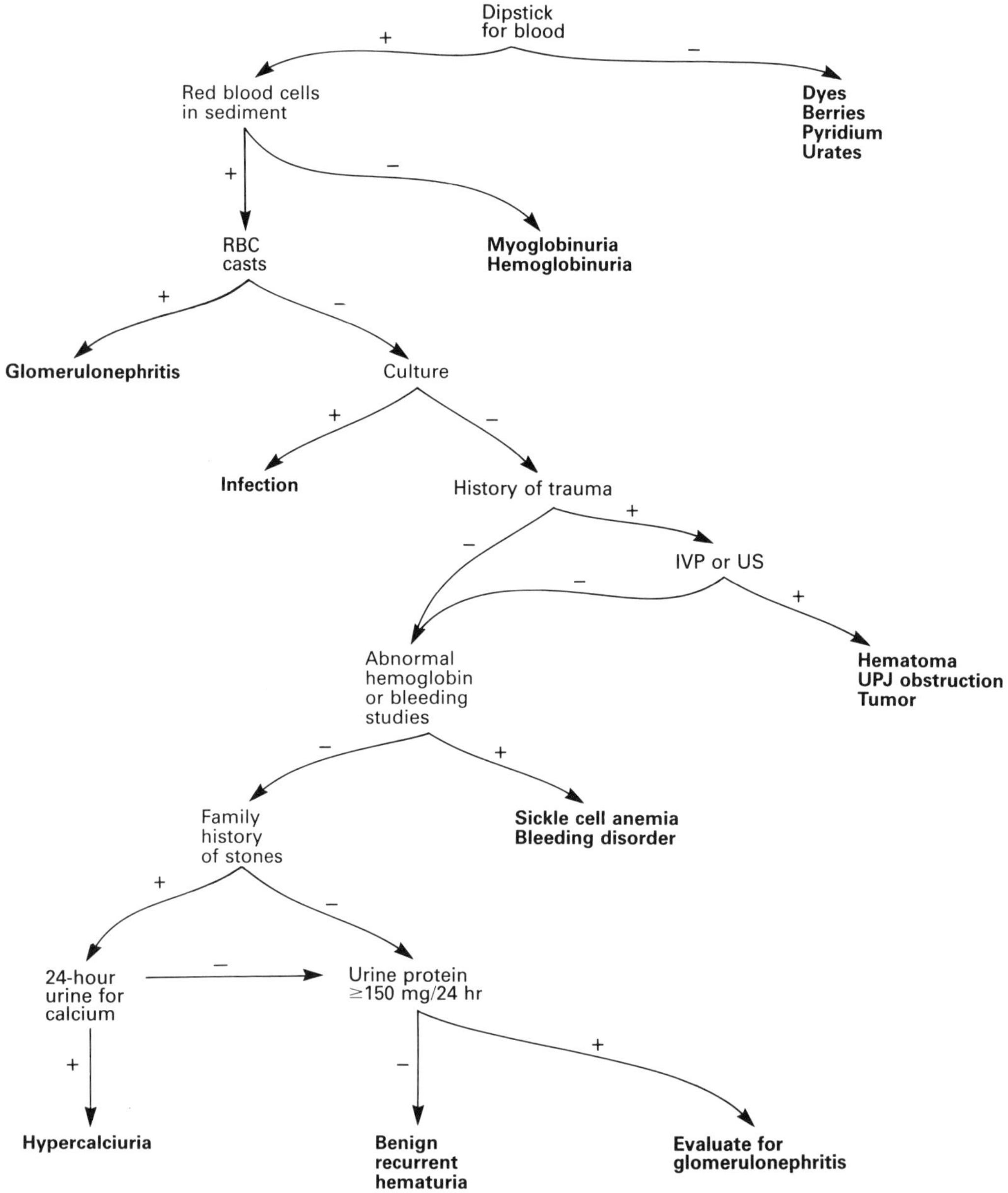

FIG 33–1
Decision tree for differential diagnosis of hematuria.
*With dipsticks, the maximum readable protein concentration in grossly bloody urine that is due to RBCs and plasma proteins is 2+.

In general, renal biopsy should be considered when significant proteinuria accompanies hematuria.

INDICATIONS FOR CONSULTATION OR REFERRAL

Consultation or referral is necessary when the following symptoms or conditions are present:

1. Fever, systemic toxicity, severe abdominal colic
2. Persistent (>48 hours) gross hematuria
3. Gross hematuria after significant abdominal or perineal trauma
4. Gross hematuria followed by urinary retention
5. Hypertension, oliguria, edema
6. Coexistent heavy proteinuria
7. Azotemia

DISCUSSION OF ALGORITHM

An algorithm for the differential diagnosis of hematuria is presented in Figure 33–1. Keeping in mind the common causes of hematuria will help guide the explanation of this problem. First, the presence of blood rather than hemoglobin or myoglobin should be established by looking at the sediment rather than relying on the dipstick detection of blood. A history of trauma should make the physician consider renal US or IVP to delineate renal hematoma, laceration, or blood clots in the bladder. The urinary sediment should be examined for RBC casts, which if present will lead to evaluation for glomerulonephritis. A positive urine culture will confirm a urinary tract infection.

BIBLIOGRAPHY

Gauthier B: Asymptomatic hematuria, in Gauthier B, Edelman CM, (eds): *Nephrology and Urology for the Pediatrician*. Boston, Little Brown & Co, 1982.

Gauthier B: Gross hematuria, in Gauthier B, Edelman CM, (eds): *Nephrology and Urology for the Pediatrician*. Boston, Little Brown & Co, 1982.

Hogg RJ, Silva F, Walker P, et al: A multicenter study of IgA nephropathy in children. *Kidney Int* 1982; 22:643.

Kitagawa T: Lessons learned from the Japanese nephritis screening study. *Pediatr Nephrol* 1988; 2:256.

Schwartz MW: Hematuria, in Fleisher GR, Ludwig S, (eds): *Textbook of Pediatric Emergency Medicine*, ed 2. Baltimore, Williams & Wilkins Co, 1988, pp 197–200.

Norman ME: An office approach to hematuria and proteinuria. *Pediatr Clin North Am* 1987; 34:545.

Stapleton FB, Roy S, Nue HN, et al: Hypercalciuria children with hematuria. *N Engl J Med* 1984; 310: 1345.

34 HOARSENESS

William Potsic, M.D.

Chronic hoarseness, a common complaint, is brought to the attention of the primary care physician when the voice is husky, breathy, or weak.

Acute onset of hoarseness is most commonly (90% of cases) associated with inflammation that occurs with viral infections of the upper respiratory tract. Croup and epiglottitis are also accompanied by hoarseness but the parents and patients are more concerned by the stridor or respiratory insufficiency. Acute voice abuse from shouting or smoking are other frequent causes of hoarseness.

DIFFERENTIAL DIAGNOSIS

COMMON CAUSES OF HOARSENESS

Trauma
Blunt neck trauma
Arytenoid dislocation from intubation
Postoperative recurrent nerve injury
  Cervical
  Mediastinal
  Thoracic
Recurrent laryngeal nerve trauma
Vocal cord nodules
Vocal polyps

Infection
Viral
Bacterial
Diphtheria
Bulbar polio
Botulism

Drug-toxin
Lead

Allergy-inflammation
  Allergic laryngitis
  Rheumatoid arthritis
  Guillain-Barré syndrome

Laryngeal tumors
Benign
  Laryngeal papilloma
Malignant (rare)
  Rhabdomyosarcoma
  Myeloma
Mediastinal masses
  Tumors
  Cysts

Congenital laryngeal disorders
Webs
  Glottic
  Subglottic
Laryngoesophageal cleft
Cysts
  Mucocele (mucus retention cyst)
  Laryngocele
Vascular lesions
  Subglottic hemangioma
  Lymphangioma
  Cri-du-chat syndrome
Unilateral vocal cord paralysis
Arnold-Chiari malformation
Gastroesophageal reflux-(GER)–chronic laryngitis

DISCUSSION

In the neonate, congenital lesions such as laryngeal webs of the larynx may cause hoarseness. This is always of concern and if it is associated with difficulty breathing or feeding, it requires immediate referral to an otolaryngologist for evaluation by laryngoscopy and bronchoscopy. If there is no respiratory distress or feeding difficulty, a lateral neck x-ray film and barium swallow should be done to rule out mass lesions. If no masses are identified, laryngoscopy should be postponed until the infant is 10 to 12 weeks old if the problem has not resolved. Laryngoscopy should be done if there is any worsening of the hoarseness in the infant prior to 12 weeks of age.

Children, aged 18 months and older, often develop progressive hoarseness. The most common cause is vocal nodules from vocal misuse and abuse. Nodules are usually indicated by hoarseness that is progressive and worse in the afternoon or evening in a child that screams or shouts frequently. Laryngeal nodules may resolve with resting of the voice or speech therapy (Fig 34–1). However, any other cause of hoarseness that may be progressive also requires a specific diagnosis.

Papillomas on the vocal cords cause increasing hoarseness and, if severe, respiratory distress. These wart-like lesions are easily visualized by laryngoscopy. Although removal of the papilloma can be carried out under direct visualization, they recur, necessitating numerous procedures. At puberty, the papillomas regress.

Rarely, unusual conditions like hypothyroidism, botulism, traumatic recurrent nerve paralysis, blunt laryngeal trauma, or mycotic infection of the larynx may cause a weak or hoarse voice.

DATA GATHERING

HISTORY

Hoarseness of acute onset suggests infection or trauma, including trauma from both direct injury and overuse from screaming. Often documentation of trauma is difficult but indirect evidence of hoarseness in an enthusiastic sports participant or fan may be enough to suggest the diagnosis.

Botulism is suggested in infants who are breast-fed or offered honey in their feedings. Hoarseness appearing in the neonate should suggest laryngeal anomalies.

PHYSICAL EXAMINATION

The physical examination requires direct visualization of the cords to make a definite diagnosis. Not all patients need this procedure if an obvious cause of hoarseness is detected on the general physical examination. The most likely positive physical finding will be evidence of upper airway infection. Other entities suggested by the physical examination include botulism with decreased or absent reflexes, hypotonia, and a weak cry. Hypothyroidism also causes hypotonia and decreased reflexes, but characteristic facies.

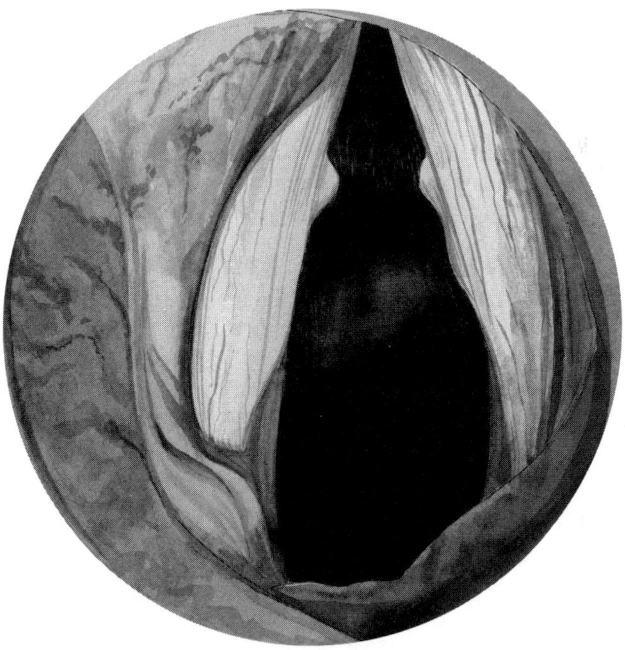

FIG 34–1
Vocal cord nodules.

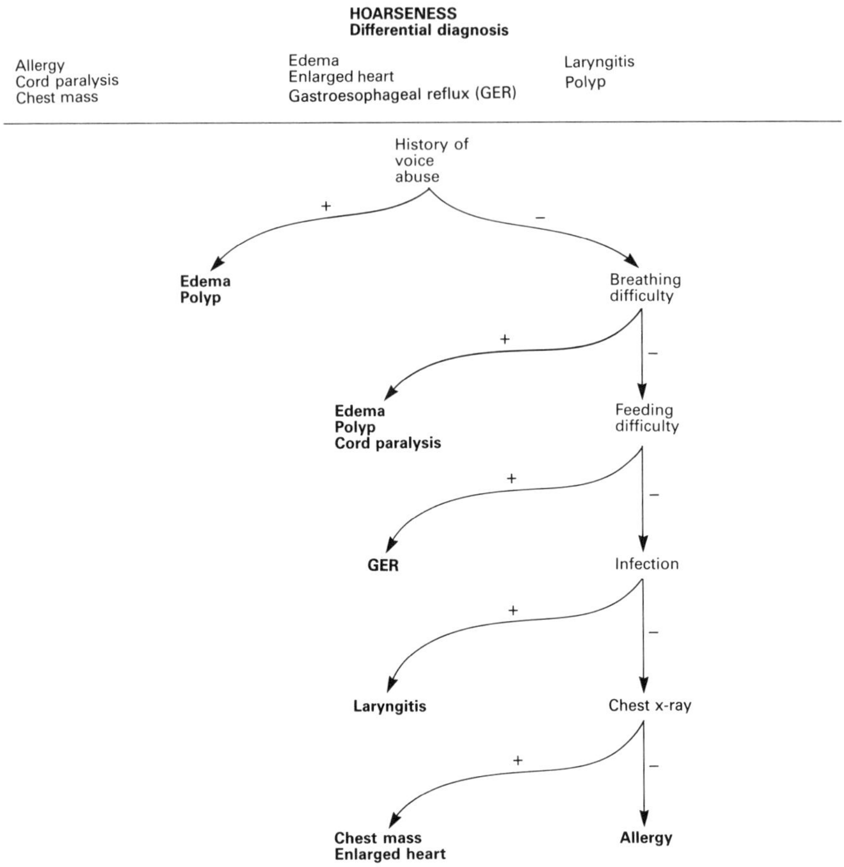

FIG 34–2
Decision tree for differential diagnosis of hoarseness.

LABORATORY EVALUATION

The laboratory tests required by the primary care physician are few since visualization of the larynx is required. This can usually be done by an otolaryngologist with a mirror or flexible fiberoptic instruments. Other tests such as lateral neck x-ray film, barium swallow, and chest roentgenogram are ordered before or after laryngoscopy as indicated.

INDICATIONS FOR CONSULTATION OR REFERRAL

Patients who do not respond to treatment of infection or voice rest should be seen by someone experienced in visualization of the larynx.

DISCUSSION OF ALGORITHM

An algorithm for differential diagnosis of hoarseness is presented in Figure 34–2. The patient should be assessed for respiratory distress or feeding difficulty. If these symptoms are present, the patient's airway should be evaluated by ordering lateral neck x-rays films, if needed, and consulting with an ear, nose, and throat specialist.

Next, the condition of the patient should be evaluated for infection and voice abuse. If these are not present, these patients need visualization of the vocal cords by a specialist.

BIBLIOGRAPHY

Ferguson CF: Congenital abnormalities of the infant larynx. *Otolaryngol Clin North Am* 1970; 3:185–200.

Hander SD: Trauma to the larynx and upper trachea. *Int Anesthesiol Clin* 1987; 26:39–41.

Holinger PH, Brown WT: Congenital webs, cysts, laryngoceles and other anomalies of the larynx. *Ann Otol Rhinol Laryngol* 1967; 76:744–753.

Holinger PH, Schild JA, Weprin L: Pediatric laryngology. *Otolaryngol Clin North Am* Oct 1970; 625–637.

Potsic WP, Handler SD: *Primary Care Pediatric Otolaryngology*. New York, Macmillan Publishing Co, 1986.

Senturia BH, Wilson FE: Otorhinolaryngic findings in children with voice deviation. *Ann Otol Rhinol Laryngol* 1968; 77:1027–1041.

Silverman E, Zimmer CH: Incidence of chronic hoarseness among school-age children. *J Speech Hear Disord* 1975; 2:211–214.

Yairi E, Currin LH, Bulian N: Incidence of hoarseness in school children over a one year period. *J Commun Dis* 1974; 7:321–328.

35 HYPERTENSION

Michael E. Norman, M.D.

Hypertension is now known to be common in children; as in adults, it is often asymptomatic even when severe. Diagnosis is usually unsuspected and made during a routine examination rather than because of specific signs or symptoms related to elevated blood pressure (BP). The diagnosis of hypertension always depends on the physician's interpretation of the patient's measurements relative to published normal values; therefore, a definition of the upper limit of normal for both the systolic and diastolic values is required (Table 35–1).

Symptoms, when present, are generally nonspecific, such as nausea, vomiting, headache, epistaxis, and abdominal pain. Blurred vision and diplopia occur with prolonged hypertension. On the other hand, frequently overlooked as related to hypertension are complaints of facial palsy, altered personality, sudden onset of deteriorating school performance, and confusion. In any child with catastrophic symptoms such as sudden blindness, seizures, cerebrovascular accident, or coma, malignant hypertensive encephalopathy must be considered.

DIFFERENTIAL DIAGNOSIS

Few major diagnoses need be considered in the child with asymptomatic hypertension. Ninety-five percent have primary or essential hypertension; the other 5% have secondary hypertension due to renal (4%), renovascular (0.5%), or miscellaneous (0.5%) causes.

COMMON CAUSES OF HYPERTENSION

Infection
Pyelonephritis
Reflux nephropathy
Toxin-drugs
Corticosteroids
Sympathomimetic drugs
Licorice
Metabolic
Hyperthyroidism
Hyperaldosteronism
Hypercalcemia
Allergic-immunologic
Glomerulonephritis
Serum sickness

TABLE 35–1
Definition of Upper Limit of Normal Blood Pressure (mm Hg)

	BOYS				GIRLS			
	95TH PERCENTILE		HYPERTENSION		95TH PERCENTILE		HYPERTENSION	
AGE (YR)	SYSTOLIC	DIASTOLIC	MODERATE	SEVERE	SYSTOLIC	DIASTOLIC	MODERATE	SEVERE
0–2	110	65	>125/80	>140/90	110	65	>125/80	>140/95
3–6	112	78	>125/95	>140/100	112	80	>125/90	>140/100
7–10	124	84	>140/95	>160/105	124	84	>144/95	>170/110
11–15	140	90	>155/105	>165/110	138	88	>144/94	>170/110

Hemolytic uremic syndrome
Tumor
Wilms tumor
Pheochromocytoma
Neurofibromatosis
Brain tumors
Congenital
Uteropelvic obstruction
Coarctation of the aorta
Renal artery stenosis
Multiple etiology
Primary (essential)
Traction immobilization

DATA GATHERING

HISTORY

Approximately 50% of children with essential hypertension have a positive family history of hypertension and are obese. While essential hypertension is more common in black adults than in white adults, the same is not true for children. Children with secondary hypertension are more likely to have symptoms referable to elevated BP such as headache and irritability. Clues to the cause may be a history of prior urinary tract infections (e.g., reflux nephropathy), red or Coke-colored urine (e.g., glomerulonephritis), or the use of excessive cold remedies containing sympathomimetic amines.

PHYSICAL EXAMINATION

The BP cuff should cover two thirds of the upper arm length. Repeated measurements are required before making the diagnosis, both for accuracy and to reduce the impact of initial patient anxiety on the observed values (see Report to the Task Force on Blood Pressure Control for details). In the physical examination, pay particular attention to the presence or absence of a cardiac murmur (e.g., coarctation of the aorta), bruits over the flanks (e.g., renal artery stenosis), the external genitalia (e.g., evidence of distal urinary tract obstruction), and evidence of target organ damage from the hypertension itself (e.g., retinopathy, cardiomegaly). Any child with severe diastolic hypertension must be considered to have renovascular hypertension until proved otherwise. In any girl with severe diastolic hypertension, reflux nephropathy must be ruled out with intravenous pyelography (IVP) and voiding cystourethrography or renal scans unless another diagnosis is obvious. Finally, always remember that severe hypertension, especially with marked diastolic elevations, may present with encephalopathy mimicking intracranial disease or congestive heart failure mimicking primary cardiac disease. A search for underlying renal or renovascular disease must be made in such cases.

LABORATORY EVALUATION

The urinalysis will often point toward primary glomerulonephritis. Subsequent studies would include a complete blood cell count (CBC), serum blood urea nitrogen (BUN) and creatinine levels, and electrolytes, including calcium, C3, antistreptolysin O, and antinuclear antibody titer. Occasionally the urine culture will be positive, but often in reflux nephropathy the urine is sterile when hypertension is discovered. In these cases, renal scarring seen on IVP or renal scanning suggests prior infection. In some patients reflux is inferred because voiding cystourethrography does not show it. Some experts prefer to begin the radiologic workup with renal ultrasound (US) rather than IVP to diagnose obstruction or scarring of the kidney. An electrocardiogram (ECG) and chest x-ray film are helpful to screen for coarctation of the aorta and to evaluate the heart for signs of hypertensive effects. Renal arteriography is recommended when the hypertension is severe, the child is young (e.g., less than 10 years), and the cause is obscure after urinalysis and urine culture, renal US or IVP, and voiding cystourethrography. Neither IVP nor renal scanning is sensitive enough to rule out renal artery stenosis. A workup for pheochromocytoma should be done only when symptoms and signs suggest excess circulating catecholamines (e.g., palpitations, sweating, pallor). These tumors are rare. The neurologic, orthopedic, and drug-related causes of hypertension are obvious from the history and physical examination and few laboratory investigations are needed. Finally, while some investigators favor measuring a random serum renin level to distinguish between primary and secondary hypertension, I do not believe that it is a particularly useful test in primary practice.

INDICATIONS FOR HOSPITAL ADMISSION

Patients should be admitted to the hospital if the following conditions are present:

1. Severe hypertension at any age, as determined by repeated BP measurements during the examination.
2. Symptomatic hypertension, whatever the BP, particularly if newly discovered.
3. Hypertension associated with a renal bruit or a nephritic urine sediment (e.g., hematuria, proteinuria, RBC casts).

A pediatric nephrologist should be consulted regarding treatment and workup. If the patient has encepalopathy or congestive heart failure,

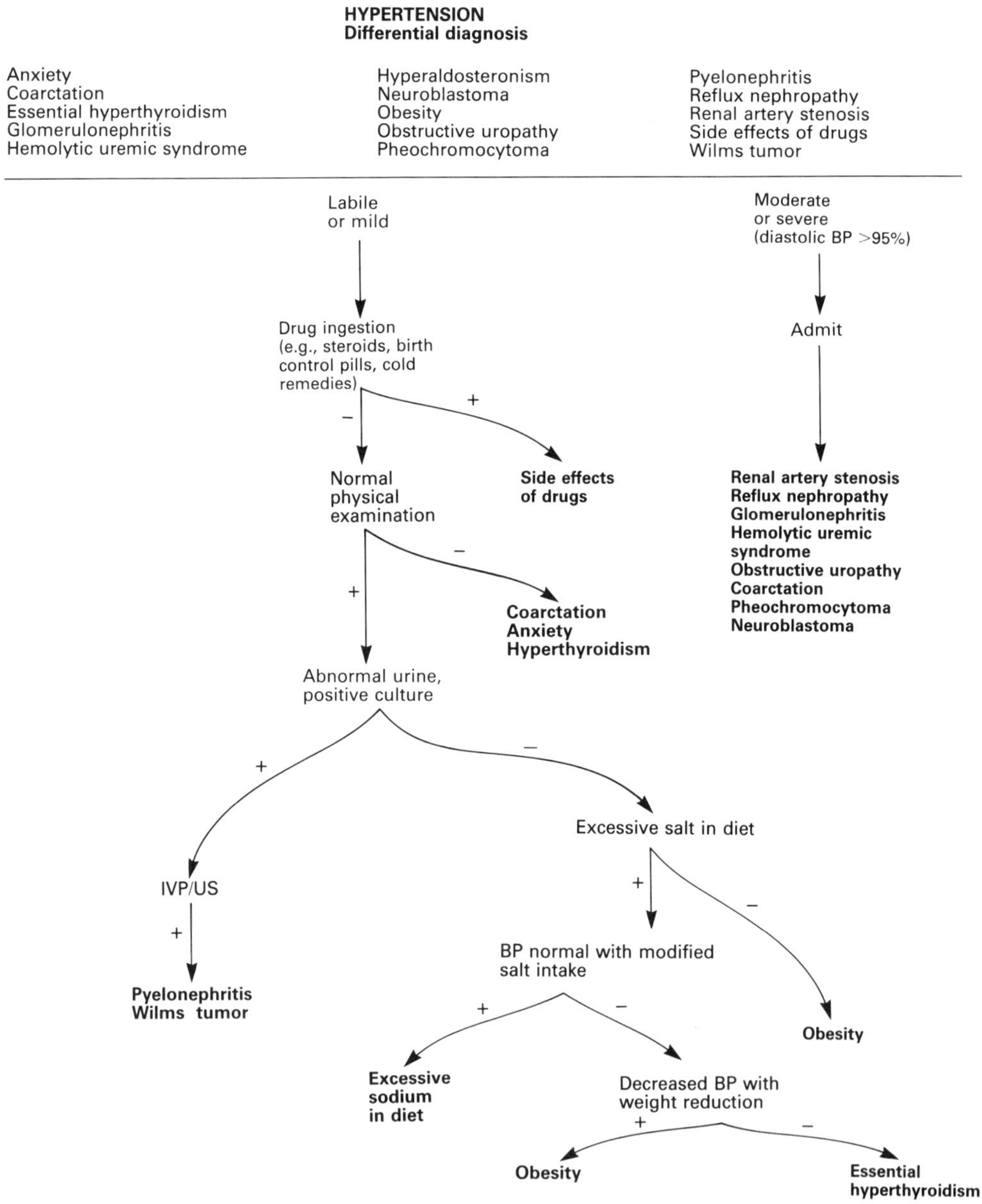

FIG 35–1
Decision tree for differential diagnosis of hypertension.

emergency intravenous therapy with diazoxide (5 mg/kg by rapid IV injection) may be given even before the cause is determined.

DISCUSSION OF ALOGORITHM

An algorithm for the differential diagnosis of hypertension is presented in Figure 35–1. The first task in the evaluation is to confirm the diagnosis of hypertension by determining the BP on at least three occasions, while trying to minimize the patient's excitement and worry. If the BP reading just exceeds the 95th percentile, the hypertension is considered mild. In this group of patients urinalysis should be done to screen for renal disease. If results of urinalysis are normal, other predisposing factors (e.g., family history, salt intake, obesity) should be identified and appropriate counseling about weight, diet, and exercise should be given.

Patients with higher BP readings require examination for renovascular disease, including arteriography if the patient is younger than 10 years old and no other disease to explain hypertension is found.

BIBLIOGRAPHY

Dillon MJ: Clinical aspects of hypertension, in Holiday MA, Barratt TU, Vernier RL, (eds): *Pediatric Nephrology*, ed 2. Baltimore, Williams & Wilkins Co, 1987.

Gauthier B, Edelmann CM, Barnett H: *Nephrology and Urology for the Pediatrician*. Boston, Little Brown & Co, 1982.

Norman ME: Renal and electrolyte emergencies, in Fleisher G, Ludwig S, (eds): *Textbook of Pediatric Emergency Medicine*, ed 2. Baltimore, Williams & Wilkins Co, 1988; p 499–506.

Report of the Second Task Force on Blood Pressure Control in Children, 1987. *Pediatrics* 1987; 79:1.

36 JAUNDICE

William R. Treem, M.D.

The primary care physician must often differentiate between physiologic and pathologic jaundice in the newborn immediately after birth. Causes of prolonged pathologic jaundice in the first week of life are familiar to physicians caring for children; however, the differential diagnosis of prolonged neonatal jaundice or of the onset of jaundice within the first few years of life may be less familiar. This chapter outlines the basic mechanisms and clinical entities responsible for jaundice during these periods. Because there exists specific therapy for certain causes of jaundice, a clear approach to diagnosis is essential to assure a more favorable long-term prognosis.

The reader is referred to Chapter 38 (Large Liver) for details concerning jaundice and liver disease in later childhood and adolescence. The primary care physician is faced with a unique developmental situation in the newborn, where several factors may combine to cause physiologic jaundice.

1. Enhanced bilirubin production due to:
   a. Larger red blood cell (RBC) mass
   b. Shortened RBC life span
   c. Inefficient erythropoiesis
2. Decreased albumin binding due to lower albumin concentration
3. Decreased hepatic bilirubin uptake and

binding due to decreased ligandin (Y protein)
4. Decreased conjugation of bilirubin due to decreased glucuronyl tranferase activity
5. Impaired intrahepatic bile secretion into the canaliculus
6. Increased enterohepatic circulation of bilirubin
   a. Decreased bacterial flora, with decreased production of fecal urobilinogen
   b. More hydrolysis of conjugated bilirubin to unconjugated bilirubin by β-glucuronidase, with subsequent reabsorption
   c. Shunting of bilirubin away from the hepatic sinusoids when the ductus venosus is patent

Pathologic perturbations in this period can exaggerate and perpetuate neonatal jaundice, resulting in delayed resolution of the problem.

DIFFERENTIAL DIAGNOSIS

COMMON CAUSES OF JAUNDICE

Increased production

Hemolytic

Fetal-maternal
  Rh
  ABO incompatibility
  Other
Hereditary spherocytosis
Nonspherocytic hemolytic anemias
  Glucose-6-phosphate dehydrogenase deficiency and drugs
  Pyruvate kinase deficiency
  Other RBC enzyme deficiencies
Infection with hemolysis

Extravasation of blood

Petechiae
Hematoma
Pulmonary, cerebral, or occult hemorrhage

Polycythemia

Maternal-fetal and fetal-fetal transfusion
Delayed clamping of the cord

Swallowed blood

Increased enterohepatic circulation of bilirubin

Pyloric stenosis
Small or large bowel obstruction or ileus
Breast milk jaundice

Diabetes in mother

Decreased clearance

Inborn errors of metabolism

Familial nonhemolytic jaundice, types 1 and 2 (Crigler-Najjar)
Gilbert syndrome

Drugs and hormones

Hypothyroidism
Hypopituitarism and anencephaly
Lucey-Driscoll syndrome

Prematurity

DISCUSSION

Unconjugated Hyperbilirubinemia in the Infant.—The differential diagnosis of unconjugated hyperbilirubinemia in the infant is summarized by pathologic mechanisms in the list of causes of indirect hyperbilirubinemia. Although usually listed under causes of direct hyperbilirubinemia, neonatal sepsis should also be considered in the young infant with indirect hyperbilirubinemia, who is lethargic, feeds poorly, is vomiting, and has a high-pitched cry, with or without fever or hypothermia.

Since most infants with prolonged neonatal jaundice and indirect hyperbilirubinemia appear well, sepsis is an unlikely cause. In these cases consideration is given to breast-milk jaundice, hemolytic disease, hypothyroidism, pyloric stenosis or other causes of intestinal obstruction, and familial unconjugated hyperbilirubinemia (Crigler-Najjar syndrome, Gilbert syndrome).

Hemolytic Disease.—The fetal-maternal blood group incompatibilities, Rh and ABO, are usually recognized in the immediate newborn period. Following severe hemolytic disease, persistent jaundice with conversion of indirect to direct hyperbilirubinemia has been reported, lasting up to 2 months. This has been called "inspissated bile syndrome," and was thought to be secondary to intrahepatic and extrahepatic bile plugs due to massive hemolysis. The scant histologic specimens available in some of these patients show hepatocyte necrosis, giant cell transformation, extramedullary hematopoiesis, portal fibrosis, and inflammation to varying degrees. These findings are similar to those of neonatal hepatitis, thus casting doubt on the cause of the jaundice in these patients and raising the possibility of posttransfusion hepatitis in these babies who have had exchange transfusions.

Other congenital hemolytic anemias can present with persistent unconjugated hyperbilirubinemia. These are either secondary to membrane defects of the RBC (e.g., hereditary spherocytosis) or inborn deficiencies of RBC enzymes (e.g., pyruvate kinase, glucose-6-phosphate dehydrogenase [G-6-PD]). G-6-PD deficiency, a genetically determined X-linked recessive condition, has its highest incidence among infants of Oriental and Mediterranean descent. In these babies the enzyme may be completely absent and hemolysis may occur even in the absence of known precipitating drugs. In the American black population the incidence of G-6-PD deficiency is estimated to be 9% to 13% in men and 2% to 3% in women, and hemolysis in the absence of drug exposure is rare except among premature babies. These defects can usually be suspected on the basis of anemia, a high reticulocyte count, careful inspection of RBC morphology, a normal white blood cell and platelet count, negative Coombs test, and a variably enlarged spleen and liver. A family history of early cholelithiasis (secondary to chronic hemolysis) or splenectomy because of ruptured or enlarged spleen is suggestive.

Breast-Milk Jaundice.—Five percent to 15% of women secrete milk capable of inhibiting glucuronyl transferase activity in vitro, but only approximately 1% to 2% of breast-fed babies develop the syndrome of breast-milk jaundice. With rare exception, the inhibitory factor in maternal milk does not result from maternal ingestion of drugs, although a search for drugs known to displace bilirubin bound to albumin in vitro should be made. Some of these are caffeine, sodium salicylate, diazepam, tolbutamide, sulfisoxazole, furosemide, digoxin, sulfadiazine, and hydrocortisone. Two intrinsic substances in breast milk have received the most attention as candidates for the inhibitors of bilirubin conjugation. First, an unusual isomer of the natural steroid in breast milk, pregnane-3,20-diol has been isolated from the milk of mothers whose nursing infants had breast-milk jaundice and has been shown to inhibit glucuronyl transferase activity in vitro. Second, breast milk contains a high level of lipase activity. Once ingested, the milk liberates large amounts of fatty acids that appear to interfere with the uptake, intracellular binding, or conjugation of bilirubin. Increased plasma free fatty acid in breast-fed infants may also result in displacement of bilirubin from albumin. Recent work has suggested a third factor in breast milk that may contribute to breast milk jaundice. Some breast milk contains β-glucuronidase activity. This enzyme leads to deconjugation of bilirubin, increased intestinal reabsorbtion, and increased indirect bilirubin load returned to the liver via the enteropathic circulation.

Clinically, the serum bilirubin concentration rises progressively from approximately the end of the first week of life and reaches a maximum level of indirect bilirubin of 10 to 27 mg/dL by the end of the second week. Maximum direct bilirubin does not exceed 2 mg/dL. If breast-feeding continues, elevated levels may persist for several weeks and then decline slowly, reaching normal levels by 4 to 12 weeks of age. If breast-feeding is interrupted, there is a prompt decline in serum bilirubin levels within 48 hours. Resumption of breast-feeding is followed by a rebound effect of 1 to 5 mg/dL, but the concentration does not reach previous levels. The appetite of the infant remains good, weight gain and growth are maintained, neurologic signs are absent, there is no evidence of hemolysis, and results of liver function tests are normal. No infant has shown any neurologic sequelae at subsequent follow-up examination. A history of a previously breast-fed sibling with unconjugated hyperbilirubinemia is helpful in suggesting the diagnosis.

Pyloric Stenosis.—Of infants with pyloric stenosis, 10% to 15% have significant elevation of indirect bilirubin. In more than half of these patients jaundice is noted to begin within the first week of life and to persist until the time of diagnosis. The levels of indirect bilirubin are usually 5 to 10 mg/dL, and drop quickly after surgical alleviation of the obstruction. Although traditionally the cause of jaundice in these infants is thought to be increased enterohepatic circulation of unconjugated bilirubin, recent work has suggested that diminished activity of glucuronyl transferase and the effects of starvation on bilirubin binding and uptake may be primarily responsible.

Hypothyroidism.—Persistent unconjugated hyperbilirubinemia is a presenting sign in approximately one third of children with congenital hypothyroidism, preceding by 3 to 6 weeks the more obvious clinical manifestations. Although many states now have mandatory screening tests, any child with persistent unexplained indirect hyperbilirubinemia should undergo repeated thyroid function studies. Jaundice clears quickly once treatment of the deficiency state is begun.

Crigler-Najjar Syndrome.—First described in 1952, Crigler-Najjar syndrome, with severe persistent unconjugated hyperbilirubinemia in neonates but without hemolysis or evidence of hepatic disease, has been attributed to an inherited absence or deficiency of bilirubin uridine diphosphate glucuronyl transferase. Two varieties have been described. The first, with complete absence of the enzyme, results in marked jaundice within hours of birth that cannot be controlled with phototherapy and requires treatment by repeated exchange transfusions. Some of these infants can also be given bilirubin binding agents such as agar or cholestyramine in conjunction with daily phototherapy. With this aggressive therapy, kernicterus may be prevented. A second less severe type is due to deficient but not absent glucuronyl transferase activity. Unconjugated bilirubin levels between 5.0 and 20 mg/dL may appear early in infancy or may be delayed until later in childhood. The bilirubin levels fall to 1.0 to 5.0 mg/dL within 2 to 4 weeks of instituting daily phenobarbital therapy.

Gilbert Disease.—In the older child, Gilbert disease is probably the most common cause of mild, chronic, or intermittent unconjugated hyperbilirubinemia occurring in the absence of overt hemolysis. It is often diagnosed at times of intercurrent illness and caloric deprivation secondary to decreased intake or vomiting, or even serendipitously by routine laboratory screening because of nonspecific complaints such as abdominal pain, fatigue, or anorexia. Although a diagnosis of hepatitis is often entertained, results of aminotransferase determinations are normal, bilirubin is unconjugated, urine has normal color, and there is no hepatomegaly. Mean postprandial levels of unconjugated serum bilirubin are 1.5 to 2.0 mg/dL but rise to approximately 3.0 to 4.0 mg/dL after 24 hours of fasting or caloric deprivation.

Conjugated Hyperbilirubinemia in the Infant.—Causes of prolonged conjugated hyperbilirubinemia, also referred to as prolonged obstructive jaundice or neonatal cholestasis, are summarized in the above list of causes of direct hyperbilirubinemia. The hallmark of these conditions is an elevated direct bilirubin level, clinical jaundice, and hepatomegaly. Prompt diagnosis is critical so that infectious causes are rapidly treated; metabolic causes are recognized and dietary restrictions applied if necessary; genetic cases are appropriately counseled; and those children with surgically amenable lesions can quickly undergo surgery. Certain rare causes, such as Dubin-Johnson syndrome or Rotor syndrome, represent pure defects in bilirubin excretion. However, all of the other entities listed under direct hyperbilirubinemia involve more profound abnormalities of hepatocyte function, resulting in a decrease in bile flow on the basis of infectious, toxic, or metabolic injury to hepatic parenchymal cells and bile duct epithelium.

Bacterial Infection.—Once direct hyperbilirubinemia is demonstrated, infection as a primary cause should be ruled out. Bacterial infection, particularly with *Escherichia coli* and other endotoxin-producing organisms, is a frequent cause of conjugated bilirubin elevation. Although positive blood cultures in a sick infant are clear-cut evidence of jaundice secondary to sepsis, direct hyperbilirubinemia has also been reported in association with bacterial infection in clinically well infants (predominantly in boys), particularly with a urinary tract source for bacteremia. Thus urinalysis should be performed, and urine, blood, stool, and cerebrospinal (CSF) fluid, as clinically indicated, should be cultured as part of the evaluation.

Known Viral Causes of Neonatal Hepatitis.—Acquired viral infection (see above list of causes of direct hyperbilirubinemia), either by transplacental spread late in the third trimester, from swallowed contaminated products in the birth canal during delivery, or later from infected breast milk or contaminated hands, can also cause early neonatal direct hyperbilirubinemia. As opposed to infants with congenital infection acquired early in pregnancy who are born small for gestational age, with microcephaly, cardiac lesions, cataracts, and intracranial calcifications, infants with late-acquired infection may have decreased appetite, vomiting, failure to thrive, jaundice, and hepatosplenomegaly during the first 3 months of life. Stool may be normal to pale, but is seldom acholic. Splenomegaly is variable. In sicker patients with certain agents, a maculopapular or petechial rash may be present in conjunction with thrombocytopenia, hemolysis, and elevated prothrombin time (PT) and partial thromboplastin time (PTT), suggesting disseminated intravascular coagulation. Screening laboratory tests include TORCH (toxoplasmosis, rubella, cytomegalovirus, herpesvirus, syphilis) titers in both mother and infant; serum IgM levels; viral stool, urine, and nasopharyngeal cultures; urinalysis for characteristic inclusion-bearing cells in cytomegalovirus (CMV) infection; acute serum spun and saved for titers against other possible viruses (coxsackievirus, echovirus); and a fluorescent treponema antibody (FTA) test or VDRL test for syphilis.

The spectrum of neonatal liver disease caused by hepatitis B virus (HBV) is extremely variable. Fulminant hepatic necrosis has been reported, particularly with the use of infected intrapartum or postpartum blood transfusions. More commonly, neonatal hepatitis B is acquired at the time of parturition from a mother who is a chronic carrier or actively infected. Since the hepatitis B virus has a long incubation period, infection results in mild or even subclinical disease at 2 to 4 months of age, with hepatomegaly and mild elevations in the levels of bilirubin and serum aminotransferases. In general, those infants born to mothers acutely infected with HBV during the third trimester or at parturition are more likely to have clinically evident mild liver disease, but also are more likely to clear hepatitis B surface antigen (HBsAg). However, infants born to mothers who are chronic carriers of HBV, particularly if those women are hepatitis B e antigen positive (HBeAg$^+$) are more likely to remain HBsAg positive if they are infected in the neonatal period. Chronic persistent hepatitis may follow for many years, with serologic evidence of persistent antigenemia (HBsAg$^+$) and mild aminotransferase elevations. Progression to cirrhosis is most unusual. However, since infants born to HBsAg$^+$ mothers are at high risk for becoming chronic carriers of HBV, they should receive hyperimmune hepatitis B serum immediately after delivery and hepatitis B vaccine in the first 24 hours of life and again at 1 month and at 6 months of age. All infants born to HBsAg-positive mothers should have such immunization irrespective of the HBeAg status of the mother.

Metabolic Liver Disease.—After infectious causes of direct hyperbilirubinemia, the physician must consider rare but important metabolic causes of neonatal liver disease. The scope of this chapter does not allow a complete discussion of these entities. However, many can present early in the neonatal period, with vomiting, poor feeding, diarrhea, and lethargy preceding jaundice, hepatomegaly, ascites, and failure to thrive. In addition, laboratory parameters of hypoglycemia, acidosis, and evidence of renal tubular dysfunction (such as aminoaciduria, proteinuria, phosphaturia, glycosuria, hypophosphatemia, and hypouricemia) may all suggest one of various metabolic causes of neonatal jaundice and liver disease.

α_1-Antitrypsin Deficiency.—One of the more common metabolic causes of neonatal conjugated hyperbilirubinemia is α_1-antitrypsin deficiency. This entity should be ruled out early, since the diagnosis may avoid the need for invasive diagnostic procedures, such as a liver biopsy or intraoperative cholangiography.

α_1-antitrypsin is the major α_1-globulin of human plasma and the principal inhibitor of destructive proteolytic enzymes such as trypsin and leukocyte elastase, which is able to cleave the connective tissue components of the extracellular tissue of various organs. Therefore, α_1-antitrypsin normally protects these tissues from destruction. Deficiency of this protein, mediated via inheritance of different alleles, can result in both liver and lung disease. In infancy, the most common presentation is obstructive jaundice, as early as 3 to 12 weeks of age, without lung disease. This is most often associated with the inheritance of the Z allele that produces an electrophoretically slower-moving protein and a total level of α_1-antitrypsin only 10% to 15% of normal. The PiZ variant protein appears to be synthesized in the hepatocyte but not secreted at a normal rate. It aggregates in the hepatocytes, and this accumulation and intracellular retention of the abnormal α_1-antitrypsin is thought to cause the liver damage.

The heterozygote state (PiMZ) exists in up to 3% of the population, and the incidence of the homozygous state (PiZZ) is approximately one in 1,500 live births in Sweden and one in 7,600 in North America. Any infant with direct hyperbilirubinemia and hepatomegaly or even hepatomegaly without jaundice should be examined for α_1-antitrypsin deficiency. Since only 10% to 20% of PiZZ infants present with obstructive jaundice in the first year of life and the jaundice resolves in most by the age of 1 year, any older child with persistent hepatomegaly or evidence of chronic aminotransferase elevations and liver disease should also have this possibility evaluated. This can be done by measuring serum α_1-antitrypsin levels and determining the phenotype of the α_1-antitrypsin present (Pi-typing) with acid-starch gel electrophoresis. If these methods are not available, the diagnosis may be suggested by the absence or marked decrease in the α_1 macroglobulin band on a serum protein electrophoresis.

Neonatal Hepatitis and Biliary Atresia.—The most important and urgent diagnosis to consider in the infant with obstructive jaundice is extrahepatic biliary atresia, which occurs with a frequency of one in 8,000 to 15,000 live births. The cause of biliary atresia is unknown. Recent efforts have centered around identifying an intrauterine viral pathogen acquired late in gestation that results in progressive obliterative sclerosis of the large bile ducts. Such a candidate virus is the double-stranded RNA virus reovirus 3. This virus damages mouse bile duct epithelium and produces a biliary atresia–like picture in weanling mice. Antibodies to reovirus 3 were identified more frequently in the sera of infants with biliary atresia or idiopathic neonatal hepatitis than in control infants or infants with other cholestatic disorders in one epidemiologic study.

An acquired ongoing insult is suggested by the following findings: the first passed stools are normal in color and become acholic. The bile ducts are progressively obliterated more distally but are more proliferative and inflamed proximally. Despite successful surgical portoenterostomy with bile drainage, the intrahepatic biliary ducts are progressively damaged. However, the variable progression and prognosis of biliary atresia suggests that genetic factors such as HLA status and immune response genes may also be important.

For the office physician, the nuances of various intrahepatic and extrahepatic cholestatic syndromes are not nearly as important as differentiating the two. An identifiable infectious, genetic, or metabolic cause can be found in no more than 25% of infants with obstructive jaundice, and once these causes have been ruled out, the primary care physician should refer the patient to a center where more definitive testing can be done. This may include abdominal US to rule out choledochal cyst or common duct disease, DISIDA or other radionucleotide biliary excretion study, 24-hour duodenal fluid collection for the presence of bile, closed liver biopsy, and if necessary, intraoperative cholangiography and open liver biopsy. For three main reasons, there is no justification for waiting and watching past 6 weeks of age to see if the direct hyperbilirubinemia clears, even with the patient receiving choleretic agents such as phenobarbital or cholestyramine. First, early surgical intervention in biliary atresia (Kasai procedure, portojejunostomy) is clearly linked to successful biliary drainage, with Japanese physicians reporting a success rate of 80% if the operation is done before the infant is 60 days old and only 20% if done after 90 days. Second, some cases of neonatal giant cell hepatitis, α_1-antitrypsin deficiency, and intrahepatic paucity of bile ducts will clinically persistently mimic complete extrahepatic obstruction, with acholic stools and similar total bilirubin levels as low as 5 or 6 mg/dL. These cases can only be differentiated from extrahepatic obstruction by the above-mentioned tests. Third, in the hands of an experienced pediatric gastroenterologist trained in the technique of closed percutaneous liver biopsy, and a pediatric pathologist, differentiation between intrahepatic and extrahepatic causes of infantile cholestasis can be made without resorting to intraoperative cholangiography in approximately 90% to 95% of patients.

DATA GATHERING

HISTORY

Jaundice is evident in most newborn infants with a serum bilirubin concentration of 5 to 7 mg/dL, whereas jaundice appears in older children when the level reaches 2.5 mg/dL. Before it is visible in the skin, jaundice can be seen in the conjunctiva, in the mucous membrane of the hard palate, or under the tongue, especially in blacks or others with darkly pigmented skin. Carotenemia, the result of a large intake of yellow or orange vegetables, can be differentiated from jaundice by its lack of involvement of the conjunctiva and prominence in the nasolabial folds and on the palms and soles.

Laboratory investigation of total and direct serum bilirubin levels should begin the sorting process for possible causes of jaundice, since this will divide and direct the workup along uniquely different paths. A direct serum bilirubin concentration greater than 2 mg/dL (even if this represents only 15% to 20% of the total bilirubin level) indicates conjugated or direct hyperbilirubinemia and should immediately be considered pathologic. If the direct fraction is less than 1.5 mg/dL, the baby has unconjugated hyperbilirubinemia, but should not be categorized as having physiologic jaundice if the total serum bilirubin concentration exceeds 13 mg/dL or if clinical jaundice has persisted for more than 1 week. In the premature infant, these guidelines translate to a total bilirubin concen-

TABLE 36–1
Features That Discriminate Intrahepatic From Extrahepatic Infantile Cholestasis

INTRAHEPATIC	EXTRAHEPATIC
Clinical Features	
Prematurity	Full-term
Small for gestational age	Appropriate gestational age
Familial incidence 15%–20%	No familial incidence
Ill appearing	Well appearing
Intermittently acholic stools	Completely acholic stools
Hepatosplenomegaly	Splenomegaly rare before 3 wk
Liver not hard	Liver firm to hard
Associated abnormalities:	Associated abnormalities:
Alagille syndrome	Polysplenia
Peripheral pulmonic stenosis	Cardiovascular
Vertebral anomalies	Malrotation
Posterior embryotoxon	
Laboratory Features	
Coombs-negative hemolytic anemia	No excretion on DISIDA scan
PT, PTT; unresponsive to vitamin K	Increased lipoprotein X, all patients
Excretion on DISIDA scan	High or normal α-fetoprotein level
Increased lipoprotein X, 15%–20% of patients	24-Hour duodenal fluid colection shows no pigment
High α-fetoprotein level	
24-Hour duodenal-fluid collection shows pigment (especially after feeding)	
Pathologic Features	
Bile ducts normal or decreased	Bile duct proliferation and inflammation
Minimal fibrosis	Portal fibrosis
Giant cell transformation	Giant cell transformation, 25% of patients
Hepatocellular necrosis	Bile lakes
Lobular disarray	Bile plugs in portal ducts
Portal inflammation	Cholestasis
Cholestasis	

TABLE 36–2
Laboratory and Radiologic Studies to Evaluate Obstructive Jaundice

BLOOD	URINE	CULTURES	SEROLOGY	LIVER FUNCTION	SPECIAL STUDIES	RADIOLOGY
CBC count	Urinalysis	Blood	TORCH	Total and direct bilirubin	Sweat test	US
Smear	Urine glucose test (Clinitest)	Urine	VDRL or FTA	ALT, AST, GGT	Stool trypsin	Hepatobiliary
Reticulocyte count	Urine metabolic screen (amino and organic acids)	CSF, as indicated	HBsAg in mother and child	Alkaline phosphatase	SPEP or α_1-antitrypsin level	Scintigraphy (DISIDA, PIPIDA)
Platelets		Urine for CMV	Hepatitis A antibody	PT, PTT	5′-nucleotidase	UGI series
Electrolytes, CO_2		Viral cultures of nasopharynx, stool	Epstein-Barr Virus serology	Total protein and albumin	Lipoprotein X, α-fetoprotein	Skull x-ray film
BUN, glucose				Cholesterol	24-Hr duodenal fluid	Long bone films
Uric acid						
Phosphate						

JAUNDICE
Differential diagnosis

Alagille syndrome
α_1-Antitrypsin deficiency
Biliary atresia
Breast-feeding
Choledocal cyst
Cytomegalovirus infection (CMV)
Common duct stone
Criglar-Najjar syndrome
Cystic fibrosis
Familial unconjugated hyperbilirubinemia
Galactosemia
Gilbert syndrome
Hemolytic anemia
Herpes
Hepatitis
Hypothyroidism
Metabolic liver disease
Rubella
Sepsis
Syphilis
Toxoplasmosis

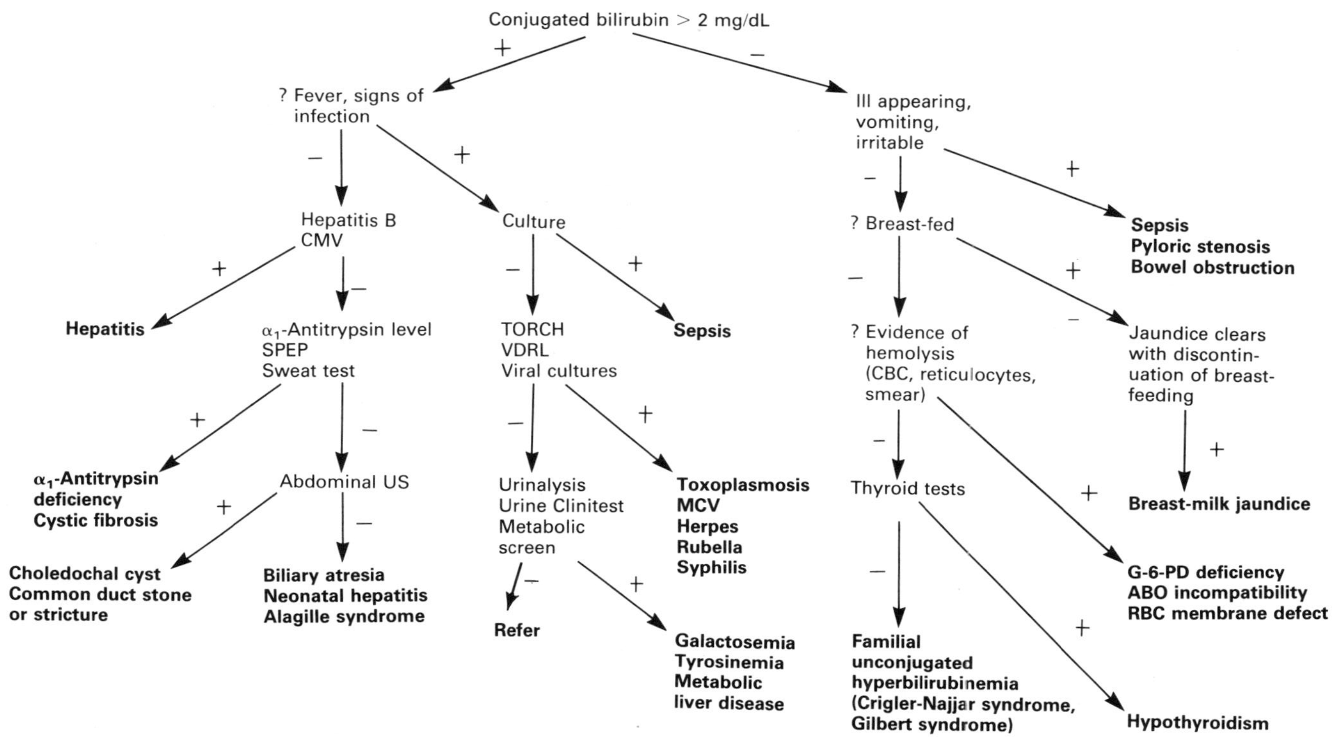

FIG 36–1
Decision tree for differential diagnosis of jaundice.

tration exceeding 15 mg/dL or clinical jaundice persisting for more than 2 weeks.

Table 36–1 offers clinical, laboratory, and pathologic guidelines that help discriminate intrahepatic from extrahepatic causes of obstructive jaundice. The diagnosis of neonatal hepatitis or intrahepatic cholestasis is suggested in a premature baby or a baby small for gestational age, who is ill appearing, has early splenomegaly (before 3 to 4 weeks of age), inconsistently acholic stools, a family history of prolonged neonatal obstructive jaundice, or any extrahepatic manifestations of familial cholestatic syndromes, such as cardiac abnormalities, vertebral abnormalities, or ocular abnormalities. In contrast, infants with biliary atresia are usually born at term, have appropriate weight for gestational age, appear well, and have a firm hard liver and consistently acholic stools. Infants with atresia may have no direct bilirubin elevation early in life, often have delayed onset of acholic stools, and may not have symptoms of clinical jaundice until 3 to 4 weeks of age.

The presence of the gallbladder on US is not a discriminating factor, because a rudimentary gallbladder filled with "white" bile can be present in biliary atresia, and US can easily miss the small empty postprandial gallbladder of an infant 1 to 3 months old.

Laboratory and roentgenologic studies useful in evaluating direct hyperbilirubinemia in neonates are listed in Table 36–2.

INDICATIONS FOR CONSULTATION OR REFERRAL

When faced with treating the infant with obstructive jaundice, the practitioner must decide whether the obstruction is intrahepatic (e.g., neonatal hepatitis, metabolic liver disease, intrahepatic paucity of bile ducts) or extrahepatic (e.g., biliary atresia, choledochal cyst, common duct stone, stenosis). This decision is critical because prevailing evidence suggests that early surgical intervention in biliary atresia is associated with a better prognosis for effective bile drainage and retardation of progressive liver disease. Many of the critical tests necessary to evaluate the nature of the obstruction can only be accomplished by pediatric gastroenterologists in major centers, so the primary pediatrician can begin the diagnostic evaluation, as outlined in the decision tree, separating self-limited or easily identifiable problems from those that need more definitive evaluation.

DISCUSSION OF ALGORITHM

The algorithm (Fig 36–1) suggests an approach to prolonged neonatal jaundice or new onset of jaundice within the first year of life, incorporating most of the entities discussed. The office clinician must differentiate direct from indirect hyperbilirubinemia and rule out the infectious, metabolic, hemolytic, and endocrine abnormalities that can cause immediate and irreversible damage and which require urgent treatment. Further workup, especially of persistent direct hyperbilirubinemia or obstructive jaundice, is best completed by referral to pediatric gastroenterologists in major medical centers.

BIBLIOGRAPHY

Alagille D, Odievre M, Gautier M, et al: Hepatic ductular hypoplasia associated with characteristic facies, vertebral malformations, retarded physical, mental, and sexual development, and cardiac murmur. *J Pediatr* 1975; 86:63–71.

Balistreri WF: Neonatal cholestasis: Medical progress. *J Pediatr* 1985; 106:171–184.

Beasley RP, Hwang LH, Chin-Yun LG, et al: Prevention of perinatally transmitted hepatitis B virus infection with hepatitis B immunoglobulin and hepatitis B vaccine. *Lancet* 1983; 2:1099–1102.

Gourley GR, Arend RA: Beta-glucuronidase and hyperbilirubinemia in breast-fed and formula-fed babies. *Lancet* 1986; 2:644–646.

Maisels MJ: Jaundice in the newborn. *Pediatr Rev* 1982; 3:305–319.

Mowat AP: *Liver Disorders in Childhood*, ed 2, London, Butterworth and Co, 1987.

Schmid R: Bilirubin metabolism: State of the Art. *Gastroenterology* 1978; 74:1307–1312.

Watkins JB, Katz AJ, Grand RJ: Neonatal hepatitis: A diagnostic approach. *Adv Pediatr* 1977; 24:399–454.

37 MACROCEPHALY

Carol Carraccio, M.D.

The child with a large head represents a diagnostic dilemma because of the spectrum of etiologies and clinical outcomes. The possibilities range from a normal familial trait to the life-threatening case of a child with increased intracranial pressure. In some cases, there is apparent head enlargement because of a small body. The evaluation of a large head requires the physician to be familiar with a standard of normal head circumferences, the concept of growth velocity, and an approach to evaluation that identifies those patients who can be safely observed versus those needing a diagnostic workup or immediate intervention.

DIFFERENTIAL DIAGNOSIS

Since parents rarely complain about large head size, the problem is detected by measuring and recording head circumference. The primary task in pursuing the differential diagnosis is to identify those children who need immediate workup and treatment. The causes of macrocephaly are listed below. Although the list is large, certain causes, such as hydrocephalus, mass lesions, congenital malformations, and intracranial hemorrhage, are more common and deserve more attention here.

COMMON CAUSES OF MACROCEPHALY

Trauma
Subdural hematoma or hemorrhage leading to hydrocephalus
Infection
Congenital
Postmeningitis hydrocephalus
Metabolic-endocrine
Metachromatic leukodystrophy
Infantile leukodystrophy
Tay-Sachs disease
Mucopolysaccharidosis
Gangliosidoses
Rickets
Hyperphosphatasia
Mass lesions
Brain tumors
Brain abscess
Cysts
Arteriovenous (AV) malformation
Congenital
Malformations associated with hydrocephalus
- Dandy-Walker syndrome
- Vein of Galen aneurysm
- Aqueductal stenosis
- Hydranencephaly
- Myelomeningocele with Arnold-Chiari malformation

Neurocutaneous syndromes
- Neurofibromatosis
- Tuberous sclerosis
- Sturge-Weber disease
- Klippel-Trénaunay-Weber syndrome

Skeletal and cranial dysplasia
- Achondroplasia
- Camptomelic dwarfism
- Osteogenesis imperfecta
- Craniosynostosis
- Cleidocranial dysostosis
- Osteopetrosis

Other
Severe chronic anemia
- Beckwith-Weidemann syndrome
- Cerebral gigantism
- Histiocytosis X

Pseudotumor cerebri
Primary megalencephaly

DISCUSSION

Hydrocephalus

Hydrocephalus results from either excessive production of spinal fluid, obstruction to flow, or decreased ability to resorb the fluid into the circulation. The causes range from congenital malformations, trauma, and intracranial hemorrhages to infection and tumors. Although some of the patients will present at birth with an obviously large head and full fontanelle, in others the condition will develop insidiously. Especially suspect are patients who recover from neonatal ventricular hemorrhage or meningitis.

Mass Lesions.—Enlarging head circumference is most likely due to primary brain lesions rather than metastatic spread. Common primary tumors include astrocytoma, ependymona, glioma and glioblastoma, medulloblastoma, meningioma, and craniopharyngioma. Neurologic deficits are usually the presenting signs. Other mass lesions such as cysts, abscesses, and vascular malformation also require consideration.

Intracranial Hemorrhage.—Intracranial hemorrhage may result from congenital defects such as arteriovenous malformations, intraventricular hemorrhage—seen in premature infants—or trauma. The latter should raise a suspicion of child abuse.

Dysplasias of the Cranium and Skeleton

Craniosynostosis or premature closure of cranial sutures, distorts the normal shape of the skull and makes the head appear enlarged. Careful inspection of the sutures should identify this problem.

Skeletal dysplasias will be obvious on inspection. The most common of these conditions is achondroplasia, which results in limb shortening as well as an enlarged head. Macrocephaly is also associated with camptomelic dwarfism and Conradi syndrome.

Systemic Diseases

Macrocephaly may be a feature of a variety of systemic conditions. The neurocutaneous syndromes will be easily recognizable by their peculiar skin manifestations: the port-wine stain of Sturge-Weber syndrome, the hypopigmented macules and ash-leaf patches of tuberous sclerosus, and the café-au-lait spots and neurofibromas of neurofibromatosis. Seizures are also a common manifestation of these disorders.

Children with metabolic causes of macrocephaly will also have other features of these disease entities on physical examination. The mucopolysaccharidoses and gangliosidoses cause characteristic coarse facial features. Tay-Sachs disease and the leukodystrophies are associated with progressive neurologic impairment. Hypophosphatasia and rickets will manifest with other deformities of the long bones and ribs.

Pseudomotor Cerebri.—Pseudotumor cerebri manifests as increased intracranial pressure without obstruction to cerebrospinal fluid flow. It may be idiopathic or secondary to such drugs and toxins as steroids, excessive amounts of vitamin A, and lead. Association with certain endocrine conditions, such as hypoparathyroidism and adrenal insufficiency, has also been found.

Primary Megalocephaly.—Megalocephaly is a diagnosis of exclusion made in a child with a negative history and normal physical examination, including developmental and neurologic assessments. It may be familial, so head circumference measurements in other family members are helpful.

DATA GATHERING

HISTORY

The age of the child is an important historical factor in the evaluation. Congenital causes of hydrocephalus as well as some cranial and skeletal abnormalities present at birth or very early in life. The neurocutaneous, metabolic, and degenerative diseases may not manifest themselves until late infancy and early childhood. Other etiologies such as mass lesions, infection, hemorrhage, and toxins may occur at any age. It is important to find out whether there are associated symptoms of headache, vomiting, or abnormal motor activity.

Developmental delay has been associated with many of the diseases that cause macrocephaly. Careful developmental assessment should be part of the evaluation.

Family history of anemia such as thalassemia or sickle cell anemia may help explain the presence of a large head secondary to increased bone marrow activity. Primary megalencephaly tends to run in families. A history of large heads in other family members should be sought.

PHYSICAL EXAMINATION

Since many of the diseases that present with a large head may also manifest signs and symptoms of increased intracranial pressure, a rapid assessment of neurologic status is necessary to differentiate the child who needs immediate treatment and referral from the child who can be approached in a more systematic fashion. Hypertension accompanied by bradycardia, change in mental status, asymmetry of pupil size, decrease in pupil reactivity, papilledema, and focal neurologic findings are all signs associated with increased intracranial pressure.

The head should be measured carefully. The measuring tape is placed from the glabella and supraorbital ridge to the most prominent part of the occiput. This circumference should be compared to that of previous measurements, if available. Head size that crosses two main percentile curves of the head growth chart raises great concern. The head size should also be compared with the height and weight percentiles. In cases of malnutrition, the normal head size may appear large in comparison with a small torso. A child with weight, length, and head circumference all greater than the 95th percentile on the growth curve is likely to be normal. A clue that hydrocephalus is the cause of macrocephaly is that the head is disproportionately large with respect to the face. A complete physical examination will reveal other signs that will be helpful in generating a differential diagnosis. This is particularly true of the congenital and metabolic causes of macrocephaly. A detailed developmental and neurologic examination must be performed.

LABORATORY EVALUATION

Children with macrocephaly who have a positive family history of large head size, a normal head growth velocity, and normal physical examination (including developmental and neurologic) do not require additional evaluation. By contrast, children with signs of increased intracranial pressure should be referred directly to a neurologist or neurosurgeon for diagnostic workup and therapeutic intervention.

Skull radiographs are helpful in determining the status of the sutures as well as calcifications that may indicate tumor, congenital infection, or a neurocutaneous syndrome. Ultrasound examination in young infants will detect hydrocephalus.

Computed tomography or magnetic resonance imaging of the head are the most sensitive tests for the detection of mass lesions. Examination of the cerebrospinal fluid will aid in determining an infectious or metabolic etiology. Determination of the hemoglobin level is important when hemorrhage or a hemoglobinopathy is suspected. Arteriograms are indicated in the evaluation of vascular anomalies and certain tumors.

INDICATIONS FOR CONSULTATION OR REFERRAL

A child with symptoms or signs of increased intracranial pressure requires immediate hospitalization for workup and treatment. The child who has a large head as part of a more global systemic process may benefit from a genetic or neurologic consultation.

DISCUSSION OF ALGORITHM

An algorithm for differential diagnosis of macrocephaly is presented in Figure 37–1. The major task in evaluating a child with a large head is determining if there is increased intracranial pressure, which requires immediate referral for therapy. If there are no signs of increased pressure, the history and physical, developmental, and neurologic examinations can be pursued in a systematic fashion. These measures will provide clues to distinguish those patients who require additional laboratory tests from those who can be observed with close follow-up.

MACROCEPHALY
Differential Diagnosis

Anemia	Familial megalocephaly	Neurocutaneous syndromes
AV malformation	Hydranencephaly	Skeletal cranial dysplasias
Congenital infection	Hydrocephalus	Storage diseases
Congenital malformation	Intracranial hemorrhage	Subdural effusion
Craniosynostosis	Mass lesions	

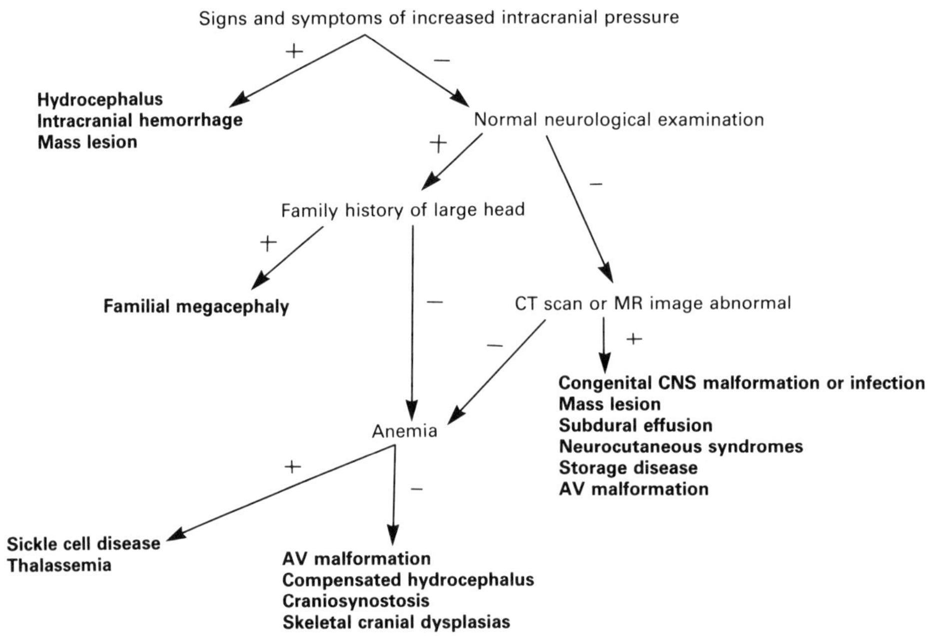

FIG 37–1
Decision tree for differential diagnosis of macrocephaly.

BIBLIOGRAPHY

Briner E, Bodensteiner J: Benign subdural collections of infancy. *Pediatrics* 1980; 67:802.

Brody AS, Goading CA: Magnetic resonance imaging. *Pediatr Rev* 1986; 8:87.

Chaplin E, Goldstein G, Myerberg D, et al: Posthemorrhagic hydrocephalus in the preterm infant. *Pediatrics* 1980; 65:901.

Horton WA, Rotter JI, Rimoin DL, et al: Standard growth curves for achondroplasia. *J Pediatr* 1978; 93:435–438.

Lemieux BG, Wright FS, Swaiman KF: Genetic and congenital structural defects of the brain and spinal cord, in Swaiman KF, Wright FS, (eds): *The Practice of Pediatric Neurology*. St Louis, CV Mosby Co, 1982, pp 402–471.

Nellhaus G: Head circumference from birth to 18 years. *Pediatrics* 1968; 41:106.

Page RB: Hydrocephalus, in Hoekelman R, Blatman S, Friedman S, et al (eds): *Primary Pediatric Care*. Washington, DC, CV Mosby Co, 1987, pp 1282–1285.

Tunnessen WW: *Signs and Symptoms in Pediatrics*. Philadelphia, JB Lippincott Co, 1988, pp 114–121.

38 LARGE LIVER

William R. Treem, M.D.

An enlarged liver is found in many diverse disease processes in infancy and childhood; thus the primary care physician must direct the workup toward the most fruitful areas of investigation and make a decision to follow-up, refer, or hospitalize the child. This chapter offers guidelines for that decision process based on the pathophysiology of hepatomegaly, review of selected diseases, careful history, physical examination, and selected screening laboratory tests.

DIFFERENTIAL DIAGNOSIS

COMMON CAUSES OF LARGE LIVER

Infection
Hepatitis A, B, nonA, nonB, δ agent
Sepsis
Epstein-Barr virus (EBV)
Syphilis
Enteroviruses
TORCH infections (toxoplasmosis, rubella, cytomegalovirus, herpes)
Parasites
Hepatic abscess
Tuberculosis, histoplasmosis
Acquired immune deficiency syndrome (AIDS)

Trauma
Traumatic cyst

Tumor
Leukemia
Lymphoma
Neuroblastoma
Hepatoblastoma
Hemangioma
Adenoma

Toxin
Drug-induced hepatitis
Hypervitaminosis A

Metabolic
Glycogen storage disease
Galactosemia
Tyrosinemia
Hereditary fructose intolerance
Sphingolipidosis (Gaucher disease, Niemann-Pick disease)
Mucolipidosis (I-cell disease)
GM_1 gangliosidosis
Mucopolysaccharidoses (Hurler syndrome, Hunter syndrome)
α_1-Antitrypsin deficiency
Wilson disease
Urea cycle disorders
Diabetes
Disorders of fatty acid oxidation
Cystic fibrosis

Inflammatory
Chronic active hepatitis
Sclerosing cholangitis
Sarcoidosis

Multiple etiologies
Malnutrition
Hyperalimentation
Obesity

Vascular
Budd-Chiari syndrome
Veno-occlusive disease
Congestive heart failure
Constrictive pericarditis

Congenital
Cyst
Hamartoma
Congenital hepatic fibrosis

Biliary obstruction
Common duct stones, stricture
Pancreatitis, cystic fibrosis
Choledochal cyst, tumors of biliary tract (rhabdomyosarcoma)

DISCUSSION

Pathophysiologic mechanisms involved in liver enlargement include (1) congestion secondary to elevated central venous pressure or localized vascular obstruction, as in congestive heart failure or Budd-Chiari syndrome; (2) inflammation with expansion of portal tracts by inflammatory cells, as in viral hepatitis; (3) storage of materials that are accumulating because of metabolic enzyme deficiencies as in glycogen storage disease; (4) accumulation of fat, as seen in malnutrition, diabetes mellitus, Reye syndrome, and disorders of fatty acid oxidation; (5) intrinsic expanding masses such as adenomas, hemangiomas, and hepatoblastomas; and (6) biliary obstruction with accompanying jaundice, as seen with common duct stones or strictures, choledochal cysts, or lesions in the head of the pancreas. Subsequent chapters cover hepatomegaly with jaundice, especially in infancy, and acute viral hepatitis. The following discussion is limited to some of the differential diagnoses of chronic hepatomegaly and chronic hepatitis in the older child who is asymptomatic or subacutely ill. A reasonable definition of "chronic hepatitis" is persistence or relapse of features of acute hepatitis beyond 3 months including elevated aminotransferase levels, hepatomegaly, hard liver, splenomegaly, ascites, anorexia, weight loss, muscle wasting, persistent fever, or jaundice.

Infections Causing Chronic Hepatitis

Although hepatitis A almost always causes an acute self-limited hepatitis, other viruses can cause a more prolonged indolent disease with chronic hepatomegaly and elevated liver enzymes. Hepatitis B virus (HBV) infection can result in chronic hepatitis and a chronic carrier state, particularly in those infected early in life. Sources of HBV infection in childhood include infection acquired at delivery or post-natally from a mother whose blood tests positive for hepatitis B surface antigen ($HBsAg^+$), close contact with saliva or blood from an $HBsAg^+$ family member, exposure to infected blood products in the setting of hemophilia or renal dialysis, and spread among institutionalized children. Most children with chronic HBV are asymptomatic, with mild elevations of aminotransferase levels and either mild chronic active hepatitis or chronic persistent hepatitis. Serologic investigation shows the presence of HBsAg and core antibody (anti-HBc) and the absence of hepatitis B surface antibody (anti-HBs). Hepatitis B e antigen may or may not be present.

Extrahepatic manifestations of HBV infection are common in children. HBV is found in up to 20% of cases of membranous glomerulonephropathy in early childhood. A specific flat erythematous nonpruritic papular eruption of the skin of the face and extremities has been described in children with acute or chronic HBV infection. This is called papular acrodermatitis of childhood or Gianotti-Crosti disease.

Cytomegalovirus (CMV) infection must also be considered in the differential diagnosis of unexplained hepatomegaly in older children, usually accompanied by only mild abnormalities in aminotransferase levels. CMV can be isolated from fresh urine or from liver tissue obtained via needle biopsy. Liver histologic findings vary from minimal chronic persistent hepatitis to granulomatous hepatitis.

Non-A, non-B hepatitis accounts for 80% to 95% of posttransfusion hepatitis in North America. The acute infection may be asymptomatic, icteric, or fulminant. Liver enzymes remain abnormal in two thirds of patients for up to 6 months; approximately half of these patients develop chronic liver disease. Since there is no commercially available serologic test as yet for non-A, non-B hepatitis, the diagnosis rests on serologic exclusion of other causes of hepatitis and prior exposure to blood transfusions.

Acquired immune deficiency syndrome (AIDS) secondary to human immunodeficiency virus (HIV) infection frequently results in hepatosplenomegaly, especially in infants. These findings often occur in the setting of failure to thrive, lymphadenopathy, persistent thrush, chronic pulmonary infiltrates, and diarrhea. Biochemical tests of liver function, including hyperbilirubinemia and prolonged prothrombin time (PT), frequently yield abnormal results.

Chronic Active Hepatitis

After the first few months of life, when liver disease is primarily caused by neonatal hepatitis or anatomic aberrations of the biliary system, the leading cause of persistent jaundice and chronic liver disease in the pediatric population is chronic active hepatitis. This clinicopathologic entity is defined by chronic elevations of liver enzyme levels, hepatomegaly, and a histologic lesion of periportal inflammation, piecemeal necrosis, and portal, septal, and intralobular bridging fibrosis or cirrhosis. Known associations include hepatitis B (but not hepatitis A, EBV, and most other viral causes of acute hepatitis), δ hepatitis, non-A, non-B hepatitis, a positive antinuclear antibody (ANA) test, or other markers of autoimmune phenomena, ulcerative colitis, or Crohn disease, Sjögren syndrome, thyroiditis, diabetes, or immunodeficiency syndromes. Girls are affected more often than boys, and patients usually have hepatosplenomegaly and jaundice. A significant proportion of patients will not have had an identifiable episode of acute hepatitis preceding the insidious onset and may show physical stigmata of chronic liver disease, such as spider angiomas, clubbing, ascites, and palmar erythema. Accompanying extrahepatic signs and symptoms may be prominent and may include epistaxis, easy bruising, urticaria, vitiligo, amenorrhea, arthralgia, arthritis, pleural effusions, iridocyclitis, and laboratory evidence of glomerulonephritis and Coombs-positive hemolytic anemia.

Chronic active hepatitis can often be distinguished from the less serious chronic persistent hepatitis only by liver biopsy. There are two major differences: (1) The inflammatory infiltrate is confined to the portal areas of the liver in chronic, persistent hepatitis and does not spread into the lobule. (2) Chronic, persistent hepatitis usually is self-limited and does not progress to either cirrhosis or liver failure. The differential diagnosis is similar to that of chronic active hepatitis except that it includes other viruses, such as CMV or even hepatitis A, which rarely cause chronic active hepatitis.

Drug-Induced Hepatitis

Drugs and toxins can cause severe hepatic damage resulting in hepatomegaly, "hepatitis," cholestasis, jaundice, and even hepatic failure. Some agents produce liver damage in a predictable dose-related fashion, usually starting at a predictable time after exposure to the drug. Other agents are unpredictable, causing an idiosyncratic reaction in only a small proportion of patients taking the drug. The list of drugs that may cause liver injury is vast, but some of the more commonly used agents are erythromycin salts, trimethoprim-sulfamethoxazole, isoniazid, ketoconazole, methotrexate, azathioprine, cyclosporin, halothane, sodium valproate, phenytoin, phenothiazines, acetaminophen, aspirin, hydralazine, anabolic steroids, oral contraceptives, vitamin A, and cimetidine. Erythromycin, anabolic steroids, and phenothiazines cause a predominantly cholestatic injury pattern with clinical jaundice; phenytoin and sulfa drugs can cause hepatocellular necrosis with features of a generalized hypersensitivity reaction, such as fever, arthralgia, rash, lymphadenopathy, and eosinophilia. Fatty infiltration of the liver can be seen with the use of corticosteroids, tetracycline, and also sodium valproate, which has also been associated with hyperammonemia and a Reye-like syndrome. Drugs such as isoniazid used in therapeutic doses predictably cause hepatotoxicity in approximately 10% of patients based on the accelerated rate of metabolism of the drug. Acetaminophen, iron, vitamin A, and salicylates are only toxic when taken in massive overdoses.

The essential clinical feature in establishing the diagnosis is a history of exposure to the drug or toxin, knowledge of the dose ingested, and the timing between ingestion and onset of symptoms. Other possible causes for liver dysfunction must be excluded. The simultaneous appearance of rash, fever, arthralgia, or eosinophilia can be helpful. Disappearance of the symptoms on discontinuation of the drug is strong confirmatory evidence. Most drug-induced hepatic injury is completely reversible with removal of the offending agent.

Wilson Disease

A rare but treatable cause of hepatomegaly in children older than 3 years is Wilson disease, an autosomal recessive disorder characterized by defective biliary copper excretion and accumulation of toxic amounts of copper in the liver, brain, kidney, and cornea. This entity frequently presents during childhood, either as asymptomatic hepatomegaly, insidious cirrhosis, or with biochemical and laboratory features that may mimic chronic active hepatitis. More than 50% of all patients with Wilson disease have symptoms before 15 years of age, and more than 50% have overt hepatic involvement.

The absence of more classic manifestations of the disease, such as tremor, dysarthria, muscular rigidity, Kayser-Fleisher rings in the cornea, and renal tubular disturbance, is common in childhood and should not prohibit consideration of the diagnosis. Neurologic abnormalities associated with Wilson disease in childhood may be subtle, and include deteriorating school performance, behavior problems, clumsiness, and particular difficulty in fine motor skills such as handwriting.

It is important, therefore, for physicians to think of Wilson disease when evaluating hepatomegaly in the school-aged child, since prompt and specific therapy with D-penicillamine affords a favorable prognosis for many and subsequent identification and treatment of asymptomatic homozygote siblings can be accomplished. The best screening tests are an ophthalmologic examination for Kayser-Fleischer rings and measurements of serum ceruloplasmin and 24-hour urinary copper excretion. Often a quantitative measure of liver copper content is necessary for definitive diagnosis.

α_1-Antitrypsin Deficiency

In addition to presenting as a neonatal cholestatic syndrome, α_1-antitrypsin deficiency may be serendipitously discovered later in infancy or childhood during evaluation because of hepatomegaly or failure to thrive, or progress insidiously through anicteric hepatitis to cirrhosis with accompanying splenomegaly and portal hypertension. The incidence of this defect ranges from one in 1,500 live births in Sweden to one in 7,000 in the United States. Only 5% to 15% of homozygote PiZZ individuals will manifest neonatal jaundice, but 25% to 50% will continue to show either clinical or biochemical abnormalities of liver function, suggesting hepatic damage. Diagnosis is made by quantitation of circulating α_1-antitrypsin levels and protease inhibitor (Pi) typing to determine if the patients' phenotype corresponds to PiZZ, the only phenotype definitely associated with liver disease.

Liver transplantation has been successful in many children with cirrhosis due to α_1-antitrypsin deficiency, with conversion to the normal donor phenotype of PiMM and restoration of normal circulating levels of the protein. No other specific treatment exists at this time, but the importance of diagnosis may be in the early institution of monitoring, prevention of exposure to hepatotoxins (alcohol), avoidance of smoking, and identification and counseling of PiMZ heterozygotes.

Other Metabolic Liver Diseases

Many metabolic liver diseases present in the neonatal period or within the first year of life and are accompanied by hepatomegaly, jaundice, and often other signs and symptoms such as vomiting, failure to thrive, seizures, hypotonia, abnormal facies, and neurologic or visual impairment. However, a few of these entities can develop later in childhood, primarily with asymptomatic hepatosplenomegaly, thrombocytopenia, bone pain, or even cirrhosis, severe liver dysfunction, and portal hypertension. Glycogen storage disease, type IV (deficiency of amylo-1, 4-1, 6-transglucosidase–branching enzyme) is a rare cause of early childhood cirrhosis in which neither fasting hypoglycemia nor acidosis is likely to be found. Type VIa and type IX glycogenoses are milder forms, both resulting in hepatomegaly in which the liver fluctuates in size, being enlarged during periods of well-being and often normal during intercurrent illnesses.

Of the sphinogolipidoses, a predominantly visceral form of Gaucher disease without neurologic involvement may develop in late childhood or adolescence, with hepatosplenomegaly and slow progression to cirrhosis. The presence of vacuolated lymphocytes in the peripheral smear, radiologic abnormalities in long bones, and an elevated acid phosphatase level are suggestive of Gaucher disease. Bone marrow examination will show foam cells, and the diagnosis is confirmed by peripheral leukocyte lipid enzyme studies.

Portal Hypertension

Many liver diseases can progress to cirrhosis, and present with primary splenomegaly, hematologic evidence of hypersplenism (thrombocytopenia, neutropenia), upper gastrointestinal bleeding from esophageal and gastric varices, or ascites. At this stage the liver may be of normal size or small, hard, and nodular on palpation. Two causes of portal hypertension without cirrhosis peculiar to the pediatric population are cavernous transformation of the portal vein and congenital hepatic fibrosis. Cavernous transformation of the portal vein usually presents with asymptomatic splenomegaly or upper gastrointestinal bleeding as the initial manifestation, between the ages of 1 and 10 years. The lesion consists of replacement of a stenotic, thrombosed, or fibrous portal vein with a collection of small portoportal recanalized collateral vessels, and is a prehepatic or presinusoidal obstruction. Therefore the liver is usually normal in size or only mildly enlarged, and the determinations of aminotransferase levels, bilirubin levels, and PT are normal. The liver is histologically normal. Although the cause of this condition remains obscure, a history of neonatal illness (respiratory distress syndrome, sepsis, omphalitis, dehydration) or umbilical vein catheterization is obtained in one third of patients. Ultrasonography can facilitate making the diagnosis, and abdominal angiography will give the clearest picture of the portal venous system.

Congenital hepatic fibrosis is an intrahepatic disorder characterized by a pathologic lesion of broad bands of mature connective tissue in portal and periportal distribution. These fibrous bands surround increased numbers of ectatic and dysplastic bile ducts within portal areas. Regenerative nodules are lacking, individual hepatocytes are normal, and cholestasis and inflammatory cells are seldom observed except in a rare variant complicated by bacterial cholangitis. Half the cases occur sporadically; the other half are associated with a family history of portal hypertension, splenomegaly, gastrointestinal bleeding, or renal disease, including polycystic kidney disease in infancy or adulthood. The coexistence of hypertension, mild azotemia, decreased urinary concentrating ability, or abnormal results of intravenous pyelography, with hepatomegaly in the young child, should alert the physician to the diagnosis.

Portal hypertension is regularly accompanied by splenomegaly and gradual reductions in the platelet account to less than 100,000/mm^3 and the white blood cell count to less than 4,000/mm^3. This has been attributed to trapping and sequestration of platelets and white blood cells in the markedly enlarged spleen and is called hypersplenism. Often this finding prompts consideration of a hematologic malignancy as the primary diagnosis and deflects attention from the possibility of primary liver disease, cirrhosis, and portal hypertension.

Intrahepatic Tumors and Space-Occupying Lesions

Benign and malignant intrahepatic tumors are exceedingly rare in childhood, but focal or asymmetric liver enlargement should alert the clinician to this possibility. Vascular lesions (hemangiomas and hemangioendotheliomas) are the most common primary benign tumors of childhood, usually presenting within the first year of life with hepatomegaly with or without cutaneous hemangiomas, or systemic symptoms such as congestive heart failure, petechiae, and thrombocytopenia. Hamartomas contain normal hepatic elements of an embryonic nature in disorderly array, tend to be solid, and present as an abdominal mass, with the only symptoms related to the pressure effects and resulting disturbances in function of neighboring structures. The prevalence of a third benign liver tumor, the highly vascular liver cell adenoma, has increased since the advent of oral contraceptives. Other nontumorous causes of asymmetric liver enlargement or abdominal masses include local abscess, hepatic trauma and resulting parenchymal hemorrhage, solitary or multiple cysts, congenital hepatic fibrosis, echinococcal cysts, and focal nodular hyperplasia.

Hepatoblastoma is the most common primary malignant liver tumor in children. Most lesions present as enlarged livers or masses and are greater than 10 cm in diameter at the time of diagnosis. Hepatocellular carcinoma, seen frequently complicating the later stages of chronic HBV infection or α_1-antitrypsin deficiency in adults, has been reported as early as the age of 7 years in a congenital carrier of HBV, in cirrhosis induced following intravenous hyperalimentation in a young child, and in children requiring long-term anabolic androgen therapy for aplastic anemia.

DATA GATHERING

The clinical disease states and the age at presentation of hepatomegaly are summarized in

Table 38–1. The clinical questions for the primary pediatrician are: Is the apparent hepatomegaly pathologic? If so, is it representative of an acute or chronic process? Does the patient's condition require immediate extensive evaluation or hospitalization? Is evaluation best accomplished by a consultant? After initial screening, can the patient be safely observed over time for any progression in liver abnormality? The preliminary evaluation should include an accurate evaluation of liver size, consistency, and contour as well as a complete history and physical examination.

HISTORY

The history is invaluable in differentiating acute from chronic processes. Careful questioning is essential about exposure to jaundiced or ill persons, possible contact with carriers of HBV or animal vectors of hepatotropic infections, previous blood transfusions, shellfish exposure, intravenous drug use, and travel history. Exposure to potentially hepatotoxic drugs such as acetaminophen, salicylate, phenytoin, sulfonamides, erythromycin, valproic acid, iron, halothane, or vitamin A should be ruled

TABLE 38–1
Clinical Disease States and Age of Presentation of Hepatomegaly*

AGE	CLINICAL DISEASE STATES
Newborn	Intrauterine and intrapartum acquired infection (TORCH, syphilis, other)
	Erythroblastosis fetalis
	Neonatal hepatitis, α_1-antitrypsin, Alagille syndrome
	Biliary atresia
	Congestive heart failure
	Congenital paroxysmal atrial tachycardia
	Sepsis
Infant	Cystic fibrosis
	Metabolic disease: glycogen storage, α_1-antitrypsin deficiency, galactosemia, tyrosinemia, hereditary fructose intolerance, other
	Neonatal hepatitis, hepatitis B
	HIV (human immunodeficiency virus) infection (AIDS)
	Histiocytosis
	Malnutrition
	Tumors (intrinsic, metastatic)
	Cholelithiasis
	Choledochal cyst
Young child (1–6 yr)	Viral hepatitis
	Drug-toxic hepatitis
	Parasitic
	Tumor
	Leukemia, lymphoma
Older child, adolescent	Viral hepatitis
	Drug-toxic hepatitis
	Wilson disease
	Chronic active hepatitis
	Congenital hepatic fibrosis
	Focal nodular hyperplasia, adenoma
	α_1-Antitrypsin deficiency
	Reye syndrome
	Sickle cell anemia
	Cholelithiasis
	Juvenile rheumatoid arthritis, lupus erythematous, sarcoidosis
	Leukemia, lymphoma
	Gonococcal perihepatitis
	Cystic fibrosis
	Diabetes

*Adapted from Walker WA, Mathia RK: *Pediatr Clin North Am* 1975; 22:929.

out, as should poisonings with tetrachlorethanes, carbon tetrachloride, mushrooms (*Amanita phalloides*), phosphorus, or arsenic.

The evolution of symptoms must be accurately understood and the rapidity of their development assessed. Disease of acute onset is more likely to be infectious, toxic, or congestive rather than infiltrative, obstructive, or metabolic (with the exceptions of the acute presentation of galactosemia and hereditary fructose intolerance in infancy or of Wilson disease in later childhood). Characteristic prodromal symptoms facilitate diagnosis. Acute hepatitis associated with EBV is preceded by fever and pharyngitis; hepatitis A infection is commonly associated with a prodrome of nausea, vomiting, anorexia, and fever; and HBV infection usually has a more gradual onset with associated malaise, arthalgia, occasional arthritis, an urticarial or maculopapular rash, or hematuria and proteinuria.

Clues to the cause of more chronic liver disease can be obtained by careful family history, past medical history, and review of systems. Patients and families should be questioned about a history of liver or lung disease, jaundice, gastrointestinal bleeding, neurologic or psychiatric disease, mental retardation, infantile renal disease, and early infant deaths. A search should be made for a medical history of prolonged neonatal jaundice and failure to thrive. Review of systems specifically focuses on dietary intake, chronic diarrhea or vomiting, chronic pulmonary problems, developmental delay, easy bruising, frequent nosebleeds, and pruritus. Pruritus is an important symptom of cholestasis, and its relationship to the appearance of jaundice should be defined. In general, pruritus before jaundice suggests extrahepatic obstruction; jaundice before pruritus is more typical of intrahepatic disease.

PHYSICAL EXAMINATION

A palpable liver is not synonymous with an enlarged liver, particularly in infants or young children. During the first 6 months of life, the palpable edge of the liver extends from 1 to 3 cm below the right costal margin in the midclavicular line. It seldom exceeds 2 cm in the child from 6 months to 4 years of age. In older children the liver edge should not be palpable 1 to 2 cm below the thoracic cage unless the upper edge is percussible below the sixth intercostal space. The normal adult liver extends from the right fifth intercostal space in the midclavicular line to the right costal margin and may descend 1 to 3 cm with deep inspiration. Liver span (height in the right midclavicular line) is obtained by percussing the upper border and palpating the lower border and is the only reliable measure of liver size. Table 38–2 offers guidelines for liver span in children aged 6 months to 20 years. Great variation is present

TABLE 38–2
Expected Liver Span of Infants and Children*

	BOYS		GIRLS	
AGE (YR)	MEAN ESTIMATED LIVER SPAN	STANDARD ERROR OF MEAN	MEAN ESTIMATED LIVER SPAN	STANDARD ERROR OF MEAN
6mo	2.4	2.5	2.8	2.6
1	2.8	2.0	3.1	2.1
2	3.5	1.6	3.6	1.7
3	4.0	1.6	4.0	1.7
4	4.4	1.6	4.3	1.6
5	4.8	1.5	4.5	1.6
6	5.1	1.5	4.8	1.6
8	5.6	1.5	5.1	1.6
10	6.1	1.6	5.4	1.7
12	6.5	1.8	5.6	1.8
14	6.8	2.0	5.8	2.1
16	7.1	2.2	6.0	2.3
18	7.4	2.5	6.1	2.6
20	7.7	2.8	6.3	2.9

*From Lawson EE, Grand RJ, Neff RK, et al: *Am J Dis Child* 1978; 132:475. Used by permission.

in infants, making interpretation difficult. Epigastric palpation revealing a liver edge below the xiphoid may be a good indication of hepatomegaly.

Perception of hepatomegaly is influenced by the relationship between the liver and adjacent structures. Anatomic variations such as narrow costal angle, pectus excavatum, flared costal margins, and Riedel lobe (downward prolongation of the right liver lobe caused by an adhesion to the mesocolon) lead to overestimation or underestimation of liver size based solely on palpation of the lower edge. Other pathologic states such as obstructive lung disease, retroperitoneal mass, perihepatic abscess, or pneumothorax may be associated with apparent hepatic enlargement.

In addition to the size of the liver, evaluation should include shape (symmetry or asymmetry), consistency (soft, firm, rock-hard), presence or absence of tenderness, and surface contour (smooth, irregular, nodular). Asymmetry suggests an intrinsic space-occupying lesion, although a choledochal cyst or hydropic gallbladder can simulate focal enlargement. Firm symmetric hepatomegaly with a rounded edge is consistent with infiltration, fibrosis, or congestion and connotes a more chronic process. Rock-hard hepatomegaly with a sharp, nontender edge favors cirrhosis or malignancy. Diffuse liver tenderness implies generalized capsular distention from acute parenchymal inflammation or congestion. Rubs and bruits should be auscultated to rule out infectious or traumatic inflammation of the liver capsule or intrahepatic vascular tumors.

Serial examinations are important to assess changes in liver size. A rapidly enlarging liver may indicate congestion associated with congestive heart failure or cardiomyopathy, or massive rapid infiltration with fat seen in malnutrition, cystic fibrosis, diabetes mellitus, and metabolic disorders of fatty acid oxidation or branched-chain amino acid oxidation. A rapidly shrinking liver may signal a resolving problem but may also indicate hepatic necrosis and collapse of hepatic parenchymal architecture, especially if accompanied by a rising bilirubin level and PT.

Careful physical examination reveals diagnostic clues in the evaluation of hepatomegaly. Some, such as spider angiomas, clubbing, and gynecomastia, indicate chronicity of liver dysfunction. Rickets or pathologic fractures, multiple ecchymoses, decreased or absent reflexes, and glossitis or gingival inflammation reflect the malabsorption of fat-soluble vitamins and malnutrition that at times accompany chronic cholestatic liver disease. Conjugated hyperbilirubinemia and jaundice characterize extrahepatic biliary tract obstruction and inflammatory hepatitis secondary to drugs, toxins, and infectious agents and are seen in the later stages of many chronic processes (e.g., Wilson disease, chronic active hepatitis, cystic fibrosis). However, jaundice is unusual in infiltrative processes (malignancies), storage diseases, or chronic congestive syndromes. The evaluation of jaundice, especially in the infant, is more fully discussed in chapter 36.

Splenomegaly associated with hepatomegaly is an important sign in the differential diagnosis. In the presence of other symptoms and signs such as fever, malaise, pharyngitis, or adenopathy, splenomegaly suggests acute viral infection such as mononucleosis or CMV. However, in the absence of systemic symptoms, a large spleen connotes chronic liver disease and portal hypertension. Massive enlargement justifies concern over storage diseases such as Gaucher disease or Niemann-Pick disease with stored material in both liver and spleen, or infiltrative disease with stored material in both liver and spleen, or infiltrative disease such as histiocytosis or hematologic malignancy.

Ascites is a manifestation of chronic liver disease secondary to increased portal vein pressure and low circulating serum albumin levels. It is also found in hepatic venous obstruction (Budd-Chiari syndrome), constrictive pericarditis, or congestive heart failure. The cardiopulmonary examination, including a search for jugular vein distention, peripheral edema, pulmonary rales, or a gallop rhythm will help exclude cardiac causes of hepatomegaly or ascites.

Careful mental status examination is particularly important in assessing the severity of liver dysfunction. The early findings of hepatic encephalopathy seen in Reye syndrome, acute severe viral or drug-induced hepatitis, or severe chronic liver disease with cirrhosis are subtle and often missed. These include inversion in the sleep-wake cycle, hypersomnia or insomnia, impaired computation, shortened attention span, euphoria or depression, irritability, impaired handwriting, muscular incoordination, and hyperventilation. In the older patient, asterixis or liver flap should be looked for. Fetor hepaticus, a sweetish odor described as fruity or musty, can occasionally be detected on the breath and urine of such patients.

LABORATORY EVALUATION

Patterns of laboratory abnormalities permit rough classification of liver disease as inflammatory, obstructive, and infiltrative and allow assessment of the extent of compromise of liver function. In conjunction with the physical findings, these tests influence the decisions about hospitalization or referral vs. office follow-up. The following studies should be performed in all infants and children with hepatomegaly: aspartate aminotransferase (AST [SGOT]) level, alanine aminotransferase (ALT [SGOT]) level, total and direct bilirubin levels, PT, partial thromboplastin time (PTT), total protein and albumin levels, alkaline phosphatase level, complete blood cell (CBC) count, sedimentation rate, differential cell count, platelet count, electrolyte levels, glucose level, and blood urea nitrogen (BUN). Inflammatory diseases resulting in hepatocyte necrosis produce dramatic elevations of AST and ALT levels, usually proportional to the extent of the damage. Extreme elevation of AST, greater than 1,000 U/L, implies severe acute viral, drug, or ischemic injury. An elevated alkaline phosphatase level (of confirmed hepatic origin) or γ-glutamyl transpeptidase (GGT) level out of proportion to elevations of aminotransferases indicates an obstructive or infiltrative disorder, the latter being more likely in the absence of jaundice and pruritus. Serum albumin levels and clotting studies more accurately reflect hepatocellular synthetic function and yield abnormal results only after profound liver injury. End-stage liver disease may occur with normal levels of serum enzyme levels and subclinical jaundice but abnormal results of serum albumin levels and clotting studies. Derangements of PT and PTT can occur with severe acute hepatitis, but when found with a low albumin level, more chronic liver disease is suggested. An attempt at correction of PT by parenteral administration of vitamin K is valuable in assessing the severity of hepatocyte synthetic dysfunction.

Hypergammaglobulinemia is characteristic of the entities that cause chronic active hepatitis. The serum IgG is usually elevated above 1.6 g/dL. Non-organ-specific IgG autoantibodies to internal components of cells are present in nearly every case of chronic active hepatitis. These include, in various combinations, antinuclear antibody (ANA), smooth muscle antibody (SMA), and liver/kidney microsomal antibody (also called endoplasmic reticulum antibody).

Depending on the prodromal illness and presenting symptoms and signs, tests for hepatitis A antibody, HBsAg, and infectious mononucleosis (Mono-spot test) should be performed. In a child younger than 3 years of age, the Mono-spot test has a very high false negative rate; thus an EBV titer is the only confirmatory test. If acholic stools, asymmetric enlargement, hepatic bruit, or abdominal mass is present, abdominal ultrasound should be performed, provided an experienced ultrasonographer is available.

Further laboratory evaluation, including technetium 99m sulfur colloid or DISIDA nuclear medicine scans, computed tomography (CT) of the abdomen, endoscopic retrograde cholangiopancreatography (ERCP), percutaneous transhepatic cholangiography (PTC), selective angiography, and closed-needle liver biopsy, should only be performed at referral centers under the direction of trained pediatric gastroenterologists. Urine and blood metabolic screens, serum α_1-antitrypsin level, serum and urinary copper determinations, ophthalmologic slit-lamp examination, ANA titer, immunoglobulin levels, α-fetoprotein, and values for fasting serum bile acids are all part of the evaluation of chronic liver disease undertaken by the consultant.

INDICATIONS FOR CONSULTATION OR REFERRAL

Patients with an enlarged liver can be divided into three groups. The first group manifests signs, symptoms, and laboratory values that dictate immediate hospitalization and consultation:

1. Persistent anorexia or vomiting
2. Mental status changes, hyperventilation, respiratory alkalosis, fetor hepaticus

3. Persistent or deepening jaundice
4. Relapse of initial symptoms after a period of improvement
5. Known toxin or hepatotoxic drug ingestion
6. Prolonged PT
7. Depressed serum albumin and fibrinogen levels
8. Bilirubin >20 mg/dL
9. AST level >2,000 IU
10. Development of ascites
11. Hypoglycemia
12. Leukocytosis and thrombocytopenia

The second group has evidence of chronic liver disease or chronic multisystem disease that requires a more extensive evaluation by a pediatric gastroenterologist but does not call for immediate hospitalization. The third group seems to have benign self-limited acute liver disease or asymptomatic hepatomegaly discovered on physical examination. These children can be observed safely, with monthly physical examinations and determinations of bilirubin, AST, ALT, and GGT levels, until liver size and chemical parameters have normalized, provided they completely recover, remain asymptomatic, liver size does not increase, and there is no development of splenomegaly or stigmata of chronic liver disease. If after 3 months hepatomegaly persists, with or without elevated

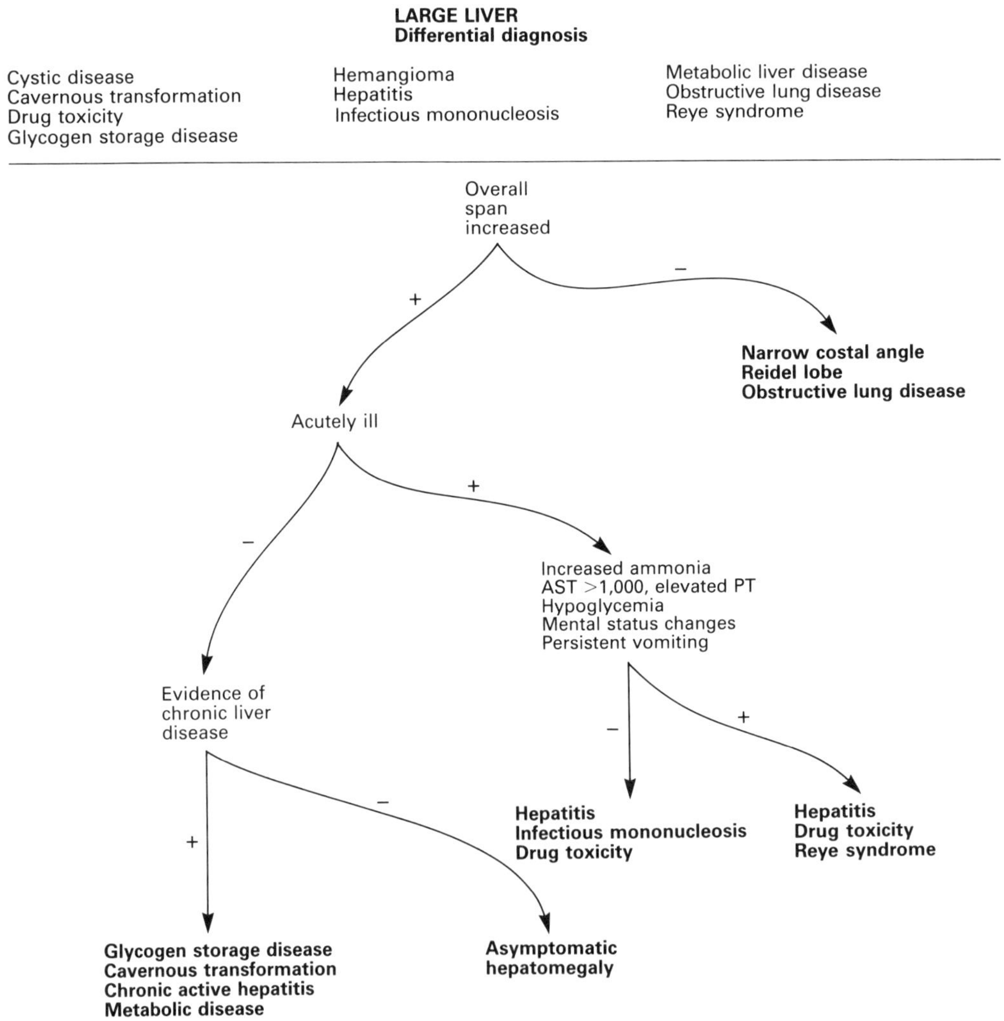

FIG 38–1

Decision tree for differential diagnosis of large liver.

transaminase levels, they should be referred to a consultant for workup of potential chronic liver disease. The decision to observe the patient may be difficult, but in the asymptomatic patient, perhaps recovering from an intercurrent viral illness, good clinical judgment and careful serial follow-up examinations may save the child and the parents many expensive and traumatic procedures.

DISCUSSION OF ALGORITHM

An algorithm for differential diagnosis of hepatomegaly is presented in Figure 38–1. The first task of the evaluation requires the primary care physician to determine if the palpable liver is really enlarged. Next, a physical examination should reveal if there is any irregularity of the liver margins. Patients with asymmetric liver require an abdominal ultrasound study; those with a smooth and large liver require blood tests to detect hepatitis or chronic liver disease. Those with asymptomatic hepatomegaly can be observed for 3 months; if the liver is still large, referral is indicated.

BIBLIOGRAPHY

Balistreri WF, Schubert WK: Liver disease in infancy and childhood, in Schiff L, Schiff ER, (eds): *Diseases of the Liver*. Philadelphia, JB Lippincott Co, 1987.

Dupuy JM, Kostewicz E, Alagille D: Hepatitis B in children. I. Analysis of 80 cases of acute and chronic hepatitis B. *J Pediatr* 1978; 92:17–20.

Maggiore G, Bernard O, Halchouel M, et al: Treatment of chronic active hepatitis in childhood. *J Pediatr* 1984; 104:839–844.

Mowat AP: Liver Disorders in Childhood, ed 2. London, Butterworth, 1987.

Sveger T: Prospective study of children with 1-antitrypsin deficiency: Eight year follow-up. *J Pediatr* 1984; 4:91–94.

Vegnente A, Larcher VF, Mowat AP, et al: Duration of chronic active hepatitis and development of cirrhosis. *Arch Dis Child* 1984; 59:330–335.

39 LARGE SPLEEN

Steven Altschuler, M.D.

Splenomegaly is detected when the spleen is increased two to three times its normal size. A palpable spleen is not always abnormal. Of normal neonates, 15% to 30% will have a palpable spleen on examination. Additionally, a palpable nonenlarged spleen can be found in children with chronic pulmonary disease secondary to increased lung volume and flattening of the diaphragm. Abdominal masses can displace an abnormal spleen to a position below the left costal margin. Massive hepatic enlargement may result in the left hepatic lobe being palpable in the left upper quadrant and mistaken for an enlarged spleen.

Functionally, the spleen plays a role in the body's immune system with the presence of lymphoid tissue and reticuloendothelial cells. Normally, the spleen produces antibodies against blood-borne antigens and acts as a filtering system removing damaged and altered blood elements. The spleen is a vascular organ, anatomically part of the liver's portal circulation. Disturbance to any splenic function or alteration in portal circulation can result in an enlarged spleen.

DIFFERENTIAL DIAGNOSIS

COMMON CAUSES OF LARGE SPLEEN

Trauma
Hematoma
Infection
Bacterial
- Sepsis
- Chronic infection
  - Bacterial endocarditis
  - Chronic pyelonephritis
- Local infection
  - Splenic abscess

Viral
- Congenital
  - TORCH
  - Hepatitis A and B
- Acute
  - Hepatitis A and B
  - Infectious mononucleosis
  - Coxsackievirus

Tuberculosis
Rickettsial
Spirochetal
Parasitic
Allergic-immunologic
Collagen-vascular
- Rheumatoid arthritis
- Systemic lupus erythematosus
- Rheumatic fever

Immune defect
- Severe combined immunodeficiency
- Chronic granulomatous disease
- Hypogammaglobulinemia

Endocrine-metabolic
Anemia
- Iron deficiency

Tumor
Leukemia
Lymphoma
Neuroblastoma
Histiocytosis
Congenital
Hemolytic anemia
- Sickle cell anemia
- Thalassemia
- Hereditary spherocytosis

Cyst
Congenital hepatic fibrosis
Cystic fibrosis
Multiple etiologic
Cirrhosis
Portal vein thrombosis–cavernous transformation
Budd-Chiari syndrome
Storage disease
- Gaucher disease
- Niemann-Pick disease
- Wolman disease
- Mucopolysaccharidoses
- Glycogen storage disease, type IV

DISCUSSION

Detection of splenomegaly requires a careful examination of the left upper abdominal quadrant. Ideally, the examination should be carried out with a patient relaxed in a supine and right lateral decubitus position. If this is impossible, as in the case of a crying infant, palpation during deep inspiration between cries is helpful. Occasionally, percussing along the anterior axillary line will reveal an enlarged spleen when palpation is unsuccessful. Abdominal x-ray film, ultrasound (US), computed tomography (CT), or a Tc-99m sulfur colloid liver-spleen scan can be used to confirm splenomegaly.

Splenomegaly is usually indicative of a systemic illness and rarely the result of a localized process within the spleen. Splenomegaly can result from five basic mechanisms: (1) activation of the immune response as occurs in infection, autoimmune disease, and immune defects; (2) increased filtering of blood-borne elements found in hemolytic anemias; (3) vascular congestion from an obstructed portal venous system in liver disease; (4) proliferative malignancy as occurs in acute leukemias and lymphoma; (5) infiltration of reticuloendothelial cells, as occurs in storage diseases. Extremely rare causes of splenomegaly include cysts and trauma resulting in splenic hematoma or rupture.

In the newborn period, splenomegaly is most commonly found in association with the syndrome of neonatal hepatitis. Neonatal hepatitis can result from many etiologies, infection being the most common. Neonates with infection will classically present with fever, hepatosplenomegaly, and direct hyperbilirubinemia. The congenital TORCH (toxoplasmosis, rubella, cytomegalovirus, herpes virus, and syphilis) and hepatitis A and B infections and bacterial sepsis are the most common causes of splenomegaly. Bacterial sepsis is diagnosed by appropriate culturing of the blood, urine, and spinal fluid. Definite diagnosis of viral infections requires serologic methods; however, the prenatal history and thorough physical examination will strongly suggest these infections. Hepatic dysfunction will be prominent in these disorders. Additional causes of neonatal hepatitis and splenomegaly include metabolic disorders such as α_1-antitrypsin deficiency, galactosemia, cystic fibrosis, and fructosemia. Storage diseases, such as Niemann-Pick disease and Wolman disease, present in later infancy. Neonatal hepatitis must always be differentiated from obstructive lesions of the liver. These include biliary atresia, congenital hepatic fibrosis, infantile polycystic disease, and congenital cirrhosis.

Thus, isolated splenomegaly is rare in the neonatal period. Splenomegaly is usually seen simultaneously with hepatomegaly and direct hyperbilirubinemia. This triad of findings requires immediate workup for etiology and, usually, admission to the hospital.

Splenomegaly in older infants, children, and adolescents usually results from a viral infection. Common viral infections include infectious mononucleosis, hepatitis A, coxsackievirus A5 or A6, and measles. Transient enlargement of the spleen occurs in these cases. Infectious mononucleosis is characterized by fever, easy fatigability, exudative tonsillitis, and diffuse adenopathy in addition to the splenomegaly. Rarely, hepatomegaly and hepatitis will be found. Diagnosis is confirmed by appropriate laboratory studies. A complete blood cell (CBC) count will show an elevated white blood cell count and an absolute lymphocytosis, with a differential cell count revealing greater than 10% atypical lymphocytes. In the patient over 10 years of age, the heterophile titer will be positive. Specific serologic methods, now available for detecting antibody against Epstein-Barr virus, provide the best means of diagnosis.

Infection with hepatitis A virus will classically present with fever, nausea, vomiting, and jaundice as indicated by the presence of scleral icterus. Both splenomegaly and hepatomegaly will be quite evident. Splenomegaly will rarely last longer than 1 to 2 months (see Chapter 36).

Splenomegaly in the older child and adolescent can occur secondary to chronic urinary tract infections. Therefore, the workup of any child with splenomegaly should usually include urinalysis and culture. The older child with heart disease who develops splenomegaly must also have his condition evaluated for bacterial endocarditis. Workup for this should include a CBC count, blood cultures, and echocardiographic examination for evidence of vegetations within the heart. Other less common causes of splenomegaly in children include tuberculosis, fungal infection, rickettsial infection, protozoal infection, and parasitic infections.

Generally, any child with splenomegaly of duration greater than 2 months who has relapsing fevers, associated hepatomegaly, failure to thrive, or evidence of anemia, neutropenia, and thrombocytopenia needs additional workup and possible referral. The presence of anemia, neutropenia, or thrombocytopenia can occur secondary to infiltration of the bone marrow from a malignancy or other infiltrative process or secondary to hypersplenism. Hypersplenism implies increased work by the spleen and removal of normal elements from the bloodstream. Hypersplenism can occur in any process in which the spleen is enlarged or in which there is an increased destruction of bloodborne elements. Common causes of hypersplenism in infancy include hemolytic anemias. In black children, the most common hemolytic anemia is sickle cell disease. Splenomegaly commonly develops within the first year of life.

Infiltrating diseases of bone marrow such as leukemia, neuroblastoma, and storage diseases may also present with evidence of anemia, thrombocytopenia, and neutropenia, in addition to splenomegaly. The basis of the cytopenia in these patients is decreased production of these elements within the bone marrow. The child with a malignancy, may also present with a history of recurrent fevers, failure to thrive, and episodes of bleeding.

Immune defects may be present in the child who has a history of failure to thrive, recurrent infections, and fever in addition to splenomegaly. Common immune defects include severe combined immunodeficiency, chronic granulomatous disease, and hypogammaglobulinemia.

In children of Mediterranean descent, thalassemia is a common hemolytic anemia. Most children with hemolytic anemias will present with hemoglobins in the 7 to 8 g/dl range. Further evaluation of these cases and chronic therapy for these children should be carried out in a center with experience.

Hypersplenism is also a common finding in any condition that affects the liver. The child with a history of neonatal umbilical vein catheterization needs appropriate workup for cavernous transformation of the portal vein. Cavernous transformation of the portal vein results in portal hypertension and secondary splenomegaly. Approximately 25% of these children present between 2 and 5 years of age with splenomegaly. Usually, there is evidence of anemia, thrombocytopenia, and, uncommonly, neutropenia. Diagnosis can usually be made with US. Additional studies that may be considered are a barium swallow study or cautious endoscopy looking for evidence of esophageal varices.

DATA GATHERING

HISTORY

The history items have been mentioned in the discussion. Important information should include history of trauma, exposure to infectious disease, any medical events that predispose to liver disease such as umbilical catheters or familial liver disease such as polycystic disease of the liver and kidney.

PHYSICAL EXAMINATION

Detection of splenomegaly requires a careful examination of the left upper quadrant. Ideally the examination should be carried out with the patient relaxed in a supine and right lateral decubitus position. If the infant is crying, a bottle or pacifier will help to relax the abdominal muscles. Occasionally, percussing along the anterior axillary line will reveal an enlarged spleen when palpation is unsuccessful.

LABORATORY EVALUATION

Laboratory aids will depend on the diagnostic pathway. A CBC count with platelet and reticulocyte count will begin the evaluation of viral illness, infectious mononucleosis, hemolytic anemia, or leukemia. More definitive testing should follow any positive screening. If there is a history of trauma, abdominal US or CT will be helpful. If the liver is also enlarged, hepatitis testing and liver function testing are indicated as the initial assessment.

INDICATIONS FOR CONSULTATION OR REFERRAL

Children with cavernous transformation of the portal vein and hypersplenism have a high instance of upper gastrointestinal bleeding from ruptured varices; thus, when this diagnosis is suspected, referral to an appropriate center is advisable. Other chronic active hepatitis or cirrhosis of undefined etiology can lead to portal hypertension and hypersplenism. As with the patient with cavernous transformation, these patients also require additional workup and referral.

The child with recurrent fevers, arthralgias, and fleeting rashes, in addition to splenomegaly, should have his condition evaluated for evidence of connective tissue disease. Common disorders presenting in childhood include: juvenile rheumatoid arthritis (JRA), rheumatic fever, and systemic lupus erythematosus. Workup of these patients may reveal anemia of chronic disease, an elevated erythrocyte sedimentation rate, and thrombocytosis.

Any child who presents with acute onset of left upper quadrant pain and splenomegaly may have an acute splenic hematoma or rupture. The most common cause of acute splenic rupture or hematoma is trauma. Other less common causes of splenic rupture or hematoma include an infectious etiology. Infectious mononucleosis would be the most common infectious cause encountered by the practitioner. When splenic rupture or hematoma is contemplated, workup and evaluation must be expedited. Effort should be made to have the patient transferred to a center where a pediatric surgeon experienced in surgery of the spleen is available.

DISCUSSION OF ALGORITHM

An algorithm for differential diagnosis of splenomegaly is presented in Figure 39–1. First the patients with an enlarged spleen should be differentiated from those with a normal-sized palpable spleen. The next task in evaluating an enlarged spleen includes detecting the spleen

LARGE SPLEEN
Differential diagnosis

Bacterial endocarditis
Chronic pulmonary disease
Collagen vascular disease
CMV
Cystic fibrosis
Hemolytic anemia
Immune deficiency
Infiltrative disease
Infectious mononucleosis
Leukemia
Neoplasm
Ruptured spleen
Sepsis
Viral syndrome

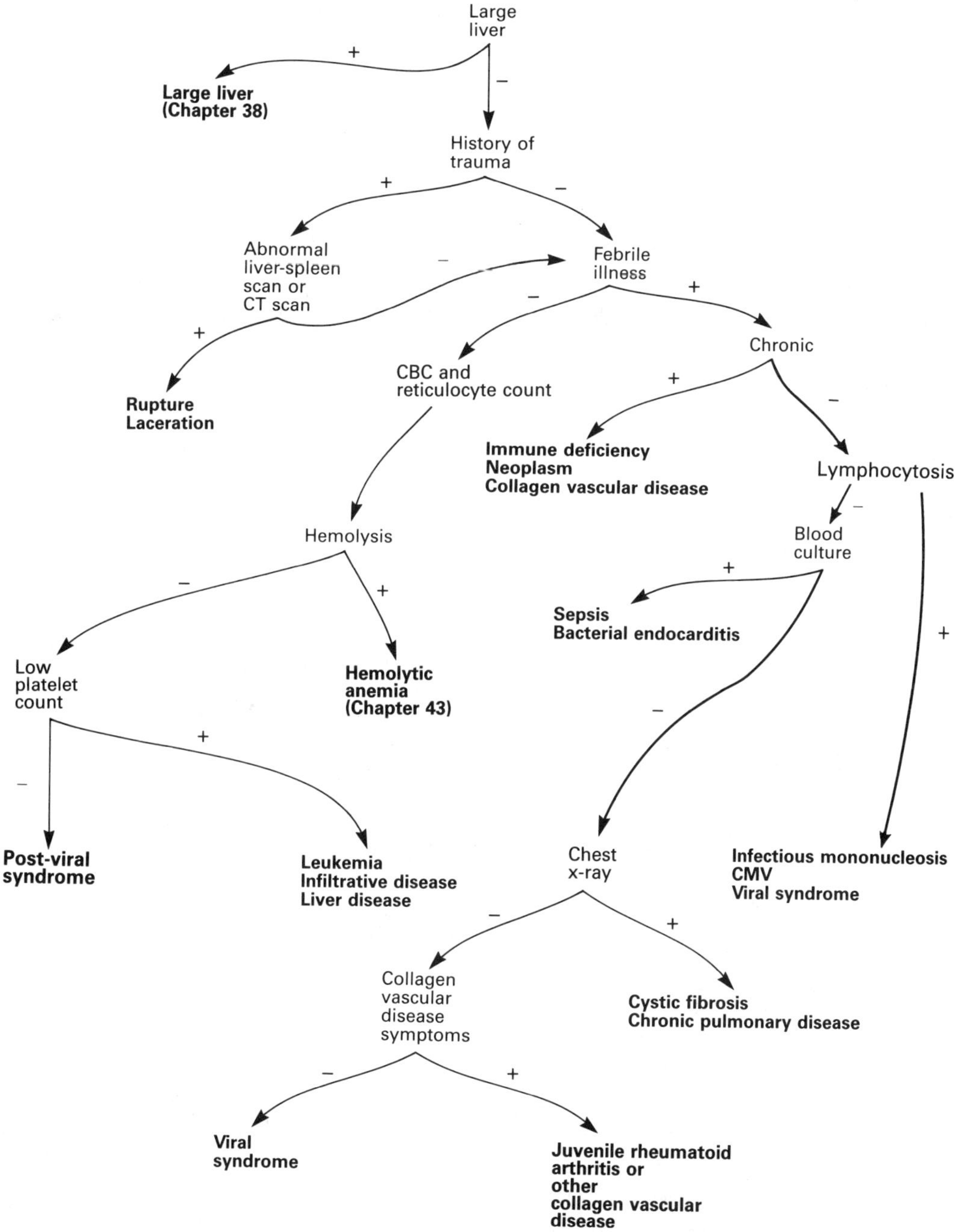

FIG 39–1
Decision tree for differential diagnosis of large spleen.

with an associated large liver, a recent trauma episode, or fever. If these factors are not positive, then anemia should be ruled out. Finally, either a search for rare diseases should be undertaken or, if the patient is making a recovery or looks well, a tentative diagnosis of viral syndrome can be made, and the patient observed for improvement or development of new problems.

BIBLIOGRAPHY

Andres JM, Mathis RK, Walker WA: Liver disease in infants. *J Pediatr* 1977; 90:686–697, 864–880.

Henle G, Henle W, Horwitz CA: Antibodies to Epstein-Barr virus: Associated nuclear antigen in infectious mononucleosis. *J Infect Dis* 1974; 130:231.

Mall JC, Kaiser JA: CT diagnosis of splenic laceration. *AJR* 1980; 134:265.

Mintzer WC, Wang WC: Sickle-cell disease: Pathophysiology and diagnosis. *Pediatr Ann* 1980; 9:287.

Odom LF, Tuburgen DG: Splenomegaly in children. *Postgrad Med* 1979; 65:191.

Perman JA, Grand RJ: Acute and chronic hepatitis in children. *Postgrad Med* 1978; 63:191.

40 LEG PAIN

Andrew Eichenfield, M.D.
Robert Doughty, M.D., Ph.D.

Aches and pains in the extremities are among the commonest childhood complaints. The vast majority of these painful episodes are self-limited and are probably related to minor trauma, physical overexertion, or intercurrent systemic illness. When limb pain becomes recurrent or when a child suddenly develops a limp or is reluctant to bear weight, medical attention is frequently sought. The primary care physician can effectively evaluate such problems through careful questioning of parent and child, thorough physical examination, and a few simple laboratory evaluations. This chapter outlines a differential diagnosis of limb pain in childhood and an approach to its evaluation.

DIFFERENTIAL DIAGNOSIS

COMMON CAUSES OF LEG PAIN

Trauma

Muscle or bone contusion; sprains and strains
Fractures, subluxations, internal derangements
Hyperextensibility
Overuse syndromes: tendonitis
Superficial irritation
Muscle injection
Child abuse

Infection

Osteomyelitis
Septic arthritis
Acute myositis
Neuritis
Pyogenic sacroiliitis and/or diskitis
Lyme disease
Retroperitoneal or pelvic infection

Toxins

Hypervitaminosis A
Acrodynia

Allergic-immunologic

"Postinfectious" arthritides or toxic synovitis
Hypersensitivity vasculitides
Juvenile rheumatoid arthritis
Systemic lupus erythematosus

Dermatomyositis or polymyositis
Polyarteritis nodosa
Inflammatory bowel disease
Kawasaki syndrome
Endocrine-metabolic
Sickle cell disease
Rickets caused by vitamin D deficiency
Renal osteodystrophy
Hypothyroidism
Hyperlipidemias
Fabry disease
Gaucher disease
Tumor
Leukemia and/or lymphoma
Metastatic neuroblastoma
Malignant bone tumors
  Osteogenic sarcoma
  Ewing sarcoma
Benign bone tumors
  Osteoid osteoma
  Benign osteoblastoma
Localized orthopedic
Slipped capital femoral epiphysis
Avascular necrosis (osteochondrosis)
  Legg-Calvé-Perthes disease
  Osgood-Schlatter disease
  Freiberg disease
  Kohler disease
  Sever disease
  Osteochondritis dissecans
Chondromalacia patellae
Multiple etiologic
"Growing pains"
Raynaud phenomenon
Reflex neurovascular dystrophy

DISCUSSION

Trauma.—The most common causes of limb pain in childhood are related to trauma. The major concern will center about differentiating soft-tissue injuries from fractures and subluxations in an anxious child in pain. Children whose extremities are hyperextensible are more prone to soft-tissue injury and may present with recurrent extremity pain and swelling even though there is little supportive history.

"Overuse" syndromes are seen in increasing numbers of school-aged children involved in organized sports activities. Localized tendonitides such as "Little League shoulder" and tennis elbow are not uncommon. Other considerations that may be elucidated through careful history-taking are superficial irritation secondary to muscle injections. Child abuse should be suspected if the degree of injury seems out of proportion to the history or is recurrent.

Infection.—Bacterial infections of the bone or joint present with the acute onset of localized pain associated with fever. *Staphylococcus aureus* is the most common organism in children over the age of 6 years; in younger children *Hemophilus influenzae* is also common. Roentgenograms and bone scans assist in diagnosis. Failure to recognize septic arthritis or osteomyelitis early can have disastrous sequelae. Myalgia associated with viral infections such as influenza and with parasitic infestations should be considered when pain appears to be diffuse and localized to muscle. Herpes zoster can present as exquisite neuritic limb pain that precedes the appearance of vesicles. Pyogenic sacroiliitis and diskitis may present insidiously with back pain that may be referred to the hip. These diagnoses are notoriously difficult to document and may require serial bone scans to be confirmed. Retroperitoneal or pelvic infection may present with hip pain as well; ultrasonography is invaluable in such cases.

Toxins.—Chronic excessive ingestion of vitamin A can result in cortical hyperostosis and limb pain. Children with chronic mercury poisoning suffer from acrodynia that is characterized by excruciating pain in the hands and feet and unusual cutaneous manifestations.

Allergic-Immunologic.—Arthralgia and arthritis may follow bacterial or viral infections, immunizations, or other antigenic stimulation (e.g., drug exposure). Toxic synovitis of the hip is probably the most common form of postinfectious arthritis in childhood. It is usually not associated with fever or systemic illness. Other well-characterized postinfectious syndromes include acute rheumatic fever and the "reactive" arthritides associated with enteric infections and parvovirus. Hypersensitivity vasculitides (i.e., serum sickness, Henoch-Schönlein purpura) are similar pathophysiologically and may present with myalgia, arthralgia, or arthritis.

Rheumatologic diseases that commonly present with inflammatory arthropathy include juvenile rheumatoid arthritis and systemic lupus erythematosus. Muscle pain is frequently the presenting feature of dermatomyositis, polymyositis, and polyarteritis nodosa. Inflammatory bowel disease can be preceded by arthralgia and arthritis for months to years. Kawasaki syndrome can occasionally occur with extremity changes (i.e., indurative edema and extremity pain) as the predominant physical findings.

Endocrine-Metabolic.—Symmetric painful swelling of the hands and feet in a black toddler suggests the hand-foot syndrome of sickle cell disease. The swelling and painful extremity occur mainly in patients under 2 years of age. The changes take about 2 weeks to appear. Extremity pain may be the presenting sign of sickle cell crisis in a previously undiagnosed case.

Bone abnormalities arising from rickets caused by vitamin D deficiency and renal osteodystrophy can lead to bone pain. Hypothyroidism may result in swelling of the extremities, which can be painful.

Tendon xanthomas associated with hyperlipidemias may result in tendonitis of the Achilles tendon and other tendons. The bone lesions of Gaucher disease are frequently symptomatic. Fabry disease "crises" are characterized by severe burning pain in the hands and feet.

Tumor.—Bone pain is a frequent early manifestation of systemic malignancy such as leukemia, lymphoma, and metastatic neuroblastoma. Pain is frequently excruciating, worse at night, and may awaken the child from sleep. Systemic signs may not be appreciated early in the disease course; exquisite night pain should call malignancy to mind.

Tumors of the bone itself present with persistent, increasing pain. Osteogenic and Ewing sarcomas commonly occur in adolescents and are diagnosed radiographically. Benign osseous tumors that can cause pain include osteoid osteoma and osteoblastoma. The former should be suspected when night pain is relieved by aspirin.

Localized Orthopedic Problems.—Slipped capital femoral epiphysis (Fig 40–1) occurs in adolescents from 10 to 17 years of age and results in a painful limp and loss of abduction and internal rotation. Since in all hip disease pain may be referred to the knee, radiographs of the hips should be performed in all patients with knee pain. The child should be hospitalized and placed in traction as soon as the diagnosis is made. Further weight bearing on the hip may result in greater deformity.

Avascular necroses of bone (osteochondroses) result in localized tenderness and pain and are known by their eponyms. Legg-Calvé-Perthes disease involves the femoral head, is more common in boys than girls, and affects younger children than does slipped epiphysis. Other osteochondroses include Osgood-Schlatter disease, affecting the tibial tubercle; Frieberg disease, affecting the second metatarsal head; Kohler disease, affecting the tarsal navicular; Sever disease, affecting the calcaneal apophysis; and osteochondritis dissecans, affecting the femoral condyle.

Chondromalacia patellae is common in adolescent girls and is the result of softening and roughening of the undersurface of the patellar cartilage. This results in an ill-defined aching within the knee. Descending stairs and prolonged knee flexion tends to aggravate the condition. Patellofemoral crepitus may be present on physical examination; occasionally a small effusion may be noted. Compressing the patella against the distal femur with the knee in extension while the patient contracts the quadriceps will usually reproduce the pain. This entity needs to be distinguished from internal derangements of the knee.

Multiple Etiologic.—"Growing pains" is an idiopathic symptom complex that affects 10% to 20% of school-aged children. The pain does not come from growing but from muscle overuse by active children. Pain is intermittent and most frequently affects the lower extremities, most commonly localized deep within the thighs or calves. Joint pain is rare. Symptoms tend to occur at night and may awaken the child from sleep. Growing pains last from 30 minutes to several hours and generally respond to analgesics, massage, and local heat. There are no associated physical or laboratory abnormalities. Although attacks may be precipitated by overexertion, emotional factors may play a role as well.

Raynaud phenomenon, characterized by the triad of pallor, cyanosis, and rubor, is fre-

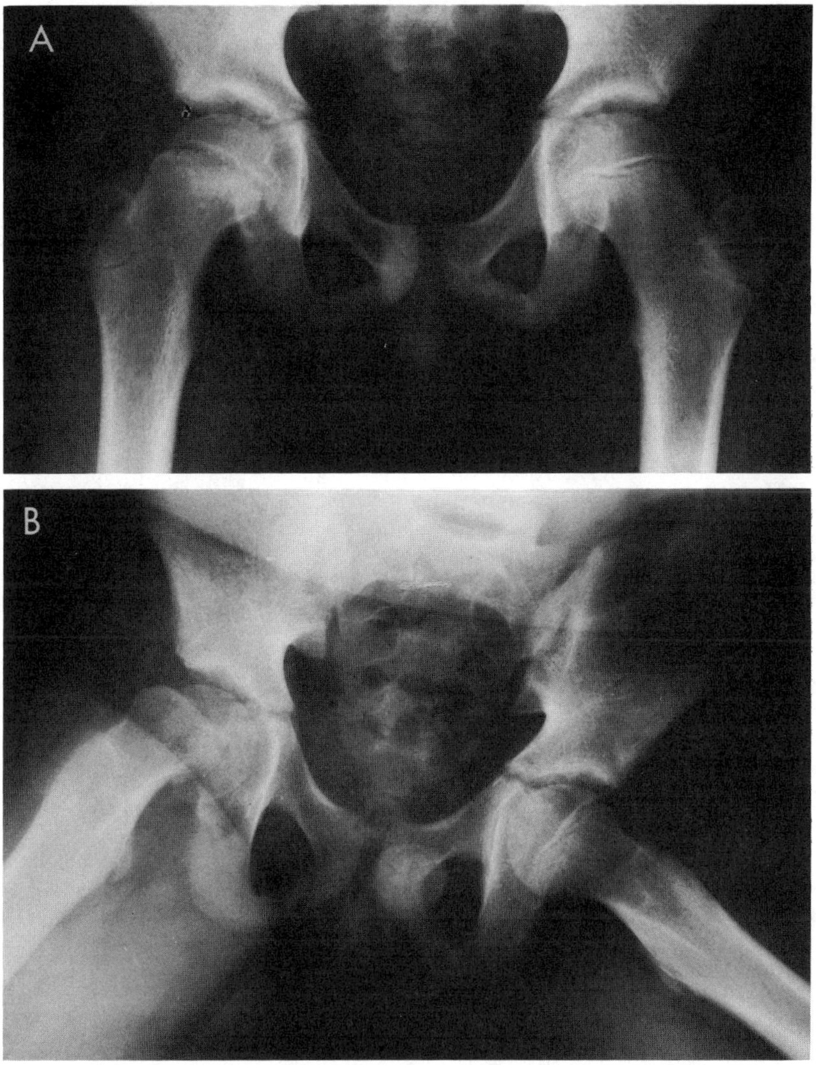

FIG 40–1

Slipped capital femoral epiphysis. **A,** this film of the hip was taken in neutral position and shows asymmetry in the physis of the femoral heads. The right appears wider, and the head appears somewhat medially displaced. In all suspected cases of slipped capital femoral epiphyses, a frog-leg lateral film is taken **(B)**. **B,** frog-leg lateral film shows complete separation of the right femoral head. This will require pinning of the head to the neck. (From Haller JO, Slovis TL: *Introduction to Radiology in Clinical Pediatrics.* Chicago, Year Book Medical Publishers, 1984, p 159. Used by permission.)

quently associated with pain, particularly during the reflex vasodilatation phase on rewarming. The hands and feet can be swollen, reddened, and extremely tender to palpation.

Reflex neurovascular dystrophy as it affects pediatric patients is a disorder characterized by complaints of severe limb pain that follows seemingly trivial trauma. The child refuses to move the affected extremity, setting up a "pain-disuse" cycle, i.e., disuse leads to further pain on attempted movement. With time, vasomotor changes can be seen with mild acrocyanosis, coolness to palpation, and hyperhydrosis. Perceived pain may be exquisite, virtually neuritic in nature. Disuse can result in marked muscle wasting. Many of these children have psychological problems that contribute to the condition. Laboratory investigations fail to reveal evidence of inflammation; bone scanning may show decreased or, less commonly, increased uptake over affected areas and mild osteopenia may be seen on x-ray film. Successful treatment consists of positive reinforcement, graded physical therapy, and judicious use of transcutaneous electronic nerve stimulation, with remarkable relief of pain and return of function in a majority of cases.

DATA GATHERING

HISTORY

Careful history taking is of paramount importance in the evaluation of the child with limb pain. A history of trauma should always be sought, but may be exceedingly difficult to document in the younger child. New hobbies and other physical activities may predispose to tendonitis. A history of "double-jointedness" should be noted. The character of the child's pain may provide clues to diagnosis: the pain of acute bone and joint infection or malignancy is most severe; the pain of the osteochondritides and juvenile arthritis is more aching in nature; the child with reflex neurovascular dystrophy may complain of pain out of proportion to objective physical findings. Night pain that does not allow sleep is suggestive of malignancy unless it is dramatically relieved by aspirin, in which case osteoid osteoma is likely. Night pain that is poorly localized and responds to massage and heat is suggestive of "growing pains." Stiffness, rather than pain, is more characteristic of chronic joint inflammation, particularly when it is worse in the morning. Other significant historical features include the presence of antecedent illness, fever, or malaise that makes infection, malignancy, and collagen-vascular disease more likely considerations.

PHYSICAL EXAMINATION

The general demeanor of the child is noted; a patient who will absolutely not allow an extremity to be touched or moved may very well be suffering from a septic arthritis or osteomyelitis. Other foci of bacterial infection (i.e., otitis, cellulitis) may be present in such cases. Rashes, generalized lymphadenopathy, and hepatosplenomegaly should be noted as markers of systemic inflammation associated with malignancy, chronic infection, or rheumatic disease. The musculoskeletal system is examined in detail, noting any swelling, tenderness, loss of range of motion, or other asymmetry. Subtle muscle wasting may become apparent on careful measurement of the thighs and calves. The gait should be observed while the child is unaware of the examiner and more informally, noting the degree of pain that ambulation elicits.

Hyperextensibility is often associated with recurrent limb pain and swelling (the benign hypermobile joint syndrome of childhood) presumably secondary to trivial trauma of which patient and parent are not aware. Hyperextensibility may be documented by attempting to approximate the thumb to the volar forearm, extending the metacarpophalangeal joints so that they parallel the forearm, and noting hyperextension at the elbows and knees. These may be the only abnormal findings in the child with recurrent pain of seemingly obscure etiology.

LABORATORY EVALUATION

Radiographs are obtained of the affected extremity and, especially in the younger child, of the opposite side for comparison. This will effectively demonstrate fractures, dislocations, and traumatic effusions. In the absence of a clear-cut history of trauma, a complete blood cell (CBC) count and erythrocyte sedimentation rate (ESR) should be obtained. The latter is a sensitive, though nonspecific, screening test for ongoing inflammation. The CBC count is helpful in revealing anemia (suggesting malignancy, chronic disease, hemoglobinopathy), leukocytosis (acute infection or inflammation) or thrombocytopenia (malignancy, severe infection). The peripheral smear is invaluable in suggesting acute infection and malignancy. If fever, systemic signs or symptoms, and/or abnormal laboratory findings are present, then hospitalization should be strongly entertained to rule out bone and/or joint infection, malignancy, or collagen-vascular disease. Radiographs may be helpful in differentiating among these disease states.

In the absence of a history of trauma, systemic illness, or abnormal laboratory findings, the musculoskeletal examination should be carefully repeated over time to reveal any focal abnormalities. Radiographs may prove helpful in revealing occult bone tumors, osteonecrosis, or slipped epiphysis. Orthopedic consultation may prove helpful at this point. If no abnormality can be documented on careful physical examination or x-ray films, then "growing pains" or muscle or tendon strain remain the most likely diagnoses of exclusion. Other entities to be considered, include reflex neurovascular dystrophy and benign hypermobile joint syndrome. Persistent or recurrent complaints should be investigated with repeated physical examination and laboratory investigations as indicated depending on the duration and severity of the problem.

INDICATIONS FOR CONSULTATION OR REFERRAL

The majority of limb pain problems clear with rest, analgesics, and time. When the pain is more severe, when there are symptoms of systemic disease, anemia, or fever, the limb pain requires additional evaluation.

LEG PAIN
Differential diagnosis

Growing pains
Juvenile rheumatoid arthritis (JRA)
Malignancy
Osteochondroses
Osteomyelitis
Rickets
Septic arthritis
Sickle cell anemia
Slipped capital femoral epiphysis
Sprain/strain
Toxic synovitis
Trauma

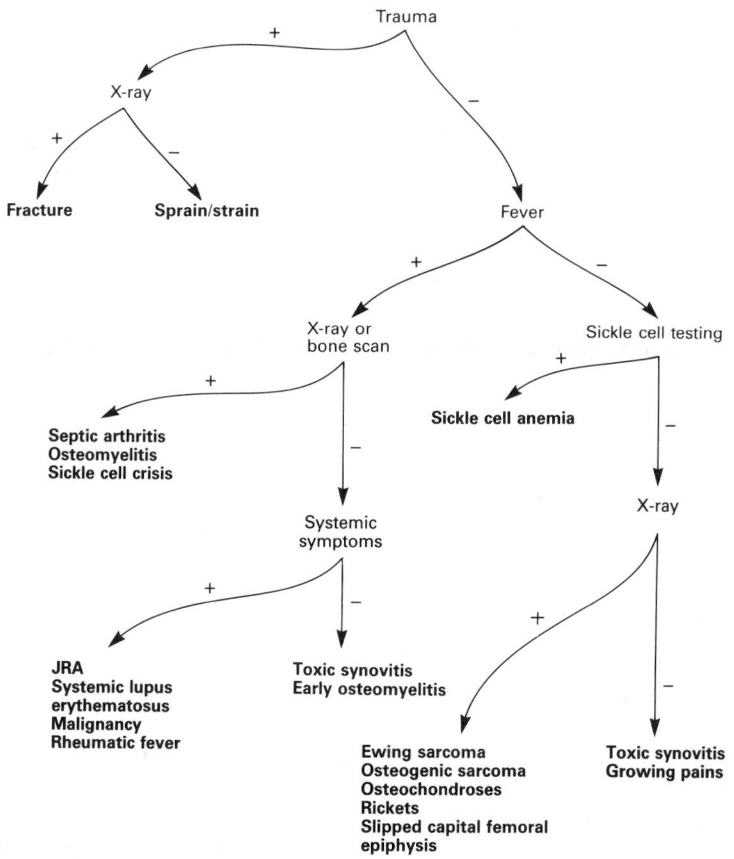

FIG 40–2
Decision tree for differential diagnosis of leg pain.

DISCUSSION OF ALGORITHM

An algorithm for differential diagnosis of limb pain is presented in Figure 40–2. Since trauma is the cause of most limb pain, this possibility should be ruled out first. Next, bone or joint infection should be considered as well as malignancy and rheumatic disease. Bone scans, radiographs, and, possibly, needle aspiration will be needed to explore these possibilities.

For the patient without fever or systemic illness, the muscle overuse syndromes or growing pains need to be considered. If the clinical picture does not fit, then radiographs need to be performed to rule out avascular necrosis, bone tumor, slipped epiphysis, or chondromalacia.

BIBLIOGRAPHY

Bernstein BH, Singsen BH, Kent JT, et al: Reflex neurovascular dystrophy in childhood. *J Pediatr* 1978; 93:211.

Committee on Sports Medicine: *Sports Medicine: Health Care for Young Athletes*. Evanston, American Academy of Pediatrics, 1983.

Gedalia A, Person DA, Brewer EJ, et al: Hypermobility of the joints in juvenile episodic arthritis/arthralgia. *J Pediatr* 1985; 107:873.

Kunnamo I, Kallio P, Pelkonen P, et al: Clinical signs and laboratory findings in the differential diagnosis of arthritis in children. *Am J Dis Child* 1987; 141:34.

Naish JM, Apley J: 'Growing pains': A clinical study of non-arthritic limb pain in children. *Arch Dis Child* 1951; 26:134.

Passo MH: Aches and limb pain. *Pediatr Clin North Am* 1982; 29:209.

Rivara FP, Parish RA, Mueller BA: Extremity injuries in children: predictive value of clinical findings. *Pediatrics* 1986; 78:803.

ter Meuten DC, Majd M: Bone scintigraphy in the evaluation of children with obscure skeletal pain. *Pediatrics* 1987; 79:589.

41 NECK MASSES

William Potsic, M.D.

Children often present to the primary care physician with the complaint of a neck mass. A systematic approach is helpful, combining the history, physical findings, and location to lead to a diagnosis. It must also be remembered that neck masses that are congenital may not be evident until the child is several years old or even a teenager.

DIFFERENTIAL DIAGNOSIS

COMMON CAUSES OF NECK MASSES

Trauma

Hematoma
Sternocleidomastoid fibrosis in neonate

Inflammatory and infection

Lymphadenitis viral
Bacterial lymphadenitis
- *Staphylococcus*
- *Hemophilus influenzae*
- Tuberculosis
- Atypical myobacteria
- Actinomycosis
- Kawasaki syndrome

Sialadenitis, parotitis

Drug-induced

Dilantin-induced lymphoid hyperplasia

Neoplasms

Benign
- Benign salivary gland tumor
- Thyroid tumors

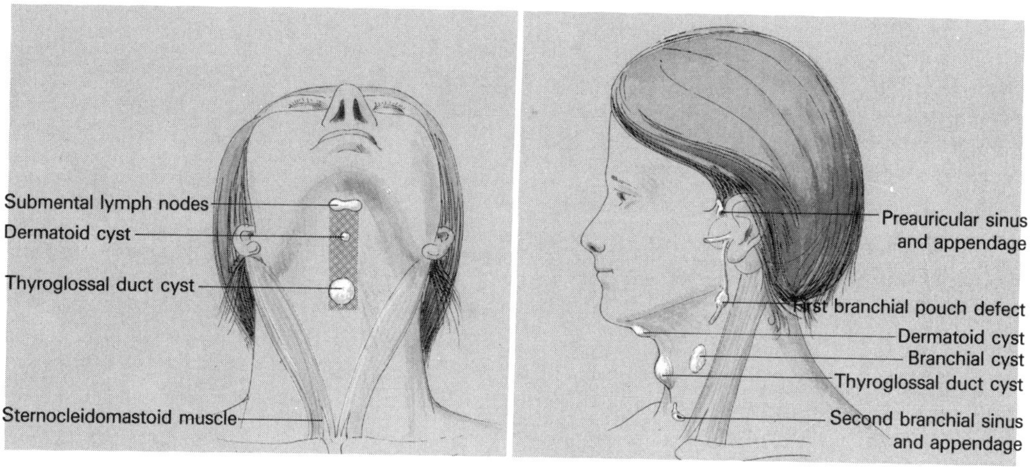

FIG 41–1
Common neck masses and their locations.

- Parathyroid tumors
- Juvenile fibromatosis
- Neurilemoma
- Carotid body tumor
- Lipoma

Malignant

- Lymphoma
- Metastatic carcinoma or sarcoma
- Primary sarcoma
- Salivary gland carcinoma
- Neuroblastoma

Congenital masses

First, second, or third branchial cleft cysts
Thyroglossal duct cyst
Cystic hygroma
Hemangioma
Dermoid cyst
Venous malformation

DISCUSSION

A history of trauma should suggest a hematoma or fibrosis following ecchymosis. Rapidly enlarging masses cause concern about malignancy or an acute inflammatory process. Inflammatory masses are usually painful and a history of recent head and neck infection can be elicited. Soft and fluctuant masses are usually cysts, vascular lesions, or secondary to inflammation. Firm neck masses suggest a possible malignant process. A mobile mass is most often benign but malignant masses as well as recently infected nodes or cysts may become fixed. Any mass associated with regional cranial nerve paralysis should immediately bring to mind a malignant process. Vascular lesions enlarge with crying and salivary lesions may enlarge with eating. Vascular lesions (i.e., hemangioma) may also cause a reddish-blue discoloration of the skin. Presence of cutaneous hemangiomas are often associated with a second lesion in the head and neck including the aerodigestive tract. Café-au-lait spots may be found on the trunk or limbs of patients with neurilemoma.

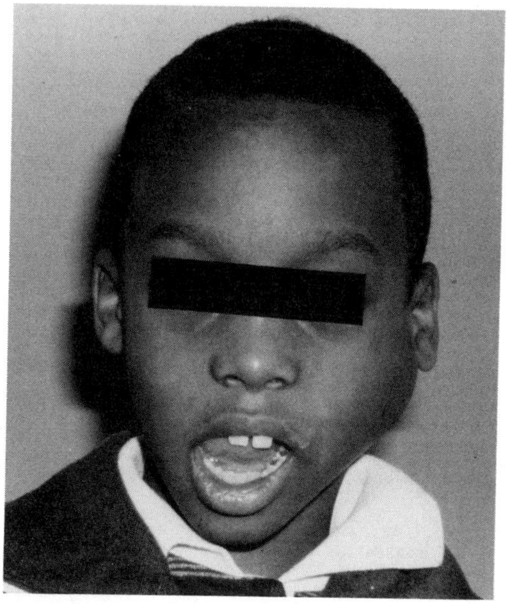

FIG 41–2
Parotid swelling, secondary to parotitis.

Most of the lesions of the neck are inflammatory or infections. The incidence of neck masses is as follows: lymph nodes, 95% (with hyperplastic nodes constituting 90% and cervical adenitis, 10%); congenital masses, 3%; and others, 2% (Fig 41–1).

DATA GATHERING

When a neck mass is evaluated, attention to a careful history and physical examination in conjunction with the location of the mass may lead to the diagnosis. Additional diagnostic studies such as a complete blood cell count, skin tests, and radiographic studies should be obtained. Computed tomography (CT) of the head and neck may be useful to determine the character of a neck mass. If the mass is in or around a salivary gland (Fig 41–2), CT can be combined with sialography to demonstrate the mass.

Inflammatory masses such as cervical adenitis that are painful, erythematous, and fluctuant can be aspirated with a needle. This is both diagnostic for material to culture and to obtain sensitivities, but also drainage aspiration hastens the resolution of the infection. Incision and drainage should be reserved for abscesses that are about to drain spontaneously.

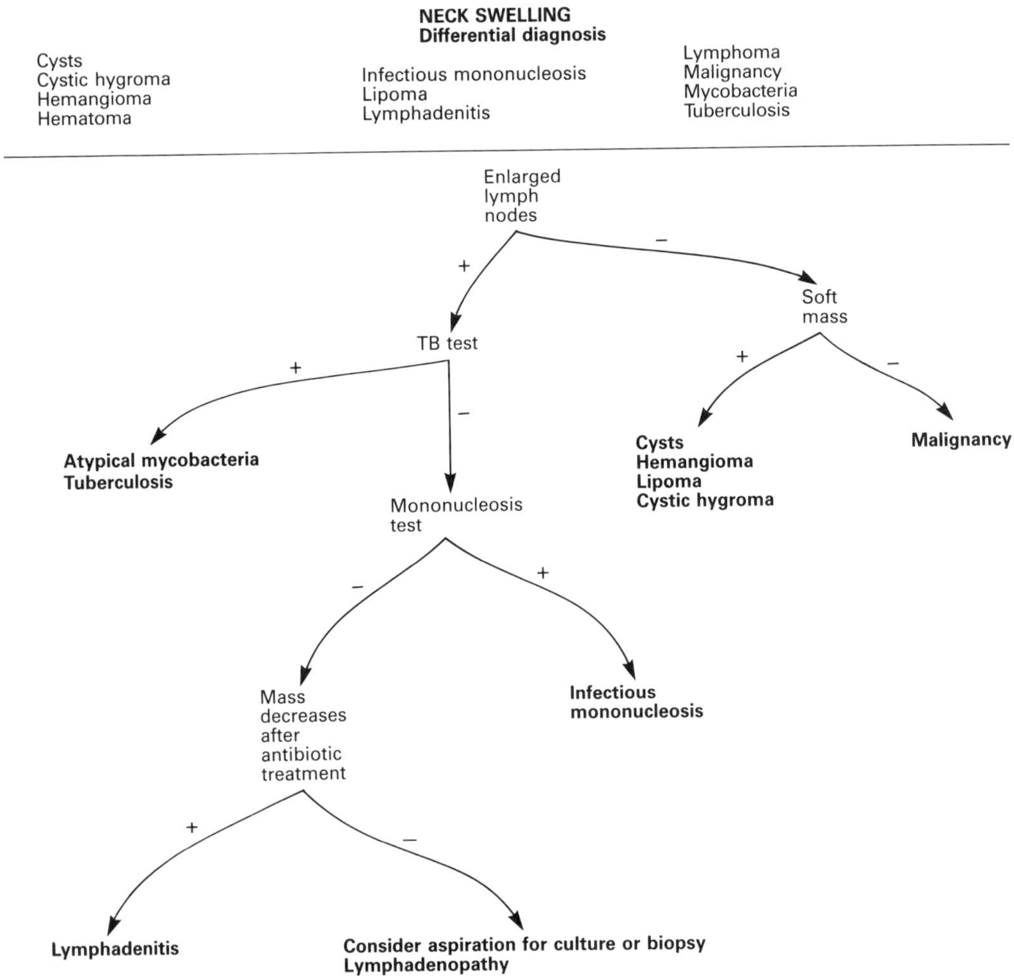

FIG 41–3

Decision tree for differential diagnosis of neck swelling.

INDICATIONS FOR CONSULTATION OR REFERRAL

Neck masses that do not appear to be inflammatory and do not resolve with antibiotic therapy should be evaluated by an otolaryngologist who will perform a complete head and neck examination including pharyngoscopy. Aspiration of masses near or in the salivary glands should be left to an otolaryngology consultant because of the potential for facial nerve injury and paralysis.

DISCUSSION OF ALGORITHM

An algorithm or decision tree for differential diagnosis of neck mass is presented in Figure 41–3. The evaluation of a neck mass initially is determined by the presence or absence of the findings associated with *inflammation*. If the lesion is not tender or erythematous, then the differential diagnosis is focused on congenital structure, hematomas, and neoplastic disease.

The patient with an inflamed, tender mass that does not involve the salivary gland may have the mass evaluated with needle aspiration and receive treatment with antibiotics. It is important to recall that congenital structures such as branchial cleft cysts may present with signs of infection.

BIBLIOGRAPHY

Goepfert H, Lindberg RD, Sinkovics JG, et al: Soft-tissue sarcoma of the head and neck after puberty. *Arch Otolaryngol* 1977; 103:365–368.

Handler S, Raney RB: Management of neoplasms of the head and neck in children. I. Benign tumors. *Head Neck Surg* 1981; 3:395–405.

Lane RJ, Keane WM, Potsic WP: Pediatric infectious cervical lymphadenitis. *Otolaryngol Head Neck Surg* 1980; 88:332–335.

Mair JW: Cervical myobacterial infection. *J Laryngol Otol* 1975; 89:933–939.

Raney R, Handler SD: Management of neoplasms of the head and neck in children. II. Malignant tumors. *Head Neck Surg* 1981; 3:500–507.

Tom LWC, Handler SD, Wetmore RF, et al: The sternocleidomastoid tumor of infancy. *Int J Pediatr Otorhinolaryngol* 1987; 13:245–55.

Torsiglieri AJ, Tom LWC, Ross AJ, et al: Pediatric neck masses: guidelines for evaluation. *Int J Pediatr Otorhinolaryngol* 1988; 16:199–210.

Traggis D: Non-Hodgkin's lymphoma of the head and neck in children. *Arch Otolaryngol* 1976; 102:244–247.

42 NOSEBLEEDS

William Potsic, M.D.

Epistaxis, a common pediatric problem, is intermittent, minor, and usually occurs during the winter when humidity is low and nasal hyperemia is present from viral upper respiratory tract infections. The vast majority of cases of epistaxis are treated at home without medical consultation.

Recurrent epistaxis is reported because it is a frightening experience. Life-threatening epistaxis is rarely a problem in otherwise normal children as it almost always occurs in hospitalized patients with disturbed coagulation from chemotherapy.

DIFFERENTIAL DIAGNOSIS

COMMON CAUSES OF NOSEBLEEDS

Trauma

Dry mucosa (low humidity)

Digital trauma (nose-picking)
Blunt trauma
Foreign body
Postsurgical bleeding
Barotrauma (self-limited hemorrhage into a sinus)

Infection and inflammation

Viral upper respiratory tract infection
Bacterial rhinosinusitis
Rare fungal infection in immune-suppressed host
- Mucormycosis
- *Aspergillus*

Parasitic infection
Nasal syphilis
Allergic rhinosinusitis

Neoplasms

Benign
- Hemangioma (Osler-Weber-Rendu disease)
- Nasopharyngeal angiofibroma
- Nasal granuloma
- Nasal glioma

Malignant
- Rhabdomyosarcoma
- Lymphoma
- Nasopharyngeal carcinoma
- Leukemia

Coagulopathy

Thrombocytopenia
- Idiopathic
- Drug-induced (chemotherapy)

Thrombosthenia
- von Willebrand disease
- Aspirin ingestion
- Hemophilia

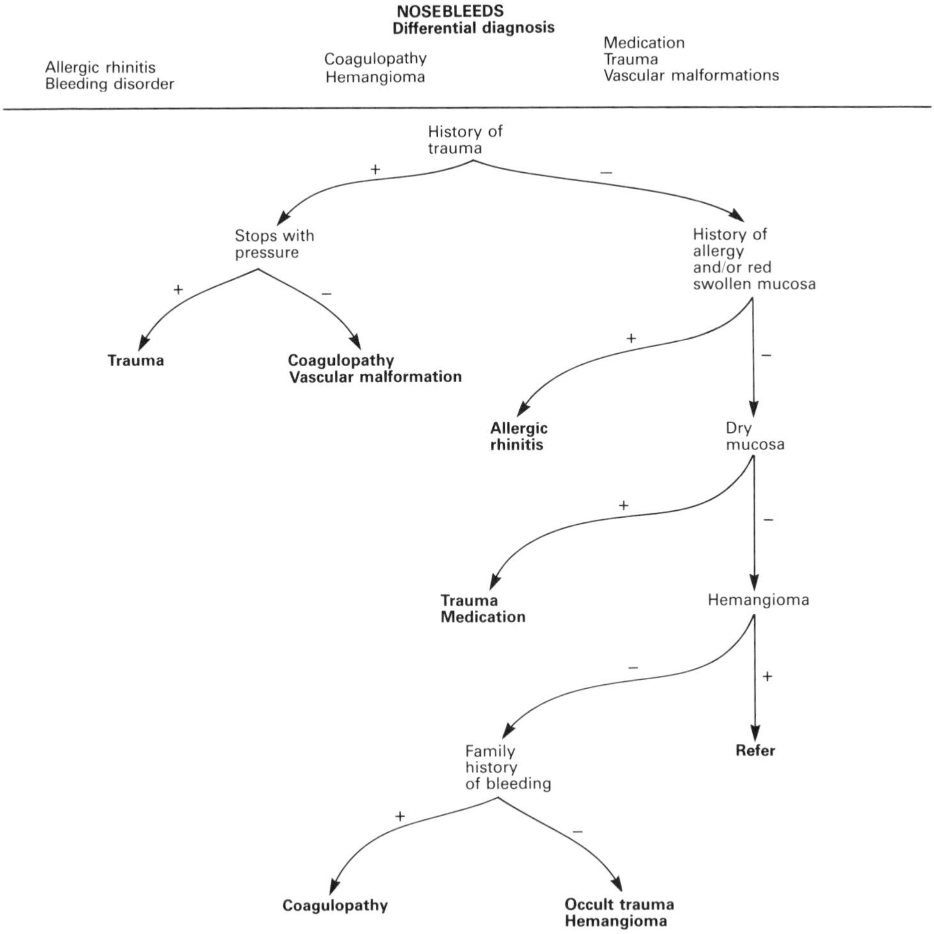

FIG 42–1
Decision tree for differential diagnosis of nosebleeds.

DISCUSSION

An algorithm for differential diagnosis of epistaxis is presented in Figure 42–1. Recurrent epistaxis can be evaluated carefully and healed by the primary care physician. The etiology of the vast majority of recurrent epistaxis is obvious after a history and an examination of the nose. One usually sees an excoriated area with crusted mucus on the anterior septum either on both sides or even more often on the side of the dominant hand (nose-picking).

Most bleeding can usually be stopped with 1½ minutes of digital compression of the soft part of the nose between the index finger and thumb. Nasal vasoconstrictor drops (Neosynephrine or Afrin) or spray can be introduced to shrink the mucosa and assist in attaining hemostasis and direct visualization. The involved area is usually near the mucocutaneous junction of the nose (Little's area). If needed, the excoriated surface can be cauterized by application of silver nitrate with a stick but this is usually not necessary. Occasionally, but rarely, a light packing of the nostril with oxidized cellulose (Surgical or Oxycel) is needed to stop the bleeding (Fig 42–2).

Management of uncomplicated epistaxis is directed toward increasing humidity and reducing trauma. Humidity can be improved at home by placing a humidifier on the heating system and in the child's room. Antibiotic ointment or Vaseline should be applied to the nasal septum bilaterally twice daily by the child. This heals the excoriated areas and gives the child something to do with his finger. Commercially prepared nonprescription saline nasal sprays are also helpful and should be used before bedtime.

DATA GATHERING

HISTORY

The best screening for a coagulopathy is a carefully obtained family history of bleeding problems. Usually inquiry about trauma is unrevealing since the most common trauma is secondary to an exploring finger, which, for social reasons, the child will deny. Rather than asking if he picks his nose, the patient could be asked "which finger do you use"? The physician should perform a general review of systems, in-

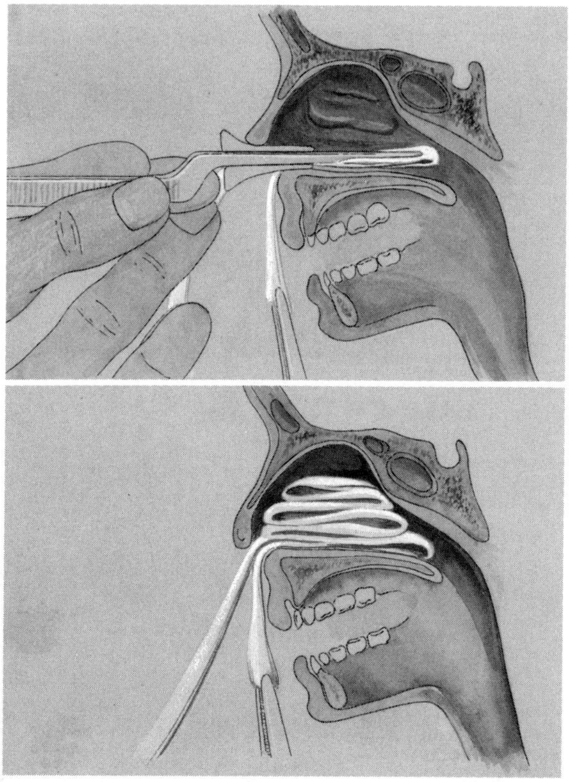

FIG 42–2
Nasal packing technique. One end of packing is held by hemostat, while the remainder is passed through speculum with forceps.

cluding looking for medication that might depress the bone marrow and cause epistaxis and evidence of allergy.

PHYSICAL EXAMINATION

The major task of the physical examination concerns the location of the bleeding so that treatment can be planned if direct pressure to the nose is not successful in stopping the bleeding.

LABORATORY EVALUATION

No laboratory tests are needed if there is no family history of bleeding and direct pressure stops the problem. If a bleeding disorder is suspected, a coagulation profile, including value of platelets, prothrombin time, and partial thromboplastin time should be ordered. On review of the other causes of epistaxis listed earlier, it is apparent that other problems require subspecialist evaluation.

INDICATIONS FOR CONSULTATION OR REFERRAL

Several factors will identify the patient whose condition needs further investigation: (1) if pressure and/or packing do not stop the problem; (2) if there is a family history of bleeding disorder, physical findings of systemic bleeding, or other symptoms of malignancy; (3) when the cause of recurrent epistaxis is found to be more complex, as in a nasal foreign body or Osler-Weber-Rendu syndrome, the child should be referred to an otolaryngologist. However, when the cause of recurrent epistaxis is not identified or is unresponsive to therapy, additional data must be gathered.

BIBLIOGRAPHY

Culbertson MC: Epistaxis, in Bluestone CD, Stool SE (eds): *Pediatric Otolaryngology*, vol 1. Philadelphia, WB Saunders Co, 1983.

Handler SD: Epistaxis, in Gellis S, Kagan B (eds): *Current Pediatric Therapy*, ed 13 (in press).

Juseliush H: Epistaxis: A clinical study of 1,734 patients. *J Laryngol Otol* 1974; 88:317.

Leslie J, Ingram GI: The diagnosis of long-standing bleeding disorders. *Semin Hematol* 1971; 8:140.

Potsic WP, Handler SD: *Primary Care Pediatric Otolaryngology*. New York, Macmillan Publishing Co, 1986.

Potsic WP, Wetmore RF: Pediatric rhinology, in Goldman J (ed): *The Principles and Practices of Rhinology*. New York, John Wiley, 1987, pp 801–845.

Quick AJ: Telangiectasia: Its relationship to the Minot-von Willebrand Syndrome. *Am J Med Sci* 1967; 154:585.

Saunder WH: Septal dermoplasty: Its many uses. *Laryngoscopy* 1970; 80:1342.

Schnelman I: The significance of epistaxis in children. *Pediatrics* 1967; 24:489.

43 PALLOR

Mortimer Poncz, M.D.

Pallor or paleness, a common parental concern, may be related to a child's fair skin or reflect a significant illness in the child that can be elucidated by an orderly diagnostic approach.

Significant pallor in a child often reflects an underlying anemia but may also indicate a circulation disorder. A brief review of the normal physiology of blood flow in the skin will illustrate these other clinical conditions associated with pallor. Besides providing nutrients and removing wastes, blood flow to the skin helps regulate body heat and acts as a blood volume reservoir. When needed, the body can shift blood flow away from the skin to conserve heat or to increase the supply of blood to essential internal organs.

The thin infant with a large surface area and little subcutaneous fat will, in a cool environment, have more vasoconstriction in order to conserve body heat. Pallor secondary to peripheral vasoconstriction can be seen with intravascular volume loss as in acute blood loss, vomiting or diarrhea, and disseminated intravascular coagulopathy (DIC). Atropinic ingestions will also cause peripheral vasoconstriction (and loss of sweating) leading to an inability to dissipate heat. At times, pallor may be due to more than one factor. For example, a child with recurrent severe epistaxis may be pale secondary to the volume of blood lost and peripheral vasoconstriction as well as from anemia due to chronic loss of blood.

DIFFERENTIAL DIAGNOSIS

COMMON CAUSES OF PALLOR

Trauma
Blood loss
Infection
Sepsis
Toxin
Atropine
Lead poisoning
Aplastic anemia
Metabolic-inherited
Iron deficiency
Thalassemia
Sideroblastic anemia
Sickle cell anemia
Hereditary spherocytosis
Glucose-6-phosphate dehydrogenase
(G-6-PD) deficiency
Allergic-immunologic
Autoimmune hemolytic anemia
Goodpasture syndrome
Hemolytic-uremic syndrome
Systemic lupus erythematosus
Tumor
Leukemia
Marrow infiltration
Congenital
Diamond-Blackfan syndrome
Multiple etiologic
Acute blood loss
Anemia of chronic illness
Recurrent blood loss (e.g., menorrhagia)
Pulmonary hemosiderosis

Pallor can also be considered in relationship to the hemoglobin level:

Normal hemoglobin level
Acute intravascular volume loss
Atropine exposure
Cold exposure
- Fair-skinned

Anemia (low hemoglobin level)
Microcytic anemia
- Iron deficiency
- Lead poisoning

- Thalassemia
- Sideroblastic anemia

Normocytic anemia
- Low reticulocyte count
  - Anemia of chronic disease
  - Transient erythroblastopenia of childhood
  - Diamond-Blackfan syndrome
  - Leukemia
  - Marrow infiltration
  - Aplastic anemia
- Elevated reticulocyte count
  - External blood loss
  - Pulmonary hemosiderosis
  - Goodpasture syndrome
  - Intraerythrocyte defects
  - Hemolytic uremic syndrome
  - Sickle cell disease
  - Hereditary spherocytosis
  - G-6-PD deficiency

Macrocytic anemia
- Low reticulocyte count
  - Folate or vitamin B_{12} deficiency
  - Preleukemia
  - Aplastic anemia
  - Diamond-Blackfan syndrome
  - Transient erythroblastopenia of childhood
- Elevated reticulocyte count
  - Hemolytic anemia and high reticulocyte count
  - Autoimmune hemolytic anemia
  - Secondary folate deficiency in hemolytic anemia

DISCUSSION

As can be seen in the previous lists, the differential diagnosis of pallor in childhood covers many aspects of pediatrics. The most common cause of significant pallor in children is iron deficiency anemia. This microcytic hypochromic anemia is most commonly seen in children under the age of 3 years and in adolescent girls. These two periods of life involve rapid growth and poor dietary iron intake. Adolescent girls also might be losing blood from menstruation. Outside of these two age groups, iron deficiency anemia is unusual and an underlying cause of blood loss should be considered if iron deficiency anemia occurs.

Microcytic anemia can also be due to lead poisoning or thalassemia. Thalassemia is found predominantly in populations from the malarial belt of the world (Mediterranean, Africa, and East Asia). Lead poisoning tends to occur in toddlers. The potential risk for environmental exposure to lead should be explored in a child with an unexplained mild microcytic anemia.

Normocytic anemias are also common causes of childhood pallor. These can be divided into those associated with increased blood destruction or blood loss and those associated with decreased blood production. The most common cause of these disorders is increased blood loss. Two caveats need be remembered about blood loss. Initially the hemoglobin level may remain high, only to fall later as volume is replaced. Initial pallor is often due to peripheral vasoconstriction. The second caveat is that significant blood loss can be occult. The child who has recurrent iron deficiency anemia despite adequate iron supplementation may have occult gastrointestinal blood loss (and needs a guaiac stool test) or internal bleeding in a site where iron cannot be efficiently reutilized as in pulmonary hemosiderosis.

Other causes of increased blood destruction leading to a normocytic anemia include autoimmune disorders, disseminated intravascular coagulation (DIC), and intraerythrocytic disorders. The first two may have other signs and symptoms besides pallor, while ethnic background (e.g., sickle cell disease), and family history (e.g., hereditary spherocytosis) may be of value in diagnosing the intracellular disorders.

Normocytic anemias may be due to decreased production. Most often these are secondary to either an anemia of chronic disease or marrow failure. Pallor secondary to decreased red blood cell (RBC) production may be the presenting symptom of a chronic illness. Hypothyroidism and inflammatory bowel disease can present in this fashion, although the latter anemia is often due to a combination of iron deficiency with anemia of chronic disease. Marrow failure in leukemia or aplastic anemia involves other cell lines besides the RBCs, although rarely only the RBC line can be predominantly affected.

Macrocytic anemias are uncommon. Most often the macrocytosis is secondary to a high number of reticulocytes. True macrocytic anemia in childhood is often due to folate or vitamin B_{12} dietary deficiency. A thorough history of the dietary habits of the child (and of the mother in a breast-fed child) may reveal an unusual diet. For example, a 1-year-old baby fed only goat's milk may become folate deficient, while the breast-fed baby of a mother who is a strict vegetarian may become vitamin B_{12} deficient.

DATA GATHERING

HISTORY

In a 1-year-old child, a detailed birth history as well as a dietary history can help in assessing the risk of iron deficiency, while in an adolescent girl the menstrual and dietary histories are of value. The acuteness of the pallor as well as the presence of other symptoms such as fever, weight loss, cough, rash, pica, change in activity, bruising, obvious blood loss, or jaundice can be of value. The child's ethnic background should be obtained as well as a family history for anemia, jaundice, splenectomy, or cholecystectomy. The latter three can be found in families with inherited hemolytic anemias.

PHYSICAL EXAMINATION

The physical examination should first determine whether the child is acutely ill. The presence of tachycardia or postural changes in pulse and blood pressure with pallor might be due to loss of significant intravascular volume, DIC, or severe anemia. If the child is stable, the degree of anemia can roughly be assessed by examining the mucosal surfaces and palmar creases. Other physical signs can suggest the cause of the pallor. Scleral icterus can be present in a hemolytic anemia, pigmented gums in lead ingestion, rales and wheezes in pulmonary hemosiderosis, spooning of nails in iron deficiency, a malar rash in lupus erythematosus, and adenopathy and hepatosplenomegaly in malignancy. Petechiae, bruising, and mouth ulcers can be seen when more than just the erythroid cell line is affected by an underlying disorder.

LABORATORY EVALUATION

The single most important laboratory test to be done in evaluating pallor is the complete blood cell (CBC) count that is preferably done by an electronic counter. The counter not only gives values for hemoglobin and hematocrit but also provides information about RBC size and size distribution (mean corpuscular volume and red cell distribution width, respectively) and the hemoglobin content of the RBC (mean corpuscular hemoglobin and mean corpuscular hemoglobin concentration). In addition, most counters give a platelet count and a white blood cell count. Thus, from a single determination information is provided about whether the child is anemic (for his age) as well as providing accurate additional information that is of significant aid in the differential diagnosis.

A child with a microcytic hypochromic anemia should have a free erythrocyte protoporphyrin (FEP) determination. The test can be done rapidly on a small blood sample. An elevated FEP level can be indicative of iron deficiency, while very high levels suggest lead poisoning. If iron deficiency is confirmed, a 2- to 4-month therapeutic trial of iron at 6 mg of elemental iron per kg per day should be instituted. In most cases further evaluation such as determination of levels of serum ferritin and serum iron and iron-binding capacity can be avoided.

If determination of FEP is normal, a microcytic hypochromic anemia can be due to thalassemia. In β-thalassemia, β-globin peptides are underproduced. Hemoglobin electrophoresis with quantitation of the various hemoglobins present should confirm the diagnosis. α-Thalassemia trait does not have any abnormalities demonstrable on hemoglobin electrophoresis. In a child of appropriate ethnic background with microcytic anemia not due to any other cause, α-thalassemia trait is a diagnosis of exclusion best made by a pediatric hematologist.

Normocytic anemia can be divided into those conditions predominantly due to increased destruction of RBCs with an elevated reticulocyte count and those due to decreased production of RBCs and a low reticulocyte count. In both categories, examination of the blood smear can often lead to a diagnosis. In anemias secondary to a hemolytic process, examination of the smear can show abnormal RBC morphology as, for example, sickle forms, spherocytes, or schistocytes. Decreased platelet numbers can be present along with a hemolytic anemia in lupus erythematosus, hemolytic uremic syndrome (Fig 43–1), and DIC. In normocytic anemias

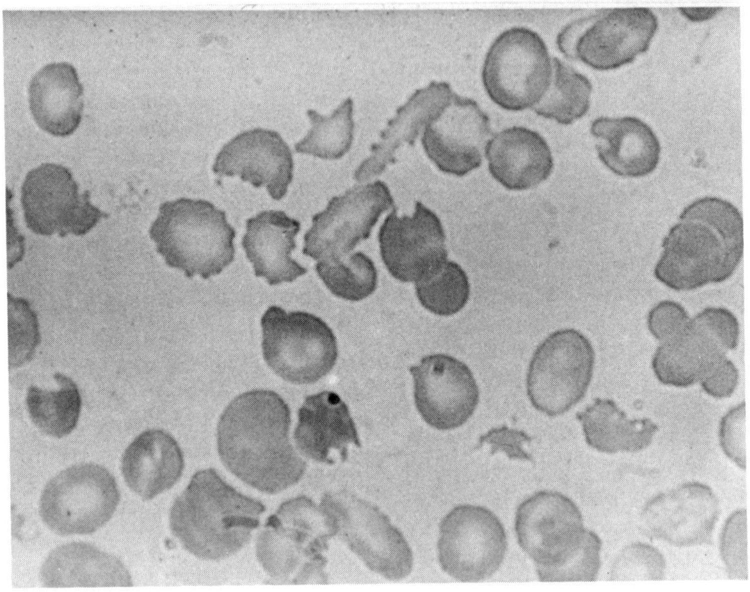

FIG 43–1
Example of RBC abnormalities. Hemolytic uremic syndrome with burr cells, fragmented cells, and a low platelet count.

with low reticulocyte counts, malignant cells (as in leukemias) and increased number of neutrophils with a shift to immature forms or toxic granulation (as in infection) can lead to the proper diagnosis.

If the blood smear is benign and there is a reticulocytosis, the most common diagnosis is acute blood loss. Internal blood sequestration such as pulmonary hemosiderosis can also cause pallor with reticulocytosis and a normal smear. Less commonly, an intraerythrocytic defect can be the cause and needs diagnostic evaluation by a hematologist.

Normocytic anemia with a low reticulocyte count and no abnormality seen on the peripheral smear may be due to an anemia of chronic disease. Determination of values for serum iron and iron binding capacity can be done to support this diagnosis. A bone marrow examination may be required to document a malignant or a congenital or acquired erythrocytic stem cell failure.

Occasionally, children with hemolytic anemias can first present in an aplastic crisis in which the reticulocyte count is low. Often a personal or family history of splenectomy or early cholecystectomy suggestive of a hemolytic anemia can be obtained. Examination of the blood smear can be of diagnostic value. However, repeated evaluation of the patient's condition and his blood smear after recovery from the aplastic crisis may be necessary to confirm the diagnosis.

Rarely, pallor is due to a macrocytic anemia. If the dietary history supports folate or vitamin B_{12} deficiency and serum levels confirm the diagnosis, appropriate supplementation and dietary manipulation can be done. Juvenile pernicious anemia and congenital folate and vitamin B_{12} malabsorptions can occur. Proper evaluation of these and other causes of macrocytic anemia shown in the second list usually requires consultation with the appropriate pediatric subspecialist.

INDICATIONS FOR CONSULTATION OR REFERRAL

The child with pallor should, in general, be hospitalized for one of three reasons: (1) The anemia is associated with congestive heart failure or shock. This is most commonly seen with acute blood loss and secondary hypovolemia. The child with a chronic anemia that has slowly developed can tolerate a very low hemoglobin level without congestive heart failure and rarely requires a blood transfusion. (2) The

PALLOR
Differential diagnosis

Acute blood loss
Aplastic anemia
Vitamin B_{12} deficiency
Chronic illness
Cold exposure
Drug exposure
Folate deficiency
Hemolytic anemia
Hemosiderosis
Iron deficiency
Lead poisoning
Leukemia
Malignancy
Red cell defects
Sideroblastic anemia
Thalassemia

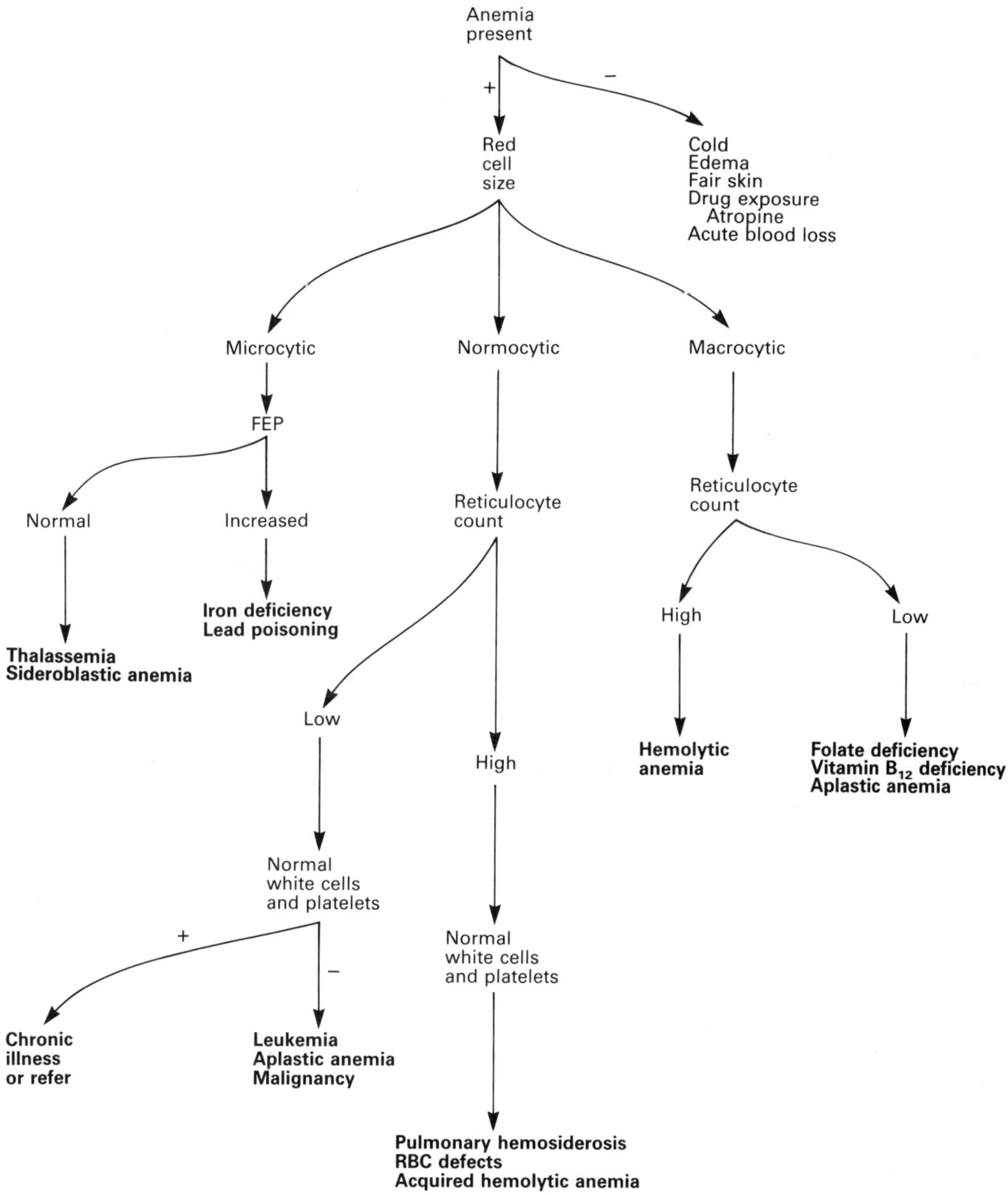

FIG 43–2
Decision tree for differential diagnosis of pallor.

cause of an anemia cannot be easily determined in the office. The majority of cases due to iron-deficiency anemia, thalassemia trait, sickle-cell disease, and a number of other disorders can be diagnosed on the basis of the CBC count and blood smear. However, a number of disorders require specialized tests. (3) An anemia associated with a severe underlying disorder may require hospitalization to confirm and treat the underlying disease.

DISCUSSION OF ALGORITHM

An algorithm for differential diagnosis of pallor is presented in Figure 43–2. In the evaluation of pallor, after documentation that the patient is anemic, the differential diagnosis is dependent upon determination of RBC size. The condition of the patient with microcytic anemia and increased level of FEP is evaluated for iron deficiency and lead poisoning. In these cases, the cause of anemia should be determined. If there is no evidence for a dietary cause, then blood loss from the gastrointestinal tract should be investigated.

Those patients with microcytic anemia and a normal value for FEP should have their conditions evaluated for thalassemia and sideroblastic anemia. If a normocytic or macrocytic anemia is present, further study by reticulocyte count aids in the differential diagnosis.

BIBLIOGRAPHY

Baehner RL (ed): Pediatric hematology. *Pediatr Clin North Am* 1980; 27:217–292, 403–486.

Crosby WH, Herbert V, Forget BG, et al: A new clinical strategy series—the anemias. *Hosp Pract*, vol 15, Feb-June 1980.

Lascari AD (ed): Symposium on pediatric hematology. *Pediatr Clin North Am* 1972; 19:841–906, 1071–1082, 1095–1112.

(Also see references for Chapter 46.)

44 POLYURIA

Andrew M. Tershakovec, M.D.

Parents often complain that their child urinates frequently, which means voiding has increased from its usual pattern. The number of times a child normally urinates varies with age: an infant may urinate 20 or more times a day, whereas an adolescent urinates about five times a day. This developmental progression can make the recognition of what is normal difficult. Frequency in children rarely stems from organic disease.

Polyuria, the production of an abnormally large amount of urine, is an unusual cause of frequency. A child who consistently produces more than 30 mL of urine per kilogram of body weight per day (with a urine specific gravity of less than 1.010 in most cases) has some pathologic condition.

When evaluating urinary frequency, the primary care physician must first determine if true frequency or polyuria exists. Although a wide variety of causes for these conditions are known, an organized approach allows for differentiation between the majority of benign complaints of frequency and those resulting from serious conditions.

DIFFERENTIAL DIAGNOSIS

COMMON CAUSES OF URINARY FREQUENCY

Trauma

Urethral trauma or irritation (masturbation, sexual abuse)

Chemical irritation (bubble bath)

Infection

Cystitis

Urethritis

Endocrine

Neurogenic or central diabetes insipidus
- Idiopathic or familial

Diabetes mellitus

Primary aldosteronism

Adrenogenital syndrome

Bartter syndrome

Catecholamine excess
- Pheochromocytoma
- Neuroblastoma/ganglioneuroblastoma

Multiple etiology

Anxiety/behavioral

Nephrogenic diabetes insipidus
- Familial/idiopathic
- Sickle cell disease
- Medullary cystic kidney disease
- Renal tubular acidosis
- Fanconi syndrome
- Hypokalemia
- Hypercalcemia
- Cystinosis
- Partial urinary tract obstruction/hydronephrosis
- Sarcoidosis

Primary polydipsia

DISCUSSION

Trauma.—Manipulation of the urethra with a variety of instruments may cause irritation and symptoms of frequency. Boys commonly induce irritation with sexual play and exploration. However, sexual abuse should always be considered a possibility in a child with irritative urethritis. Examination of the urethral meatus may show signs of trauma or irritation, which can produce hematuria. Although a child will rarely admit self-manipulation, this may be assumed if other causes are ruled out.

Infection.—Cystitis is one of the most common causes of frequency. The child and parent may note any combination of the classic symptoms of frequency, dysuria, and cloudy, malodorous urine. Viral cystitis presents with gross hematuria and fever and lasts less than a week. Bacterial cystitis may also cause hematuria and systemic signs (e.g., diarrhea, vomiting), but fever is less likely unless the infection has progressed to pyelonephritis (see Chapter 60). *Neisseria gonorrhoeae* (gonococcus), *Chlamydia trachomatis, Ureaplasma urealyticum, Trichomonas vaginalis,* and herpes simplex virus have been identified as causes of urethritis in children. Although a child may be infected by innocent means, culture should be performed in all cases of suspected infectious urethritis and the cause considered to be sexual abuse until proved otherwise.

Endocrine.—The basic types of neurogenic or central diabetes insipidus are familial and acquired. The uncommon familial forms occur as both autosomal dominant and X-linked recessive conditions. Most cases of acquired diabetes insipidus can be attributed to a specific cause, involving some injury to the pituitary region. Intracranial injury (e.g., head trauma, surgery, intracranial hemorrhage, meningitis, encephalitis, tumor) can cause immediate or delayed onset diabetes insipidus through direct injury to the pituitary region or indirectly by increasing intracranial pressure. After the primary process causing the increased pressure or inflammation resolves, most of these cases remit spontaneously. Idiopathic cases of central diabetes insipidus also occur. Care must be exercised in making this diagnosis, because diabetes insipidus may be the first manifestation of an intracranial tumor, preceding the onset of other signs or symptoms by many years. Of the tumors that cause diabetes insipidus, craniopharyngiomas, histiocytomas, and optic gliomas are most often found. The examining physician must carefully evaluate the child for signs of papilledema, optic atrophy, or other neurologic deficits induced by the malignant process. Chemotherapeutic agents may also induce central and nephrogenic diabetes insipidus in children receiving treatment of a malignant disease.

Hyperglycemia associated with diabetes mellitus causes osmotic diuresis, the most frequent cause of true polyuria that the primary care physician will see. The physician should screen all such cases for the classic history of the three "polys" (polyuria, polydipsia, and polyphagia), weight loss, and a family history of diabetes mellitus (see Chapter 57.)

Multiple Etiology.—*Anxiety/Behavioral.*—Anxiety and behavioral problems can cause intermittent frequency, as in the child who is overcome by a need to urinate when entering the physician's examining room. When a child complains of frequency unrelated to a urinary tract infection, the physician should investigate the timing and setting of the complaints and recent changes in the child's life or environment. The cause of most cases of behavioral frequency are thus identified. More obscure cases and those involving more significant psychopathology (such as daytime wetting) may require psychiatric evaluation and intervention. School teachers will attest to the high number of young children who have brief episodes of frequency that is secondary to mild anxiety or pressure.

Nephrogenic Diabetes Insipidus.—By a broad definition of the term, all children with polyuria due to an inadequate renal response to anti-diuretic hormone (ADH) have nephrogenic diabetes insipidus. Familial forms occur, but acquired forms are much more common. Familial nephrogenic diabetes insipidus usually presents in infancy or early childhood. Although it seems to be inherited as an X-linked recessive trait, the disorder has been reported in girls.

Chronic pyelonephritis can significantly alter renal function, especially concentrating ability and tubular reabsorption. Affected children produce a large volume of dilute urine containing increased amounts of electrolytes and glucose.

Drugs may contribute to tubular dysfunction through a variety of mechanisms. Methicillin and related penicillin antibiotics, analgesics, and mercury poisoning can induce interstitial nephritis. Other agents (e.g., diuretics) directly affect tubular function. Such drugs as lithium and demeclocycline interfere with antidiuretic hormone (ADH)–stimulated cyclic adenosine monophosphate production, indirectly influencing tubular function. Drug-induced tubular dysfunction may be transient, as with diuretics, whereas agents such as analgesics and mercury cause permanent dysfunction. Amphotericin can cause permanent tubular dysfunction that is significantly worsened when the agent is administered.

Electrolyte abnormalities may cause tubular dysfunction and polyuria. Hypercalcemia inhibits adenyl cyclase activity, which interferes with the response to ADH. Hypokalemia also alters renal response to ADH. The polyuria independently seen in some conditions (e.g., diabetic ketoacidosis, Bartter syndrome, primary aldosteronism, Fanconi syndrome) may be exacerbated by the hypokalemia also common in these conditions.

Interstitial nephritis may be idiopathic or related to conditions such as autoimmune diseases, ureteral reflux, and drug reactions. Acute cases ordinarily present with oliguria, and progress to polyuria when permanent tubular damage occurs. Hypokalemia and hypercalcemia may also cause interstitial nephritis when allowed to continue for an extended time.

Children with sickle cell disease acquire renal concentrating defects after the age of 5 years. The poorly oxygenated medullary region of the kidney is predisposed to recurrent local sickling crises and infarcts, significantly altering concentrating ability.

Urinary tract obstruction and hydronephrosis also damage renal concentrating ability. Neonates with polyuria should be examined for the presence of posterior urethral valves or other obstructions. It should be noted that significant urinary tract dilatation has been seen in children with polyuria in the absence of any anatomic obstruction.

Medullary cystic kidney disease, an autosomal recessive condition, presents in early childhood with polyuria, renal loss of sodium and calcium, and anemia. Renal failure usually develops over a period of years.

Primary Polydipsia.—The diagnosis of primary polydipsia is sometimes difficult to make. Infants develop primary polydipsia in response to an inappropriate feeding pattern (e.g., the child who displays any signs of distress is given a bottle of water instead of having his or her needs appropriately assessed). In older children, the search for recent changes or disturbances in the child's life may yield precipitating factors for psychogenic polydipsia. Some cases have been reported in households in which family members have true diabetes insipidus or a history of polydipsia or polyuria. A slightly low serum sodium level may be a clue to the diagnosis. Rare cases of primary polydipsia have been reported secondary to a reset osmolality control mechanism. Affected persons continue to be thirsty until serum osmolality drops to their new "normal" value.

Long-standing polyuria dilutes renal medullary solute concentration, limiting the concentrating ability of the otherwise intact kidney and ADH system. As a result, laboratory evaluation of primary polydipsia (e.g., water deprivation test) may not be diagnostic and is potentially dangerous. If considered, this evaluation should be performed in a hospital under carefully monitored conditions.

Miscellaneous.—Conditions causing urinary tract irritability (e.g., bladder masses, renal calculi) can cause urinary tract spasm and feelings of urgency and dysuria.

DATA GATHERING

When evaluating a child because of frequent urination, the primary care physician should initially focus on the most common causes, including frequency associated with anxiety and behavioral factors, urinary tract infection, mucosal irritation, and diabetes mellitus. If indicated, the physician should then study the information obtained for clues leading to a more obscure diagnosis.

HISTORY

As a first step it must be determined if the child has frequency or if the parent misinterpreted a normal pattern of urination. Specifically asking how many times the child goes to the bathroom to urinate (or has episodes of enuresis) per night and estimating the volume produced at each void is useful. Although it is difficult to estimate urinary volume unless the child regularly urinates into a small container, the physician can ask if the urinary stream is strong for a significant length of time. Frequency unrelated to polyuria presents with small volumes of urine and a weak stream. Dysuria, darkened or cloudy urine, hematuria, or a change in odor of the urine are consistent findings of a urinary tract infection.

Variations in the pattern of urination associated with behavior or activity may indicate psychological influences. However, even children with frequency due to organic causes urinate more frequently at times of stress or excitement. Significant changes in the child's life and behavior should be investigated, along with the reaction of the child and family to the problem. Extremes in response may be indicative of psychopathology. For example, if the parent makes a major issue of the child's enuresis there may be a disturbed parent-child relationship.

Children with frequency and fever may have an infection (cystitis or pyelonephritis), but central temperature instability (associated with hypothalamic-pituitary dysfunction) or severe dehydration related to large free water losses in the urine should be considered. The latter occurs in young children with diabetes insipidus who do not have adequate access to drinking water.

Historic evidence of diabetes mellitus should be explored; a history of polyphagia or weight loss and a family history of diabetes mellitus may be diagnostic.

PHYSICAL EXAMINATION

Although the physical examination is rarely diagnostic in cases of frequency, a thorough examination should be performed. Specific attention should be directed toward neurologic defects and the presence of irritation or injury at the urethral meatus.

LABORATORY EVALUATION

The examination begins with urinalysis and urine culture. The urinalysis provides evidence of concentrating ability (specific gravity), diabetes mellitus (glycosuria, ketonuria), urinary tract infection (pyuria, hematuria), urinary tract abnormalities (hematuria), and renal disease (e.g., glycosuria, hematuria, proteinuria). A serum glucose level should be determined if glycosuria is present. Serum electrolyte levels may provide evidence for metabolic, endocrinologic, renal, neurologic, or emotional disease but are not a necessary part of the initial evaluation.

If a child is suspected of having frequency related to polyuria, a 24-hour urine sample can be collected. A child normally produces less than 30 mL of urine per kilogram of body weight per day (2 L in adults). However, because accurate 24-hour samples are difficult to obtain in children, this collection should not be undertaken initially. Measuring the specific gravity of a first morning urine sample is the most useful test to grossly evaluate renal concentrating ability. Normally this sample will have a specific gravity greater than 1.010. It would be unusual to have true polyuria and a urine specific gravity above 1.010.

Any child suspected of having diabetes in-

POLYURIA
Differential Diagnosis

- Anxiety or behavioral
- Cystitis
  - Chemical
  - Viral
- Diabetes mellitus
- Primary polydipsia
- Trauma
- Urethritis
- Urinary tract abnormality

- Nephrogenic diabetes insipidus
  - Familial
  - Idiopathic
  - Sickle cell anemia
  - Renal tubular acidosis
  - Interstitial nephritis
  - Chronic pyelonephritis
  - Hyperkalemia
  - Hypercalcemia
  - Fanconi syndrome
  - Cystinosis

- Neurogenic (central) diabetes insipidus
  - Familial
  - Idiopathic
  - Head trauma or intracranial injury
  - Encephalitis or meningitis
  - Tumor or malignancy

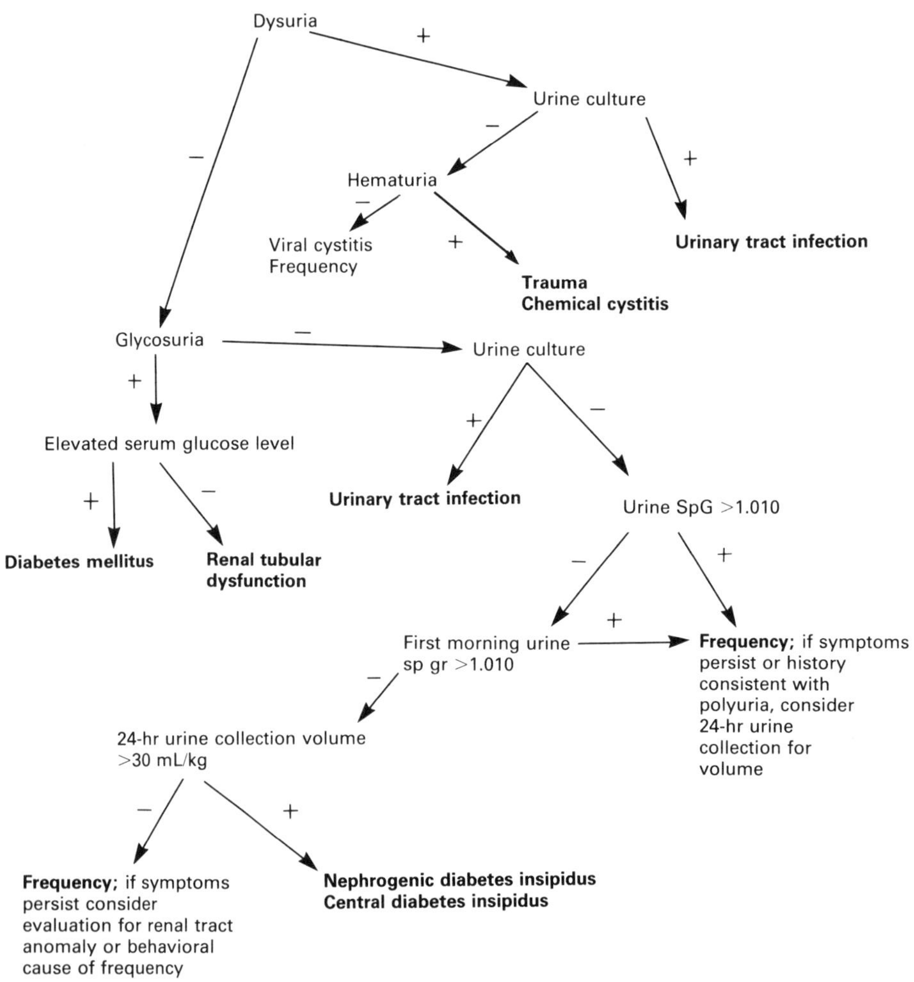

FIG 44–1
Decision tree for differential diagnosis of polyuria.

sipidus must have free access to water at all times. A water deprivation test should be undertaken only in a controlled and monitored environment.

INDICATIONS FOR REFERRAL OR CONSULTATION

The primary care physician should refer children with true polyuria or an inability to concentrate urine for renal or endocrinologic evaluation. Children with frequency unrelated to cystitis or urethritis may have a urinary tract abnormality that is causing bladder irritation. If urinalysis yields normal results, however, most cases of frequency are related to mild trauma, behavior, or anxiety. If the problem persists, urologic or psychologic evaluation may be considered.

DISCUSSION OF ALGORITHM

An algorithm for the differential diagnosis of frequency is presented in Figure 44–1. The outlined method seeks to eliminate common causes of frequency with screening tests that are readily available to primary care physicians. This begins with the evaluation of dysuria.

After eliminating dysuria, the physician should identify those children with glycosuria associated with diabetes mellitus or renal tubular dysfunction. In the absence of glycosuria, the urine sample should be cultured. (Although the steps are listed separately in the flow chart, urinalysis and urine culture should be performed simultaneously as part of the initial evaluation). As a urinary tract infection is being eliminated, the specific gravity of the urine should be evaluated as a gross screen of renal concentrating ability. A first morning urine sample is more indicative of true concentrating ability. Those children with continued dilute urine samples should have a 24-hour urine collection completed. Those with polyuria should then be referred for evaluation of nephrogenic or neurogenic diabetes insipidus. In most cases, children with urine specific gravity above 1.010 do not have polyuria.

With this protocol, most causes of urinary tract infections, diabetes mellitus, and diabetes insipidus will be identified. In the face of persistent signs or symptoms, other causes of frequency, such as trauma, anxiety, and primary polydipsia, should be considered. If the cause is still not evident, more obscure causes involving neurologic, endocrinologic, renal, or psychologic disease may be present.

BIBLIOGRAPHY

Leiken S, Caplan H: Psychogenic polydipsia. *Am J Psychiatry* 1967; 123:1573–1576.

Linshaw M, Hipp T, Gruskin A: Infantile psychogenic water drinking. *J Pediatr* 1974; 85:520–522.

McMillan JA, Nieburg PI, Oski FA: *The Whole Pediatrician Catalog*. Philadelphia, WB Saunders, 1977.

Robertson GL: Differential diagnosis of polyuria. *Ann Rev Med* 1988; 39:425–442.

Siegel N, Gaudio K: Disorders of urine volume in the critically ill child. *Yale J Biol Med* 1984; 57:29–47.

Vaamonde CA: Differential diagnosis of polyuria. *Pediatr Nephrol* 1974; 1:261–175.

45 PURPURA

Mortimer Poncz, M.D.

Purpura or bruising represents the presence of extravasated blood in the superficial layers of the skin. Excessive bruising is a common complaint seen in children in the primary care office and often simply reflects their high level of physical activity. Since purpura might also be the first sign of a significant systemic illness, proper office evaluation is of great importance in the diagnosis and management of the child with purpura.

The integrity of the vascular system depends on three interacting factors: platelets, the plasma coagulation factors, and the vessels and their supporting tissues. Decreased platelet counts or defective platelets can lead to extravasation of blood, resulting in either extensive hemorrhages, called ecchymosis, or fine pinpoint hemorrhages, called petechiae. Defects in the serum coagulation pathway and in the vascular system can also present with ecchymosis, although petechiae are rarely seen.

In addition, to properly understand the pathophysiology of a patient's purpura, the degree and the nature of the trauma suffered by the child must be taken into account. A 1-month-old infant with severe thrombocytopenia may have no ecchymosis or petechiae since the infant spends most of his time quietly in the horizontal position. In contrast, a 2-year-old with the same degree of thrombocytopenia will have multiple bruises as a result of his active lifestyle.

DIFFERENTAL DIAGNOSIS

COMMON CAUSES OF PURPURA

Trauma
Child abuse
Self-inflicted
Easy bruisability
Infection
Congenital infections
AIDS
Toxin
Aspirin exposure
Drug-induced platelet depression
Metabolic-genetic
von Willebrand disease
Hemophilia
Scurvy
Cushing disease
Uremia
Allergic-immunologic
Idiopathic thrombocytopenic purpura
Lupus erythematosus
Henoch-Schönlein purpura
Vasculitis
Tumor
Bone marrow infiltration
Congenital
Kasabach-Merritt syndrome
Thrombocyotopenia, absent radii
Multiple etiologies
Hemolytic-uremic syndrome
Aplastic anemia
Disseminated intravascular coagulation

DISCUSSION

The major cause of excessive unprovoked purpura in childhood is thrombocytopenia. The normal range of platelet counts is 150,000 to 400,000 mm^3. Increased bruising can be seen with a count below 100,000 mm^3, while significant purpura is seen when the count is under 20,000 mm^3. Thrombocytopenia can be due to either increased destruction, decreased production, or both. The most common cause of increased destruction is immune thrombocytopenic purpura (ITP) in which the platelets are destroyed secondary to an autoimmune antiplatelet antibody. Frequently ITP occurs after a viral illness or the taking of certain medications (e.g., a sulfa drug). It must be distinguished from the often more virulent autoimmune disorder, Evans syndrome, in which other hematologic cell lines are involved. Most frequently ITP occurs in younger children. In older children, especially in girls, an autoimmune-based thrombocytopenia may represent the onset of systemic lupus erythematosus (SLE). Hemolytic-uremic syndrome may also present with purpura in which there is increased platelet destruction. Often the purpura and other bleeding manifestations are excessive for the degree of thrombocytopenia reflecting the effect of the uremia on platelet function. In Kasabach-Merritt syndrome increased platelet destruction occurs within a large hemangioma. Disseminated intravascular coagulation (DIC) and hypersplenism represent other medical conditions associated with increased platelet destruction and potential bruising. DIC is a complicated syndrome and the bleeding manifestations not only reflect thrombocytopenia but also consumption of the plasma coagulation factors and loss of vascular integrity.

In neonates, sepsis should be considered whenever thrombocytopenia is present. In an otherwise well newborn, thrombocytopenia may be due to increased destruction secondary to transplacental transmitted antiplatelet antibodies. These can be secondary to an isoimmune disorder, maternal SLE, or maternal ITP. Decreased platelet production can also underlie neonatal purpura. Congenital infections such as cytomegalovirus or rubella can cause thrombocytopenia due to decreased production ("blueberry muffin baby").

AIDS may present with thrombocytopenia. Often the degree of thrombocytopenia is moderate, but can be severe. The decrease in platelets is due to the combination of decreased production of HIV-infected megakaryocytes and an immune-related increased destruction.

In older children, decreased platelet production can be seen when the marrow is infiltrated with another cell line as in leukemias and neuroblastoma. Decreased production can also be seen when there is defective production of megakaryocytes, as can occur following a viral illness or in aplastic anemia and in congenital disorders such as thrombocytopenia absent radii syndrome.

Platelet dysfunction can account for excessive bruising. Platelet counts are normal or near normal. The platelet dysfunction may be intrinsic to the platelet as in the congenital disorder of Bernard-Soulier syndrome, which is also associated with giant platelets. It may be extrinsic to the platelet as in von Willebrand disease, uremia, or aspirin ingestion. In addition, hemophilia and related plasma coagulation factor defects are rare, but can present with purpura.

Vasculitis and other causes of decreased vascular integrity can result in purpura. In Henoch-Schönlein purpura, there can be recurrent waves of purpura often confined to the lower extremities and buttocks. The diagnosis depends on the history, the characteristic rash, and the other signs of arthritis, nephritis, and intestinal vasculitis. Purpura fulminans is a rare, often postviral, vasculitis of the skin, leading to large purpuric areas of skin associated with systemic DIC. Vascular integrity can also be decreased either secondary to scurvy, excessive steroids (Cushing syndrome), or due to an inherited elastic defect (such as that seen in pseudoxanthoma elasticum, osteogenesis imperfecta, and Marfan syndrome).

Unusual trauma may underlie the purpuric lesions in a child. Petechiae limited to the face and chest of a child with a cough may be secondary to the intravascular pressure exerted during the accompanying Valsalva maneuver. Purpuric lesions that are inconsistent with the described trauma or that have an unusual distribution may be secondary to child abuse. Occasionally, in the older child, self-inflicted bruises can be seen. These, too, tend to be associated with an unusual history or physical distribution. Finally, easy bruisability after minor trauma with no underlying disorder is seen fairly frequently in adolescent women. Extensive evaluation of bruises in these patients when there is no other history of a bleeding disorder is not often productive.

DATA GATHERING

HISTORY

A thorough history and physical examination is important for the proper evaluation of purpura.

Questions should be asked concerning the duration, severity, and location of the purpura; recent viral illness; the occurrence of any significant trauma; and the presence of any other symptoms such as fever, weight loss, or joint involvement. A history of drug ingestion (such as aspirin) and a family history of bleeding manifestations or drug abuse by a parent are also important.

PHYSICAL EXAMINATION

Physical examination should be directed first to determining how acutely ill the child is. Next, the location and severity of ecchymosis and petechiae should be noted. The fundi and mucosal surfaces should be examined for hemorrhages. Signs of associated illness such as pallor, adenopathy, or hepatosplenomegaly should be sought.

LABORATORY EVALUATION

In the child with excessive unprovoked purpura, the most important single test is a complete blood cell (CBC) count including a quantitative platelet count and examination of the peripheral smear by experienced personnel. If the platelet count is low and values for the rest of the CBC count and smear are normal, ITP is the most likely diagnosis. However, since other diseases such as leukemia and SLE are still possible, the patient should be referred to a pediatric hematologist for further evaluation of the purpura, possibly including a bone marrow aspiration. If other abnormalities are present on the peripheral blood smear, further appropriate diagnostic workup based on the given abnormality should be done.

When the platelet count is normal, a bleeding time test should be performed. This test should be done by an experienced laboratory so that it can be relied on as a true indicator of both platelet function and vascular integrity. A prolonged bleeding time can be found in von Willebrand disease and in other inherited or acquired defects of platelet function. Several medical disorders affecting subcutaneous tissue such as Cushing syndrome, scurvy, and Marfan syndrome can prolong bleeding time. Usually the history and physical examination will help establish these diagnoses.

INDICATIONS FOR CONSULTATION OR REFERRAL

Purpura associated with a normal platelet count and a normal bleeding time can be seen in Henoch-Schönlein purpura and in inherited or acquired coagulation disorder. Usually the characteristic history and physical examination together with plasma coagulation studies will lead to an appropriate diagnosis. If the evaluation does not produce a diagnosis, consultation with a pediatric hematologist may be of value, as a number of the above-mentioned diagnoses such as von Willebrand disease may require either special laboratory tests or repeat testing.

Patients with purpura associated with low platelet counts should be evaluated within the hospital, often under the care of a pediatric hematologist. The patient with thrombocytopenia may require a bone marrow aspiration depending on the history, physical examination, degree of thrombocytopenia, and the blood count results.

In addition, the child is at increased risk of significant internal bleeding and his condition should be monitored in the hospital at least until the diagnosis is established, the child's clinical course understood, and the parents educated to the potential risks associated with thrombocytopenia.

Patients without thrombocytopenia but with excessive bruising should be hospitalized if there is a possibility of child abuse. In addition, patients with abnormal coagulation studies (either a prolonged bleeding time or prothrombin time or partial thromboplastin time) should have the purpura evaluated by a hematologist. They may or may not need hospitalization depending on the clinical state.

DISCUSSION OF ALGORITHM

An algorithm for differential diagnosis of purpura is presented in Figure 45–1. If the physician evaluating purpura is assured that trauma has not played a significant role, the cause of the condition is frequently defined by use of the platelet count. The child with purpura who has a low platelet count in association with other hematologic abnormalities of the CBC count needs to have the purpura evaluated for malignancy, hemolytic-uremic syndrome, DIC,

PURPURA
Differential diagnosis

Anaphylactoid purpura
Aplastic anemia
Child abuse
Drug reaction
Hemolytic anemia
Hemolytic uremic syndrome
Hemophilia
Hypersplenism
Idiopathic thrombocytopenic purpura (ITP)
Leukemia
Lupus
Malignancy
Trauma
von Willebrand disease

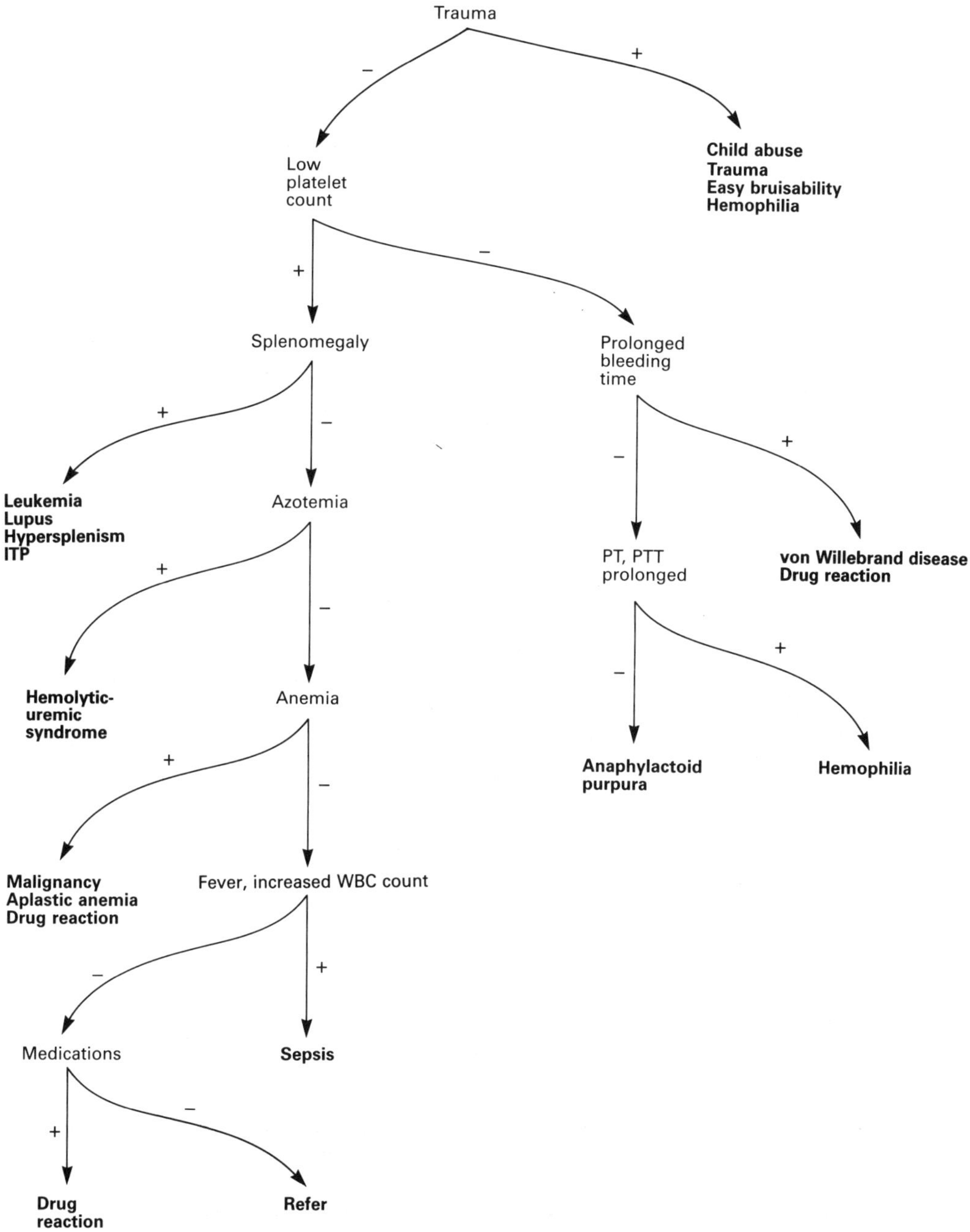

FIG 45–1
Decision tree for differential diagnosis of purpura.

or other conditions listed under differential diagnosis.

If a patient has a low platelet count without other hematolgic abnormalities, ITP is most likely. The patient with a normal platelet count requires determination of bleeding time and other laboratory studies to rule out von Willebrand disease, uremia, or congenital platelet or plasma coagulant dysfunction.

BIBLIOGRAPHY

Baehner RL (ed): Pediatric hematology. *Pediatr Clin North Am* 1981; 27:309–344.

Lascari AD (ed): Symposium on pediatric hematology. *Pediatr Clin North Am* 1972; 19:1009–1070.

46 RED EYE

Stephen D. Kronwith, M.D., Ph.D., and
David B. Schaffer, M.D.

The term "red eye" is used to denote a myriad of ocular entities, including trauma, infection, allergy, and underlying systemic processes. Parents of children with discoloration, swelling, itching, pain, excessive tearing, photophobia, decreased vision, and frank trauma all seek medical advice and help. The purpose of this chapter is to help the clinician recognize and identify the specific location and probable cause of the eye disorder, understand its immediate significance and potential complications, institute appropriate initial and even definitive therapy, or refer the patient to an ophthalmologist for more involved diagnostic techniques and treatment.

DIFFERENTIAL DIAGNOSIS

COMMON CAUSES OF RED EYE

Ocular adnexa

Trauma

- Blunt
  - Lid swelling or discoloration
    - Hyphema
    - Ruptured globe
    - Iris or lens abnormality
    - Retinal abnormality
    - Orbital bone fracture
    - Suspected child abuse or neglect
- Sharp
  - Lacerations of lid
  - Underlying lacerations of globe

Inflammation

- Localized
  - Blepharitis
  - Hordeolums and chalazions
  - Dacryocystitis
- Generalized
  - Periorbital (preseptal) cellulitis
  - Orbital cellulitis
- Other
  - Viral
  - Allergic
    - Insect bites
    - Contact dermatitis
  - Systemic
  - Reactive blepharospasm

Conjunctiva

Trauma

Subconjunctival hemorrhage

Foreign body

Inflammation

Conjunctivitis

Neonatal (ophthalmia neonatorum)
  Chemical
  Bacterial
  Viral
  Obstructed nasolacrimal duct
Older children
  Bacterial
  Viral
  Allergic
    Vernal catarrh
    Limbal catarrh
Systemic reaction
Phlyctenular
Other systemic disease
Physical or chemical irritant

Cornea
Trauma
Foreign body
Abrasions
Physical or chemical irritant
Inflammation
Ulceration
Keratitis

Anterior segment
Trauma
Inflammation

Posterior eye
Decreased visual acuity
Abnormal findings on ophthalmoscopy

DISCUSSION

Ocular Adnexa (Orbit and Lids).—Nonpenetrating trauma to the ocular adnexa may belie its seriousness. Under a swollen, intact but discolored, traumatized lid could be a ruptured globe, painful iridocyclitis, anterior chamber bleeding (hyphema), retinal detachment, or a blowout fracture of one of the orbital bones. If the eye is intact, visual acuity and pupillary size and reactivity should be compared with those of the uninjured eye. Patients who have obviously decreased vision, a hyphema, an unresponsive pupil, restricted motility, inferior orbital skin anesthesia, periorbital crepitus, or lack of visualization of a normal posterior fundus on ophthalmoscopy should be referred.

If there is even suspicion that the integrity of the brain or the eye has been violated, the child should not ingest any food or liquids and should be transported for definitive care. Both eyes should be taped closed under soft eye pads, with a protective hard shield over the injured eye.

Inflammatory discoloration and swelling of the adnexal structures can also denote trivial or significant disease. Scaling at the lid margins, styes (hordeolums) or chalazions, dacryocystitis, allergic reactions, and superficial or deep orbital cellulitis are collectively more common adnexal problems than is trauma.

Inflammation of the lid margins (blepharitis) frequently is seen in the pediatric population. The typical findings consist of waxy scaling at the base of the lashes (Fig 46–1); red, irritated, slightly swollen lid margins; loss of lashes; and even lid margin ulceration in the more severe forms. Mild to moderate conjunctivitis is common, and occasionally there is corneal involvement (keratitis). Treatment consists of daily cleansing of the lid margins with baby shampoo and warm water. If needed, an antimicrobial ophthalmic ointment is also massaged onto the lid margins. Once resolved, the medication is titrated to the least frequent application that keeps the condition quiescent. Recurrence is common.

Rarely, pediculosis can mimic seborrheic blepharitis. With proper magnification, visualization of black lice eggs attached to the cilia confirms the diagnosis. Manual removal of the lice and their eggs is required.

Styes are acute, often painful, localized bacterial infections arising in either a gland of the lid's fibrous tarsal plate or in the glands located around the eyelashes. The causal organisms are usually *Staphylococcus aureus* or nonhemolytic *Streptococcus*. Most styes cause erythematous swelling of the involved lid, with a localized tender mass that may point, rupture, and drain through the palpebral conjunctival surface, at the lid margin, or through the external skin (Fig 46–2). Treatment consists of frequent application of hot compresses.

The oil secreted by each meibomian gland may break out of the gland into the lid tissue and produce a granuloma called a chalazion. Although acute meibomitis is painful, the chronic granulomatous chalazion slowly undergoes painless enlargement and can be palpated as a firm, nonmovable nodule, often presenting on the palpebral surface of the lid as a

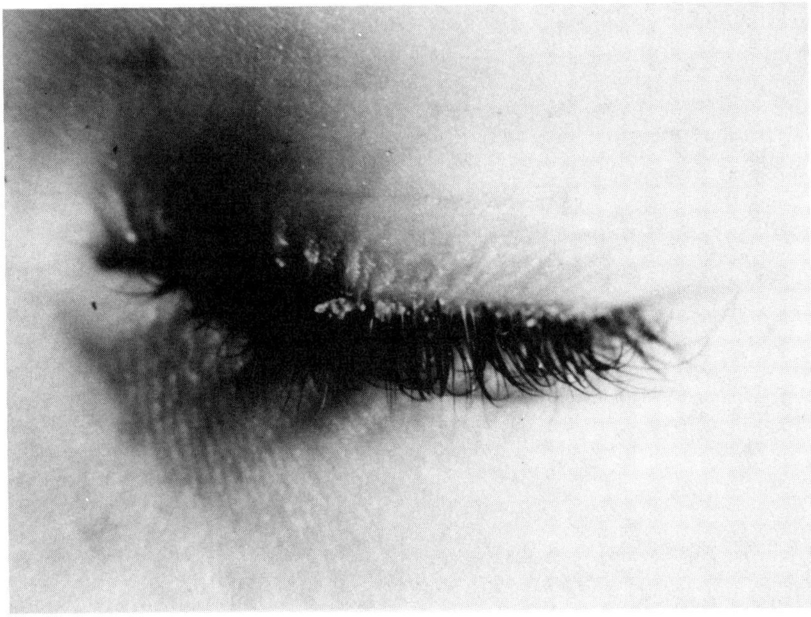

FIG 46–1
Encrustations at base of lashes and wrinkling of the eyelid in blepharitis.

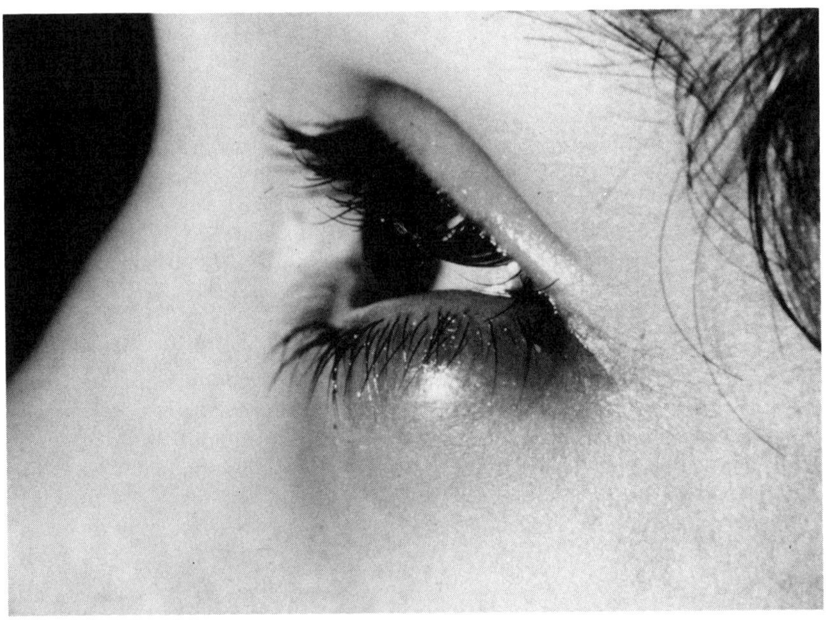

FIG 46–2
External hordeolum (stye) of the inferior lid just before spontaneous rupture and drainage.

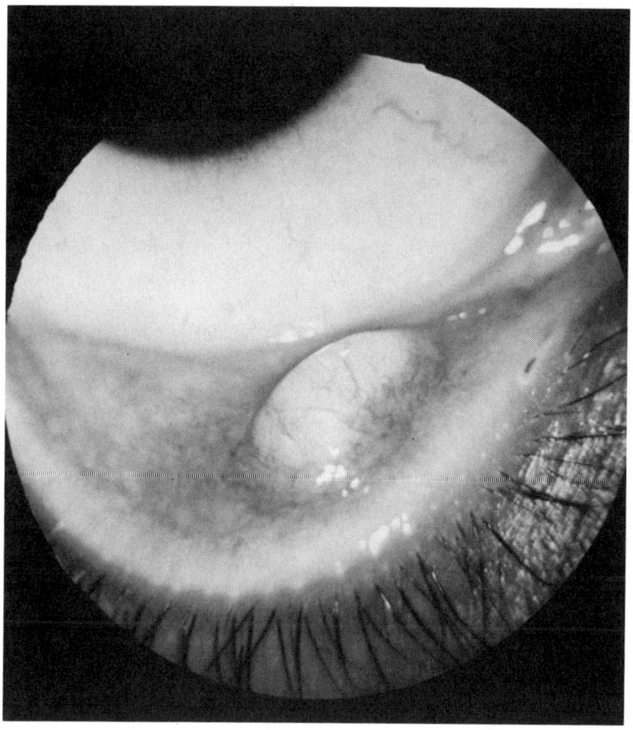

FIG 46–3
Chronic chalazion; note the large, raised yellowish granuloma on the internal aspect of the lower eyelid.

yellowish-white area (Fig 46–3). In time, large chalazions may produce significant astigmatism because of chronic pressure on the cornea. Although hot compresses decrease its size, a chalazion usually must be surgically incised.

In neonates and very young infants, acute dacryocystitis can also produce inflamed, tender, localized swelling in the lid, typically at the inferonasal border of the bony orbital rim (Fig 46–4). These abscesses can be associated

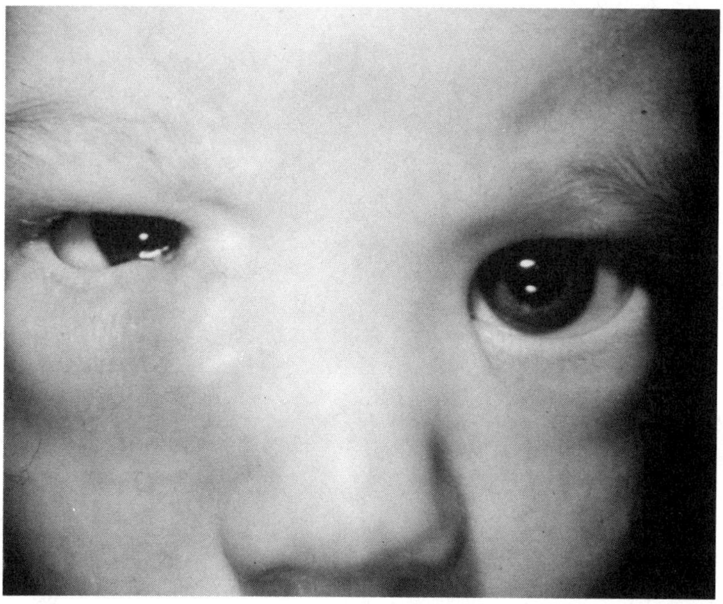

FIG 46–4
Swollen, inflammed lacrimal sac (dacryocystitis) at the inferonasal border of the orbit. (Courtesy of Dr. James A. Katowitz.)

with fever and elevated white blood cell (WBC) counts. The abscessed sac can be decompressed by aspiration of its purulent contents with a fine needle, which relieves symptoms and produces a specimen for culture and sensitivity tests. Appropriate intravenous antibiotics should be started. Once under control, definitive irrigation and probing of the lacrimal drainage system must be performed.

By far the most serious inflammatory processes involving the ocular adnexa are preorbital and orbital cellulitis, both of which are almost invariably unilateral. Either condition may result in a number of significant complications (e.g., orbital or subperiosteal abscesses, cavernous sinus thrombosis, extradural brain abscess, meningitis, and osteomyelitis of the skull), and therefore requires hospitalization. Predisposing factors for either disease include sinusitis (most commonly ethmoid and maxillary), coryza, otitis media, local trauma, and local skin infections. Many patients have a history of a recent cold that was partially treated. The most frequent causal organisms are *Haemophilus*, parainfluenza virus, *S. aureus*, β-hemolytic *Streptococcus*, and *Streptococcus pneumonia*.

Local findings of periorbital (preseptal) cellulitis consist of painless erythema and edema of the eyelids (Fig 46–5). The conjunctiva usually is not congested or chemotic, there is little to no discharge, and ocular motility and vision are normal. Rhinorrhea is frequent; the patient is often alert, irritable, febrile, and has significant leukocytosis. There is often a previous history of recent trauma to the involved lid.

In contrast, orbital cellulitis presents with marked pain, redness, and swelling of the lids, with marked conjunctival injection, chemosis, and obviously decreased ocular motility. Proptosis may be present (Fig 46–6). A dilated pupil with abnormal responsiveness and decreased visual acuity may occur from inflammation surrounding the eye and from compression of the optic nerve. The fundus may reveal retinal vascular engorgement and low-grade papilledema, both grave findings heralding the beginning of cavernous sinus thrombosis. The patient is not always alert, is very irritable, may have a stiff neck, is febrile, and has a markedly elevated WBC count.

Not all swollen or erythematous eyelids are due to trauma or cellulitis. Insect bites (Fig 46–7), contact dermatitis, varicella-zoster reactions, and primary herpes simplex (Fig 46–8) can all present with swollen lids. However, the possible underlying ocular involvement is a far more important consideration. If the eye itself is involved, referral is necessary.

Recurrent painless ecchymosis of the lids may occur in children with hemophilia and can even be the hallmark of a nonpalpable orbital neuroblastoma. Furthermore, any recurrent traumatic finding around the eye must suggest child abuse or neglect.

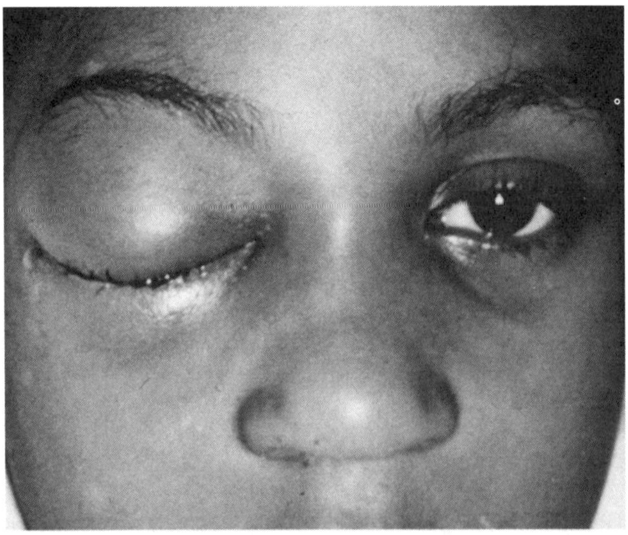

FIG 46–5
Preorbital cellulitis; note that child appears alert and eye is not proptosed.

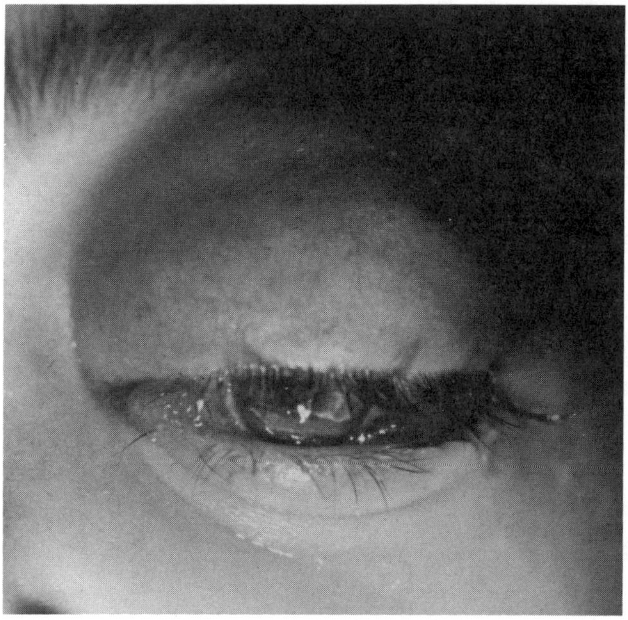

FIG 46–6
Orbital cellulitis; lids are swollen but eye is proptosed. Conjunctiva is chemotic and engorged, and cornea is exposed.

Conjunctiva.—Rupture of a small bulbar conjunctival vessel can result in extravasation of blood (Fig 46–9) between the transparent conjunctiva and the sclera. This bright red subconjunctival hemorrhage frequently is caused by hard coughing, sneezing, vomiting, or other action that produces a Valsalva-like maneuver. It can also occur from the innocent rubbing of the eye, from foreign bodies on the conjunctiva,

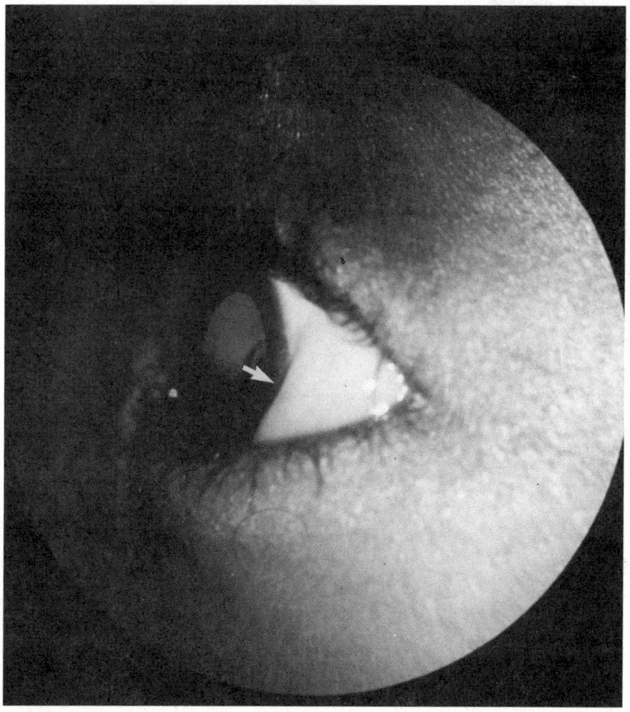

FIG 46–7
Pale chemosis of conjunctiva *(arrow)* from an insect bite.

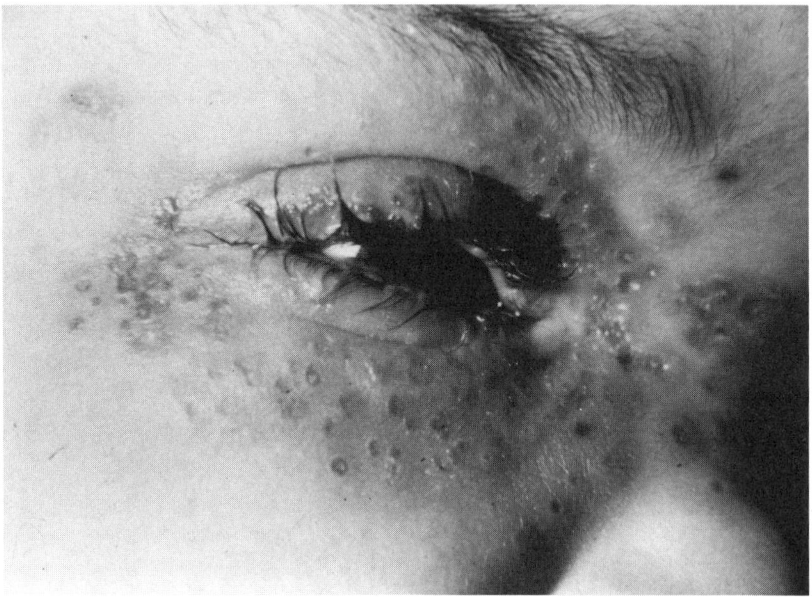

FIG 46–8
Primary herpes simplex causing periorbital cellulitis; secondary bacterial invasion is causing purulent discharge and the eye itself is not involved.

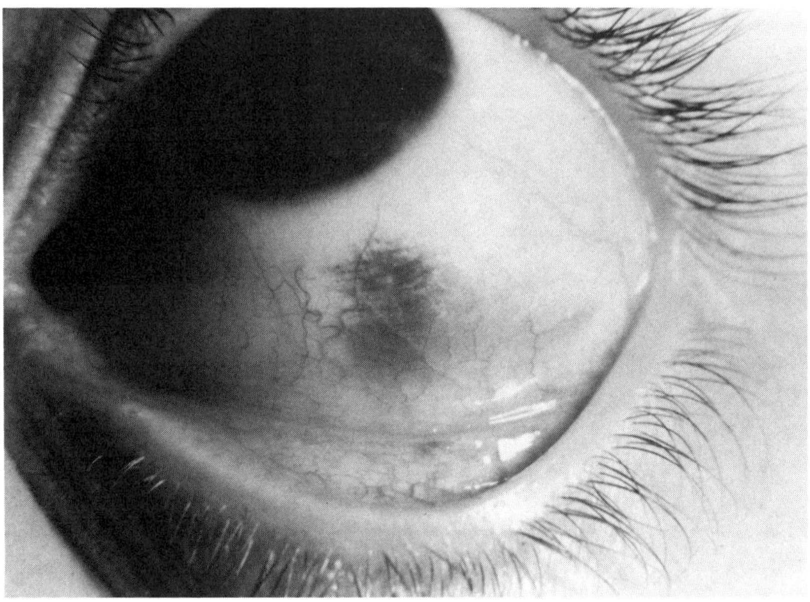

FIG 46–9
Subconjunctival hemorrhage from sneezing.

and from more serious injuries. Simple subconjunctival hemorrhage is asymptomatic, requires no treatment, and will absorb spontaneously in days to weeks, depending on its extent. Recurrent subconjunctival hemorrhages may be a sign of a blood dyscrasia or hypertension.

Foreign bodies in the conjunctiva cause various degrees of discomfort, congestion, lacrimation, and photophobia. If a foreign body is suspected and not immediately visible, the upper lid should be everted and its surface inspected. Once located, a foreign body is usually easily removed with a sterile, moist cotton swab. After removal of the foreign body the cornea should be checked with fluorescein. If staining is noted, local antibiotic drops should be used until the cornea heals (1 to 2 days). Topical anesthetics should never be prescribed, because they retard healing and mask the pain of either a worsening condition or incidental injury.

Conjunctivitis (pink eye) is the commonest ophthalmologic problem. It consists of a minimally painful conjunctival hyperemia associated with some type of discharge. The cornea is clear, the pupil is normal, and the vision is only slightly, if at all, decreased. Conjunctivitis is caused by many infectious agents, allergy, or chemical or gaseous irritants.

Newborn infants are prone to a few particular types of potentially serious conjunctividities, grouped under the term "ophthalmia neonatorum." Chemical ophthalmia neonatorium results from silver nitrate (Credé ointment). Frequently unilateral, it occurs on the first day of life and is characterized by blepharospasm and injected, swollen conjunctiva and lids with occasional rapidly clearing corneal haze. In the absence of any secondary bacterial infection, this common conjunctivitis resolves rapidly and is rarely seen in an outpatient office.

In children between 2 days and 1 month of age, ophthalmia neonatorum usually presents with markedly swollen eyelids, hemorrhagic chemotic conjunctiva, and a purulent discharge (Fig 46–10). This appearance can be caused by any acute bacterial infection, by *Chlamydia trachomatis*, and by the herpes simplex viruses (HSV-1 or HSV-2). The most immediate need is to rule out *Neisseria gonorrhoeae*, which can penetrate an intact cornea and rapidly result in destruction of the eye. The heavy purulent discharge should be rinsed away, followed by a rigorous scraping of the palpebral conjunctival epithelium for specimens to be smeared with both Gram and giemsa stains and inoculated directly onto Thayer-Martin medium or chocolate agar. Viral cultures for HSV and *Chlamydia* should also be obtained.

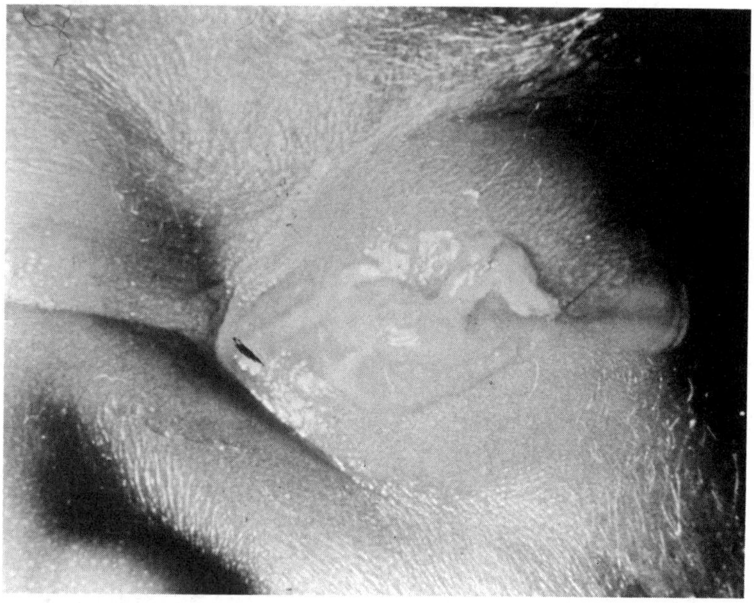

FIG 46–10
Marked lid edema and massive purulent discharge common with gonococcal ophthalmia neonatorum.

The finding of intraepithelial gram-negative diplococci on the smear is enough for a presumptive diagnosis of gonococcal conjunctivitis, and topical gentamycin or bacitracin should be applied every 2 hours until the results of the culture and sensitivity test are known. More important, saline lavage of the infected area should be done as often as needed to remove purulent discharge. Hospitalization is mandatory, along with intravenous administration of appropriate antibodies.

C. trachomatis is the most frequent cause of ophthalmia neonatorum. Although its onset is usually later than gonococcal infections (5 to 30 days postpartum), it can produce a purulent hemorrhagic picture (Fig 46–11) similar to any acute bacterial involvement or milder variant. Treatment consists of local sulfonamides, erythromycin, or tetracycline given four times daily for 2 weeks. Chlamydial pneumonitis occurs occasionally, and some clinicians use systemic erythromycin along with topical drugs. Gonococcal and chlamydial conjunctivitis can occur concomitantly, and treatment for one organism may not be effective against the other.

Severe ophthalmia neonatorum occurs in over 5% of neonates infected with HSV. Onset begins between 3 to 14 days after birth. Unilateral or bilateral, it starts with lid edema, followed quickly by conjunctival hyperemia and swelling with a serosanguineous exudate. Early HSV is indistinguishable from chlamydial infections, and secondary bacterial invasion causes a heavy purulent discharge similar to gonorrhea. Keratitis is a common complication, ending in corneal scarring. Availability of specific antiviral drugs makes it imperative to establish the presence of the virus as well as its type. Because of the frequency of corneal involvement, HSV infections should be followed up by an ophthalmologist.

Persistent or recurrent conjunctivitis in the newborn should raise the question of an obstructed nasolacrimal system. Tearing (epiphora) and a mucopurulent discharge may be present without obvious swelling of the lacrimal sac (Fig 46–12). Simple pressure on the sac usually causes the expulsion of purulent material. The discharge should be cultured and appropriate local antibiotics started; frequent, firm downward massage of the sac often results in opening of the obstructed tear duct without

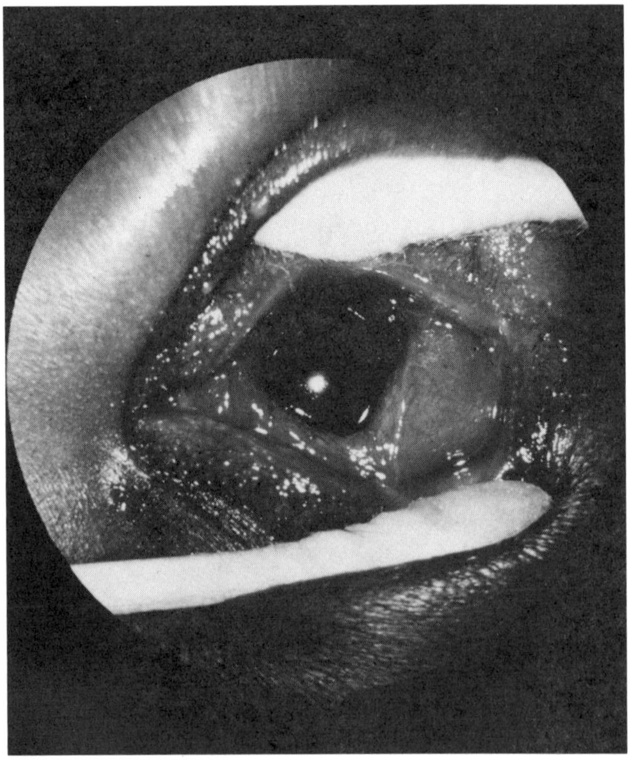

FIG 46–11
Nine-day-old infant with severe hemorrhagic chemotic ophthalmia neonatorum from *C. trachomatis.*

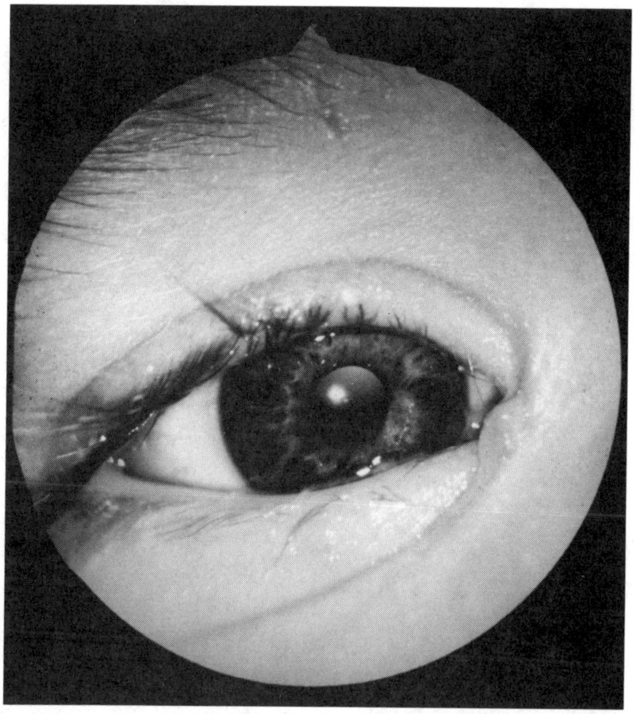

FIG 46–12
Purulent discharge and matted lashes in infant with recurrent conjunctivitis from an obstructed tear duct without acute dacryocystitis.

the need for surgical probing. If symptoms persist to 1 year of age, probing is recommended.

In contrast to ophthalmia neonatorum, bacterial conjunctivitis in older children rarely requires a workup. Most clear within 48 to 72 hours with antibacterial preparations. Bacterial conjunctivitis is often unilateral and not associated with fever. The palpebral conjunctiva is more injected than the bulbar conjunctiva, and there is usually a mucopurulent or purulent discharge (Fig 46–13). The lashes are often matted, especially in the morning, and both preauricular and submandibular lymph node swelling can occur. There should be no pain or photophobia, no corneal involvement, no change in pupillary size or response, and no decrease in vision beyond that thought reasonable as secondary to the blurring caused by the purulent discharge.

Viral conjunctivitis occurs more frequently than bacterial conjunctivitis, is often bilateral with a watery discharge, and is frequently associated with upper respiratory tract symptoms and fever. Resistant to treatment, the infection usually lasts longer than bacterial disease. The lack of response to therapy, the annoying tearing and gritty sensation, and the prolonged course are often the reasons these patients are improperly given local steroid-antimicrobial preparations, with the hope of symptomatic relief. Except for a local pure decongestant or antibiotic, no medication is indicated for viral conjunctivitis. Local steroids can have serious ocular side effects, and the antiviral agents are usually saved for specific viruses (HSV). Some strains of adenoviruses can cause corneal scarring, and viral conjunctivitis with obvious corneal opacities or a decrease in visual acuity not seemingly attributable to tearing should be referred to an ophthalmologist.

Allergic reactions are often seasonal or associated with a particular contact. The itching and tearing are often disproportionate to the findings, which consist of pale, edematous bilateral conjunctival and lid swelling. In its mildest form, the lower lids are most involved (Fig 46–14). However, severe allergic conjunctivitis (vernal catarrh) can have large cobblestonelike papillary hypertrophy, best seen by everting the upper lids. There may also be pronounced photophobia and circumcorneal injection. A third type of allergic conjunctivitis is limbal vernal catarrh, in which the palpebral reaction may be minimal, but there are white

FIG 46–13
Diffuse conjunctival injection and heavy purulent discharge in 10-year-old child with acute *H. influenzae* conjunctivitis.

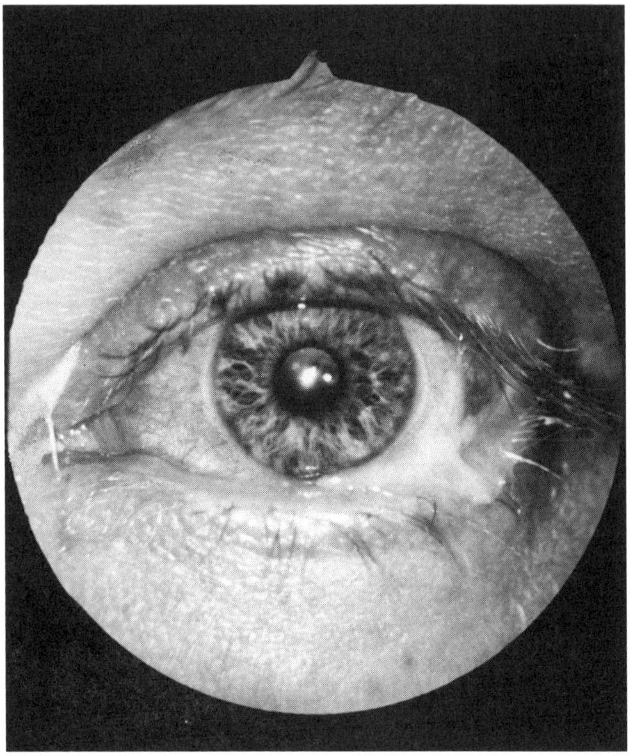

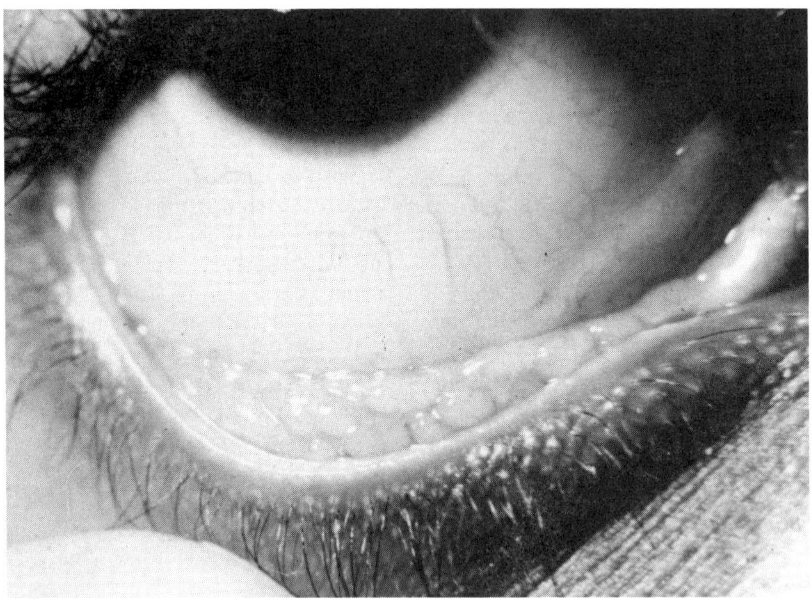

FIG 46–14
Allergic papillary response of lower palpebral conjunctiva.

infiltrates within the limbus (Fig 46–15). Mild allergic conjunctivitis may respond to local and systemic antihistamines; the more severe forms usually require referral to both an allergist and an ophthalmologist, because systemic desensitization is needed as well as rather extensive use of local steroids.

A somewhat similar reaction is phlyctenular conjunctivitis, a localized allergic response in the conjunctiva at or close to the limbus (Fig 46–16). The phlyctenule results from an antigenic stimulus arising somewhere in the body. In the past it was almost synonymous with tuberculosis, but in the United States today it most often occurs as an allergy to some underlying bacterial infection, usually *S. aureus*. Topical steroids are indicated.

Chemical and gaseous conjunctivitis also occur commonly. The principal and most important treatment is immediate irrigation with water. Contact lenses, if present, should be removed immediately. Once the patient reaches any medical facility, further irrigation must be continued. This is best accomplished by instilling a local anesthetic, retracting the lid, and pouring 1 to 2 L of sterile saline solution directly onto the eye. The upper lid and lower fornix should be inverted and swept with a cotton swab to remove any particulate matter. Never try to neutralize acids with bases or vice versa. These patients should be referred to an ophthalmologist.

Cornea and Anterior Segment.—Trauma to the cornea most commonly results from small airborne particles, and includes blepharospasm, tearing, local sharp pain, and photophobia. Conjunctival congestion is rapid and followed by a deeper circumcorneal (limbal) flush. Secondary spasm of the muscles of the iris and ciliary body causes pupillary constriction and even severe headache. If not removed, the foreign body can cause edematous clouding and even vascularization of the cornea (Fig 46–17). Removal of corneal foreign bodies requires a local anesthetic to break the blepharospasm. A sterile, moist cotton swab should be tried first, and sharp instrumentation (sterile metal spud or syringe needle) used only if the swab fails. After removal, there will always be a residual corneal defect that stains with fluo-

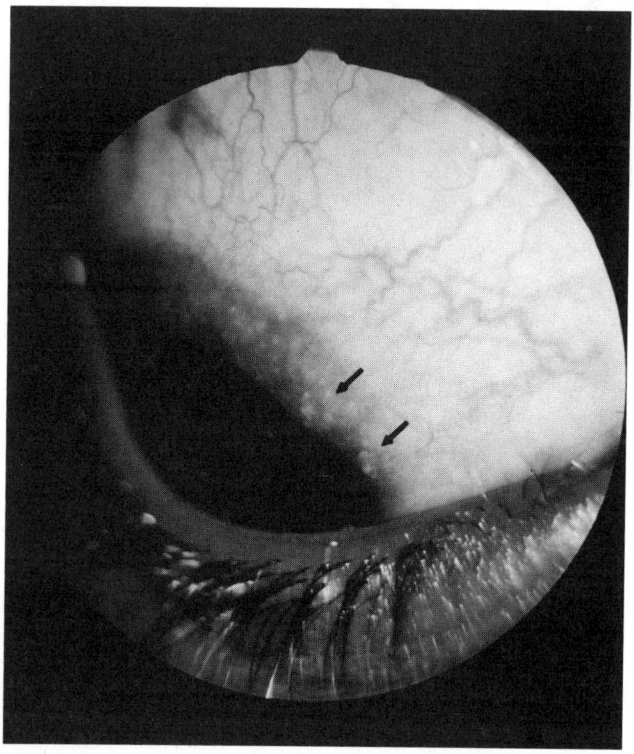

FIG 46–15
Limbal vernal catarrh. The white dots *(arrows)* in the superior limbal area are focal collections of degenerated eosinophils.

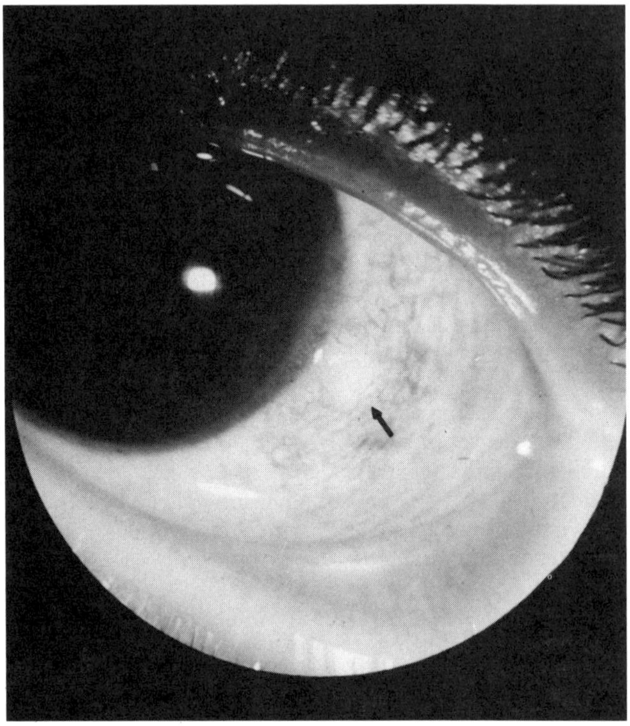

FIG 46–16
Pearl-white, raised phlyctenule *(arrow)* surrounded by red conjunctival injection and chemosis. Underlying diagnosis was pneumonia from *S. aureus.*

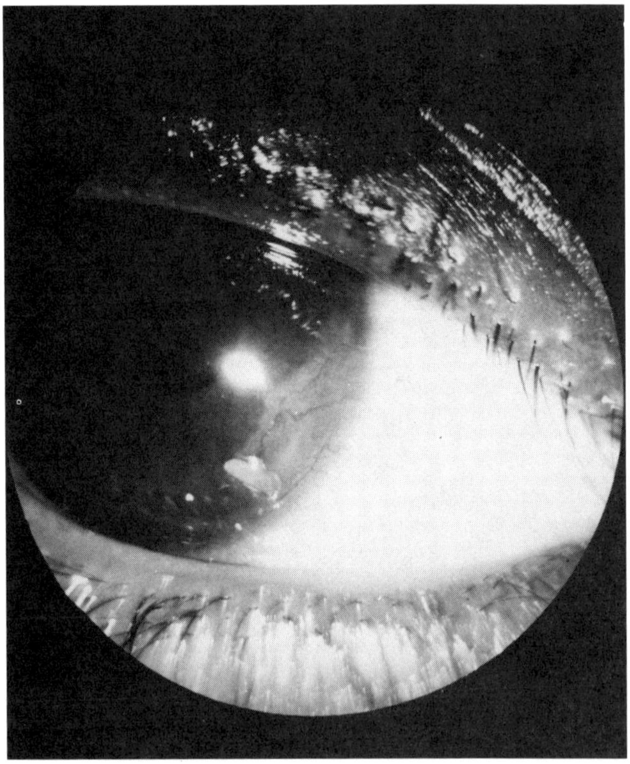

FIG 46–17
Chronic foreign body of the cornea producing hazy white edema as well as early corneal neovascularization.

rescein, so prophylactic local antibiotic drops should be used until the abrasion heals. A simple soft eye patch can be taped over closed lids to promote comfort, but if there is marked ciliary spasm, a cycloplegic agent is needed to stop the pain. Continued use of a local anesthetic for comfort while healing takes place should never be prescribed.

Primary corneal abrasions and scratches from fingernails, pets, branches, cigarette burns, and other objects can be treated as for a foreign body. However, these abrasions tend to be large and more contaminated, and healing can take several days. Any evidence of corneal clouding during the acute or healing phase of an abrasion should warrant referral, because it is the earliest sign of onset of a corneal ulcer. Repeated trauma, especially cigarette burns, should alert the clinician to the possibility of child abuse.

Exposure to excessive ultraviolet light, chlorine in swimming pools, many aerosol sprays, tear gas, and other noxious gases can all cause diffuse superficial punctate corneal abrasions that are painful. The history, severe pain, photophobia, excessive lacrimation, and circumlimbal flush are diagnostic; immediate relief with a drop of local anesthetic helps confirm the diagnosis. Once the eyes are irrigated with sterile saline solution, periodic instillation of a cycloplegic agent combined with patching of both eyes should allow enough comfort during healing (less than 24 hours).

Inflammation of the cornea (keratitis) may not be quite so symptomatic as trauma, but decreased vision, photophobia, and especially limbal flush (Fig 46–18) associated with any visible corneal lesion are reason enough for referral.

Anterior segment (aqueous, iris, lens, ciliary body) disorders mimic symptoms and signs of corneal disease, and once detected demand appropriate consultation. Irritation of the iris and ciliary body (iridocyclitis) can result from trauma or infection; the telltale sign is ciliary flush (Fig 46–19 to 46–22).

Posterior Segment.—Purely posterior (vitreous, retina, optic nerve) problems commonly cause decreased vision. Without obvious anterior trauma or inflammation, the eye is usually

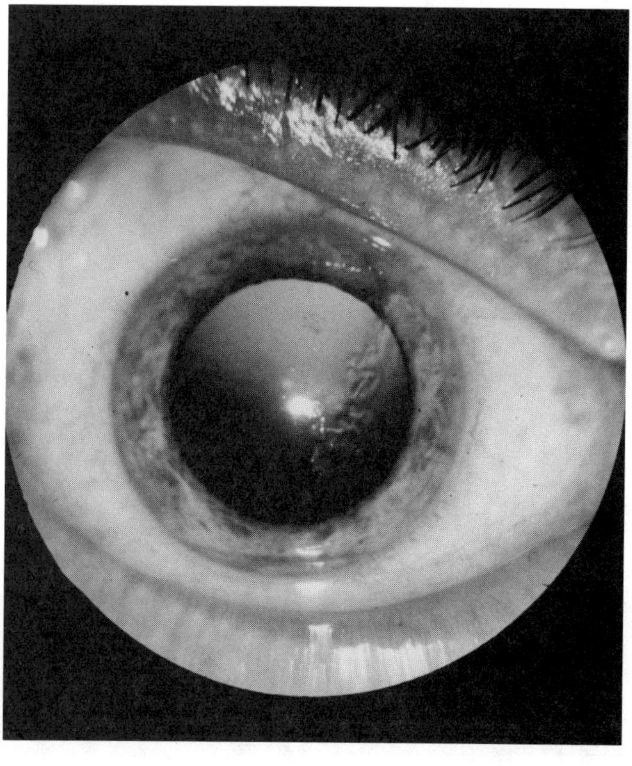

FIG 46–18

Fine circumcorneal (limbal) flush with acute herpes simplex keratitis. The dendritic nature of the acute herpes lesion can be seen within the dilated pupil by using the red reflex as viewed through a direct ophthalmoscope.

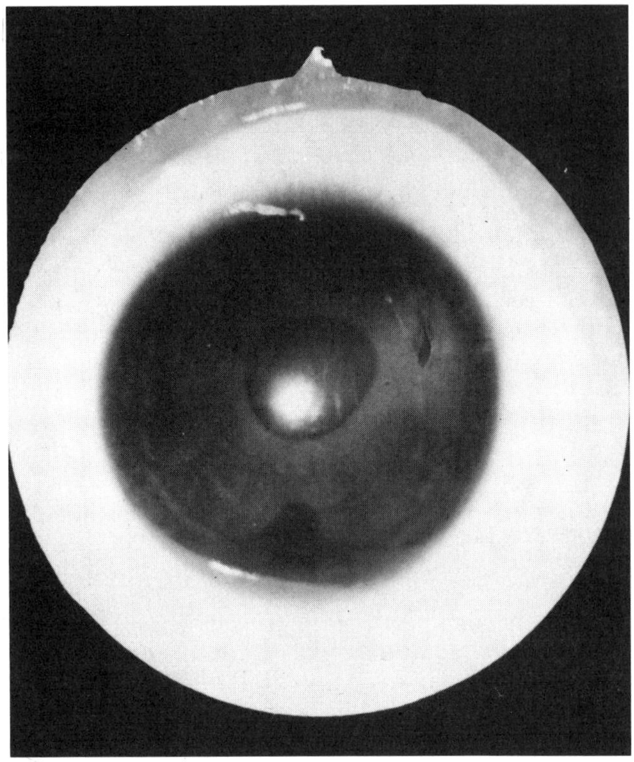

FIG 46–19
Layered hyphema (blood) in the anterior chamber. Note the corneal lesion (by fluorescein staining) and irregular pupil. The eye was struck while open.

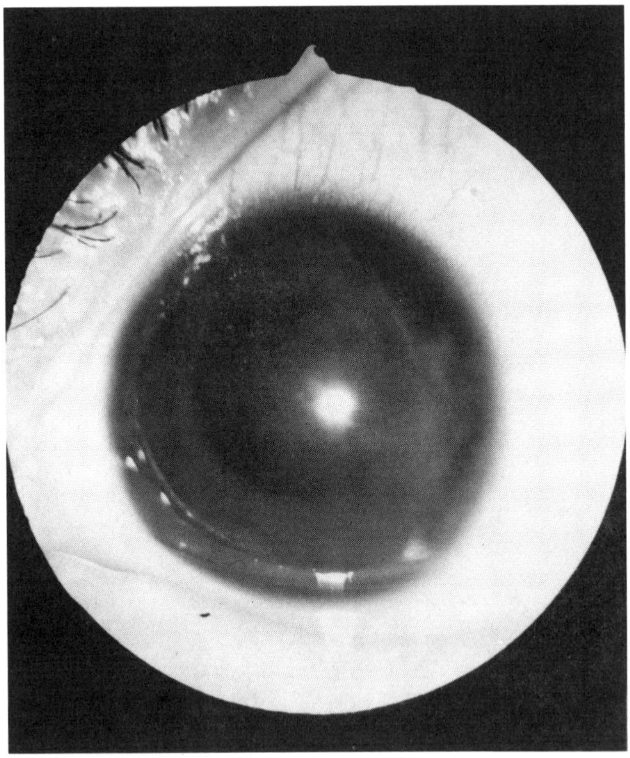

FIG 46–20
Acute hyphema before settling of the blood. Child was hit in the eye by a fist while lids were closed.

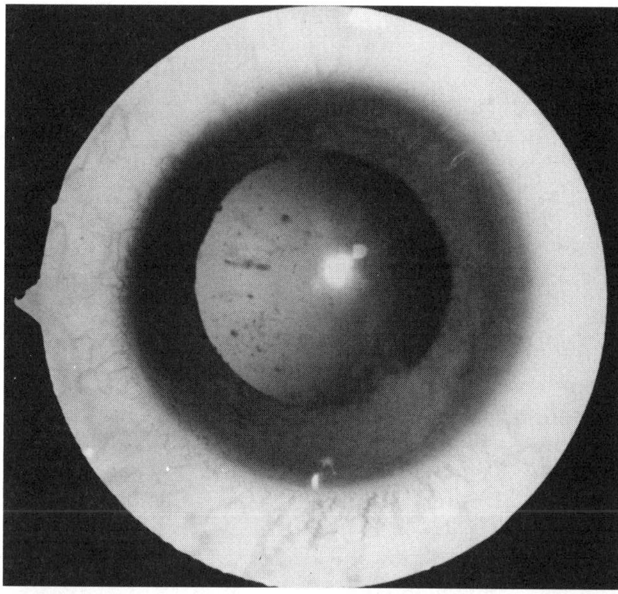

FIG 46–21
Juvenile rheumatoid arthritis with ciliary injection and heavy deposit of inflammatory cells on the corneal endothelium. The pupil is dilated from cycloplegic agents.

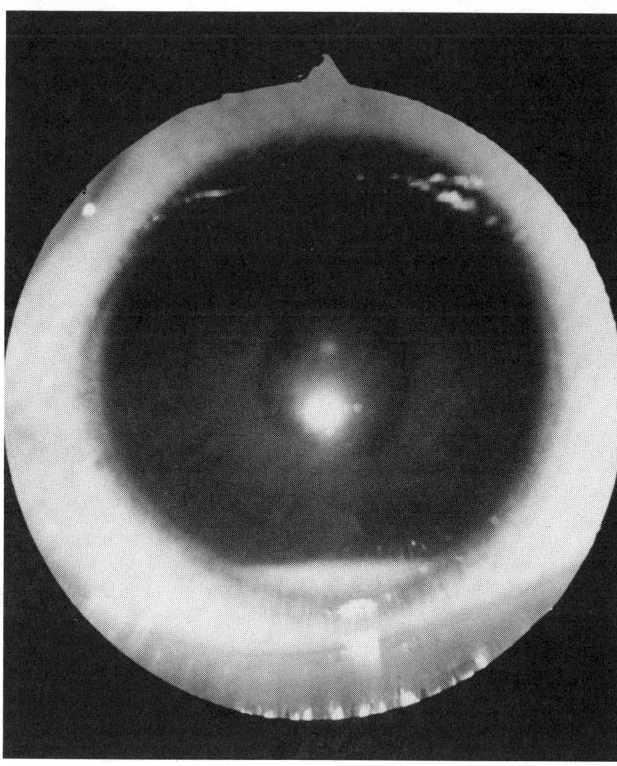

FIG 46–22
Red ciliary flush, irregular pupil, and layer of white blood cells (hypopion).

asymptomatic. The patient who has unexplained decreased vision in one or both eyes should see an ophthalmologist.

DATA GATHERING

For any acute eye problem, history taking is often quickly accomplished and usually governed by the immediate appearance of the child as he or she enters the office. First, was there trauma? Was it physical, chemical (acid or alkali), or thermal? Is there decreased vision, foreign body sensation, or pain? The answers to the questions can tell the examiner at once if the child needs direct referral. In the absence of trauma, history taking can be accomplished more leisurely and in more detail. Is there decreased vision, pain, or other uncomfortable sensation (photophobia, tearing, itching)? Is it acute, chronic, or recurrent; unilateral or bilateral? Are there associated acute systemic findings such as fever, irritability, upper respiratory tract or gastrointestinal tract symptoms? Does the child have any primary disease or syndrome associated with ocular changes (e.g., prematurity, juvenile rheumatoid arthritis, Marfan syndrome, homocystinuria, phakomatosis, tuberculosis, sarcoidosis, allergic or immunologic disorder)?

INDICATIONS FOR REFERRAL OR CONSULTATION

The following causes of red eye require that the patient be referred to an ophthalmologist (compare with the differential diagnosis).

OCULAR PROBLEMS REQUIRING REFERRAL

Ocular adnexa

Trauma

Punctures and lacerations

Orbital blow-out fractures

Inflammation

Persistent chalazions

Acute dacryocystitis

Periorbital cellulitis

Orbital cellulitis

Intractable blepharospasm

RED EYE
Neonate

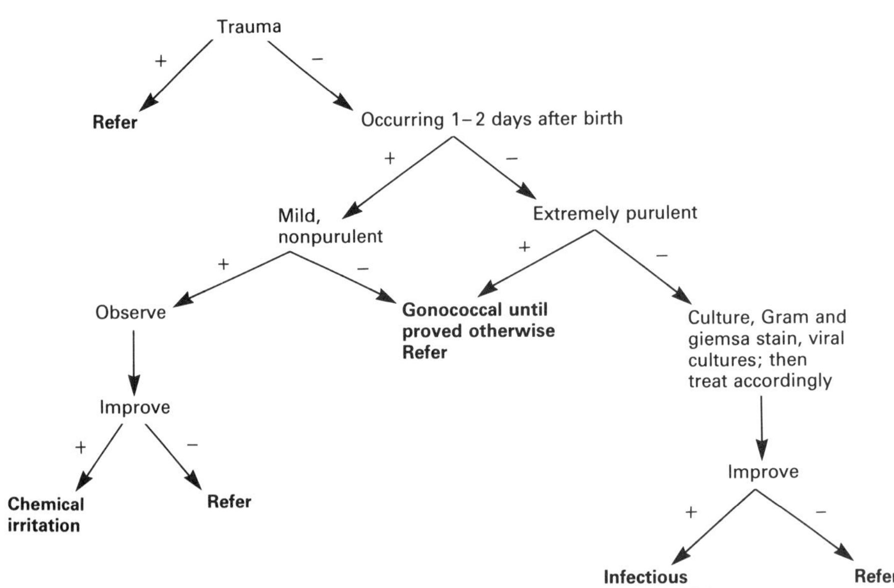

FIG 46–23
Decision tree for red eye in the neonate.

RED EYE
Older child

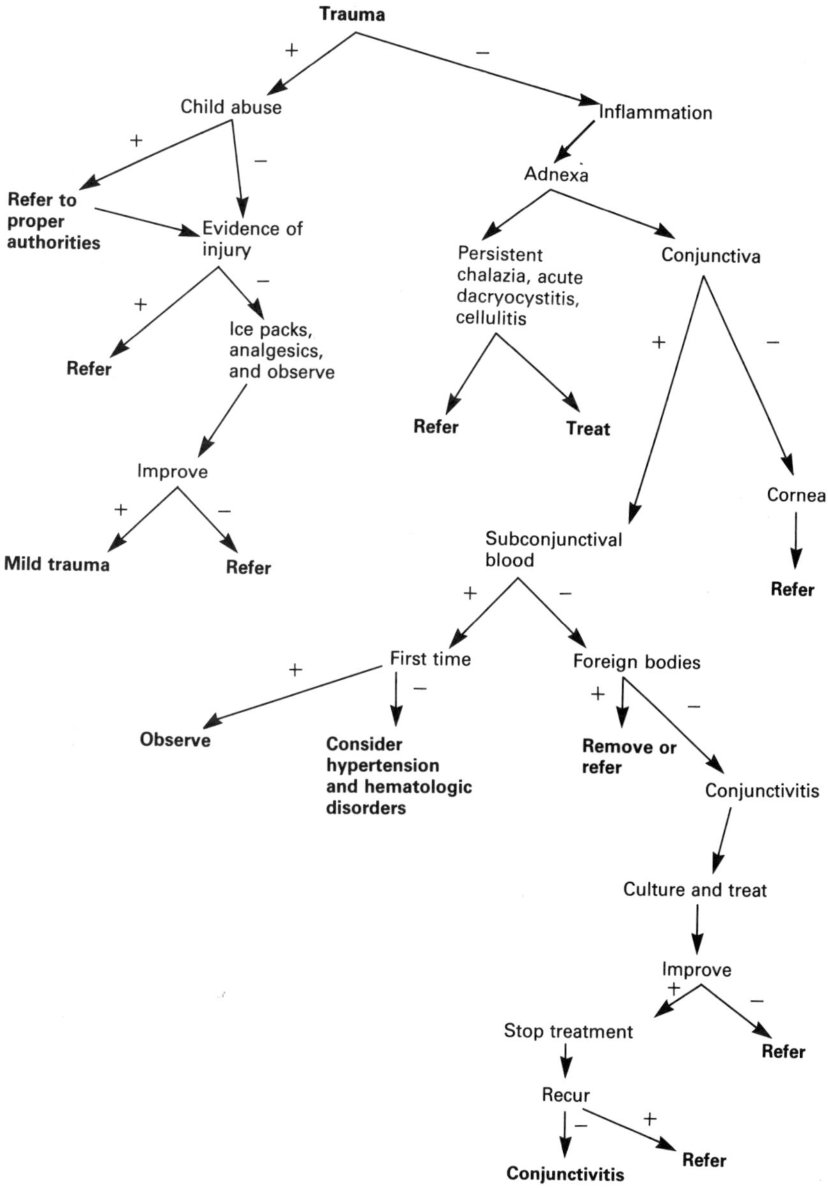

FIG 46–24
Decision tree for red eye in the older child.

Conjunctiva
Trauma
Lacerations >5 mm
Chemical or gaseous burns
Inflammation
Ophthalmia neonatorum
Gonococcal
Herpes simplex
Recurrent conjunctivitis

Cornea
Trauma
Large abrasions (more than one-fourth corneal diameter)
All lacerations
Chemical burns
Thermal burns
Inflammation
All keratitis
All cloudy corneas

Anterior segment
Trauma
Hyphema
Torn iris
Dislocated lens
Steamy cornea (glaucoma)
Inflammation
Hypopion
Bound-down pupil
Hazy cornea (endothelial debris)

Posterior eye
Unexplained decrease in vision
Abnormal findings on ophthalmoscopy

CONCLUSION

It is important to realize the extreme range of diagnoses that red eye brings to mind (Figs 46–23, and 46–24). An orderly approach involves proper history taking, rapid in instances of obvious trauma and in-depth when time allows. Attention to all the symptoms, an accurate assessment of the visual acuity, a logical step-by-step examination of the ocular adnexa and thorough and gentle evaluation of the globe should afford most clinicians with sufficient and appropriate data to identify the cause and location of the ocular irritant. Once done, the ability to treat or the need to refer should be immediately clear.

BIBLIOGRAPHY

Katowitz JA: Trauma to the eye and adnexa, in Kelly VC, (ed): *Practice of Pediatrics*, vol 10. Philadelphia, Harper & Row Publishers, 1983, pp 1–13.

Katowitz JA: Lacrimal drainage surgery, in Duane TD, (ed): *Clinical Ophthalmology*, vol 5. Philadelphia, Harper & Row Publishers 1983, pp 1–32.

Raucher RS, Newton MJ: New issues in the prevention and treatment of ophthalmia neonatorum. *Ann Ophthalmol* 1983; 15:1004–1009.

Rubenstein JB, Handler DS: Orbital and periorbital cellulitis in children. *Head Neck Surg* 1982; 5:15–21.

Schaffer DB: Eye findings in intrauterine infections, in Plotkin SA, Starr SE (eds): *Clinical Perinatology*. Philadelphia, WB Saunders Co, 1981; pp 415–443.

Schaffer DB: Pediatric ophthalmology, in Scheie HG, Albert DM, (eds): *Textbook of Ophthalmology*, ed 9. Philadelphia, WB Saunders Co, 1977; pp 279–358.

Scheie HG, Albert DM, (eds): Ophthalmic overview: An introduction to ophthalmic diseases and their terminology, in *Textbook of Ophthalmology*, ed 9. Philadelphia, WB Saunders Co, 1977; pp 3–44.

47 RECTAL BLEEDING

David A. Piccoli, M.D.

Rectal bleeding, a common manifestation of gastrointestinal (GI) disease, is the final pathway of hemorrhage from any site along the GI tract or nasopharynx, and may, in the neonate, represent blood of foreign origin. A common, and often unsuspected cause of rectal bleeding is an upper GI tract hemorrhage, originating above the ligament of Treitz. Factors such as volume of the hemorrhage and intestinal transit time may lead to the mistaken clinical impression of lower GI tract bleeding. Lower GI tract bleeding that originates from sites below the ligament of Treitz, most frequently from the distal ileum and colon, may result from a discrete anatomic lesion or diffuse mucosal disease. The degree of rectal bleeding depends on the site and severity of the lesion.

DIFFERENTIAL DIAGNOSIS

COMMON CAUSES OF RECTAL BLEEDING

All causes of upper GI tract bleeding
Lower GI tract bleeding
Trauma
Anal fissure
Child abuse
Foreign body
Infection
Bacterial: *Salmonella, Shigella, Yersinia, Campylobacter, Aeromonas,* enteropathogenic *Escherichia coli, Clostridium difficile* (antibiotic-associated colitis)
Protozoal: amebiasis *(Entamoeba histolytica)*
Parasitic: *Trichuris,* hookworm
Viral (rarely)
Inflammatory
Necrotizing enterocolitis
Ischemic colitis
Acute colitis
Ulcerative colitis
Crohn disease
Henoch-Schönlein syndrome
Hemolytic-uremic syndrome
Nodular lymphoid hyperplasia
Vascular-tumor
Hemangiomas
Arteriovenous (AV) malformations
Telangiectasias
Hemorrhoids
Congenital
Meckel diverticulum
Duplications
Structural
Intussusception
Juvenile polyp
Polyposis syndromes
Midgut volvulus
Allergic
Cow milk (soy milk) protein allergy

DISCUSSION

Pseudoblood.—It is important in the well child to verify rectal bleeding biochemically. A number of substances can be mistaken for blood in its various states including food coloring, fruit-flavored drinks, beets, grapes, colored antibiotics, iron, and other medications. Even the most dramatic diaper should be tested for heme positivity. Several biochemical tests are currently available for the detection of blood in feces.

The guaiac reagent in cards or paper strips (e.g., Hemoccult) utilizes a heme-catalyzed color change in a phenolic compound for detection. This has good sensitivity, excellent reproducibility, and rare false-positive results. There is only minimal effect of specimen storage, and iron will not cause a false-positive result. An added advantage of the guaiac cards is the ability to test the stool specimen that is obtained by the parent or patient at home and delivered or sent to the physician's office. This not only improves the detection of intermittent bleeding but may also obviate the need for repeated rectal examinations. The tablet tests utilizing the peroxidation of the chromogen orthotoluidine (e.g., Hematest) have higher false-positive rates.

Foodstuffs causing false-positive reactions in various tests include iron, high-meat diets, bananas, horseradish, turnips, and tomato skins. Black stools that give a negative guaiac reaction may result from ingestion of iron preparations, bismuth (Pepto-Bismol), lead, licorice, charcoal, coal, or dirt. False-negative reactions may occur with prolonged storage in some reactions, and with high vitamin C intake that interferes with the color change normally produced by peroxidase.

"Red diaper syndrome" may occur with storage of soiled diapers for 24 to 36 hours, and is due to *Serratia marcescens*, which produces the red pigmentation. The stools give a negative guaiac reaction.

Type and Color of Bleeding.—A description of the color, location, and amount of blood in feces may provide valuable information. Bright red blood or blood streaking of the stool is most often due to distal lesions such as fissures or polyps. In the newborn, an upper GI tract hemorrhage may present with bright red rectal bleeding. The bleeding of a Meckel diverticulum may produce red or dark bleeding. An ileocolic intussusception classically produces a "currant jelly" stool.

Mucus-associated bloody stools may be due to infection, milk and/or soy protein allergy, ischemia, hemolytic-uremic syndrome, or Hirschsprung enterocolitis. Melena is generally a sign of upper GI tract bleeding but may rarely occur with a Meckel diverticulum.

A comprehensive list of the causes of GI bleeding in all pediatric age groups was provided under differential diagnosis. The more frequent etiologies are listed by age group in the following sections. The focus of the initial evaluation should be guided by the patient's age, associated symptoms, and the magnitude of blood loss (Table 47-1).

MOST FREQUENT CAUSES OF RECTAL BLEEDING

NEWBORN TO 3-MONTH-OLD INFANTS

Swallowed maternal blood
Nasopharyngeal trauma
Anal fissure
Upper GI tract sources
Hemorrhagic disease of the newborn
Anatomic abnormalities

Swallowed Maternal Blood.—A well newborn or breast-fed infant with red or tarry rectal bleeding but no other signs of hypovolemia or systemic disease may have swallowed maternal blood from the time of delivery or from breastfeeding. The Apt-Downey alkali denaturation test should be performed to determine if the blood is of maternal origin. A specimen of emesis, nasogastric aspirate, or stool is mixed with 5 to 10 parts water to lyse the red blood cells. Black coffee-grounds material or melena cannot be used because the hemoglobin has been changed to hematin. The pink suspension is then centrifuged and decanted or filtered.

A specimen from the infant's blood and a control (child or adult) blood lysate is also prepared. One milliliter of 0.25N (1% solution) NaOH is mixed with five parts hemoglobin solution. Adult hemoglobin changes from pink to brown-yellow over 2 minutes, while fetal hemoglobin remains pink (undenatured).

Nasopharyngeal Trauma.—Suctioning following delivery of the newborn or nasopharyngeal trauma may cause upper GI tract bleeding that can manifest itself as rectal bleeding. A careful physical examination will be useful, and history in the older child is helpful.

Anal Fissure.—Anal fissure is the most common cause of rectal bleeding in children less than 2 years old. It presents with recurrent small amounts of bright red blood coating the stool. It may be associated with hard stools or pain during defecation. Visual inspection or anoscopy will identify the lesion. In the older child a fissure or fistula may be associated with systemic symptoms in inflammatory bowel disease.

TABLE 47–1
Etiologies of Rectal Bleeding Based on Age and Common Clinical Presentation

SIGNS	NEONATAL	INFANCY	CHILDHOOD	ADOLESCENCE
Occult blood	Milk or soy allergy; gastric outlet obstruction; oropharyngeal trauma	Milk/soy allergy; esophagitis; peptic disease; gastric outlet obstruction	Esophagitis; peptic disease; gastric outlet obstruction; hemangiomas/ telangiectasias	Peptic disease; esophagitis; vascular malformations
Visible blood, well child	Anal fissure; swallowed maternal blood; fissure; milk/soy allergy; bleeding disorders	Anal fissure; colonic polyp; swallowed epistaxis; foreign body; nodular lymphoid hyperplasia; gastric heterotopia in ileum	Anal fissure; polyps; foreign body; epistaxis; nodular lymphoid hyperplasia	Polyps; anal fissure; hemorrhoids; foreign body; epistaxis
Evidence of systemic disease	Infections; sepsis; necrotizing enterocolitis; gangrenous bowel; midgut volvulus; intussusception; hemorrhagic disease of the newborn; Hirschsprung disease enterocolitis; tumor; colitis with immune deficiency	Infections; milk/soy allergy; esophagitis; intussusception; gangrenous bowel; antibiotics; parasites; Henoch-Schönlein syndrome; acute colitis	Infections; parasites; antibiotics; esophagitis; Crohn disease; intussusception; hemolytic uremic syndrome; Henoch-Schönlein syndrome; ulcerative colitis; acute colitis	Infection; ulcerative colitis; Crohn disease; acute colitis; parasites
Massive hemorrhage	Hemorrhagic gastritis; peptic ulcer; Meckel diverticulum; duplications; vascular malformations	Meckel diverticulum; gastritis; peptic ulcer; vascular malformations; duplications	Meckel diverticulum; gastritis; peptic ulcer; varices; vascular malformations	Meckel diverticulum; varices; peptic ulcer; gastritis; vascular malformations

Upper Gastrointestinal Tract Sources.—The newborn is susceptible to a variety of perinatal stresses that may result in gastric ulceration or hemorrhagic gastritis. Although the usual presentation is hematemesis and hypovolemia, rectal bleeding may be the only symptom. The diagnosis is suggested by prolonged labor, fetal bradycardia, meconium staining, hypoxemia, acidosis, sepsis, or low Apgar scores. Primary CNS disease has been associated with peptic ulcers, as have trauma, systemic illness, and burns. A nasogastric tube should always be placed to identify the site of bleeding and to provide accurate ongoing assessment of the extent of current hemorrhages. In older children and adolescents, an upper hemorrhage may present with occult heme positivity or melena without hematemesis. There may be associated nausea, heartburn, or epigastric pain.

A history of aspirin ingestion should be aggressively pursued. All over-the-counter preparations should be reviewed, as the patient and parent may be unaware of the salicylate content in decongestant and cold preparations.

Hemorrhagic Disease of the Newborn.—Deficiency of vitamin K results in the most commonly acquired coagulation abnormality in the newborn. There is a normal transient depression of the four clotting factors dependent on vitamin K. Newborns and especially premature infants are at risk. Vitamin K is routinely given in delivery rooms but may be neglected in some situations and in home deliveries. Breastfeeding has also been implicated because of the lower concentration of vitamin K in human milk. The GI tract hemorrhage may be large and is associated with other signs of bleeding or bruising. The neonate generally appears well unless there are signs of hemodynamic compromise.

Other acquired coagulopathies occur in sepsis with disseminated intravascular coagulation in an ill-appearing infant. Coagulation abnormalities may be secondary to fat malabsorption in the older child but rarely present with GI tract bleeding.

Hereditary coagulopathies are less common but must be considered in a well-appearing child with GI tract bleeding and abnormal prothrombin and partial thromboplastin times.

Anatomic Abnormalities.—Structural lesions of the GI tract may present as rectal bleeding, often with catastrophic results. A midgut volvulus may produce red or tarry stools in an irritable or lethargic infant with a distended abdomen, who appears to be in shock. Volvulus is frequently secondary to an intestinal malrotation with malfixation of the mesentery. Prompt diagnosis based on examination and radiographs is critical for the preservation of viable bowel.

Another structural abnormality is intestinal duplication, which usually presents early in life. The stool may be red to tarry, in variable amounts, and a mass or obstruction may be suspected on examination. Diagnosis is made by upper GI tract series, isotope scans, ultrasound, or laparotomy.

CHILDREN—3 MONTHS TO 3 YEARS OLD

Infection
Anal fissure
Milk or soy protein allergy
Colonic polyp
Intussusception
Antibiotic-related colitis
Meckel diverticulum
Esophagitis
Lymphoid hyperplasia
Peptic ulcer or gastritis
Structural abnormalities
Hemolytic uremic syndrome
Vascular abnormalities

Infection.—Infection of the GI tract is common at all ages and frequently presents with bloody stool, often associated with mucus. Culturing for *Salmonella* and *Shigella* alone is inadequate for diagnosis. *Campylobacter* is increasingly recognized as a cause of bloody diarrhea and requires special microbiologic techniques for its isolation. *Yersinia, Aeromonas,* and enteropathogenic *Escherichia coli* may produce a colitis and require special isolation techniques. Parasitic infections such as amebiasis may cause a colitis, mimicking a bacterial infection. Multiple fresh ova and parasite examinations and specific serum counterimmunoelectrophoresis establish the diagnosis. Viruses may cause heme-positive diarrhea, especially in infancy and in acquired immunodeficiency syndromes. Nematode parasites (hookworms, *Trichuris*, or *Strongyloides*) cause occult heme positivity without mucus and are associated with anemia and eosinophilia.

Milk or Soy Protein Allergy.—Protein allergy can cause occult or small amounts of visible rectal bleeding and may be associated with mucus in the stool. The onset of disease occurs from the first week of life to 2 years of age. Associated symptoms may include colic, chronic diarrhea, vomiting, rhinitis, wheezing, rash, eczema, or edema. Up to 30% of atopic children may have formula protein allergies. A family history of atopy, early exposure to cow milk protein, or a recent enteritis may be predisposing factors. In younger infants, the syndrome includes severe diarrhea with enteric bleeding, distention, and emesis following exposure to milk protein antigens. Symptoms resolve with elimination of the offending antigens. Since soy and goat milk can have cross-reactivity, an elemental protein formula may be necessary. Other infants present only with chronic mucoid heme-positive diarrhea. Anemia, iron deficiency, hypoproteinemia, and failure to thrive may occur. No laboratory test is totally diagnostic and the clinical response to withdrawal and rechallenge is frequently employed, with clinical remission followed by a recrudescence within 48 hours of rechallenge on repeated trials. Lactose intolerance may simulate diarrheal aspects, but does not cause protein or blood loss in the stool.

Polyp.—Juvenile polyps are the most common cause of enteric bleeding in children 2 to 5 years old (Fig 47–1). They frequently present with intermittent, mild-to-moderate, bright or dark red blood. This may persist over months to years and is usually unassociated with pain or failure to thrive. The juvenile polyp is a benign colonic lesion that rarely causes signifi-

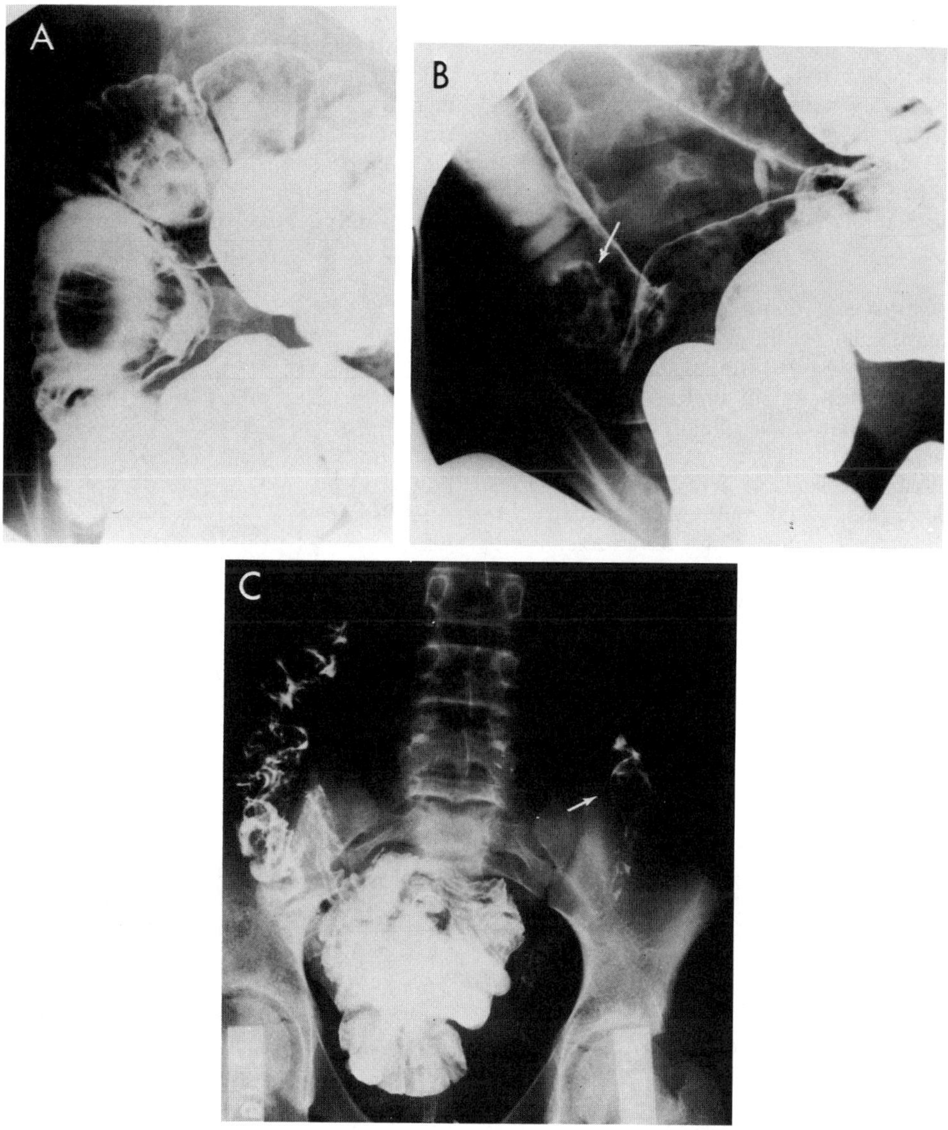

FIG 47–1
Juvenile polyp of the colon. **A,** coned-down view of the ascending colon reveals a large lesion, well outlined by contrast medium. **B,** when the patient is positioned so that there is contrast material in this portion of the colon, the lesion *(arrow)* is seen with its irregular margins. **C,** evacuation films are most helpful to show polypoid lesions. Note how a large juvenile polyp (on another patient) distends the otherwise collapsed descending colon *(arrow)*. (From Haller JO, Slovis TL: *Introduction to Radiology in Clinical Pediatrics.* Chicago, Year Book Medical Publishers, 1984. Used by permission.)

cant bleeding and may undergo spontaneous autoamputation. Chronic significant bleeding or associated symptoms may necessitate colonoscopic polypectomy. The majority are solitary and located in the rectum or sigmoid. Diagnosis is made on rectal examination, via air contrast barium enema in a well-prepared colon or via colonoscopy. All resected polyps should be examined microscopically because of the very rare occurrence of adenomatous change.

Other polyposis syndromes present in childhood. Peutz-Jeghers syndrome consists of diffuse polyposis of the GI tract and is associated with melanotic areas on the buccal mucosa and lips. The polyps are hamartomas and most frequently occur in the small intestine but may be found from the stomach to the rectum. A small number of the polyps may undergo malignant transformation. The polyps may cause obstruction or serve as a lead point for intussusception.

The autosomal dominant familial polyposis coli, with a late childhood onset, is clearly a premalignant lesion. The majority of polyps, which may number up to thousands per patient, are in the colon. Therapy is colectomy, and genetic counseling is advised.

Gardner syndrome is familial adenomatous polyposis associated with subcutaneous tumors, cysts, and bone lesions. Inheritance is autosomal dominant. The polyps have a high frequency of malignant transformation in early adulthood and colectomy is advised.

Intussusception.—Intussusception occurs most commonly during the first 2 years of life. It occurs three times as frequently in boys and is usually ileocolic. Only rarely is there a specific lesion (Meckel diverticulum, polyp, hematoma, or tumor) initiating the intussusception. Gastroduodenal, ileoileal, and colocolic intussusceptions are rare and may present atypically. Intussusception is the most common cause of intestinal obstruction in infants. There may be recurrent attacks of abdominal pain, colic, crying, and drawing up the knees that can progress to vomiting, lethargy, irritability, and "red currant-jelly" stools late in the course. Examination may demonstrate a mass or an empty right lower quadrant. Abdominal tenderness may proceed to peritonitis with perforation. Hydrostatic reduction, the initial treatment of choice, is successful in three-fourths of cases. Failure of hydrostatic reduction, significant bleeding, obstruction, peritonitis, or recurrent intussusception necessitates surgery.

Meckel Diverticulum.—Usually asymptomatic, Meckel diverticulum, the remnant of the omphalomesenteric duct, is the most common anomaly of the GI tract. Less than half actually contain gastric mucosa. Significant bleeding is more frequent in boys and usually presents below 2 years of age. The bleeding is painless, may be massive, and is usually red or maroon. Meckel diverticulum may lead to obstruction, intussusception, or volvulus. Diagnosis may be suggested by a radionuclide scan with ^{99}Tc pertechnetate that is taken up by gastric and heterotopic gastric mucosa. Surgery is indicated for a bleeding Meckel diverticulum.

CHILDREN AND ADOLESCENTS—3 TO 18 YEARS OLD

Infection
Polyps
Anal fissure
Inflammatory bowel disease
Peptic ulcer disease and/or gastritis
Varices
Lymphoid hyperplasia
Vascular lesions

Inflammatory Bowel Disease.—Crohn disease or ulcerative colitis may present with occult or visible rectal bleeding. There are frequently associated systemic complaints including diarrhea, abdominal pain, tenderness, weight loss, anorexia, malaise, fatigue, joint pain, or reduction in linear growth velocity. Family history is positive in about one-sixth of cases. Laboratory signs include a microcytic anemia, thrombocytosis, elevated erythrocyte sedimentation rate, hypoalbuminemia, low levels of serum minerals (zinc, magnesium, copper, iron), water-soluble (folate) and fat-soluble (carotene) vitamins. The final diagnosis will be based on specific colonoscopic and radiographic findings (Fig 47–2).

Vascular Lesions of the Intestine.—Telangiectasias, angiodysplasia, and hemangiomas of the GI tract are rare causes of rectal bleeding in pediatric populations but may be responsible for occasional significant bleeding episodes undiagnosed by other testing. Arterial aneurysms may be seen on arteriography. Several syndromes, including Turner, Osler-Weber-Rendu, blue rubber nevus, and Ehlers-Danlos, may have GI vascular abnormalities with associated bleeding.

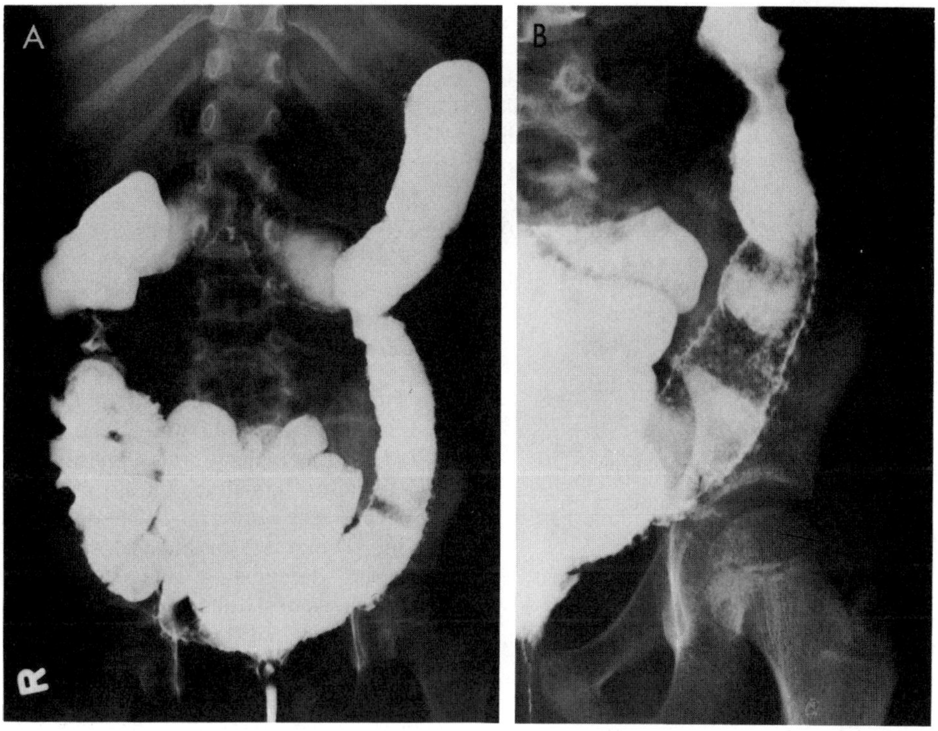

FIG 47–2
Ulcerative colitis. **A,** frontal film from a barium enema reveals contrast material outside the lumen and in the wall, particularly evident in the descending colon. Note "collar-button" ulcerations. **B,** close-up shows the "collar-button" ulcerations to advantage. The key to diagnosis in this case is the abnormal *contour* of the bowel. (From Haller JO, Slovis TL: *Introduction to Radiology in Clinical Pediatrics.* Chicago, Year Book Medical Publishers, 1984. Used by permission.)

DATA GATHERING

HISTORY

The most useful diagnostic test in the evaluation of rectal bleeding is a careful history and physical examination. The age of the patient and the associated symptoms will guide the investigation. The initial evaluation should determine if the child has had cardiovascular compromise or if a surgical condition may exist, which would necessitate immediate hospitalization and consultation. The association of bleeding with systemic symptoms such as abdominal pain, diarrhea, weight loss, or fever may be due to infectious or inflammatory conditions of short duration or secondary to inflammatory bowel disease over months or years. Terminal pain with defecation unassociated with abdominal pain suggests fissure or hemorrhoids. Bleeding from a Meckel diverticulum, juvenile polyp, or vascular malformation is nonpainful. Massive bleeding suggests a Meckel diverticulum, vascular anomaly, or upper GI tract hemorrhage.

The presence of other child care or family members with similar concurrent illness suggests an infectious etiology. A family history of polyps, colitis (but not irritable or "spastic" colitis), bleeding disorders, or severe food allergy is useful. Patients with chronic constipation may have a fissure or Hirschsprung enterocolitis (a very rare but serious complication of Hirschsprung disease). Increasingly, an adolescent's sexual activity must be considered in cases of infectious proctitis or anorectal trauma. Anorectal or perineal trauma in a younger child mandates a careful evaluation for child abuse by family or nonfamily caretakers.

All prescription and over-the-counter medications should be reviewed. Antecedent viral infections may not only be treated with aspirin or antibiotic-containing medications leading to GI bleeding, but also may be the prodromal phase of diseases that may present with a colitis (hemolytic-uremic syndrome). Recent anorexia, hypoglycemia, hypoperfusion, or intrinsic cardiac disease may result in ischemic colitis.

The following information should be gathered at history-taking:

Age of patient
Estimation of the quantity of blood loss
Condition of the patient
Character of blood
Association with abdominal or rectal pain
Association with diarrhea or mucus
Association with fever
Association with other systemic symptoms (arthritis or uveitis)
Failure to thrive or to grow
Recent illnesses
Family history of GI diseases
Family history of bleeding disorders
Travel history
Drinking water

PHYSICAL EXAMINATION

The initial assessment should determine the extent and duration of recent and ongoing blood losses. Attention to vital signs is more reliable than estimation of blood loss, which may be exaggerated. Evidence of skin lesions or bruising may support coagulopathy, vasculitis (Henoch-Schönlein syndrome), or inflammatory bowel disease (pyoderma gangrenosum, erythema nodosum). Pallor may be due to decreased perfusion or anemia. Abdominal pain, distention, or an "acute" abdomen may be present in intussusception or midgut volvulus, or may indicate infection or inflammatory bowel disease. A careful perirectal examination will reveal fissures or fistulae. The digital rectal examination will confirm the presence of blood and may reveal a distal polyp. Physical examination should include determination or evaluation of the following:

Vital signs (heart rate, blood pressure, temperature)
General condition
Skin vascular lesions, pallor, or bruising
Evidence of oropharyngeal trauma or epistaxis
Cardiac abnormalities
Abdominal pain
Organomegaly
Rectal examination to verify blood in stools and identify fissures, fistulae, and distal polyps

LABORATORY EVALUATION

The laboratory tests, outlined in this section, help organize an evaluation. The first stage, guided by the history and physical examination, contains hematology tests and cultures. The second stage involves direct observation or imaging. The sulfur colloid test or tagged RBC scans may demonstrate active bleeding. The technetium scan will be concentrated in gastric mucosa, which will help identify a Meckel diverticulum.

LABORATORY EVALUATION

First stage (guided by history and physical examination)
Complete blood cell count, differential cell count, platelet count
Reticulocyte count
Erythrocyte sedimentation rate
Stool cultures
Stool ova and parasites
Apt-Downey test
Serologic evidence of chronic malnutrition
Second stage
Nasogastric aspiration to rule out upper GI tract bleeding
Sigmoidoscopy or colonoscopy
Sulfur colloid or RBC bleeding scan
Technetium Meckel scan
Abdominal x-ray for "thumbprinting," obstruction
Barium enema with air contrast
Pentagastrin-stimulated scan for Meckel diverticulum
Upper GI tract barium series with small bowel follow-through
Third stage
Arteriography
Surgical exploration

RECTAL BLEEDING
Differential diagnosis

Arteriovenous (AV) malformation
Colitis
Constipation
Duplication
Fissures
Enteritis
Inflammatory bowel disease
Intussusception
Meckel diverticulum
Milk protein allergy
Necrotizing enterocolitis (NEC)
Polyp
Swallowed blood
Stricture
Viral enteritis
Volvulus

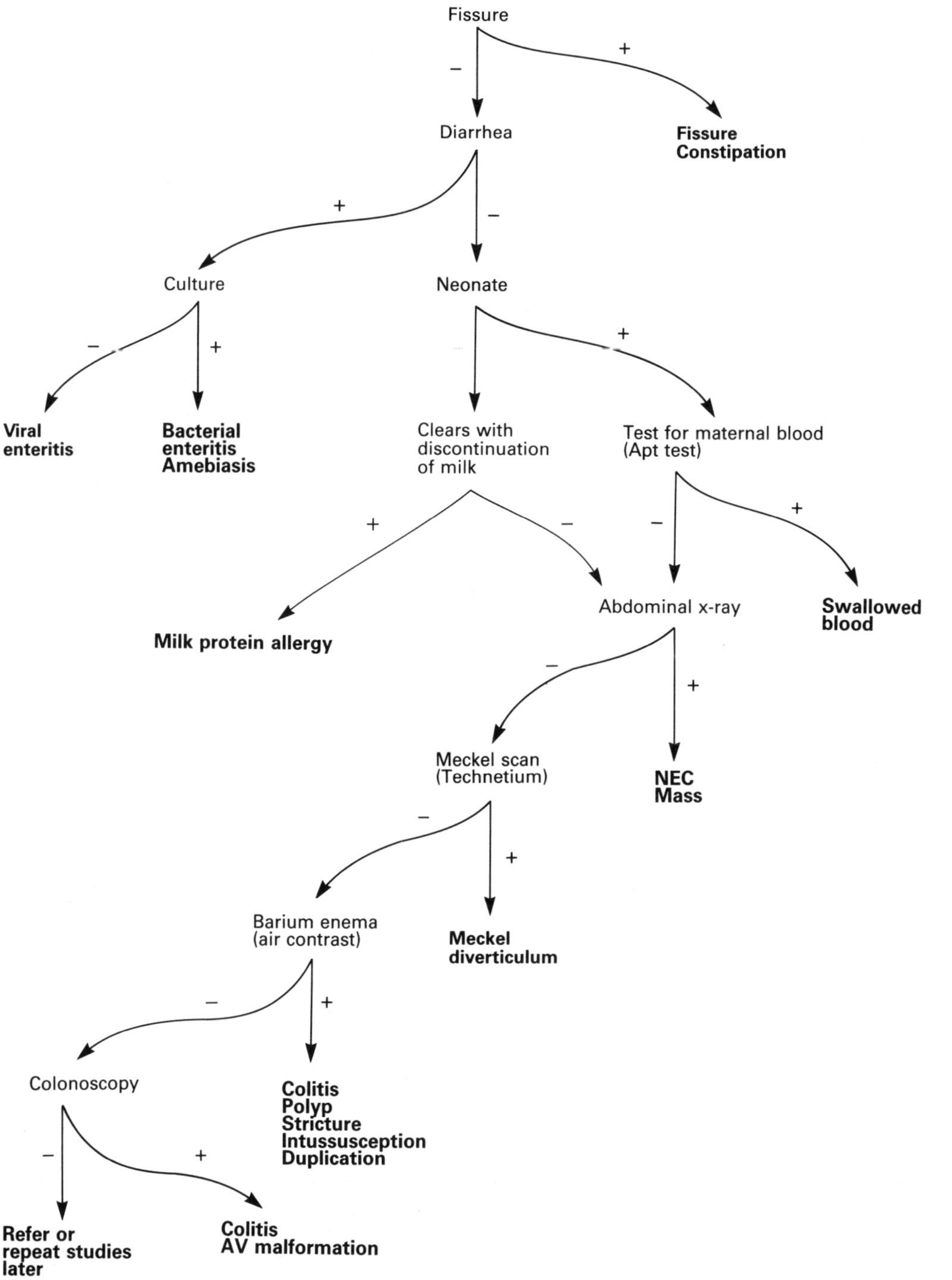

FIG 47–3
Decision tree for differential diagnosis of rectal bleeding.

INDICATIONS FOR CONSULTATION OR REFERRAL

The evaluation of rectal bleeding can usually be coordinated in the outpatient setting. Screening serologic studies and stool cultures should be performed before an advanced evaluation is performed. Radiographic, sigmoidoscopic, and nuclear medicine scans can be performed on most patients on an ambulatory basis.

DISCUSSION OF ALGORITHM

The evaluation of rectal bleeding is guided by the age of the patient in association with the particular symptoms and signs. The decision tree (Fig 47–3) stresses a differential diagnosis based on the age of the patient and knowledge of the circumstances under which the blood loss is identified. Table 47–1 stresses the large number of conditions that may result in rectal bleeding. Categorization based on whether blood loss is occult, visible but in a well child, associated with systemic findings, or a result of massive hemorrhage will aid narrowing the diagnostic consideration.

BIBLIOGRAPHY

Boley SJ, et al: Severe lower intestinal bleeding: Diagnosis and treatment. *Clin Gastroenterol* 1981; 10:65–91.

Collins REC: Some problems of gastrointestinal bleeding in children. *Arch Dis Child* 1971; 46:110.

Franken EA Jr.: Gastrointestinal bleeding in infants and children: Radiologic investigation. *JAMA* 1974; 229:1339.

Hyams JS, Leichtner AM, Schwartz AN: Recent advances in diagnosis and treatment of gastrointestinal hemorrhage in infants and children. *J Pediatr* 1985; 106:1.

Liebman WM: Diagnosis and management of upper gastrointestinal hemorrhage in children. *Pediatr Ann* 1976; 5(11):690–699.

Motil KJ, Grand RJ: Ulcerative colitis and Crohn disease in children. *Pediatr Rev* 1987; 9:109.

Sherman NJ, Clatworthy HW Jr: Gastrointestinal bleeding in neonates. A study of 94 cases. *Surgery* 1967; 62:614.

Spencer R: Gastrointestinal hemorrhage in infancy and childhood. 476 cases. *Surgery* 1964; 55:718.

Stanley-Brown EG, Stevenson SS: Massive gastrointestinal hemorrhage in the newborn infant. *Pediatrics* 1965; 35:482.

Wagner ML: Acute gastrointestinal bleeding in infants and children. *Pediatr Ann* 1975; 5:663.

48 STIFF NECK

Carol Carraccio, M.D.

Stiff neck may be either a presenting complaint or an accompanying sign of a more generalized illness. The diagnostic possibilities make it a challenge for the primary care physician, since some cases run a self-limited course, while others require immediate intervention.

DIFFERENTIAL DIAGNOSIS

COMMON CAUSES OF STIFF NECK

Trauma
Vertebral
  Subluxation
  Dislocation
  Fracture
Intracranial hemorrhage
Muscle spasm
Infection
Cervical adenitis
Meningitis
Brain abscess
Epidural abscess
Encephalitis
Epiglottitis
Retropharyngeal abscess
Tonsillitis
Cervical osteomyelitis
Diskitis
Pneumonia
Otitis media
Poliomyelitis
Tetanus
Other systemic infections
  Infectious mononucleosis
  Influenza
Immunologic
Collagen diseases
Intoxications
Phenothiazines
Tumor
Brain or spinal cord
Meningeal
Vertebral
Congenital
Bony deformities of the spine
Spastic cerebral palsy
Congenital torticollis
Cerebral aneurysms

DISCUSSION

The differential diagnosis of neck stiffness includes such benign conditions as muscle spasm and such life-threatening conditions as meningitis. Typically, the more serious causes of neck stiffness, such as significant trauma, epiglottitis, and central nervous system (CNS) disease will present with other historical and physical features suggestive of the cause.

Any infection that causes significant cervical adenopathy may also cause a patient to present with a chief complaint of neck stiffness. Included in this category would be streptococcal pharyngitis manifested by fever, tonsillar exudate, and cervical adenopathy and also infectious mononucleosis manifested by fever, generalized adenopathy, pharyngitis, and, possibly, hepatosplenomegaly. Cat-scratch disease may also cause neck stiffness on the basis of cervical adenitis or the myeloradiculopathy that may be part of its clinical spectrum. The scratch should be visible on physical examination. There may be a pustule at the site of the scratch with involvement of the regional lymph nodes. The atypical mycobacteria cause cervical adenopathy that is oftentimes suppurative. Other local infectious processes such as upper lobe pneumonia, cervical osteomyelitis, and dental abscess may be associated with neck stiffness. The child with osteomyelitis usually has low-grade fever and point tenderness over the involved cervical vertebra. Dental abscess may be detected by examination of the oral cavity for erythema and swelling of the alveolar ridge or sensitivity to percussion of the involved tooth. Viral infections, particularly influenza, have been associated with neck stiffness. Children with these infections will usually have other respiratory signs as well as fever and myalgias to go along with this stiffness.

Children with a complaint of stiff neck secondary to drug reactions usually have severe nuchal ridigity and often opisthotonic posturing and facial grimacing. Reactions to phenothiazine may be treated with intravenous diphenhydramine.

Nuchal rigidity secondary to cervical arthritis is one of the findings in juvenile rheumatoid arthritis (JRA) and also in ankylosing spondylitis. Since neck stiffness is usually not a presenting complaint in these diseases, a past history of joint involvement with limitation of motion are consistent with the diagnosis. Likewise, most congenital causes of neck stiffness will be readily diagnosed on the basis of history and physical examination.

DATA GATHERING

HISTORY

Typically, with the more serious injuries, the acute onset of pain immediately follows the injury. The type of activity that the child was engaged in when the injury occurred will also be helpful in determining the sequelae of the injury. For children with Down syndrome, ligamentous laxity involving the upper cervical spine causes atlantoaxial instability. Whether this actually predisposes these children to cervical dislocations with lesser degrees of trauma remains controversial. Minor trauma leading to muscle strain or spasm is usually more insidious in onset and thus more difficult to pin to a specific traumatic event. In the young infant, a history of birth trauma is important since a hematoma may form within the sternocleidomastoid muscle. Irritation of the meninges by blood, as occurs in a subarachnoid hemorrhage, causes nuchal rigidity. Likewise, tumor cells can cause similar meningeal irritation.

Once a history of serious injury has been explored, symptoms of serious infections must be addressed. Fever and stiff neck with change in mental status or seizure activity suggests meningitis, encephalitis, or brain abscess. Fever and stiff neck with respiratory difficulty suggests epiglottitis, retropharyngeal abscess, or pneumonia.

There are numerous other less severe infections that may be associated with neck stiffness, and specific complaints must be sought. Does the child have a sore throat? Cervical adenitis associated with pharyngitis, whether bacterial (as in streptococcal infection) or viral (as in Epstein-Barr virus infection), may cause neck stiffness. Cervical adenitis unassociated with pharyngitis may also cause neck stiffness. Multiple pathogens may be implicated. These include bacteria such as *Staphylococcus aureus* and *Streptococcus* as well as mycobacteria, especially the atypical types, and the etiologic agent of cat-scratch disease. Mouth pain and cervical adenopathy are seen with dental abscesses. Upper respiratory tract symptoms accompanied by fever and headache suggest influenza infection. Back pain accompanying the neck stiffness may be indicative of diskitis, cervical osteomyelitis, or a vertebral tumor such as osteoid osteoma. Other tumors associated with stiff neck are those that infiltrate the meninges by local spread or metastasize to the meninges, as occurs with leukemia. Joint involvement with a history of pain and stiffness should alert the physician to explore other features consistent with collagen diseases.

A medication history is also important since drugs such as phenothiazines and metoclopramide may cause dystonic reactions of which neck stiffness is a major manifestation. Since ingestions are not always witnessed, the acute onset of nuchal rigidity associated with facial grimacing and, oftentimes, opisthotonic posturing in an otherwise healthy child should alert the physician to the possibility of drug toxicity. Phenothiazine derivatives are a common ingredient in cough medications. Metoclopramide, a new antiemetic drug, has also been implicated in causing these reactions. Lead poisoning may cause an encephalopathy characterized by cerebral edema that has neck stiffness as one of its manifestations. A history of pica as well as associated symptoms of ataxia and change in mental status should be sought.

PHYSICAL EXAMINATION

A rapid assessment for signs of respiratory distress, significant traumatic injury, and change in mental status is indicated. In these cases, immediate diagnostic and/or therapeutic procedures should be initiated. A child with epiglottitis or a retropharyngeal abscess will present in respiratory distress. Classically, patients with these disorders have difficulty swallowing; thus, drooling is a classic sign of these diseases. The neck is rigidly held in a position that allows maximal air entry into the trachea.

If significant traumatic injury to the head and/or neck is suspected, physical examination of this area should be deferred. Neck immobilization is indicated while appropriate x-ray studies are obtained.

Children who have a stiff neck secondary to CNS pathologic conditions usually have other signs on physical examination. There may be an altered mental status as well as abnormal neurologic findings or seizure activity.

Cervical adenitis is manifested by erythematous, swollen, hot, tender lymph nodes. Children with cervical adenitis are typically febrile. Cervical adenopathy may accompany systemic illnesses such as infectious mononucleosis or influenza; generalized adenopathy, pharyngitis, and splenomegaly should be sought in the former and other signs of respiratory infection in the latter. Cervical lymph nodes, providing lymphatic drainage to the pharynx, will respond to an infection in this area by becoming swollen and tender.

Since neck stiffness secondary to cervical arthritis in the rheumatologic disorders is typically not a presenting complaint but a later manifestation, the physical examination will usually reveal stiffness in other joints and possibly joint deformity with some limitation of motion.

Neck stiffness as a result of congenital anomalies is quite evident on physical examination. Klippel-Feil syndrome, which is characterized by failure of segmentation of the cervical spine, is usually associated with other skeletal anomalies. Likewise, Arnold-Chiari malformations, which consist of abnormal development and displacement of cerebellar and medullar tissue, are usually associated with aqueductal stenosis and thus hydrocephalus. Spastic cerebral palsy will be evident by a generalized increase in tone, not just neck stiffness, and possibly contractures resulting in significant impairment of motor skills. Congenital torticollis is, however, usually found in otherwise healthy infants. It is associated with unilateral shortening of the sternocleidomastoid muscle with subsequent tilting of the head to the shortened side.

LABORATORY EVALUATION

For some patients, such as those suffering from minor trauma or minor infectious processes, laboratory tests may not be indicated. However, for more severe pathologic conditions, laboratory tests may be quite helpful in diagnosis.

When indicated, the most useful laboratory aid in establishing a diagnosis is radiography of the neck. X-ray studies are useful in determining the severity of a traumatic injury. They will also be helpful in diagnosing epiglottitis, retropharyngeal abscess, some tumors, arthritic changes, osteomyelitis, pneumonia, and congenital anomalies. A bone scan is more sensitive in detecting osteomyelitis and diskitis.

Computed tomography (CT) provides excellent resolution of bone and the paraspinal soft tissues, making it a useful diagnostic tool for injuries, congenital malformations, and tumors. The ability of magnetic resonance imaging (MRI) to complement CT with excellent resolution of processes involving the marrow and soft tissues allows detection of lesions within the spinal cord.

A high white blood cell count and sedimentation rate will support the suspicion of an infectious cause of neck stiffness. Examination of the cerebrospinal fluid is critical when CNS infection is considered. Screening tests for toxins are useful when such an ingestion is suspected.

DISCUSSION OF ALGORITHM

An algorithm for differential diagnosis of stiff neck is presented in Figure 48–1.After documentation of the absence of trauma as a causation of neck stiffness, signs of fever and toxicity should be sought.

The febrile, toxic-appearing patient demands prompt evaluation so that treatment of such medical emergencies as meningitis, epiglottitis, and retropharyngeal abscess may be initiated.

In the afebrile patient who appears toxic,

STIFF NECK
Differential diagnosis

Brain abscess
Cervical adenitis
Collagen disease
Congenital anomaly
Dental abscess
Diskitis
Drug
Encephalitis
Epiglottitis
Intracranial hemorrhage
Juvenile rheumatoid arthritis (JRA)
Lumphadenitis
Meningitis
Mononucleosis
Muscle strain
Osteomyelitis
Pneumonia
Retropharyngeal abscess
Rotary subluxation
Trauma
Tumor
Vertebral fracture

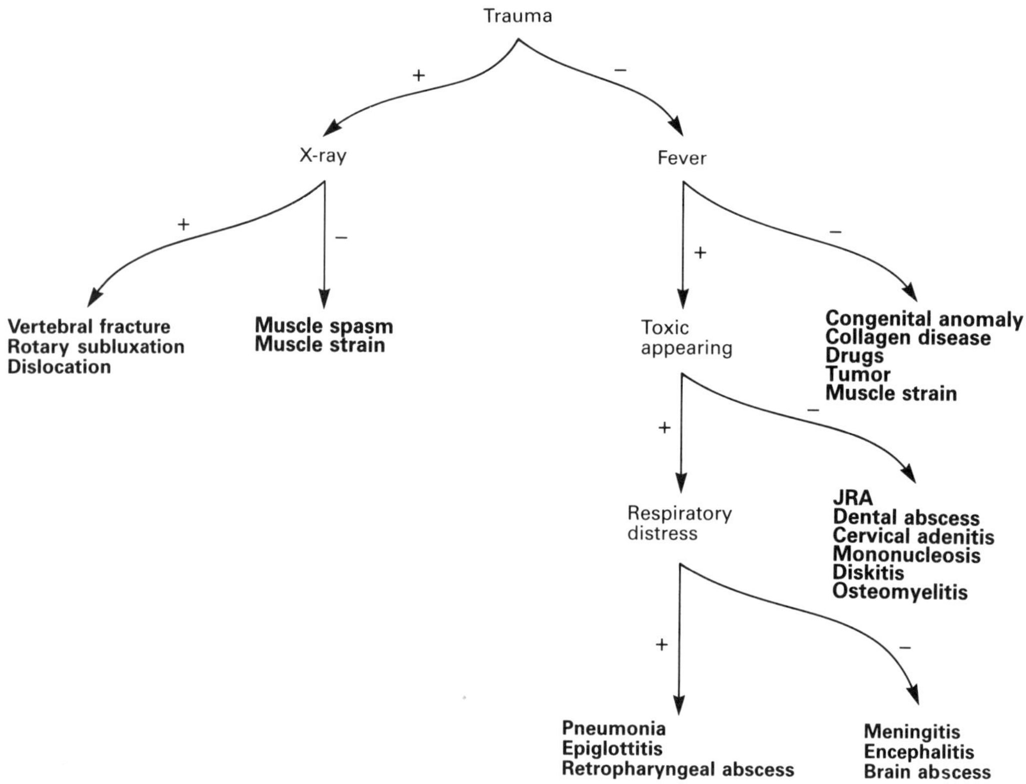

FIG 48–1
Decision tree for differential diagnosis of stiff neck.

consideration centers on drug reaction and intracranial catastrophies.

The febrile patient who is not toxic-appearing can be evaluated for the less serious infections associated with neck stiffness.

BIBLIOGRAPHY

Davidson RG: Atlantoaxial instability in individuals with Down syndrome: A fresh look at the evidence. *Pediatrics* 1988; 81:857–865.

Doughty RA: Stiff neck in Fleisher G, Ludwig S, Henretig F, et al (eds): *Textbook of Pediatric Emergency Medicine*, ed 2. Baltimore, Williams & Wilkins, 1988; pp 219–222.

Fitz CR: Diagnostic imaging in children with spinal disorders. *Pediatr Clin North Am* 1985; 32:1537–1558.

Menkes J: *Textbook of Child Neurology*. Philadelphia, Lea & Febiger, 1974.

Weiner HL, Bresnan MJ, Levitt LP: *Pediatric Neurology for the House Officer*. Baltimore, Williams & Wilkins, 1977.

49 WEAKNESS OR FATIGUE

Stephen Ludwig, M.D.

Children sometimes complain of feeling weak or tired; more often, however, parents of young children note the loss of developmental milestones or increased lassitude. At other times when a child's cranky behavior is analyzed by parents, fatigue is the presumed cause. In preschool-aged children, parents may note decreased athletic ability or lack of stamina in comparison with the child's peers. The school-aged child and adolescent demonstrates weakness or fatigue by diminished school performance and excessive sleeping despite a psychological desire to participate in activities. Once the parent raises the question of weakness, the child may confirm. This invariably prompts concern and an immediate visit to the primary care physician.

DIFFERENTIAL DIAGNOSIS

COMMON CAUSES OF WEAKNESS OR FATIGUE

Trauma
Extremity trauma, fracture, dislocated radial head
Vertebral or spinal cord trauma
Child abuse
Post head trauma
Infection or post infection
Viral myositis
Poliomyelitis
Guillain-Barré syndrome
Transverse myelitis
Epidural abscess
Botulism
Mononucleosis
Hepatitis
Tuberculosis
Toxic
Tick paralysis
Drug reaction (e.g., antihistamine)
Drug abuse
Allergy or inflammation
Allergic fatigue
Adenoidal hypertrophy
Dermatomyositis
Polymyositis
Rhabdomyolyis
Endocrine or metabolic
Hypothyroidism
Hyperthyroidism
Adrenal insufficiency
Hypokalemia
Hypercalcemia
Tumor
Leukemia
Diffuse malignant disease
Congenital or genetic
Duchenne muscular dystrophy
Myotonic dystrophy
Central core disease of muscle
Nemaline myopathy
Myotubular myopathy
Werdnig-Hoffmann disease
Multiple etiologies
Anemia
Sleep disturbance
Chronic illness
Psychogenic

DISCUSSION

Acute Onset of Symptoms

If onset of weakness or fatigue is acute, determine if there is associated infectious disease or post infection. Diseases that have rapid onset can be subdivided into those associated with signs of infection, such as fever and prodromal illness, and those not. Infectious or postinfectious causes include viral myositis, Guillain-Barré syndrome, transverse myelitis, epidural abscess, and poliomyelitis.

Viral myositis, the most common reason for acute onset of weakness, is caused by influenza virus, enteroviruses, and other viruses. It is associated with weakness, muscle pain, and tenderness to palpation. The laboratory finding of a high creatine kinase level (which may be as high as several thousand units per liter) is supportive of the diagnosis. The inflammation resolves spontaneously after a period of rest and pain control.

In *Guillain-Barré syndrome,* the muscle weakness has a characteristic pattern, as flaccid weakness or frank paralysis ascends from feet to head over several hours or several days. Sensory changes also may be found on examination. The child should be immediately referred for inpatient care because of the possibility of respiratory distress. On lumbar puncture the CSF shows the classic finding of albumin-cytologic dissociation (i.e., protein level elevated, number of leukocytes normal or slightly elevated).

Transverse myelitis is another serious condition that requires hospitalization. It may be recognized in the office in a child with lower extremity weakness or paralysis with associated sensory abnormality and urinary retention or loss of bowel control. Myelitis may occur at any site along the cord, producing variations of the typical presentation. The CSF has increased cells and protein. Transverse myelitis has been associated with other infections such as varicella, hepatitis A, cytomegalovirus and *Mycoplasma pneumoniae.*

Epidural abscess is caused by bacterial agents, usually staphylococci. It arises from a spreading local infection or from osteomyelitis of a vertebra. The abscess impinges on nerve roots and in turn causes weakness. The CSF examination usually shows a marked increase in white blood cells. The diagnosis is confirmed by computed tomographic scan.

Poliomyelitis also causes acute onset of weakness. It begins with an infectious prodrome of fever, lethargy, and irritability. These may be signs of diffuse central nervous system involvement and clinical and laboratory finding of aseptic meningitis. Poliomyelitis is accompanied by asymmetric paralysis.

Several disorders with acute onset not associated with typical infectious prodromal symptoms are trauma, tick paralysis, and botulism.

Trauma should be considered when weakness has acute onset, particularly in the infant or the preverbal child. Fractures, dislocations (particularly of the radial head), and soft tissue injury to an extremity may cause weakness and disease. Trauma to the cervical spine may also produce weakness or paralysis. Children with cervical instability are at increased risk for this type of injury, particularly those with juvenile rheumatoid arthritis or Down syndrome. The trauma may be accidental or inflicted, and it is important that the physician make this determination (see Chapter 52, Child Abuse and Neglect).

Tick paralysis, an uncommon cause of acute onset of paralysis, results from a toxin elaborated by either the dog tick or the wood tick. The pattern of paralysis is similar to that in Guillain-Barré syndrome: the weakness is ascending and symmetric. Careful examination may reveal a tick, removal of which will promptly reverse the paralysis. Unlike Guillain-Barré syndrome, there is no viral prodromal illness.

Botulism, a condition with acute onset, has two forms: infantile and adult. The infantile form has moderate spread of onset, and often begins with constipation, lethargy, and generalized weakness. The descending pattern of weakness includes facial and airway stabilizing musculature. These infants, usually 1 to 5 months of age, should be immediately referred for hospitalization. The progression of symptoms and electromyographic features are diagnostic. The adult form of botulism may also be seen in children. It is acquired from eating contaminated (canned) foods. It too progresses in a cephalocaudal pattern, often beginning with diplopia secondary to ocular muscle weakness, dysphagia, and dysarthria. The peripheral muscles are involved later, and occasionally the respiratory and cardiac muscles.

Subacute Onset of Symptoms

Conditions with a subacute, chronic, or more indolent onset include a group that affect the young infant and are related for the most part to disorders of neurologic innervation, muscle structure, and metabolism. The major entities in this category are diseases of anterior horn cells, such as *Werdnig-Hoffmann disease;* diseases of the myoneural function, such as *myasthenia gravis;* congenital muscle disease, such as *central core disease* and *nemaline* or *myotubular myopathy;* and *muscular dystrophies,* such as Duchenne.

The second subgroup with chronic onset includes conditions that produce weakness through electrolyte, metabolic, and hormonal disturbance: *hypokalemia* and *hyperkalemia;* endocrine causes of weakness, such as *hypothyroidism* and *Addision disease;* and rare conditions such as *polymyositis, rhabdomyolysis, paroxysmal myoglobinuria,* and *acute intermittent porphyria.*

DATA GATHERING

HISTORY

The first step in evaluating fatigue or weakness is to clarify the patient's and family's use of the terms. Fatigue refers to a subjective feeling of being tired, unable to maintain a normal level of activity, a desire to have more rest. Weakness on the other hand is an objective and quantifiable state characterized by diminished muscular strength and inability to exert force. Those patients who demonstrate weakness usually feel fatigued. However, the opposite is not true. Many children have no true weakness, yet feel and act fatigued. The clinician must distinguish between the objective and subjective in working through the differential diagnosis. In the history, it is important to look for functional impairment, which gives the physician an indication of how rapidly the evaluation must be pursued.

Once it has been established that true muscular weakness is present, it must be determined whether this symptom is of acute or slow onset. Rate of onset should be easy to determine by history. However, in some cases, because of the age of the child, the observation skills of the parents, or the nature of the disorder, the point of symptom onset is difficult to determine. Those diseases that have rapid onset can also be subdivided into those associated with signs of infection, such as fever and prodromal illness, and those not.

If the child is young and weakness clearly is present, several other historical points are important, including pregnancy history, labor and delivery history, family history, genetic history, and careful developmental history.

When fatigue is present without objective weakness, exploration of the sleep history, social history, and family history may yield important clues to the diagnosis. Also inquire how the child is functioning in relationships at home, in school, and in the community. Often the patient is not getting enough rest or is using the acceptable excuse of fatigue to avoid responsibilities or social interactions.

PHYSICAL EXAMINATION

The examination begins by observing how the child walks into the office, or in the case of an infant how the child moves when placed prone and supine on a flat surface. In addition, the physical examination should isolate and test specific muscle groups and test for proximal, distal, or diffuse muscle weakness. The examiner must also determine the size, shape, and symmetry of muscles and palpate for tenderness, induration, and bulk of muscle mass. For example, in proximal muscle weakness there may be wasting of the thigh muscles and appearance of pseudohypertrophy of the calf muscles. It is important to grade muscle strength using standard nomenclature:

Grade 5: Normal; full range against gravity and normal resistance.
Grade 4: Good; full range against gravity and moderate resistance.
Grade 3: Fair; full range against gravity.
Grade 2: Poor; full range against gravity eliminated.
Grade 1: Trace; no movement of joint.
Grade 0: No motion, flaccid.

Careful examination of the integument may reveal lesions of dermatomyositis or other collagen vascular diseases. Examine the joints for signs of arthritis and the presence of skin contractures. A thorough neurologic examination is also essential, because many causes of weakness are nerve related.

LABORATORY EVALUATION

The evaluation of true weakness is based on three primary studies: muscle enzymes (creatine kinase and aldolase), electromyography, and muscle biopsy. For the office practitioner, muscle enzyme studies are available, but the others usually must be ordered and interpreted by a specialist. Additional studies may be ordered to search for infection or toxicologic disease.

In evaluating fatigue, a complete blood cell count, reticulocyte count, sedimentation rate, mononucleosis test, and toxicologic studies are useful. More complex studies are usually not indicated unless the history and physical examination raise the possibility of a specific line of inquiry.

INDICATIONS FOR CONSULTATION OR REFERRAL

Consultation and referral will depend on the cause discovered or suspected. Consultants in neurology, genetics, infectious diseases, rheumatology, or psychiatry may be needed. Consultations are needed in the minority of actual cases. The primary physician, using the approach presented here and time as a modifier, most often will arrive at a benign diagnosis for fatigue. The finding of true weakness occurs less often, and usually referral is necessary. When weakness appears to be progressive over hours to days, prompt referral to a hospital is necessary, particularly because of potential progression to respiratory seizures.

DISCUSSION OF ALGORITHM

The evaluation begins by distinguishing between true muscular weakness and fatigue (Fig 49–1). The entities that cause true weakness have been classified on the basis of acuteness of onset and association with signs and symptoms of infection.

In the second major group to be considered are children who complain of feeling weak yet have no objective muscular weakness that is detectable. The first issue to be addressed is the finding of pallor. If pallor is present, it needs to be elucidated by obtaining a complete blood cell count and reticulocyte count. Most of these children will be found to have anemia. By using the CBC and in particular the red blood cell indices and reticulocyte count, the cause of anemia may be determined (see Chapter 59, Anemia). These studies will elucidate a common problem, such as simple iron deficiency anemia, or sequestration crisis in a patient known to have sickle cell anemia. In some cases the finding of pallor and anemia may lead to the diagnosis of a malignant lesion. The most common childhood malignancies can be detected if the laboratory test is accompanied by a thorough physical examination (see Chapter 63, Malignancy).

The next decision point is made by determining if the child has significant functional impairment. If there is a sense of fatigue but the child continues to function or simply requires a bit more sleep to function, the child can be observed. However, if the symptom is accompanied by decreased function, lack of participation in usual activities, lack of appetite, or actual weight loss, it needs prompt evaluation. The cause of functional impairment usually is infectious, allergic, or psychophysiologic. In the infectious category are primarily prolonged infections such as *mononucleosis, hepatitis,* or *tuberculosis.* The child with severe *asthma, allergic rhinitis,* or *"allergic fatigue" syndrome* may have fatigue, as may children who are receiving allergy medications such as antihistamines. In the psychophysiologic category are significant *depression, school avoidance,* or *drug abuse.* Each of these conditions is a psychosocial emergency and requires prompt referral to a mental health specialist.

Those children who were initially observed may have both physiologic and psychologic reasons for feeling fatigued. Observation may continue for 1 to 3 weeks, after which another visit and further evaluation may be required. In the physiologic realm, the reason for fatigue is most often an actual sleep disturbance, something that keeps the child from getting a complete night's sleep, thus producing the feeling of fatigue. Conditions such as recurrent minor infections, adenoidal hypertrophy, and gastroesophageal reflux are common causes. In the psychological realm the mechanism is the same: Something is keeping the child from falling asleep, for example, anxiety, or from staying asleep, for example, recurrent nightmares, phobias, or parental behavior such as frequent checking or too rapid parental response to the normal stirrings of the infant at rest. With the watching-waiting method of treatment many of these minor situations resolve themselves. If fatigue persists, the primary care provider may

WEAKNESS OR FATIGUE
Differential Diagnosis

Anxiety	Electrolyte disturbance	Myositis
Asthma	Endocrinopathy	Poliomyelitis
Botulism	Fears	Polymyositis
Chronic Infection	Family dysfunction	School avoidance
Depression	Guillain-Barré syndrome	Tick paralysis
Drug abuse	Hepatitis	Transverse myositis
Epstein-Barr virus (EBV)	Myelitis	Trauma
Epidural abscess	Myasthenia gravis	Viral myositis

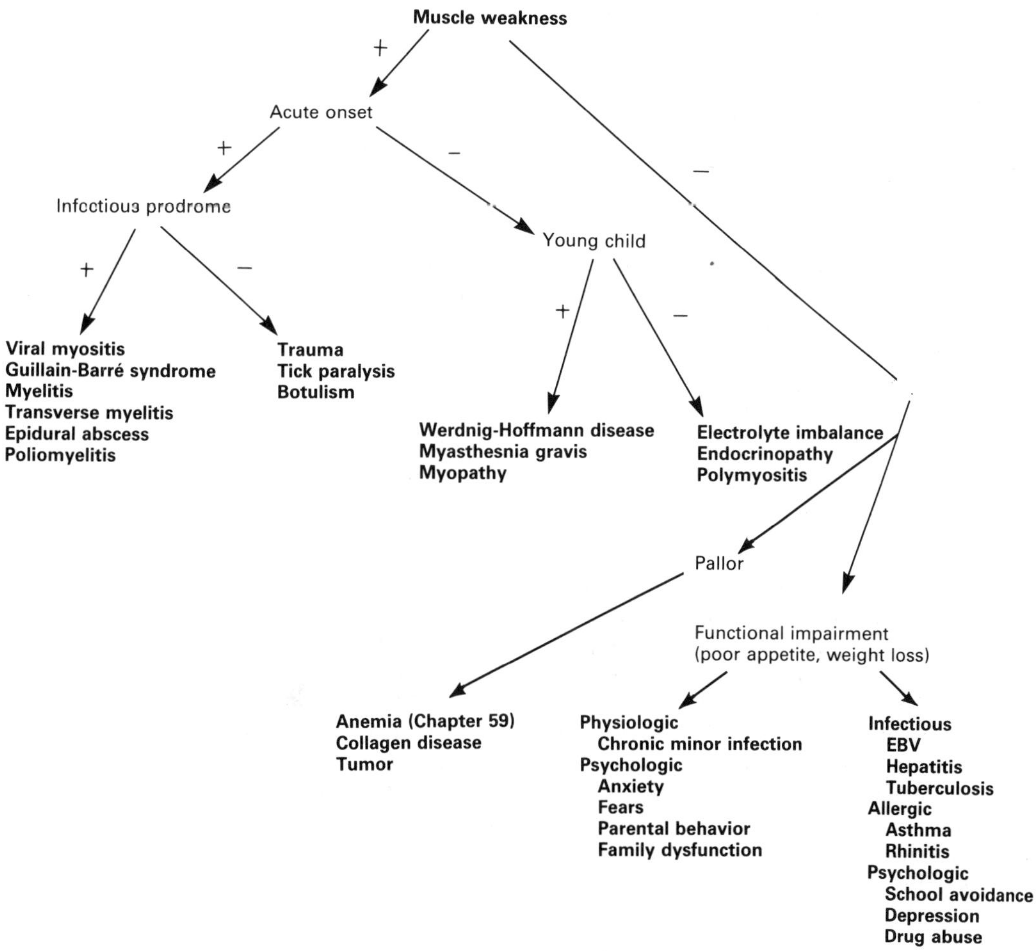

FIG 49–1
Decision tree for differential diagnosis of weakness or fatigue.

need to hold a long office visit to track down the elusive cause.

BIBLIOGRAPHY

Antony JH, Procupis PG, Oririen RS: Benign acute childhood myositis. *Neurology* 1979; 29:1068–1072.

Bellett PS: The diagnostic approach to common symptoms and signs in infants, children and adolescents. Philadelphia, Lea & Febiger, 1989.

Fenichel GM, Swaiman KF, Wright FS, et al: The practice of pediatric neurology, ed 2. St Louis, CV Mosby Co, 1982.

Hadley G: Pediatric spinal trauma. *J Neurosurg* 1988; 68:1824.

Ruff RL, Weissman J: Endocrine myopathies. *Neurol Clin* 1988; 6:575–592.

50 VOMITING

Jeffrey R. Avner, M.D.

Vomiting is defined as forceful expulsion of matter from the stomach through the mouth. This action is often preceded by nausea and accompanied by gastric and abdominal contractions. These various components are coordinated by a vomiting center located in the reticular formation of the medulla. Physicians need to differentiate true vomiting from spitting up or regurgitation, common in young infants. Unlike the rhythmic and coordinated action of vomiting, regurgitation refers to nonforceful reflux of stomach contents, which tend to roll out rather than being expelled from the mouth and is usually of little significance.

The clinical findings in a child with acute vomiting relate to both the underlying cause and the duration of the vomiting. For example, fever, diarrhea, abdominal pain, headache, and other systemic complaints may predominate initially, but as the vomiting continues the signs and symptoms of dehydration, such as lethargy, tachycardia, and poor skin turgor, become increasingly apparent. Associated symptoms that should serve as warning signs of more serious illness include age less than 6 months, intractable or projectile vomiting, bloody or bilious emesis, severe abdominal pain, and abdominal distention.

DIFFERENTIAL DIAGNOSIS

COMMON CAUSES OF VOMITING

Infectious

Gastroenteritis
Otitis media
Upper respiratory tract infection
Sepsis
Meningitis
Urinary tract infection or pyelonephritis
Pneumonia
Pertussis
Appendicitis
Hepatitis

Gastrointestinal

Esophageal
- Gastroesophageal reflux
- Chalasia
- Hiatus hernia
- Esophageal stricture

Gastric
- Pyloric stenosis
- Peptic ulcer disease
- Gastric bezoar

Intestinal
- Intussusception
- Incarcerated hernia
- Postoperative adhesions
- Malrotation
- Volvulus
- Cholelithiasis

Central nervous system

Head trauma
Increased intracranial pressure
Brain tumor
Hydrocephalus
Migraine
Seizure

Metabolic-endocrine

Inborn errors of metabolism
Diabetic ketoacidosis
Congenital adrenal hyperplasia
Hypercalcemia
Renal tubular acidosis
Reye syndrome

Genitourinary-renal

Urinary tract obstruction
Renal stones
Renal failure
Pregnancy

Allergic-immunologic
Cow's milk allergy
Celiac disease
Toxic
Drugs
Toxins
Food poisoning
Psychosocial
Inappropriate feeding
Psychogenic vomiting
Cyclic vomiting

DISCUSSION

Infection.—Viral infection of the gastrointestinal tract is the most common cause of acute vomiting. There may be associated low-grade fever and diarrhea, but the child usually appears well unless the vomiting is prolonged and signs of dehydration ensue. Bacterial gastroenteritis is more abrupt and is accompanied by abdominal pain, fever, anorexia, and bloody diarrhea. *Salmonella, Shigella,* and *Yersinia* are the common bacterial agents. Vomiting may be a symptom of parasitic infection, such as giardiasis, amebiasis, ascariasis, and hookworm; other symptoms include abdominal pain, poor weight gain, and bloody diarrhea.

Infections that occur outside the GI system may present with vomiting. Otitis media, for example, is one of the most common causes of vomiting. Upper respiratory tract infections may produce vomiting when postnasal drip or swallowed mucus cause gastric irritation. However, in the young child, in whom clinical signs are often absent or difficult to ascertain, vomiting may herald the onset of a more serious underlying infection. A child with meningitis often has vomiting, irritability, and lethargy before other meningeal signs appear. Urinary tract infection and pyelonephritis often present with the same constellation of findings seen in gastroenteritis (vomiting, fever, abdominal pain, back pain) and may not include urinary tract symptoms. A young child with pneumonia may have vomiting and dehydration as a result of fever and tachypnea. The child with paroxysmal cough and posttussive emesis should alert the physician to the possibility of pertussis.

Infection of the abdominal organs usually begins with anorexia and vomiting and may progress to severe abdominal pain and peritonitis. Appendicitis may occur at any age, and typically begins with nausea, vomiting, periumbilical abdominal pain, and low-grade fever. As the inflammation of the appendix progresses, peritoneal irritation occurs and the abdominal pain shifts to the right lower quadrant. There is marked tenderness at McBurney's point (one-third the distance from the right iliac crest to the umbilicus), but this varies depending on the position of the appendix (e.g., retrocecal, pelvic, retroileal). Prompt diagnosis of appendicitis is important because appendiceal abscess or perforation may occur.

Hepatitis usually presents with jaundice in addition to nausea, vomiting, and right upper quadrant tenderness. In the infant, hepatitis is usually due to congenital infection, whereas in the older child viruses and toxins predominate.

Gastrointestinal.—GI disorders that lead to vomiting are related to abnormal anatomy in the GI tract that interferes with normal peristalsis. It is useful to think of these disorders based on the presence or absence of intestinal obstruction.

An abnormality of esophageal or gastric motility usually presents in the first few months of life with recurrent vomiting or regurgitation after feeding. Chalasia is poor tone in the lower esophageal sphincter and may be accompanied by physiologic gastroesophageal reflux in as many as one third of all healthy newborns. Anything that increases intraabdominal pressure, and thus intragastric pressure, will exaggerate gastroesophageal reflux. Thus it is common for an infant to vomit or regurgitate after eating, coughing, or exercising. The position of an infant in an infant seat also tends to increase intraabdominal pressure and lead to reflux. In some cases the child may exhibit spasms of head, neck, and back arching (Sandifer syndrome) in response to the reflux, as a mechanism to prevent aspiration. While severe cases of reflux may be associated with aspiration pneumonia, failure to thrive, or esophagitis, most cases resolve by the end of the first year of life as the child spends more time upright and esophageal sphincter tone increases.

Hiatal and paraesophageal hernias, which involve prolapse of a portion of the stomach into the thoracic cavity, present with recurrent gastroesophageal reflux. Intermittent colicky abdominal pain, often associated with fatty foods, point to cholelithiasis, especially in children with risk factors for the development of biliary stones (e.g., patients with sickle cell disease and recurrent hemolysis develop bilirubin stones).

Any projectile, nonbilious vomiting should raise a high suspicion of pyloric stenosis. The infant usually has an unremarkable birth history, but episodes of vomiting begin by the first month of life. The vomiting is at first intermittent, but soon becomes projectile (often described as "shooting across the room"). The symptoms depend on the duration of the vomiting. Initially the infant appears well, but as the illness progresses, may appear irritable or lethargic. With prolonged vomiting, metabolic changes (hyponatremia, hypochloremia, hypokalemia, alkalosis) become evident. On physical examination, there may be a palpable olive, the hypertrophied muscle, just to the right of the midline above the umbilicus. Visible abdominal peristaltic waves may also be seen.

Intussusception is the telescoping of an intestinal segment and usually involves invagination of the ileum through the ileocecal valve into the colon. It is characteristically seen in children between 3 and 24 months of age and begins with the sudden onset of crampy abdominal pain during which the child screams and pulls the knees up to the abdomen. Vomiting follows shortly thereafter, and the child becomes increasingly lethargic or demonstrates paradoxic irritability. An abdominal mass, usually in the right lower quadrant, and heme-positive or currant jelly stools may be seen later in the course of the disease.

Gastric bezoars can present with intermittent vomiting, an abdominal mass, and weight loss. In children the bezoar usually consists of large quantities of matted hair in the stomach. Other causes of vomiting associated with small bowel obstruction include inguinal hernia, intestinal volvulus, or if there was previous abdominal surgery, intestinal adhesions.

Central Nervous System.—Any process that causes irritation of the central nervous system may result in vomiting. Cerebral edema, increased intracranial pressure, or changes in cerebral vascular flow may cause hypersensitivity of the vomiting center. The vomiting is often forceful, at times projectile, and may not be preceded by nausea.

It is common for head trauma to cause vomiting. Even minor head trauma, without any loss of consciousness, may cause vomiting for 6 to 8 hours after the initial injury. However, persistent vomiting or any associated neurologic change should alert the physician to the possibility of more serious injury (i.e., epidural, subdural, or subarachnoid bleed).

The vomiting associated with increased intracranial pressure from brain tumors, hydrocephalus, or pseudotumor cerebri is usually worse in the morning or when lying down and is accompanied by headache. Over time, other signs of increased intracranial pressure develop, such as increasing head circumference, bulging fontanelle, sunsetting, cranial nerve palsies, ataxia, or papilledema.

Certain types of headache, especially migraine, have vomiting as a prominent symptom. The typical migraine headache is pulsatile, preceded by an aura, and accompanied by nausea, vomiting, abdominal pain, and the desire to rest or sleep. Vomiting is occasionally seen with seizures, either during the acute event or in the early postictal period.

Metabolic-Endocrine.—Recurrent or persistent vomiting may be a sign of an underlying defect in amino acid, organic acid, or carbohydrate metabolism. These inborn errors of metabolism usually present as either acute decompensation or failure to thrive. In the acute setting, there is often a mild preceding illness, which is followed by rapid production of a metabolic acidosis or hyperammonemia. These metabolic derangements are accompanied by persistent, forceful vomiting. The child becomes progressively lethargic, and seizures or coma may ensue. On a more chronic basis, there is growth retardation and slowly progressive neurologic deterioration.

Diabetic ketoacidosis often presents with nausea, vomiting, and abdominal pain, although there is usually a history of tiredness, polyuria, polydipsia, and anorexia. As the vomiting, osmotic diuresis, and acidosis proceed, the child becomes more dehydrated and shock may ensue. The fruity smell of ketones on the breath reflect ketoacidosis.

Vomiting can be seen in acute adrenal insufficiency, which may be precipitated in a child with congenital adrenal hyperplasia who is under stress, noncompliant, or undiagnosed. Hypercalcemia usually produces anorexia, vomiting, dehydration, headache, polydipsia, and polyuria.

The abrupt onset of protracted vomiting, lethargy, and sleepiness after varicella or a flu-like illness should immediately alert the physician to the possibility of Reye syndrome. The vomiting usually starts within 1 week of the prodrome and is present in more than 80% of cases. Rapidly progressive encephalopathy and increased intracranial pressure can lead to altered mental status, stupor, and coma. Rapid evaluation and immediate referral to an intensive care unit should be the rule.

Genitourinary-Renal.—Infections of the genitourinary system, such as pelvic inflammatory disease, urethritis, cystitis, and pyelonephritis, are often accompanied by vomiting. In addition, any process that causes obstruction usually has vomiting in association with abdominal pain. Obstruction in the urinary tract can be caused by a variety of problems including posterior urethral valves, congenital or anatomic anomalies, calculi, or trauma. Typically there is nausea, vomiting, abdominal pain, and flank pain that is colicky in nature. Overflow incontinence and poor urinary stream may be noted as well. Obstructive renal insufficiency can lead to vomiting, diarrhea, and failure to thrive. Other causes of acute renal failure may be accompanied by anemia, edema, hypertension, and lethargy.

Pregnancy is a commonly overlooked diagnosis when an adolescent girl complains of nausea, vomiting, or morning sickness. A teenage girl should be questioned without her parents present about sexual activity, and a urine pregnancy test performed if there is the slightest suspicion of pregnancy.

Allergic-Immunologic.—Cow's milk allergy usually manifests itself within the first 2 months of life, and is more common in boys and children with a family history of allergies. There is an abnormal GI response probably related to the protein in cow's milk. Vomiting, diarrhea, and abdominal pain predominate, and may progress to gastric outlet obstruction. In addition there is often GI blood loss and protein malabsorption leading to anemia, edema, and failure to thrive.

Toxins.—Several drugs may cause vomiting when toxic levels are achieved either by inappropriate dosing, accidental ingestion, or suicide attempt. Theophylline is the most common medication used for reversible bronchospasm in the pediatric age group. The recommended oral dose is 16 to 24 mg/kg/day to maintain a serum concentration of 10 to 20 mg/L. Changes in theophylline metabolism are commonly seen in children during certain illnesses or when used in combination with certain drugs (e.g., erythromycin). As the toxic level is approached, nausea, vomiting, and abdominal cramping become apparent, and at high levels seizures may ensue.

Digitalis toxicity is often first manifested by nausea and vomiting, and may progress to weakness, worsening heart failure, and cardiac arrhythmias. With aspirin and iron toxicity, GI upset usually predominates the clinical picture and may be severe enough to cause GI hemorrhage. Lead poisoning is classically seen in children younger than 6 years old who often have a history of pica. As blood lead levels rise, there is the onset of forceful vomiting, irritability, and weight loss. At very high levels the signs of increased intracranial pressure and encephalopathy (personality change, seizures, coma) become more apparent.

Food poisoning usually presents with the abrupt onset of vomiting, cramps, and diarrhea. These symptoms are mediated by emetic and necrotizing toxins produced by bacteria in contaminated food. Staphylococci are found in dairy and cream preparation; *Vibrio* is associated with fish, shellfish, and crabs; toxigenic *Escherichia coli, Clostridium,* and *Bacillus* are found in a variety of contaminated meats and food.

Psychosocial.—Overfeeding and inappropriate feeding are common causes of regurgitation and vomiting during the first year of life. Excessive amounts of formula given at each feeding or given too frequently will result in gastric distention and lead to vomiting of small amounts of formula. High-fat diets result in delayed gastric emptying, causing vomiting, distention, and discomfort. Inappropriately mixed formula resulting in a high caloric content can cause gastric irritation, vomiting, and diarrhea.

Psychogenic vomiting is related to stress, fear, depression, or anticipation of unpleasant events. In these situations the medullary vomiting center probably receives afferent stimuli from the sensory organs. Cyclic vomiting is recurrent episodes of forceful vomiting without an apparent cause. There may be associated nausea, headache, and abdominal pain as well as a family history of migraine.

DATA GATHERING

The most common diagnosis in a child with vomiting is gastritis or gastroenteritis, often viral. However, this is usually a diagnosis of exclusion. A careful history and physical examination are necessary to narrow the long list of differential diagnoses and rule out more serious illness.

HISTORY

The history should concentrate on several areas: age of the child, time course and characteristics of the vomiting, associated abdominal and extraabdominal symptoms, and state of hydration. First, it is necessary to ascertain that the complaint is truly one of vomiting and not just regurgitation. The age of the child will help narrow the diagnosis, as many disorders are seen almost exclusively in certain age groups. A detailed history about the vomiting should be sought. Is the vomiting nonforceful or is it projectile? When did it start? How many times a day? Is it related to eating? Vomiting immediately after eating points to infection. Recurrent vomiting 1 to 4 hours after eating is consistent with intrinsic gastric or duodenal lesions. When during the day is the vomiting worse? Early morning vomiting is usually seen with increased intracranial pressure, pregnancy, uremia, or postnasal drip. Is there associated nausea? Vomiting without nausea is common in CNS lesions. The characteristics of the vomiting are important. Blood or bile in the vomitus may be related to prolonged vomiting or to obstruction. Is there vomiting of mucus or food particles?

Associated symptoms may help further define the cause of the vomiting. Abdominal pain, obstipation, and abdominal distention are seen in intestinal obstruction. Diarrhea is consistent with a gastroenteritis. Headache, stiff neck, blurred vision, mental status change, or a history of head trauma are suggestive of a CNS injury. Paradoxic irritability, a high-pitched cry, and convulsions suggest meningitis. A sore throat, cough, or earache point to other infectious causes.

Finally, a detailed dietary history should be obtained. Is the child tolerating clear fluids? Have normal urine output? Is the child taking any medicines or have any predisposing illness?

PHYSICAL EXAMINATION

The general appearance of the child often reflects the severity of the underlying illness. A toxic-appearing or inconsolable child usually has a serious infection. Paradoxical irritability (i.e., the child cries more when held by parent) is commonly seen with meningitis or intussusception. A chronically ill child may have metabolic or renal disease.

A careful and thorough examination is necessary to detect a source of infection. Next, attention should be directed to an orderly and complete abdominal examination. Inspection of the abdomen for distention and visible peristalsis may help diagnose an intestinal obstruction. Auscultation of all four quadrants is necessary to assess bowel sounds. Percussion should be used to determine liver size. Tenderness to percussion is often used as a clinical predictor for rebound tenderness. Finally, the abdominal examination should concentrate on palpation. It is helpful to identify which quadrant has guarding, tenderness, or rebound. A patient with jaundice may have hepatitis or cholelithiasis. A palpable olive in the right upper quadrant just to the right of midline above the umbilicus suggests pyloric stenosis (Fig 50–1). Intussusception often presents with a palpable mass in the right lower or right upper quadrant. Finally, a rectal examination and stool heme test should be performed.

Assessment of hydration is best done by serial weights, but in their absence, clinical parameters are often helpful. Tachycardia, rapid respirations, poor skin turgor, dry mucous membranes, and sunken eyes are indicators of dehydration.

LABORATORY EVALUATION

The majority of cases of vomiting are benign. The child usually appears well, and no further laboratory tests are needed. Otherwise, the physician should direct the workup based on the

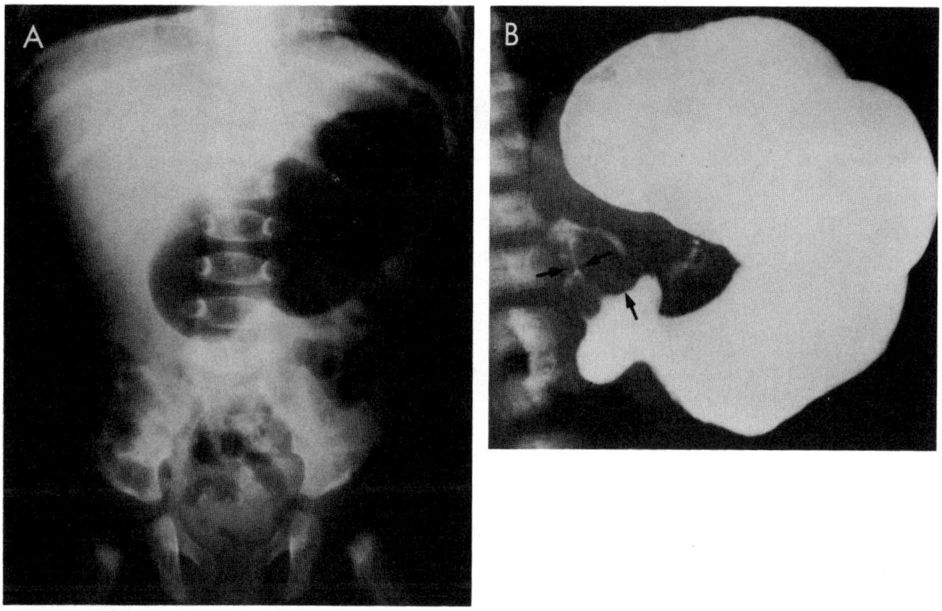

FIG 50–1

Pyloric stenosis. **A,** supine film of the abdomen reveals distention of the stomach. Multiple peristaltic waves (contractions) are visible. This is one of the plain-film findings of gastric outlet obstruction. **B,** oblique view of this patient shows the elongated upturned pyloric channel with a single track (contrast in a compressed lumen) above the arrows, and a double, or railroad-track, configuration (contrast in two asymmetric lumens) below the arrows. In addition, there is an impression of the pyloric muscle on the base of the duodenal bulb and on the antral surface of the stomach *(single arrow).* (From Haller JO, Slovis TL: *Introduction to Radiology in Clinical Pediatrics.* Chicago, Year Book Medical Publishers, 1984. Used by permission.)

history and physical examination. If a child is febrile and ill-appearing, it may be necessary to sample blood, urine, stool, or cerebrospinal fluid to identify a source of infection. Upright and supine abdominal x-ray films are the first step in evaluation of intraabdominal disease. Ultrasound is useful in diagnosing pyloric stenosis, and a barium enema study is often both diagnostic and therapeutic for intussusception. Other specific tests should follow from positive assessment. Any child in whom the status of hydration is in question should undergo tests for urine specific gravity and serum electrolyte levels.

MANAGEMENT ISSUES

Most vomiting is caused by an underlying disease. Therefore, prompt treatment of the primary illness is the most effective therapy. In addition, appropriate symptomatic treatment will stop most vomiting in 8 to 12 hours.

The basic treatment is frequent meals, which produce less distention and stress on the stomach. At first, all feedings, including formula, liquids, and solids, should be stopped. When no vomiting has occurred for 2 hours or after 24 hours, a clear liquid diet should be started. The child should be allowed only 1 ounce every hour. This approach is often difficult, because the child usually wants more fluid; but if allowed, the vicious cycle of gastric distention causing vomiting causing hunger causing increased intake causing gastric distention will ensue. Commercial rehydration solutions may be given to infants; flat soda, juices, tea, or popsicles are appropriate for the older child. Plain water should be avoided. If there is no vomiting for 8 to 12 hours, a BRAT diet may be started (bananas, rice, applesauce, toast). If no vomiting occurs after 24 hours, breast-feeding, formula, and milk products may be added slowly.

The parent should understand the importance of these guidelines and not be tempted to give the child large amounts to drink; this will

VOMITING
Differential Diagnosis

Appendicitis	Metabolic disease	Psychogenic
CNS injury	Migraine	Pyloric stenosis
Diabetes mellitus	Otitis media	Regurgitation/reflux
Food poisoning	Peptic ulcer	Renal disease
Hernia	Postoperative adhesion	Toxin
Inappropriate feeding	Pregnancy	Viral gastroenteritis
Intussusception		

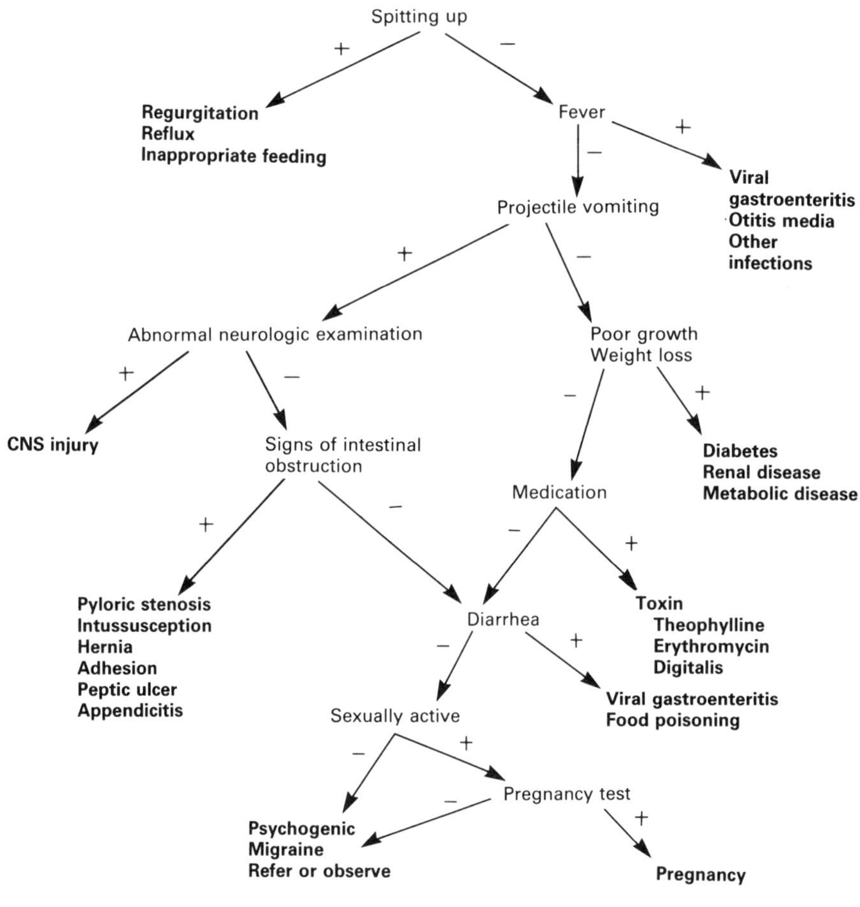

FIG 50–2
Decision tree for differential diagnosis of vomiting.

only increase the vomiting. It should also be stressed that a clear liquid diet should not be given for more than 2 days, because reactive loose stools or starvation stools may result.

Antiemetic therapy in the form of antihistamines and anticholinergics is occasionally used, but the associated side effects are often more troubling than any relief it offers and may mask intraabdominal disease. Furthermore, antiemetics should be avoided in the young or ill-appearing child. Proper hygiene and hand-washing techniques should be stressed to help prevent spread of disease.

INDICATIONS FOR CONSULTATION OR REFERRAL

Most vomiting can be treated in the outpatient setting by frequent telephone follow-up calls or office visits. If the child is ill-appearing or has signs of moderate to severe dehydration, referral for intravenous fluids and assessment of acid-base status is indicated. Any child with projectile vomiting or an abnormal abdominal examination should be seen by a surgeon. In addition, bloody, feculant, or bilious vomiting suggests an anatomic etiology.

Children with persistent vomiting for more than 12 hours and infants younger than 6 months are at high risk for rapid development of dehydration and may need in-hospital observation. Finally, any child with a severe underlying illness, such as serious infection, CNS injury, or a suspected metabolic disorder, should be admitted to the hospital and appropriate consultation sought.

DISCUSSION OF ALGORITHM

An algorithm for the differential diagnosis of vomiting is presented in Figure 50–2. The first step is to make sure that the problem is not just "spitting-up." Next, a careful history will help differentiate acute and chronic causes. If the vomiting is acute, then infectious, CNS, and intraabdominal causes should be ruled out. Recurrent vomiting associated with failure to thrive suggests chronic disease. Finally, if these pathways are not productive, viral gastroenteritis, food poisoning, or psychogenic vomiting are the more likely causes.

BIBLIOGRAPHY

Gryboski J: *Gastrointestinal Problems in the Infant.* Philadelphia, WB Saunders, 1975.

Roy CC, Silverman A, Cozzetto FJ: *Pediatric Clinical Gastroenterology.* St Louis, CV Mosby, 1975.

section III

The Ill or Injured Child

Section III offers information on the treatment of the ill or injured child. It includes chapters that detail the management of childhood illness and injuries: acute and chronic, biomolecular and psychosocial, self-limiting and life-threatening. The goal of this section is to provide the primary care physician with clinical information that will be useful in the office setting. A limited amount of background information has been included with the expectation that this section will be used as an immediate practical desk reference rather than as a shelved volume used for interest reading. Obviously in a book of this size, we could not include every rare condition and syndrome. Thus, we have limited ourselves to the most common illnesses (e.g., fever, pneumonia, minor trauma) and the ones that bring the primary care provider and subspecialist in frequent communication (e.g., epilepsy, hemophilia, diabetes).

We have also limited the scope of management guidelines to what can be done in the office. The authors have provided clear indications for when and in what situations a referral to the hospital or to the specialist should be made. Many of the chapters in this section have been written by primary care providers. Other chapters, written by pediatric subspecialists or pediatric surgeons, stress not what the subspecialist knows but what the primary care provider may want to know and be able to do.

The chapters are arranged in alphabetical order for easy reference. There are two major chapter clusters; one having to do with infections and the other with traumatic injuries. These two areas consume the greatest percentage of the primary care physician's time beyond that devoted to well-child care.

51 ASTHMA AND OTHER ALLERGIC DISORDERS

Robert Anolik, M.D.

Asthma, allergic rhinitis/conjunctivitis, and urticaria are among the more common diseases seen in the primary care physician's office. All are a cause of significant morbidity. Recently the mortality rate of asthma has been rising. Among chronic illnesses, asthma is the number one cause of school absenteeism. This chapter presents the more common allergic problems seen by the primary care physician in an attempt to facilitate diagnosis and subsequent treatment.

DIAGNOSIS OF ALLERGY

As is the case in most areas of medicine, a thorough history and complete physical examination are prerequisite to the diagnosis of atopy. Atopic diseases are IgE mediated, resulting in an immediate hypersensitivity reaction. This sensitivity develops in an individual who has a genetic predisposition to IgE antibody formation directed against allergens or antigens. Then there must be repeated exposure to the allergen, resulting in sensitization, with the formation of antigen-specific IgE. Numerous IgE antibodies bind to mast cells. Subsequently, when the individual is exposed again to the allergen, a bridging reaction occurs at the surface of the mast cell and results in the release of various chemical mediators, such as histamine and leukotrienes. These mediators in turn affect various target organs.

When pursuing a diagnosis of allergy by history, clues should be sought to help differentiate allergic from other causes of the child's problems. One needs to know the kind of illness, its duration, and factors that affect its course. It is particularly important to link clinical symptoms and signs in time with events or exposure to potential allergens. Particular attention should be placed on examining the home and especially the child's bedroom. Exposure outside of the home such as in school, in a babysitter's home, or at a job may also play a significant role. The presence of a familial history of atopy also lends support to the diagnosis of allergy.

A number of features can be found on the physical examination that lend support to the diagnosis of atopy. The examination of the face should include evidence of "allergic shiners" (dark circles below the eyes), eyelid edema, conjunctival injection, and cobblestoning from lymphatic hyperplasia. Examination of the nose should consist of checking for allergic creases on the anterior surface. The interior of the nose can be examined easily in most children by bending the tip of the nose upward with one's finger and illuminating the interior surfaces with an otoscope. In most children it is not necessary to actually insert the otoscope head in the nose. The presence of pale, boggy, enlarged nasal turbinates supports the presence of an allergic diathesis. Associated eustachian tube dysfunction contributes to the production of fluid in the middle ears. In examining the oropharynx, one should look for enlarged tonsils and a cobblestoned appearance to the posterior pharyngeal wall. The presence of a gaping habitus and maxillary overbite (allergic facies) supports the diagnosis of atopy. Examination of the chest should include a check for a barrel-chest deformity due to chronic airway obstruction. During auscultation, one should pay attention to the inspiratory to expiratory ratio. With subtle airway obstruction, there often is a prolonged expiratory phase. The presence of wheezing, rhonchi, or end-expiratory wheezing should also be sought. The skin examination should include a search for eczematoid changes and the presence of dermatographism.

A number of techniques both in vivo and in vitro have been developed to aid in the diagnosis of allergy. An elevated total eosinophil count is helpful but it is not diagnostic of allergy. In addition, many children with severe atopic problems do not have an elevated peripheral eosinophil count. Likewise, the presence of eosinophils in nasal secretions can provide evidence of allergy but in children the specimens are difficult to obtain and eosinophils are not always found when allergic rhinitis is present. In addition, in the entity, non–allergic rhinitis with eosinophilia (NARES), nasal eosinophilia is present even though a link with specific allergens cannot be found. Elevated IgE levels can provide support to the diagnosis of allergy, but other illnesses can elevate the total IgE level. In addition, a child might have a high level of allergen-specific IgE with a normal total serum IgE level.

The major in vitro test for diagnosis of allergy is the RAST (radioallergosorbent test), or modifications of it. The RAST is generally more expensive and less sensitive than properly performed skin tests. In children with severe dermatitis, RAST can offer an advantage. The RAST, unlike skin tests, is not altered by prior use of an antihistamine.

There are two major types of in vivo skin testing. Epicutaneous testing includes the prick, the scratch, and the multi-test methods, in which only the epidermis of the skin is stimulated. Intradermal testing involves the injection of allergen into the dermis.

Epicutaneous testing can be accomplished either on the back or on the forearm. The back is preferable since it is less accessible to the child and is a more sensitive skin test site. In the prick test, the allergen or antigen is placed on the skin and the skin is subsequently pricked by a sterile needle. This is done so superficially that blood is not drawn. The scratch test is similar but involves abrading the skin after the antigen is applied. The scratch test is less sensitive, and consistency is more difficult to attain. The multi-test technique involves the use of a disposable sterile device that has eight test heads so multiple antigens are applied simultaneously in a uniform fashion. Studies have shown that the sensitivity of this technique correlates well with intradermal testing and the presence of clinical disease. The technique has advantages that include speed of application and consistent application of allergen to the skin.

Intradermal testing involves the use of a more dilute form of allergen in a larger dose. The intradermal technique is more sensitive than the epicutaneous technique, but there is a greater likelihood of false-positive results.

Skin testing should be done with appropriate positive and negative controls. Histamine is normally used as a positive control and the dilutent that is used in preparing the testing material is used as a negative control. This helps rule out reactions that might be due to an irritant effect. When scoring skin tests, one is primarily interested in the wheal or the amount of edema that develops. The skin test response can be altered by antihistamines and therefore the patient should not be given antihistamines for several days before the testing is performed. Steroids and all asthma medications presently available do not interfere with the skin test response.

Allergy testing by one of the skin test methods or by RAST is most sensitive and specific for inhalant and stinging insect sensitivities. Food testing materials are not very pure, and false-positive results occur more frequently. Therefore, all positive food test results must be correlated with clinical history, and should be confirmed by two or three challenges (unless there is a history of anaphylaxis).

A number of other testing techniques being used have not been proved valid by controlled studies. These include the Rinkel skin test titration technique, provocative testing by sublingual and subcutaneous techniques, and leukocytotoxic testing. The American Academy of Allergy and Immunology in a position statement has recommended that these techniques be abandoned until proper studies are done.

ASTHMA

BACKGROUND

Prevalence figures for asthma are difficult to obtain, but estimates range from 3% to 8% of school-age children. Prior to puberty, asthma in boys outnumbers asthma in girls by a ratio of 2:1. After puberty, this ratio evens out and in adults is actually reversed. This section will emphasize the new understanding of the pathophysiology of asthma and changes in treatment modalities. A comprehensive discussion of emergent treatment, and the treatment of hospitalized patients is beyond the scope of this section.

PATHOPHYSIOLOGY

Asthma can be classified in a number of ways. Extrinsic asthma is triggered by allergic (i.e., IgE mediated) mechanisms. Intrinsic asthma includes those reactions in which allergy does not play a role, such as bronchospasm triggered by viral infections, irritants, and changes in barometric pressure. Exercise-induced asthma is triggered by sports activities, or in children, by play. Airway cooling and moisture loss during exercise are primarily responsible for the subsequent bronchospasm. Mixed asthma, the predominant form in childhood, can be triggered by both intrinsic and extrinsic factors. In the very young, viral infections are often the initial event. As the child becomes older, indoor inhalants such as dust mites, mold spores, and animal dander and hair subsequently play a role. When the child is in school, outdoor inhalants, such as pollens and mold spores, can be responsible for aggravation of asthma.

Asthma has been characterized by hyperresponsiveness of the airways and reversible airway obstruction. A number of pathophysiologic changes have been found in asthma, including smooth muscle contraction, submucosal edema, and increased mucus production. These all lead to various degrees of airway obstruction. Most recently, asthma has been viewed as a disease of diffuse airway inflammation. The inflammation is induced by a number of chemical mediators. It has similarities to other inflammatory reactions that occur in the body. The early asthmatic reaction or acute phase reaction is one characterized by changes in the airway within minutes or several hours of exposure to a trigger. The late asthmatic reaction or late-phase reaction can occur 6 to 8 hours after exposure to an inciting agent. A late asthmatic reaction can occur whether or not there has been an early asthmatic reaction. Unlike the early phase reaction, which is quite transient and normally easily reversed, the late-phase reaction tends to persist for a longer period of time and is often more difficult to treat. Since it does not occur with an obvious temporal relationship to the inciting agent, triggers are often missed.

MANAGEMENT

Drug therapy for asthma should include consideration of the late-phase reaction as well as airway inflammation. Table 51–1 summarizes the actions of a number of asthma medications on the airway.

Theophylline, a methylxanthine, has been available for more than 50 years for the treatment of asthma and has been the primary first-line drug therapy in the United States. Even though controversy exists as to how theophylline acts at cellular and metabolic levels, it induces smooth muscle relaxation and inhibits submucosal edema formation. It does not prevent the late-phase reaction nor decrease airway hyperirritability or responsiveness. Recently, concerns have been raised about the effect of theophylline on cognitive behavior and its subsequent effect on school performance. In addition, some children develop persistent central nervous system stimulatory side effects that prohibit routine theophylline treatment. A number of good long-acting theophylline preparations are now available, both in tablet and bead-filled capsule formulations, so it can be used in children of all ages. The good absorption and long-acting properties of these formulations allow most children to be maintained on a twice-a-day dosing schedule. These same long-acting properties can result in pitfalls for the primary physician. When treatment is started with a long-acting preparation without a loading dose, it can take several days to reach a steady state level and at the same time, a therapeutic theophylline level. In addition, when a child is treated for status asthmaticus, one must remember that a long-acting theophylline preparation might be absorbed for as long as 24 hours after it is taken.

β-Agonists have also been available for a number of years for the treatment of asthma. They are available in oral (both syrup and tablet), metered-dose inhaler, and nebulizer forms. The more commonly used β-agonists include albuterol, terbutaline, metaproterenol, and isoetharine. Oral β-agonists have the advantage of ease of administration, but concerns have

TABLE 51–1
Pharmacotherapy of Asthma

DRUG	BRONCHODILATOR	↓ NONSPECIFIC REACTIVITY	BLOCK EARLY-PHASE REACTION	BLOCK LATE-PHASE REACTION
Theophylline	Yes	No	Yes	No
β-agonists	Yes	No	Yes	No
Anticholinergics	Yes	No	Yes	No
Cromolyn sodium	No	Yes	Yes	Yes
Corticosteroids	No	Yes	No	Yes

been raised about drug tolerance with long-term use. Recently, a long-acting oral form has become available. Tolerance is much less likely to occur with an inhaled form. None of the inhaled forms have a therapeutic duration greater than 4 to 6 hours. Like theophyllines, the β-agonists induce relaxation of smooth muscle and decrease submucosal edema. They do not prevent the late asthmatic reaction nor do they decrease airway hyperresponsiveness. In most children, β-agonistic therapy plays its primary role in short-term treatment of acute asthma or as a secondary or tertiary drug in the treatment of chronic asthma.

Anticholinergic agents such as ipratromium bromide have been found to have a limited role in the treatment of childhood asthma. They also are bronchodilators but do not decrease airway hyperirritability nor do they prevent the late asthmatic reaction. Both theophyllines and β-agonists are more potent bronchodilators. Anticholingergic agents are probably of greater value in the treatment of chronic bronchitis and chronic obstructive pulmonary disease.

The use of cromolyn sodium as a first line drug in the treatment of childhood asthma has recently increased. It is now available in a number of forms, including nebulizer solution, metered dose inhaler, and a capsule that is administered with a spinhaler. Studies comparing the efficacy of theophylline to cromolyn sodium have found them to be similar. Cromolyn sodium, a nonabsorbable drug, offers the advantage of not inducing any cognitive side effects. It is more expensive than theophylline, though, and somewhat more cumbersome to administer. In young children with asthma, nebulized cromolyn sodium can be quite efficacious at home. In infants with recurrent bronchospasm who are subsequently diagnosed as having asthma and in children with bronchopulmonary dysplasia, nebulized cromolyn sodium has been found by some to be of greater therapeutic benefit than theophylline. Cromolyn sodium offers advantages from at least a theoretical point of view as a drug that decreases airway inflammation and hyperresponsiveness. In addition, the early and late asthmatic reactions are blocked by cromolyn sodium.

Corticosteroids, which have been used for many years in the treatment of asthma, are potent anti-inflammatory drugs that do decrease airway edema and mucus release. Like cromolyn sodium, steroids cause a decrease in airway hyperirritability. Corticosteroids are effective in preventing or decreasing the late-phase reaction but do not have a significant effect on the early-phase reaction. The main disadvantage of this class of drugs is untoward side effects.

CORTICOSTEROID SIDE EFFECTS

Increase in appetite
Cushingoid facies
Acne
Hirsutism
Electrolyte abnormalities
Myopathy
Cataracts
Increase in susceptibility to infection
Peptic ulcers
Delay in sexual development
Menstrual changes
Adrenal suppression
Mood/behavioral changes
Hypertension
Osteoporosis
Diabetes mellitus

Daily oral corticosteroid use is most commonly associated with these problems. Alternate day steroid use, or preferably the use of a steroid metered dose inhaler significantly decreases the risk of side effects. Since all presently available inhaled preparations do have some, albeit small, systemic absorption, the potential exists for side effects, especially in the growing child. The risk of side effects must be weighed against the benefits of controlling a child's asthma that is still problematic despite treatment with first and second line medications. Inhaled steroids can result in oral and/or esophageal candidiasis and therefore a spacer should always be used. The child should also rinse his or her mouth immediately after a steroid inhaler is used.

To summarize, in the treatment of chronic asthma, cromolyn sodium or theophylline are appropriate first-line therapy. When one agent is used, the other can also be used as a second-line drug. β-agonists, preferably via inhalation, serve a role as a secondary or tertiary drug. Corticosteroids, though extremely effective, should be reserved as a tertiary line of treatment in children.

In addition to the pharmacologic treatment of asthma, precipitating and aggravating factors must be considered. Among those listed, sinusitis and gastroesophageal reflux are common precipitating triggers. In situations in which asthma becomes difficult to control, allergic bronchopulmonary aspergillosis (ABPA) in addition to reflux and sinusitis must be considered.

ASTHMA PRECIPITATING AND AGGRAVATING FACTORS

- Infections
  - Viral
  - Mycoplasma
- Allergy
  - Inhalants
  - Foods
- Irritants (including tobacco smoke)
- Weather changes
- Emotions
- Sinusitis
- Gastroesophageal reflux
- ABPA (allergic bronchopulmonary aspergillosis)
- Aspiration
- Immune compromise

The recognition of subclinical or chronic cough asthma is important. Children with low-grade airway inflammation sometimes have a chronic cough without evidence of bronchospasm. Pulmonary function tests at rest in these children sometimes show evidence of airway obstruction, and most children show evidence of airway obstruction after exercise. The cough, often precipitated by crying, laughter, and sports activity, is frequently intense in the early morning hours. If spirometry is not available, then the measurement of peak expiratory flow rates before and after exercise might be helpful. In children who have been coughing for more than several weeks, a trial with a rapid-acting bronchodilator such as a β-agonist might also be warranted.

Sinusitis can result in asthma that appears resistant to normal medical therapy. Suggested mechanisms for this include direct soiling of the tracheobronchial tree, heightening of airway hyperirritability, and stimulation of irritant or cholinergic receptors. Prolonged antibiotic therapy is often needed for control of sinusitis.

Gastroesophageal reflux can also trigger asthma through direct soiling of the tracheobronchial tree if gastric contents are refluxed into the pharynx and subsequently aspirated. A number of studies also suggest that reflux without aspiration that results in esophageal inflammation can also trigger acute and chronic bronchospasm. This occurs through stimulation of irritant or cholinergic receptors and subsequent reflex bronchospasm and airway inflammation.

As will subsequently be discussed, immunotherapy does play a role in the treatment of asthma in a very specific patient population. It should not be viewed, though, as a primary modality of treatment.

Children with asthma should lead normal lives. They should be able to participate in sports both casually and competitively. Children with asthma should not be routinely restricted from normal activities. In addition, the parents of a child with asthma should not live with the constant fear that wheezing might develop. The fact that a child wheezes should not be used as an excuse for lack of discipline or school absence at examination time.

ALLERGIC RHINITIS/CONJUNCTIVITIS

BACKGROUND

The terms "hay fever" and "rose fever" are misnomers that describe fall and spring upper airway allergy symptoms, respectively. In temperate zones, fall allergies typically are due to weed sensitivities, and in the spring, seasonal allergies are caused by tree and grass sensitivities. Flowering plants are usually not significant aeroallergens since their pollens are heavy and are spread by insects rather than by air currents.

DATA GATHERING

Allergic rhinitis/conjunctivitis can be grouped into perennial and seasonal types. It is not uncommon for many children to have both varieties. Perennial allergic rhinitis-conjunctivitis is caused by allergens that are present year-round. The most commonly identified allergens are as follows:

INHALANT ALLERGENS

- Perennial
  - House dust mite
  - Animal dander and hair
  - Mold spores
  - Horse hair
  - Cotton linters
  - Kapok
  - Pollens: trees, grasses, weeds (tropics, subtropics)
- Seasonal
  - Pollens: trees, grasses, weeds (temperate regions)
  - Mold spores (temperate regions)

The pollens, including trees, grasses, and weeds, are the most important seasonal allergens. In temperate zones, molds can also contribute to seasonal difficulties. Pollen counts are usually highest in the late afternoon and evening and can therefore affect the way in which upper airway allergies present.

Common features of allergic rhinitis include allergic shiners (dark circles below the eyes), Dennie's lines (creases below the lower eyelids), gaping habitus or adenoid faces (long drawn-out face with open mouth), allergic salute (upward rubbing of the nose), and allergic creases (transverse lines on the nose). In the examination of the nose, white, pink, or pale blue boggy enlarged nasal turbinates are often seen. Presentations of allergic rhinitis include sneezing, sniffing, throat clearing, nose rubbing, congestion, and clear rhinorrhea. Signs and symptoms of allergic conjunctivitis include eye rubbing, pruritis, edema of the conjunctival tissues, erythema of the conjunctiva and sometimes the sclera, and a pebbly appearance of the conjunctival sac known as cobblestoning.

Vasomotor rhinitis, uncommonly seen in children, appears similar to perennial allergic rhinitis. It is caused by irritants such as tobacco fumes, perfumes, deodorants, as well as changes in temperature. Some individuals have allergic rhinitis and vasomotor rhinitis.

Chronic allergic rhinitis/conjunctivitis are not without consequences. Chronic nasal congestion combined with eustachian tube dysfunction can result in serous otitis media or sinusitis. The chronic mouth breathing associated with allergic rhinitis can also result in maxillofacial abnormalities including maxillary overbite and associated malocclusion. Nasal obstruction leading to mouth breathing can also complicate asthma or lead to exercise-induced asthma since the air is not warmed or humidified.

TREATMENT

A number of treatment modalities are available for allergic rhinitis and allergic conjunctivitis. First and foremost, avoidance of environmental factors should be established. Efforts should be undertaken to remove the offending allergens in the home. This is obviously more easily accomplished with horse hair in an old couch than with a dog or a cat that has been with the family for a long period of time. Avoidance of outdoor allergens is more difficult but the closing of windows and the use of air conditioning during periods of high pollen counts in the spring and fall, and during periods of high mold spore counts during the mid-summer can be quite helpful.

H_1 antihistamines usually in combination with a decongestant have been the hallmark of treatment for years. Most patients find that oral antihistamines or decongestants will afford them with some relief but usually will not eliminate all symptoms. In the more severe cases, adequate relief is often not attained. If an oral antihistamine or decongestant is not effective in the treatment of ocular allergy, then a topical antihistamine/decongestant ophthalmic solution can be used.

Cromolyn sodium is available in nasal and ocular forms for the treatment of allergic rhinitis and allergic conjunctivitis, respectively. Since 2 to 3 weeks of treatment is needed for maximum drug benefit, treatment on an as-needed basis is not useful. If a specific time of year can be identified as problematic, treatment can be started prior to the onset of symptoms, often with good success. Since cromolyn sodium is not absorbed, it is almost devoid of side effects.

A more potent means of treatment of allergic rhinitis are the topical steroid nasal sprays. They are available both as powders propelled by an inert gas as well as aqueous preparations. Some have been approved by the Food and Drug Administration for children as young as 6 years old. Even though systemic absorption is limited and many of the drugs are deactivated in their first pass through the liver, they should be used cautiously. The smallest possible dose that alleviates the child's symptoms should be used only after antihistamines and/or cromolyn sodium have failed. Topical steroid preparations are also available for treatment of ocular allergies. Since significant risks also exist, corticosteroids should be prescribed with caution.

Immunotherapy does play a role in the treatment of allergic rhinitis and allergic conjunctivitis. Studies support the use of desensitization primarily for pollen and dust mite sensitivities. Therefore, children with a strong seasonal pattern in temperate zones or significant dust mite sensitivity who have a perennial pattern are those who would benefit most from this course of treatment. Like the topical steroids, they are not first-line treatment and should be reserved for those cases that do not respond well to avoidance and the use of antihistamines and decongestants or cromolyn sodium. Long-term studies in children have demonstrated that immunotherapy has an excellent safety profile. In the warmer climates such as the tropics and subtropics, pollen sensitivities occur in all seasons. Treatment decisions, therefore, cannot be based on the presence of a seasonal pattern alone.

Treatment of allergic rhinitis and allergic conjunctivitis should not be trivialized. In addition to the above described sequelae of nasal obstruction, individuals with significant upper airway allergic reactions do not feel well. Severe congestion can result in mood and behavioral changes and can affect a child's performance in school. School performance can also be affected by the sedative or stimulatory side effects seen with antihistamines and decongestants. Given the wide array of treatment modalities available, children should not have to suffer.

URTICARIA AND ANGIOEDEMA

BACKGROUND

Urticaria (hives) and angioedema (swelling) are similar lesions caused by mediator release from mast cells. Urticaria is manifest as a wheal and flare reaction of the upper portion of the dermis while angioedema involves changes in the deeper subcutaneous tissues. In the prevention and/or treatment of urticaria and angioedema, an attempt must first be made to classify the type of lesion and determine its cause.

Urticaria and angioedema can be induced by three distinct mechanisms. In an IgE-mediated or true allergic reaction, allergen binds to mast cells inducing a change in the membrane of the cells and mediator release follows. Immune complex reactions such as those seen in acute serum sickness can also induce formation of hives and angioedema. Lastly, mast cells can be induced to release chemical mediators by the direct effect of a number of agents that are not IgE mediated. Examples include foods (strawberries, tomatoes), drugs (opiates, antibiotics), and radiographic dyes.

DATA GATHERING

Urticaria can be divided into three major categories. The first is acute urticaria in which hives occur transiently. By definition, they cannot last more than 6 weeks. Although in most cases the cause for acute urticaria is not determined, the common known causes include viral illnesses, drugs, and foods.

Chronic urticaria persists for longer than 6 weeks. It is an entity that occurs much more commonly in adolescents and adults than in younger children. Most studies have shown that in over 80% of the cases, the cause for chronic urticaria remains elusive. Since chronic urticaria can be the first manifestation of an underlying illness such as occult infection, cancer, or collagen vascular disease, these problems should be included in the assessment of the patient. The first and probably most important part of the evaluation process is a thorough history and complete physical examination. Suggested laboratory tests include complete blood cell (CBC) count, differential, erythrocyte sedimentation rate, liver function tests, antinuclear antibody (ANA), total hemolytic complement, urinalysis, and urine culture. If these tests are unremarkable, the focus of attention then turns to the treatment of the lesions. In most situations, allergy testing by either an in vivo or in vitro technique will not be helpful.

Physical urticarias are those in which the hives are induced by physical stimuli. The most common manifestation is dermatographism where stroking of the skin, particularly the back, will induce a wheal and flare reaction. Less commonly, exposure to cold water or cold air will induce hives in an individual with cold urticaria and in cholinergic urticaria, heat and/or exercise can precipitate very small pruritic hives. Less commonly seen physical urticarias include solar urticaria, aquagenic urticaria, vibratory angioedema, and delayed pressure urticaria.

TREATMENT

Acute urticaria should be treated with an H_1 antihistamine such as diphenhydramine or hydroxyzine. In most children, the drug can be used on an as-needed basis. In persistent cases, routine use of the medication until the lesions resolve is often helpful. In refractory cases, a short course of corticosteroids in conjunction with an H_1 antihistamine can be used.

Chronic urticaria is somewhat more difficult to treat. Often a single antihistamine is not effective. Treatment options include the use of two H_1 antihistamines from different classes, or the combination of an H_1 antihistamine and an H_2 antihistamine. Doxepin hydrochloride is a tricyclic antidepressant medication that has been shown to be helpful in severe cases. Doxepin exerts both H_1 and H_2 antihistamine effects. Given that chronic urticaria is a prolonged problem, corticosteroid use should be reserved for the most refractory of cases to avoid side effects. In most instances, salicylate- and tartrazine-free diets or other dietary changes have not been consistently demonstrated to be beneficial.

The treatment of physical urticaria is determined by the specific type. Dermatographism usually does not warrant treatment. Terfenadine and brompheniramine have both been shown to be effective. Cholinergic urticaria is more difficult to treat, but hydroxyzine has been shown to be the drug of choice. Often high doses are needed, and the dose has to be titrated to the individual patient's need. Cyproheptadine, on the other hand, has been shown to be the most effective antihistamine for the treatment of cold urticaria. Individuals with cold urticaria are at risk for acute anaphylaxis with intense cold exposure such as that which occurs when jumping into cold water. Pretreatment is necessary and the child or family should be educated so that acute changes in temperature are avoided. Some individuals with cholinergic urticaria also are at risk for systemic anaphylaxis. In these instances, there is an exaggeration of the cholinergic response, which has been termed exercise-induced anaphylaxis. Again, caution must be exercised and pre-treatment is helpful.

STINGING INSECT ALLERGY

BACKGROUND

The stinging insects, honeybees, bumblebees, wasps, hornets, and yellow jackets, tend to invoke fear in patients and physicians alike. Fortunately, true anaphylactic sensitivity to the stinging insects is uncommon. Nonetheless, stinging insect allergy accounts for approximately 40 deaths in the United States per year.

In most cases of stinging insect anaphylaxis the responsible insect is not identified by history. In addition, some children present with acute anaphylaxis without a history or skin lesion to suggest an insect sting as the triggering factor.

DATA GATHERING

The order Hymenoptera contains the insects responsible for anaphylaxis. The honeybee and bumblebee are members of the superfamily Apoidea. Despite its impressive size, the bumblebee is a rare cause of insect sting and in turn anaphylactic reaction. Honeybees are also mild-mannered insects, but will sting to protect themselves or the hive. The superfamily Vespoidea includes wasps, white-faced and yellow hornets, and yellow jackets, which are much more common causes of anaphylactic reactions. Wasps tend to build their nests in the overhangs of buildings or under other sheltered areas and will sting when they are disturbed. Hornets build dome-shaped nests that hang from trees and shrubs and occasionally from buildings, and will also sting when bothered. Yellow jackets build their hives at ground level, usually under logs, branches, or in the ground itself. They are more commonly disturbed, therefore, and are the number 1 cause of insect sting reactions. Recently, a member of the superfamily Formicidae, the imported fire ant, has been recognized as a cause of anaphylactic reactions due tc both its bite and sting. The imported fire ant has been identified primarily in southeastern and south central states.

Reactions to the stinging insects can be classified as follows:

STINGING INSECT REACTIONS

Local: Erythema and edema at sting site
Large local: Extensive swelling contiguous with sting site
Dermal anaphylaxis: Urticaria or angioedema anywhere on body
Systemic anaphylaxis: Respiratory, gastrointestinal, or vascular compromise

Local reactions occur within minutes or several hours of the insect sting and are characterized by pain, pruritis, swelling, and erythema. Large local reactions are characterized by extensive swelling, but the erythema and edema are always contiguous with the insect sting site. If the sting occurs on the foot and the leg is swollen to the knee this would be classified as a large local reaction. If, on the other hand, the sting occurred on the foot and there was swelling of the face, the reaction would be classified as dermal anaphylaxis. Systemic or anaphylactic reactions can be divided into two categories. The first, as suggested by the example above, is anaphylaxis involving only the skin. Urticaria or angioedema anywhere on the body following an insect sting would be included in this category. An anaphylactic reaction that results in respiratory compromise, such as laryngeal edema or bronchospasm, gastrointestinal reactions including vomiting, cramps, or diarrhea, or a change in sensorium due to vascular instability need to be considered separately. Children in this latter category have true life-threatening anaphylactic sensitivity.

MANAGEMENT

Local, large local, and dermal anaphylactic reactions can be managed with antihistamines, especially diphenhydramine, ice to the insect sting site, and if necessary a short course of corticosteroids. Children in all of these categories are not at significant risk for life-threatening reactions with subsequent stings. Despite the ominous appearance of diffuse urticaria and angioedema, subsequent sting risks do not warrant insect testing or consideration of immunotherapy in children.

Children who have a history consistent with life-threatening anaphylaxis should undergo venom insect testing as potential candidates for venom immunotherapy. All five insects need to be tested for, since cross-reactivity does occur. Sensitivity to each insect is tested with a series of prick and intradermal tests. Several companies have marketed kits for this purpose. A child who has a positive skin test reaction to one or more of the stinging insects and a history that correlates with it should receive venom immunotherapy. Venom immunotherapy has been shown to be extremely protective through deliberate and inadvertent sting challenges. Immunotherapy can be given for each individual insect if there is more than one sensitivity, but a mixed vespid extract for yellow hornet, white-faced hornet, and yellow jacket is available. The risks for both local and systemic reactions from venom immunotherapy are greater than those with inhalant immunotherapy, and therefore the shots should be given in an office with personnel experienced in administering insect venom and treatment of potential reactions. At present the optimal duration of venom immunotherapy has not been determined; consensus is that it be continued for a minimum of 5 years. If at the end of a 5-year period an individual's skin test reaction has become negative, then venom immunotherapy likely can be discontinued. If the reaction is still positive, it is not clear how long immunotherapy needs to be continued.

The imported fire ant causes sensitivity both by biting and stinging. Like other members of the order Hymenoptera, it can cause large local, dermal anaphylactic, and systemic anaphylactic reactions. For children who have had previous life-threatening reactions to the imported fire ant bite or sting, immunotherapy with a whole-body extract has been effective.

Despite the efficacy of venom immunotherapy, the potential for anaphylaxis must still be realized. Children should wear an identification bracelet that indicates their sensitivity. In addition, epinephrine and an H_1 antihistamine should be available at all times.

The treatment of stinging insect allergy also includes avoidance. Children who are sensitive to insects should not be allowed outdoors barefoot and should avoid wearing brightly colored clothing as well as scented toiletries. Caution should also be exercised in doing yardwork, as this often disturbs the yellow jacket. Many stinging insects are attracted to food, and precautions should be taken in orchards, at picnics, and around trash containers.

ATOPIC DERMATITIS

BACKGROUND

Atopic dermatitis, an intensely pruritic form of eczema, is often associated with other allergic conditions, especially asthma, allergic rhinitis-conjunctivitis, and urticaria. Even though the pathophysiologic mechanisms involved in atopic dermatitis have not been well defined, most cases are amenable to treatment.

DATA GATHERING

Atopic dermatitis can be characterized by the age at which it presents and the areas of the skin that are affected. In the infantile type of atopic dermatitis, the rash presents by 4 to 6 months of age and often involves the cheeks. The lesions can spread to other parts of the face, neck, upper trunk, and sometimes onto extensor surfaces. Even though the lesions result in discomfort, especially intense pruritis, many children improve by 2 to 3 years of age. Childhood atopic dermatitis generally presents between 2 and 4 years of age. In contrast to the areas involved in the infantile stage, flexor surfaces are most intensely affected. Unlike the infantile type of atopic dermatitis, this eczema often persists for many years. In the adult phase of atopic dermatitis, flexor surfaces are also involved. In addition, discrete areas such as the neck, wrists, hands, ankles, and feet might also be affected. Investigations that have attempted to define the pathophysiology of atopic dermatitis have found abnormalities of the immune system, cellular biochemical defects, and abnormal skin physiologic responses. Despite these studies, a thorough understanding of the disease process is lacking. Nonetheless, in all children with atopic dermatitis, dry skin, intense pruritis, and a tendency for secondary infection are seen. The issue of specific allergic triggers is controversial. Some studies have shown a very low incidence of food allergies contributing to flares of atopic dermatitis but other studies have shown an incidence as high as 20% to 30%. In addition, recently there has been documentation that airborne allergens, such as the dust mite, can also trigger the disease process.

MANAGEMENT

Basic management principles are important to emphasize though details are discussed elsewhere (Chapter 56). Irritants should be kept away from the skin as they can serve as triggers for the vicious cycle where irritants (or allergens) stimulate pruritis and subsequent scratching followed by more pruritis. The skin must also be well hydrated by avoiding baths or by applying emollients to the skin immediately after bathing. Soaps, even those with a neutral pH, tend to dry the skin and should be used sparingly. Topical corticosteroid preparations as well as oral corticosteroid preparations play a role in management depending on the severity of the lesions. Any sign of secondary infection should be treated aggressively, as acute flares often will not resolve without systemic antibiotics.

The search for allergic trigger(s) need not be undertaken in children in whom atopic dermatitis can be controlled well with appropriate irritant avoidance, bathing techniques, topical emollients, and mild steroid preparations. For the more difficult-to-control cases, allergy testing for possible food and/or inhalant sensitivities is appropriate. In some children, skin testing is more problematic than in those without atopic dermatitis, given the hyperirritable state of the skin. In most instances, though, it can be accomplished. If necessary, the RAST can be used as a substitute though it is not as sensitive. The most common foods involved in aggravating atopic dermatitis are eggs, milk, and wheat. Recent studies have demonstrated that dust mite contact with the skin can also trigger pruritis and a flare of atopic dermatitis. There is less convincing evidence for other inhalants, but it is likely that a number of them also play a role.

To date, immunotherapy has not been shown to be effective for atopic dermatitis. In a child with severe respiratory allergies as well as atopic dermatitis, treatment with immunotherapy is reasonable for the former problem. However, immunotherapy as the sole treatment of atopic dermatitis is not appropriate given our present knowledge.

FOOD ALLERGY AND INTOLERANCE

BACKGROUND

Reactions to foods can be characterized as either immunologic or nonimmunologic. The immunologic reactions are true IgE-mediated phenomena. Nonimmunologic food reactions or food intolerances can be classified as pharmacologic, toxic, metabolic, or idiosyncratic.

DATA GATHERING

Food allergy is less common than one would expect, given reactions that are coincidental or nonimmune mediated. Food reactions are most likely to occur with early introduction of cow's milk or of solid foods. The most commonly seen food allergies are to milk, egg, peanut, and soy. The majority of children lose their sensitivity by 2 to 3 years of age. Once a diagnosis of food allergy has been established, the offending allergen should be strictly avoided. Since allergic reactions result from proteins in the food, heating or cooking the food decreases its allergenicity. For example, peanut oil is usually not allergenic in peanut-sensitive individuals. After 2 years of age, it is reasonable to periodically challenge the child with the offending food(s) to see if the sensitivity has dissipated. If a child has a history of an anaphylactic reaction to a food, then challenges should be done in a physician's office where rescusitative equipment is available. It is better that challenges be done in a physician's office than in a school lunchroom when sandwiches are traded.

The nonimmune reactions or food intolerances are often mistaken for allergic reactions. Pharmacologic reactions are those due to chemicals inherent in the food such as caffeine in cola, theobromine in chocolate, and tyramine in cheese. Toxic reactions are characterized by food-induced release of histamine, or by histamine already present in a contaminated food. In both instances, a true allergic or immediate hypersensitivity reaction does not occur. There is an abnormality in the normal breakdown and processing of a food in metabolic reactions. Examples of this include lactose intolerance and phenylketonuria. Idiosyncratic reactions are unexpected, non-dose related reactions that occur from very small amounts of the food. Adverse reactions to food dyes and preservatives fall in this category.

Food allergies can result in respiratory, dermatologic, gastrointestinal, occasionally neurologic, and systemic anaphylactic reactions. Claims that occult food allergy are the cause of hyperactivity, developmental delay, enuresis, and seizures are unsubstantiated in controlled, blinded studies.

MANAGEMENT

Most children with food allergy will outgrow their sensitivity by 2 to 3 years of age. Therefore, avoidance of the offending food(s) is the treatment of choice. Foods are classified on the basis of plant families and cross-reactivity can occur within families. If reactions to a member of a specific family have been severe, caution should be exercised in eating all foods in that particular family. Clearly, the fewer allergens an infant's immature gastrointestinal tract is exposed to, the less likely the child is to develop food allergy. The introduction of cow's milk should be delayed to 9 to 12 months of age, and the introduction of solid food should be delayed to at least 4 to 6 months of age. Breastfeeding has also been advocated as a means for preventing food allergy, and should be recommended in highly atopic families for this reason, even though clear-cut documentation does not exist.

Desensitization (orally, sublingually, or parenterally) plays no legitimate role in the treatment of food allergy. Recently, prophylactic administration of oral ketotifen and cromolyn sodium have been studied and show some promise. At present, the value of this modality of treatment has not been established.

Most food intolerances can be treated by avoidance of the offending foods and associated agents. Unlike food allergy, though, many of these reactions will persist throughout childhood and into adult years.

ADVERSE REACTIONS TO DRUGS

BACKGROUND

Adverse reactions to drugs occur commonly in children, but true IgE-mediated allergic reactions are rare. Reactions ascribed to a medication are often a result of the underlying illnesses, as many viruses can cause an exanthem. It is important to be able to differentiate true allergic from nonallergic reactions so that appropriate medications can be administered. Penicillin allergy has been the best studied drug reaction. Given the availability of alternate antibiotics, the need for penicillin testing and desensitization has significantly decreased.

DATA GATHERING

Drug reactions can be classified as allergic, toxic, intolerance, and idiosyncratic. Toxic reactions are those due to an overdose of the medication and are therefore dose related. The side effects are predictable. Drug intolerances result in predictable side effects, but only a very small dose of the drug is needed to precipitate the reaction, which is the result of an individual's susceptibility to the side effects and is not an allergic reaction. Idiosyncratic reactions are unpredictable, non-dose-related side effects. Again, an IgE-mediated mechanism for this kind of reaction has not been shown. Anaphylactoid reactions mimic a true allergic reaction without an immediate hypersensitivity reaction occurring. A prototypic reaction in this category is one induced by radiologic contrast material.

MANAGEMENT

Penicillin allergy occurs infrequently in children, although late-onset rashes often lead to an inappropriate label. Sensitivity to penicillin can be confirmed by testing but this should only be undertaken if the drug is needed immediately and there are no alternatives available. Penicillin testing makes a statement about sensitivity only at the time testing is done. It is not predictive of what might ensue if the drug is given at a later date. A number of good protocols have been developed for penicillin testing, though testing material is somewhat limited. Desensitization protocols by both the oral and parenteral routes have been well established, and can be undertaken in an intensive care unit when appropriate.

Reactions to radiologic contrast material occur much more commonly in adults than children. Recent developments in the field of radiology have produced contrast media with fewer side effects. If there is a history of reactions to contrast material, then pretreatment with corticosteroids and diphenhydramine (or corticosteroids and cimetidine) will prevent subsequent reactions in most instances.

Insulin allergy also is more commonly seen in adults than children. With the availability of synthetic human insulin, the incidence of both local and systemic reactions has decreased. Nonetheless, in incidences of true sensitivity, desensitization can be accomplished with a subcutaneous protocol.

IMMUNOTHERAPY

Immunotherapy, hyposensitization, or desensitization is only part of the total treatment of the child with allergies. Immunotherapy cannot be viewed as a substitute for the pharmacologic management of allergies or for allergen avoidance. Indeed, immunotherapy should only be used in those instances in which allergen avoidance is not possible. Immunotherapy has been used since the early 1900s with various degrees of success. Recently the immunologic mechanisms involved have been better defined and a true science is evolving. Immunotherapy induces a decrease in clinical sensitivity or tolerance to the allergen for which treatment is being given. This is accomplished by a number of mechanisms including an increase in IgG blocking antibody levels, a reduction in white blood cell sensitivity to allergens, and suppression of the seasonal rise in IgE antibody levels.

Controlled studies have shown efficacy for immunotherapy in specific disease states for specific allergens as indicated in Table 51–2. The efficacy of immunotherapy in allergic rhinitis-conjunctivitis has been shown for pollens (trees, grasses, weeds), house dust mites, and recently, a standardized cat dander extract. Immunotherapy has also been shown to have a role in the treatment of asthma that is exacerbated by dust mites, pollens, and cats if cats are unavoidable. Immunotherapy blunts the late-phase reaction as well as the early-phase reaction.

Mold immunotherapy in some studies has been shown to have benefit in the treatment of allergic rhinitis-conjunctivitis but not as consistently and not to the degree that has been shown for other allergens. Immunotherapy at the present time does not play a role in the treatment of food allergy, urticaria-angioedema, atopic dermatitis, or vasomotor rhinitis. Immunotherapy has also been shown to be effective in the management of stinging insect allergy. A long-term prospective study in young children has also suggested that immunotherapy started when only allergic rhinitis is present might prevent the subsequent development of asthma.

Immunotherapy or allergy shots should be given deep subcutaneously, preferably over the triceps brachii muscle. The closer the shot is to the muscle, the more local discomfort will be experienced. Small local reactions that resolve within 24 hours are not of concern and the child's immunotherapy schedule can be followed. Reactions that are large, do not resolve within 24 hours, or induce systemic side effects should not be repeated without consultation with the prescribing physician. Even though the risks of immunotherapy for inhalant sensitivities are small, the shot should always be given with physician supervision, and with oxygen, a tourniquet, epinephrine, and diphenhydramine readily available.

Over a period of several months, immunotherapy injections are advanced from initial concentrations diluted to as low as 1:100,000 of the offending allergen to concentrations at maintenance of approximately 1:100 to 1:50. Improvement in the child's symptoms should be seen after the maintenance dose has been attained. This normally takes a period of several months with injections being given weekly. After the maintenance dose of immunotherapy has been attained, shots can be normally given on a monthly schedule. Recent studies with more purified allergy extracts suggest in the future that a series of less than ten injections will be needed to reach maintenance immunotherapy. At present, very few allergy extracts have been standardized. It is therefore very important that the extracts are supplied by a reliable company.

TABLE 51–2
Indications for Immunotherapy

ALLERGENS	DISEASE	PROVED
House dust mite	Allergic rhinitis/conjunctivitis	Yes
	Asthma	Yes
Pollens: trees, grasses, weeds	Allergic rhinitis/conjunctivitis	Yes
	Asthma	Yes
Standardized cat extract	Allergic rhinitis/conjunctivitis	Yes
	Asthma	Yes
Stinging insect venom	Systemic anaphylaxis	Yes
Molds	Allergic rhinitis/conjunctivitis	Controversial
	Asthma	Controversial
Foods	Allergic rhinitis/conjunctivitis	No
	Asthma	No
	Behavioral changes	No

Severe reactions to immunotherapy are uncommon. The most commonly experienced reaction is local swelling, erythema, and pruritis. Systemic reactions in children are infrequently seen. At present, there are no well-documented cases of long-term, adverse effects from immunotherapy in children. Allergy shots are usually given for a 3- to 5-year period and then discontinued. Most children will show prolonged benefit from allergy shots after they are stopped. If within 1 or 2 years of initiation of immunotherapy improvement is not apparent, the treatment should be discontinued and the situation reassessed. The child might be receiving treatment with the wrong allergens or possibly an incorrect dose is being used. Nonetheless, a response is usually apparent by the end of the first year of treatment. Treatment for more than 5 years does not offer any documented advantages.

BIBLIOGRAPHY

Anderson TA, Sogn DD, (eds): *Adverse Reactions to Foods*. Rockville, Md, American Academy of Allergy and Immunology Committee on Adverse Reactions to Foods and the National Institute of Health and Human Services, NIH Publication No 84–2442.

Blumenthal MN, Selcow J, Spector S, et al: A multicenter evaluation of the clinical benefits of cromolyn sodium aerosol by metered-dose inhaler in the treatment of asthma. *J Allergy Clin Immunol* 1988; 81:681–687.

Bock SA: A prospective appraisal of complaints of adverse reactions to foods in children during the first 3 years of life. *Pediatrics* 1987; 79:683–688.

Correo WM, Bramen SS, Irwin RS: Chronic cough as the sole presenting manifestation of bronchial asthma. *N Engl J Med* 1979; 300:633–637.

Eggleston PA: Immunotherapy for asthma: Don't count it out. *J Respir Dis* 1988; 9:13–21.

Furukawa CT, Shapiro GG, Bierman CW, et al: A double blind study comparing the effectiveness of cromolyn sodium and sustained-release theophylline in childhood asthma. *Pediatrics* 1984; 74:453–459.

Goldstein RA, Patterson R: Drug allergy: Prevention, diagnosis, treatment (II). *J Allergy Clin Immunol* 1984; 74:549.

Johnstone DE, Dutton A: The value of hyposensitization therapy for bronchial asthma in children—a 14-year study. *Pediatrics* 1968; 42:793.

Larsen GL: The pulmonary late-phase response. *Hosp Pract* 1987; 22:155–169.

Lichenstein LM, Valentine MD, Norman PS: A reevaluation of immunotherapy for asthma. *Am Rev Respir Dis* 1984; 129:657–659.

Lieberman P: Rhinitis. Allergic and nonallergic. *Hosp Pract* 1988; 23:117–145.

Marks MB: Physical signs of allergy of the respiratory tract in children. *Ann Allergy* 1967; 25:310.

Matthews KP. Management of urticaria and angioedema. *J Allergy Clin Immunol* 1983; 72:1.

Ormerod AD, Greaves MW: Physical urticaria and angioedema, in Lichenstein LM, Fauci AS, (eds): *Current Therapy in Allergy, Immunology, and Rheumatology*, ed 3. Toronto, BC Dekker, Inc. 1988.

Rachelefsky GS, Katz RM, Siegel SC: Chronic sinus disease with associated reactive airway disease in children. *Pediatrics* 1984; 73:526–529.

Rachelefsky GS, Wo J, Adelson MA, et al: Behavior abnormalities and poor school performance due to oral theophylline use. *Pediatrics* 1986; 78:1133–1138.

Rasmussen JE: Recent developments in the management of patient with atopic dermatitis. *J Allergy Clin Immunol* 1984; 74:771.

Reisman RE: American Academy of Allergy position statement—controversial techniques. *J Allergy Clin Immunol* 1981; 67:333.

Reisman RE: Insect sting allergy in children, in Lichenstein LM, Fauci AS, (eds): *Current Therapy in Allergy, Immunology, and Rheumatology*, ed 3. Toronto, BC Dekker, Inc, 1988.

Sampson HA: Role of immediate food hypersensitivity in the pathogenesis of atopic dermatitis. *J Allergy Clin Immunol* 1983; 71:473.

Sheffer AL, Rachelefsky GS, (eds): Asthma '84: Pharmacologic update. *J Allergy Clin Immunol* 1985; 76:249.

Van Metre TE: Critique of controversial and unproven procedures for diagnosis and therapy of allergic disorders. *Pediatr Clin North Am* 1983; 30:807.

52 CHILD ABUSE

Stephen Ludwig, M.D.

Child abuse, a major medical and social problem, accounts for significant mortality and unmeasurable morbidity in children. The primary care physician has the challenge to suspect and detect child abuse, as it is a pervasive phenomenon in our society, occurring in every community.

Physicians have been accused of underreporting abuse. The possible reasons for failure to report are many. Helfer has indicated that some of the reasons are: (1) unfamiliarity with the problem and how to manage it; (2) not wanting to get involved in court; (3) fear of reputation damage in the community; (4) fear of reaction from parents; and (5) lack of training for working with professionals in other disciplines (e.g., social workers).

Another barrier to reporting is questioning of the ultimate good that comes from reporting. In other aspects of their work, physicians must perform many tasks that are difficult, unpleasant, discouraging, and emotionally painful. Most physicians will perform in these matters if they are sure a positive outcome will ensue. With child abuse, there is a mistaken presumption that reports always result in an adversarial relationship, and that the physician reports to punish a family that has failed to protect their child. The physician may feel that once this report is made the physician-patient relationship must end, and that the child protective service department of a public agency will take over or perhaps may do nothing anyway. So why report? The physician will lose a patient and the child will still be in danger.

This negative mind-set lends a sense of futility that dampens any initial intentions to do good. The primary care physician not only represents the first line of recognition and reporting, but the important hub of ongoing management and monitoring. The physician must recognize that the relationship need not be adversarial, that good does come from intervening with these families, that public welfare agencies profit from our support and crumble as the result of our condemnation. However, a positive outcome can only occur if the abuse is recognized and an initial report is made. This chapter will emphasize these early initial steps.

BACKGROUND

INCIDENCE AND EPIDEMIOLOGY

The incidence of child abuse has been steadily increasing in the United States. Currently, there is an incidence of 25.2 cases per 1,000 children in the population. Not only has the total number of cases increased, but the severity of abuse has escalated. Child homicide has become the fourth leading cause of death in the 1-year-old to 14-year-old age group and the second most common cause of death in adolescence. It is estimated 2,000 to 5,000 children are killed each year by their parents or caretakers. Most of the homicides involving children are caused by family members. At the Children's Hospital of Philadelphia, over 600 cases of abuse/neglect are reported per year. This makes the recognition and reporting of an abuse case more than a once per day occurrence. Thus, child abuse is a modern-day plague—a problem of epidemic proportion. Unfortunately, unlike other conditions that are suffered at one point in time, the cyclic nature of abuse has the potential to make today's abused child the future's abusive parent. Our failure to prevent abuse now may further elevate the already high level of violent crime in society for years to come.

There are no adequate studies of the epidemiology of abuse. Reporting of abuse cases does not match the incidence of occurrence. Best estimates are that reports represent 50% of the actual number of cases. Thus, there is a general belief that those using public facilities, e.g., lower socioeconomic groups are overrepresented in reports. Many authors have written that abuse occurs across all ethnic groups, socioeconomic status, and educational levels. The studies of David Gill show that this is indeed true. However, without knowing the universe of abusive episodes, we cannot relate the prevalence of abuse to epidemiologic factors. Faced with suspicion of abuse in a given case, the parents' background should neither encourage nor dissuade the reporter.

FORMS OF ABUSE

Abuse may be manifest in many forms; these are summarized below. The general categories are (1) physical, (2) sexual, (3) emotional, and (4) neglect.

MANIFESTATIONS OF CHILD ABUSE

Physical abuse
Soft tissue trauma
Skeletal trauma
Central nervous system trauma
Visceral injury
Sensory organ injury
Dental trauma
Poisoning
Starvation

Sexual abuse
- Rape
- Statutory rape
- Deviate sexual intercourse
- Indecent assault
- Incest
- Sexually transmitted diseases
- Child pornography
- Child prostitution

Emotional abuse
Depression
Fear
Aggressive behavior
Agitation
Social withdrawal
Pseudosophistication

Neglect
Nutritional neglect (failure to thrive)
Psychosocial neglect
Medical neglect
Educational neglect
Abandonment

Each form of abuse has a specific definition, yet there is a great deal of overlap between the forms. An abused child never sustains a single form of abuse. For example, with every episode of physical abuse, there is a negative message to the child such as, "You are no good." Such messages constitute emotional abuse. There have been great debates in the literature whether abuse and neglect are subsets of the same phenomenon or entirely different entities. From the child's perspective, this debate seems moot. Either acts of omission or acts of commission cause injury to the child. Whether the parents' behavior was active or passive does not seem terribly important. Neglect and emotional abuse are very difficult to define. Both definitions require that significant value judgments be made. Both are hard to define in the context of a single emergency department or office encounter. The physician reporting emotional abuse needs in-depth knowledge and a long-term perspective on the family. The primary care provider is well equipped for this task.

CAUSES OF ABUSE

Like the forms of abuse, the causes of abuse are many and often there are overlapping contributory factors. The factors that cause abuse can be grouped into four categories: (1) parental pathologic states, (2) family interaction problems, (3) external stressors, and (4) societal factors.

Individual parental factors include problems that are primarily linked to one parent or parent figure, although such problems clearly affect all family members. This category includes parental drug/alcohol abuse, parental depression, and parental retardation. Some parents simply have weak impulse control.

Family interaction problems are defined as difficulties in parents relating to each other and difficulty in parents relating to children. Within this class of problem, we see many unsupportive marital relationships. Also, there are individual children who seem to be incompatible with their parents. This may be due to differences in temperament or differences due to the child being particularly different or difficult (whether in reality or in the mind of the parent). In some families there seem to be many conflict-laden relationships: husband with wife, wife with children.

External stresses contribute greatly to abuse. If nothing else, stress seems to often be the spark that ignites an abusive explosion, albeit the potential may have been caused by other factors. Stress is felt in many forms. In our patients, housing, economic, and work-related stresses are prominent. Stress without release seems to be another common factor present. Stated simply, it is a feeling of being trapped and without hope. This is an unfortunate human condition that results in anger and primitive aggressive behavior toward others or toward oneself.

The fourth set of causative factors is labeled societal. These are circumstances within our society that form some of the background or matrix conditions for abuse. Within this cluster of factors are three very important ones: (1) social isolation; (2) lack of preparation for parenthood; and (3) widespread use of corporal punishment. Many families in the United States find themselves living in social isolation. The American family is subject to many housing moves for employment-related reasons. Few people live in the same location as their extended family. Also, sociologic factors such as the development of surburban living and shopping, the high rate of urban crime, and a high societal value on independence have contributed to this trend of isolation. Independence is a desirable trait—except when families are in trouble. Then a state of independence becomes isolation, an additional stress factor.

Most first-time parents have had little preparation for parenthood. For most parents the time to have children becomes more often based on conforming to one's peer group than on the achievement of a level of child care competence. Parents who do not prepare themselves for parenthood find that they are stressed by their children. These parents harbor unrealistic expectations of their children that are formed without regard for, or knowledge of, the child's developmental level. Thus, the unprepared parent expects that when his 14-month-old soils his diaper, it is purposeful and defiant. Our society expects that to have children is equivalent to knowing how to care for them, yet to perform in other areas (e.g., driving a car, practicing medicine, selling real estate) there are some minimum competency requirements. Without any preparation or education from outside our own experience, we tend to behave as our parents behaved toward us. If our parents were competent and caring, we have a chance to repeat those positive qualities. If our parents were abusive in their approach, we are likely to repeat that pattern, particularly when stressed.

The final important factor that contributes to abuse is our societal belief in the value of corporal punishment, which leads to the philosophy of "spank your children regularly whether they need it or not." Our belief is that when corporal punishment is the discipline technique of choice, many individuals escalate their punishment to the point that abuse occurs. There is a continuum between "normal" corporal punishment and reportable abuse. The point of excess along this continuum is a vague one. One person's concept of acceptable punishment is another's abuse. This lack of precision in definition makes the primary physician's task a difficult one. The physician must be the one to draw the line.

DATA GATHERING

In the case of physical abuse, how does the physician "draw the line"? What does the "line" mean? Each state in the United States has adopted child abuse legislation. Each state describes what constitutes child abuse as well as what should be reported, when, and how to report. Most states also include a definition of a mandated reporter, as well as a penalty for failure to report and protection for reporting in good faith. All states require that there be a demonstrable injury in order for physical abuse to exist. There must be *injury*. If we observe unusual or even distasteful child-rearing practices, but those practices do not result in injury, then we have not witnessed abuse. Each state law also indicates the age that defines the term "child." In most state laws the physician is *required* to report the *suspicion* of abuse. The line that must be drawn then is the one that defines suspicion. The physician should have suspicion of abuse for every traumatic episode encountered. Granted, for the vast majority of injuries, abuse will be a fleeting consideration. In other cases, the physician will ponder the possibility of abuse. In yet others, the physician will be virtually convinced of abuse. The line of suspicion to be drawn is the threshhold at which the physician is ready to report the case as suspected abuse. The physician may reach this threshhold by using a combination of building blocks. The blocks include: (1) physical findings; (2) history; (3) laboratory data; and (4) observed interaction. The blocks are of different value and may be stacked in different combinations: for example, a 2-year-old child is brought to the office with multiple bruises over the buttocks and chest (Fig 52–1). The physical findings are suspicious in that accidental injury does not usually involve multiple bruises in such a central location. Thus, there is one building block in place. The history given is that the parent does not know how this injury occurred—a second block. A normal coagulation profile provides the third block. In the observed family interactions, the child seems fearful and withdrawn. The parents are fighting with each other. This final datum is enough to reach a threshhold and for the physician to decide to report these injuries as suspected abuse. In another case (Fig 52–2), a 6-year-old girl is seen for a cold. In examining her back, the physician finds multiple red linear and looped-shaped whip marks. In this case the physical examination block is sufficient to meet the threshhold. There are many different combinations that can lead to making a diagnosis. Some of the specific observations the physician should make are listed in the sections that follow.

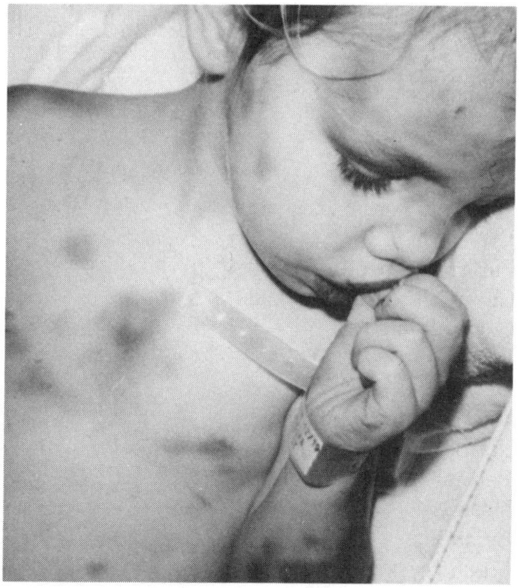

FIG 52–1
Patient with multiple bruises in a central distribution.

HISTORY

In obtaining a history suspicious of abuse, the key process is to compare the history to the physical findings. Does the history make sense? Does it explain the findings? For the most part the physician must use common sense and experience with accidental trauma situations to make some judgments. Also helpful is a knowledge of child development, as many abuse his-

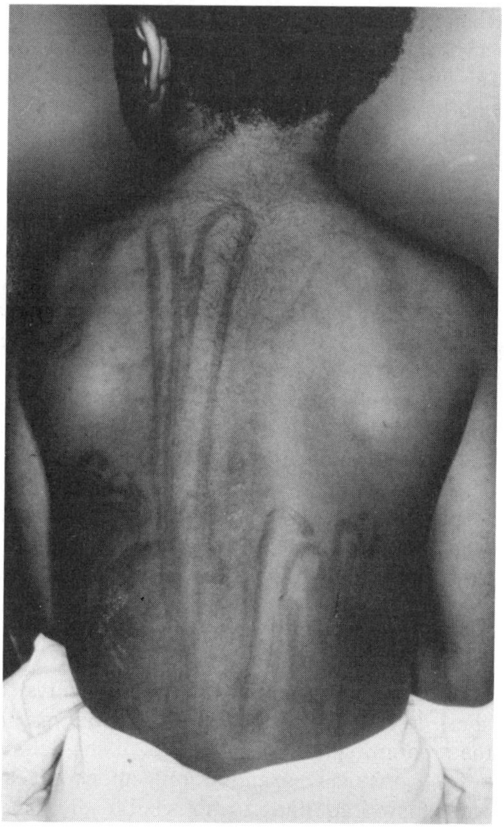

FIG 52–2
Multiple looped-shaped marks caused by beating with an electric extension cord.

tories will attribute remarkable motor skills to young children.

When a parent can provide no history for an injury involving a young child, this is also worrisome. When the parent states, "I just found him that way in his crib," in reference to a 4-month-old with a fractured femur, the history is suspect. Parents may also be inconsistent in the giving of the history. The physician must decide if this inconsistency is based on fabrication of the story or "normal" inconsistency that occurs when telling and retelling a history and using supposition to fill in gaps in an unwitnessed history.

Parents who have abused will often misgauge the severity of the child's injury. Guilt may be a major factor in this dynamic. Another factor may be an unconscious desire to be detected and controlled. A parent who has inflicted a minor facial bruise may magnify the injury to the point that they feel the child needs to be examined in the emergency department. Thus, when the parent gives a history of severe injury and only minor injury exists, consider abuse. The opposite situation may also exist. Parents who have severely injured their child may underestimate the injury and, thus, may not seek medical attention in a timely fashion. In studies of several different forms of abuse, time delays in coming to the hospital have been documented. Perhaps the delay represents a period of time that the parent expends in conflict, asking the following questions: Is the injury severe or not severe? Will I be detected? Will being detected keep me from injuring my child again?

The parent who admits to abusing his child but floods the physician with indications of remorse should not divert the physician from reporting the case. When the parent admits to inflicting the injury, the reporting threshhold has been met, no matter how sincere the parent may seem about never repeating the abuse.

PHYSICAL EXAMINATION

Since there must be injury in order for physical abuse to have occurred, physical findings are the predominant building blocks of suspicion.

The physical examination often reveals pathognomonic signs of abuse. Linear marks, looped-shaped marks, and some pattern injuries are themselves sufficient to diagnose abuse. Other findings are less specific and must be evaluated in conjunction with the history. Injuries that are multiple, are in various stages of healing, or vary pathophysiologically, are suspicious. Unusual or unexplained physical findings must also be considered suspicious. Emergency physicians have the advantage of seeing many children who have sustained accidental trauma. This serves as an important data base on which to make judgments.

Integument injuries are the most common manifestations of abuse; these are summarized in the list below.

INTEGUMENT INJURIES

Pattern marks (e.g., buckle imprint)
Linear whip marks
Loop marks (e.g., electric cord)
Hand prints
Punctures (e.g., fork marks)
Binding of wrist or ankles
Multiple bruises
Bruises in various stages of healing
Unusual location
  Central distribution
  Protected areas (e.g., neck)
Human bite
Hair loss
Burns
Pattern burn (e.g., cigarette, iron)
Immersion burn
  Stocking or glove distribution
  Buttocks and feet pattern
Splash burn

INJURY TO SENSORY ORGANS

Ear
"Boxed" ear
Hemotympanum
"Cauliflower" ear
Eye
Periorbital ecchymosis
Conjunctival hemorrhage
Corneal abrasion
Hyphema
Dislocated lens
Vitreous hemorrhage
Retinal detachment
Retinal hemorrhage
Nose
Epistaxis
Fracture
Mouth
Lip trauma

Frenulum tear, "bottle jamming"
Posterior pharyngeal trauma
Airway obstruction

TIMING OF HEALING

Color of skin—time after injury

Red/blue—first 24 hr
Dark purple—1 to 4 days
Green—5 to 7 days
Yellow—7 to 10 days
Normal tint—1 to 3 weeks

In particular, linear welts and bruises are visible after excessive punishment with a belt or electric cord. The physician may see a clear outline of a belt buckle or the looped end of a doubled electric cord. Other findings of significance are pattern injuries. These are bruises or burns that form a pattern (e.g., hand print on the side of the face; symmetric bruises on the upper arm from being grasped). Burns may take the pattern of a hot object or may occur in a stocking or glove distribution following hot-water immersion; immersion burns are summarized as follows:

IMMERSION BURNS

Etiology

Child placed in hot water. Many tap water sources yield water 130° F. Exposure for 30 seconds yields full-thickness burn.

Target group

Children of toilet-training age; most burns occur in children younger than 3 years old.

Physical findings

Symmetric burns on buttocks and feet and over entire lower extremity.

If child is clothed, burn severity is increased in clothed area.

Palms and soles relatively spared.

Look for bruises elsewhere on body.

Other findings

Delay in seeking treatment greater than 2 hours.

Child brought by caretaker not present at time of burn.

Family stress easily identified.

Nonspecific bruising can be a more difficult physical finding for raising the suspicion of abuse. Children often acquire accidental bruises from the rough nature of their play. Also, as they drive themselves to achieve new developmental milestones, they are likely to sustain accidental injuries. Accidental bruising occurs mainly on extremities and forehead. When bruises become multiple and move toward a central distribution, they raise more suspicion. A skin lesion that looks like a bruise may in fact be a fixed hyperpigmented lesion. The correct diagnosis can be made when the lesion is observed over time. Normal mongolian spots are sometimes thought to be abuse. The normal progression of a bruise through stages of healing will not be seen in a hyperpigmented lesion.

Skeletal injuries (summarized below) are also frequent manifestations of abuse. Fractures of the ribs and of other infrequently injured bones (e.g., scapula, vertebral bodies) are particularly worrisome. Fractures of long bones need to be examined for the mechanism of injury and estimation of the extent of force sustained by the bone. All fractures in children younger than 1 year old are suggestive of abuse.

SKELETAL INJURY

Etiology

Skeletal trauma, either direct or bending trauma to bone, traction to an extremity, or rotational force.

Target group

Any age

Physical findings

Direct trauma: transverse fracture, periosteal elevation

Bending force: transverse fracture, plastic deformity

Rotational trauma: spiral fracture

Traction force: metaphyseal chip fracture, periosteal elevation, bucket-handle fracture

Subacute trauma: callus formation

Unusual locations: fractures of ribs, scapula, spine

Diagnostic studies

Skeletal survey for trauma

Radionuclide skeletal scintigraphy

Normal levels of serum calcium, phosphorus, and alkaline phosphatase

Head trauma is another frequent form of abuse. We see two forms of head trauma: (1) direct trauma, and (2) shake injury. Direct trauma results in scalp hematoma, skull fracture, and intracranial bleeding. Intracerebral injury without major external manifestations is called "shaken baby syndrome." In this form of abuse, intracranial bleeding may be subdural hemorrhage, subarachnoid hemorrhage, cerebral con-

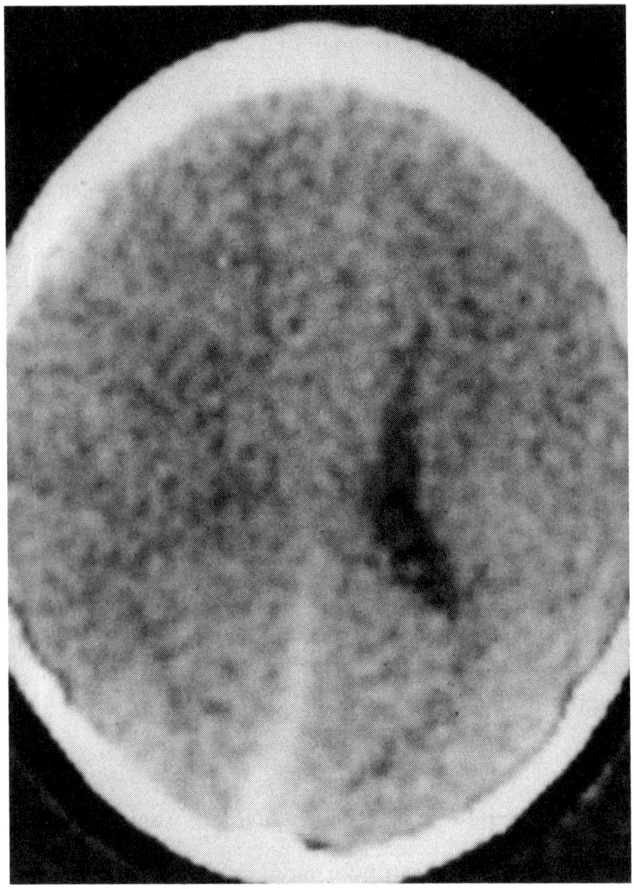

FIG 52–3
Shaken baby syndrome. Computed tomography scan showing left-sided cerebral edema and interhemispheric subdural bleeding. Ventricle obscured due to edema.

tusion, or cerebral infarction. Computed tomography (CT) aids the diagnostic process greatly, as it defines specific lesions and makes some estimation of the chronology of the injury (Fig 52–3). These children will generally be seen in the hospital.

Another form of abuse that must be recognized quickly to preserve life is *abdominal trauma*. With this form the child is punched, kicked, or stepped on. The factors of relatively weak abdominal musculature and relatively large organ size contribute to serious injury of a variety of types. The abdominal wall is pliable enough that it does not sustain evidence of trauma or at worst only shows minor bruising at the same time that major organ injury is sustained.

Failure to thrive is a term used to describe children who are not growing according to norms established for our population. The cause may be organic or nonorganic.

NONORGANIC FAILURE TO THRIVE

Etiology

Failure of the child to receive adequate calories in appropriately stimulating environment.

Target group

Usually children younger than 18 months old.

Physical findings

Growth parameters below standards for age.
Weight more severely affected than length.
Head circumference relatively spared.
Dull, lackadaisical look to eyes.
Flat occiput, passive "frog-leg" posture.
Other signs of neglect (e.g., severe diaper rash).
Other than growth failure, normal findings of physical examination.

Other findings

No history of abnormal losses (e.g., vomiting, diarrhea).
Idealized feeding history.
Timing of growth failure with life stress.
Caretakers fail to perceive growth failure.

Diagnostic studies
Weight gain in hospital.
Normal routine laboratory studies.

Nonorganic failure to thrive frequently is reportable as a form of abuse or gross physical neglect. Outcome studies have shown high rates of morbidity and mortality for this group of children, thus, prompt recognition and reporting are important. Failure to thrive is discussed in more detail in Chapter 30.

Many *miscellaneous forms of abuse* that we have seen and reported are listed below.

UNUSUAL MANIFESTATIONS OF ABUSE

- Intoxication
  - Salt—hypernatremia
  - Water—hyponatremia
  - Alcohol—hyperosmolality, hypoglycemia
  - Other drugs or toxins
- Confinement
- Münchausen's syndrome by proxy
- Sleep deprivation
- Dehydration or starvation
- Fetal abuse

In general, any unusual physical finding should lead one to consider the possibility of abuse. Entertaining the diagnosis early will allow the physician to gather more historical information, laboratory data, and to observe interactions in a way that may add building blocks high enough to reach a reporting threshhold. An important caution is that the extent of the trauma does not correlate with the seriousness of abuse. Minor injury may be the result of abuse perpetrated with extreme intent but fortunately not much physical result. A child recently seen had the finding of a superficial skin abrasion on his chest. This was not impressive as far as extent of injury, yet it was caused by a psychotic mother who was attempting to cut his heart out with a knife. Fortunately, the child was able to escape with only minor injury.

LABORATORY EVALUATION

The clinical laboratory may be used in many different ways to support the diagnosis of abuse and to add building blocks of suspicion. The most frequently used laboratory information is the radiograph. Radiography may be helpful in dating an injury, documenting skeletal injury, and in determining the type of force and mechanism of injury. Skeletal surveys should not be obtained in every case of suspected abuse. We use the following criteria:

1. An infant (< 1 year) with any form of injury.
2. An infant or toddler with one fracture.
3. A child with failure to thrive.
4. A child with extensive bruising.
5. A child with oral trauma.

In some institutions, radionuclide scans have been used and are reported to be more sensitive than roentgenograms.

Other laboratory studies include those summarized in Table 52–1. There have been no studies of the sensitivity or specificity of individual tests. The emergency physician must use clinical judgment in determining the need for laboratory information. There are times when the medical-legal nature of abuse will re-

TABLE 52–1
Laboratory Studies for Physical Abuse

STUDY	DOCUMENTATION
Complete blood cell count (CBC)	Blood loss, nutritional anemia
Platelet count, prothrombin time, partial thromboplastin time (PT/PTT)	Coagulation status
Blood urea nitrogen (BUN), urine specific gravity	Dehydration
Toxic screen serum urine, gastric contents	Poisoning
Urine hematest	Urinary tract trauma, myoglobinuria
Creatinine phosphokinase (CPK)	Muscle trauma
Bullae culture	Pyoderma
Serum amylase determination	Pancreatic trauma
Determinations of serum calcium, phosphorus, alkaline phosphatase	Bone disease

quire that laboratory tests be ordered to document the normal state. For example, the child with obviously inflicted bruises may require a coagulation profile to prove the absence of a coagulopathy.

Physicians may overlook the urinalysis as an important test. Urine specific gravity determines hydration status. The presence of blood may indicate renal trauma. When urine dipstick testing is positive for blood, yet there are no visible red blood cells, consider myoglobinuria from muscle breakdown. The finding of myoglobin in the urine is important as it may be a signal of impending renal failure from acute tubular necrosis.

INTERACTION

The final building block to be used in determining the level of suspicion is interaction. The physician must be aware of the relationship of the patient and his caretakers, as well as the relationship between the parents and the physician. Are the parents open? Are they tense and withholding? Many parents express concern, some remorse. Thus, it should not surprise the physician to see the parents demonstrate concern and caring. Other parents may more fit the stereotype of the hostile, suspicious, difficult parents. Parents may be feeling guilty, which is easily transformed into anger directed toward the physician or the hospital. Is the child wary? Some have described the abused child as withdrawn; others report a more clinging, dependent child who will form immediate attachments with anyone. Some children may exhibit "radar eyes," which cautiously follow the movements of the adults in the room. The older abused child may be very engaging and pseudosophisticated as a result of having assumed parental responsibility at a young age.

In cases of suspected abuse, the physician should make a specific point of thinking about the interaction. The more the abusive parent is like the physician, the more difficult an objective assessment will be. Parents who are educated and articulate and live in the same neighborhood as the examining physician are less likely to stimulate suspicion. This is a natural defense mechanism. The unconscious line of reasoning is, "If those parents abused a child, and they are like me, then I could also abuse." The simple fact is that anyone under sufficient volume of stress is capable of injuring a child.

SEXUAL ABUSE

PHYSICAL EXAMINATION

Although the majority of sexually abused children have no physical findings that would indicate abuse, the physician needs to perform a thorough physical examination of the genital and rectal areas. For prepubertal children, inspection of the genitalia, with the child in the froglike or knee-chest position, is sufficient. A speculum examination should not be attempted. If vaginal bleeding is the predominant finding on examination, the child must be referred to the emergency department, where the pediatric surgeon or gynecologist should be consulted immediately. We have seen cases where a small trickle of blood was the presenting sign for major vaginal lacerations that required extensive repair.

If the child is not bleeding from the vaginal orifice, then the genitalia may be examined for trauma, signs of sexually transmitted disease, and the presence of seminal fluid. Evidence of trauma may appear not only on the genitalia; the entire skin surface must also be examined for evidence of a forceful attempt. Bruises on the upper thighs and lower abdominal wall are suggestive. Hand prints on the upper arms or facial trauma may be clues to the diagnosis. Due to common nonmedical beliefs, there is always concern about the state of the hymenal structures. The term intact or nonintact hymen should not be used. A fully intact hymen is an imperforate hymen, a very rare anatomic variation. The state of the hymenal ring may have no bearing on whether a child was abused, unless it shows evidence of acute trauma (e.g., bleeding from the hymenal ring). There are currently no agreed on standards for the width of the labial opening. Some investigators use a 4mm transverse opening as the maximum size in a prepubertal child. If the labia appear to be distended, measure the opening rather than using vague descriptors such as "gaping."

The physician must also carefully inspect the rectum. Again, one must make an estimation of the opening of the rectum. The presence of any traumatic fissures or lacerations should be noted. The physician must also examine the oral cavity for signs of trauma.

In looking for sexually transmitted diseases (STD; see Chapter 60), careful inspection is crucial. The physician should be looking for vaginal or urethral discharge, or the presence of any scabbed or vesicular lesions. The laboratory tests will be critical in establishing a firm diagnosis of STD. The child should be carefully examined for the presence of seminal fluid in the genital, rectal, and oral cavity, as well as on upper thighs, lower abdominal wall, and on underclothing. In looking for seminal fluid, some have suggested the use of a Wood's lamp. With a Wood's lamp, seminal fluid is a fluorescent dark-green color. Laboratory confirmation of the presence of sperm is also important.

One physical finding that should always raise the possibility of sexual abuse is teenage pregnancy. Often, in the flurry of activity around diagnosing pregnancy in a young teenager, the question of paternity is forgotten. There is an assumption that the consort is a peer. However, with careful exploration, the physician may reveal a pregnancy resulting from an incestuous relationship.

SPECIAL ASPECTS OF SEXUAL ABUSE CASE MANAGEMENT

The management of sexual abuse has many of the characteristics of the management of physical abuse. Once a threshhold of suspicion is reached, a report should be made. More often the report will be made to the police as most states have specific criminal statutes for sexual abuse crimes. Reaction from family members will vary depending on many factors. If the perpetrator is a family member or equivalent (e.g., boarder, neighbor), one can expect more reaction and more turmoil. If the perpetrator is a stranger outside the family system, there is expressed anger but usually reaction is more focused toward the perpetrator. The parents should understand how important their reaction is to the ultimate recovery of the child. If parents "fall apart," make sudden changes in life-style, or blame the child, the child's psychological morbidity will be increased. If family members can provide protection and support the child, then there should be improved outcome.

It is important that the child is not made to feel a victim any more than has already occurred at the hands of the abuser. The examination must be conducted with care so as not to commit the so-called "second rape." The child should be made as comfortable as possible. For example, the child may hold the moistened swab while the physician guides the child's hand to obtain the cultures. This allows the child some sense of control and reduces fear. In line with this reasoning, hospitalization of the sexually abused child is unusual unless there is a medical indication (i.e., vaginal or rectal bleeding).

Another treatment issue concerns the need to treat or provide prophylaxis against sexually transmitted disease, in particular *Neisseria gonorrhoeae*. Obtaining a detailed history is important in deciding. In some cases of child sexual abuse, there will have been no genital contact and, thus, treating for gonorrhea is unnecessary. There are situations in which the child has been used as a source of sexual stimulation without much physical contact. In other situations, one may obtain the history of more physical contact either genital-genital, genital-oral, or genital-rectal. In those situations, the physician may wish to treat the possibility of gonorrhea by using probenecid (25 mg/kg, orally for a maximum of 1 g) and amoxicillin (50 mg/kg, orally for a maximum of 3 g). We prefer this regimen because it is administered in the office, and we can ensure compliance. Also, it is a nonpainful regimen that complements our philosophy of not injuring the victim further. Any prophylaxis should be given after adequate cultures have been obtained. In areas where penicillinase-producing organisms are predominant, an IM cephalosporin must be used (see Chapter 60).

All children who have been sexually abused need a specific plan for follow-up care. At the follow-up visit, culture results are reviewed. The physician also reviews the state of the family and their ability to cope with this crisis.

MANAGEMENT

CONSIDER THE DIFFERENTIAL DIAGNOSIS

On paper, the differential diagnosis of abuse is complex (Table 52–2). In reality, the majority of conditions listed are quite rare and can be

TABLE 52–2
Differential Diagnosis of Abuse

DIAGNOSIS	CONFIRMATORY STUDY
Accidental trauma	History, physical examination, laboratory studies, observed interaction of child and parents
Scurvy	Long bone roentgenogram
Rickets	Wrist roentgenogram, determination of levels of calcium, phosphorus, alkaline phosphatase
Secondary hyperparathyroidism	BUN, creatinine, long bone roentgenogram
Kinky hair syndrome	Long bone, skull, rib roentgenograms, hair analysis
Mucolipidosis II (I-cell disease)	Long bone, rib roentgenograms, analysis of facial features, fibroblast studies
Congenital syphilis	VDRL
Osteomyelitis	Bone culture, blood culture, sedimentation rate
Osteogenesis imperfecta	Skeletal roentgenograms, bone biopsy
Infantile cortical hyperostosis	Long bone, mandible roentgenograms
Skeletal sclerosis	Long bone roentgenogram

eliminated by simple laboratory tests and roentgenographic studies. The most frequent, and perhaps most difficult differentiation is between accidental trauma and inflicted trauma. If this differential diagnosis is unclear at the time of the initial visit, the physician must err on the side of overreporting. The physician may find that discussing the case with another health care professional will in itself be instructive. Thus, confidentially discuss the case with a colleague, a child abuse specialist at a nearby center, or a social worker from a local public or private agency.

REPORTING SUSPECTED ABUSE

State and local laws and regulations will dictate the method of reporting. In some places the physician reports to the child protective services division of the welfare department or another social service agency. In other jurisdictions, abuse must be reported to the police department. Some communities have established joint reporting to both child welfare and law enforcement personnel. This third reporting alternative offers the best combination of investigative and supportive services. Reporting should be done promptly and directly. The physician must state the degree of injury, the rationale for suspecting abuse, and an estimation of the volatility of the home environment. The physician should also determine whether there are other children at risk whose conditions need immediate evaluation.

NOTIFY THE PARENTS

We think it is very important to notify parents that an official suspected child abuse report is being filed. This step is perhaps the most difficult for most physicians. As a result, some tend to omit it. Others soft-pedal the information to the point that the message to the parents is unclear. There are certain key elements of notification. First, the physician must be making the report in the spirit of support. Reporting is not a vindictive act. It is a therapeutic step. Reporting is not done to punish the parent. It is done to help the child. Most physicians and parents can find common ground in their desire to help the child. Concern for the child is the cornerstone of all actions. If the physician is openly angry, this will cause the parents to become entrenched in their position of denial or to become hostile. Second, parents need to be told what will be the consequences of the report. Because many parents are already feeling guilty, they tend to exaggerate the consequence of the report. Give parents a clear idea that this is a report of *suspected* abuse and what will be happening. It is important to use the word "abuse." For some parents this is a startling word that they need to hear. At the same time, present a picture of the spectrum of abuse from well-intentioned yet over-vigorous punishment to prolonged torture. Doing this allows the parents to see where they fit in the spectrum while clearly stating that they have entered the "abuser" category. If indicated, they should be informed of the existence of services of which they might avail themselves to avoid problems in the future. It is not necessary for the physician to obtain an admission of guilt on the part of the parent. Societal stigma and personal shame are so forceful that it is unusual for a parent to admit to abuse even when the findings are obvious.

HOSPITALIZATION

Some children will require hospitalization for the treatment of their injuries. However, the emergency physician will need to hospitalize some children solely for protection. The key question to be answered is: "Is the home safe?" Factors that may play a role in this determination are summarized below.

FACTORS TO CONSIDER IN HOSPITALIZATION OF THE ABUSED CHILD

Is the home safe?
Is the perpetrator still in the home?
Is the perpetrator known?
Are caretakers abusers of drugs or alcohol?
Are caretakers psychotic? Psychopathic?
Response time of police or welfare agency.
Nature of crisis that triggered abuse.
Are there supportive relatives or neighbors?
Is the child capable of calling for help?
Age of child.
Has abuse been repetitive?
Is there an alternative setting (e.g., emergency foster care)?

If the physician believes that the home is unsafe or if there is any question about it, the child should be protected by hospitalization. Some communities have established crisis shelters and immediate response of child welfare personnel. These capabilities are preferable over that of placing the child in the frightening environment of the hospital. However, many communities cannot provide such services and the hospital must fill the gap.

MEDICAL-LEGAL CONSIDERATION

The final aspect of management is medical-legal. Medical records are always both medical and legal documents. In the case of suspected abuse, the legal nature of the record is more apparent. Documentation needs to be meticulous. The nature and extent of the injuries must be detailed. Drawings or color photographs are helpful in documenting a complex injury that cannot be vividly reported by description alone. Photographs in most states can be taken without parental permission. It is important to have good photography that realistically shows the nature and extent of injury. Poor-quality photographs may hurt a case more than help it. The statements of the parents and child should be recorded verbatim and recorded in quotation marks. The observations of the interaction should also be reported. List the names of all consultants. Remember that this chart may be vital to you if the case comes to court in 6 months to a year later. Don't speculate in writing—but record objective observations and conclusions. Other aspects of court testimony techniques are discussed later in this chapter.

MAINTAINING A RELATIONSHIP

It is important to make it clear to the family that in reporting suspected abuse you are not intending to end your relationship. If you believe that what you are doing is therapeutic, you will be able to continue your working with the family. It is in this ongoing care that the physician can see the positive benefits of the reporting. Many families will voice positive changes. Others will continue to need close monitoring and frequent periods of support. Many physicians mistakenly feel that they can provide ongoing care without establishing an initial report. This mistaken notion may lead to denial on the part of the family and, perhaps, legal action directed toward the physician. It is akin to treating a condition without informing the patient of the diagnosis or having the patient accept the diagnosis. The attitude often professed—"I can work with my patients. No one needs to be reported. No outsiders need to be involved"—is a dangerous one.

BIBLIOGRAPHY

Burgess AW, et al: *Sexual Assault of Children and Adolescents.* Lexington, Mass, Lexington Books, 1978.

Ellerstein NS: *Child Abuse and Neglect: A Medical Reference.* New York, C Wiley, 1981.

Gelles RJ: Violence toward children in the United States. *Am J Orthopsychiatry* 1978; 48:580.

Gill D: *Violence Against Children: Physical Abuse in the U.S.* Cambridge, Mass, Harvard University Press, 1970.

Green FC: Child abuse and neglect: A priority problem for the private physician. *Pediatr Clin North Am* 1975; 22:329.

Helfer RE: Why most physicians don't get involved in child abuse cases and what to do about it. *Child Today* 1975; 4:28.

Homer C, Ludwig S: Categorization of etiology of failure to thrive. *Am J Dis Child* 1981; 135:848.

Ludwig S: Child abuse and neglect, in Fleisher G, Ludwig S (eds): *Textbook of Pediatric Emergency Medicine*, ed 2. Baltimore, Williams & Wilkins Co, 1988.

Ludwig S: Prevention of child abuse, in *Critical Issues in Emergency Medicine*. New York, Churchill Livingstone, 1988.

Ludwig S, Warman M: Shaken baby syndrome. *Ann Emerg Med* 1984; 13:2, 104.

National Incidence and Prevalence of Child Abuse and Neglect. Rockville, Md, US Department of Health and Human Services, DHHS Publication No 10585–1702.

O'Neill JA, Meacham WF, Griffin PP, et al: Patterns of injury in the battered child syndrome. *J Trauma* 1973; 13:332.

Sgroi SM: Sexual molestation of children: The last frontier in child abuse. *Child Today* May, June 1975; 4:18–21, 44.

PHYSICIAN'S ROLE IN FAMILY COURT

For most families there is a relative balance between the rights of parents, the rights of their children, and the rights of the family unit. The individuals involved usually have overlapping goals, aspirations, and values. However, there are times when the rights of the various family members are in conflict. One clear example of this occurs when a child has been abused. In such a situation the child's rights to be free from physical harm and the parents' rights to discipline their child as they see fit are in conflict. Other examples include rights to health care, rights to education, and rights to live with the parent of their choice in the case of divorced parents.

When the rights of the child are in conflict with those of the parent or the family unit, frequently the primary care physician is asked to provide information to the "resolver of conflict," the family court. This chapter will review some of the principles to be used when appearing in court on behalf of a child. Throughout this chapter, the example of a child abuse case is used, as this will be the most frequent situation encountered. Many of the basic concepts may be applied to other child advocacy situations.

PREPARING TO GO TO COURT

Define the Purpose.—The first step in the process is defining the reason for going to court. The simple reason is because you have been issued a subpoena. However, once subpoenaed, you should consider why you are going to court. There are many different reasons, such as (1) to effect placement of a child outside his or her natural home; (2) to establish an official record of facts; (3) to institute or enforce a treatment plan for parents or for the child; (4) to ensure that someone repays society for a crime committed; and (5) to request that a judge hear the facts of a case and make an impartial decision. In some cases you may have more than one objective in mind when you go to court. Importantly, you must have at least one objective in mind. Otherwise, your experience will be an unsatisfactory one.

Know the Setting.—Before you go to court, it is helpful to know the setting in which you will appear. Will you be in a small conference room with all the parties seated around a table, or will you be in a large, imposing courtroom facing a jury? Knowing the setting will help you to prepare what you need to say and how you must say it.

Beyond the physical setting, you will want to know the kind of case in which you are to testify: civil or criminal. Table 52–3 outlines the differences between the two systems. There are many legal differences; however, in nonlegal terms these may be divided into differences in the issues, the penalties, the parties, and the rules of evidence. These differences are important in that they determine what you must prove and how you must go about proving it. For the perpetrator of abuse, these differences are also critical.

TABLE 52–3
Comparison of Civil vs. Criminal Child Abuse Proceedings

PARAMETER	CIVIL	CRIMINAL
Laws	State Child Protection Law	State criminal codes for specific crimes (e.g., assault, endangerment, murder)
Need to prove	The child was injured by nonaccidental means	That a specific individual injured the child at a particular time
Fact finder	Judge	Judge or judge and jury
Maximum penalty	Removal of the child from parents	Sentence of incarceration or probation dependent on specific crime
Rules of evidence and formality	Lenient	Strict
Burden of proof	Predominance of the evidence (51%)	Beyond a reasonable doubt (95%)

Understand the Context.—It will also be helpful if you can determine from the lawyer or lawyers involved how they see your testimony contributing to the case. As physicians, we often feel that the entire weight of the case depends on our findings and opinions. Although this is often true, it is not always so. The legal counsel should give us the context of our testimony. How will our testimony meld with the testimony of other witnesses in making the entire case? Attorneys will take this to the point of formulating each question to be asked in advance of the trial.

Review Documentation.—Nothing will relieve the anxiety of the expert witness more than a thorough review of all existing documents, medical records, radiographs, and pertinent medical literature. The witness who is ill-prepared will find that his objectives in going to court will be easily foiled by a defense counsel who is prepared. Although medical records may be introduced as evidence to be read from in court, the witness will gain a psychological advantage by committing some details to memory. This leaves the judge and jury with the impression that this was an important case in your mind and that you remember it as distinct from the many cases of children you encounter each day.

Know the Parties.—It is also important to know all the parties involved. You will of course know the child and the parents. However, it is also good to know the lawyers and their assistants. In a given case there may be legal counsel for the parents, for the public welfare agency, and for the child. One question that comes up often is "Should I talk to the lawyers?" There is fear that in speaking with the defense counsel somehow the case will be ruined. This fear is an exaggeration of reality. Telling the lawyers what you will say during the court session is not harmful. Vague speculation and going beyond what will be said is dangerous and should be avoided.

Establish an On-Call System.—The court process is often bogged down by delays, continuances, out-of-court settlements, etc. Thus, you should try to establish an on-call system in such a way that if your testimony is needed you will be called and you will respond promptly to that call. This system will save you countless hours of wasted time in court waiting rooms. If you cannot make such arrangements, be aware that one of defense counsel's strategies will be to frustrate with delays to the point where you will refuse to testify. This strategy will have you abdicating your role as child advocate. If you are forced to appear at a set time, bring material with you that can make your waiting time more profitable.

THE HEARING

The typical family court hearing consists of three parts: the qualification, direct examination, and cross-examination. Each of these sections will be explored separately.

Qualification.—The prosecution or the defense may call you as a witness. Usually, it will be the prosecution who will seek to qualify you as an expert. There may be various kinds of expert testimony. For example, most physicians may be qualified as medical experts based on their completion of formal medical training and licensure. A physician may also be qualified in his/her field of specialty, for example, pediatrics. Additionally, the physician may be qualified as an expert in "child abuse and neglect." Being qualified as an expert allows the physician to not only report on findings but to draw conclusions as well.

During the qualification section of the hearing, the physician will be asked to display his training, experience, and qualifications to testify in a specific area. It is helpful to have supplied the lawyers with your curriculum vitae. The opposition lawyer may attempt to "stipulate" to your qualification. In doing this, the defense attempts to agree to the level of expertise, usually in order that the judge and jury do not hear the full details of your qualification. From the psychological perspective, it is better that the fact finders hear just how qualified you are. Be sure to mention previous court experiences. Having been qualified as an expert once makes it easier the second time. Sometimes physicians are more qualified than they think. In the case of a sexual abuse matter, the qualification is the physician's previous examination of many normal genitalia, rather than an extensive past experience with sexual abuse. In this example the primary care physician is far more qualified than the gynecologist who rarely examines the genitalia of the normal prepubertal female.

Direct Examination.—The goal of this part of the hearing is to present all the material that is relevant to the case. With this in mind, the physician should review in advance all the information deemed important. By doing this, one can make sure that all the important facts are brought forth. Nothing is more frustrating than completing testimony and knowing that the court has not been told a salient feature of the case. For example, lawyers may not know enough to ask you about the child's development. At the same time, the child's developmental delay may be at the heart of a case. By planning in advance what is important, you may bring out the child's developmental delay even when asked about the physical findings. During the direct examination the expert will reveal the findings of the case and the conclusions drawn from those findings. In the ideal situation, the lawyer and the expert witness will have planned the relevant questions needed to bring to the court all the important features of the case. During the testimony, the expert is wise to discuss only those issues for which he is an expert. Be careful not to delve into areas of speculation or areas of peripheral knowledge. Remember that any area brought out during the direct examination is subject to cross-examination. If a doctor expounds on the mental health status of the parents, this may come back to haunt him in the cross-examination. Usually, as one crawls out on a limb, the sound of sawing is clear.

Throughout the direct examination, remember the psychological aspects of your court appearance. A good expert witness is present merely to present objective data to the court. The expert must be impartial and fair. The physician in this role must not appear to be "out to get the parents." The expert must appear to have special knowledge and ability. To this end it may be helpful to use a certain amount of jargon in a professional way. At the same time translate those technical terms in order to be understood. Always keep in mind that the court is a nonmedical arena. The level of medical sophistication is much lower than that of many of your well-read patients.

During the direct examination, the expert may refer to notes and medical records. Usually the defense will have access to the same medical records. In front of a jury, being a good witness is like being a good teacher. Being clear and concise and using graphs, charts, x-rays, and photographs are important. The old adage that a picture is worth a thousand words is a truism in court. Even the most articulate witness cannot describe the child with multiple lash marks of a beating, either in terms of the number of marks on the child or the quality of the child's affect.

At any point during the testimony, the lawyers may raise objections. When something is objected to, the witness should stop speaking. This is a signal there is a legal objection that must be resolved by the lawyers and the judge.

The objecting lawyer is not indicating that the witness did or said anything wrong or incorrect. However, there are certain rules to which the law must adhere. How strictly these rules of law are followed will vary depending on the type of hearing, the point of the testimony, and the mind-set of the lawyers and the judge.

At the end of the direct examination, the physician will usually be asked about probable cause. The lawyer will ask, "Doctor, what is the probable cause of these findings?" As physicians we are trained to always be on the lookout for the one unusual circumstance, the one possible cause that is rare. Because of the nature of our training, the answer to this final question may pose a challenge. What the lawyer is asking is, "What is the most likely cause?" The lawyer is not asking for the one and only cause. Thus, the expert must answer in this light. Tell the court the probable cause, the most likely cause. The defense is likely to bring out the other possible although unlikely causes.

As a last step in the direct examination, the expert should bring forth recommendations for the case. Frequently, in the turmoil of bringing forth evidence, the overview is lost. What, in your opinion, should result from your findings? This is the essence of the case and should not be forgotten.

Cross-examination.—The nature of the legal process requires that the attorney representing the parent challenge the statements of the expert. The attorney may do this by attacking the facts or by making it appear that testimony of the expert has not been objective and fair. By increasing the expert's level of anxiety, these goals may be realized. The first step in preparing for cross-examination is to lower one's anxiety level. The expert will have taken the first step in this regard by careful precourt preparation. The second step is to realize that the expert is not the one on trial. Remember that a rigorous cross-examination is not a personal vendetta against the witness, it is the normal conduct of legal process. On many occasions, two lawyers who have harassed one another all day shake hands at the conclusion of a trial. Whenever you are asked a question, think about the question itself but also the purpose behind the question. If questions are being asked in a rapid-fire manner, they do not have to be answered with equal speed. Take time to consider your answer and how it might affect the question behind the question.

There are certain cross-examination techniques of which one should be aware. The defense lawyer may pose a question in a yes-or-no format. However, some questions cannot be answered yes or no, they require some qualification or modification. Thus, the witness should attempt to make this known by saying, "I cannot answer that 'yes' or 'no' " or "Yes, but with the following reservation." There will be times that modification will not be allowed and the judge will instruct the witness to answer with "yes" or "no." Nonetheless, in protesting you have let the judge and jury know your reservations. There are some questions that will be asked that you simply cannot answer. All questions need not be answered. The expert should feel free to say, "I do not know" or "That is outside my area." The lawyer may ask a very complex multifaceted question that is so convoluted that the point is lost. For this type of question or for any question that you do not understand, ask for the question to be repeated.

Whenever you hear the phrase, "In other words . . . ," be very cautious. These words signal that the attorney has taken your words and is about to modify them slightly. In that slight modification the essence of what you have said may be turned completely opposite to your intent. Thus, at the utterance of that phrase, keep your ears open and be sure that you are being paraphrased correctly.

An expert witness is allowed to be given a hypothetical situation. This may be used by the defense counsel to make the expert appear as a biased reporter. In the hypothetical case, circumstances will be presented that parallel the real matter before the court with some important exceptions. For example, the problem is an abused child with a large area of vaginal laceration and positive examination findings for the presence of seminal fluid. The question asked is, "Doctor, is it not true that little girls who fall on the crossbar of their bicycle will sustain a vaginal laceration?" The answer to this must be "yes." The inexperienced witness can easily be infuriated that an analogy is being drawn. Some will fail to admit to situations that any layman knows as possibilities. Thus, the defense will show the expert in an unflattering light. Always recall that the entire case does not rest on your shoulders. The expert is there as a friend of the court to present information and expert interpretation of that information.

A final area that may be used to cross-examine the expert is the written charts and notes. The defense may wish to know why something was written or why another detail was omitted. The answer here is that the interactions we have with patients and their parents are very complex. Even the most meticulous note taker cannot include every detail. Thus, some items will be omitted, others will be weighed disproportionately, and others will be indicated appropriately. Undergoing this part of the cross-examination gives the expert resolve to become more exacting in the use of the medical record. Good record keeping is a skill that is vital to the entire medical-legal process. Its importance cannot be stressed too heavily.

CONFLICTS WITHIN THE SYSTEM

The court system contains many conflicts. There are many problems and dilemmas that the physician must face when entering the foreign territory of the courthouse. These problems go beyond the fact that in court there are foreign policies and procedures and a different technical language is spoken. There are many procedural problems that make delays and continuances a common problem. In many areas the courts are so backlogged that cases do not come up for weeks or months.

Perhaps the most important conflict is the fact that the court system has been established to determine right and wrong, guilt and innocence. The matters that we bring to court can often not be resolved in these terms. Which parent should have custody of a child is not a matter of right or wrong. Thus, sometimes the system does not fit the purpose for which we are applying it. The heart of the system is an adversarial system that we are trying to apply to a family in which there is often already too much conflict. There are many situations in which the court process widens the distances between family members rather than bring the family to a solution.

Many of the concepts with which we are working (child abuse, neglect, child custody, to name a few) are concepts in transition. What child abuse is today is not what it was 500 years ago or even 50 years ago. In the future we will have even different concepts. This leaves room for differences between what the court believes is abuse, what the expert considers abuse, and what the family would label as abusive. With conflicts, even in our definitions, it is not surprising that conflict ripples through the system. Conflict can lead to frustration and frustration to avoidance. If we avoid our responsibilities as child advocates, who will assume them?

BIBLIOGRAPHY

Bell C, Mlyniec WJ: Preparing for a neglect proceeding: A guide for the social worker. *Public Welfare*, Fall, 1974.

Brent RL: The irresponsible expert witness: A failure of biomedical graduate education and professional accountability. *Pediatrics* 1982; 70:754–762.

Caffey J: On the theory and practice of shaking infants. *Am J Dis Child* 1972; 124:161.

Derdeyn AP: Child abuse and neglect: The rights of parents and the needs of children. *Am J Orthopsych* 1977; 47:377–387.

Kempe HC, Helfer RE: *Child Abuse and Neglect. The Family and the Community*. Cambridge, Mass, Ballinger Publishing Co, 1976.

Ludwig S, Heiser A, Cullen TR, et al: You are subpoenaed. *Clin Proc Childrens Hosp Natl Med Center* 1974; 30:133–147.

Torrey S, Ludwig S: Emergency physician's role in the courtroom. *Pediatr Emerg Care* 1987; 3:50–53.

Wilkerson AE (ed): *Rights of Children*. Philadelphia, Temple University Press, 1974.

53 THE CROSSED EYE

Graham Quinn, M.D.

Strabismus, a general term for describing eyes that are not parallel, is apparent in approximately 2% of children, and twice that number of children may have latent eye muscle imbalances. The recognition of eye muscle problems is often the responsibility of the primary care physician, while classification and treatment depends on the ophthalmologist. This chapter will deal with the basic types of strabismus seen in the pediatric age groups and how to screen for these problems in the outpatient office practice.

If there is a possibility of strabismus, the primary care physician can examine the child initially in the office to see if a referral should be made. Depending on the interest and expertise in using the tests to be described, the examiner can make an informed judgment concerning the presence or absence of strabismus and characterization of the problem. Further evaluation and treatment of the condition should be carried out by the ophthalmologist who has the necessary equipment to conduct a full eye examination and the experience in treating these problems in children.

BACKGROUND

Fundamental to a discussion of binocular function is an assessment of the visual acuity in each eye and the presence or absence of amblyopia. Amblyopia or poorer vision in one eye when compared with that of the other eye has many causes, including strabismus, anisometropia (difference in refractive error between the two eyes), and structural ocular abnormalities such as macular scars and cataracts. Since many 2-year-old and 3-year-old children are able to read a simple chart like the HOTV or E-game with a little review and encouragement, it is frequently possible to document vision acuity objectively in this age group. In the examination of the preverbal (or more likely precooperative) child, one may simply have to observe the child's reaction to occlusion with the examiner's thumb or an eye patch to see if there is objection or a marked change in behavior when each eye is covered individually. Be suspicious of ambylopia of the uncovered eye if different behavioral changes are noted with occlusion.

TYPES OF STRABISMUS

Disturbances of fine sensory and motor forces may cause strabismus to be either manifest or latent. The manifest deviation is always present and observable. There is no need for the observer to bring the deviation out with manipulation of the eye or by altering the use of two eyes together. Such deviation is called heterotropia. The prefix *hetero* may be deleted in favor of a prefix that has directional value and more accurately describes the deviation, for example, *eso*tropia (in-turning), *exo*tropia (out-turning), or *hyper*tropia (one eye higher).

Phoria, on the other hand, is exhibited only when fusional mechanisms have been disrupted. This type of deviation usually remains latent in normal visual functioning, but may cause symptoms of eye fatigue or blurring when the patient "breaks down" from a latent to manifest deviation.

In-turning of the eyes is called esotropia if it is constant and esophoria if fusion must be broken to demonstrate it. Exotropia and exophoria refer to out-drifting of one eye with respect to the other eye in a similar manner. The prefixes, *hypo* and *hyper* refer to one eye being on a different vertical plane from the other; for example, left hypertropia means that the vertical alignment of the left eye is higher than that of the right eye.

One last set of terms is necessary to accurately define strabismus: comitant and noncomitant. A deviation is comitant when the amount of the deviation is the same in all directions of gaze. For example, a patient who has sixth nerve palsy cannot have comitant strabismus, because he or she is unable to fully abduct the affected eye, and therefore has noncomitant strabismus.

Strabismus may be constant or intermittent, congenital or acquired, and an effort should be made to determine which category the condition fits, since therapy, prognosis, and outcome depend on these variables.

DATA GATHERING

Several basic tests for screening for suspected strabismus are available. In all of these tests, the examiner must be confident that the child is fixating on the target and has useful vision in each eye.

To understand if a patient has "straight" eyes, it is essential to know what the child is focusing on at any given moment. One must use an object of sufficient interest to the child to be able to control where he or she is looking and how much accommodation or focusing power the child is using. For this reason, the best circumstance for screening strabismus is to have the child focus on a letter or target some distance away (preferably infinity). Realistically in the young age group, controlling near-fixation with a small puppet or toy that is sufficiently interesting is adequate for most purposes.

The Hirschberg test or corneal light reflex test is done by holding a small light source about 33 cm directly in front of the patient. By noting where the light reflex is on each cornea, one may get a rough measurement of the degree of strabismus. The light reflex is normally in mirror-image position from one eye to the other (Fig 53–1), and each millimeter of horizontal or vertical disparity corresponds to 7 degrees of squint. An in-turned (esotropic) eye will usually demonstrate a light reflex that is displaced temporally from the center of the pupil, and the out-turned eye (exotropic) will have a nasally displaced light reflex.

A more accurate way of assessing alignment is the cover-uncover test (Fig 53–2), which demonstrates the presence or absence of tropia of any type. The child with heterotropia has one eye that is not aligned with the object of interest and, when one covers the fixating eye, the deviating eye will move to take up fixation.

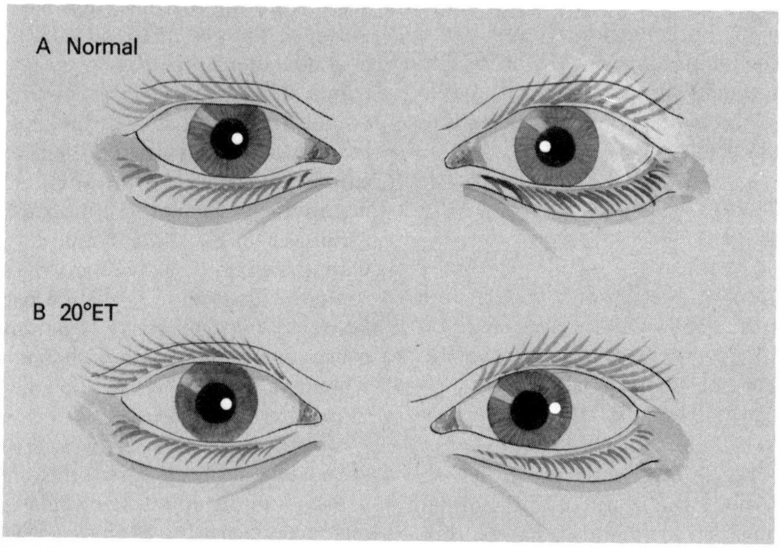

FIG 53–1
Hirschberg or corneal light reflex test. **A,** normal light reflex. **B,** light reflex demonstrating 20° esotropia.

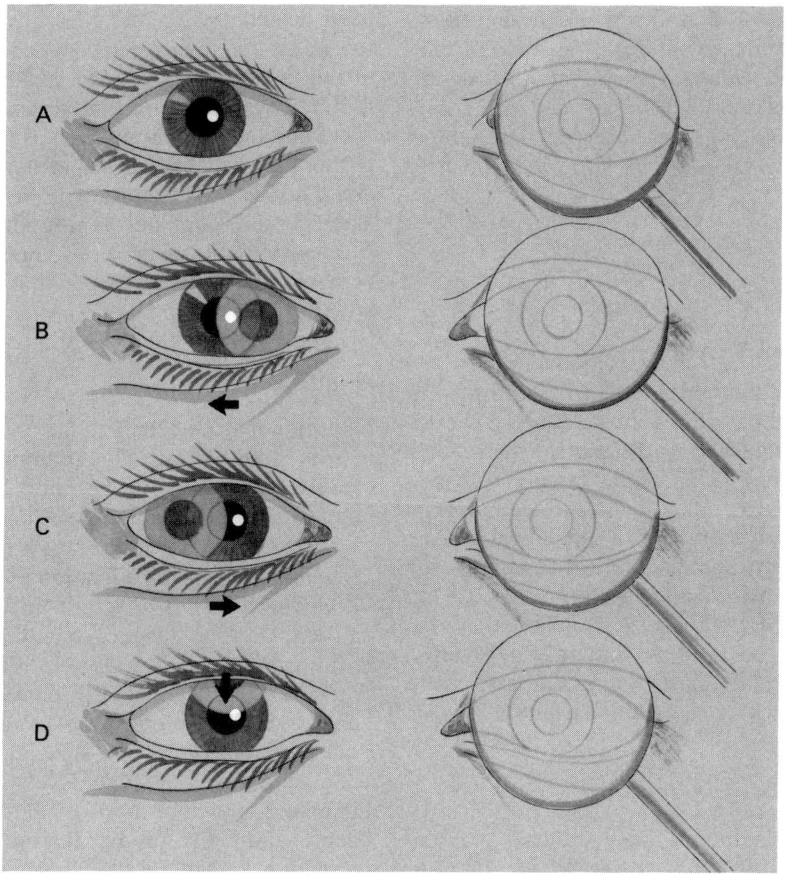

FIG 53–2

Cover-uncover test. **A,** left eye covered elicits no movement of right eye. **B,** left eye covered elicits outward movement of right eye, suggesting esotropia. **C,** left eye covered elicits inward movement of right eye, demonstrating an exotropia. **D,** left eye covered gives downward motion; right hypertropia is present.

Each eye must be covered in turn because the examiner may not know which is the fixing eye initially.

First, cover the right eye and observe for a fixation movement in the left eye. Remove the cover and after a few seconds move to cover the left eye and observe the right. If no movement occurs, there is no tropia; if movement is noted, the direction of the movement should be noted and the diagnosis of heterotropia made (Fig 53–2). Outward movement of the eye as it takes up fixation suggests esotropia; inward movement, exotropia; and upward movement, hypotropia.

The alternate cover test demonstrates phorias and tropias. As in the cover-uncover test, each eye must be tested in turn, but here the cover is quickly moved to occlude the other eye. Fusional mechanisms (coordinated binocular function) are thereby disrupted. The examiner covers one eye and then rapidly moves the cover to the other eye. If no movement is noted, then no tropia or phoria has been demonstrated. If movement is noted, then a phoria, tropia, or both have been elicited. Based on the outcome of the cover-uncover test, the examiner knows the presence of tropia and then can interpret the results of the alternate cover test.

The ophthalmologist will quantitate the degree of misalignment by using the same tests while introducing prisms of increasing strength to change the angle of incident light to one eye.

A funduscopic examination is an integral part of any evaluation for strabismus. Cataracts, corneal clouding, and chorioretinal abnormalities from trauma, infection, or congenital malformation, as well as life-threatening conditions such as retinoblastoma, may present as strabismus and may be observed first with a careful funduscopic examination by a primary care physician.

MANAGEMENT

PSEUDOSTRABISMUS

Pseudostrabismus, or false impression of esotropia related to facial configuration of the infant, is sometimes very difficult to distinguish from true esotropia. A broad, flattened bridge of the nose and prominent epicanthal folds can make the most experienced examiner hesitate on examination, and many of these families can be reassured by a demonstration of the Hirschberg corneal light reflex test. When there remains a question, the child should be referred to an ophthalmologist for examination and care.

ESOTROPIA

Esotropia in infants or older children is abnormal. Constant esotropia in early infancy must be differentiated from bilateral sixth nerve palsy or extraocular muscle abnormalities. Once other ocular and systemic pathologic conditions are ruled out, the child may be said to have a congenital esotropia, and unless the child has proper visual alignment prior to 2 years of age, he or she has little chance of ever acquiring binocular capabilities. As more than one surgical procedure or other therapy may be necessary to align the eyes, the child should be referred as early as possible to allow for properly paced therapy. Most ophthalmologists suggest performing surgery as early as the angle of the strabismus is reproducible and the infant can safely tolerate a surgical procedure, usually at 4 to 6 months of age.

Esotropia in the child from 1 to 7 years of age can be quite different in presentation from infantile esotropia and is usually related to a focusing imbalance caused by either hyperopia or abnormal accommodative powers. Regardless of the cause, the fusional mechanisms that allow the child to keep the eyes straight have been overcome and the child turns the eyes in too much for the object distance. The amount of the in-turning is variable. After referral, the child will most likely receive some sort of antiaccommodative therapy, such as glasses for hyperopia or certain drugs that help control accommodation. The child with esotropia is at significant risk for developing amblyopia, and if untreated will usually develop an unvarying component to the esotropia that does not respond to antiaccommodative therapy.

EXOTROPIA

Exotropia may be constant, latent, or most commonly, intermittent. The intermittent type is usually seen in a child between 1 and 4 years of age and is noticeable when the child is daydreaming, recently ill, or very fatigued. It is most noted at distance fixation at first, and can be very difficult to diagnose in the office because obtaining distance fixation in a young child is difficult. Suspect intermittent exotropia when the child constantly closes one eye in sunlight or the parent gives a vague history of poor eye contact and eye muscle problems.

Constant exotropia is relatively uncommon at birth, and sufficient numbers of cases have not been examined to predict the optimal time for correction. In general, the ophthalmologist seeing a child with congenital exotropia will approach the problem in a manner similar to that used for the patient with infantile esotropia. In older children, constant exotropia is usually acquired or, more rarely, a sequel to untreated intermittent exotropia. Treatment belongs in the hands of an ophthalmologist.

OTHER TYPES OF STRABISMUS

Vertical deviations often present with an abnormal head posture, and a child with a consistent head tilt or chin position without obvious skeletal or neck muscle abnormalities should be examined for a vertical eye muscle problem. The most common problem is a fourth nerve palsy, which manifests as a head tilt to the opposite side from the affected muscle. Other noncomitant strabismus problems that may present in the office include A and V patterns, oblique muscle problems, muscle palsies, and certain developmental defects such as Duane's syndrome and Möbius' syndrome. These problems require a complete ophthalmologic examination for documentation and should be referred for evaluation.

BIBLIOGRAPHY

Ehrlick MI, Reinecke RD, Simons K: Preschool vision screening for amblyopia and strabismus: Programs, methods, guidelines, 1983. *Surv Ophthalmol* 1983; 3:145–163.

Friendly DS: Preschool visual acuity screening tests. *Trans Am Ophthalmol Soc* 1978; 76:383–480.

Ing MR: Early surgical alignment for congenital esotropia. *Ophthalmol* 1983; 90:132–135.

Moody E, Gibson G: Ophthalmic examination of infants and children, in Harley RD (ed): *Pediatric Ophthalmology.* Philadelphia, WB Saunders, 1975; pp 59–85.

Parks MM: *Ocular Motility and Strabismus.* New York, Harper & Row, 1975, Chapters 2, 5, 6, 7, 10, 12, 13.

Schaffer DB: *Disorders of Ocular Motility in Practice of Pediatrics,* vol 4. New York, Harper & Row, 1977, Chapter 57.

von Norden GK, Maumenee AE: *Atlas of Strabismus,* ed 2. St Louis, CV Mosby, 1973.

54 CYSTIC FIBROSIS

Thomas F. Scanlin, M.D.

Cystic fibrosis (CF), the most common lethal inherited disease in white populations, has an incidence of 1 in 2,000 live births. One in 20 persons is a carrier of the CF gene. Cystic fibrosis does occur in blacks, although the incidence is significantly less among blacks in this country. Most homozygotes for the disease have the "classic triad" of clinical findings: (1) chronic pulmonary disease, (2) malabsorption secondary to pancreatic insufficiency, and (3) elevated concentration of sweat electrolytes. Although there is a great variability in the severity and the clinical course of the disease, the course of CF is generally a chronic progression of the pulmonary disease.

Many more CF patients are now surviving to adulthood; the mean age of survival in the United States is now approximately 25 years. More effective antibiotics, earlier diagnosis, comprehensive care in CF centers, and aggressive treatment of complications contribute to this improved survival time. The goal of this chapter is to provide guidelines for the practitioner in the treatment of patients with CF. The discussion of this treatment will necessarily be rather brief; however, the reader is referred to several excellent and comprehensive reviews for further details. The primary care practitioner is also encouraged to form a close working relationship with a CF center and to freely use the CF center for consultation on the management of this complicated chronic disease.

DIAGNOSIS

The diagnosis should be considered in children who present with a variety of acute and chronic problems listed below:

COMMON SIGNS AND SYMPTOMS OF CF

Neonates
Meconium ileus
Prolonged obstructive jaundice
Infants and children
Persistent cough
Recurrent pneumonia, bronchitis, or wheezing
Failure to thrive

Frequent, bulky stools
Rectal prolapse
Intussusception
Edema, anemia, and hypoprothrombinemia
Hepatomegaly
Nasal polyps
Heat intolerance
Metabolic alkalosis

Failure to thrive and a history of chronic respiratory or gastrointestinal symptoms is a fairly typical presentation of CF. The respiratory symptoms may vary from a mild but persistent cough to recurrent pneumonia and atelectasis. Expiratory rhonchi and low-pitched wheezes are sometimes found on auscultation of the chest in CF patients. The atypical asthmatic who has digital clubbing, bronchiectasis, or a cough productive of purulent sputum may also have CF.

Frequent passage of pale, bulky, loose, and excessively foul-smelling stools is characteristic of CF. Patients with this presentation are often misdiagnosed as having chronic diarrhea or milk allergy and are treated with repeated formula changes. Other intestinal problems include rectal prolapse and intussusception or volvulus.

CF should also be considered in cases of dehydration in warm weather, especially if diarrhea alone cannot account for the dehydration or if a metabolic alkalosis occurs. In a typical case, anorexia followed by lethargy are the predominant symptoms. The electrolytes usually show a slight hyponatremia with a profound hypochloremia. Examples of the electrolyte abnormalities that were seen in two infants are shown in Table 54–1.

The cornerstone of the diagnosis of CF is a carefully performed sweat test. The sweat test should be done by the quantitative pilocarpine iontophoresis method. If there is not an accredited CF center nearby where the sweat test can be done, then the patient should be sent to the laboratory that has the most experience with this quantitative method. Sweat tests done by other methods are not reliable since they produce too many false-positive and false-negative results. All siblings of CF patients should have a sweat test performed. First cousins of CF patients should have sweat tests if they have any symptoms that could possibly be due to CF.

Although the basic defect in CF has not yet been elucidated, important advances in molecular genetics have recently localized the CF gene to the long arm of chromosome 7. By using DNA probes that are linked to the CF locus, it is now possible to perform accurate prenatal diagnosis of CF for families in which there is an affected child with CF. Since the CF gene has been defined, prenatal diagnosis and carrier detection will soon be available to the general population.

CF is a complex and varied disease and a number of presentations that are less common than those listed earlier have been described. These are described in the general references and will not be discussed. The symptoms of CF may remain mild for many years, and the diagnosis of CF should not be excluded because "the child looks too good to have CF."

At the time of diagnosis, each patient should have a thorough evaluation to assess the functions of the lungs, pancreas, and liver as well as a careful assessment of nutritional and developmental status. Often this is best accomplished in the hospital setting. Hospitalization also provides a good opportunity to monitor the response of the patient to each component of the therapeutic regimen and to counsel the entire family on the diagnosis, prognosis, and treatment of CF.

TABLE 54–1
Electrolyte Abnormalities in Two Infants With Cystic Fibrosis*

		Electrolytes				
Patient	Age (mo)	Na	K	Cl	CO_2	Serum pH
1	9	123	2.2	49	48	7.60
2	6	125	2.4	55	41	7.63

*From Scanlin TF: Cystic fibrosis, in Fleisher G, Ludwig S (eds): *Textbook of Pediatric Emergency Medicine*, Baltimore, Williams & Wilkins, 1988. Used with permission.

APPROACH TO GENERAL MANAGEMENT

NUTRITION

The following aspects of nutritional care will be considered: salt replacement, vitamin supplementation, diet, enzymes, and nutritional supplementation.

Because of the defect in the reabsorption of sodium and chloride by the sweat glands in CF, patients with CF are at risk for the development of salt depletion during febrile episodes and periods of warm weather. For these reasons, patients with CF must have a continuous salt replacement program established. Because of recent changes in guidelines and recommendations, many infant formulas and infant foods have less salt than they did a few years ago; therefore the salt replacement program must be established in infancy. Since infants may need an extra gram of salt each day, this can be done by adding approximately one quarter teaspoon of salt to the infant formula over the course of the day, usually by adding a pinch to each feeding. When vegetables are introduced to this diet they should be salted. Older children are encouraged to salt their food liberally and salty snacks are encouraged.

As a minimum, CF patients should take a double or twice daily dose of a standard multivitamin preparation to ensure an adequate absorption and maintenance of adequate levels of vitamins. During the first year of life, infants should receive a supplement of vitamin K, 1.25 mg twice weekly. After the first year of life, supplementation is usually only necessary for patients with known liver involvement or those receiving continuous antibiotics. The need for vitamin K supplementation is guided by prothrombin time determination. Because many CF patients have low serum tocopherol levels despite taking multivitamins, vitamin E supplementation is recommended. However, exact requirements and recommended dosages have not been well established.

The concept has emerged in recent years that patients with CF need more than 100% of the recommended daily allowance of calories. The older notion that patients with CF all had voracious appetites has not been borne out by clinical experience. Although some centers have recommended severe fat reduction and/or a special elemental diet, our experience is that good growth can be achieved with an adequate intake of a well-balanced diet and enzyme supplementation for those patients in need of pancreatic enzymes. Many infants with CF will do well on a standard cow's milk formula or breast milk if they receive supplementation with pancreatic enzymes. Soybean formulas are generally not recommended for CF patients because of the increased risk for developing hypoproteinemia and anemia. Some infants who have had an episode of severe failure to thrive or who have had meconium ileus and subsequent surgery will require an elemental formula such as Pregestimil for at least several months. All patients with CF will benefit from frequent evaluation for nutritional assessment by an experienced nutritionist. Newly diagnosed patients with CF and their parents should have a complete nutritional assessment and have a nutritional program outlined that will enable them to achieve the necessary caloric intake in a well-balanced diet to ensure adequate growth and nutrition.

The development of an enteric-coated pancreatic enzyme preparation in the past few years has been a major advance in the therapy of CF. These specially coated preparations (Pancrease or Cotazym S) have allowed CF patients to achieve better absorption and to reduce the symptoms and the complications of malabsorption while taking a much lower total amount of pancreatic extract. For infants and children who cannot swallow the whole capsules, the microspheres may be given in a small amount of applesauce immediately before or during the meal. Besides being more effective at a lower dose, the newer preparations have eliminated some of the other problems that occur from using the powder preparations, such as irritated mucosal surfaces and respiratory allergy from inhaling the powder preparations. The goal of therapy should be to ensure adequate absorption for growth while reducing bowel symptoms. Fat restriction is only recommended if a patient is required to take an excessively high dose of enzymes and still has bulky stools.

Although the general nutritional program outlined above works well for most patients with CF, there may be several categories of patients who will have nutritional problems despite such a program, and these patients may require special supplementation measures. One such patient is the infant with meconium ileus who has undergone a resection of a significant portion of the small or large bowel. Intravenous hyperalimentation for several weeks postoperatively has resulted in a good outcome for many of these patients. A special formula such as Pregestimil and a pancreatic enzyme preparation can be introduced slowly while the patient is receiving intravenous hyperalimentation. Patients who have severe failure to thrive prior to diagnosis may require additional supplementation. Some centers have recorded success with either continuous or intermittent nasal gastric tube feedings at night. An advantage to the nasal gastric tube feedings at night is that the patient can continue to eat regular meals during the day and use a formula such as Vivonex, which does not require enzyme supplementation. Some older patients with moderately severe lung disease also reach a point at which there is either no weight gain or weight loss over a period of many months, despite what appears to be adequate nutritional therapy. If there is no response, even after treating the pulmonary disease, aggressive nutritional supplementation either by gastrostomy or by nasal gastric tube feedings may be of benefit to these patients.

PULMONARY THERAPY AND ANTIBIOTICS

Most patients with CF have some degree of small airway abnormality, although the degree of severity of the small airway disease may vary greatly from patient to patient. Two factors, mucus viscosity and infection, are most important. The respiratory tract mucus in CF is more viscous because of abnormal physiochemical properties, and this mucus is responsible for the airway obstruction, whether it is complete or partial, focal or diffuse. This thickened mucus results in either hyperinflation or atelectasis of lung segments distal to either a partial or a complete obstruction of the airway (Fig 54–1). Chronic recurrent pulmonary infection also contributes to airway disease. The respiratory tract in CF is commonly colonized with bacterial pathogens. Early in the course of the disease, *Staphylococcus aureus* and later *Pseudomonas aeruginosa* are the most characteristic organisms in CF but other gram-negative bacteria may also be found, such as *Klebsiella, Hemophilus influenzae,* and *Escherichia coli.* The combination of obstruction with thickened mucus and colonization and infection with bacterial pathogens produces a gradual destruction of airways resulting in both diffuse and focal bronchiectasis.

Therapy for the lung disease in CF is designed to clear the obstructing mucus from the airways and to treat the bacterial infection. An important part of the therapy of CF is chest physiotherapy or percussion and postural drainage, which is aimed at clearing these thickened mucus secretions from the lungs. Although adequate controlled studies to determine the optimum regimen of physiotherapy for either prophylaxis or therapy have not been done, most CF centers use physiotherapy as the cornerstone of their pulmonary therapy. If it is to be effective, it is important that the parents, caregivers, or other family members are carefully trained in the technique and that they administer it conscientiously and thoroughly. We generally recommend that most patients who are diagnosed as having CF begin a twice-daily chest physiotherapy treatment in early morning and evening. During exacerbations of pulmonary symptoms we usually recommend that an additional treatment be given each day, and often for exacerbations we recommend that an intermittent aerosol be used prior to the percussion and postural drainage, although these are not generally prescribed for regular use. Chest physiotherapy is a difficult and time-consuming treatment. Periodic assessment of technique is helpful because the therapy needs to be modified as the patient grows. Since parents and patients often have difficulty complying with this therapy, the review of procedures serves to reinforce and support the parents in administering this home therapy.

Many CF centers now use an intermittent aerosol therapy as part of their therapy for the pulmonary disease in CF. While some of the intermittent aerosol therapy seems to provide a clear benefit for many patients, controlled studies to provide exact guidelines as to which agent should be used and whether the treatment should be prophylactic or therapeutic, continuous or intermittent, are not available. Although it was a common practice a decade ago, very few CF centers now prescribe nocturnal mist tent therapy for their CF patients. We recommend that a dilute 5% solution of N-ace-

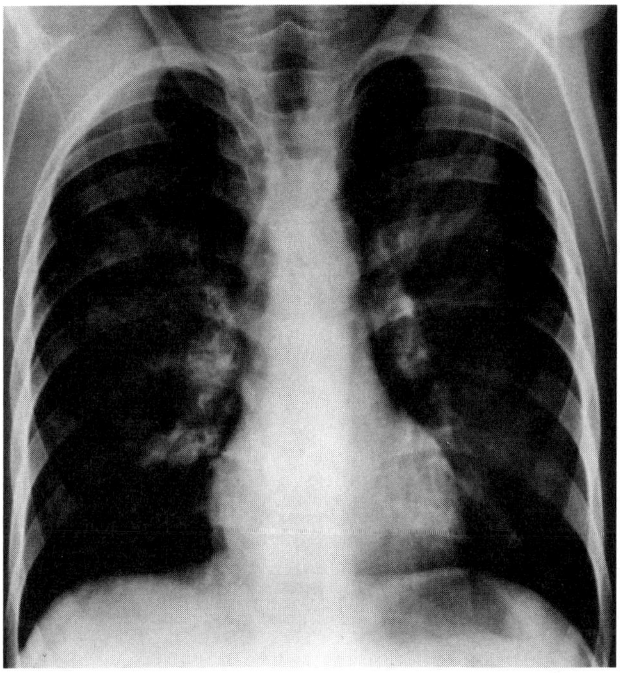

FIG 54–1
Chest radiograph of patient with CF demonstrating hyperaeration, increased bronchial markings, and nodular cystic densities.

tylcysteine be given by nebulizer prior to percussion and postural drainage in those patients who have copious, thickened pulmonary secretions or only during periods of exacerbation of pulmonary symptoms. Most cases of bronchial irritation occur when a 20% solution is used. We have found very few side effects and reasonable efficacy using a 10% solution diluted 1:1 in saline solution, resulting in a 5% solution. Although many centers routinely use bronchodilators for patients with CF, some patients with CF do not need bronchodilators and some may even have adverse reactions to them. We therefore evaluate the need for bronchodilators on an individual basis, and patients who have reversible bronchospasm are treated with either oral or inhaled bronchodilators using guidelines that are established for the therapy of asthma.

Corticosteroids have been used with good results in infants with severe obstructive airway disease that does not respond to antibiotics and bronchodilators, and in patients with CF in whom the pulmonary disease is complicated by either severe asthma or allergic bronchopulmonary aspergillosis. Preliminary observations suggest that patients with CF may benefit from the long-term administration of corticosteroids on alternate days. The presumed effect of the corticosteroids is decreased inflammatory response of the airways; this treatment regimen is currently being evaluated in a multicenter trial.

The development of newer and more effective antibiotics has resulted in a marked improvement in survival of CF patients and a decrease in pulmonary morbidity. However, once again, controlled studies on the most effective antibiotic regimens, whether continuous or intermittent, have not been established. Our general approach is to treat with antibiotics during exacerbations of pulmonary symptoms, that is, when patients show an increased cough, an increased amount of purulent sputum, when there are new or increased rales on chest auscultation or when respiratory rate and effort increase. The decision of which antibiotic to use is guided by the results of sputum culture.

Even in young infants, some useful information can be obtained by culture of sputum obtained by a cough swab. In patients who have *S. aureus* colonization and in whom symptoms are not too severe, treatment with an oral antistaphylococcal penicillin and an increase in the chest physiotherapy and intermittent aerosol use at home are usually adequate to treat an exacerbation. Cephalosporins are useful antibiotics for both *Staphylococcus* organisms and some of the gram-negative organisms. Trimethoprim-sulfamethoxazole combination is used if *H. influenzae* is cultured or in combination with cephalosporin (Keflex) if *Staphylococcus* plus a gram-negative organism is present.

The choices are more difficult when *P. aeruginosa* or other species are cultured in the sputum and the patient is having increased symptoms. There are no effective oral antibiotics for *Pseudomonas*. For some patients, chloramphenicol may be useful as some percentage of the *Pseudomonas* strains are sensitive to it. Many centers will use trimethoprim-sulfamethoxazole for long-term or suppressive therapy in patients who have *Pseudomonas* in their sputum. However, patients who are showing an increase in symptoms who are not responsive to oral antibiotics and who are culture-positive for *Pseudomonas* will probably have to be treated with intravenous antibiotics. The preferred regimen is a combination of an aminoglycoside and a semisynthetic penicillin such as gentamicin and carbenicillin or tobramycin and ticarcillin given for 10 to 14 days. Longer courses of antibiotics (i.e., 2 to 4 weeks in duration) are occasionally necessary for the CF patient with severe pulmonary involvement.

The decisions regarding the initiation and duration of intravenous antibiotic therapy are often best guided by pulmonary function testing when serial data on pulmonary performance can be used to document deterioration and improvement in pulmonary function.

Recent reports from several large centers have indicated an increasing incidence and prevalence of infections with *P. cepacia* in CF patients. Most of these organisms are highly resistant. Many CF patients will improve after treatment with a combination of antibiotics, which includes newer drugs such as piperacillin or ceftazidime.

PSYCHOSOCIAL SUPPORT

Skilled psychosocial support for the patients and families of those affected by this chronic and ultimately fatal disease are required. Psychosocial support should be started while the diagnosis of CF is being made and should continue throughout the course of the patient's lifetime. At the time of diagnosis, the facts concerning CF should be explained thoroughly to the patient and parents of the newly diagnosed patient. These conferences are best conducted in several long sessions separated by an interval of several days so that the patients and family have time to ask questions concerning what they have previously been told and to clarify any misconceptions they may have. This sequence also provides an initial opportunity for the physician and social worker to assess how the family is beginning to cope with the diagnosis of CF. As soon as the diagnosis of CF is confirmed, it is important that the family be educated in the details, techniques, and rationale of the care regimen for CF. This is best accomplished in individual sessions with skilled health care professionals from medicine, nursing, physical therapy, nutrition, and respiratory therapy departments. While the seriousness of the diagnosis of CF cannot be ignored in these educational sessions, it is important to emphasize that the average survival of patients with CF has improved dramatically over the last two to three decades because of the effective care regimen that has been developed during this time. The combination of a thorough educational program along with the facts concerning the improved survival of patients with CF and the ever more realistic hope that basic research may provide better answers for patients with CF provide the patient and the family with a realistically optimistic attitude and a positive approach to living with CF.

We encourage all patients and families to provide a conscientious home care regimen for the CF patient but to otherwise encourage the child to live an unrestricted and active life. We encourage the parents to plan for their child to participate in all the activities of his peers. A skilled and experienced team of CF care providers can help the family and provide support by anticipating some of the common problems that CF may create as the child progresses through normal developmental stages and moves through the different stages of the educational process. The patient and the family should be given guidance and assistance in answering questions and explaining the diagnosis of CF to friends and family. We recommend that all the relatives be informed of the diagnosis of CF because of its autosomal recessive pattern of inheritance. And we encourage patients and family to inform close friends and those who need to know, such as teachers and school nurses, of the diagnosis of CF. They should also be informed that the patient is being cared for regularly in a CF center and that other than providing the opportunity to take the prescribed medications and treatments, no preferential treatment need be given to the child.

During periods of exacerbations of the disease, patients and parents often become anxious and depressed. It is important to provide a skilled assessment of the patient and family as the disease progresses, and should serious emotional or psychiatric symptoms develop, an appropriate referral should be made for psychiatric care. However, by providing support during periods of exacerbation, a physician, social worker, and experienced CF health care professionals can usually provide the necessary support. Often, when the condition of the patient improves in response to medical therapy, the anxiousness and depression abate considerably, and psychiatric intervention will not be required.

As long as is reasonably possible, we encourage patients and families to set goals and work with the medical team to achieve them. However, where it becomes evident that the patient's pulmonary insufficiency is increasing despite an aggressive medical regimen, the patient and family should be prepared for impending death. The possibility of a fatal outcome and the way in which the patient and family would be most comfortable in facing this must be discussed. Many patients and families prefer to remain in the hospital, even when medical therapy can no longer improve the increasing respiratory failure. However, this does not mean that extreme or heroic measures must be provided for what is obviously progressive and irreversible respiratory failure. Instead, every effort should be made to make the patient and family comfortable and able to face the patient's death in a dignified and humane fashion. Some families and patients will prefer to have the patient at home if oxygen and other therapies to ensure the patient's comfort can be provided. However, support of the CF center team is not withdrawn when the patient is discharged to home. It is extremely helpful if a physician, nurse, and social worker are able to visit the home; to assess the situation, strengths, and support that the family has; and to provide guidance in what to expect and how to cope with the signs and symptoms of terminal respiratory failure. Guidance in how to comfort and support the patient and each other should also be provided to family members.

APPROACH TO SPECIFIC SYMPTOMS AND COMPLICATIONS

RECTAL PROLAPSE

Rectal prolapse occurs most commonly in younger children with CF when pancreatic enzyme therapy has been inadequate. Although the appearance of the first prolapse may be quite frightening, it can usually be easily reduced by placing the infant in a comfortable position and using a lubricated glove for manual reduction. It is extremely unusual that an intussusception will be associated with the prolapse or that there will be a danger of bowel strangulation. Surgery will rarely be needed to correct a recurrent rectal prolapse. By adjusting the patient's intake of fat and matching the fat intake with appropriate pancreatic enzyme dosages, the recurrent prolapse can usually be controlled.

ABDOMINAL PAIN

Patients with CF frequently give a history of either acute or chronic crampy abdominal pain. If the examination of the abdomen is normal, the pain usually can be treated by adjusting the pancreatic enzyme dosage to meet the intake of fat and protein. A careful history will often uncover the fact that the patient is eating significant amounts of food between meals but is taking pancreatic enzymes only with meals.

If the physical examination reveals a tender fecal mass in the right lower quadrant, more aggressive therapy is necessary. In this instance, we recommend that the patient be given a Fleet's enema to clear the rectum. The patient is placed on clear liquids for 24 hours, and mineral oil followed by *N*-acetylcysteine (30 mL in 30 mL of cola) are given orally. This is usually effective in clearing the inspissated fecal material. If there are signs and symptoms of abdominal obstruction either on physical examination or on a radiograph of the abdomen, a barium enema will be necessary. If a nonreducible volvulus or intussusception is seen, emergency surgery is necessary. If only a fecal mass is present without an associated volvulus or intussusception, medical management using Gastrografin (diatrizoate meglumine) and saline enema usually results in dissolution of the impacted feces. Pressure other than hydrostatic should not be used to instill the Gastrografin. External pressure to the abdomen is also contraindicated. These procedures should be done in consultation with surgeons so that they may be prepared to intervene.

HEAT INTOLERANCE

Patients with CF have high concentrations of sodium and chloride in their sweat. They are at risk to develop vascular collapse during periods of hot weather when the amount of sweating increases. We recommend that patients salt their food liberally, take salty snacks, and drink liquids such as Coca-Cola and Pepsi Cola, which contain electrolytes, during periods of warm weather. However, during an intercurrent illness in a period of warm weather, symptoms such as an abrupt decrease in oral intake may be followed by lethargy. In this situation, patients may become dehydrated rapidly and may have serum electrolytes similar to those shown for the two patients in Table 54–1. For such patients, prompt fluid replacement with isotonic saline is critical; 20 to 30 mL/kg should be given within 15 minutes if there are signs of shock or within 1 hour in less severely ill patients. Potassium chloride should be administered as soon as urine output is established. Frequent determinations of serum electrolyte levels will be necessary to guide further therapy until fluid and electrolyte correction has been completed.

PULMONARY EXACERBATION

Patients with CF may have an increase in respiratory symptoms such as cough and in the rate and effort of breathing shortly after the onset of a mild upper respiratory tract infection. These patients require careful evaluation. A chest radiograph should be obtained to determine if pneumothorax or local consolidation or atelectasis are present. However, in many cases the radiograph will show only diffuse peribronchial thickening with a varying amount of fluffy infiltrates and hyperinflation. It is most helpful in assessing the degree of acute change in the symptoms and radiograph if comparison can be made in consultation with medical personnel who are familiar with the patient's previous course. Establishment of the network of CF centers by the Cystic Fibrosis Foundation for the comprehensive care of CF patients has helped to ensure that such information will be available even on an emergency basis.

If such guidance is not available and if lobar atelectasis, significant respiratory distress, or hypoxia is present, the patient should be treated in a hospital setting with vigorous chest physiotherapy and antibiotics effective against *S. aureus* and *P. aeruginosa* (until the results of sputum culture are available). Oxygen therapy should be guided by arterial blood gas determination.

PNEUMOTHORAX

Pneumothorax is being reported with increasing frequency in older CF patients. It usually presents as the sudden onset of chest pain often referred to the shoulder and sometimes is associated with the acute onset of dyspnea and cyanosis. It is most important to realize that recurrences are very common in CF patients. Therefore, after the pneumothorax has been treated by tube thoracostomy by an experienced surgeon or chest physician, some attempt should be made to use either chemical sclerosis (e.g., with a high concentration of tetracycline) or open thoracostomy and pleural abrasion to prevent further recurrences.

HEMOPTYSIS

For many patients with CF, a small amount of blood streaking in the sputum is a fairly common occurrence. Although the first such episode may be very alarming to the patient and parents, there is no need for a major change in the patient's usual home care regimen other than considering an appropriate course of antibiotic therapy to treat any intercurrent pulmonary infection. Significant hemoptysis (arbitrarily defined as the expectoration of at least 30 to 60 mL of fresh blood) should be treated in the hospital setting. The proposed mechanism is the erosion of an area of local bronchial infection into a bronchial vessel. If the bleeding persists or increases after hospitalization, vitamin K (5 mg initially) and antibiotics should be administered. The patient's blood type should be determined in the event that transfusion is necessary. Some patients with CF occasionally present with an episode of massive hemoptysis with volumes of blood loss ranging from 300 mL to 2,500 mL. Massive hemoptysis is a life-threatening situation and in addition to instituting the measures described above, the intervention of a skilled team including a bronchoscopist, anesthesiologist, and thoracic surgeon may be necessary to maintain an airway and to locate and ligate the bleeding vessel. When an experienced angiographer is available, bronchial artery embolization has been shown to be an effective procedure to treat recurrent or persistent hemoptysis in patients with CF.

RESPIRATORY FAILURE

When a patient presents with respiratory failure (i.e., hypercarbia, Pa_{CO_2} greater than or equal to 55 mm Hg), the management decisions are extremely difficult. If the respiratory failure is complicated by cor pulmonale and if this is the first such episode, the patient may respond well to the regimen described for pulmonary exacerbation with the addition of oxygen and diuretics. However, if the patient does not respond to medical therapy, the management decisions become extremely difficult. Patients with CF in general do not respond as well to mechanical ventilation and have more complications from mechanical ventilation when they are compared to patients with other forms of chronic obstructive pulmonary disease.

If an acute episode, such as viral pneumonia or status asthmaticus, precipitates respiratory failure in a patient who has had a history of good pulmonary function prior to the episode, mechanical ventilation should be considered. There are many factors that must be considered in making this decision; however, objective guidelines are not currently available. One large retrospective study found that a history of prior hypercarbia indicated a poor prognosis. It seems reasonable that good pulmonary function prior to the acute episode provides an opportunity for a good result. However, when mechanical ventilation is used for a patient with CF, a skilled intensive care team must be prepared for a potentially difficult course. When respiratory failure with increasing hypercarbia occurs in a CF patient after a course of progressive pulmonary insufficiency despite adequate medical therapy, mechanical ventilation is not indicated. However, consultation with the physicians providing the chronic care for the patient is important before choosing this course. Some of the factors that must be considered in supporting the family and the patient who is in irreversible respiratory failure are discussed in the previous section on psychosocial support. Members of the family must be educated about signs and symptoms of terminal respiratory failure and also given guidance in how to comfort and support the patient and each other.

Since most patients with CF eventually die of respiratory failure, consideration has been given to the possibility of heart-lung transplantation for these patients. To date, only a few heart-lung transplants have been attempted in patients with CF. In the first attempt in the United States the patient survived for 2 months but died of complications of immune suppression. Recently there have been several apparent successes. However, these procedures will require careful evaluation before a general recommendation can be made for patients with CF.

BIBLIOGRAPHY

Boat TF, Welsh MJ, Beaudet AL: Cystic fibrosis, in Scriver CR, Beaudet AL, Sly WS, et al (eds): *The Metabolic Basis of Inherited Disease*, ed 6. New York, McGraw-Hill Book Co, 1989, pp 2649–2680.

Davis PB (ed): Cystic fibrosis. *Semin Respir Med* 1985; 6:243–333.

Desmond KJ, Schwenk WF, Thomas E, et al: Immediate and long-term effects of chest physiotherapy in patients with cystic fibrosis. *J Pediatr* 1983; 103:538–542.

Fellows K, Khaw KT, Schuster S, et al: Bronchial artery embolization in cystic fibrosis. Technique and long-term results. *J Pediatr* 1979; 95:959–963.

Isles A, Maclusky I, Corey M, et al: *Pseudomonas cepacia* infection in cystic fibrosis. An emerging problem. *J Pediatr* 1984; 104:206–210.

Lloyd-Still JD, (ed): *Textbook of Cystic Fibrosis*. Boston, Wright PSG, 1983.

McLaughlin FJ, Matthews WJ, Strieder DJ, et al: Pneumothorax in cystic fibrosis: Management and outcome. *J Pediatr* 1982; 100:863–869.

Newmark P: Testing for cystic fibrosis. *Nature* 1985; 318:309.

Redding GJ, Restuccia R, Cotton EK, et al: Serial changes in pulmonary functions in children hospitalized with cystic fibrosis. *Am Rev Respir Dis* 1982; 126:31–36.

Ruddy R, Scanlin T: Abnormal sweat electrolytes in a case of celiac disease and a case of psychosocial failure to thrive. Review of other reported causes. *Clin Pediatr* 1987; 26:83–89.

Ruddy R, Anolik R, Scanlin TF: Hypoelectrolytemia as a presentation and complication of cystic fibrosis. *Clin Pediatr* 1982; 21:367–369.

Scanlin TF: Cystic fibrosis, in Fleisher G, Ludwig S (eds): *Textbook of Pediatric Emergency Medicine*, ed 2. Baltimore, Williams & Wilkins, 1988; pp 665–687.

Scanlin TF: Cystic fibrosis, in Fishman AP (ed): *Pulmonary Diseases and Disorders*, ed 2. New York, McGraw-Hill, 1988; pp 1273–1294.

Stern RC, Borkat G, Hirschfeld SS, et al: Heart failure in cystic fibrosis. *Am J Dis Child* 1980; 134:267–272.

Stern RC, Wood RE, Boat TF, et al: Treatment and prognosis of massive hemoptysis in cystic fibrosis. *Am Rev Respir Dis* 1978; 117:825–828.

Taussig LM, (ed): *Cystic Fibrosis*. New York, Theime-Stratton, 1984.

55 DEHYDRATION

Susan B. Torrey, M.D.

A thorough understanding of fluid and electrolyte homeostasis and derangements is important to the practice of medicine. Children are unique both because of differences in physical size and physiology and in the etiology of pathologic states. In addition, infants and children frequently experience illnesses that alter fluid and electrolyte balance. Consequently, in the primary care setting it is important to identify the child at risk and to institute appropriate treatment. For the most part, fluid problems involve volume dehydration and related electrolyte abnormalities. The typical scenario involves a young infant with fever, vomiting, and diarrhea who becomes mildly dehydrated over a period of a few days. This chapter includes a discussion of the normal physiology of fluids and electrolytes in infants and children and provides a description of the pathophysiologic states. Discussion focuses on the office treatment of patients.

BACKGROUND

BASIC FLUID AND ELECTROLYTE REQUIREMENTS

Total body water is estimated as 60% to 70% of body weight. Of this, about two thirds, or 40% to 45% of body weight, is intracellular fluid, and one third, or 20% to 25% of body weight, is extracellular. The extracellular fluid compartment can be further divided into the intravascular space, about one fifth of extracellular fluid, or 4% to 6% of body weight, and the interstitial space, about four fifths of extracellular fluid, or 16% to 19% of body weight. The electrolyte composition of these compartments is similar in all children regardless of size (Table 55–1).

Adequate treatment of the sick child requires familiarity with maintenance fluid and electrolyte requirements and with the electrolyte composition of body fluids. Maintenance water requirements are calculated in terms of caloric expenditure, because metabolic rate determines both the amount of heat dissipated as insensible loss and the amount of solute that the kid-

TABLE 55–1
Electrolyte Composition of Body Fluid Compartments

COMPARTMENT	CATION (MEQ/L)	ANION
Extracellular fluid	Sodium (144)	Bicarbonate, chloride
Intracellular fluid	Potassium (154)	Phosphate
Intravascular	Sodium (142)	Bicarbonate, chloride, proteins

ney must excrete daily. Thus, for each of the first 10 kg of body weight, 100 calories/kg are required for maintenance of homeostasis, with 50 calories/kg for each of the next 10 kg, and 20 calories/kg for each subsequent kilogram (Table 55–2). This maintenance requirement will increase 12% per degree centigrade (7% per degree Fahrenheit) when the child is febrile. Tachypnea will increase insensible loss and thereby increase maintenance requirements. For example, an 11 kg infant has a maintenance fluid requirement of 1,050 calories/day or mL/day, and a 24 kg child would require 1,580 calories or mL/day. If this 24 kg patient has a body temperature of 40° C, he or she will require an additional 475 mL of maintenance fluid. The electrolyte composition of gastric contents and stool varies over a wide range in both normal and pathologic states. Some of this variation is related to dietary intake, and some to the cause of the pathologic state (Table 55–3). For example, water, sodium, and chloride losses are increased in secretory diarrheal diseases such as those caused by *Vibrio cholerae* and enterotoxigenic *Escherichia coli*. In all but the most complex situations, electrolyte losses can be estimated based on the range of values presented here.

MAJOR CLINICAL PROBLEMS

ISOTONIC DEHYDRATION

Because of the prevalence of gastrointestinal disease in young infants and children and the vulnerability of these patients to dehydration, isotonic dehydration is the most common fluid and electrolyte problem encountered in primary practice. In isotonic dehydration water and sodium salts are lost in approximately equal amounts from the gastrointestinal tract. Although the electrolyte composition of diarrheal losses is quite variable, compensatory body mechanisms maintain relative electrolyte homeostasis.

In the patient with equal losses of electrolytes and water, intracellular and extracellular fluid losses are similar, and the severity of illness is directly related to the degree of dehydration. Also, since the illness is usually acute, weight loss reflects loss of total body water. When the weight has dropped by 5%, there is about a 7% to 8% loss of body water and the patient is mildly dehydrated. Clinical signs include thirst, tacky mucous membranes, and decreased tears. As weight drops further, signs of cardiovascular compromise become evident; therefore, with a 10% drop in body weight (14% to 15% body water), tachycardia and orthostatic changes are present, with changes in skin turgor (Fig 55–1), sunken eyes and fontanelle, and oliguria. When weight loss is

TABLE 55–2
Maintenance Caloric Requirements

PATIENT WEIGHT	REQUIREMENT (CALORIES/KG/24 HR OR ML/KG/24 HR)
First 10 kg	100
11–20 kg	50
Each kg over 20	20

TABLE 55–3
Electrolyte Composition of Body Fluids in Normal and Pathologic States

ELECTROLYTE	GASTRIC CONTENTS (MEQ/L)	STOOL (MEQ/L)
Normal		
Sodium	35–60	Minimal
Potassium	10	Minimal
Chloride	80–180	Minimal
Pathologic		
Sodium	20–80	5–150
Potassium	5–20	12–120
Chloride	100–150	4–130

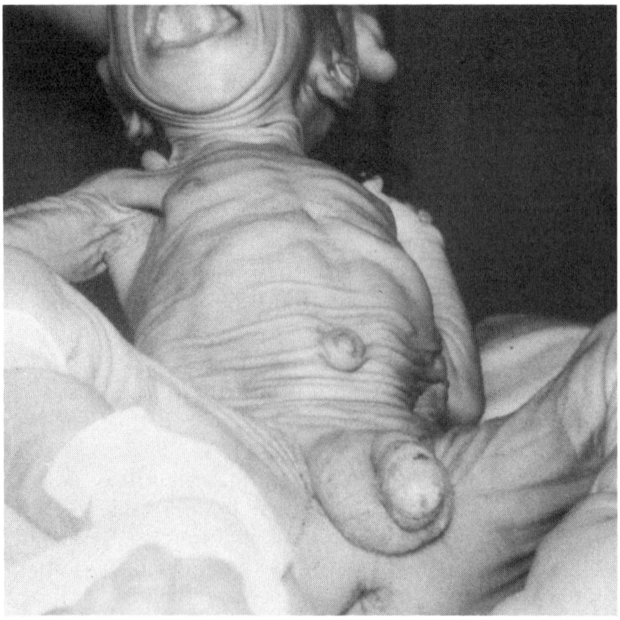

FIG 55–1
Severe dehydration in an infant. Note loss of skin turgor.

greater than 10%, the child is severely dehydrated, with physical signs of shock, including hypotension, a rapid respiratory rate, and poor peripheral perfusion (Table 55–4).

The key decision in the treatment of the young child with isotonic dehydration is whether it can be managed on an outpatient basis. In general, half of the deficit must be replaced over the first 8 hours of therapy, and the remainder over the next 16 hours. If this cannot be accomplished enterally or ongoing losses (including those from fever and vomiting) are large, outpatient treatment will not be successful. Successful home care depends on the parents' resources, which should be taken into consideration when deciding whether to hospitalize the child.

HYPONATREMIC DEHYDRATION AND WATER INTOXICATION

About 10% of children with dehydration will be hyponatremic, because losses are replaced with free water in excess of sodium. The child is thus dehydrated and water intoxicated. Hyponatremia can also occur with excessive losses of sodium. These circumstances are more unusual and include children with cystic fibrosis exposed to high environmental temperatures and children with gastrointestinal loss through tubes or ostomies. Hyponatremia results in relative preservation of the intracellular fluid volume at the expense of extracellular fluid. The cardiovascular signs of dehydration are exaggerated and the deficit is overestimated. Other clinical manifestations of hyponatremia include lethargy, coma, and hypothermia. Seizure activity may occur particularly if the level of serum sodium is less than 120 mEq/L or if there has been a rapid decrease in the serum sodium level.

Treatment must be directed toward the underlying mechanism that resulted in hyponatremia. For instance, one could use diuretics for the child with pure water intoxication and replace the sodium deficit of a child with excessive sodium loss. When seizures complicate the clinical presentation, 3% sodium solution can be used to acutely increase the level of serum sodium. Administration of 2 mL/kg of 3% sodium solution will safely raise the serum sodium and stop the seizure. As with many primary care problems, prevention in the form of parent education is the most effective treatment. Parents need instructions about providing adequate electrolyte levels and water for the treatment of simple gastroenteritis. Specific information regarding oral rehydration and refeeding is provided in the next section.

TABLE 55–4
Estimation of Percent Dehydration

	% DEHYDRATION			
CLINICAL PARAMETERS	<5	5	10	15
Appearance	Normal	Normal	Lethargic	Obtunded
Mucus membranes	Moist	Tacky	Parched	Parched
Eyes	Normal	Less tears	Sunken	Sunken
Fontanelle	Normal	Normal	Sunken	Sunken
Skin turgor	Normal	Normal	Decreased	Poor
Heart rate	Normal	Orthostatic	Increased	Increased
Respiratory rate	Normal	Normal	Increased	Increased
Blood pressure	Normal	Normal	Orthostatic	Markedly

HYPERNATREMIC DEHYDRATION AND HYPERNATREMIA

A hypernatremic state can develop either because of a disproportionate loss of free water producing dehydration or an excess of sodium from increased intake or a failure of excretion. Most hypernatremic states in children involve dehydration. In fact, 20% of children with dehydration will have a level of serum sodium greater than 150 mEq/L. This results from lack of access to water and greater insensible water loss related to a larger surface area. Defects in the thirst mechanism, inadvertent replacement with excess salt, and diarrheal loss with water in excess of solute will also result in hypernatremic dehydration.

Hypernatremia has a clinical effect on the central nervous system (CNS). Hyperosmolarity and resultant fluids shifts result in cerebral edema as well as hemorrhage and thrombosis. These CNS insults occur in both hypernatremic dehydration and salt poisoning, and frequently result in permanent neurologic damage. One response of the CNS to hypernatremia of greater than 24 hours is the formation of idiogenic osmoles from the breakdown of peptides and protein. These osmotically active amino acids remain inside of cells, maintaining intracellular fluid osmolality and, therefore, preserving cell volume. This probably prevents brain shrinkage and subsequent hemorrhage. However, the persistence of these idiogenic osmoles during therapy for dehydration can result in cerebral edema if the serum osmolality is lowered too rapidly.

Since the extracellular fluid is relatively preserved, the degree of dehydration is often underestimated. Doughy skin is frequently seen rather than tenting. Fever, irritability, and seizures are prominent problems. Clinical suspicion of hypernatremia is very important since therapy must include decreasing the serum osmolarity slowly. A specific goal is to decrease the level of serum sodium by no more than ½ mEq/L hour or 10 mEq/L in 24 hours. Seizures and hypocalcemia may also occur.

ORAL REHYDRATION

Traditionally, in developed countries, children in whom dehydration is severe enough to warrant treatment have been rehydrated parenterally. This is believed to be a more reliable route for both restoration of volume status and preservation of electrolyte homeostasis. Glucose solutions produce active glucose absorption in the small bowel that promotes the absorption of sodium. These solutions have most often been used early in a diarrheal illness to prevent dehydration or following parenteral replacement as part of a refeeding regimen. Concern about using the oral route for rehydration stems from the susceptibility of young infants to dehydration and to hypernatremia. Most reports of hypernatremia during oral rehydration involved errors in mixing the electrolyte solutions. In developing countries, diarrhea and subsequent dehydration are a major cause of morbidity and mortality among young infants and children. Intravenous fluid replacement is often not feasible in these settings. As a result, there has been much work in developing nations over the past 10 years indicating that oral therapy for dehydration is both safe and effective. Similar success has also recently been demonstrated in well-nourished populations.

Glucose and electrolyte solutions currently available are described in Table 55–5. Use of these solutions must be appropriately tailored to the clinical setting. In developing countries or in situations in which no hospital or physician is available, oral rehydration can be lifesaving. For children with access to more sophisticated medical care, oral rehydration at home should be reserved for those in whom dehydration is less than 5% and whose care can be adequately supervised. Also, early intervention with glucose-electrolyte solutions may be used as a preventive measure. When the patient is more than 5% dehydrated, oral rehydration can still be prescribed, but it should be carried out in a closely monitored setting. Intake and ongoing losses should be recorded frequently and the level of serum electrolytes should be measured periodically.

Specific suggestions for treating dehydration orally are described below:

1. The preferred solution for rehydration in both the United States and developing countries is the World Health Organization (WHO) formulation containing 90 mEq/L of sodium and 2% glucose. Infants should be offered an amount equivalent to the calculated deficit, or at least 150 mL/kg, in the first 24 hours. If the infant finishes this in less than 24 hours, free water should be offered to prevent the development of hypernatremia.

2. If the WHO formula is going to be used as a maintenance solution, following rehydration, or to prevent dehydration, additional free water must be offered. This can be in the form of ad lib breast milk or as free water (one free water feeding: two feedings of the WHO solution).

3. When the goal of therapy is maintenance of hydration or prevention of dehydration, a commercially available solution of 50 to 60 mEq/L sodium and 111 mmol/L glucose can be used alone. Again, the volume offered should be restricted to 150 mL/kg/day. Any additional fluid offered should be free water (tap or juice) or breast milk.

Finally, diarrhea and vomiting are usually the precipitating events when a child becomes dehydrated. When treating these problems, one must take care not to starve the child; however, limited data are available which suggest optimal nutritional treatment of the infant with diarrhea. It does appear that patients who are fed either breast milk or a soy-containing formula in addition to glucose-electrolyte solutions have diarrhea of lesser duration or severity. Therefore, it is recommended to continue breast-feeding whenever possible and, for the formula-fed infant, to use a soy-based formula is suggested until the diarrhea has resolved.

CONCLUSION

The clinician in primary practice seldom needs sophisticated calculations to care for children with fluid and electrolyte problems that are most often caused by gastrointestinal disturbances and aggravated by fever. However, familiarity with maintenance fluid and electrolyte requirements as well as specific recommendations for oral rehydration and maintenance therapy will assure a favorable outcome. In addition, the sicker child or the one who fails to improve with this regimen will be identified quickly and appropriately referred. Finally, patients with extreme electrolyte imbalance, profound disturbances in fluid volume, or

TABLE 55–5
Glucose-Electrolyte Solutions

Solution		Ingredients (mEq/L)			
		Na^+	K^+	Cl^-	Carbohydrate (g/L)
ReSol (Wyeth-Ayerst)	Liquid; ready to use	50	20	50	Glucose 20
Lytren (Mead Johnson)	Liquid; ready to use	50	25	45	Dextrose 20
Pedialyte (Ross)	Liquid; ready to use	45	20	35	Dextrose 25
Rehydralyte (Ross)	Liquid; ready to use	75	20	65	Dextrose 25
WHO oral rehydration salts	Powder	90	20	80	Glucose 20

other unusual manifestations may have underlying disease. Here the primary practice physician plays a key role in identifying the sick child and suspecting a more serious problem.

BIBLIOGRAPHY

Cleary TG, Cleary KR, DuPont HL, et al: The relationship of oral rehydration solution to hypernatremia in infantile diarrhea. *J Pediatr* 1981; 99:739.

Finberg L, Harper PA, Harrison HE, et al: Oral rehydration for diarrhea. *J Pediatr* 1982; 101:497.

Finberg L, Kravath R, Fleischman A: *Water and Electrolytes in Pediatrics.* Philadelphia, WB Saunders Co, 1982.

Gruskin A: Parenteral fluid therapy and therapy for electrolyte disorders for children, in Goldsmith H (ed): *Practice of Surgery.* New York, Harper & Row, 1981.

Isolauri E, Vesikari T, Saha P, et al: Milk versus no milk in rapid refeeding after acute gastroenteritis. *J Pediatric Gastroenterol Nutr* 1986; 5:254.

Khin-Maung-u, Nyunt-Nyunt-Wai, Myo Khin, et al: Effect on clinical outcome of breast feeding during acute diarrhoea. *Br Med J* 1985; 290:587.

Listernick R, Zierseri E, Davis AT: Outpatient oral rehydration in the United States. *Am J Dis Child* 1986; 140:211.

Oral rehydration solutions. *Med Lett* 1983; 25:629.

Pizarro D, Posadz G, Mata L: Treatment of 242 neonates with dehydrating diarrhea with an oral glucose-electrolyte solution. *J Pediatr* 1983; 102:153.

Santosham M, Daum RS, Dilman L, et al: Oral rehydration therapy of infantile diarrhea: A controlled study of well-nourished children hospitalized in the United States and Panama. *N Engl J Med* 1982; 306:1070.

Santosham M, Foster S, Reid R, et al: Role of soy-based, lactose-free formula during treatment of acute diarrhea. *Pediatrics* 1985; 76:292.

Santosham M, Brown K, Sack RB: Oral rehydration therapy and dietary therapy for acute childhood diarrhea. *Pediatr Rev* 1987; 8:273.

56 DERMATOLOGY

Herbert B. Allen, M.D.
Paul J. Honig, M.D.

This chapter covers a number of common dermatologic disorders seen by the primary care provider. Diagnostic characteristics and treatment issues are stressed for each condition.

ATOPIC DERMATITIS

Atopic dermatitis or eczema, a common skin disease of unknown cause, is found predominantly in children who have a personal history or family history of allergies such as hay fever, allergic rhinitis, or sinusitis. Intense pruritus is the predominant symptom. In fact, atopic dermatitis has been termed "the itch that rashes."

BACKGROUND

The onset of atopic dermatitis is early in life; 60% of the cases will occur by the age of 1 year. In the early months of life, a severe diaper dermatitis may be the harbinger of future skin trouble. The condition is usually not lifelong, however; 90% of all children recover by adolescence.

In infancy, the rash appears on the cheeks and extensor surfaces of arms and legs as red exudative plaques. Similar lesions may be present in the diaper area. By the age of 2 years, the more characteristic flexural involvement (Fig 56–1) has generally evolved, with the common sites being the neck, antecubital, and

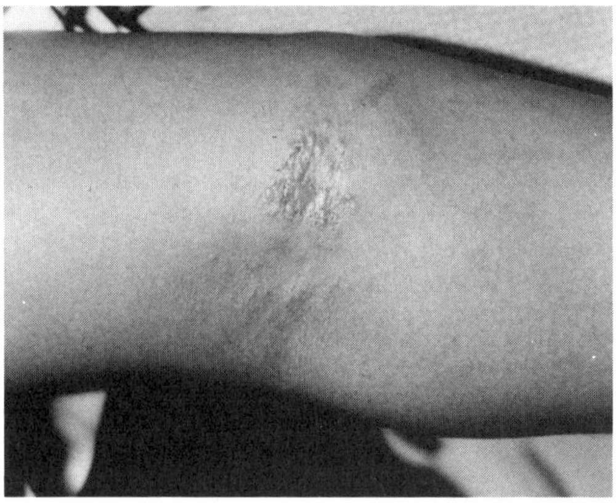

FIG 56–1
Mild atopic dermatitis.

popliteal spaces (Fig 56–2). Lesions include erythema, edema, papules, vesicles, papulovesicles, and lichenification. Weeping, oozing, and crusting may be present. The course of the eruption may wax and wane, with chronic relapses being quite common.

In atypical locations the findings are different. If the feet become involved, the soles usually have shiny, peeling skin with painful fissures. Diffuse follicular accentuation, scaling in the scalp (with or without alopecia), hyperlinear palms and soles, pityriasis alba, or fissured or crusted plaques in the auricular folds may variably be present.

Children with atopic dermatitis have poor resistance to superficial viral infections. For example, such children are frequently infected with warts, molluscum contagiosum, and herpes simplex. Eczema herpeticum (Fig 56–3) can be a serious complication of atopic dermatitis that requires hospitalization and intravenous acyclovir.

The diagnosis of atopic dermatitis is based solely on clinical findings. The laboratory yields no diagnostic assistance. On occasion, elevated IgE, eosinophilia, or positive scratch tests may be found, but these are nonspecific and do not truly confirm the diagnosis.

MANAGEMENT

The major therapy for atopic dermatitis is topical corticosteroid application. The potency of the preparation depends on the amount of inflammation, the age of the patient, and the severity of involvement. As the condition improves (generally within 2 to 3 weeks), it is judicious to shift to a moderate or mild topical agent, with 1% hydrocortisone being the mildest of the effective preparations. If there is prominent crusting or erythema, antibiotics such as erythromycin may be employed for 1- to 2-week intervals. These lesions tend to be heavily colonized with *Staphylococcus aureus*. Antihistamines may be helpful in controlling pruritus.

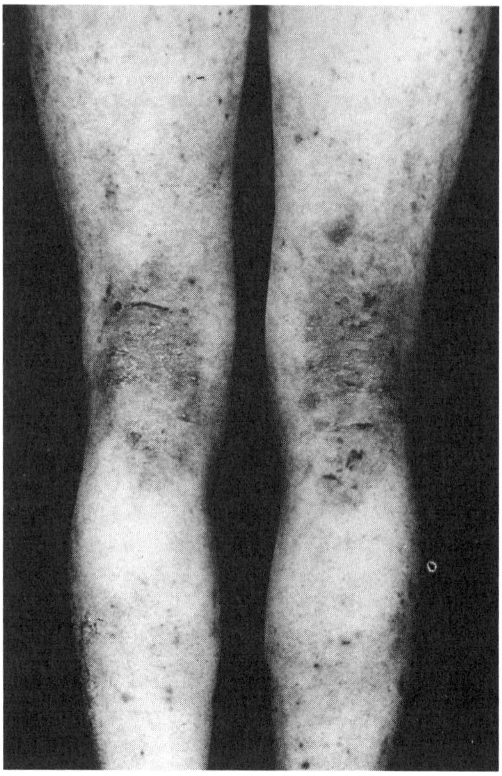

FIG 56–2
Atopic dermatitis. Note the diffuse erythema and excoriated lesions concentrated on flexor surfaces.

General prevention measures are probably as important as specific treatment and include: (1) decreased bathing; (2) the use of mild soaps—and even these must be used sparingly; (3) the avoidance of irritants, such as quaternary ammonium in perineal wipes; and (4) the generous use of emollients. Soaks (tap water; tea water, especially for feet; Burow's solution; saline solution) are useful if considerable weeping and oozing are present. Lotions, creams, and pastes are also preferable in this instance. For

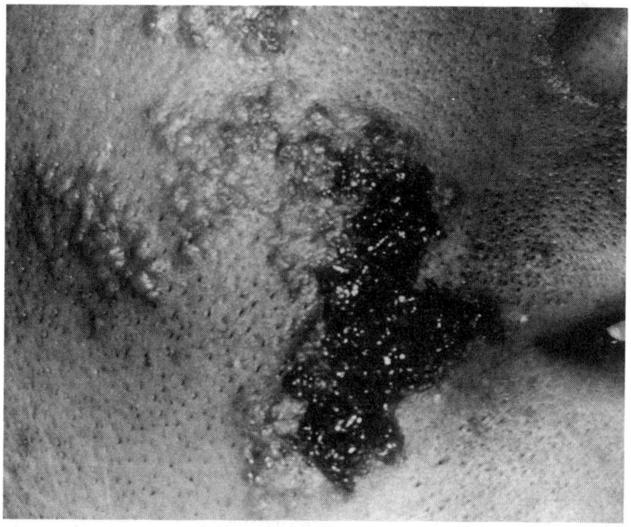

FIG 56–3
Herpes simplex showing grouped vesicles on an erythematous base.

the drier, more lichenified lesions, ointments are generally more effective. Dietary measures may be helpful if the offending food can be identified; however, hyposensitization is not usually indicated in "purely" skin disease. For scalp disease, decreased use of even mild shampoos and topical steroid lotions is helpful. When the feet are involved, topical steroid ointments and liberal use of petrolatum (whenever the shoes are removed) are helpful.

Recently, primrose oil, which contains linoleic acid, has been advocated as an oral treatment for atopic dermatitis. This has met with various degrees of success and is quite costly. Its use should be cautiously considered.

URTICARIA

Urticaria is a skin condition characterized by "hives and itching." It is very common and many children have had at least one episode in their lives. In the allergic type of hives, a type I immunologic reaction occurs that may be induced by drugs, foods, infections, or other allergens. The classic examples are: for the drug-induced variety, penicillin; for foods, shellfish; and for infections, viral hepatitis.

BACKGROUND

The clinical lesions are widely distributed pink wheals, which may be small or large. Individual lesions usually last less than 24 hours. When involvement of the respiratory passages occurs, a medical emergency exists.

In general terms, if the hives are of relatively short duration, the offending allergen may be identified. The longer the hives persist and become chronic, the more difficult it is to find the antigenic stimulus. In fact, in chronic urticaria, multiple antigens may be provocative. Subtle antigens such as dyes, salicylates, and preservatives may assume a large role; carefully taken dietary and activity history may be revealing.

Cholinergic urticaria is a condition to be distinguished from allergic hives. In cholinergic urticaria the wheals are tiny at first, then enlarged by coalescing. Adolescents and young adults are more at risk than infants or children. The lesions tend to be distributed on the trunk and are not preceded by an allergen. Dermographism is usually easily demonstrated. Cholinergic urticaria may be provoked by exercise, sweating, rubbing, scratching, emotions, or exposure to either cold or hot temperatures.

MANAGEMENT

If respiratory symptoms are present, treatment with subcutaneous epinephrine, antihistamines, and careful observation should help to alleviate the symptoms. Ordinary treatment involves antihistamines and, possibly, even a short, tapering course of oral corticosteroids. If it does not work, another antihistamine of a different class (i.e., cyproheptadine) may be added for concurrent administration. This treatment usually needs to be given for 1 to 2 months, and patients are advised to avoid known precipitating factors and activities.

ERYTHEMA MULTIFORME

Erythema multiforme (EM) is a reaction pattern in the skin somewhat similar to urticaria. It differs in the type of clinical lesion that arises (the iris or "target" lesion [Fig 56–4] vs. the wheal) and in the minimal pruritus present. The skin reaction may be secondary to drugs (such as penicillin, sulfonamides, hydantoin, and barbiturates) or to viral infections. Herpes simplex virus is the most common. Other drugs and other infections may also precipitate the phenomenon.

BACKGROUND

Lesions generally begin on the distal surfaces of feet and spread centrally; however, they may arise in generalized fashion de novo. The findings may include macules, papules, vesicobullae, and the iris lesion, which has a red or dark center surrounded by pale pink and red rings. When mucous membranes are involved and constitutional symptoms are present, the designation Stevens-Johnson syndrome is used (Fig 56–5). The lips and oral cavity are most commonly affected. The lips show marked hemorrhagic crusting. Moreover, the conjunctivae, urethra, vagina, perianal area, and even the tracheobronchial and esophageal membranes may be involved.

MANAGEMENT

The treatment for EM in mild cases is symptomatic. Severe involvement may require corticosteroids to treat systemic effects. Given early (i.e., in the prodromal phase), a short course (5 to 7 days) of prednisone can even obliterate the development of EM. This is characteristic in the EM following herpes simplex infection. If eye changes are present, consultation with an ophthalmologist is necessary. For severe crusting of the lips, intermittent warm water compresses should be followed by application of an ointment such as petrolatum. As in urticaria, if a drug is the provoking agent, it should be discontinued. Antihistamines may benefit the patient who is itchy.

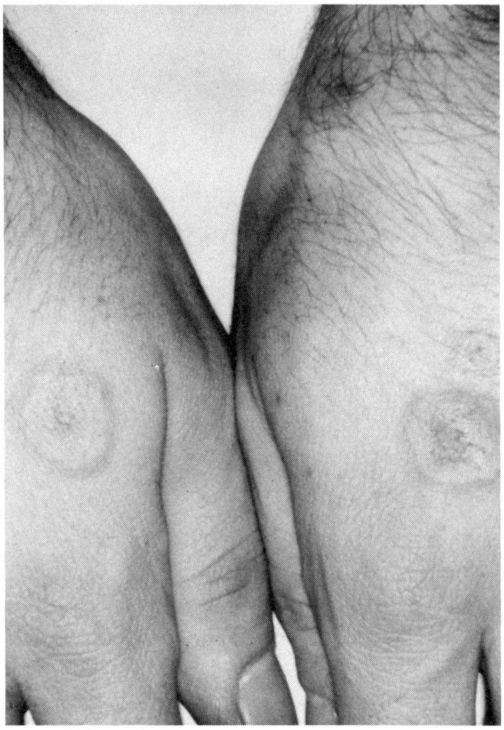

FIG 56–4
Target lesion of erythema multiforme.

DRUG ERUPTIONS

In addition to urticaria and EM, drugs may induce maculopapular eruptions, bullous (diffuse or fixed) lesions, vasculitis, nodular lesions, photosensitivity, and toxic epidermal necrolysis. In fact, drugs are an important differential diagnosis in almost all types of skin eruptions.

In managing drug eruptions, the offending agent must be discontinued; in cases in which multiple agents are being used, all should be stopped, if possible. When the eruption clears, the least likely agent may be reintroduced followed by the next agent every 3 to 5 days. If the eruption recurs after a drug is taken, that agent is presumed to be the agent producing the rash. As multiple allergens may be present, a persistent search may be necessary. Subtle allergens may be responsible, i.e., dyes in liquids, capsule coatings, preservatives, or flavorings. Drug eruptions may be induced by agents patients do not ordinarily term "drugs," for example, nose drops, nose sprays, suppositories, lozenges, and others. A complete review of all such agents is necessary. Frequently, other family

Feigin RD, Shearer WT: Fever of unknown origin in children. *Curr Probl Pediatr* 1976; 6:3–64.
Jaffe DM, Tanz RR, Davis AT, et al: Antibiotic administration to treat possible occult bacteremia in febrile children. *N Engl J Med* 1987; 317: 1175–1180.
Kleinman MB: The complaint of persistent fever: Recognition and management of pseudo fever of unknown origin. *Pediatr Clin North Am* 1982; 29:201.
Kluger MJ: Fever. *Pediatrics* 1980; 66:720.
Marshall R, Teele DW, Klein JO: Unsuspected bacteremia due to *Hemophilus influenzae*: Outcome of children not initially admitted to the hospital. *J Pediatr* 1979; 95:690.
McCarthy PL: Controversies in pediatrics: What tests are indicated for the child under 2 with fever? *Pediat Rev* 1979; 1:51.
McCarthy PL, Sharpe MR, Spiesel SZ, et al: Observation scales to identify serious illness in febrile children. *Pediatrics* 1982; 70:802.
McCarthy PM, Jekel JF, Dolan TF: Temperature greater than or equal to 40° C in children less than 24 months of age: A prospective study. *Pediatrics* 1977; 59:663.
Pearson HA: Splenectomy: Its risks and its roles. *Hosp Pract* 1980; 15:85.
Pizzo PA, Lovejoy FH Jr, Smith DH: Prolonged fever in children: Review of 100 cases. *Pediatrics* 1975; 55:468.
Roberts KB: Blood cultures in pediatric practice. *Am J Dis Child* 1979; 133:996.
Stern RC: Pathophysiologic basis for symptomatic treatment of fever. *Pediatrics* 1977; 59:92.
Teele DW, Marshall R, Klein JO: Unsuspected bacteremia in young children: A common and important problem. *Pediatr Clin North Am* 1979; 26:773.

59 HEMATOLOGY

ANEMIA

Mortimer Poncz, M.D.

The differential diagnosis of anemia in children has already been described under "Pallor" in Chapter 43. In this section, four common causes of anemia in childhood are discussed in detail: iron deficiency anemia, the thalassemias, hereditary spherocytosis, and glucose-6-phosphate dehydrogenase (G-6-PD) deficiency. Sickle cell anemia is discussed in the following section.

IRON DEFICIENCY ANEMIA

Background

Prevalence and Etiology.—The most common cause of childhood anemia is iron deficiency. Approximately 3% of white children and 15% of black children 1 year of age have iron deficiency anemia, while another 20% are iron deficient but without anemia. Two major factors account for the high rate of anemia due to iron deficiency in childhood: the rapid increase in body size (and blood volume) and the relative insufficiency of iron in the diet. The two periods of greatest body growth are the first 2 years of life, in which a child more than triples his birth weight, and the adolescent years; both periods are also associated with poor dietary iron intake. In infancy, if the formula is not iron-fortified or if whole cow's milk is introduced too early, total dietary iron intake may be inadequate. Poor iron intake may again occur in adolescence because of erratic eating habits or fads that do not include a food source rich in iron.

Blood loss during these two time periods can further stress the limited iron reserve and lead to iron deficiency anemia. For example, a term infant who had significant perinatal blood loss due to transplacental bleeding will be more likely to develop iron deficiency anemia and

8. Antinuclear antibody titers
9. Rheumatoid factor determination
10. C3, C4, and total hemolytic complement measurement
11. Platelet count

The sequence in which these are performed will be determined by the differential diagnosis. For example, if the child is having vague abdominal complaints and/or diarrhea, gastrointestinal contrast radiography should be performed early in the investigation. If, on the other hand, the history and physical examination are totally unhelpful in pointing to a diagnosis, then the tests should be done in whatever order is convenient. If these tests are nondiagnostic, one may wish to consider a bone marrow aspiration, both for cytologic examination and bacterial culture.

After the laboratory and radiologic evaluation is completed, most life-threatening or treatable diseases will have been detected. Most of the remaining children will either have a self-limited infectious process or never have a diagnosis made with ultimate resolution of the febrile process. For children who continue to be febrile but appear healthy on examination with no focal physical signs, it is appropriate to reassure the parents and not pursue test after test. These children, however, must be carefully followed up, with additional tests (or previously ordered tests redone) as the clinical condition changes.

The emotional state of the parents of children with fever of unknown origin must be recognized. In general, these parents are anxious and frustrated because of the unknown diagnosis. The physician should put the dilemma on a perspective that they are not the only parents to have faced this problem and that as long as the child looks well and does not develop a new sign or symptom, he can be observed. This will serve to reassure the parents by indicating that they are undergoing the same emotional responses as other parents and preclude the parents from "doctor shopping." The physician must continue to see these patients frequently, both to assure that no previously unrecognized disease process is becoming clinically manifest and to continue to reassure the parents and the child that the child is not seriously ill.

For those children who continue to have a fever, appear ill on physical examination, or who may have sustained weight loss, it is important to assure the parents that the physician will continue to see the child frequently until either a diagnosis is made or the fever disappears. At times, it may be helpful to seek a second opinion by a physician who can view the entire situation with a fresh perspective. Physicians should also recognize that children with fever of unknown origin often induce feelings of anxiety and frustration in the physician. Physicians often allow themselves to believe that there must be an answer to every clinical problem, and that it is the physician's task to make a diagnosis. This is obviously untrue, particularly in cases of children with fever of unknown origin. It is essential that the physician recognize his inability to make a diagnosis in the cases of many of these children. This allows the physician to establish appropriate self-expectations. With this mindset, fever of unknown origin becomes a fascinating, challenging, and rewarding part of a physician's office practice.

BIBLIOGRAPHY

Bellanti JA, Boner AL: Immunology of the fetus and the newborn, in Avery GB (ed): *Neonatology: Pathophysiology and Management of the Newborn*. Philadelphia, JB Lippincott, 1981.

Bratton L, Teele DW, Klein JO: Outcome of unsuspected pneumonococcemia in children not initially admitted to the hospital. *J Pediatr* 1977; 90:703.

Carroll WL, Farrell MK, Singer JI, et al: Treatment of occult bacteremia: A prospective randomized clinical trial. *Pediatrics* 1981; 72:608.

Caspe WB, Chamudes O, Louis B: The evaluation and treatment of the febrile infant. *Pediatr Infect Dis* 1983; 2:131.

Committee on Infectious Diseases of the American Academy of Pediatrics: Aspirin and Reye's syndrome. *Pediatrics* 1982; 69:810.

DeAngelis C, Jaffe A, Wilson M, et al: Iatrogenic risks and financial costs of hospitalizing febrile infants. *Am J Dis Child* 1983; 137:1146.

Dechovitz AB, Moffett HL: Classification of acute febrile illnesses in childhood. *Clin Pediatr* 1968; 7:649.

Dinarello CA, Wolff SM: Pathogenesis of fever in man. *N Engl J Med* 1978; 298:609.

Done AK: Treatment of fever in 1982: A review. *Am J Med* 1983; 74:27.

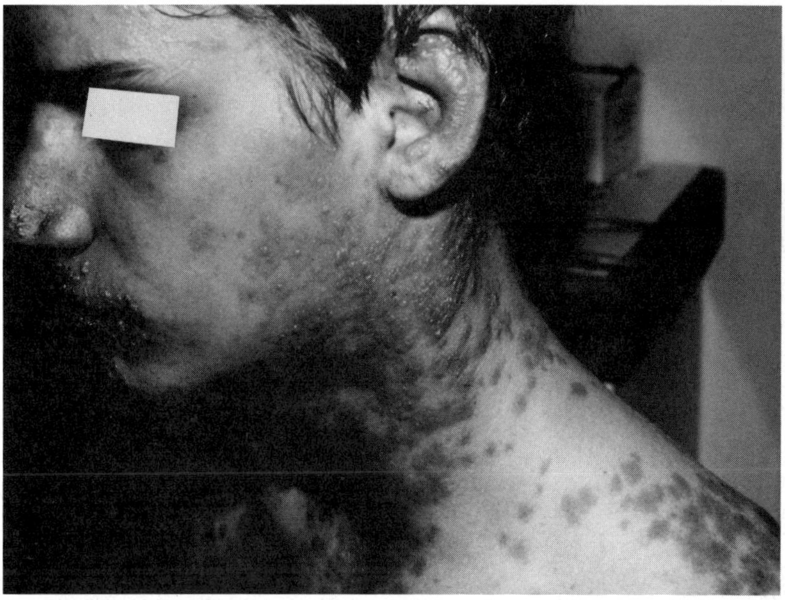

FIG 56–5
Erythema multiforme.

members are able to fill in the total picture of ingestants and inhalants.

Other treatments are symptomatic, ranging from antihistamines for control of pruritus to corticosteroids for systemic symptoms. Topical corticosteroids may or may not be useful in drug eruptions because of the diffuse nature of the condition. Soothing baths or compresses (mineral oil or oilated oatmeal) may be used, and, for oozing eruptions, shake lotions (calamine or calamine mixed with equal parts of a moisturizing lotion) may be helpful.

CONTACT DERMATITIS

Allergic contact dermatitis is a form of delayed, cell-mediated hypersensitivity and is less common in children than adults. The incidence below the age of 1 year is rare.

BACKGROUND

The offending allergen is deposited on the skin, penetrates the stratum corneum, is transcribed or modulated by Langerhans' cells, joins with a carrier protein, and travels to the regional lymph node; after processing by macrophages, it gets recognized by T cells, which then become sensitized. The T cells enter the circulation, migrate to the skin, react with the allergen, and release lymphokines. Six to 24 hours later, dermatitis erupts.

The distribution of the dermatitis may be an important clue to the provoking allergen, for example, contact dermatitis on the neck from perfume or earrings; the mouth, due to dentifrices or bubble gum; the feet, due to shoes or rubber. The pattern of linear vesicles (Fig 56–6) in rhus dermatitis (poison ivy) is virtually diagnostic of this form of contact dermatitis.

Clinically, one sees vesicles, bullae, papulovesicles, edema, erythema, crusting, and excoriations. With airborne contactants, there is severe involvement of the eyes. Both upper and lower lids are markedly swollen and there is generalized facial edema and erythema. Photocontact dermatitis is distinguishable by its presence in areas where sunlight strikes the skin and its absence in nonexposed areas. Nonspecific factors such as trauma, pressure, heat, and sweating may play a role during both the initiation and elicitation phases of contact sensitivity.

MANAGEMENT

Topical steroids are helpful in most cases of contact allergy. In rhus and airborne dermatitis, oral prednisone may be necessary; a dose of 1 to 2 mg/kg/day for 1 week, with tapering off over 2 to 3 weeks to prevent rebound. Usually

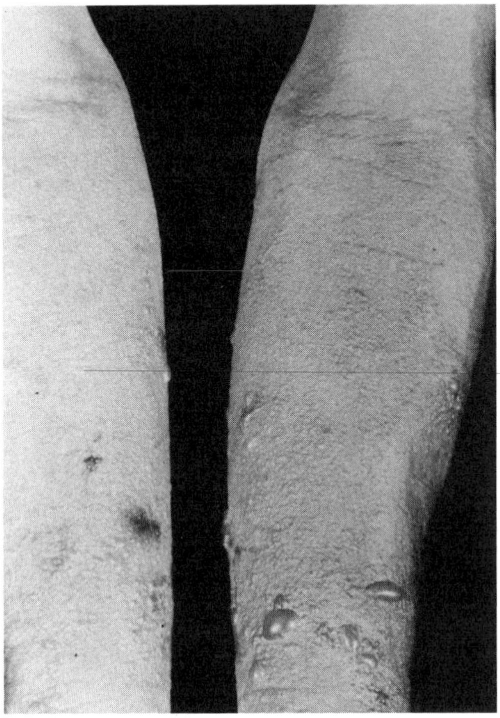

FIG 56–6
Contact dermatitis edematous. Vesicobullous lesions that have sharply demarcated margins.

the pruritus will disappear 36 hours after the initial dose of prednisone. Then the lesions will flatten, fade, and, ultimately, scale. Soaks, compresses, and shake lotions are useful in the early vesicular, bullous, and weeping eruptions and should be used for 3 to 5 days. Avoid antihistamine-containing lotions because of possible secondary contact sensitization. Ice-water compresses to the eyelids are soothing and beneficial in lessening the edema of airborne reactions and in photocontact sensitivities. Oral antihistamines may be prescribed to reduce pruritus.

Avoidance of the offending allergens is a must or the eruption will recur with repeated exposure. Some "hardening" may occur during the season such that the first case of rhus is ordinarily the worst of the year. Vectors such as pets, clothing, wood, or smoke may carry the allergen to a sensitive person. Secondary contact dermatitis such as sensitivity to the antihistamine in shake lotions or to vitamin E rubbed on the skin may obscure the primary disease. The history and the clinical appearance of the rash are important in recognizing a secondary sensitivity. Patch testing may be useful in all varieties of contact allergy and is especially useful when the specific allergen is unclear.

INSECT BITE REACTION

The common insects that bite children are mosquitoes and fleas. Chiggers, gnats, black flies, "no-see-ums," and others cause bite reactions that are also bothersome but are less common compared to mosquitoes and fleas.

To make the diagnosis, consider the time of year, the location of the lesions, and the type of lesion. Mosquitoes appear in the warmer months, as do sand fleas. Animal fleas are present year-round on pets or in rugs or furniture.

Exposed surfaces are involved with pink and red papules with a central punctum, papulovesicles, vesicles (Fig 56–7), and even bullae in highly sensitized patients. Pruritus, intense at times, is the main symptom. Crusting and secondary infection may appear.

Treatment is symptomatic with utilization of ice for acute lesions, antihistamines for pruritus, and shake lotions for soothing. Lotions and creams containing antihistamines may be sensitizing.

The prior use of insect repellents (particularly those that contain *N,N*-diethylmetatoluamide [DEET]) helps prevent bites, but must be applied every 3 to 4 hours because the substance wears off or evaporates. Ingestion of garlic may also help ward off attackers. Avoidance of perfume or perfumed shampoos, rinses, or lotions is also helpful.

DIAPER DERMATITIS

Diaper rash is a common problem in young children. The disorder has many causes, including occlusion, bacterial overgrowth, monilial proliferation, friction, and innate susceptibility (atopic or seborrheic diatheses) having more or less importance in individual cases. Differing types of rashes may be noted when one factor predominates: candidal, atopic, seborrheic, and primary irritant. Mixed types, for example, irritant with monilial overgrowth, are also seen.

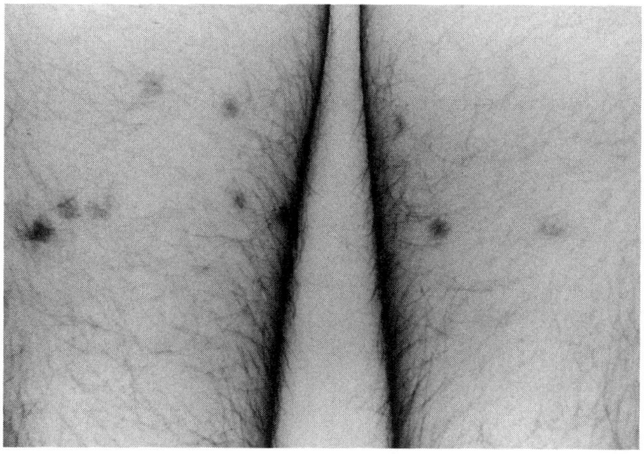

FIG 56–7
Flea bites. Erythematous lesions on exposed surface.

Candidal types are recognized by their "beefy red" plaques associated with satellite papules and pustules. Primary irritant eruptions may wax and wane and, when present, have shiny glazed skin that may become macerated. Atopic and seborrheic eruptions generally are associated with body rashes in typical locations and have appropriate family histories. Bacterial superinfection may occur and if blistering is present, *S. aureus* infection should be considered.

Treatment of diaper dermatitis consists of allowing the skin to dry as much as possible via air exposure. Candidal infections may be treated with nystatin or the imidazoles such as clotrimazole. Secondary bacterial infections may be treated with triple antibiotic topical agents; inflammation may be reduced by topical corticosteroids. Mixtures of the above may be employed or an already prepared compound (Mycolog) may be selected. Note that the ointment formula is far less sensitizing than the cream. The use of soap and water should be decreased and mild soaps should be used. Perineal wipes, especially those containing quaternary ammonium compounds, may be irritating. An alternative to wipes or soap-and-water cleaning for soiled buttocks is the use of a lotion (Keri, Nutraderm, Baby Magic, etc.).

Another useful compound is "triple" paste applied at bedtime (formula: 10 gm of Burow's solution 1:40, 20 gm of aquaphor, 30 gm of zinc oxide paste). This may be removed in the morning by mineral oil, if necessary. The compound itself is soothing, gently drying, and remarkably protective because of its water-impervious nature. A very light dusting of powder may be utilized to make the substance an even better barrier. Caution must be used with talc-containing powders to prevent inhalation of the substance.

"Id" (diffuse disseminated papules and papulovesicles) reactions generally respond to topical corticosteroids, with 1% hydrocortisone being the safest. Oral nystatin may be necessary to clear an intestinal focus of *Candida albicans*.

TINEA CAPITIS

Tinea capitis is a *dermatophytic* infection of the scalp. It is most common before puberty. The organisms that usually cause tinea capitis are *Microsporum* species and *Trichophyton tonsurans*. There has been a gradual increase in the percentage of cases caused by *T. tonsurans*. Most tinea capitis lesions will not demonstrate fluorescence on Wood's lamp examination due to this changing etiology. Clinically, there are several different forms of tinea capitis. These include: (1) patchy, scaling alopecia; (2) boggy, purulent-appearing kerion; (3) diffuse chronic scaling or "dandruff"; and (4) "blackdot," in which the hair is broken off at the scalp, giving the appearance of multiple black dots. These forms vary depending on the infecting organism, the site of infection, the patient's immune response, and state of treatment. The diagnosis of tinea capitis is made by culturing the affected scalp area with dermatophyte test medium.

The management of tinea capitis includes

treatment with oral griseofulvin 10 to 20 mg/kg/day in two divided doses for a period of 6 to 8 weeks. It is useful to give the medication with a fatty meal (e.g., ice cream) to aid absorption. Topical application of selenium sulfide suspension 2.5% (Selsun) in the form of shampoo twice weekly will also decrease the spore count, and thus decrease infectivity. Topical antifungal medications should not be used; they are ineffective. Some dermatologists will treat a painful kerion with steroids, but if the patient requires this therapy, he/she should be referred. The differential diagnosis of tinea capitis includes seborrhea, alopecia areata, trichotillomania, and traction alopecia.

TINEA PEDIS

Tinea pedis is decidedly rare before the age of 11 years but increases in frequency during adolescence. Sweating and occlusion or partial occlusion play large roles in allowing this infection to occur. The ordinary causative organisms are *T. rubrum, T. mentagrophytes,* and *Epidermophyton floccosum.*

The fourth interspace is the most common site of involvement although other sites may also be troublesome. If the dorsal toes or the ball of the foot is involved at an early age, it is almost never caused by a fungus. Contact or atopic dermatitis are more likely diagnoses. The fungal eruption is characterized by pruritus, which may be intense at times. Scaling maceration and fissuring between toes may be present. Nails are seldom involved early. The diagnosis may be confirmed by potassium hydroxide examination or culture.

Treatment consists of topical antifungals—tolnaftate, miconazole, clotrimazole, econazole, and ciclopirox olamine are all effective. Ordinarily, oral griseofulvin need not be administered. Keeping the foot dry helps prevent recurrences.

ACNE

Acne affects over three-fourths of the population during adolescence and early adult life. Although usually mild and self-limited, the disorder can leave many physical and emotional scars. In most instances, these scars can be prevented by control of the disease. Although the pathogenesis of acne is not completely clear, knowledge of current theories makes therapy more understandable.

BACKGROUND

The target skin appendage is the sebaceous follicle. With initiation of puberty, adrenal androgenic influences cause sebaceous enlargement and secretion. Due to abnormalities in the keratinization process of the follicular lining, epithelial cells are not shed normally. This leads to obstruction within the follicle and retention of sebum. Obstruction then leads to the next step in the cycle, i.e., overgrowth of the follicle with *Propionibacterium acnes.* Although most sebaceous follicles are colonized with this organism, acne patients have greater numbers of the bacteria and respond to its presence in an exaggerated fashion. It is this idiosyncratic inflammatory response to *P. acnes* that leads to most inflammatory papules, pustules, and cysts that are seen.

The classic lesions seen in acne are the open and closed comedone (i.e., blackhead and whitehead), inflammatory papules and pustules, and cystic lesions (some with connecting sinus tracts). Acne is found wherever sebaceous follicles are present, i.e., the face, chest, back, upper arms, upper thighs, and buttocks.

On occasion, infants are found to have acne within the first several months of life or later in the first year. Transplacental maternal hormones are the cause. Spontaneous resolution usually occurs with early onset disease.

MANAGEMENT

All treatment is directed toward (1) relieving follicular obstruction, (2) reducing the number of *P. acnes* organisms, and (3) preventing the inflammatory response.

GUIDELINES FOR TREATMENT OF ACNE

Put acne in perspective by discussing the problem, the treatment, and usual outcomes.
Early acne (comedone)
  Retinoic acid: Start with use every other day, then progress to daily treatments.
Mild to moderate acne
  Benzoyl peroxide
Moderate to severe acne
  Benzoyl peroxide

Retinoic acid
Add oral antibiotics (tetracycline, erythromycin)
Additional options if no improvement:
Can increase benzoyl peroxide or retinoic acid to twice a day, combine the two treatments, or add topical antibiotics (clindamycin, erythromycin, tetracycline)
Refer: Problem cystic acne

Therapy begins with the education of patients as to proper skin care. Mild soaps should be used and vigorous scrubbing avoided. The skin should be patted dry and treated gently at all times. Patients should be instructed to avoid squeezing lesions. Certain commonly used cleansers and moisturizers should be avoided because of their comedogenic potential.

Topical retinoic acid is used for open and closed comedones (Table 56–1). This preparation decreases the adhesiveness between cells and relieves obstruction. Topical benzoyl peroxide is used when inflammatory lesions are present as well. Benzoyl peroxide has antibacterial activity as well as acting as an exfoliant and a comedolytic agent. It may cause redness and scaling. With other than mild involvement with inflammatory lesions, systemic antibiotics are required. Severe involvement (i.e., diffuse cystic and nodulocystic lesions and sinus tracts) requires the use of 13-*cis*-retinoic acid. Because of the many side effects (including teratogenicity) of this preparation, only physicians experienced with this medication should prescribe it.

When attempts to control acne vulgaris are unsuccessful, referral to a dermatologist is advisable.

TABLE 56–1
Rank order of Irritancy of Retinoic Acid Preparations*

DEGREE OF IRRITATION	VEHICLE	RETINOIC ACID CONCENTRATION (%)
High	Solution	0.05
	Gel	0.05
	Gel	0.025
	Gel	0.01
	Cream	0.10
	Gel	0.005
Low	Cream	0.05

*From CM: The cutaneous safety of topical tretinoin. *Acta Derm Venereol* [Suppl] (Stockh) 1975; 128. Used by permission.

LICE

BACKGROUND

The incidence of pediculosis is gradually increasing in the United States, especially pediculosis capitis. Although crowding and poor hygiene favor infestation, it is now clear that social class is not a factor.

The female louse can lay eggs at a rate of eight to 12 per day, producing large populations of lice within 3 to 4 months. Eggs (nits) are glued to hairs or fibers of clothing. Once hatched, the lice depend on blood meals for survival and therefore cannot exist for more than a few days away from humans.

During feeding periods, toxins released into the skin cause small red or purpuric spots. Continued exposure to these bites results in sensitization, with formation of papules and wheals. Pruritus becomes a major symptom, and secondary eczema occurs due to vigorous scratching.

Three forms of lice infest humans: the head louse, the body louse, and the pubic or crab louse.

Head Louse.—The major louse infestation in children involves the scalp. Children are more susceptible to pediculosis capitis than are adults, with girls more often infested than boys. For unknown reasons, blacks are not usually affected. Infestation occurs by direct contact with another individual or indirectly from hats, brushes, or combs. The female louse attaches her eggs to the hair shaft near the scalp surface. The egg hatches and the nit is left behind. The numerous nits attached to hair shafts (usually behind the ears or on the occiput) resemble dandruff. Pruritus of the scalp is common. Secondary excoriations and infection with cervical lymphadenopathy frequently occur from vigorous scratching.

Diagnosis is made by differentiation of the nits (which do not easily pull off or move freely along the hair shaft) from dandruff scales or artifacts in the hair (which do). The presence of nits is confirmed by removing a hair and looking for the attached nit under the microscope.

Pubic Louse.—Pubic lice infest the hairs and skin of the genital area, the lower abdomen, thighs, and occasionally the axilla. Preadolescents, especially, may have pubic lice in their eyelashes, eyebrows, and scalp lines. Transmission is usually venereal in adolescents and by close contact with infested adults (for example, the mother) in preadolescents. On occasion, indirect transmission occurs from clothing, bedding, and towels.

Excoriations secondary to pruritus frequently occur. With severe infestation, blue macules (maculae caeruleae) can be seen on the thighs, abdomen, or thorax. The exact cause is unknown, but they are thought to result from a substance released by the feeding louse.

Diagnosis is made by identification of nits attached to the hair shaft. Since hair grows slowly in the areas infested by the pubic louse, nits are usually found close to the skin surface.

Usually it is the pubic louse that attaches to eyelashes or eyebrows; on occasion, the head or body louse will. Crusting blepharitis, produced by the infestation, is often misdiagnosed because lice are not considered as a cause.

Body Louse.—The body louse lives in clothing or bedding and is found on the body only when feeding. Body lice feed frequently during the day or night when the host is quiet or inactive. They hide in the seams of clothing and attach their eggs to the cloth fibers.

Primary skin lesions are frequently obliterated by scratching. Pruritus is severe. Pressure points beneath collars, belts, and underwear are the usual sites for identifying bites. The face, scalp, hands and feet are usually spared.

Since body lice are not usually found on the body surface, diagnosis is made by searching the seams of clothing for nits or parasites.

MANAGEMENT

Head Lice

Treatment is carried out with 1% lindane (gamma benzene hexachloride) shampoo, 1% permethrin, 1% pyrethrin, or 10% crotamiton.

1% Lindane shampoo (Kwell)

1. Protect eyes with towel.
2. Apply enough shampoo to wet hair and scalp.
3. Work thoroughly into hair using water to produce lather and leave in place for 5 minutes.
4. Rinse hair thoroughly and towel briskly.
5. Allow hair to dry naturally (do not blow dry).
6. Repeat application of 1% lindane in 7 to 10 days.
7. Remove nits: Soaking hair with 3% to 5% acetic acid solution (NOTE: Regular vinegar is 5% acetic acid; therefore 1 part vinegar plus 2 parts water yields 3% acetic acid.); cover with towel saturated with this solution or apply mineral oil; comb hair with fine-toothed comb (special metal combs available include Medi Comb, Nitex Labs, Boston; Derboc Comb, Johnson Manufacturing, Boonton, N.J.; Innomed Comb, Innomed Inc., Greenwich, Conn.).

1% Permethrin creme rinse (Nix)

1. Shampoo hair and towel dry.
2. Saturate hair with creme rinse.
3. Leave on hair for 10 minutes.
4. Rinse off with water.
5. A single application is sufficient.

1% Pyrethrin (RID, R & C Shampoo, A-200, Cuprex) with piperonyl butoxide

1. Apply to scalp for 10 minutes.
2. Rinse out.
3. Let hair dry naturally.
4. Repeat in 7 to 10 days.
5. Remove nits.

10% Crotamiton (Eurax) cream or lotion

1. Apply to entire scalp.
2. Leave on for 24 hours.
3. Shampoo out.
4. Remove nits.

Pubic Lice

Each of the preparations used to treat head lice is also effective against pubic lice. Contacts must be treated as well. Lice on the eyelashes can be treated with a thick layer of white petrolatum applied two to five times per day for 8 days. Alternatives include 0.25% physostigmine (Eserine) four times a day for 3 consecutive days and 10% fluorescin drops.

Body Lice

Since body lice reside in clothing, patients do not need therapy; however, their clothing must be treated. Clothing and linens should be sterilized by boiling, steam under pressure, or the use of a hot iron over seams. The patient should be told to bathe frequently, change clothing frequently, and change bed clothes often. Symptomatic treatment of the skin can be accomplished with antipruritics (antihistamines or topical corticosteroids) and systemic antibiotics for infection.

SCABIES

Scabies has pruritus as its major symptom and a nonspecific skin eruption as its major sign. Frequent misdiagnosis is attributed to the variability and nonspecificity of the skin changes. The astute clinician will think of this disorder when a patient has uncontrolled itching.

BACKGROUND

The causative organism, *Sarcoptes scabiei*, completes its life cycle in humans. Fertilized female mites burrow into the stratum corneum, laying several eggs per day during a 1- to 2-month life span. Within 2 weeks the ova become adults. It is unusual for pruritus, the major symptom of this disorder, to occur earlier than 1 month after initial infestation. The duration of this latent period seems to indicate that pruritus is a result of sensitization to the organism.

The skin lesions include nonspecific papules, pustules, and vesicles (especially in infants). Linear burrows, rarely longer than 1 cm, occur in only 10% of patients and are frequently distorted by vigorous scratching and eczematization. Therefore, aside from the cardinal symptom of pruritus, one must rely on two major clues when making the diagnosis of scabies. Despite diffuse involvement, lesions are concentrated on the skin of the hands and feet (including the palms and soles in infants and young children) and in the folds of the body (axillae, groin, and especially the fingerwebs). Infants are more likely to develop blisters. They also will frequently have involvement of the skin of the face and head, in contrast to adolescents. The second point to elicit is whether family members and caretakers have pruritus and skin lesions.

The primary dermatitis of scabies can become secondarily infected. Persistent reddish brown pruritic nodules may develop. These remain despite adequate treatment and probably represent a reaction to dead mite parts. Norwegian scabies is that form of scabies infestation that produces thick, crusted lesions. It is usually seen in institutionalized, retarded, debilitated, or immunologically deficient individuals.

The diagnosis is made by examination of skin scrapings under the 10X objective for mites, ova, or fecal concretions. Mites are difficult to isolate, but persistence usually yields positive results. The materials required for examination of the skin for scabies includes a glass slide, immersion oil, and a No. 15 scalpel blade. A drop of immersion oil is placed on a glass slide and the edge of the No. 15 blade is dipped into it (the mite sticks to the oil). The skin is scraped and the material obtained is placed back into the drop of oil on the glass slide. A cover slip is placed over the oil, and the slide examined under the microscope.

MANAGEMENT

The most effective treatment for scabies at present is gamma-benzene hexachloride (GBH). It is available by prescription as a 1% cream, lotion, or shampoo. Reports of adverse effects have led some to question the safety of this chemical. There is no doubt that this medication is absorbed through the skin. Because of the large surface area of infants and young children relative to weight, the potential for significant absorption and toxic blood levels exists. A major concern is central nervous system toxicity (due to preferential concentration of lindane in brain substance). Although convulsions have been associated with topical application of lindane in children, in most cases use was excessive or prolonged or the insecticide was ingested. Therefore, some believe that when properly applied and not abused, GBH can be used safely.

Alternate drugs are also available, including crotamiton and sulfur ointment. Crotamiton is not as effective as GBH. Five percent sulfur in petrolatum has an unpleasant odor and stains clothing and bedding. Therapy for pruritus includes the use of oral antihistamines, medium-strength topical corticosteroids, and crotamiton.

1% Lindane (Kwell) lotion or cream

1. Avoid using on children younger than 1 year of age and on pregnant women.
2. Be certain that the patient's skin is cool and dry before applying lindane.
3. Apply from the neck down (all skin creases and between toes).
4. Wash off with soap and water.
5. Do not reapply lindane sooner than 1 week after the last treatment.
6. Treat all family members and close contacts simultaneously to prevent reinfestation.
7. Keep lindane out of reach of children to prevent accidental ingestion and poisoning.

10% Crotamiton lotion or cream

1. Apply from the neck down.
2. Leave on for 24 hours.
3. Reapply after 24 hours without removing the previous application.
4. Wash medication off with soap and water 48 hours after the initial application. Retreatment is frequently required.
5. Crotamiton is probably safe for use in children younger than 1 year of age and in pregnant women; however, safety has not been established is clinical trials.

5%–10% Sulfur in petrolatum

1. Apply from the neck down.
2. Reapply for three consecutive nights.
3. Wash off with soap and water after 72 hours.
4. Preparation is probably safe for use in infants younger than 1 year of age and in pregnant women.

BIBLIOGRAPHY

Atopic dermatitis

Caputo RV, Frieden I, Krafchik BR, et al: Diet and atopic dermatitis. *J Am Acad Dermatol* 1986; 15:543–545.

Hanifin JM, Lobitz WCJ: Newer concepts of atopic dermatitis. *Arch Dermatol* 1977; 113:663.

Krafchik BR: Atopic dermatitis. *Pediatr Clin North Am* 1983; 30:669.685.

Urticaria

Mathews KP: A current view of urticaria. *Med Clin North Am* 1974; 58:185.

Schuller DE, Elvey SM: Acute urticaria associated with streptococcal infection. *Pediatrics* 1980; 565:592.

Erythema multiforme

Edmond BJ, Huff JC, Weston WL: Erythema multiforme. *Pediatr Clin North Am* 1983; 30:631–640.

Howland WW, Golitz LE, Weston WL, et al: Erythema multiforme: Clinical, histopathologic and immunologic study. *J Am Acad Dermatol* 1984; 10:446.

Shelley WB: Herpes simplex as a cause of erythema multiforme. *JAMA* 1967; 201:53–156.

Drug eruptions

Arndt KA, Jick H: Rates of cutaneous reactions to drugs: A report from the Boston Collaborative Drug Surveillance Program. *JAMA* 1976; 235:918.

Contact dermatitis

Fisher AA: *Contact dermatitis*, ed 2. Philadelphia, Lea & Febiger, 1975.

Insect bite reactions

Honig PJ: Arthropod bites, stings and infestations: their prevention and treatment. *Pediatr Dermatol* 1986; 3:189.

Marks MB: Stinging insects, allergy implications. *Pediatr Clin North Am* 1969; 16:177–191.

Athlete's foot

Leyden JJ, Kligman AM: Aluminum chloride in the treatment of symptomatic athlete's foot. *Arch Dermatol* 1975; 111:1004–1010.

Diaper dermatitis

Berg RW, Buckingham KW, Stewart RL: Etiologic factors in diaper dermatitis: The role of urine. *Pediatr Dermatol* 1986; 2:102–106.

Honig PJ: Diaper dermatitis: Factors to consider in diagnosis and treatment. *Postgrad Med* 1983; 74: 79–88.

Weston WL, Lane AT, Weston JA: Diaper dermatitis: Current concepts. *Pediatrics* 1980; 66:532.

Acne

Atton AC, Tunnessen WN Jr: Acne update: Help your patients help themselves. *Contemp Pediatr* 1988; 5:18–50.

Lucky AW: Update on acne vulgaris. *Pediatr Ann* 1987; 16:29–38.

Schachner L: The treatment of acne: A contemporary review. *Pediatr Clin North Am* 1983; 30:501–510.

Scabies and lice

Honig PJ: Bites and parasites. *Pediatr Clin N Am* 1983; 30:563–581.

Honig PJ: Arthropod bites, stings, and infestations: Their prevention and treatment. *Pediatr Dermatol* 1986; 3:189–197.

Rasmussen JE: The problem of lindane. *J Am Acad Dermatol* 1981; 5:507–516.

Rasmussen JE: Pediculosis and the pediatrician. *Pediatr Dermatol* 1984; 2:74–79.

57 DIABETES MELLITUS

Barry S. Marx, M.D.
Charles A. Stanley, M.D.

Diabetes mellitus is one of the most common chronic diseases of childhood. In the United States, one in 350 to 600 children will develop diabetes by the age of 18 years. The most frequent form of diabetes in childhood, by current nomenclature, is called type I diabetes mellitus (formerly, juvenile or insulin-dependent diabetes), while that seen most frequently in adults is type II diabetes mellitus (formerly, maturity-onset or non-insulin-dependent diabetes). During the past decade, an increasing focus has been placed on efforts to maintain plasma glucose levels close to normal, particularly in adolescents and adults with type I diabetes. This trend derives not only from evidence linking metabolic control to the development of long-term diabetic complications, but also from the development of practical methods to measure blood glucose levels at home) and to objectively measure long-term blood glucose control (glycosylated hemoglobin). Efforts to improve glucose control have emphasized the role of the family as primary decision-makers in managing diabetes. The physician's responsibilities are to provide support and supervision for the family as educator, counselor, and medical consultant. This chapter will provide an outline of the approaches to outpatient management and common crises that the primary care physician encounters in children with diabetes.

BACKGROUND

Although type I diabetes can be considered a genetic disease, the inheritance does not follow classic mendelian recessive or dominant patterns. The concordance rate in identical twins is estimated to be only about 25%; the risk of diabetes in first-degree relatives (siblings, parents, or offspring) is also low, approximately 5%. As is true of other autoimmune diseases, the inheritance of type I diabetes is closely linked to the major histocompatibility loci of chromosome 6, particularly HLA antigens DR_3 and DR_4. The actual gene defect for type I diabetes is not known.

The current model for the development of type I diabetes mellitus involves some inherited predisposing factor that, in association with an environmental insult, leads to autoimmune destruction of the pancreatic β cells. Evidence for an autoimmune process includes the inflammatory round cell infiltrate of the islets of Langerhans seen in children who have died shortly after the onset of disease, and the recent demonstration of circulating antibodies directed against pancreatic β cells. Anti-islet cell antibodies can be demonstrated in most patients with type I diabetes at diagnosis. In a few patients, anti-islet cell antibodies have been found several years prior to diagnosis. This suggests that islet-cell destruction may be a chronic process in which clinically apparent diabetes does not occur until late in the disease, when most of the β cells are already destroyed.

There continues to be interest in the nature of the environmental insult responsible for initiating the autoimmune islet cell destruction in the genetically predisposed individual. Circumstantial evidence suggests that viral infections might play such a role. Coxsackie virus, mumps, and rubella have been linked to the incidence of type I diabetes historically and by demonstration of specific autobodies. This is an area of much uncertainty, however, particularly in view of the reports noted above, that the autoimmune process may begin years before the onset of clinical diabetes.

Long-term complications of type I diabetes include neuropathy, nephropathy, retinopathy, and accelerated coronary vascular disease. While few of these problems manifest in the pediatric patient, the more closely one looks for early changes, the more likely one is to see them. The current statistics for complications of type I diabetes are grim: 30% of patients show early changes of retinopathy within 5 years; 50% within 7 years; and 95% within 25 years of disease. Approximately one-half of patients with type I diabetes in the United States will develop renal failure caused by nodular or diffuse glomerulosclerosis within 20 years. While the impact of "tight control" on the incidence of complications is under study, experimental data from animal models link complications to hyperglycemia and show clinical improvement with better regulation of blood glucose.

DIAGNOSIS

The diagnosis of diabetes in childhood is usually straightforward. The onset of symptoms is most often acute, with a 1- to 2-week history of polydipsia and polyuria. Weight loss of 5% to 10% is common, but the parents may not be aware of it. Although polyphagia is classically part of the triad of symptoms of diabetes, the appetite may decrease as ketosis develops. The majority of patients are now recognized prior to the development of the severe hyperosmolar dehydration and metabolic acidosis that lead to diabetic coma.

The diagnosis of diabetes mellitus should be confirmed quickly to prevent further progression of dehydration and acidosis. A positive urine test for glucose and ketones provides presumptive evidence of diabetes. This can be confirmed by a random or postprandial blood glucose level over 200 mg/dL. Because most children already have markedly elevated blood glucose levels at the time of diagnosis, formal glucose tolerance testing is unnecessary. Stress-induced hyperglycemia may be distinguished from diabetes with serial postprandial blood glucose determinations for several days following presentation. Intravenous glucose tolerance testing should never be used.

MANAGEMENT

In considering strategies for managing type I diabetes, it is helpful to consider "closed-loop" and "open-loop" systems. The normally functioning pancreas provides an example of a close-loop system. Insulin need (due to changes in the levels of plasma glucose, amino acids, hormonal and neural inputs, etc.) is detected by the pancreatic β cell; insulin secretion rate is appropriately altered; and the effect of the change in insulin secretion is continuously monitored to make further adjustments on a minute-to-minute basis. This closed-loop system maintains plasma glucose levels in a narrow range of 80 to 120 mg/dL despite the wide variations in insulin requirements imposed by meals, exercise, and fasting. By contrast, all of the current methods for long-term management of insulin-dependent diabetes are open-loop systems, in which there is no direct connection between insulin requirement, insulin dose, and insulin effect. This absence of autoregulation explains why type I diabetes has been termed "brittle." To achieve optimal blood glucose control in children with diabetes, it is necessary to focus attention on three areas: (1) insulin administration in a manner that approximates normal β-cell secretion, (2) a diet plan designed to minimize variability in insulin requirements, and (3) methods of monitoring blood sugar responses to provide a basis for making decisions about changes in insulin dose, diet, etc. The patient and his/her family can be viewed as the external decision-makers responsible for working to match insulin dose with insulin requirement in "closing the loop." The sections that follow discuss the three components of the open-loop regulatory system: insulin dose regimens, diet, and monitoring.

INSULIN DOSE REGIMENS

Table 57–1 shows the time of peak effect and duration of action of the most commonly used insulin preparations. Familiarity with a short-acting insulin (insulin injection) and an intermediate-acting insulin (isophane insulin suspension or insulin zinc suspension) is usually sufficient, since most insulin regimens now being recommended use a combination of these two preparations. Three forms of insulin preparations are available: mixed beef and pork insulin, pure pork insulin, and human insulin.

TABLE 57–1
Action Profiles of Commonly Used Insulin Preparations

TYPE	TIME (HR)		
	ONSET OF ACTION	PEAK	DURATION OF EFFECT
Insulin injection	½–1	1½–2	4–6
Isophane insulin suspension	1–2	6–12	24–28
Prompt insulin zinc suspension	½–1	2–4	10–12
Insulin zinc suspension	1–2	6–12	24–28
Extended insulin zinc suspension	6	18–24	36+

There is little practical difference between these preparations. Anti-insulin antibody titers tend to be higher with mixed beef-pork insulin, but significant insulin resistance due to such antibodies is rare. Pure pork and human insulins are less antigenic, but cost about twice as much as beef-pork insulin.

The goal of insulin therapy is to approximate pancreatic insulin secretion with a low basal level between meals and overnight, and peaks of insulin to coincide with meals. The closest approximation of this pattern is provided with a subcutaneous insulin infusion pump. This device delivers a "background rate" of insulin infusion, and boluses of insulin prior to meals on command of the patient. In combination with close monitoring of blood glucose levels, it is possible to achieve very good diabetic control with insulin-infusion pumps; however, they are cumbersome and subject to malfunction and should be considered experimental in the pediatric age-group. Intensive programs, with three or four injections a day of insulin, with intermediate insulin to provide a background level during the night, achieve nearly as good diabetic control. These "tight control" regimens are usually reserved for highly motivated patients and are rarely used in children under the age of 13 years.

Currently, most diabetologists suggest twice daily injections of insulin for diabetic children of all ages. As a rough guide, the total daily insulin requirement equals 1 U/kg (range, 0.5–2.0). Two-thirds of the total is given 10 to 30 minutes before breakfast in a ratio of one part insulin injection to two parts isophane insulin suspension; the remaining third is given before supper in a ratio of one part insulin injection to one part isophane insulin suspension. This distribution must be individualized for each patient, based on experience. Single daily injections of insulin offer less flexibility in achieving control. With one shot a day, the total dose is again approximately 1 U/kg, given before breakfast as a mixture of one part insulin injection to three to five parts isophane insulin suspension.

All patients can now use U100 insulin preparations (100 U/mL). Patients taking less than 50 U can use 0.5-mL syringes; those taking over 50 U use 1 mL syringes. Injection sites should be rotated to avoid lipoatrophy or hypertrophy, using the skin over the triceps brachii, quadriceps, and gluteus medius muscles, and over the abdomen.

DIET

In the context of "open-loop" systems for regulating diabetes, the diet plan can be viewed as an effort to minimize day-to-day differences in insulin requirements. This is obviously an approximation, and a consideration of other factors affecting insulin requirements (such as exercise, growth, intercurrent illness, emotional stress, and variable rates of insulin absorption) may be important, particularly in programs designed to achieve "tight" diabetic control. The major elements of any diet plan for type I diabetes are: (1) regularity in the timing of meals, and (2) consistency in the amount of carbohydrate, fat, and protein eaten at each meal.

The American Diabetes Association (ADA) diet provides a convenient way of teaching patients and their families how to plan meals. The ADA diet groups foods into six "exchange" categories according to their content of carbohydrate, fat, and protein. Common household measures are used to determine the size of portions. This diet is sufficiently accurate that weighing of foods is unnecessary. It provides a basis for a high degree of flexibility in planning meals. Details on the ADA diet are provided in the references at the end of the chapter.

The diet for children with diabetes should be identical in total calories to that required by nondiabetic children of similar age and size (approximately 1,000 calories plus 100 calories per year of age). All diabetic children should have at least four meals a day: breakfast, lunch, supper, and a bedtime snack. The latter is important in avoiding nocturnal hypoglycemia, due to the effects of the evening isophane insulin suspension dose. A midmorning and midafternoon snack may be used in younger children and toddlers or in children who are prone to hypoglycemia in the late morning or afternoon.

It should be emphasized that the diet plan for children with diabetes is not aimed at restricting calories and need not eliminate sugar; with the ADA exchange lists, it is possible to incorporate all types of foods into the diet and plan "treats" of ice cream and cake, etc.

MONITORING

The goal of monitoring is to obtain sufficient data on levels of plasma glucose to permit appropriate decisions about changes in insulin dose. Until recently, only urine tests for glucose and ketones were available for use at home. Now, blood glucose testing at home is the preferred method of monitoring diabetes control. Some of the commonly used methods for home glucose monitoring are listed in Table 57–2. All use test strips impregnated with glucose-oxidase to measure the glucose level in a single drop of blood. Readings can be made by visual comparison with a color chart or by reflectance meter. Spring-loaded devices with fine lancets make obtaining a drop of blood by finger-prick nearly painless.

In addition to blood sugar testing, patients with diabetes should also know how to test urine for glucose and ketones with one of the methods shown in Table 57–2. The simplest methods use dip-sticks that test both glucose and ketone levels (Keto-Diastix, Chemstrip uGK).

The routine times for testing are before breakfast, lunch, dinner, and bedtime snack (i.e., when blood glucose levels are likely to be lowest). A useful time to check for possible nocturnal hypoglycemia levels is between 1 A.M. and 3 A.M. Records of test results should be kept to guide adjustments in insulin dose. Although patients are encouraged to test four times a day, when control is stable, it is reasonable to test less frequently but at least 14 times per week. A practical system for school-aged children uses breakfast and suppertime testing on weekdays, and four tests each day on the weekend. Urine should be tested for ketones during illness, or if blood sugar is above 240 mg/dL.

TABLE 57–2
Methods for Blood Glucose and Urine Testing at Home

METHOD	COMMENTS
Blood glucose test strips	
Chemstrip bG, Glucostix, etc.	May be used with meter or read visually
Glucoscan strips, etc.	Use with meter only
Visidex II	Read visually only
Finger-prick devices	
Monoject, Autoclix, Penlet, Glucolet, Autolet, etc.	Use same lancet (e.g., Monoject Lancet)
Autolance	Uses special lancet
Urine test strips	
Chemstrip uGK, Keto-Diastix	Measure ketones (0–large), glucose (0–5 or 2 g/dL), glucose specific
Chemstrip K, Ketostix	Measure ketones only
Chemstrip uG, Diastix,	Measure glucose only
Tes-Tape	Measure glucose only
Urine test tablets	
Acetest	Measures ketones (0-large)
Clinitest	Test-tube test for reducing sugars (0–2 g/dL)

GOALS FOR HOME MANAGEMENT AND GUIDELINES FOR DOSE ADJUSTMENT

The primary goals of diabetes management are:

1. Resumption of normal physical and social activities
2. Normal rates of growth and sexual maturation
3. Avoidance of episodes of hypoglycemia
4. Avoidance of symptoms of hyperglycemia
5. Avoidance of ketoacidosis

The secondary goal is to maintain plasma glucose levels as near normal as practical within the limitations imposed by the age of the child, the characteristics of the family, and the intensity of the "open-loop" system used to manage the diabetes. For example, in infants and children under the age of 10 years, it is necessary to accept higher levels of plasma glucose to avoid hypoglycemia. The degree of blood sugar control that can be attempted also depends on whether control is monitored with blood glucose or urine testing and on the frequency of insulin injections. For patients using only urine testing, it is usually possible to have about 50% of tests negative for glucose without seeing frequent hypoglycemic episodes. With blood glucose testing at home and twice-daily insulin injections, it should be possible to have about half of the readings in the range of 80 to 180 mg/dL. To get the majority of blood glucose readings between 80 and 150 mg/dL requires intensive regimens such as the use of multiple daily insulin injections or subcutaneous infusion pumps.

Adjustments in insulin dose for persistent hyperglycemia should be made gradually to avoid overshooting. Changes equal to about 5% of the total daily insulin dose can be made at intervals of 2 to 3 days. Recurrent hypoglycemia should be corrected aggressively by lowering the insulin dose by 20% each day until mild hyperglycemia persists and then readjusting the dose upward in small increments. This avoids the phenomenon of rebound insulin resistance with hyperglycemia, which lasts for several hours following a hypoglycemic episode. Such a "Somogyi phenomenon" should be suspected in a patient who has morning ketonuria with little or no glycosuria or in a patient taking more than 1 U/kg/day of insulin in whom control does not improve on higher doses.

CRISIS MANAGEMENT

HYPOGLYCEMIA

Hypoglycemia, the most common and most acute medical crisis in home management of diabetes, is the problem that children and parents understandably fear the most.

Hypoglycemia may occur as a result of exercise, a delay in eating, or as a complication of attempts at "tight control." Symptoms of hypoglycemia fall into two groups: those related to central nervous system (CNS) glucose deprivation and those related to adrenergic stimulation. Symptoms related to CNS glucose deprivation include hunger, lethargy, irritability, or confusion and may progress to generalized seizures. Adrenergic symptoms include tachycardia, sweating, pallor, and a feeling of anxiety and tremulousness.

Hypoglycemia must be treated promptly. Mild insulin reactions can be treated orally with the equivalent of 10 to 20 g of glucose. Liquids are preferred, such as 8 oz of fruit juice or soft drink. In emergencies, any source of carbohydrate will do: candy, bread, fruit, cookies, etc. Patients should be instructed to carry some form of sugar with them at all times. The use of hard candies should be discouraged, because they dissolve too slowly and present the risk of aspiration. Convenient packages of glucose tablets are now available at drugstores. Plastic tubes of cake icing (Cakemate), available in most supermarkets, are a reasonable substitute.

Families of children with diabetes should have glucagon available at home for treatment of severe insulin reactions if the child cannot readily eat or drink. Glucagon for injection is available in kits containing 1 mg of glucagon with a vial of diluent. The dose is 1 mg for children of all ages and can be given subcutaneously with an insulin syringe of either the 0.5-mL or 1-mL size. Plasma glucose level will rise within a few minutes and remain elevated for at least 60 to 90 minutes. Clinical improvement is usually rapid, but may be slower if the duration of hypoglycemia was prolonged. If the child is not fully alert and oriented within 15 to 30 minutes, the parents should consult with the physician.

KETOACIDOSIS AND INTERCURRENT ILLNESS

Ketoacidosis is a much less common crisis in home management of children with diabetes than hypoglycemia. The most frequent precipitating event, an intercurrent viral or bacterial infection, leads to an increase in insulin requirements. Less frequent causes include deliberate omission of insulin or emotional stress. Mild ketoacidosis can be corrected with appropriate therapy at home, if recognized early and treated before severe dehydration and acidosis develop.

Patients and parents should be instructed to monitor levels of plasma glucose and urine glucose and acetone more closely during intercurrent illnesses. As a general guide, the specific illness can be treated in the same way as in a nondiabetic child. Medications containing sugar need not be avoided, as the amount of extra sugar consumed is small compared to that already in the diet. Decongestants containing adrenergic drugs may cause mild hyperglycemia; this can be readily managed with small increases in the doses of short-acting insulin (see below). It is safest not to make increases in the dose of intermediate or long-acting insulin.

For moderate hyperglycemia leading to

symptoms of polyuria and for ketonuria, treatment should be started promptly to (1) provide supplemental short-acting insulin and (2) correct any dehydration. In addition to the usual dose of insulin, extra insulin injection should be given every 4 hours until the plasma glucose level falls to 200 mg/dL or less and ketonuria disappears. If ketonuria persists with the plasma glucose level below 200 mg/dL, carbohydrate-containing liquids should be given in addition to supplemental regular insulin until the ketones clear. The initial dose of supplemental regular insulin should be 10% to 20% of the usual total daily dose; this can be modified upward or downward depending on the degree of hyperglycemia and ketonuria and response to previous doses. Oral fluids should be encouraged to correct deficits and to replace ongoing urine losses (initially, at least 8 to 16 oz hourly). The child's thirst usually provides a good indication of fluid need. Parents should be carefully instructed to seek medical advice if significant improvement is not seen within 4 to 8 hours or if the child is vomiting.

WELL-PATIENT CARE

Regular office visits provide the physician an opportunity to (1) review the diabetes management by the family and the physiologic effects on the patient; (2) determine if there are areas in which the family needs additional education; and (3) assess the psychosocial adaptations of the patient and family. The family should present their blood glucose and urine test monitoring records to the physician and discuss adjustments they have made in the home regimen, including diet, activity, and insulin dose. The physical examination includes careful documentation of weight, height, and blood pressure. The funduscopic examination may reveal changes of diabetic retinopathy, although early changes may only be appreciated by an experienced ophthalmologist. The thyroid gland should be palpated routinely, as children with type I diabetes have an increased incidence of Hashimoto thyroiditis. Hepatomegaly may be seen with poor control (Mauriac syndrome). Injection sites should be examined for evidence of lipoatrophy or hypertrophy. Contractures of the interphalangeal joints of the fingers have been described in diabetic patients in poor control. The hands and fingers are placed flat together with the fingers spread. The patient with contractures is unable to bring the palmar surfaces of the fingers into contact along their entire length.

Measurement of glycosylated hemoglobin level is very useful as an objective indicator of glycemic control during the preceding 3 months, a period of time corresponding roughly to red blood cell life span. Normal ranges vary depending on whether total glycosylated or specifically HbA_{1c} is measured and must be obtained from the laboratory.

We recommend that the condition of a child with diabetes be evaluated periodically by a pediatric endocrinologist or diabetologist. There is no substitute for experience in the management of type I diabetes, and the diabetologist may be a valuable resource for the primary care physician both in routine management and crisis care. Children who have had diabetes for more than 5 years should have an annual ophthalmologic evaluation by an ophthalmologist with experience evaluating diabetic patients for retinopathy. This group of patients should also have a urine test for protein annually.

The psychosocial aspects of diabetes are critical to successful long-term management. Behavioral counseling begins at the time that the diagnosis of diabetes is made. The manner in which the child and family adjust to the diagnosis and education and the resources they are able to mobilize give important indications of potential problem areas. Parenting skills surrounding control vs. autonomy issues must be assessed and discussed in terms of the impact that the patient's disorder may have on family dynamics. Strategies for coping with such crises as refusal to test blood glucose level, administer insulin, or follow the meal plan should be worked out by the parents in consultation with the physician.

Behavior problems at home are often attributed to hypoglycemia, and therefore excused by parents. While we stress that unexplained irritability or lethargy may be a symptom of hypoglycemia, the behavior needs to be addressed in an appropriate manner by the family.

Invariably, there are families whose needs cannot be adequately met with office counseling. Referral to an appropriate psychological or psychiatric therapist should be initiated as quickly as possible. If therapy is to be effective, the primary physician and the therapist must coordinate their efforts to provide the patient and family with unambiguous goals and expectations. The inclusion of the therapist within the health care team emphasizes the importance of the family's involvement in counseling.

Implantable closed-loop pumps and pancreas transplants of β cell may ultimately become the therapy for type I diabetes. Until then, the family's decision-making skills and understanding of diabetes are the key to diabetic management. The family is supported in this by the primary care physician, in the role of educator, counselor, and consultant. The resources of other health care personnel, including dieticians, nurse-educators, and subspecialists such as diabetologists, ophthalmologists, and nephrologists are coordinated by the primary physician. Our goal in this chapter has been to provide a framework for the comprehensive approach to the care of the child with type I diabetes. Managing diabetes is not an easy task. It is time-consuming for the physician and requires an alteration of life-style for the family. With support from the primary care physician and other professionals, the quality of life of the family and child with diabetes can be greatly improved.

BIBLIOGRAPHY

1987 Buying guide: Diabetes supplies. *Diabetes Forecast* 1987; 32:46.

Castells S (ed): Symposium on juvenile diabetes. *Pediatr Clin North Am* 1984; 31:519–753.

MacDonald M (ed): Symposium on diabetes mellitus in children. *Primary Care* 1983; 10:529–760.

Travis L: *An Instructional Aid on Insulin-Dependent Diabetes Mellitus*, ed 8. Fort Worth, Texas, Stafford-Lowdon, 1988 (distributed by American Diabetes Association Texas Affiliate, 8140 N Mopac, Bldg 1, Suite 130, Austin, TX, 78759).

58 FEVER

David Jaffe, M.D.
A. Todd Davis, M.D.

While fever is not a disease itself, it is the most common sign of disease that causes parents to seek medical evaluation and advice. Since children with high fevers may appear uncomfortable, many parents worry that fever may harm their children, particularly that brain damage may result. The physician, knowing that a variety of treatable diseases are accompanied by fever, often determines whether and how soon a patient needs to be seen on the basis of the presence and height of fever, thereby adding, perhaps inadvertently, to parental anxiety about fever. Every parent of every child will eventually have to confront problems caused by fever: What has caused the fever? Will my child be harmed by the fever? How can I help my child to feel better and to get rid of the fever for good (or at least until next time)? The care with which the physician responds to these concerns at the time of a febrile illness often affects not only the level of trust that parents develop for the physician, but also the level of confidence that parents develop in their own ability to cope with their children's illnesses.

BACKGROUND

Body temperature is regulated by the hypothalamus. "Normal" temperature varies diurnally, with the high temperature occurring in the early evening and low in the early morning. Children show even more variability than adults, 0.9° C (1.6° F) between the ages of 2 and

6 years, and 1.1° C (2° F) in children over 6 years. There is also variability of "normal" set point temperature among individuals. In the appropriately clothed child, a rectal temperature greater than 38.0° C (100.4° F) is defined as fever.

To provide appropriate therapy, it is useful to distinguish between fever and heat illness when considering the pathophysiology of elevated body temperature. Heat illness (heat prostration, heat stroke) occurs when the normal temperature-regulating mechanisms are overwhelmed, usually by extraordinary environmental conditions such as strenuous exercise in hot, humid weather, prolonged sauna exposure, or accidental enclosure in hot automobiles.

In contrast, fever is a *regulated* elevation of body temperature. A variety of infectious agents, such as bacteria and viruses, as well as other substances such as antigen-antibody complexes and etiocholanolone act as *exogenous pyrogens*. These exogenous pyrogens stimulate both fixed and mobile phagocytic leukocytes to produce endogenous pyrogen, a small molecular weight protein, now thought to be identical to interleukin 1, which promotes lymphocyte proliferation as part of the inflammatory process. Endogenous pyrogen acts on thermoregulatory areas in the preoptic area of the hypothalamus, perhaps by stimulating production of prostaglandins of the E series. These thermoregulatory areas can be conceptualized as a thermostat that, when reset, causes physiologic and behavioral responses that change the core body temperature. When the thermostat is "reset" at a higher temperature, the organism suddenly "feels cold" and a variety of physiologic and behavioral responses occur. Metabolic rate and oxygen consumption increase. Mammals shiver and seek warmer environmental conditions. While these changes are occurring, the organism is developing a fever. Because they are regulated, febrile temperatures rarely, if ever, reach levels that are hazardous to the organism. In humans, fevers rarely reach 41.7° C (107° F).

APPROACH TO THE FEBRILE PATIENT

There is an extensive differential diagnosis for acute onset of fever. Before considering individual diagnoses, the primary care physician must assess the child's overall clinical appearance or "toxicity" and ascertain the immune status. These determinations will affect both the diagnostic focus and the management plan.

TOXICITY

No single clinical skill is more important to the management of acute febrile illness than the ability to recognize ill-appearing, or "toxic," children. While observational skills are subjective and based mainly on the examiner's clinical experience, there have been several recent attempts to develop quantitative observation scales to assist in initial assessment. The Acute Illness Observation Scale (AIOS) uses the following six variables: (1) quality of cry; (2) reaction to parent stimulation; (3) state variation; (4) color; (5) hydration; and (6) responses to social overtures (Table 58–1). Since toxic-appearing febrile children are likely to have life-threatening infections (Table 58–2), the physician must respond rapidly. In addition to a physical examination, "toxic" patients require complete blood cell (CBC), differential cell, and platelet counts; chest x-rays; urinalysis; and cultures of blood, urine, and cerebrospinal fluid. Assessment of arterial blood gases and of the status of the coagulation system may also be needed. Subsequently, these children should be admitted to the hospital. In general, broad-spectrum intravenous (IV) antibiotic therapy (e.g., ampicillin and chloramphenicol) is initiated until cultures either reveal a specific organism or are negative after 48 to 72 hours. In selected circumstances, however, the physician may elect to observe the patient closely in the hospital without starting antibiotics until the clinical diagnosis becomes evident or the culture results are known.

SPECIAL SITUATIONS

Immune Compromise.—Patients who are immune-compromised also require special diagnostic and therapeutic approaches. There are, of course, rare congenital immune deficiency syndromes such as Bruton agammaglobulinemia, DiGeorge syndrome, Wiskott-Aldrich syndrome or severe combined immune deficiency disease. Much more commonly, however, the physician will encounter children with ac-

TABLE 58–1
Predictive Model: Six Observation Items and Their Scales*

OBSERVATION ITEM	1 NORMAL	3 MODERATE IMPAIRMENT	5 SEVERE IMPAIRMENT
Quality of cry	Strong with normal tone *or* content and not crying	Whimpering *or* sobbing	Weak *or* moaning *or* high-pitched
Reaction to parent stimulation	Cries briefly then stops *or* content and not crying	Cries off and on	Continual cry *or* hardly responds
State variation	If awake → stays awake *or* if asleep and stimulated → wakes up quickly	Eyes close briefly → awake *or* awakes with prolonged stimulation	Falls to sleep *or* will not rouse
Color	Pink	Pale extremities *or* acrocyanosis	Pale *or* cyanotic *or* mottled *or* ashen
Hydration	Skin normal, eyes normal *and* mucous membranes moist	Skin, eyes-normal *and* mouth slightly dry	Skin doughy *or* tented *and* dry mucous membranes *and/or* sunken eyes
Response (talk, smile) to social overtures	Smiles *or* alerts (≤ 2 mo)	No smile, face anxious, dull, expressionless *or* no alerting (≤ 2 mo)	

*From McCarthy PL, et al: *Pediatrics* 1982; 70:802. Used by permission.

quired or age-related immune deficiency states.

Loss of splenic function is most commonly associated with sickle cell anemia, but it also occurs in congenital asplenia syndromes and in patients who have had therapeutic splenectomies either for control of hemorrhage in abdominal trauma or for treatment of idiopathic thrombocytopenic purpura, hereditary spherocytosis, or Hodgkin disease. Asplenia impairs the ability to fight polysaccharide-encapsulated organisms such as *Streptococcus pneumoniae* and *Hemophilus influenzae*. Systemic infections caused by these organisms account for the majority of childhood deaths in sickle cell anemia. Children with sickle cell anemia are 300 times as likely as normal children to acquire bacterial meningitis.

Children with cancer also often have compromised immunity. Many cancers affect the immune system primarily, especially lymphoma and leukemia. Most importantly, however, aggressive chemotherapy usually results in periods of time during which significant granulocytopenia occurs. Infection has become the proximal cause of death in 60% to 80% of children with leukemia and lymphoma and in 40% of children with solid tumors. Fever may be the only early sign of life-threatening infection in these unfortunate patients.

Acquired immune deficiency syndrome (AIDS) is another illness that is occurring with increasing frequency among children, especially in urban areas where illicit intravenous substance usage is prevalent. These children are susceptible to a wide range of infections, both opportunistic and non-opportunistic.

Other conditions associated with the impaired ability to fight infection include cystic fibrosis, nephrotic syndrome, and conditions that require chronic steroid therapy such as asthma, inflammatory bowel disease, or collagen vascular disease. While febrile reactions may be suppressed in children with such conditions, fevers that do occur must be taken seriously.

Management of fever in immune-compromised children must, of course, be tailored to suit the particular immune deficiency. In general, however, the physician's search for infection will be more intense and accelerated than for children with normal immune function. Chest x-rays may reveal pneumonia even in absence of classic physical signs, especially in younger children. Urinalysis may suggest urinary tract infection, especially if nitrites are discovered. However, normal urinalysis can occur in children who have urinary tract infections. Cultures of blood and urine provide the

TABLE 58–2
Selected Life-Threatening Conditions Associated With Fever*

- Infection
  - Central nervous system
    - Bacterial meningitis
    - Encephalitis
    - Brain abscess
  - Upper airway
    - Acute epiglottitis
    - Retropharyngeal abscess
    - Laryngeal diphtheria (rare)
    - Croup (severe)
  - Pulmonary
    - Pneumonia (severe)
    - Tuberculosis (miliary)
    - Bronchiolitis (severe)
  - Cardiac
    - Myocarditis
    - Bacterial endocarditis
    - Suppurative pericarditis
  - Gastrointestinal tract
    - Acute gastroenteritis (fluid/electrolyte losses)
    - Appendicitis
    - Peritonitis (other causes)
  - Systemic
    - Meningococcemia
    - Other bacterial sepsis
    - Rocky Mountain spotted fever
    - Toxic shock syndrome
- Collagen-vascular
  - Acute rheumatic fever
  - Systemic lupus erythematosus
  - Polyarteritis nodosa
  - Polymyositis
  - Kawasaki disease
  - Stevens-Johnson syndrome
- Miscellaneous
  - Thyrotoxicosis
  - Heat stroke
  - Acute poisoning: atropine, aspirin, amphetamine

*Adapted from Henretig F: Fever, in Fleisher G, Ludwig S (eds): *Textbook of Pediatric Emergency Medicine.* Baltimore, Williams & Wilkins, 1983, pp 149–158.

most definitive information about the presence of bacterial and fungal pathogens. Opportunistic organisms such as *Pneumocystis carinii,* fungal abscesses or fungemia, and a host of "nonpathogenic" bacteria must be suspected. Other laboratory tests and hospitalization will usually be required. Febrile children with neutropenia should receive broad-spectrum antibiotic coverage that is effective against *Pseudomonas aeruginosa* and enteric pathogens, as well as more common bacteria. A widely accepted regimen is cefazolin, ticarcillin, and tobramycin. Febrile children with splenic dysfunction, especially those with congenital asplenia or with sickle cell anemia, require an intensive search for encapsulated bacterial disease. All asplenic children with temperatures greater than 39.5° C should be hospitalized and receive intravenous antibiotic therapy effective against *S. pneumoniae* and *H. influenzae.* Febrile children under the age of 2 years with sickle cell hemoglobinopathy or asplenia and even very low-grade fevers (greater than 38.0° C) are often also admitted and treated pending culture results.

Neonate.—Neonates, defined here as children less than 2 months of age, have maturational deficiencies in immune function that render them susceptible to serious infection. Nonspecific immune mechanisms such as chemotaxis and opsonization for gram-negative organisms are developmentally immature. In addition, there may be as yet undiscovered immune abnormalities. Neonates often manifest fewer and more subtle signs of serious infection than do older children. Indeed, fever itself is not a consistent response to infection in the neonate due to a relative resistance of the hypothalamus to endogenous pyrogen. When fever occurs, the possibility of infection must be seriously considered. One recent study found 20% of febrile neonates (under 60 days) had a serious infection, although only 4% had bacteremia.

Mottling of skin, temperature instability, lethargy, and alteration of feeding are all clues to serious neonatal illness and should prompt a rapid response. Much more often, however, there will be a paucity of clinical signs of serious illness. Both because of this and the increased susceptibility of neonates to overwhelming serious infection, many institutions recommend that all febrile infants under 2 months of age receive a complete "sepsis workup" as outlined above for toxic-appearing children. In addition, broad-spectrum antibiotics are generally prescribed for all febrile neonates who appear ill or are less than 1 month of age. The choice of antibiotic should include coverage for gram-negative enteric organisms group B streptococci and *Listeria.* Ampicillin and an aminoglycoside are a suitable combination. In neonates between the ages of 1 and 2 months, *H. influenzae* becomes a potential cause of meningitis. Thus, for treating meningitis in the child over 1 month of age, we recommend ampicillin and chloramphenicol or penicillin and ceftriaxone, rather than ampicillin and an aminoglycoside.

DeAngelis and associates have recently documented iatrogenic complications in 20% of hospitalized febrile neonates. These included intravenous infiltrates, fluid overload, antibiotic overdosage, isolette malfunction, diarrhea, thrush, and chloramphenicol-induced bone marrow suppression. Many office-based physicians elect to treat well-appearing febrile neonates as outpatients. After completing the "sepsis workup," this strategy is acceptable provided that careful follow-up contact is assured.

TABLE 58–3
Common Infectious Causes of Fever in Children Seen in the Emergency Department*

Central nervous system
Acute bacterial meningitis
Viral meningoencephalitis
Oral cavity
Dental abscess
Herpangina
Herpetic gingivostomatitis
Mumps
Upper respiratory tract
Common cold
Pharyngitis
Cervical adenitis
Epiglottitis
Croup
Sinusitis
Otitis media
Pulmonary
Bronchiolitis
Pneumonia
Gastrointestinal tract
Acute gastroenteritis
Appendicitis
Genitourinary
Urinary tract infection
Acute salpingitis
Musculoskeletal
Septic arthritis
Osteomyelitis
Cutaneous or *systemic* with prominent rash
Cellulitis
Scarlet fever
Viral exanthems
Rocky Mountain spotted fever
Meningococcemia

*Adapted from Henretig F: Fever, in Fleisher G, Ludwig S (eds): *Textbook of Pediatric Emergency Medicine.* Baltimore, Williams & Wilkins, 1983, pp 149–158.

DATA GATHERING

ASSESSMENT

The vast majority of children with acute onset of fever will be neither toxic-appearing nor immune-compromised. While chronic fever (duration greater than 2 to 3 weeks) must begin at some time, the differential diagnosis and diagnostic approach to chronic fever differs considerably from that of acute fever and will be considered separately in this chapter.

Table 58–3 contains a list of the common infectious conditions causing acute fever in children. While most of the children with life-threatening infections such as meningitis, epiglottitis, acute appendicitis, meningococcemia, and Rocky Mountain spotted fever will appear "toxic" or can be identified with specific physical findings, occasionally these life-threatening conditions present more subtly, especially early in their course. In addition, a variety of less serious but treatable bacterial diseases such as pneumonia, otitis media, and streptococcal pharyngitis may be discovered. Thus, the search for specific signs and symptoms of infection is routine and important.

HISTORY

The history should include information about the duration and pattern of fever and associated symptoms such as cough, vomiting, and diarrhea. The volume of urine output will help estimate adequacy of fluid intake. Alteration in the child's activity level (i.e., sleeping, eating, and playing patterns) provides clues to the severity of illness. If old enough, the child may be able to provide specific information about ear pain, sore throat, or dysuria. In younger children, paradoxical irritability, manifest as increased irritability during attempts to rock or comfort the child, is a particularly important symptom suggesting meningitis. A history of exposure to others with similar illness may be useful. The physician should also inquire about recent immunizations, because fever can be caused by diptheria-pertussis-tetanus vaccine for 24 to 48 hours and by measles-mumps-rubella vaccine 7 to 10 days after immunization.

Toxic ingestions can also cause acute onset of fever, especially salicylates, atropine, phenothiazines, amphetamine, and tricyclic antidepressants. Generally, the child's caretaker discovers an ingestion; however, when fever and altered mental status are present, ingestion should be suspected even in the absence of a positive history.

The physician may use the time during the history taking to *observe* the child both for overall toxicity and for specific signs of illness. The respiratory rate is best counted prior to touching the child. Similarly, the presence and color of a rash can be observed. Also, notice peculiar postures assumed by the child that might indicate the presence of localized pain or airway compromise.

PHYSICAL EXAMINATION

The physical examination, already begun during the observation period, must then focus on specific important areas. Since otitis media is frequently found in febrile infants, the tympanic membranes must be examined. If necessary, remove cerumen to achieve adequate visualization. Mild redness of the tympanic membrane may be erythema secondary to the fever. In addition to redness, there should be dullness and poor mobility. The mouth may contain characteristic signs: anterior ulcers suggesting herpes stomatitis; posterior ulcers suggesting herpangina caused by coxsackievirus; Koplik's spots suggesting measles, etc. Evidence of pus on the tonsil does not always indicate a *Streptococcus* infection. Examination of the chest may be surprisingly benign in the presence of pneumonia, especially in children under 12 months old. Often, tachypnea and cough will be the only signs of pneumonia. The triad of tachypnea, flaring of the alae nasi, and end-expiratory grunting are signs of more advanced pneumonia. Meningism and/or a bulging anterior fontanelle are obviously important, but infants with meningitis who are under 12 to 18 months of age may have neither of these signs. Examine the abdomen for distention, localized rigidity, or tenderness. Again, appendicitis in the 2- to 3-year-old child may present few abdominal signs. Inspect extremities thoroughly for rashes, redness, and/or bony tenderness suggesting cellulitis, arthritis, or osteomyelitis.

If the history and physical examination fail to reveal a focus of infection, several possibilities remain:

1. A clinically silent focal bacterial infection exists that will be discovered with appropriate laboratory tests. Examples include urinary tract infection, pneumonia, and sinusitis.
2. The patient has a nonspecific, self-limited viral syndrome. This category accounts for 85% to 98% (depending on age and height of fever) of patients with acute onset of fever who have no discernible focal infection.
3. The patient does not have an infectious disease but rather is manifesting early signs of other entities associated with chronic fever such as collagen vascular disease or cancer.
4. The patient has bacteremia.

LABORATORY EVALUATION

There are no universally established indications for use of the various laboratory investigations that may assist in diagnosis of febrile illness. The younger or more ill-appearing the child and the higher the fever, the stronger are the indications to order laboratory tests. Many children will require no laboratory tests, either because the physical examination yields a specific diagnosis, or because, despite the failure to reach a specific diagnosis, the children appear relatively well, have exposure histories, and have rectal temperatures less than 40.0° C.

Complete Blood Cell Count.—On average, children with bacterial disease have higher total white blood cell (WBC) counts than do those with viral disease. Indeed, the phenomenon of transient bone marrow suppression by viral disease has been well described. However, the problem for the clinician arises when trying to interpret the meaning of the total WBC count in an individual child. Although the child with an elevated WBC count is more likely than one with a low WBC count to have bacterial disease, that same child is still even more likely to have self-limited disease, with no detectable bacterial pathogen than to have bacterial disease. In one series, 88% of children with WBC counts over 30,000/mm^3 had no bacterial disease. In other words, the background rate of bacterial disease is so low that, although an elevated WBC count raises the probability of bacterial disease somewhat, viral disease is still the most likely cause among febrile children with high WBC counts.

Radiography.—Radiography of the chest and, less commonly, of the paranasal sinuses will occasionally reveal unsuspected infections. Although normal respiratory rates vary with age, a convenient guide is that a chest radiograph is absolutely indicated for resting respiratory rates over 50/min (in absence of wheezing) and relatively indicated for rates between 40 and 50/min in febrile children.

Cultures.—Cultures of blood urine, cerebrospinal fluid, oropharynx, and stool will yield definitive diagnoses when positive. However, most cultures require 1 to 3 days to incubate. Positivity rates are fairly low and seem to depend to some extent on age and degree of fever.

When no apparent focus of infection is present, but the child appears ill enough to obtain cultures, the blood and urine will yield bacterial pathogens about 3% to 5% of the time. Pharyngitis in children under 2 years old is rarely caused by group A β-hemolytic streptococci. Nonetheless, throat culture is indicated in selected children less than 2 years of age and in all children over 2 years of age with pharyngitis.

The decision to perform a lumbar puncture remains one of the hallmarks of the "art" of pediatrics. Because meningitis can present subtle signs in young infants, it is generally recommended that all febrile neonates (under 8 weeks old) undergo cultures of cerebrospinal fluid. For infants over 8 weeks old, clinical judgment becomes the decisive factor. Meningism and/or a bulging anterior fontanelle in any febrile child are indications for a lumbar puncture. A febrile seizure in children under 18 months old is also a strong indication to obtain a culture of cerebrospinal fluid. Some children, however, receive lumbar punctures either because of a history of paradoxical irritability or because they appear either more lethargic and/or irritable than would be expected for their age and degree of fever.

MANAGEMENT

TREATING THE SOURCE OF THE FEVER

Treatment of febrile children encompasses two separate issues. First, of course, treatable sources of fever must be managed, in general, by prescribing appropriate antibiotic therapy for focal bacterial infection. Newer antiviral agents are available for certain serious viral infections such as herpes encephalitis and respiratory syncitial virus pneumonitis. Such cases, when suspected, should generally be referred to tertiary care centers for diagnosis and management. Most viral diseases, however, require no specific antibiotic therapy. Noninfectious causes of fever such as collagen vascular disease or cancer will also require specific management strategies in conjunction with appropriate specialty consultants.

Occult bacteremia in febrile infants has received much attention during the past decade. Approximately 5% of children between the ages of 3 and 36 months with high fevers (greater than 39.0° C) have bacteremia. *S. pneumoniae* causes at least 70% of such cases, while *H. influenzae*, *Salmonella* species, and others cause the rest.

Depending on the organism, bacteremia resolves in as many as 50% of untreated children without any sequelae. Bacteremia can, however, lead to both serious and minor focal sequelae such as meningitis, pneumoniae, arthritis, osteomyelitis, and otitis media.

Research has focused on two major issues: (1) Are there variables that permit the primary care physician to predict with accuracy which children are likely to have bacteremia? (2) Are the serious sequelae of bacteremia preventable by early expectant use of oral antibiotics, and, if so, at what cost?

Age, temperature, total WBC count, erythrocyte sedimentation rate, and clinical observational scales have all been used as variables to increase detectability of bacteremia. The contribution of "high-risk" values of each individual variable to the detection of bactermia appears to be small. One excellent prospective study demonstrated bacteremia in 15% of children under 2 years old, with rectal temperatures greater than 40° C and total WBC counts greater than 15,000/mm^3 (or sedimentation rates greater than 35 mm/hr). Unfortunately, however, in the same group of children, half of those with bacteremia had total WBC counts of less than 15,000/mm^3.

Long before occult bacteremia was well-defined, physicians had been prescribing antibiotics for children with fevers but no localizing signs of infection. More recently, some retrospective studies have suggested that "expectant" use of oral antibiotics may benefit a subset of young, highly febrile children who carry a small but finite risk of having bacteremia.

Two prospective studies, both small with respect to the number of bacteremic children studied, have yielded somewhat conflicting results. Carroll et al. reported that parenteral penicillin hastened recovery and prevented infectious morbidity. Jaffe et al., however, reported that oral amoxicillin hastened clinical recovery but did not prevent infectious morbidity. While larger multicenter clinical trials of amoxicillin and ceftriaxone are under way, the office physician may choose from several acceptable management alternatives.

When careful follow-up is assured, most children can be treated as if they have viral illness. They require neither antibiotic therapy nor outpatient blood cultures. Well-appearing children under the age of 24 months with rectal temperatures over 40.0° C probably should have blood cultures. It is then a matter of preference whether "expectant" antibiotic therapy is used. Amoxicillin is currently the drug of choice for this situation. If the blood culture is negative at 48 to 72 hours, the amoxicillin should be stopped.

TREATING THE FEVER

In addition to treating the underlying cause of fever, the pediatrician should develop an approach to the treatment of fever itself. Three issues arise: (1) establishing a threshhold temperature above which antipyretic therapy is instituted; (2) determining the best antipyretic regimen; and (3) managing parental concerns about fever.

There is some disagreement in the pediatric literature about when and whether to provide antipyretic therapy for fever. Proponents of early and vigorous treatment cite patient comfort and prevention of febrile seizures as reasons for treatment. Opponents of this approach refer first to the phylogenetic argument that fever represents an adaptation of the organism to fight infection. Some animal research has shown improved response to experimentally induced infection at higher body temperatures; however, neither the application of these findings nor the precise mechanism of action has been established. Regarding febrile seizures, opponents of vigorous antipyretic therapy emphasize that febrile seizures often occur within the first 24 hours of a febrile illness, before parents are aware of their child's fever. Another hazard of vigorous therapy is potential overdosage with either aspirin or acetaminophen by anxious, well-intentioned, but overzealous parents. There is also concern that pharmacologic fever control will mask important signs of illness and obscure diagnosis.

A middle course between the two extreme positions seems reasonable. Low fevers (under 38.5° C) unaccompanied by apparent discomfort may be left untreated. Children with temperatures of greater than 38.5° C or any child appearing uncomfortable should be treated. Both aspirin and acetaminophen will lower the hypothalamic "set point" temperature effectively for 3 to 4 hours. Alternating aspirin and acetaminophen on a 2-hour schedule often confuses parents and leads to overdosage. This regimen is rarely, if ever, indicated. Recent epidemiologic data linking aspirin use to Reye syndrome has led the American Academy of Pediatrics to recommend against the use of aspirin for treating fever associated with varicella or influenza. A safe and reasonable approach is to recommend acetaminophen (or aspirin, except as noted above) in a dose of 10 to 15 mg/kg every 4 to 6 hours for fever while the child is awake.

Sponge bathing in tepid water will reduce body temperature. If no antipyretic medication is provided, however, the child will experience discomfort and the benefit will be temporary. Alcohol bathing is hazardous because hypoglycemia may result.

Finally, parental concerns about fever must be addressed. Many parents believe that fever may harm their children. It is often useful for the physician to explore parental concerns specifically. Discussion can then begin with a review of the diagnostic effort that has occurred. If a specific cause of the fever has been discovered, then, of course, its nature, course, and management should be discussed. Those antipyretic measures selected should be explained. Most important, parents often require specific reassurance that fever is a transient state that will not cause any permanent harm to their children.

FEVER OF UNKNOWN ORIGIN

In some instances, fever may persist and cause parents to be concerned about the presence of a serious underlying disorder. One must be certain to detect and treat serious infections or potential life-threatening disease while at the same time recognizing that many children with fever of unknown origin have a benign self-limiting process and should not be subjected to extensive, painful, or unnecessary laboratory investigation.

The most commonly used definition for fever of unknown origin in childhood was expounded by Dechovitz and Moffett. This definition includes a fever of 101° F or more for 2 weeks without a recognized site of infection. When this definition is *not* met, one usually uses the term "fever without localizing findings."

Broad categories of disease processes frequently found in children with fever of unknown origin include infections, collagen vascular disease (including inflammatory bowel disease), malignancies, miscellaneous conditions, and, finally, undiagnosed illness. The relative distribution of these disease processes varies with the age of the child (Table 58–4). At all ages, infectious diseases are the most

TABLE 58–4
Final Diagnoses in 100 Patients With Fever of Unknown Origin*

<6 YR (N = 52)		≥6 YR (N = 48)	
DIAGNOSIS	NO. OF PATIENTS	DIAGNOSIS	NO. OF PATIENTS
Infectious	34	Infectious	18
Viral syndrome	13	Viral syndrome	4
Urinary tract infection	3	Endocarditis	3
Bacterial meningitis	3	Infectious mononucleosis	2
Pneumonia	3	Streptococcosis	2
Tonsillitis	3	Osteomyelitis	1
Septicemia	2	Sinusitis	1
Sinusitis	2	Tonsillitis	1
Generalized herpes simplex	1	Tuberculosis	1
Malaria	1	Typhoid fever	1
Peritonsillar abscess	1	Urinary tract infection	1
Osteomyelitis	1	Pneumonia	1
Enteric fever	1		
Collagen-inflammatory	4	Collagen-inflammatory	16
Rheumatoid arthritis	3	Rheumatoid arthritis	7
Henoch-Schönlein purpura	1	Lupus erythematosus	3
		Regional enteritis	4
		Ulcerative colitis	1
		Vasculitis (undefined)	1
Malignancy	4	Malignancy	2
Leukemia	3	Lymphosarcoma	1
Reticulum cell sarcoma	1	Leukemia	1
Miscellaneous	7	Miscellaneous	3
Central nervous system fever	2	Behçet syndrome	1
Agranulocytosis	1	Hepatitis, anicteric	1
Lamellar ichthyosis	1	Ruptured appendix	1
Milk allergy	1		
Aspiration pneumonia	1		
Agammaglobulinemia	1		
Undiagnosed	3	Undiagnosed	9

*From Pizzo PA, et al: *Pediatrics* 1975; 55:468–473. Used by permission.

common cause. Among the collagen vascular diseases, rheumatoid arthritis is more common than inflammatory bowel disease in children less than 5 or 6 years of age, whereas the reverse is true in children more than 6 years old. In all pediatric age groups, malignant disorders account for less than 10% of cases.

In evaluating children with fever of unknown origin, it is important to remember that 75% or more will have common pediatric diagnoses. An extensive history is required to begin sifting through the various diagnostic possibilities. The early events in the disease process should be sought, including signs and symptoms, the epidemiologic setting, and season of the year. It is important to determine other past diseases that the child may have encountered such as a urinary tract infection, or previously documented but undiagnosed fever that might indicate a relatively clinically silent source of infection. Previous behavioral or psychiatric difficulties might indicate the possibility of a factitious fever. Reservoirs of infection must be ascertained such as an undiagnosed contagious case of tuberculosis; a grandparent who might be a typhoid carrier; attendance in a daycare center that might be sustaining an unrecognized outbreak of hepatitis; unusual food habits in the family such as preference for raw meat, a potential source of toxoplasmosis; or a pet bird that might harbor *Chlamydia psittaci*, the etiologic agent of psittacosis. If pica is present, one should consider the diagnosis of *Toxocara canis* or *Toxocara cati*. Since many children with regional enteritis have absent or vague gastrointestinal tract symptoms, the physician must inquire specifically about anorexia, changes in bowel habit, weight loss, or intermittent abdominal pain.

The most important part of the physical examination is the observation of the general appearance of the child and the comparison of current weight with previous weight. Weight loss should be viewed as a serious sign that mandates a comprehensive evaluation with laboratory and radiologic studies. Examination of each organ system is frequently rewarding. Tenderness may be detected over the sinuses, although this is not an invariable sign of sinusitis. Sinusitis is a frequently overlooked cause of fever of unknown origin. It is important particularly to observe the skin for evidence of a heliotrope rash, suggestive of dermatomyositis, or a facial rash that might indicate systemic lupus erythematosus or a mixed collagen vascular disease. Heart murmurs must be sought to detect the occasional case of endocarditis. Examination of the abdomen may reveal splenic enlargement that may indicate malignancy or unrecognized mononucleosis. Pain or a mass in the right lower quadrant of the abdomen suggests the possibility of inflammatory bowel disease. There may be generalized lymphadenopathy with a lymphoma or with an infectious process such as cytomegaloviris, toxoplasmosis, or some other viral pathogen. Muscle pain may indicate polymyositis. Bone pain may be seen with osteomyelitis or tumor infiltration.

After completion of the history and physical examination, the physician must make an assessment about the likelihood of making a definite diagnosis and whether a treatable or a life-threatening condition is present. If the patient appears chronically ill or has sustained weight loss, hospitalization and a full diagnostic evaluation should be considered. If, on the other hand, the child appears healthy, has had little or no weight loss, and has normal findings on physical examination, the likelihood of serious illness or a treatable bacterial disease is diminished, and a less extensive outpatient evaluation is appropriate. In the latter circumstance, the following tests should be ordered:

1. CBC count, with WBC and differential cell count
2. Erythrocyte sedimentation rate
3. Sinus and chest radiographs
4. Urine culture

Other tests can be added, depending on the history. For example, if mononucleosis is occurring in the community, then rapid test for heterophil antibodies (Mono-spot test) and an Epstein-Barr virus titer are indicated.

For more worrisome signs or symptoms, the same screening tests need to be done along with some or all of the following procedures:

1. Bone scan
2. Gallium scan
3. Abdominal ultrasound
4. Upper and lower gastrointestinal tract series
5. Blood cultures
6. Stool cultures
7. Febrile agglutinin titers

should receive earlier iron supplementation than a child without a similar perinatal history. After menarche, the adolescent girl will have a greater risk of developing iron deficiency and should receive adequate iron supplementation to her diet. The development of iron deficiency in a child whose age is outside the two major risk ages should lead to a vigorous search for a source of blood loss as body growth is slow and the diet should be sufficiently varied to contain adequate sources of iron. The blood loss often occurs from an obvious source such as menorrhagia or recurrent epistaxis or rectal bleeding as might be seen in a child with Meckel diverticulum or polyp.

Data Gathering

Most commonly, iron deficiency anemia is diagnosed either from a routine complete blood cell (CBC) count or from a patient's pale appearance. Iron deficiency may result in neurologic dysfunction with increased irritability, shorter attention span, and poor scholastic performance. Well-controlled clinical studies have shown behavioral and scholastic improvements when iron-deficient children are appropriately treated. Whether iron deficiency can result in permanent long-term neurologic impairment is unknown.

Other unusual manifestations of iron deficiency include the presence of pica, a persistent or purposeful ingestion of material with no nutritive value. Often the pica disappears with adequate iron replacement. It is presently uncertain whether severely iron-deficient children have an increased incidence of infections reflecting a decrease in the bactericidal activity of polymorphonuclear cells in iron deficiency.

Results of physical examination are often normal although signs of pallor may be present. The child may be irritable and restless although often this aspect of the child's iron deficiency is only noticed in retrospect after treatment. Physical examination rarely reveals tachycardia and congestive heart failure, as the anemia develops slowly allowing sufficient time for compensation. Examination of the hands in severe iron deficiency may reveal spooning of the nails (koilonychia). In children with iron deficiency, atrophic glossitis is not seen.

Iron deficiency anemia is a microcytic hypochromic anemia with a low reticulocyte count (Fig 59–1). An elevated free erythrocyte protoporphyrin (FEP) level in the range of 40 to 160 μg/dL provides sufficient laboratory data to support the diagnosis of iron deficiency. An FEP level over 200 μg suggests lead poisoning. The test to determine the FEP level is a rapid spectrophotometric test that can be done on 20 μL of whole blood. Other laboratory tests determining the body's iron status such as obtaining values for serum ferritin, iron, and iron binding capacity, or bone marrow aspiration either require larger amounts of blood or are more invasive.

Management

In a child with findings of a history and physical examination consistent with iron deficiency anemia and in whom laboratory data reveal a hypochromic microcytic anemia and an elevated FEP level, it is proper to administer a trial of iron supplementation and observe the patient carefully for a therapeutic response under the assumption that the patient has iron deficiency anemia.

Since treatment can be accomplished by the oral supplementation of iron, blood transfusion or intramuscular iron-dextran can be avoided in virtually all cases. The most common iron salt used is ferrous sulfate that is 15% by weight elemental iron. In treating iron deficiency anemia, 6 mg/kg/day of elemental iron should be given, divided into three doses. Larger doses will have increased side effects (mainly constipation) without improved speed of therapeutic recovery. Changes in behavior are often noted by the second day of treatment. At the end of 1 week of therapy, a reticulocytosis occurs that is followed by a rise in the hematocrit level of about 1% per day. A normal hematocrit value for age is achieved during the first month of treatment. Full dose iron supplementation should be continued for a total of 2 months to ensure adequate iron stores. In addition, therapy should include appropriate dietary counseling and analysis for potential sources of iron loss to avoid a recurrence of the iron deficiency.

Failure to respond to oral iron supplementation is often due to poor compliance or inadequate dosage. This can often be verified by finding that the child's stools are not black (as would occur if the iron was properly adminis-

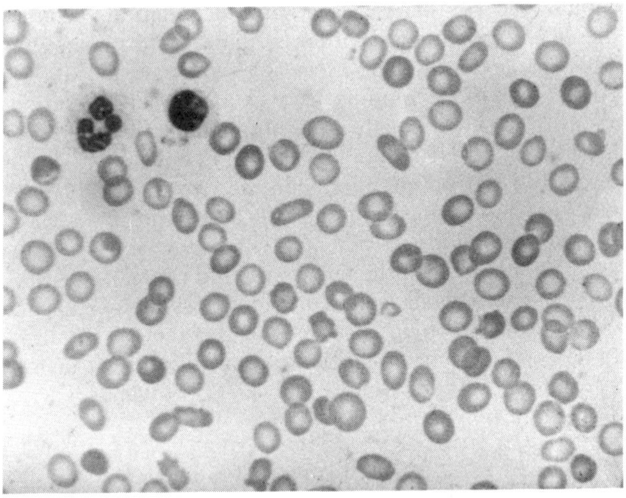

FIG 59–1
Blood smear from patient with iron deficiency anemia showing microcytic hypochromic cells with some misshapen red cell forms.

tered). If on-going blood loss is present, the child may only partly respond to the iron treatment. The presence of a concurrent chronic illness may also interfere with the body's ability to respond to the iron supplementation. Rarely, impaired gastrointestinal absorption may underlie a poor response. Finally, the diagnosis of iron deficiency anemia may have been incorrect. Often children with thalassemia trait are misdiagnosed as having iron deficiency anemia and receive prolonged courses of unnecessary iron therapy. Any child treated for iron deficiency based on a CBC count and an elevated level of FEP should be followed up to ensure that there is an appropriate response. If there is not an adequate response, part of a further evaluation should be a more extensive evaluation of the child's iron status, including determination of a serum iron level and iron binding capacity.

THALASSEMIA

Background

Hemoglobin is a tetramer of 2 α-like and 2 β-like globin chains, each of which is bound to a heme moiety. Thalassemia refers to a decreased production of a globin chain (e.g., β-thalassemia refers to an underproduction of β-globin chains and α-thalassemia refers to an underproduction of α-globin chains).

The incidence of both α-thalassemia and β-thalassemia are highest in ethnic groups originating from the world's malarial belt. This includes people from the Mediterranean region, Africa, the Near East, India, and Southeast Asia. In some groups, the incidence of the thalassemias can be surprisingly high. In blacks, the α-thalassemia gene can be found in 30% of the population; while in Cypriots, the incidence of the β-thalassemia gene is about 10%.

Data Gathering

Depending on the exact thalassemia syndrome inherited, the hematologic consequence can vary from an inapparent carrier state, to a mild hypochromic microcytic anemia, to a severe life-threatening anemia, and even to hydrops fetalis and stillbirth. The following discussion will first describe the β-thalassemias and then the α-thalassemias, the two most common thalassemia syndromes. Their pattern of inheritance, clinical manifestations, ethnic groups affected, and laboratory diagnosis are sufficiently different to warrant separate discussions.

There are two β-globin genes in every person, one on each chromosome 11. There are, therefore, three possible patterns of inheritance: (1) completely normal, having inherited two functional β-globin genes; (2) β-thalassemia trait in which one of the two β-globin genes is dysfunctional; and (3) homozygous β-thalassemia in which both of the β-globin genes are dysfunctional. The child with β-thalassemia trait is often of Mediterranean origin (although he may belong to any of the other ethnic groups mentioned above). The anemia is mild (e.g., the hemoglobin level is usually 9 to 11 g/100 mL), with a significant degree of hypochromia and microcytosis. There is a greater degree of microcytosis in thalassemia trait compared to that in a child with iron deficiency and a similar degree of anemia. Laboratory evaluation for iron deficiency anemia should be normal. A CBC count of the parents should reveal that at least one of them has hypochromic microcytic red blood cell (RBC) indices, although the parent may not be anemic, as adults with β-thalassemia trait can have a normal hemoglobin level. A quantitative analysis of the hemoglobins present in the child's blood will confirm the diagnosis of β-thalassemia trait revealing an increased level of hemoglobin A_2 (a minor adult hemoglobin). This quantitation cannot be reliably done by photometric scanning of a hemoglobin electrophoresis gel as performed in many hospitals but must be quantitated in a laboratory with an appropriate technique such as column chromatography.

Homozygous β-thalassemia (thalassemia major) is very often a severe life-threatening anemia that becomes clinically apparent after about 6 months of age when the fetal blood is replaced by adult blood. Usually the child has a severe hypochromic microcytic anemia (Fig 59–2), often with hepatosplenomegaly that in part is secondary to extramedullary hematopoiesis. Hemoglobin electrophoresis will reveal a predominance of hemoglobin F (fetal hemoglobin) with little or no adult hemoglobin A. The proper management of such a child's condition should be done by a pediatric hematologist trained in the management of such cases.

Every person inherits four α-globin genes, two on each chromosome 16. There are, therefore, five potential clinical states as shown in Table 59–1. In blacks, virtually all the α-thalassemia chromosomes involve a single α gene deletion (α–) and therefore only the silent carrier (α–/αα) or α-thalassemia trait (α–/α–) are seen. In contrast, both the single gene deletion chromosome (α–) and the double deletion (– –) are seen in Southeast Asians. This is the reason that in Southeast Asians, hemoglobin H disease (α–/– –) and hydrops fetalis (– –/– –) are seen as well as the silent carrier and α-thalassemia trait.

The diagnosis of the silent carrier and α-thalassemia trait cannot be made by hemoglobin electrophoresis except in the newborn period in which hemoglobin Bart (consisting of tetramers of the fetal β-like globin chain called γ) can be detected. The most reliable method at present to detect the majority of α-thalassemia syndromes involves DNA analysis. These studies are done in referral centers and should only be necessary in those cases in which an actual or potential risk exists of having a severely affected child. In a well black child with a mild hypochromic microcytic anemia not due to iron deficiency or lead poisoning (as screened by an FEP determination) or to β-thalassemia trait (shown by a normal hemoglobin A_2 level), the diagnosis of α-thalassemia trait is made by exclusion and no further testing need be done,

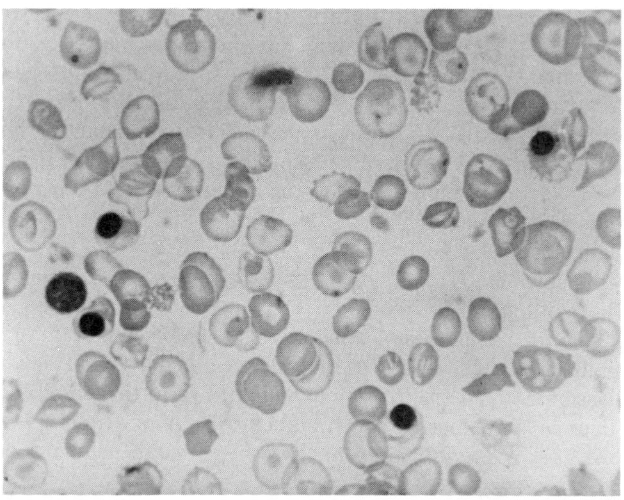

FIG 59–2
Blood smear from a splenectomized patient with thalassemia major showing severe hypochromia, microcytosis target cells, and nucleated red blood cells.

TABLE 59–1
Thalassemia Syndromes, Clinical State, and Diagnosis

DIAGNOSIS	ARRANGEMENT OF α GENES*	HEMATOLOGIC STATUS AND LABORATORY DIAGNOSIS
Normal	αα/αα	Normal
Silent carrier	α−/αα	Clinically normal. Less than 2% hemoglobin Bart (γ_4) in the newborn period.
α-Thalassemia trait	α−/α− or αα/−−	Mild hypochromic microcytic anemia. 2% to 10% hemoglobin Bart in the newborn period.
Hemoglobin H	α−/−−	Moderately severe anemia, significant α/β globin chains synthesis imbalance.
Hydrops fetalis	−−/−−	Often stillborn. Incompatible with long-term survival except with a chronic RBC transfusion program.

*In the table "α" refers to a functional α gene, while "−" refers to a nonfunctional gene. The "/" separates the maternal and paternal chromosomal pattern.

while in an Oriental patient, the risk of having more affected children should lead to a more complete genetic evaluation of the family.

Management

Genetic Counseling.—The importance of establishing the diagnosis of thalassemia trait in a child is multifold. By confirming the proper diagnosis, unnecessary and potentially harmful administration of iron therapy can be avoided. In addition, proper genetic counseling can be done. In β-thalassemia, the parents of a child with the trait should be tested to be sure that both are not carriers of the thalassemia trait. If both parents are carriers, then there is a one in four risk of having a child with severe homozygous β-thalassemia. The potential risks of the child with the trait marrying another person with the trait should also be discussed. Prenatal diagnosis for the thalassemias is now available and should be offered to the parents if a child severely affected with thalassemia is a potential outcome.

In blacks with α-thalassemia, there is virtually no risk of having a severely affected child. Genetic counseling should emphasize this point. However, in Oriental families with α-thalassemia the risks of having a severely affected child exists, and the pediatric hematologist who confirms the α-thalassemia diagnosis should also provide genetic counseling.

HEREDITARY SPHEROCYTOSIS

Background

Hereditary spherocytosis, the most common intrinsic red blood cell (RBC) membrane defect known, is an autosomal dominant disorder. It results in a hemolytic anemia with spherocytosis. Approximately 15% of cases are sporadic, with neither parent affected. In the United States, the incidence is one in 5,000, occurring most commonly in people of Northern European descent.

Recent studies have shown that hereditary spherocytosis is a defect in the RBC membrane's skeleton. The membrane's skeleton contains four proteins: spectrin, actin, protein 4.1, and ankyrin. At least several cases of hereditary spherocytosis are due to a defective spectrin molecule. The membrane abnormality results in an increased influx of sodium ion into cells and in a greater utilization of energy by the RBC to maintain its electrolyte balance. The cells are more susceptible to destruction inside the spleen, resulting in a shortened RBC life span.

Data Gathering

Hereditary spherocytosis can present at any age. In the neonatal period, early and severe hyperbilirubinemia should raise the possibility of hereditary spherocytosis. A palpable spleen is often present. However, in the newborn period, spherocytes can also be seen in other common disorders such as ABO incompatibility. Examination of the peripheral blood smears of the parents can assist in the proper diagnosis.

In older children, the diagnosis is made while evaluating a mild normochromic normocytic anemia. Occasionally, the patients' initial presentation is due to an acute severe anemia. The etiology of this severe anemia can be either an aplastic crisis with no RBC production or a hemolytic crisis with increased RBC destruction. Both can follow a viral illness. The child has a rapid and significant drop in hemoglobin level, sometimes resulting in heart failure. Deficiency of G-6-PD and autoimmune hemolytic anemia can also present in a similar fashion, and enzyme quantitation studies and Coombs' test, respectively, should help in the differential analysis. Again, family studies, with the physician looking at the peripheral blood smears for spherocytes and performing osmotic fragilities on family members, can be of value during the child's acute episode.

Very often the diagnosis of hereditary spherocytosis is suggested by the child's peripheral blood smear on which numerous spherocytes are seen. Spherocytes are small round erythrocytes that lack central pallor. The size of the average cell as measured by the Coulter counter is often normocytic as a result of the balancing influence of the large reticulocytes, although often the mean corpuscular hemoglobin concentration is elevated to over 35 g/dL. The red cell distribution width (RDW) on the Coulter counter will be very high as a result of the double population of small spherocytes and large reticulocytes.

Bone marrow examination is rarely indicated but shows erythroid hyperplasia unless the patient is in the midst of an aplastic crisis.

In hereditary spherocytosis, the RBCs have an increased osmotic fragility. RBCs from patients with hereditary spherocytosis hemolyze at a higher osmotic concentration than normal RBCs. This test is the cornerstone on which the diagnosis of hereditary spherocytosis is made. In addition, RBCs from a patient with hereditary spherocytosis have a higher rate of autohemolysis when incubated for 48 hours at 37° C. This is secondary to the greater energy depletion caused by the membrane's increased permeability to sodium ion influx. The addition of glucose to the incubating RBCs corrects the degree of autohemolysis.

Management

Splenectomy prolongs the half-life of RBCs in hereditary spherocytosis to 80% of normal, resulting in a disappearance of the anemia and the reticulocytosis. Splenectomy should be performed on all symptomatic patients and on all asymptomatic patients in whom the reticulocyte count is consistently greater than 5%, as they have an increased risk of bilirubin stones and biliary colic. The decision to perform a splenectomy should be made in conjunction with a pediatric hematologist.

If possible, splenectomy should be postponed until the child is more than 5 years old. The risk of life-threatening bacterial infections is much higher in children under 5 years of age who have had their spleen removed. At least 1 month prior to splenectomy, the child should receive a pneumococcal vaccine and *Hemophilus influenzae* vaccine. After splenectomy, the child should receive prophylactic penicillin, 250 mg twice a day. After splenectomy, febrile episodes should be vigorously treated. A splenectomized child with a fever over 101.5° F without an obvious source should be hospitalized and treated with intravenous antibiotics until blood cultures prove to be negative.

In addition, until splenectomy, the child with hereditary spherocytosis should receive 1 mg of folic acid daily. The increased hemolysis results in an increased need for folic acid. In some cases of aplastic crisis, folate deficiency may be a contributory factor.

GLUCOSE-6-PHOSPHATE DEHYDROGENASE DEFICIENCY

Background

The most common intraerythrocyte enzymatic defect is G-6-PD deficiency. It is a recessive sex-linked disorder; thus the vast majority of patients are men. The exact clinical picture seen depends on the enzyme mutation present and on the oxidizing stress to which the RBC is exposed.

G-6-PD is the first enzyme in the hexose

monophosphate shunt and plays a major role in preventing oxidation of the hemoglobin and membrane components of the RBC. In G-6-PD deficiency, when a RBC is exposed to an oxidizing agent, denatured hemoglobin precipitates in the cell as Heinz bodies, resulting in a shortened RBC life span.

G-6-PD deficiency occurs in the malarial belt of the world, where gene frequency for the disorder can be greater than 20%. In blacks, the most common form of G-6-PD deficiency has a level of enzyme activity that is 10% to 20% of normal. The G-6-PD level is higher in young RBCs. The common Mediterranean form of G-6-PD deficiency has 0% to 5% of the normal activity and is not found at a higher level in reticulocytes. The end result is that given a continued oxidizing stress, a black child with G-6-PD deficiency has a more limited fall in hemoglobin level, with the younger RBCs being protected from further hemolysis, while the child with the Mediterranean form of G-6-PD deficiency has a greater fall in hemoglobin level and is not protected from recurrent hemolysis with continued exposures.

Data Gathering

Unless exposed to an oxidizing stress, most patients with G-6-PD deficiency have a normal hemoglobin level. A G-6-PD deficiency may, however, lead to a severe neonatal hyperbilirubinemic state. In Thailand, for example, 65% of infants with a bilirubin level above 15 mg/dL have G-6-PD deficiency. In the United States, the G-6-PD deficiency seen in the black population is associated with an increased incidence of hyperbilirubinemia only in premature infants.

Another common presentation of G-6-PD deficiency is acute hemolytic anemia secondary to ingestion of an oxidizing agent. In the United States, ingestion of moth balls made from naphthalene is the most common ingestion leading to a hemolytic anemia in G-6-PD–deficient children. Other oxidizing agents include several antipyretics and analgesics (but not aspirin or acetaminophen), antimalarials, sulfa drugs, sulfones, fava beans, nalidixic acid, toluidine blue, phenylhydrazine, and methylene blue. After ingesting an oxidizing agent, the G-6-PD–deficient patient has a precipitous drop in hemoglobin level, often associated with jaundice. Congestive heart failure could develop if the fall in hemoglobin level is sufficiently acute and severe.

Rarely, a G-6-PD deficiency can cause a chronic hemolytic anemia. Virtually all such cases are in men, and in 80% of the cases, steady state hemoglobin values are greater than 10 g/dL. Infections and exposure to oxidant drugs exacerbate the hemolysis. Like other hemolytic anemias, aplastic crisis can occur.

During an acute hemolytic episode, the G-6-PD–deficient patient will have spherocytes, polychromasia, and sometimes eccentrocytes with a clear "blister" area under the cell membrane in the peripheral smear. Special stains such as methyl violet stain are needed to show the presence of precipitated hemoglobin (Heinz bodies) in the peripheral blood. A Coombs test to rule out autoimmune hemolytic anemia and an osmotic fragility test to rule out hereditary spherocytosis may be necessary.

The definitive test is a quantitative measurement of G-6-PD level. In severe deficiency, the level should be low or absent in spite of the resultant reticulocytosis. However, in black children with G-6-PD deficiency, after an oxidizing stress the presence of reticulocytes with their higher level of G-6-PD could result in a borderline or even normal level. Therefore, the degree of reticulocytosis should be taken into account when deciding whether a child has G-6-PD deficiency. A low normal G-6-PD level with an elevated reticulocyte count should be considered suspicious, and the quantitative G-6-PD level should be repeated when the reticulocytosis has resolved.

Management

Other than avoidance of oxidizing stresses and supportive measures during acute hemolysis, there is no specific treatment for G-6-PD deficiency. Severe neonatal jaundice exacerbated by G-6-PD deficiency may require phototherapy or exchange transfusion.

BIBLIOGRAPHY

Massaro TF, Widmayer P: The effects of iron deficiency on cognitive performance in the rat. *Am J Clin Nutr* 1981; 34:864.

Poncz M, Cohen A, Schwartz E: Thalassemia. *Adv Pediatr* 1984; 31:43.

Sadowitz PD, Oski FA: Iron status and infant feeding in an urban ambulatory center. *Pediatrics* 1983; 72:33.

Shannon K, Buchanan GR: Severe hemolytic anemia in black children with glucose-6-phosphate dehydrogenase deficiency. *Pediatrics* 1982; 70:364.

Walter T, Kovalsky J, Staked A: Effect of mild iron deficiency on infant mental development scores. *J Pediatr* 1983; 102:519.

Wolfe LC, John KM, Falcone JC, et al: A genetic defect in the binding of protein 4.1 to spectrin in a kindred with hereditary spherocytosis. *N Engl J Med* 1982; 307:1367.

SICKLE CELL DISEASE

Frances M. Gill, M.D.

BACKGROUND

Normal adult hemoglobin (hemoglobin A) is composed of two alpha (α) and two beta (β) globin chains. Their production is controlled by autosomal recessive genes. Hemoglobin disorders can result from the inheritance of genes for structurally abnormal hemoglobins, such as sickle hemoglobin, or of thalassemia genes that produce decreased amounts of α- or β-globin (see preceding section). In hemoglobin S (HbS) the sixth amino acid of the β-chain is a valine instead of a glutamic acid residue. The biophysical effects of this single substitution cause the sickling phenomenon. In hemoglobin C (HbC) the sixth amino acid of the β-chain is lysine instead of glutamic acid. The genes for HbS and HbC are common in the American black population, sickle cell trait being found in about 7% of American blacks and HbC trait in about 3%. The person with sickle cell trait (HbAS) is normal, although some people with sickle cell trait will have transient hematuria. People with HbC trait may have transient hematuria but are generally asymptomatic. Homozygous HbC causes a mild hemolytic anemia that requires no treatment (Fig 59–3).

The term sickle cell disease refers to all disorders due to sickle hemoglobin and its interaction with other abnormal genes. Sickle cell disease affects about one in every 400 to 500 black Americans. It occurs much less frequently in people of Mediterranean, Arabic, and Indian origin.

There are three common forms of sickle cell disease. The most frequent and most severe is sickle cell anemia (HbSS) due to the inheritance of two β^s genes. Patients with HbSC disease have one gene for β^s and one for β^c. HbSC disease is generally milder than sickle cell anemia. Patients with HbSC comprise about 30% of the sickle cell disease population. In the β-thalassemias, β-chain production is either decreased (β^+-thalassemia) or absent (β°-thalassemia). A sickle gene interacting with a β°-thalassemia gene produces sickle-β°-thalassemia, which is similar to HbSS in clinical severity. Sickle-β^+-thalassemia is milder, resembling HbSC disease in severity. Patients with both forms of sickle-β-thalassemia comprise about 10% of sickle cell patients. Other structurally abnormal hemoglobins (such as D and O_{Arab}) can interact with HbS to produce a significant disorder. These are much rarer, however. Unless otherwise noted, the discussions here refer to all the sickling disorders.

The pathophysiology of the sickling disorders may be thought of in terms of three clinical problems: (1) hemolytic anemia and its consequences; (2) occlusion of vessels by the sickled red blood cells (RBC); and (3) increased susceptibility to infection. Serious infections are the most significant problem in children under 5 years of age. With advancing age the problems of chronic organ damage increase in importance.

The amino acid substitution in hemoglobin S results in a shortened life span of RBCs, and all patients with sickle cell disease have a hemolytic anemia. The usual hemoglobin level is between 7 and 10 g/dL in patients with sickle cell anemia and with S-β°-thalassemia and between 10 and 13 g/dL for those with HbSC and S-β^+-thalassemia. Cardiac enlargement is routinely seen on chest radiographs of even young children with sickle cell anemia. The hemolysis may result in the formation of bilirubin gallstones. Gallstones may be present in children with sickle cell anemia in the first 5 years of life, and by 20 years of age, 40% of SS patients may have gallstones.

When HbS is deoxygenated, it polymerizes, and the RBC assumes the sickled form. In this rigid state the RBC cannot deform enough to pass through small capillaries. Occlusion of

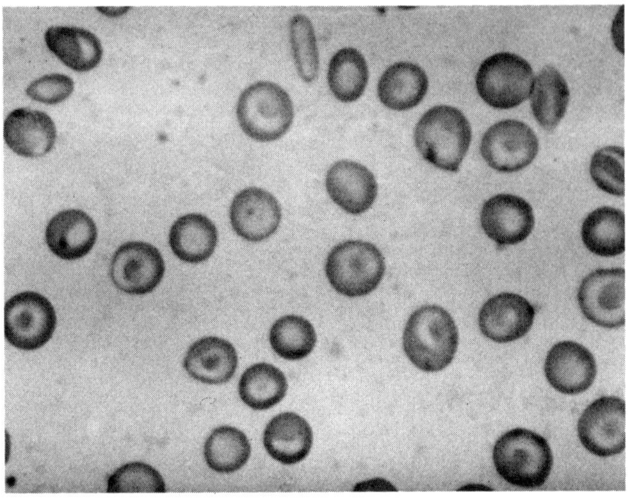

FIG 59–3
Target cells seen in SC or C-trait disease.

small vessels is felt to cause tissue hypoxia and pain. This is seen most characteristically in the vaso-occlusive or painful crisis. Repeated episodes of occlusion and infarction lead to permanent organ damage.

The high level of hemoglobin F present in the RBCs in the newborn seems to protect the cells from sickling in the first few months of life. By about 4 months of age, however, the child is susceptible to most of the acute problems encountered in older patients. The most important effect on the young child is the increased susceptibility to serious infection, particularly sepsis and meningitis. The risk of meningitis is 300 times higher for the child with Hb SS than the normal child and the risk for pneumococcal meningitis is 500 times higher.

Although many defects in the immune defenses of the sickle cell patient have been found, the most important seems to be the loss of the reticuloendothelial function of the spleen, termed functional hyposplenism. This function can be lost even while the spleen is enlarged. The spleen's filtering function is most important for encapsulated organisms, such as *Streptococcus pneumoniae* and *Hemophilus influenzae*. The young patient who has not developed many antibodies is most susceptible, particularly to sepsis and meningitis, but the increased risk of infection persists throughout life.

DATA GATHERING

All black children should undergo electrophoresis, preferably at birth but certainly by 2 months of age, to determine if they have sickle cell disease. The diagnosis can be made in the first 6 months of life with citrate agar gel electrophoresis. Family studies help delineate the exact form of sickle cell disease. The child should undergo a G-6-PD assay, since G-6-PD deficiency is common in the black population and may influence the choice of antibiotic therapy at some point.

Early diagnosis is essential, particularly now that penicillin prophylaxis begun by 4 to 5 months of age has been shown to decrease markedly mortality from infection. The early months are an important period for family education and formation of a strong family-physician bond. The family should receive genetic counseling about the risk of having another affected child and about the availability of prenatal diagnosis with amniotic fluid fibroblasts or chorionic villi samples.

MANAGEMENT

General Care

The baby in the first 4 months of life may be treated normally as far as immunizations, diet, and general care are concerned. By the age of 4 to 5 months, most infants with sickle cell anemia and S-β°-thalassemia have a mild anemia and reticulocytosis. Some have even lost the reticuloendothelial function of the spleen. Penicillin prophylaxis must be started by the age of 4 to 5 months in all children with Hb SS and Hb S-β°-thalassemia. A double-blinded, randomized study showed a significant reduction in mortality rate from infection in young children with Hb SS who received 125 mg of penicillin-V twice daily compared to the mortality rate in children who received placebo. The role of prophylaxis in SC and S-β-thalassemia has not been studied. Prophylaxis should continue at least to 5 years of age. Even with the use of prophylaxis, children with fever must be handled with special care.

Good pediatric care is important for children with sickle cell disease. Screening for iron deficiency and lead poisoning are done as for normal children. Diet should be appropriate for the patient's age. Folic acid, 1 mg daily, may help maintain adequate RBC production.

In addition to routine immunizations, a polyvalent vaccine against pneumococcus should be given. Antibody response is best when the vaccine is given to a child after the age of 2 years. However, since many serious pneumococcal infections occur before this age, many clinics give the infant an initial vaccination at 6 or 12 months of age and then repeat the immunization at 2 years of age. Booster immunizations are given every 4 years until the patient is an adult. Vaccination with conjugated *H. influenzae* B vaccine should be given at 18 months. Children older than 5 years who have not been vaccinated should also receive the *H. influenzae* B vaccine, since children with sickle cell disease are at increased risk of infection with this organism throughout life. It is important that parents realize that penicillin prophylaxis and appropriate immunizations are not guarantees against infection. The child must be brought for immediate medical attention when fever occurs, and his illness must be treated aggressively by physicians.

Baseline determinations of hemoglobin and reticulocyte levels and spleen size are important, since they are helpful in assessing the condition of the ill child. Yearly urinalysis and assessment of hepatic and renal function can reveal early changes of chronic organ damage.

Intelligence is not affected by sickle cell disease unless the patient develops neurologic complications. Although more severely affected patients may miss some school days because of their disease, they should be expected to attend regular class and to perform well. Rarely does a child require tutoring at home.

The patients are generally well adapted to their lower hemoglobin levels. The children should be able to play active games and take gym classes at school. They should be allowed to rest when tired, however, and should not be pushed to perform when fatigued. Because of the loss of the ability to concentrate urine, the children may need to leave class to get water or to urinate.

Nocturnal enuresis is common past the age of 5 years because of the development of isosthenuria. Parents should be counseled that this is physiologic and will resolve as the bladder capacity increases and the child learns to wake to urinate. Fluid intake should not be restricted because of this obligate water loss, but other usual methods of managing enuresis are helpful.

Education of the patient and family is extremely important. The significance of fever or pallor as a danger signal must be emphasized. Older patients need help in understanding the implications of the disease for their life. Genetic counseling is important for parents and for older patients. The education should be provided both by personnel from the sickle cell center and by the primary physician.

As in other chronic disease, patients and their families may need specialized support services from social workers, psychologists or psychiatrists, and vocational guidance counselors. These services can usually be provided by the sickle cell center working with the patient's own physician.

Examination of the Ill Child

Certain symptoms or complaints that might be minor in normal children may herald a more difficult problem in children with sickle cell disease. These include fever (which might herald a serious infection), unusual fatigue and loss of appetite (aplastic crisis, sequestration crisis), abdominal pain (vaso-occlusive crisis, pneumonia, biliary disease), pain in the extremities (vaso-occlusive crisis), headache or weakness (stroke), or a limp (stroke, aseptic necrosis).

A careful history is important in evaluating the condition of the sick child. Does the child have fever? Duration and height of the fever as well as any accompanying symptoms should be noted. It is important to note whether the child receives penicillin prophylactically and whether the child has received a pneumococcal vaccine. Although neither of these measures surely protects against a pneumococcal infection, the antibiotic coverage in these cases might be broadened.

The history of fluid intake should be noted. Vomiting, diarrhea, and increased sweating during the summer can lead rapidly to dehydration in the sickle cell patient, since the ability to concentrate urine is lost by 4 or 5 years of age. Persistent diarrhea or bloody diarrhea warrants a stool culture, since *Shigella* and *Salmonella* dysentery are more common in sickle cell disease.

A careful examination should be performed on any ill patient with sickle cell disease. A site of infection may be found in the febrile child. The degree of pallor and jaundice should be noted. Particular attention should be paid to the chest and abdominal examinations. The size of the spleen should be noted carefully and compared to the usual size in the patient. Swelling of joints or extremities may be due to vaso-occlusion but may also signal infection. Signs of neurologic deficit require further neurologic evaluation.

Laboratory studies helpful in evaluating the ill child's condition are the CBC count with differential cell count. In addition, the reticulocyte count should be determined to be sure that the child does not have an aplastic crisis. If the child has any respiratory symptoms or signs or has abdominal pain with the fever, a chest radiograph should be obtained. It is common for an infiltrate to be found on the radiograph of a child who has no rales or wheezing.

Transfusions of RBCs play an important role in the care of the sickle cell patient. Although transfusions are not used routinely in the care of the patients, they are essential for the treatment of some acute and chronic problems. The formation of alloantibodies is high in this group of patients. Prior to the first transfusion a complete RBC typing should be done. The patient receiving long-term RBC transfusions must be monitored for the development of excessive iron stores. Hepatitis B immunization should also be considered.

Acute Problems

The most common acute problems in sickle cell disease are listed below. Those that can be managed on an outpatient basis are discussed in more detail. Those requiring hospitalization are outlined only sufficiently so that their importance and differential diagnosis can be understood. Sickle cell patients who develop a major complication are best referred to a sickle cell center.

ACUTE PROBLEMS IN SICKLE CELL DISEASE

- Infection
- Acute anemic episode
  - Splenic sequestration
  - Aplastic crisis
- Vaso-occlusive crisis
- Right upper quadrant syndrome
- Stroke
- Hematuria
- Priapism

Infections.—*Infection* is the major cause of death in the child less than 5 years of age. Fever must be recognized as a danger signal in patients of every age but particularly in the young child. The infections that have an increased incidence in sickle cell disease are listed in Table 59–2.

The most serious infections in children are sepsis and meningitis. The risk is greatest for patients with Hb SS or S-β°-thalassemia but is also increased for the other sickling disorders. The most common cause of sepsis and meningitis is *Streptococcus pneumoniae*, but *H. influenzae* and other gram-negative organisms also cause serious disease. Meningitis occurs predominantly in the young child. Sepsis can occur in older children and adults and is more commonly due to gram-negative organisms. Since sepsis often cannot be separated clinically from a viral febrile illness, guidelines for hospitalization of children with sickle cell disease with fever have been developed. These are discussed below.

The most common infection in patients with sickle cell disease is pneumonia. This increased risk persists throughout life and is true for all forms of sickle cell disease. All sickle cell patients with pneumonia should be hospitalized. Although no cause is found in most children, the infection can be due to *S. pneu-*

TABLE 59–2
Common Infections in Sickle Cell Disease

INFECTION	COMMON ORGANISMS	COMMENTS
Sepsis	*Streptococcus pneumoniae* *Hemophilus influenzae* *Escherichia coli*	More frequent in young children
Meningitis	*S. pneumoniae* *H. influenzae*	Almost always in young children
Pneumonia	*S. pneumoniae* *H. influenzae* *Mycoplasma pneumoniae*	Often no organism identified
Urinary tract infection	*E. coli* *Klebsiella*	Often associated with positive blood culture
Osteomyelitis, pyogenic arthritis	*Staphylococcus aureus* *Salmonella* species *S. pneumoniae*	Multiple sites possible
Dysentery	*Salmonella* species *Shigella* species	Bloody diarrhea common

moniae, H. influenzae, M. pneumoniae, or viral organisms.

Osteomyelitis may occur at any age and is most commonly due to *Salmonella* organisms or *Stataphylococcus aureus*, but other organisms may be responsible (Fig 59–4). These patients usually have a high fever, appear to be in a toxic state, and have localized bone pain. A bone infarct may also produce localized pain, swelling, and warmth, but the patient does not usually appear as ill. Hospitalization is necessary to establish the correct diagnosis and to provide treatment. The hand-foot syndrome is usually easy to differentiate from osteomyelitis, but if there is a question, the child should be hospitalized.

Urinary tract infections occur more commonly in patients with sickling disorders than in normal people. Patients with pyelonephritis usually have a high fever, a positive urine culture, and signs of toxicity. Since pyelonephritis is frequently accompanied by sepsis, sickle cell patients with findings of urinary tract infection and fever should be admitted for treatment. Bacteriuria not accompanied by fever may be managed on an outpatient basis, with antibiotic coverage based on the organism's sensitivity. The guidelines for investigative studies and suppressive antibiotic coverage are the same as for patients who do not have sickle cell disease.

Salmonella and *Shigella* dysentery are fairly common in patients with sickling disorders. Hospitalization is not needed if the diarrhea is mild, the patient afebrile, and fluid intake can be maintained. Despite not receiving antibiotic therapy, most children recover without complications.

The patient with a fever and no discernible source is a problem. Although most of these episodes will be due to viral infections, some represent sepsis. In the young child sepsis may progress to irreversible septic shock within a few hours. For this reason young children are frequently hospitalized and treated with antibiotics before culture results are known. The scheme used at our center is outlined below.

Management of the Febrile Patient.—Children less than 5 years of age with a rectal temperature above 38.5° C are admitted and treated prophylactically with antibiotics after cultures of blood, throat, urine, and cerebrospinal fluid (if indicated) are obtained. Older children who have a high fever or who appear to be in a toxic state should also be admitted and treated expectantly.

The child over 5 years old who has low-grade fever may be treated as an outpatient in almost all cases if he or she feels well and is in a stable hematologic state. Evaluation of fever includes a thorough history as outlined above, a complete and careful examination, a CBC count with differential cell count and reticulocyte

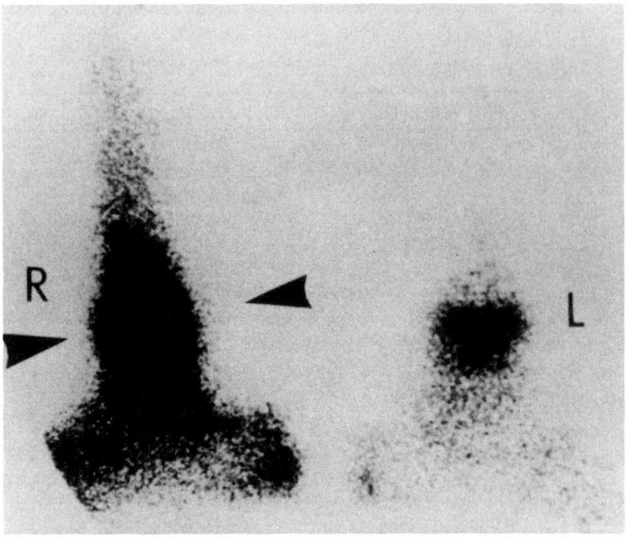

FIG 59–4
Bone scan of ankle demonstrating increased uptake in area of osteomyelitis.

count, and appropriate cultures. Even with apparently minor infections it may be necessary to hospitalize the patient if the fever is over 39° C, if vomiting or diarrhea may lead to insufficient oral fluid intake, if the fever is accompanied by a vaso-occlusive crisis that cannot be managed at home, or if the CBC count reveals a marked decrease in the hemoglobin level or the reticulocyte count.

If a minor infection is found, the child over 5 years of age may be treated as an outpatient with an appropriate antibiotic. Pharyngitis due to group A β-hemolytic *Streptococcus,* otitis media, and asymptomatic bacteriuria are the most common infections treated at home. Diarrhea not leading to dehydration may also be managed at home, as can influenza, chickenpox, and other viral diseases.

Acute Anemic Episode.—Increased pallor and/or increased fatigue may be due to a fall in the hemoglobin level. This can be caused by an *aplastic crisis* or by a *splenic sequestration crisis.*

Since RBC survival is shortened, and markedly so in Hb SS and S-β°-thalassemia, cessation of bone marrow production of RBCs for even a few days can cause a marked fall in the hemoglobin level. Viral infections, particularly infections with the parvovirus, can cause an aplastic crisis in a patient of any age.

The fall in hemoglobin level occurs over several days. Initially, the child may be more tired than usual and play less. As the hemoglobin level drops farther, the child may lose interest in eating and may refuse to walk. Eventually, usually at hemoglobin levels of 2 to 3 g/dL, congestive heart failure occurs.

If the parents report any of these changes in activity or if the child appears to be paler, a CBC count with reticulocyte count should be obtained. The hemoglobin level will be lower than normal and the reticulocyte count will be 0 or extremely low. If marrow recovery has begun, nucleated RBCs and reticulocytes will be present in the peripheral blood. If the aplasia persists long enough, the white blood cell (WBC) and platelet counts may also be low.

Treatment depends on the degree of anemia and the stage of recovery. If the hemoglobin value is more than 2 g below the usual level, the patient should be hospitalized for observation and possible transfusion of packed RBCs. If the hemoglobin level is only mildly reduced and, particularly, if there are signs of marrow recovery, the child may be reexamined and the hemoglobin and reticulocyte values determined every day or two until the marrow recovers. The child should rest during this period. If the hemoglobin level continues to fall, the child should then be admitted. The aplasia generally lasts only a few days.

In the splenic sequestration crisis, the spleen enlarges and blood pools within, resulting in hypovolemia that may be severe enough to cause shock and death. This is a medical emergency, since shock may occur within a few hours. The parents usually report that the child seems irritable and pale. There may be abdominal pain as the spleen enlarges. On physical examination the spleen will be larger than usual and very firm. The CBC count shows a decreased hemoglobin level and sometimes decreased WBC, platelet, and reticulocyte counts. The child should be hospitalized immediately and given a transfusion of packed RBCs that replaces volume and usually reverses the sequestration.

Vaso-Occlusive Crisis.—The most common acute event in sickle cell disease is the *vaso-occlusive crisis,* also called the painful event. Many events, even some of the more painful ones, can be managed at home. Increased intake of fluids may be helpful. Analgesics ranging from aspirin and acetaminophen to codeine or occasionally oral meperidine may be used at home. Warmth to the painful areas gives comfort to some patients.

If these measures do not give adequate relief, if the vaso-occlusive crisis is accompanied by a significant fever, or if vomiting or diarrhea limits the amount of fluid that can be taken, the patient should be seen by a physician. A parenteral analgesic, usually meperidine, is given. Infections, if present, should be treated. If relief is obtained and oral fluid intake is adequate, the patient can probably be treated at home with further analgesia. If relief is not obtained, the patient is hospitalized.

A crisis usually involves pain in one or more bones, particularly in the extremities. Bone infarcts, particularly in young children, may produce localized swelling, erythema, and tenderness, suggesting an underlying osteomyelitis. The child with these findings should be hospitalized for observation and appropriate testing.

The child may have vaso-occlusion in the small bones of the hand and/or feet, producing the hand-foot syndrome. Swelling is usually present in several extremities at once but may be unilateral, and fever is usually present. Most of these episodes can be managed at home with increased fluid intake and oral analgesics. If the fever is high or the findings suggest an osteomyelitis, the child should be hospitalized. In our experience almost every child with Hb SS has the hand-foot syndrome at some point. No permanent damage to the bones results.

Vaso-occlusive crises in some areas may mimic more serious problems such as an "acute" abdomen that requires surgery or orbital cellulitis. In such cases the patient must be hospitalized for observation and appropriate consultation and testing.

Right Upper Quadrant Syndrome.—Pain in the abdomen may result from vaso-occlusive crisis, pneumonia, urinary tract infection, intrahepatic sickling, acute or chronic cholecystitis, or biliary tree obstruction by gallstones. Careful physical examination and appropriate laboratory tests will help sort out these causes. Pain in the right upper quadrant is often due to biliary or hepatic disease. Children with such pain, particularly if it is accompanied by fever or vomiting, should be admitted for evaluation of their condition.

Because of the hemolytic anemia, gallstones are very common in sickle cell patients. In many patients the gallstones will not produce symptoms but they can cause chronic gallbladder symptoms as well as acute problems. Children with recurrent abdominal pain and gallstones demonstrated on ultrasonography or plain radiography may need referral to a surgeon for consideration of a cholecystectomy.

Cerebrovascular Accident.—Chronic damage to the large cerebral vessels leads to vessel narrowing and occlusion in some patients with sickle cell anemia. The occlusion produces an acute cerebrovascular accident (CVA). In older patients, intracranial hemorrhage is more frequently the cause of CVA. Patients with neurologic symptoms must be hospitalized immediately. Further discussion of CVA is contained in the section on chronic problems.

Hematuria.—Hematuria is common in both sickle cell disease and sickle cell trait. Other causes, such as infection and kidney stones, must be investigated. Blood loss is rarely significant enough to require transfusions. Mild episodes that last only a few days may be managed at home with bed rest and increased fluid intake. If pain or costovertebral-angle tenderness is present or if the hematuria persists beyond several days, the patient should be hospitalized for renal studies and observation. Nephrectomy should not be performed.

Priapism.—Painful, prolonged erection is an acute problem in some boys with sickle cell disease. This may occur before puberty but seems to be more frequent around the time of puberty. Almost all episodes of persistent priapism require hospitalization. In a mild episode, increased fluid intake and oral analgesia may be sufficient treatment.

Chronic Problems

Almost any organ system can be damaged by repeated occlusion of small vessels by sickled cells. Regular evaluation by the primary care physician may diagnose chronic complications at an early stage. The following are the most common sites of chronic organ damage; specific chronic problems are discussed below.

CHRONIC ORGAN DAMAGE

CNS: CVA, occlusive and hemorrhagic
Eye: Retinal vessel proliferation
Bone: Aseptic necrosis
Skin: Leg ulcer
Heart: Congestive heart failure
Liver: Chronic liver disease
Kidney: Nephrotic syndrome, chronic renal failure
Lungs: Pulmonary insufficiency

Although chronic damage occurs in the heart, lungs, liver, and kidneys, there is no specific therapy available for these complications. The patient should receive appropriate care for the specific problem. For example, renal transplantation has been successful in sickle cell patients.

Central Nervous System.—CVA is a major complication of sickle cell anemia. Those that are due to occlusion of large cerebral vessels are common in patients in the first two decades of life and affect 8% to 12% of children with Hb SS. Hemorrhagic CVA is more common in older patients and often is due to rupture of the circle of Willis but may be intracerebral.

Occlusive CVA is most commonly manifest as hemiparesis, aphasia, and/or facial palsy. Sickle cell patients with these findings must be hospitalized for immediate transfusion and studies. Some completed CVAs are preceded by transient neurologic abnormalities, such as limp or temporary aphasia. The findings may be explained on a vascular basis and correspond to transient ischemic episodes. Such symptoms and findings must be taken seriously, and the child's condition must be evaluated by a neurologist. If the diagnosis is transient ischemic attacks (TIA), the patient should receive transfusions. A computed tomography (CT) scan of the brain several days after a transient attack may demonstrate an area of infarction. If not, the child should be referred to a sickle cell center for further studies.

The occurrence of nonspecific neurologic symptoms such as headache or fainting is much more difficult to evaluate. These are sometimes warning symptoms of cerebral artery disease but may occur for other, more usual reasons. Referral of the child with recurring neurologic symptoms to the sickle cell center is advised.

Recurrence of CVA, which has been reported to be as high as 60%, can essentially be prevented by a chronic transfusion program in which the hemoglobin S level is kept below 30%. Such a program can be done on an outpatient basis.

Intracranial hemorrhage is more common in the adolescent and adult. Warning symptoms such as a severe headache may occur, although some patients are first seen in coma. CT should demonstrate the hemorrhage. Some patients survive, and immediate diagnostic studies and hospitalization are essential.

Eye.—Proliferative retinopathy may threaten the vision of sickle cell patients. Evaluation by a retinal specialist is necessary to detect the early lesions, which can be treated, if necessary, by laser phototherapy. Significant retinal disease is rare before 10 years of age. Thereafter, it increases in frequency and is particularly common in patients with Hb SC disease. These patients should be seen yearly after 10 years of age by a retinal specialist. Patients with Hb SS and S-β-thalassemia may be seen every other year unless significant abnormalities are found.

Bone.—Avascular necrosis occurs in as many as 8% of patients, usually in the second and third decades of life. The femoral heads and, less frequently, the humeral heads are involved, either unilaterally or bilaterally. It is usually discovered when the patient complains of pain or develops a limp. The pain is usually chronic but may be acute if synovitis is present. Examination of the involved joint usually shows limitation of motion and pain. Diagnosis is facilitated with radiography of the bones.

The patient should be referred to an orthopedist for treatment, which usually involves non-weight-bearing and may entail surgery. The acute symptoms of synovitis are usually controlled by bed rest with traction. Many patients are able to resume normal activities after a period of non-weight-bearing. In some older patients, total hip replacement has been successful, although later revisions will probably be necessary.

Leg Ulcers.—Leg ulcers are rare in the first decade of life but increase in frequency in patients after the age of 15 years. Although they are not a major health threat, ulcers result in much time lost from school or work. The exact cause of the ulcers is unknown, but therapy is similar to that for stasis ulcers. Good local care with soaking, dressing changes, and antibiotic ointment, if indicated, is extremely important. Bed rest and elevation of the affected limb may help. In children, an infected cut often leads to ulcer formation; oral antibiotic therapy combined with vigorous local care usually results in rapid resolution of the ulcer. In older patients recovery is often very slow. For resistant ulcers, RBC transfusions given over a period of months and other measures such as grafting may be necessary. Once the ulcer has resolved, the area should be protected with support hose or socks. Recurrence is very frequent.

General Growth and Development.—Infants with sickle cell disease grow and develop normally in the newborn period. A minority of children will later have height and/or weight gains below the normal limits. No specific cause has been found. The physician should be sure that food intake is adequate and that other causes of poor growth have been excluded. Some patients have delayed onset of the pubertal growth spurt and sexual maturation. Bone age is delayed, and endocrine studies suggest a prepubertal state. It is very important to reassure the teenager that puberty will occur in a few years. Infertility is not a problem in sickle cell disease.

Birth control is important in sexually active women, since pregnancy is associated with higher risks for the mother and fetus. There is concern that oral contraceptives may increase the risk of vascular occlusion and that there is an increased incidence of infection with intrauterine devices in sickle cell women. Most gynecologists recommend low-dose estrogen pills or barrier methods for these women.

Because of the problems of pregnancy in sickle cell disease, pregnant women should be under the care of obstetricians who specialize in high-risk pregnancies.

Consultations

If possible, the child with sickle cell disease should be seen at a sickle cell center at least twice yearly. This allows the child to be seen by hematologists experienced in the care of chronic complications and also allows the family to take advantage of the educational and psychosocial services of the center. Personnel in centers recognize the valuable role of the primary physician and are willing to work with him or her by telephone. For certain problems, however, the patient is treated best in the center's hospital. Patients with CVA, severe and frequently recurring vaso-occlusive CVA, and ocular disease are among the patients best followed up in conjunction with the center.

Because sickle cell disease affects so many organ systems, many medical and surgical specialists are essential for the best care of the patients. Routine evaluations by a retinal specialist are needed as described above. Regular dental examinations are also important.

Referrals to surgeons are often necessary for acute or chronic problems such as abdominal pain, gallbladder problems, and leg ulcers. Surgery may be successfully performed for sickle cell patients. It is the feeling of most sickle cell center personnel that patients should be prepared for most surgical procedures by partial exchange transfusions or a series of simple transfusions to produce an Hb S level of less than 30%.

Social workers and psychologists or psychiatrists are extremely helpful in the long-term care of sickle cell patients. They provide educational and vocational advice, emotional support, and family and patient counseling.

BIBLIOGRAPHY

Charache S, Lubin B, Reed CD (eds): *Treatment of Sickle Cell Disease*. US Department of Health, Education and Welfare publication no 84–2117, 1984.

Gaston MH, Verter JI, Woods G, et al: Prophylaxis with oral penicillin in children with sickle cell anemia. A randomized trial. *N Engl J Med* 1986; 314:1593.

Gill FM: Treatment of sickle cell disease, in Rakel RE (ed): *Conn's Current Therapy*. Philadelphia, WB Saunders Co, 1984, pp 252–257.

Platt OS, Nathan DG: Sickle cell disease, in Nathan DG, Oski FA (eds): *Hematology of Infancy and Childhood*. Philadelphia, WB Saunders Co, 1987; pp 655–698.

Powars DR: Natural history of sickle cell disease: The first ten years. *Semin Hematol* 1975; 12:267.

HEMOPHILIA

Frances M. Gill, M.D.

Inherited deficiencies are known for each of the coagulation factors. Deficiency of factor XII does not result in abnormal bleeding. For all other coagulation factors, deficiency of the factor or the presence of an abnormally functioning factor causes a bleeding disorder.

The term hemophilia is restricted to the inherited deficiency of factor VIII (hemophilia A) or factor IX (hemophilia B). Since the genes for factor VIII and factor IX are sex-linked and recessive, hemophilia affects men primarily, but women may rarely be affected. Hemophilia occurs in all races. About one of 10,000 men in the United States is affected; hemophilia A is five to seven times more common than hemophilia B.

von Willebrand disease, the most common of the coagulation disorders, is inherited autosomally, usually in a dominant fashion. In the classic form the levels of factor VIII coagulant (VIII), von Willebrand-related antigen, and von Willebrand factor are all low. Since the latter is necessary for the normal adhesion and aggregation of platelets, the bleeding time is prolonged. Many variants of von Willebrand disease occur.

The other factor deficiencies are much rarer. Since they are autosomally inherited, they occur in men and women with equal frequency.

PATHOPHYSIOLOGY

The absence or deficiency of the coagulation factor causes prolonged bleeding. Hemorrhage may occur spontaneously from small vessels, particularly those in the joint synovia, kidneys, or gastrointestinal tract, or may result from trauma of even a minor degree. In the absence of factor replacement, the vessels will continue to bleed. In closed areas (such as joints), pain and swelling develop early. In noncontained areas (such as the retroperitoneal space) pain and other symptoms may not appear until the hemorrhage is large. Continued hemorrhage, either internally or externally, results in anemia and eventually in hypovolemic shock. The clinical severity of the disorder is closely related in almost every patient to the measured level of the factor. The clinical classification of severity is given in Table 59–3.

The advances in the care of the hemophiliac patient can be attributed to the development of better factor replacement products, the establishment of hemophilia centers where comprehensive care by multiple specialists is available, and the development of home therapy programs. Home care eliminates the need for frequent visits to a treatment site for minor bleeding episodes and reduces the financial costs of treatment.

The median age, life expectancy, and age at death of hemophiliac patients have increased markedly in recent years. Therapy cannot prevent all deaths; bleeding (particularly intracranial hemorrhage) is still a major cause of death.

Recurrent joint bleeding can lead to crippling joint deformities and chronic arthritis. Modern replacement treatment has decreased the severity and frequency of joint deformity and has ap-

TABLE 59–3
Severity of Hemophilia

SEVERITY	FACTOR LEVEL (%)	CLINICAL MANIFESTATIONS
Severe	<1	Frequent, spontaneous hemorrhages; hemarthroses common
Moderate	1–5	Occasional hemorrhages; hemarthroses uncommon
Mild	>5	Spontaneous hemorrhages rare; hemarthroses only after trauma

parently slowed the development of arthritis. All damage cannot be prevented, however, in severely affected patients.

The therapeutic materials themselves, being derived from blood, carry some risks. Hepatitis (both B and non-A, non-B) occurs frequently. Chronic hepatitis results in some patients. Infection with human immunodeficiency (HIV) virus is unfortunately frequent in those children who were exposed to large numbers of donors before the use of heat-treated concentrates and updated blood donor screening tests. Both acquired immunodeficiency syndrome (AIDS) and AIDS-related complex have developed in these patients, although many remain asymptomatic. The clinical picture is that seen in other patients who received HIV from blood transfusions. Opportunistic infections are common in AIDS patients, but Kaposi's sarcoma has been extremely rare. The guidelines for precautions issued by the Centers for Disease Control should be followed in caring for patients with hepatitis or HIV infection.

DATA GATHERING

The diagnosis of hemophilia may be made at birth if there is a family history. Since neither factor VIII nor factor IX crosses the placenta, a citrated blood sample of cord blood may be used to measure the factor level. Because factor VIII is present at normal levels (greater than 50%) in premature and term infants, the diagnosis of any degree of deficiency may be made at birth. The level of factor IX, a vitamin-K-dependent coagulation factor, is lower than normal at birth in normal infants. Although severe factor IX deficiency can be diagnosed, it may be necessary to repeat measurements over a period of several months if the initial value is low and the family history suggests mild or moderate disease. The degree of factor deficiency is consistent throughout affected family members, although the clinical severity may vary somewhat.

In the absence of a family history, the diagnosis of severe hemophilia is usually made when the family or physician notices unusual bruising or bleeding. Prolonged bleeding from a circumcision site or laceration, particularly in the mouth; multiple, elevated bruises; and large ecchymoses following trauma should suggest the presence of a bleeding disorder. In mildly affected patients, the diagnosis may not be suspected until excessive bleeding occurs after dental extractions or surgery.

The studies necessary for diagnosis depend on the deficiency suspected, e.g., a partial thromboplastin time (PTT) and factor VIII assay if hemophilia A is suspected or a prothrombin time (PT) and factor VII assay for factor VII deficiency. Diagnosis should be confirmed at a hemophilia treatment center. Choice of the proper replacement product depends on the precise identification of the deficient factor.

MANAGEMENT

General Care

Ideally, all patients with hemophilia should be enrolled in a hemophilia treatment center where periodic comprehensive evaluations can be made by a hematologist, orthopedist, dentist, and psychosocial worker. Family education and home care training are offered. Genetic counseling and referral of the mother for carrier testing and prenatal diagnosis, if desired, can be arranged. Prenatal diagnosis with a fetal blood sample has been extremely successful for factor VIII deficiency. Amniocentesis is initially done to determine if the fetus is a boy and, therefore, at risk for hemophilia.

In many families, prenatal diagnosis of factor VIII deficiency is now possible by DNA analysis. In these families, chorionic villi sampling or amniocentesis provides the material necessary for the diagnostic studies. The hemophilia center or a genetic center can provide the latest information on prenatal diagnosis of factor VIII or IX deficiency.

The primary physician is central to the care of the hemophiliac patient, providing well-child care and treating all nonbleeding related problems. If the patient lives a long distance from the hemophilia treatment center, the willing primary physician can participate actively in the treatment of minor bleeding episodes and in the initial treatment of major bleeding. Patients should be referred to the center for life-threatening bleeding and for surgical procedures.

Regular well-child care can be given. Immunizations are important but should be given subcutaneously rather than intramuscularly. A 26-gauge needle should be used, and firm pressure exerted at the injection site for several minutes. Immunization for hepatitis B is now available and should be begun early in infancy. The initial immunization is followed with booster doses 1 and 6 months later.

Young children with severe bleeding disorders often require iron therapy in the dose of 6 mg of elemental iron/kg/day to replace the iron lost from bleeding.

Aspirin should never be used for the child with a bleeding disorder. Its interference with platelet function can markedly increase bleeding. Other drugs that can interfere with coagulation, such as the newer antibiotics like moxalactam, should be used with caution.

Patients with severe and moderate hemophilia may participate in outdoor activities and in physical education classes. Contact sports (such as football and soccer) and activities with a high risk of trauma (such as motor-biking) should be avoided. Many sports, including swimming, golf, and tennis, can be safely pursued.

Hemophilia should not interfere with placement in a regular school. Homebound tutoring is only rarely needed. The child should be encouraged to participate fully in those activities that are not specifically prohibited.

Evaluation of Acute Problems

In the discussion of problems below, the minor bleeding episodes that can be readily managed in the office or emergency room or at home by families on home treatment programs are discussed. Those problems requiring hospitalization will be mentioned briefly. The discussion of treatment in more detail is beyond the scope of this book but can be found in the suggested references. The physician who is willing to provide care for minor bleeding episodes should discuss the case of the patient in detail with the center personnel to decide on treatment protocols and referral patterns.

Some bleeding problems may mimic other disorders. The primary physician must keep in mind at all times that the child has hemophilia and must question whether any acute problem, particularly pain or anemia, can be due to bleeding. In case of doubt, treatment for the bleeding disorder should be given while other considerations are still entertained. For example, the young hemophiliac with abdominal pain should receive replacement therapy. The physician must be alert, however, to the possibility that the child has a nonbleeding problem, such as appendicitis or urinary tract infection.

Bleeding episodes can be divided for purposes of management into those that are minor and not life-threatening and those that do threaten life or function.

Bleeding can be prevented or stopped by replacement of the missing factor. The levels required to treat bleeding depend on the extent and location of the injury. Most minor injuries can be treated by raising the factor level to 20% to 30% for a brief period. Life-threatening bleeding or surgical wounds require higher levels of factor for more prolonged periods and hospitalization. The common bleeding episodes are listed below according to severity.

COMMON HEMORRHAGES

Minor

Skin lacerations
Subcutaneous bruises
Muscle hemorrhages
Joint hemorrhages
Mouth bleeding
Epistaxis
Nontraumatic hematuria

Major

Intracranial hemorrhage
Retroperitoneal hemorrhage
  Iliopsoas muscle hemorrhage
  Uncontained bleeding
Hemorrhage threatening the airway
Muscle hemorrhage with nerve compression
Traumatic hematuria
Gastrointestinal tract hemorrhage
Surgical procedures

Blood products available for treatment of factor VIII deficiency are cryoprecipitate and factor VIII concentrate. For factor IX deficiency fresh-frozen plasma or concentrate containing factor IX are effective. Since cryoprecipitate contains von Willebrand factor and fibrinogen, it is effective treatment for patients with von Willebrand disease and congenital fibrinogen deficiency. Fresh-frozen plasma, which contains all the coagulation factors, can be used to treat the other coagulation disorders.

Concentrates containing VIII and IX are now heat-treated by the manufacturer to kill the HIV. It is not known if heat treatment will decrease the incidence of hepatitis B or non-A, non-B hepatitis in recipients. Screening of donors with self-exclusion questionnaires and with HIV antibody testing has increased the safety of the blood supply. Patients requiring frequent factor replacement should receive heat-treated concentrates. At present some centers are treating young, severe hemophiliacs with single-donor products (cryoprecipitate or fresh-frozen plasma), and others are using heat-treated concentrates. Physicians treating hemophiliacs should keep abreast of the current recommendations of the National Hemophilia Foundation and the Centers for Disease Control for treatment products.

In some patients it is possible to avoid the use of blood products by using desmopressin (intravenous vasopressin), which raises the plasma level of factor VIII, von Willebrand factor, and von Willebrand antigen threefold to fivefold. Since desmopressin probably acts by releasing stored factors, it is not effective in patients with severe or moderate hemophilia who have very low VIII levels or in patients with those types of von Willebrand disease in which von Willebrand factor is absent or defective. It should be used to treat most bleeding episodes in patients with mild factor VIII deficiency or with the common type of von Willebrand disease. It is necessary to determine which type of von Willebrand disease the patient has to know if desmopressin therapy will be effective and safe. The specialized testing needed to determine the type of von Willebrand disease can be done at hemophilia centers.

Most *skin lacerations* require no treatment. Firm pressure will generally stop the bleeding. If the cut is larger and particularly if sutures are necessary, treatment should be given. Occasionally treatment is needed when sutures are removed.

Subcutaneous bruising is the most common bleeding manifestation. Application of a cold pack, if the child will tolerate it, may decrease the bleeding. If, however, the bruise continues to enlarge or is in a tight area such as the buttock, one treatment may be needed.

Muscle bleeding responds in most cases to one infusion of the factor to raise the level to 30%. Immobilization with a posterior splint is sometimes necessary to prevent reinjury and rebleeding. Cold applications may help limit the hemorrhage.

Bleeding in some muscles requires special precautions. Hemorrhage in the gastrocnemius muscle usually requires several treatments. Exercises, and even physical therapy, may be necessary after the acute bleeding has stopped to prevent tightening of the heel cord. Iliopsoas muscle hemorrhage is treated in the hospital because rebleeding is frequent unless the patient receives multiple infusions. Since bleeding into the thigh can be massive, often resulting in a drop in hemoglobin level of 3 to 4 g/dL, the patient needs repeated treatment in the hospital. Bleeding into muscle compartments, such as the forearm or gastrocnemius, may cause nerve compression. If there is appreciable swelling in these areas, the patient should be hospitalized for aggressive treatment.

Joint hemorrhages are the most common form of bleeding requiring treatment. Since chronic damage can occur, treatment of all hemarthroses is recommended. Knees, elbows, and ankles are most commonly involved. Even slight bleeding causes pain. As the amount of blood in the joint increases, swelling, warmth, and decreased range of motion follow. One treatment to raise the factor level to 20% is sufficient for treatment of most hemarthroses, but elbow bleeding requires a level of 30%. If the patient has recurrent bleeding into one specific joint, a more aggressive treatment program may be designed in conjunction with the hemophilia center. Other measures that are helpful are application of cold to the joint and immobilization of painful joints. Pain will usually cease within several hours of treatment. Continued pain or progression of swelling is indication for further therapy. Patients with hip bleeding should be admitted for bed rest and repeated treatment.

Mouth bleeding from a cut or a torn frenulum is very common in the young child. Such bleeding formerly fell into the major category because many days of treatment were required. With the use of antifibrinolytic agents, however, one treatment with factor to raise the level to 50% is usually sufficient. Epsilon-amino-caproic acid (EACA) or tranexamic acid is used as adjunct therapy to prevent lysis of the clot that forms. EACA is given orally in the dose of 100 mg/kg every 6 hours (400 mg/kg every 24 hours) with a maximum dose of 24 g/day. The dose of tranexamic acid is about 25 mg/kg/dose. Treatment needs to be continued for several days until the wound is well healed. EACA or tranexamic acid must not be given in the presence of hematuria or concurrently with factor-IX containing products. One treatment dose of factor is usually sufficient, but more should be given if the clot is poor or oozing persists. Dry topical thrombin applied with an applicator to the bleeding site is also helpful. The physician should be aware that significant hemorrhage can occur from the tonsils during acute tonsillitis.

Epistaxis is usually mild and readily controlled by pressure. Prolonged bleeding warrants factor replacement. An occasional patient will have recurrent, severe epistaxis with significant blood loss. Such a patient should be hospitalized for treatment.

Hematuria unrelated to trauma is very common. Although most episodes probably result from tears in small vessels, other causes such as infection, tumor, and kidney stones should be considered, particularly if the hematuria persists for more than a few days. Most episodes can be managed by bed rest alone. One treatment with factor may help resolve the bleeding. Blood loss is rarely significant, even if the bleeding lasts for days. In hemophiliac patients, EACA should not be used for hematuria since extensive clotting with renal compromise has been reported. If there is a history of trauma, costovertebral angle tenderness, or passage of large clots, the patient should be hospitalized for close observation, diagnostic studies, and frequent factor replacement.

Major bleeding episodes are still a major cause of death in severely affected hemophiliac patients, and particularly in those who have developed an inhibitor to factor VIII or IX. Patients with an inhibitor do not respond to usual factor replacement. They should be treated through the hemophilia center.

Intracranial hemorrhage accounts for most of the hemorrhagic deaths in all age groups. Other serious hemorrhages include retroperitoneal hemorrhage (signaled by the presence of abdominal pain and often by the development of guarding and ileus); hemorrhage in the mouth or throat area that may threaten the patency of the airway; bleeding into muscles in tight compartments that can produce permanent nerve damage; hematuria following trauma; and gastrointestinal tract hemorrhage that can result in massive blood loss.

All major hemorrhages require hospitalization for close observation and repeated treatment. If the patient lives a distance from the hemophilia center, the primary physician may give the first treatment dose calculated to raise the factor to 100% and then arrange for local hospitalization or transfer to the center.

Since *intracranial hemorrhage* is so serious a threat, injuries to the head should be treated as soon as possible to prevent bleeding. Any injury in which significant force is exerted on the head should be treated. This includes minor trauma such as occurs from falls or blows from hard, thrown objects, as well as the more traumatic injuries sustained in automobile or other accidents. In the young child, frequent falls may result in many prophylactic treatments. Any blow that the patient or family feels is significant enough to report to the physician should be treated even if there is no external sign of injury and even if there are no neurologic signs. Treatment should not be withheld to see if symptoms will appear. Tears in small vessels can be sealed immediately if factor replacement is given. If it is not given, continuing oozing can occur until the hemorrhage is large enough to cause symptoms. By this time, loss of function and death may be imminent.

Only those injuries that are very minor and not associated with neurologic symptoms or findings can be managed in the outpatient setting. In such minor injuries a single dose of factor is given to raise the factor level to 100%. Although a 70% level is probably adequate, the higher dose is given to allow for extravascular extravasation. The family can be instructed to observe the patient closely. Further doses are not given if the patient remains well, and repeat examination by the physician is usually not necessary unless symptoms develop.

If the injury is more severe, e.g., an automobile accident or a fall down stairs, the patient receives the initial dose to raise the factor level to 100% and is admitted for repeated replacement therapy, diagnostic studies, and close observation.

Intracranial hemorrhage can occur in the absence of trauma. The development of neurologic symptoms such as headache or signs including drowsiness and repeated vomiting must in the hemophiliac be assumed to be due to intracranial hemorrhage. Careful evaluation by a neurologist or neurosurgeon and diagnostic studies, such as CT scanning or magnetic resonance (MR) imaging, are necessary to exclude the presence of CNS or epidural cord bleeding. Patients with neurologic findings should be treated immediately to raise the factor level to 100% and then hospitalized for evaluation of their condition and further treatment.

CONSULTATIONS

The role of the hemophilia treatment center is discussed briefly above. The value of this comprehensive approach cannot be overemphasized. Since family disruption and psychological problems are so common in this chronic disorder, the resources of the social worker and child psychologist or psychiatrist are particularly important.

It is extremely important for the child with hemophilia to receive regular dental care and fluoride administration. Although it is possible to do even extensive dental surgery under factor coverage and with the use of EACA, it is much preferable to prevent dental caries and gum disease. No factor coverage is necessary for cleaning or for placement of fillings if anesthesia is not needed. If local infiltrations are to be used, one treatment to raise the factor level to 30% is given prior to the dental appointment. Regional block anesthesia should not be used since hemorrhage in the loose tissue can extend to obstruct the airway. Extensive gum surgery, dental extractions, and any procedure involving the bone require careful planning, factor replacement, and close observation. These are best done at the hemophilia center.

The orthopedist is an essential partner in the evaluation and treatment of the severely affected patient. The child without apparent problems should be seen yearly by an orthopedist. More frequent evaluations are necessary for the child with frequent hemarthroses and chronically affected joints. Physical therapists and physiatrists also make important contributions to the preservation of joint function and the rehabilitation of affected joints.

Other surgical specialists are needed to evaluate and treat specific problems, such as intracranial hemorrhage or abdominal pain. If elective or emergency surgery is necessary, prolonged treatment with high levels of factor replacement is essential. Surgery without coverage can result in massive bleeding in even the mildly affected patient. Close cooperation between the surgeon, primary physician, and hematologist will assure adequate hemostasis and successful surgery.

BIBLIOGRAPHY

Gill FM: Treatment of hemophilia and von Willebrand's disease. *Med Clin North Am* 1984; 68:601.

Hiltgartner MW (ed): *Hemophilia in the Child and Adult.* New York, Masson Publishing, 1982.

Jones PA: *Living with Hemophilia.* Philadelphia, FA Davis, 1974.

Lusher JM: Diseases of coagulation: The fluid phase, in Nathan DG, Oski FA, (eds): *Hematology of Infancy and Childhood,* vol 2. Philadelphia, WB Saunders Co, 1987; pp 1293–1342.

COMMON PROBLEMS IN HEMATOLOGY

Steven E. McKenzie, M.D.

The primary care physician will often be the first to see and evaluate patients with hematologic conditions, ranging from mild anemias to easy bruisability to neutropenia. The purpose of this section is to provide a framework for evaluating common office problems and for identification of those patients that might benefit from the advice of a pediatric hematologist. The primary care physician may also choose to share in the long-term care of children with known hematologic disorders. This section will cover some common issues for these children that arise during primary care.

The conditions that primary care physicians may face include: (1) neutropenia, (2) possible bleeding disorders, (3) leukocytosis, (4) questions about inheritance patterns and screening tests, and (5) managing infection in the asplenic child.

NEUTROPENIA

The definition of neutropenia, the most common WBC abnormality a primary care physician will encounter, depends on the age and ethnic origin of the patient. In patients greater than 1 year old, the lower limit of normal for the neutrophil count is 1,500/mm^3. (The absolute neutrophil count is the percentage of band forms plus mature segmented neutrophils times the total WBC count.) Infants will normally have greater than 2,500 neutrophils/mm^3. Up to 30% of black infants may have neutrophil counts between 500 and 1,500/mm^3 without adverse consequences. The concern with neutropenia is the risk of life-threatening infection. While the risk of infection depends on the specific cause of the neutropenia, in general, only severe neutropenia (<500/mm^3) that lasts for more than several days confers a substantial risk of life-threatening infection.

Differential Diagnosis

COMMON CAUSES OF NEUTROPENIA

Congenital
Benign chronic neutropenia
Cyclic neutropenia
Severe congenital neutropenia (Kostmann syndrome)
Reticular dysgenesis
Decreased marrow storage pool
Malignant
Leukemia, lymphoma, solid tumor (e.g., neuroblastoma)
Toxic
Drugs
Radiation
Heavy metals
Organic compounds
Infectious
Viral
Bacterial
Rickettsial
Idiopathic
Aplastic anemia
Immune
Isoimmune neonatal neutropenia
Autoimmune neutropenia
Drug-induced neutropenia
Complement-mediated
Collagen-vascular disease
Miscellaneous syndromes
Schwachman-Diamond (neutropenia and exocrine pancreatic insufficiency)
Fanconi's anemia
Chediak-Higashi

In an ill-appearing neutropenic child with a fever or history of fever, prompt evaluation is needed. The hemoglobin level, platelet count, and other elements of the blood smear must be carefully assessed. Even if these elements are normal, diagnosis and treatment may depend on a bone marrow examination coupled with expeditious consultation with the hematologist. In a child with a history of good health without frequent infections, isolated neutropenia is rarely a major problem. Furthermore, rarely is neutropenia found to be the culprit in a child with recurrent infection.

In a healthy child, neutropenia will usually be discovered because a concurrent viral syndrome or focal bacterial infection such as otitis media has led to a CBC count. Occasionally neutropenia is discovered when a routine CBC count has been done. This is most often a transient neutropenia, associated with either viral infection itself (as in varicella, rubella, influenza, mononucleosis, and hepatitis) or with frequently prescribed antibiotics (such as penicillins, cephalosporins, and sulfa agents). All drugs that can be safely stopped should be stopped, and serial neutrophil counts obtained at least weekly. In 3 to 6 weeks, a normal count should return.

Neutropenia in the newborn may be associated with serious underlying infection, such as bacterial sepsis, meningitis, or congenital viral infection with an agent like cytomegalovirus. Transient neutropenia has been reported with maternal hypertension, birth asphyxia, and in preterm infants in association with copper deficiency. After these causes, congenital or familial neutropenia should be considered.

The patient with congenital neutropenia will benefit from evaluation by a pediatric hematologist. The current prognosis in these individuals ranges from excellent (isoimmune neonatal neutropenia and benign chronic neutropenia) to good with supportive care (cyclic neutropenia) to grim (Kostmann syndrome and reticular dysgenesis). New trials of hematopoietic hormones, such as granulocyte-colony-stimulating factor, may improve the prognosis in severe congenital neutropenia.

Screening Tests.—Evaluation of a neutropenic patient begins with a thorough history including recent viral illnesses, drug exposures, and family history. One reassuring, useful, and inexpensive step is to check the results of any prior CBC counts the child had. The physical examination starts by considering if this is a well child: is he growing well, is he febrile? In performing the physical examination, extra attention should be devoted to the skin and mucosal surfaces, especially the mouth, and the lymph nodes, liver, and spleen. The primary laboratory test is the CBC count with differential and platelet count. The blood smear should be examined carefully for several reasons. Sometimes the neutrophils clump together and are missed, giving a falsely low neutrophil count. Bizarre neutrophil appearances may provide a clue to a specific syndrome. Finally, even with relatively normal hemoglobin and platelet counts, leukemic blasts might be seen. The diagnosis of leukemia is rarely made when neutropenia is present alone.

Because most primary care physicians will see transient neutropenia in a healthy child, serial CBC counts twice weekly at first and then weekly for 6 to 8 weeks will establish the pattern. If the neutrophil count returns to and remains normal, no further tests are needed. If drug exposure is implicated and there are adequate alternatives, that drug should be avoided in the future.

Anticipated Complications.—Neutropenic patients commonly have infections of the skin, oral mucosa, nasopharynx, gingiva, and perianal areas. Often the classic signs of inflammation are diminished or absent. More severe infections include pneumonia, sepsis, meningitis, and septic arthritis caused by *Staphylococcus* species, the gram-negative enteric organisms especially *Escherichia coli* and *Pseudomonas*, and fungi especially *Candida* species. These infections may present without fever but with mild redness, tenderness, or fluctuance or they may present with fever only in an ill-appearing child.

Primary Care Treatments.—Regardless of the cause of neutropenia, infection must be approached carefully. The use of prophylactic oral antibiotics has not been established. There is no role for prophylactic granulocyte transfusions. The afebrile child with focal infection, such as otitis or pharyngitis, should be treated with broad-spectrum oral antibiotics with mandatory close follow-up for resolution. The febrile, neutropenic child should be admitted to the hospital for at least 48 to 72 hours of broad-spectrum intravenous antibiotics pending clinical resolution and negative results on cultures. At the Children's Hospital of Philadelphia we use an anti-staphylococcal penicillin, an anti-pseudomonal cephalosporin, and an aminoglycoside. Cultures of blood, throat, urine, and any lesion sites for bacteria and fungus are needed. If a positive result on a culture is found, specific intravenous antibiotic therapy continues for an acceptable duration, for example 7 days after the first negative result on a blood culture in a clinically improved child with bacteremia. These guidelines are essential to the care of children with a known neutropenic disorder. A generally well child with a viral syndrome or on oral antibiotics for otitis media can be watched closely, with serial physical examinations and CBC counts as outlined previously.

Indications for Referral or Consultation.—Congenital neutropenia, persistent or cyclic neutropenia, severe infection at the time of neutropenia, other cell lines affected, or phenotypic abnormalities of the child or his neutrophils are indications for referral or consultation. If a self-limited process is not evident, further evaluation begins with a bone marrow aspirate and biopsy coupled with serologic and culture screening for infection. Further useful tests include a Coombs' test, serum folate levels, and serum B_{12} levels. CBC counts in other family members are sometimes revealing. To make a specific diagnosis and prognosis, the hematologist might also consider the anti-neutrophil antibody assay, antinuclear antibody assay, quantitative immunoglobulins, in vitro neutrophil colony forming assays, a hydrocortisone stimulation test, or tests of exocrine pancreas function, which are abnormal in Schwachman-Diamond syndrome.

POSSIBLE BLEEDING DISORDERS

The question of a bleeding disorder usually arises because of frequent nosebleeds, easy bruising, excessive bleeding after minor trauma, or before elective surgery. The approach to the child with acute onset of clinical bruising and/or bleeding is covered elsewhere in an earlier section. Briefly, those children will be ill and will have one or more abnormalities of the platelet count, PT, or PTT. Important diagnostic categories include idiopathic thrombocytopenic purpura, leukemia, and disseminated intravascular coagulation. Likewise, the presentation of the common hemophilias (factor VIII and factor IX deficiency) is discussed in an earlier section. There the predominance of affected men and manifestations that may include bleeding with circumcision and into deep muscles and joints are distinctive.

The differential diagnosis of possible bleeding disorders in a generally well child is listed below, by area of the circulation primarily involved. Severe bleeding under stressful circumstances can certainly occur in these conditions.

Differential Diagnosis

COMMON CAUSES OF BLEEDING DISORDERS

Plasma

von Willebrand disease
Acquired inhibitors of coagulation
Drug use (coumarins, heparin notably in flush solutions)
Other factor deficiencies

Platelets (qualitative or functional abnormalities)

Drug use (aspirin, indomethacin, non-steroidal agents, occasionally penicillins)
Storage pool disease
Glanzmann thrombasthenia
Other platelet defects

Vascular

Vasculitis (with or without systemic collagen vascular disease)
Ehlers-Danlos syndrome
Other connective tissue abnormalities (e.g., scurvy)

Screening Tests.—A good personal and family history helps screen for the possibility of a bleeding disorder. Scoring systems and forms that incorporate the major historical questions have been devised. A list of relevant questions includes the following:

1. Does anyone in the family have a known bleeding disorder?
2. What skin manifestations of bleeding does the patient have: petechiae, spontaneous bruising, easy traumatic bruising, or prolonged (>1 hour) bleeding from lacerations?
3. Does the patient have nosebleeds lasting more than 30 minutes? Has he or she ever sought emergency care for these or required packing?
4. Is there mouth bleeding: spontaneous, with tooth brushing, after minor trauma, after loss of baby teeth, or after dental work?
5. Is there any deep muscle bruising, spontaneous or with immunization injections?
6. Is there joint bleeding, spontaneous or with minor injury?
7. What operations has the patient had and was there excessive bleeding or need for transfusion (include circumcision, tonsilectomy, tooth extraction)?
8. Is there excessive vaginal bleeding, with menses, between menses, during pregnancy, or with childbirth?
9. Was there excessive bleeding or delayed separation (after 18 days) with the umbilical cord?
10. Is there any hemoptysis, hematemesis, melena, or hematuria without an identified anatomic abnormality?

A positive family history has one or more relatives (including parents, siblings, grandparents, aunts, uncles, and first cousins) with the same bleeding manifestations sought in the personal history. An epistaxis scoring system has recently been proposed and tested to identify which children with nosebleeds will benefit from further laboratory tests.

An algorithm for evaluating a possible bleeding disorder is presented in Figure 59–5. All individuals with a suspected bleeding disorder should have a CBC count with differential and platelet count, a PT, and a PTT. Screening for disseminated intravascular coagulation is not necessary in an essentially well child. If the CBC count, PT, and/or PTT are reproducibly abnormal, the advice of a hematologist should be sought. If the CBC count, PT, and PTT are normal and the personal and family histories are not highly suspicious, no further testing is needed, with the exception of before major surgery. If the CBC count, PT, and PTT are normal but the personal or family history is highly suspicious or major surgery is planned, a bleeding time test should be done. Other tests, such as clotting time, do not add to the evaluation.

The bleeding time test examines how long it takes a stable clot to form at the site of a small

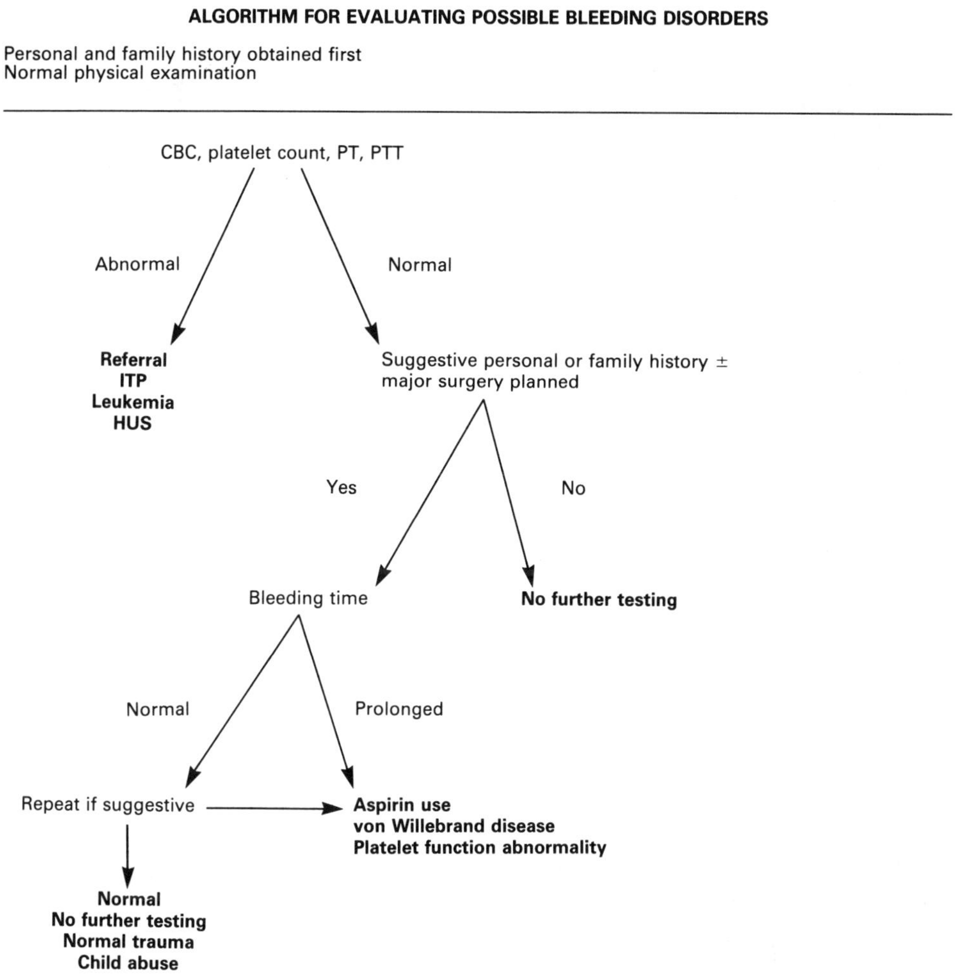

FIG 59–5

Decision tree for differential diagnosis of possible bleeding disorders.

puncture or linear wound. It is done usually on the undersurface of the forearm with a blood pressure cuff inflated to 40 mm Hg on the upper arm, and it may leave a small scar. The result of the test depends on the skill of the technician. Therefore the test is best done by experienced personnel. Normal ranges are established by the specific method and the testing lab. To have a normal bleeding time means that virtually all aspects of clotting are functional: plasma factors important to platelet adhesion and aggregation, platelet function, and vascular integrity. This feature makes the bleeding time a quite sensitive, though not specific, test. More importantly, the chances of significant bleeding with a properly performed normal bleeding time are very small.

The evaluation of a prolonged bleeding time begins by ruling out recent drug ingestion. As little as 80 mg of aspirin within as many as 7 days of the test may prolong the bleeding time. Many over-the-counter medications include aspirin. The test should be repeated when no medications have been ingested for a week. If no medications are implicated in a prolonged bleeding time, the hematologist will perform further testing directed initially at detecting von Willebrand disease or a platelet function abnormality.

Von Willebrand disease is the most common

identifiable disease with a prolonged bleeding time. Its incidence is probably close to that of hemophilia A (about one in 10,000 individuals in the general population), but its variable clinical manifestations have made precise calculations difficult. Men and women are affected equally. The defect is in the plasma factors needed for platelet adhesion to damaged endothelial surfaces and for platelet aggregation. These factors circulate with the factor VIII molecular complex. They are distinct molecules from the portion that is deficient in hemophilia A. As a result, in von Willebrand disease, the PTT is most often normal. There are several subtypes of von Willebrand disease, which vary in genetics and severity. The predominant subtype, type I, has autosomal dominant inheritance and mild-to-moderate severity. Patients may have mucosal and gastrointestinal bleeding, nosebleeds, bleeding after surgery and dental extractions, and menorrhagia in women. Other less common subtypes have autosomal recessive or dominant inheritance and may be more severe, with similar bleeding as type I but also bleeding into muscles and joints. The diagnosis of von Willebrand disease is made by measuring factor VIII coagulant activity, factor VIII antigen levels, and ristocetin cofactor activity. In the most common type of von Willebrand disease, these are low. The von Willebrand multimer distribution identifies other subtypes. These levels vary over time in the same individual, since some behave as so-called acute phase reactants. Hence when the clinical or family history is suspicious, repeat testing is needed. Testing the bleeding time in other family members can be helpful.

Anticipated Complications.—The problems with the various bleeding disorders include spontaneous bleeding and bleeding during procedures and trauma. Should inexplicable significant bleeding occur with a procedure or trauma, consultation with a hematologist is recommended. There are cogent reasons for this recommendation. First, advances have made the use of blood products unnecessary in some bleeding disorders. For instance, the drug epsilon-aminocaproic acid (Amicar) can be of great use in oral bleeding and DDAVP (1-deamino-8-D-arginine vasopressin) in type I von Willebrand disease. There are major limitations to the use of DDAVP which make initial use by the primary care physician inadvisable. Second, the choice of the optimal blood product requires either a specific diagnosis or recognition of a pattern of clinical bleeding.

Primary Care Treatments.—In those patients with an identified bleeding disorder, treatment can be provided by primary care physicians in concert with a hematologist. Topical care is indicated for superficial bleeding, such as packing or cautery for nosebleeds in conjunction with the otolaryngologist. Finally, appropriate family counseling and avoidance of high-risk situations can be offered to those families with heritable bleeding disorders.

Indications for Referral or Consultation.—The algorithm serves as a guide for referral based on an office evaluation. In general, treatment decisions for bleeding patients benefit from the advice of a hematologist.

LEUKOCYTOSIS

The primary care physician may find an elevated WBC count during routine screening, a febrile episode, or the newborn period. The elevation may be exaggerated in one specific element, hence the concern will be neutrophilia, lymphocytosis or atypical lymphocytosis, monocytosis, or eosinophilia. The definition of leukocytosis requires knowledge of the upper limits of normal, which depend on the patient's age (Table 59–4). Once true leukocytosis is identified, an orderly evaluation can proceed.

Screening Tests

The history and physical examination are paramount to this workup, because the broad range of diagnoses precludes testing all possibilities. Infection of all types, drug reactions, and systemic diseases outnumber hematologic entities. Table 59–5 summarizes the differential diagnosis of each type of elevated WBC count, noting some shared and some distinct causes.

The primary distinguishing features of leukemia and leukemoid reactions are the appearance of the cells and the presence or absence of changes in other cell lines. Increased leukocyte alkaline phosphatase has been reported as a marker for the leukemoid reaction. However,

TABLE 59–4
Normal Leukocyte Counts*

	TOTAL LEUKOCYTES		NEUTROPHILS			LYMPHOCYTES			MONOCYTES		EOSINOPHILS	
AGE	MEAN	RANGE	MEAN	RANGE	%	MEAN	RANGE	%	MEAN	%	MEAN	%
Birth	18.1	9.0–30.0	11.0	6.0–26.0	61	5.5	2.0–11.0	31	1.1	6	0.4	2
12 hr	22.8	13.0–38.0	15.5	6.0–28.0	68	5.5	2.0–11.0	24	1.2	5	0.5	2
24 hr	18.9	9.4–34.0	11.5	5.0–21.0	61	5.8	2.0–11.5	31	1.1	6	0.5	2
1 wk	12.2	5.0–21.0	5.5	1.5–10.0	45	5.0	2.0–17.0	41	1.1	9	0.5	4
2 wk	11.4	5.0–20.0	4.5	1.0–9.5	40	5.5	2.0–17.0	48	1.0	9	0.4	3
1 mo	10.8	5.0–19.5	3.8	1.0–9.0	35	6.0	2.5–16.5	56	0.7	7	0.3	3
6 mo	11.9	6.0–17.5	3.8	1.0–8.5	32	7.3	4.0–13.5	61	0.6	5	0.3	3
1 yr	11.4	6.0–17.5	3.5	1.5–8.5	31	7.0	4.0–10.5	61	0.6	5	0.3	3
2 yr	10.6	6.0–17.0	3.5	1.5–8.5	33	6.3	3.0–9.5	59	0.5	5	0.3	3
4 yr	9.1	5.5–15.5	3.8	1.5–8.5	42	4.5	2.0–8.0	50	0.5	5	0.3	3
6 yr	8.5	5.0–14.5	4.3	1.5–8.0	51	3.5	1.5–7.0	42	0.4	5	0.2	3
8 yr	8.3	4.5–13.5	4.4	1.5–8.0	53	3.3	1.5–6.8	39	0.4	4	0.2	2
10 yr	8.1	4.5–13.5	4.4	1.8–8.0	54	3.1	1.5–6.5	38	0.4	4	0.2	2
16 yr	7.8	4.5–13.0	4.4	1.8–8.0	57	2.8	1.2–5.2	35	0.4	5	0.2	3
21 yr	7.4	4.5–11.0	4.4	1.8–7.7	59	2.5	1.0–4.8	34	0.3	4	0.2	3

*Numbers of leukocytes are in thousands per mm^3, ranges are estimates of 95% confidence limits, and percentages refer to differential counts. Neutrophils include band cells at all ages and a small number of metamyelocytes and myelocytes in the first few days of life. (From Dallman, PR: In Rudolph AM (ed): *Pediatrics,* ed 16. New York, Appleton-Century-Crofts, 1977, p 1178. Used by permission.)

TABLE 59–5
Differential Diagnosis of Leukocytosis

ETIOLOGY	NEUTROPHILIA	LYMPHOCYTOSIS	MONOCYTOSIS	EOSINOPHILIA
Infection				
Bacteria	x	x(A)		x(D)
Virus		x(B)	x	x(E)
Parasite				x(F)
Mycobacteria	x	x	x	
Other		x(C)		
Systemic illness				
Allergy/asthma				x
Atopic skin disease				x
Collagen vascular			x	
Ulcerative colitis			x	
Hyperthyroidism		x		
Drug reaction				
Steroid	x			
Antibiotic				x
Idiosyncratic				x
Post-splenectomy	x		x	
Malignancy				
Hodgkin disease			x	x
Leukemia	x	x		x
Leukemoid reaction	x			
Down syndrome	x			
Congenital syndromes				
Lofflers				x

A=pertussis, parapertussis; B=EBV, CMV, many others; C=toxoplasmosis; D=scarlet fever; E=*Chlamydia;* F=helminths.

definitive distinction may require bone marrow aspirate and biopsy. This is particularly true for children with Down syndrome in whom the risks of leukemoid reactions and leukemia are greatly increased over the general population.

Anticipated Complications and Primary Care Treatments

The breadth of diagnoses precludes any generalizations here, except that treatment of the underlying disorder is the most appropriate approach. Individual references are devoted to specific abnormalities, such as eosinophilia.

Indications for Referral or Consultation

Those causes of leukocytosis beyond identifiable infection, drug reaction, or systemic illness may benefit from the advice of a hematologist.

QUESTIONS ABOUT INHERITANCE PATTERNS AND SCREENING TESTS

The primary care physician may be asked about inherited hematologic disorders. Prospective parents may inquire before pregnancy or during pregnancy, or their questions may arise in the newborn period. An important related question is the availability of prenatal and newborn screening for these disorders. In obtaining the family history, the presence of the disorder or trait for that disorder if such exists can be sought in parents, siblings, and other relatives. This may well be the reason that inheritance information is sought, though public education has progressed to the point that members of certain ethnic groups are aware of risks for common genetic diseases.

Table 59–6 lists the common RBC and coagulation factor inherited disorders, the most likely populations at risk, their inheritance and frequency, and the availability of prenatal and newborn screening. WBC and platelet inherited disorders are uncommon enough that interested primary care physicians are referred to primary hematology sources. This information is not provided to act as replacement for formal genetic counseling, an essential service to families at risk that works best when primary care physicians, hematologists, obstetricians, and human geneticists work together. Rather, the intent is to indicate to the practitioner how disorders are inherited and for which disorders screening can and should be done.

Screening Tests, Anticipated Complications, and Primary Care Treatments

The value of newborn screening for sickle cell disease has been amply demonstrated: it saves lives. The risk of death from sepsis is high, up to 5% of unidentified patients. The risk is greatly decreased by enrollment before the age of 4 months at the sickle cell center with its use of prophylactic antibiotics, immunization, and probably most importantly education about the illness and febrile episodes. Many states have made newborn screening for sickle cell disease mandatory; hopefully other states will follow. These tests have the additional benefit of identifying essentially all clinically relevant inherited hemoglobin disorders. Electrophoresis with agar gel at an acid pH (6.0) is the method of choice at Children's Hospital of Philadelphia because of the ability to distinguish abundant fetal hemoglobin from normal and sickle hemoglobin. The test can be performed with 1 mL of anticoagulated blood (purple top tube).

Indications for Referral or Consultation

Any individual whose family history places them at risk for an inherited hematologic disorder may benefit from consultation with a hematologist. All individuals found through screening to have a RBC or coagulation factor inherited disorder will need referral to a hematologist. For the much larger numbers of individuals who are identified with traits for these disorders, i.e., heterozygotes for recessive disorders, appropriate counseling can be coordinated by the primary care physician with input as needed by the hematologist and geneticist.

THE ASPLENIC CHILD

The primary care physician may encounter a child who is without spleen function for one of three reasons: the spleen was removed surgically, the spleen is in place but not working, or the child was born without a spleen. The most common reasons for surgical removal include traumatic rupture and certain hematologic processes. This latter group includes splenectomy

TABLE 59–6
Hematologic Disorders: Inheritance Patterns and Screening Tests

DISORDER	POPULATION	DISEASE FREQUENCY	INHERITANCE	SCREENING
RBC				
Sickle cell anemia	A	1 in 600 (blacks)	Autosomal recessive	Newborn (a), prenatal
Thalassemia				
alpha	A^{+}	b	Autosomal recessive	Newborn, prenatal
beta	A	1 in 20,000 (c)	Autosomal recessive	Newborn, prenatal
G-6-PD deficiency	A^{+}	1 in 5,000	X-linked recessive	Newborn
Hereditary spherocytosis	White primarily	1 in 5,000	Autosomal dominant (some recessive)	Newborn
Coagulation factor				
VIII (hemophilia A)	All	1 in 10,000–12,000	X-linked recessive	Newborn, prenatal
IX (hemophilia B)	All	1 in 40,000–50,000	X-linked recessive	Newborn, prenatal
von Willebrand disease	All	Unknown (of order 1 in 10,000)	Autosomal dominant (>90%)	Newborn

A=the "malaria belt" populations: Africa, Mediterranean, Middle East, Indian subcontinent, and Southeast Asia; +=genotypes differ in black and oriental forms with significant consequences; a=this screening is strongly encouraged, and legally mandated in increasing numbers of states; b=because there are two genes for alpha globin on each chromosome 16, the inheritance is complex; however, 3% of the American black population lacks two of the four genes and has microcytosis and mild anemia, absence of four genes causes hydrops fetalis and is lethal; c=the incidence varies widely with ethnic group and location, up to one in ten in some Greek and oriental locales.

for ITP, hereditary spherocytosis, homozygous beta-thalassemia, and Hodgkin disease. Functional asplenia occurs in sickle cell disease, after splenic radiation, and with immunodeficiencies. Syndromes with congenital absence of the spleen exist but are very rare.

The danger with reduced or absent splenic function is overwhelming bacterial infection. The spleen serves as a principal filter for bacteria that reach the blood and as a site of antibody synthesis. The risk of fulminant sepsis depends on the cause of diminished function and the age of the child, but the relative risk of death from sudden onset of sepsis ranges from 50 to 1,000 times that of the general population. Before the age of 5 years, the risk appears to be the highest, regardless of the cause. Much of our current knowledge about treating asplenic children comes from the natural history after surgical removal and the efforts of the National Collaborative Study of Sickle Cell Disease.

Screening Tests

In almost all cases the functional or anatomic asplenia of the individual is known. Specialized tests can often identify individuals with impaired spleen function, including the search for Howell-Jolly bodies on the peripheral blood smear and microscopic examination with Nomarsky optics for pitted RBCs.

Anticipated Complications and Primary Care Treatments

Sepsis in the asplenic individual is characterized by the rapid onset of fever and malaise followed by deterioration that can be fatal in hours. The encapsulated organisms are the major offenders, with pneumococcus as the most common offender. Other major pathogens include *H. influenzae* b and meningococcus. The febrile asplenic child is an emergency case, and evaluation and treatment must be prompt, regardless of oral antibiotic prophylaxis or immunization status. When the temperature exceeds 38.5° C, a careful examination, CBC count, and cultures of the blood, urine, and throat should be followed up with intravenous antibiotics effective against the likely organisms. There is no need to wait for any test results before treating; in fact, this would be dangerous. Intravenous antibiotics should continue for 48 to 72 hours until the culture results are negative and the patient is improved. Viral syndromes will occur in these children, but all fevers must be evaluated and those above 38.5° C treated as above. Fever of 38.0° to 38.4° C warrants increased oral antibiotic prophylaxis to four times a day for 5 to 7 days and close observation. However, if the child is ill-appearing, intravenous antibiotics are indicated.

Elective splenectomy should be deferred until the age of 5 years or above. It should be preceded by immunization against pneumococcus and *H. influenzae* b. Because the potential benefits outweigh the minor risks, lifelong penicillin prophylaxis is recommended. A program of immunization and penicillin prophylaxis is standard care for the sickle cell patient. If in an emergency the spleen is removed without vaccination against pneumococcus, the vaccination should be given as soon as possible after splenectomy.

BIBLIOGRAPHY

Dickerman JD: Splenectomy and sepsis: A warning. *Pediatrics* 1979; 63:938–941.

Gaston MH, et al: Prophylaxis with oral penicillin in children with sickle cell anemia. *N Engl J Med* 1986; 314:1593–1599.

Katsanis E, Luke KH, Hsu E, Li M, Lillicrap D: Prevalence and significance of mild bleeding disorders in children with recurrent epistaxis. *J Pediatr* 1988; 113:73–76.

Lukens JN: Eosinophilia in children. *Pediatr Clin North Am* 1972; 19:969–981.

Lusher JM: Diseases of coagulation: The fluid phase, in Nathan DG, Oski FA, (eds): *Hematology of Infancy and Childhood*, ed 3. Philadelphia, WB Saunders Co, 1987; pp 1293–1342.

Manroe BL, Weinberg AG, Rosenfeld CR, Browne R: The neonatal blood count in health and disease. I. Reference values for neutrophilic cells. *J Pediatr* 1979; 95:89–98.

Stockman JA: Hematologic manifestations of systemic diseases, in Nathan DG, Oski FA, (eds): *Hematology of Infancy and Childhood*, ed 3. Philadelphia, WB Saunders Co, 1987; pp 1632–1676.

Vichinsky E, Hurst D, Earles A, et al: Newborn screening for sickle cell disease: Effect on mortality. *Pediatrics* 1988; 81:749–755.

Weetman RM, Boxer LA: Childhood neutropenia. *Pediatr Clin North Am* 1980; 27:361–375.

Zarkowsky HS, Gallagher D, Gill F, et al: Bacteremia in sickle hemoglobinopathies. *J Pediatr* 1986; 109:579–585.

60 INFECTIOUS DISEASES OF CHILDHOOD

Louis M. Bell, M.D.

The infant, toddler, and child are faced with a vast array of infectious diseases. The child's maturing immune system must control the spread of primary infections, as well as provide the amnestic response needed to attenuate or prevent repeated infections from causative agents.

Despite the development of vaccines that prevent many of the once "common childhood diseases," the physician who cares for children must still be able to recognize a variety of different infections that are unique to this age group.

This chapter describes some of the infectious diseases seen in children beginning with the six childhood exanthems which were known by numbers in the late 19th century. Measles, scarlet fever, and rubella were the first three. The "fourth disease" is no longer recognized. Erythema infectiosum was named the fifth disease and roseola infantum has been referred to as the sixth disease.

MEASLES

Measles, a highly contagious disease, is spread by the airborne route and has an incubation period of 8 to 12 days. Vaccination with killed measles vaccines from 1963 to 1968 and then attenuated live measles virus vaccine since 1968 has made this a rare infection in the United States, with on average 3,000 cases of measles reported each year since 1981. However, the number of cases doubled in 1986 and continues to increase. In 1989 the CDC received reports of 56 outbreaks of measles, which accounted for an increase of more than 300% in cases over the number reported in 1988. In addition, measles is still prevalent in developing countries and therefore can be seen in the immigrant population of the United States, especially in children under 5 years of age.

DATA GATHERING

The prodrome of measles lasts about 2 to 4 days and begins with symptoms of an upper respiratory infection and fever up to 104° F. General malaise, conjunctivitis with photophobia, and cough increase in severity over this period. It is during this time that Koplik spots (white spots on the buccal mucosa) appear.

Appearance of rash on the face and abdomen occurs classically 14 days following exposure. The rash is erythematous and maculopapular and spreads from the head to the feet. After 3 to 4 days, the rash begins to clear, leaving a brownish discoloration and fine scaling. Fever is usually absent 3 days after the rash appears. Pharyngitis, cervical lymphadenopathy, and splenomegaly may accompany the rash. Diarrhea and vomiting may be seen in the young.

Modified and Atypical Measles.—Classic measles as described above is relatively rare. One is more likely to see either modified measles (occurring in a partially immune individual) or atypical measles (primarily in individuals vaccinated with killed vaccine between 1963 to 1967).

Modified measles occurs naturally in infants less than 9 months because of the presence of transplacental acquired maternal antibody or as a result of the administration of immune globulin to an exposed susceptible child. The illness follows the progression outlined above but is generally mild. Conversely, individuals (young adults) with atypical measles are quite ill with a sudden onset of fever to 103° F to 105° F associated with headache. Unlike typical measles, Koplik spots are rare, and the rash appears first on the distal extremities progressing in a cephalad direction. In addition, virtually all patients have respiratory distress with clinical and radiographic signs of pneumonia, often associated with pleural effusion.

Diagnosis depends on recognition of the progression of the clinical illness and on results of acute and convalescent measles antibody serologies, collected 1 to 3 weeks apart.

COMPLICATIONS

Pneumonia, myocarditis, pericarditis, encephalitis and disseminated intravascular coagulation (Black measles) have been associated with measles virus infection.

Subacute sclerosis panencephalitis (SSPE) occurs in one per 100,000 children with naturally occurring measles. After an incubation period of several years, a progressive encephalopathy develops among vaccinated children. The incubation period is shortened and occurs in one in 1,000,000 vaccinees.

MANAGEMENT

In an attempt to control the measles outbreaks in the United States, new recommendations for measles immunization have recently been published by the American Academy of Pediatrics. These recommendations include routine vaccination against measles, mumps, and rubella (MMR) at 15 months and a second MMR vaccination at entrance to middle school or junior high school. In addition, MMR vaccination at 12 months is recommended for preschool children in high-risk areas. In outbreak situations, monovalent measles vaccine may be given to infants as young as 6 months.

If aggressive vaccination programs around the world are pursued, elimination of measles as a cause of human disease is possible. There is no specific antiviral therapy available.

SCARLET FEVER

Scarlet fever is caused by group A β-hemolytic streptococci. The disease is spread by close contact of primarily school age children and is rare in infants. Because immunity is short-lived, it may recur every 3 to 5 years during childhood. The rash is a result of hypersensitization to the erythrogenic toxins produced by the organism, which has established a focus of infection. The most likely site of invasion by the organism is the pharynx or tonsils, but other sites such as the skin (impetigo) or perianal area also can be infected.

DATA GATHERING

The typical course of scarlet fever begins with complaints of sore throat after an incubation period of 1 to 4 days. The pharynx may appear reddened with petechiae on the soft palate, with a swollen uvula and reddened tonsils, often with a whitish exudate. However, the pharyngitis may be subclinical. The tongue may also have swollen papillae giving the appearance of a strawberry.

The rash is typically erythematous with closely grouped fine papules, giving a sandpaper feel to the skin. The rash starts on the face and trunk and is most prominent in the folds of the skin. The rash blanches with pressure. The skin will usually peel after the rash fades in 4 to 7 days. Just as the skin peels, the tongue will typically peel to a smooth surface.

Positive results of a throat culture or from other suspicious skin lesions helps to confirm the diagnosis of scarlet fever. An alternative to cultures are the numerous rapid diagnostic tests that detect the group A carbohydrate antigen. Although the specificity of the tests is usually good, they lack sensitivity, so all negative results should be confirmed with traditional culture methods. One should confirm a group A streptococcus infection because a scarlatiniform rash is sometimes associated with enteroviral infections.

MANAGEMENT

Treatment prevents the suppurative and nonsuppurative complications of group A streptococci infections.

COMPLICATIONS OF GROUP A β-HEMOLYTIC STREPTOCOCCI PHARYNGITIS

Suppurative
Peritonsillar abscess
Otitis media
Mastoiditis
Osteomyelitis of the skull
Nonsuppurative
Acute rheumatic fever
Glomerulonephritis

Treatment consists of Benzathine penicillin G or penicillin VK in appropriate doses. Penicillin prevents rheumatic fever, even if therapy is started 7 to 9 days after the onset of acute illness, so even delayed therapy is indicated.

RUBELLA (GERMAN MEASLES)

Rubella is usually a mild erythematous infection spread by infectious droplet with minimal morbidity. However, infection during pregnancy may have devastating effects on the fetus. Vaccination programs, which started in 1969, are aimed at reducing the rubella activity in women of child-bearing age.

DATA GATHERING

Symptoms of malaise, a sore throat, and low-grade fevers may precede the rash. The rash may start in the malar region of the face, then spread to the trunk and limbs. The rash, which blanches with pressure, clears after 3 to 4 days. The spleen may also be palpable. Enlarged occipital and postauricular lymph nodes in association with a morbilliform rash should raise the suspicion of rubella. Rubella can be confirmed by the presence of anti-rubella IgM antibodies in the serum.

Complications of rubella includes polyarthritis, especially in older girls; encephalitis in one of 5,000 cases; and congenital deformities in infants born to mothers with the disease. Commonly described anomalies associated with congenital rubella include cataracts, microophthalmia, chorioretinitis, sensorineural deafness, microcephaly, and mental retardation.

MANAGEMENT

If rubella infection occurs, treatment consists of supportive measures only.

ERYTHEMA INFECTIOSUM (FIFTH DISEASE)

Erythema infectiosum or fifth disease is caused by parvovirus B19, a virus first discovered in asymptomatic blood donors in 1975. The infection is probably spread by respiratory secretions. Secondary spread among susceptible family members is common and occurs in 23% to 62% of children and 14% to 38% of adults. The incubation period is 6 to 16 days.

DATA GATHERING

Erythema infectiosum is a mild childhood illness characterized by prodromal symptoms of low-grade fevers, malaise, and occasionally a sore throat. This prodrome may last 1 to 4 days, followed by a facial rash ("slapped cheeks") over the malar areas of the face. This is followed by a diffuse macular or maculopapular rash on the extremities and trunk, which is sometimes described as reticulated or lacelike. Rubella-like, vesicular and purpuric rashes have also been associated with parvovirus B19 infection. The rash may last for up to 10 days and is pruritic in 30% to 50% of cases. The rash may fade but reappear after sun exposure or exercise.

Other common associated symptoms include arthralgias and arthritis. Arthritis is rare in children but can occur in up to 90% of symptomatic adults. The most common joints affected are the knees and hands. There may be only mild swelling of the painful joint. Serologic tests for detecting a specific IgM antibody response to parvovirus are available only in research laboratories. The Centers for Disease Control will make these tests available on a limited basis.

COMPLICATIONS

In children, erythema infectiosum is a mild, self-limited illness during which the child usually remains alert and playful. Adults may have prolonged complaints of joint symptoms. In addition, parvovirus B19 infections have been associated with aplastic crisis in patients with chronic hemolytic anemia, hydrops fetalis, and chronic bone marrow suppression in immunocompromised individuals.

MANAGEMENT

Treatment is supportive. Parents of the child should be counseled concerning secondary spread of this infection among family members. The potential risks of this infection to the fetus are being studied.

ROSEOLA INFANTUM (SIXTH DISEASE)

Roseola infantum (exanthema subitum) is a common acute illness of young children with a year-round incidence. Ninety percent of those infected are less than 2 years old. It is rare before the age of 3 months. Roseola-like illnesses have been associated with enteroviruses, adenoviruses, and parvovirus B19. Most recently, human herpes virus 6 has been identified in a small number of cases. Apparently, roseola is a syndrome due to many different viral agents.

DATA GATHERING

The basic clinical pattern of the roseola syndrome is the sudden onset of fever (usually above 38.9°C [102°F]) which lasts for 3 to 5 days and may rapidly return to normal. Only after defervescence does a rash appear, predominantly on the trunk. The rash is characterized by discrete erythematous, macular or maculopapular lesions that blanch with pressure. The rash, which lasts for 24 to 48 hours, is not usually associated with pruritis or desquamation. Although febrile, the child is frequently happy and playful. A number of other signs and symptoms have been occasionally associated with roseola, including inflammation of the pharynx and tonsils, infection of the tympanic membranes, suboccipital and postauricular adenopathy, palpebral edema, and bulging of the anterior fontanelle.

Many patients will have leukopenia (with a relative lymphocytosis), which reaches its nadir on the third to sixth day of illness.

Presumably because of the often rapid onset

of fever, febrile seizures are the most common of complications associated with roseola. Roseola rarely produces encephalitis, occasionally with permanent central nervous system (CNS) sequelae.

MUMPS

Mumps, caused by a paramyxovirus, was a common childhood infection prior to the introduction of vaccine. Infection affects primarily pre-school and grade-school age children, occurring in late winter and early spring. Spread of the infection is via airborne droplets. The incubation period can be from 12 to 22 days. Asymptomatic infection is common, occurring in 20% to 40% of children.

DATA GATHERING

Rarely is mumps a severe systemic illness. A prodrome of fever, malaise, and headache may precede the parotid gland swelling. Pain and swelling may occur in one or both parotid glands. In trying to differentiate between parotid gland swelling and lymphadenopathy, the examiner should remember that the parotid gland lies in front of the ear, and the uncinate lobe of the gland wraps itself underneath and in back of the ear. Swelling in this area will result in elevation of the earlobe. After unilateral parotid gland swelling, the second parotid gland may become swollen after 1 to 2 days. At times, the submandibular glands may be involved concomitantly with the parotid gland or alone. Redness and swelling of Stenson or Wharton ducts of the affected glands may occur. Eating or drinking may cause discomfort. The swelling may last for 1 week to 10 days.

In addition, patients with mumps usually are febrile for 3 to 4 days. Headache, photophobia, and other signs of meningeal irritation are more common in older children (>15 years). The disease is considered noninfectious 1 week after the onset of parotid gland swelling.

Other infectious causes of parotid swelling should be considered in the differential diagnosis.

INFECTIOUS DISEASES ASSOCIATED WITH PAROTID SWELLING

Viruses
Mumps
Enterovirus (coxsackie A)
Parainfluenza virus
Cytomegalovirus
Epstein-Barr virus
Bacterial (suppurative)
Staphylococcus aureus
Streptococcus species
Tuberculosis
Histoplasmosis
Cat scratch disease

COMPLICATIONS

Orchitis is probably the most feared complication of mumps. Up to 35% of postpubertal men with mumps may be affected. A new onset of fever with unilateral pain, swelling, and tenderness of the testicle occurs at the end of the first week of illness with mumps. Bilateral involvement is less common but may lead to sterility. Analgesics, support of the testicle and the application of ice may help to relieve the discomfort. There is no indication for the use of steroids.

Other complications include aseptic meningitis, epididymitis, oophoritis, pancreatitis, mastitis, thyroiditis, arthritis, and deafness.

MANAGEMENT

Supportive therapy is recommended in the treatment of mumps. Analgesics may be necessary, especially if severe headaches are noted. The physician caring for the child may be asked advice concerning the father who has no history of symptomatic infection who is exposed to mumps. Although administration of the live attenuated mumps vaccine is not protective, it may prevent infection due to future exposure. In many cases, the father may have had a subclinical infection as a child.

INFLUENZA VIRUS

Influenza viruses A, B, and C are responsible for acute respiratory tract infections, which have occurred in epidemics throughout history. Although attack rates are highest in children, the major mortality and morbidity rates associated with this infection occur in the elderly or in those with underlying illness such as heart disease, chronic lung disease, chronic renal disease, and in patients with neoplasm or neuromuscular illnesses. Improvements in living standards and the ability to treat the secondary bacterial infections associated with influenza have led to a gradual decline in mortality rates. Influenza viruses A and B cause the majority of human disease. Occurring in the winter months, the infection is spread by inhalation of aerosolized nasal secretions or by direct contact. The incubation period is 2 to 3 days with viral shedding lasting up to 5 days after the onset of clinical symptoms.

DATA GATHERING

The symptoms of influenza have a rapid onset characterized by fever up to 104° or 106°C with chills, headache, and myalgias. Cough, nasal congestion, and complaints of photophobia or pain with eye movements are also common. In younger children, symptoms of bronchiolitis or the croupy cough of laryngotracheitis may predominate. Symptoms will last from 3 to 7 days. Gastrointestinal symptoms of nausea, vomiting, or diarrhea have been described for both influenza virus A and B epidemics.

Outbreaks of influenza occurring in the winter months along with the characteristic constellation of symptoms facilitate the diagnosis. Virus can be isolated from respiratory secretions to confirm the diagnosis. Generally, isolation takes 1 to 3 days. Currently, new rapid diagnostic techniques are being tested which will allow same day results. The sensitivity and specificity of these tests remain to be seen.

COMPLICATIONS

Secondary bacterial infections especially in the elderly, may complicate influenza infections. Myositis with myoglobinemia requiring careful fluid management is seen more commonly in children. Reye syndrome has been associated with influenza virus A infections and aspirin therapy. Other more rare complications include encephalitis, pericarditis, myocarditis, and acute parotitis.

MANAGEMENT

Treatment for influenza is mainly rest, fluids, and temperature control with acetaminophen. Aspirin is not recommended because of its association with the development of Reye syndrome. Amantadine has been shown to be effective against only influenza A and is most efficacious if used as prophylaxis against infection.

VARICELLA-ZOSTER INFECTIONS (CHICKENPOX AND ZOSTER)

The primary infection of the varicella-zoster virus results in chickenpox, while reactivation of latent virus results in a unilateral vesicular eruption localized to the sensory dermatomes, called zoster or "shingles." Chickenpox occurs in the late winter and early spring. The illness is transmitted by respiratory spread and will infect susceptible persons with an 85% attack rate among household contacts. The incubation period of varicella is 11 to 21 days. Most cases of infection occur in children between 5 and 10 years of age. The children are contagious until the vesicular rash is crusted. Although zoster or shingles are more common in the elderly, it is not uncommon in children and may be seen in infants whose mothers had chickenpox in the third trimester. Susceptible individuals exposed to a patient with zoster may become infected.

DATA GATHERING

In children, chickenpox is usually a mild illness characterized by a low-grade fever (temperature 38.4° to 38.9°C) and a vesicular rash. The hallmark of the rash is that one can observe lesions in different stages of evolution. Individual lesions progress from macules to papules, then to vesicles, and finally to crusted lesions on an erythematous base. The rash starts on the scalp or trunk and may involve the mucous membranes and sclera. It is often pruritic. Crops of lesions may appear over the first 3 to 5 days spreading to the extremities.

Varicella in immunocompetent children is almost always benign. However, in immunocompromised children or infants born to mothers whose rash appeared within 5 days before delivery or within 48 hours after delivery, the infection may be progressive and severe with a mortality rate of 20%. In addition, chickenpox in adolescents and adults tends to be more severe with systemic symptoms and a confluent rash.

The rash of zoster consists of grouped vesicles on an erythematous base. The vesicles are confined to one to three sensory dermatomes. If the vesicles are seen on the tip of the nose, the ophthalmic branch of the facial nerve is affected, and repeat examinations to rule out ocular involvement are necessary. Prior to eruption, there may be a prodrome of pain or tingling.

COMPLICATIONS

Secondary bacterial skin infections with streptococci or staphylococci are the most common complication.

CNS manifestations occur as well. Meningoencephalitis can occur and may be severe, appearing early in the course of chickenpox. An acute cerebellar ataxia, which usually appears after 5 to 10 days of the rash, is the most common CNS complication. The prognosis with this type of isolated cerebellitis is good. Reye syndrome appears to occur more frequently in children with chickenpox or influenza.

Idiopathic thrombocytopenic purpura can be associated with varicella infection, occurring after a week of illness. Purpura fulminans is a rare phenomenon characterized by an inflammatory vasculitis and necrosis of the tissues, predominantly the extremities and buttocks.

MANAGEMENT

Uncomplicated chickenpox or zoster in children requires only supportive therapy. Daily bathing will help decrease secondary skin infections, but soap detergents may be irritating. Some recommend oatmeal baths (one cup oatmeal with three cups cold water in a quart jar and shake well) as a soothing cleansing bath. Pruritus can be controlled with antihistamines. Fingernails should be trimmed to prevent secondary skin infections from scratching.

Acyclovir is indicated for immunocompromised children with chickenpox or zoster. The use of acyclovir in immunocompetent children with zoster is probably not necessary, but can be considered in children with involvement of the ophthalmic branch of the facial nerve. Situations in which varicella-zoster immune globulin is indicated are published by the American Academy of Pediatrics. Passive immunization has been shown to prevent or modify illness in normal and high-risk individuals. Currently, a live varicella vaccine is being considered for licensure in the United States.

HERPES SIMPLEX VIRUS

Herpes simplex virus (HSV, types 1 and 2), a ubiquitous virus, infects a majority of people. The wide spectrum of illness includes cutaneous, mucous membrane, ocular, and nervous system infection. Like other herpes viruses (cytomegalovirus, Epstein-Barr virus, and varicella-zoster virus), HSV is able to induce a state of latency in the infected individual which may lead to recurrences of disease. The mechanism leading to recurrence is unknown. People of all ages are susceptible to HSV infection, which can be symptomatic or asymptomatic. The infection is spread among individuals via close contact and is present without regard to socioeconomic group. The incubation period is not well defined but is related to the size of the inoculum and has been estimated to be 2 to 14 days.

Serologically, there are two types of HSV infection. HSV type 1 infection is found in children and adults, with 90% exhibiting HSV-1 antibodies by adulthood. HSV type 2 accounts for the majority of HSV genital infection in adults. As might be expected, HSV-2 infections are the predominate cause of neonatal disease.

DATA GATHERING

The clinical manifestation of HSV infection can be primary or recurrent, as a result of reactivation of a latent virus infection.

Mucosal Infection

Acute herpetic gingivostomatitis is one of the most frequent manifestations of a primary HSV infection. Young children are usually affected (10 months to 3 years). The child may develop fever 24 to 48 hours prior to the development of gingivirus or mucous membrane ulcers, which involve the anterior tongue and hard palate. The gingiva will be swollen and red, often with exudate at the gum line which may bleed with gentle pressure from a tongue blade. Vesicles may appear around the mouth and on the chin. In children who suck their fingers, the infection can be transferred to the digit causing herpetic whitlow. Fever may last up to 10 days. Associated cervical and submental lymph nodes are often swollen and tender. The most important complications of this infection is refusal to drink fluids with subsequent dehydration.

HSV gingivostomatitis is differentiated from herpangina (see next section) by the placement of the ulcers. The patient with herpangina, a manifestation of enteroviral infection, has ulcers on the posterior palate and anterior tonsillar pillars.

Skin Infection

HSV infections of the skin are common and may develop in apparently unbroken skin. More commonly, minor skin trauma in a child becomes infected with HSV by the common habit of "kissing it better." Grouped vesicles on an erythematous base may appear 24 to 48 hours after inoculation. Herpetic whitlow, sometimes confused with bacterial felon or paronychia, can be secondary to autoinoculation in the child with herpetic stomatitis or may be seen in sexually active patients. Health care workers (dentists, nurses, physicians) are also at risk, as they come in contact with oral secretions during care of their patients. Careful hand washing and gloves will prevent such exposure.

Interestingly, erythema multiforme may occur in some patients with recurrent HSV skin eruptions. Thought to be an allergic response, the typical rash appears 7 to 10 days after the HSV eruption. In addition, sports involving close physical contact have been associated with cutaneous HSV infection. Wrestling (herpes gladiatorum) and rugby (scrum pox) are two examples. These infections must be differentiated from impetigo.

Any child with chronic dermatitis, such as eczema, is at risk for secondary infection with HSV. The infection may spread extensively and is recognized as eczema herpeticum, otherwise known as Kaposi varicelliform eruption. Finally, HSV-2 infection can be manifest in the genitalia of both boys and girls (see section on Sexually Transmitted Disease, later in this chapter).

Herpes Simplex Infection in Neonates

Neonatal herpes infection occurs in infants after exposure either intrauterine, perinatally, or postnatal spread from the mother, father, or hospital nursery personnel. Intrauterine infection is rare but is associated with chorioretinitis, mental retardation, and microcephaly. Postnatal acquisition is also rare but is well described in the literature. The overwhelming majority of infants became infected perinatally. However, many mothers will not have any prior history of HSV infection.

The risk of HSV infection to the infants born vaginally is much higher in those mothers with primary genital HSV infection. The clinical presentation of HSV infection in neonates occurs in three patterns. The infant, usually in the first week of life, may develop a generalized sepsis involving the liver and CNS. Only one-third of these infants will necessarily have HSV skin lesions associated with sepsis. Mortality is high. Some infants may have isolated CNS symptoms, while some have localized skin and mucocutaneous infection alone.

Central Nervous System Infections

HSV infections may cause encephalitis. In the majority of cases, the encephalitis is caused by a recurrent infection with HSV-1 and can affect people of all ages. The encephalitis may not be associated with cerebrospinal fluid (CSF) pleocytosis but consistently involves the temporal lobe. HSV encephalitis is an acute illness beginning with fever and irritability, which progresses rapidly to CNS symptoms with focal neurologic or altered mental status, coma, and death in the majority of cases if untreated. HSV-2 causes aseptic meningitis usually associated with a primary genital infection. Signs of meningitis (unlike HSV-I encephalitis) are commonly observed.

Eye Infections

Primary HSV infection of the eye may cause an acute superficial conjunctivitis. This may proceed to cause ulceration of the cornea. Deep lesions of the cornea and iris are also possible and may be caused in part by a hypersensitivity to the herpes virus.

DIAGNOSIS

Diagnosis of cutaneous herpes infections can be made by the appearance of grouped vesicles on an erythematous base. Clinical suspicion can be confirmed by isolation of the virus in tissue culture from vesicles, genital lesions, CSF, urine, and blood. Fortunately, HSV grows quickly and can be identified in most cases by 3 days. More rapid diagnostic techniques include the Tzank test with the modified Wright stain. In this test, the base of a vesicle is gently scraped and the stained cells are examined for evidence of multinucleated giant cells. The test is nonspecific and will be positive in 60% to 70% of cases. A more sensitive fluorescent antibody test again depends on obtaining HSV infected cells at the base of the vesicle.

Although the diagnosis of herpes encephalitis can be difficult, contrast-material-enhanced computed tomography (CT) will often reveal involvement of the temporal lobe. The electroencephalogram (EEG) will show a characteristic spike wave pattern in the affected temporal lobe. Brain biopsy and isolation of HSV is the gold standard for diagnosis, and is necessary in some cases to confirm the HSV infection or to identify other treatable causes of encephalitis.

MANAGEMENT

In neonates with HSV infection, acyclovir and/or vidarabine have been used to treat both localized mucocutaneous lesions and CNS or systemic infections. Acyclovir has less toxicity and is easier to administer and is preferred. Acyclovir is the drug of choice for encephalitis in older patients.

Patients with HSV ocular involvement should receive a topical ophthalmic drug (1% or 2% trifluridine, 1% iododeoxyuridine, or 3% vidarabine) as well as systemic acyclovir therapy. Topical steroids are contraindicated in HSV infections of the eye.

ENTEROVIRUS INFECTIONS

The genus enterovirus includes coxsackie viruses, echoviruses, polioviruses and any newly identified enterovirus, which are now classified only by number and not assigned any particular name or grouping. The non-polio enteroviruses, which are responsible for a variety of human illness, will be discussed in this section.

In general, the peak time of enteroviral illness in temperate climates is late summer and early fall. In tropical regions, no seasonal pattern is apparent. The spread of enterovirus infections is thought to occur only among people usually by the fecal-oral route. Fecal viral excretion may continue for several weeks after the onset of infection. Insects and animals which come in contact with human excreta may spread the infection, especially among people with poor sanitary systems. The primary illnesses occur in infants and children. Many infections are asymptomatic. The incubation period is 3 to 6 days.

DATA GATHERING

Coxsackie viruses groups A and B, echoviruses, and enteroviruses are associated with specific illnesses that are outlined below.

Coxsackie Viruses, Group A

These viruses are associated with infections of the mouth and skin and are rarely serious. Herpangina is one such infection often caused by subtypes A4, A5, A6, or A10. This illness is characterized by fever and painful vesicles and ulcers on the soft palate and anterior tonsillar pillas. Sometimes ulceration on the buccal mucosa occurs. The illness lasts 4 to 5 days.

Hand-foot-and-mouth disease often occurs in epidemics, usually in children under 4 years of age. The causative agents are subtypes A16, A5, A7, or A9. Scattered vesicles appear in the mouth that quickly ulcerate. In addition, many children develop vesicular lesions on the palms and soles. Occasionally, scattered vesicles appear on the proximal extremities and buttocks. Rarely, a generalized vesicular or macular papular rash occurs that resembles varicella but occurs in only one crop. Several group A subtypes are associated with a febrile disease in infants and young children characterized by a maculopapular rash that begins on the face and spreads to the trunk. The palms and soles are usually spared.

Coxsackie Viruses, Group B

Illnesses associated with group B infections are, in general, more serious and include pleurodynia, sepsis in the neonate, myocarditis and pericarditis, and CNS infections.

Pleurodynia (Bornholm disease, devil's grip) is characterized by an acute onset of severe paroxysmal pain referred to the lower ribs. The pain is made worse by coughing or motion. In some patients, there is a prodrome of headache, malaise, and myalgia. The severe pleuritic pain may radiate to the neck and scapular region and be accompanied by upper abdominal pain and splinting of abdominal muscles. The patients are usually febrile and may have other symptoms such as headache, diarrhea, and vomiting. The illness lasts about 4 days, although recrudescence occurs frequently.

Myocarditis and pericarditis have been associated with subtype B1-5. The patient will present with symptoms of congestive heart failure, and/or pericarditis often about 2 weeks after a nonspecific febrile or respiratory tract illness.

CNS infection can occur in any age group and be caused by any of the enteroviruses. Aseptic meningitis is the most common illness, but a poliolike paralysis and encephalitis may occur as well.

Neonates may develop any of the manifestations of enterovirus infection outlined above. However, the neonate will commonly present with a nonspecific sepsislike illness. Subtype B1-5 has been associated with a fulminating encephalomyocarditis in this age group.

Echoviruses

Echoviruses can cause many of the diseases described above, but certain specific associations of virus subtype and disease are recognized. A petechial exanthem and aseptic meningitis is seen in epidemics, usually among families and is caused by an echovirus 9 infection. There may be a prodrome of fever, sore throat, anorexia, and vomiting followed by an asymptomatic period. This is followed by fever, signs of meningitis (headache, stiff neck), and a maculopapular rash. The rash is especially frequent in children under 3 years old. The rash starts on the face and spreads to the trunk and extremities. The rash may become petechial, which raises the differential diagnosis of meningococcemia. The disease lasts 3 to 5 days.

Neonatal hepatic necrosis has been associated with echovirus 11 infection. Hepatitis can be seen in infections with many different enterovirus infections.

Enteroviruses

These newly isolated viruses can cause similar illnesses described above. However, enterovirus 70 may cause acute hemorrhagic conjunctivitis. Recognized in epidemic form only in the past 20 years, this illness has a sudden onset. Symptoms include severe eye pain, photophobia, blurred vision, lacrimation, and edema of the eyelids. Systemic symptoms are rare. Preauricular lymphadenopathy is often present on examination. Recovery is usually complete without sequelae by 7 to 12 days. This disease must be differentiated from epidemic keratoconjunctivitis due to adenovirus type 8.

DIAGNOSIS

Diagnosis is based on the season of the year and the clinical presentation. The suspicion of enterovirus infection can be confirmed by isolation of the virus in tissue culture from the appropriate body fluid or biopsy. Enterovirus can be excreted for weeks in the feces. For that reason, serum antibody titers may be necessary to prove acute infection.

INFECTIOUS MONONUCLEOSIS

The association between Epstein Barr virus (EBV) and infectious mononucleosis was made more than 20 years ago. EBV infection is spread among human beings by close personal contact. Infection is common early in life, especially among lower socioeconomic groups, as evidenced by serologic studies. EBV infection in the young child may be asymptomatic or a mild illness resembling an upper respiratory tract infection. However, the development of classic mononucleosis seems to be age-related and is most often described in adolescents and young adults. Infected individuals may excrete virus for many months, and approximately 20% of individuals are asymptomatic carriers. The incubation period is estimated to be from 14 to 50 days.

DATA GATHERING

Symptoms of malaise and spiking fevers (to 40° or 40.5° C), anorexia, and easy fatigability are usually the first symptoms of mononucleosis. The fevers may be associated with chills and sweats. Generalized lymphadenopathy (especially posterior cervical) appears within the first week. The term anginose mononucleosis is used to describe the illness in the patient with exudative pharyngitis, marked tonsillar enlargement, petechiae on the hard palate, and cervical adenopathy as a prominent early feature of the disease. The face and eyelids may appear swollen and the conjunctivae infected. Diffuse erythematous macular skin rashes are occasionally seen, particularly in patients treated with ampicillin. Hepatosplenomegaly is often noted as well. Other causes of a mononucleosis-like illness include cytomegalovirus and toxoplasmosis.

DIAGNOSIS

The suspicion of clinical mononucleosis, as described above, is strengthened if the WBC counts show a lymphocytosis of over 50% with 20% atypical lymphocytes. In addition, there may be abnormalities of liver function tests.

Confirmation of the diagnosis depends on either the measurement of heterophil antibodies (Monospot test) or specific antibodies to the EBV. In children over 4 years of age, the Monospot test will detect approximately 84% of those infected. In children less than 4 years, the sensitivity decreases with age from 50% to 5% in the child less than 1 year of age. In children less than 4 to 5 years or in older patients with clinical mononucleosis, specific antibodies to EBV should be measured if the Monospot test is negative.

There are specific antibodies to various components of EBV that appear in the blood at a predictable sequence during recovery from an acute infection. The pattern of positivity to these antibodies can determine current, recent or past infection in any given patient (Table 60–1).

MANAGEMENT

Treatment of mononucleosis is supportive only. Rarely, short-term steroid therapy is considered if tonsillar enlargement leads to respiratory embarrassment or if rupture of an enlarged spleen is possible. Patients receiving steroids for these conditions warrant admission to the hospital for close observation. Others have advocated the use of a tapering dose of steroids over 7 to 10 days for more moderate symptoms of mononucleosis given as outpatient therapy.

ROCKY MOUNTAIN SPOTTED FEVER

The cause of Rocky Mountain spotted fever (RMSF) is *Rickettsia rickettsii*, named after Howard Ricketts, who in 1906 proved that ticks transmit the disease. Although first described in the Rocky Mountain region, the disease is predominant in the eastern coastal and southeastern states. The organism is a natural parasite of the dog tick *(Dermacentor variabilis)* in the eastern region and of the wood tick *(Dermacentor andersoni)* in the west. Humans are infected by the bite of an infected tick. The disease occurs in the spring, and approximately 45% of cases occur in children younger than 14 years of age. The incubation period ranges from 3 to 12 days.

DATA GATHERING

Initially, the patient develops nonspecific features of malaise, headache, and fever that may be high (40° C). Myalgia and muscle tenderness are common complaints. A maculopapular rash will appear within the first 3 days in 50% to 60% of cases. The rash usually starts on the ex-

TABLE 60–1
EBV Infection Status According to Antibody Titer

	NONE	CURRENT	RECENT	PAST
IgM anti-VCA	−	++	−	−
IgG anti-VCA	−	++	++	+
Anti-Ea	−	+	− or ±	−
Anti-EBNA	−	−	− or ±	+

VCA = viral capsid antigen; EA = early antigen; EBNA = EBV nuclear associated antigen; + = positive; − = negative.

tremities and later involves the trunk and the palms and soles. The rash may become petechial or hemorrhagic in 50% of cases. Edema in the face or extremities is a late sign, indicating that vascular endothelial damage has begun. The patient may progress to shock with disseminated intravascular coagulation. Severe headache with symptoms of meningoencephalitis (restlessness, irritability, confusion, and delirium) are common and may progress to coma.

Mortality rates of 3% to 6% persist despite prompt recognition and therapy. Long-term neurologic sequelae of RMSF include behavioral disturbances and learning disabilities. Finally, cardiac involvement with electrocardiogram (ECG) abnormalities is frequently present.

Hyponatremia (in 88%) and thrombocytopenia (in 76%) is reported in children with RMSF. Therefore, a history of tick bite, fever, and rash with laboratory abnormalities as noted above should alert the physician to the possibility of RMSF. Unfortunately, serologic confirmation of infection with the nonspecific Weil-Felix test (which depends on the common antigens of rickettsia and two strains of *Proteus* bacteria, OX-19 and OX-2) cannot be used as a rapid diagnostic test. This test becomes positive 10 to 14 days after the onset of the illness. Specific serologic tests available on acute and convalescent serum specimens are now the preferred method of diagnosis, but once again cannot be relied on for rapid early diagnosis. The most commonly used specific tests are the complement fixation or indirect fluorescent antibody tests.

MANAGEMENT

Early recognition and treatment with effective antibiotic therapy will ensure the best possible outcome. For this reason, the decision to treat cannot be based on the results of serologic tests but should be based on clinical suspicion alone. Chloramphenicol or tetracycline (for children over 9 years) is the drug of choice. Antibiotics should be continued until the patient is afebrile for 2 to 3 days; a usual course is 5 to 7 days. Management of the hyponatremia, shock, and DIC is also necessary in severe cases.

RABIES PROPHYLAXIS

The number of reported cases of rabies in domestic animals (cattle, cats, and dogs) has dropped over the second half of this century. Conversely, rabies in wild animals began to increase in the 1970s, particularly in the midwestern and mid-Atlantic states. An increase in rabies cases among raccoons and skunks constitute the major reason for this increase.

An estimated 18,000 Americans are treated for exposure to rabies each year. The majority of these occur in children under 15 years of age. The decision to immunize the individual who has been bitten is based on the location in which the bite occurred, the circumstances surrounding the attack (i.e., unprovoked), and whether the animal can be observed.

MANAGEMENT

Bites by domestic animals should be handled according to circumstance. An apparently healthy animal should be observed for 10 days. If it remains well, no treatment is needed. If the animal appears sick, it should be killed and its head removed and sent in ice (not frozen) to a qualified laboratory for examination, and immunization procedures should be initiated (see below). If the examination proves negative, the immunization can be discontinued. If the state of the animal is unknown (e.g., escaped animals) consultation with the local health department can indicate the risk from data of the presence or absence of rabies in the community.

Bites by wild animals, such as skunk, fox, coyote, raccoon, bat, or other carnivores, should be considered as potentially infected. If the animal can be captured, it should be handled as above for sick animals. If the animal cannot be examined in the laboratory, the individual should be immunized (see below).

If immunization procedures are decided on, both passive and active immunization should be given. Passive immunization consists of human rabies immune globulin (HRIG), with a standardized antibody content of 150 IU/mL. The dose is 20 IU/kg of body weight; one-half should be used to infiltrate the wound(s) and the rest administered intramuscularly. Wounds in mucous membranes should not be infiltrated; administer the entire dose intramuscularly. Concurrently, active immunization should be started with intramuscular injection of 1 mL of human diploid cell vaccine (HDCV). If the laboratory report is negative, no further vaccine need be given. If positive or if the animal is suspected of being rabid, another 1 mL of HDCV should be given intramuscularly on the 3rd, 7th, 14th, and 28th days.

Prophylaxis is advisable for animal handlers or those living in areas where animal rabies is prevalent. Three IM doses of HDCV are given on days 0, 7, and 21 or 28. In addition, an intradermal pre-exposure vaccine is available, given on the same time schedule. After exposure, these individuals need no HRIG and only two doses of vaccine on the 1st and 3rd day.

BIBLIOGRAPHY

Anderson LJ: Role of parovirus B19 in human disease. *Pediatr Infect Dis J* 1987; 6:711–718.

Annunziato D, Kaplan MH, Hall WW, et al: A typical measles syndrome: pathologic and serologic findings. *Pediatrics* 1982; 70:203–209.

Balfaur HH, Bean B, Laskin OL, et al: Acyclovir halts progression of herpes zoster in immunocompromised patients. *N Engl J Med* 1983; 308: 1448–1453.

Bloch AB, Orenstein WA, Ewing WM, et al: Measles outbreak in a pediatric practice: Airborne transmission in an office setting. *Pediatrics* 1985; 75:676–683.

Cherry JD: Enteroviruses, in Feigin RD, Cherry JD (eds): *Textbook of Pediatric Infectious Diseases*, ed 2. Philadelphia, WB Saunders Co, 1987.

Cherry JD: Roseola infantum, in Feigin RD, Cherry JD (eds): *Textbook of Pediatric Infectious Diseases*, ed 2. Philadelphia, WB Saunders Co, 1987.

Corey L: Infections with herpes simplex viruses. *N Engl J Med* 1986; 314:686–690, 747–756.

Denny FW: Current problems in managing streptococcal pharyngitis. *J Pediatr* 1987; 111:797–806.

Helmick CG, Bernard KW, D'Angelo LJ: Rocky mountain spotted fever: Clinical, laboratory and epidemiological features of 262 cases. *J Infect Dis* 1984; 150:480–488.

Hull HF, Montes JM, Hays PC, et al: Risk factors for measles vaccine failure among immunized students. *Pediatrics* 1985; 76:518–523.

Jubeliner D: Suppurative parotitis, in Feigin RD, Cherry JD (eds): *Textbook of Pediatric Infectious Diseases*, ed 2. Philadelphia, WB Saunders Co, 1987.

Krajden S, Middleton PJ: Enterovirus infections in the neonate. *Clin Pediatr* 1983; 22:87–92.

Nahmias AJ, Whitley RJ, Visintine AN, et al: The collaborative antiviral study group. *J Infect Dis* 1982; 145:829–836.

Nelson JD: The effect of penicillin therapy on the symptoms and signs of streptococcal pharyngitis. *Pediatr Infect Disease* 1984; 3:10–13.

Plummer FA, Hammond GW, Forward K, et al: An erythema infectiosum-like illness caused by human parvovirus infection. *N Engl J Med* 1985; 313:74–79.

Rabies Surveillance, United States, 1987, *Morbidity Mortality Weekly Rep* 1988; 37:SS–4.

Report of the Committee of Infectious Diseases, ed 21. Red Book. *American Academy of Pediatrics* 1988.

Sullivan-Bolyai JZ, Hull HF, Wilson C, et al: Presentation of neonatal herpes simplex virus infections: implications for a change in therapeutic strategy. *Pediatr Infect Dis J* 1986; 5:309–314.

Sumaya CV, Ench Y: Epstein-Barr virus infectious mononucleosis in children. *Pediatrics* 1985; 75:1003–1019.

Weller TH: Varicella and herpes zoster. *N Engl J Med* 1983; 309:1362–1368, 1434–1440.

Yeager AS, Ashley RL, Corey L: Transmission of herpes simplex virus from father to neonate. *J Pediatr* 1983; 103:905–910.

BACTERIAL MENINGITIS

Joseph W. St. Geme III, M.D.

Bacterial meningitis is defined as inflammation of the meninges and evidence of a bacterial pathogen in the CSF. Despite the relative rarity of this disease during infancy and childhood, it remains a major cause of morbidity and mortality. Sequelae from meningitis occur in 25% to 50% of survivors and include hearing deficits, language disorders, mental retardation, motor impairments, and seizures. While the mortality rate for many infections in children has declined dramatically in recent years, case fatality rates for bacterial meningitis have not substantially changed, remaining at 10% to 20% in the neonate and 5% to 10% in older infants and children.

The attack rate for this infection is highest in newborn infants, with an incidence as high as one per 1,000 live births in some nurseries.

Most neonatal meningitis occurs during the first week of life (early-onset disease) and results from contact with contaminated amniotic fluid near the time of delivery (ascending amniotic infection syndrome). Susceptible infants either inhale or swallow contaminated amniotic fluid and develop septicemia with bacterial seeding of the meninges. Common neonatal pathogens responsible for early-onset meningitis include group B streptococci, *Escherichia coli, Listeria monocytogenes,* enterococci, and *Klebsiella and Enterobacter* species. Late-onset neonatal meningitis occurs between 1 week and 3 months of age and is caused by the same group of pathogens as well as *Hemophilus influenzae, Neisseria meningitidis,* and *Streptococcus pneumoniae.* Late-onset infection may result from colonization at the time of birth (vertical transmission) or via postnatal transmission from nursery personnel, caregivers at home, or community contacts (horizontal transmission). During the past decade, improvements in neonatal intensive care have permitted the survival of a population of very low-birth-weight infants who are hospitalized for many months and are at increased risk for nosocomial infection. Meningitis developing in these infants is caused by a different spectrum of microorganisms, including *Staphylococcus aureus,* coagulase-negative staphylococci, and *Pseudomonas aeruginosa* in addition to the bacteria causing early-onset meningitis.

Among older infants (>3 months) and children, *H. influenzae* type b, *N. meningitidis,* and *S. pneumoniae* are the agents responsible for approximately 95% of cases of bacterial meningitis. Of these three pathogens, *H. influenzae* type b represents the most common cause in children between 3 months and 5 years of age. In patients 5 to 19 years old, *N. meningitidis* is the most frequent bacterial CSF isolate. Infection with all three of these encapsulated bacteria usually begins with colonization of the nasopharynx followed by invasion of the bloodstream and hematogenous dissemination to the meninges. Rarely infection may occur from direct extension complicating otitis media, sinusitis, mastoiditis, or fracture through the paranasal sinuses, usually due to *H. influenzae* or *S. pneumoniae.* Other less common infectious causes of CSF pleocytosis in children include mycobacterial meningitis, Rocky Mountain spotted fever, Mycoplasma infection, parameningeal infection, and spirochetal disease such as syphilis, leptospirosis, or Lyme disease. In the immunocompromised child unusual bacteria, certain viruses (especially the herpes viruses), and fungi deserve serious consideration.

In children with bacterial meningitis, several clinical and laboratory findings are predictive of neurologic sequelae. Patients with delayed sterilization of the CSF have significantly more acute complications and a higher incidence of permanent neurologic abnormalities. The presence of focal neurologic deficits at the time of diagnosis and increased bacterial counts in the CSF also correlate with poor outcome. Other factors that may have some bearing on prognosis include seizures for longer than 3 days, CSF protein concentration greater than 1,000 mg/dL, CSF WBC count greater than 10,000/mm^3, and CSF glucose concentration less than 10 mg/dL.

DATA GATHERING

The presentation of bacterial meningitis is variable. It may be acute and fulminant in association with overwhelming septicemia or insidious, beginning with a nonspecific febrile illness and progressing over a few days. The former mode of presentation is most commonly due to meningococcal infection while the latter is more typical for *H. influenzae* disease, but there is considerable overlap.

History

Common symptoms in children with meningitis include fever, neck stiffness, photophobia, headache, anorexia, and mental status abnormalities such as lethargy, irritability, or confusion. Neonates and young infants generally present with a history of poor feeding, respiratory distress, irritability, and inconsolability; up to one-half of them may lack fever, making this finding an unreliable predictor of bacterial meningitis in this population. Approximately 20% to 30% of patients of any age will experience a seizure prior to presentation.

Knowledge about infectious contacts, status of immunization against *H. influenzae* type b, presence of other medical problems, and chronic medications such as immunosuppressing agents may provide clues about the likelihood of specific pathogens. Recent antimicrobial therapy may explain a sterile CSF culture despite CSF cell counts and chemistry values that suggest a bacterial cause. Information about family composition and daycare or nursery school attendance facilitates formulation of a plan for prophylaxis if infection is due to *H. influenzae* type b or *N. meningitidis*. A detailed history of the child's level of development establishes a baseline against which to evaluate recovery.

Physical Examination

In toddlers and older children, classic findings on physical examination reflect meningeal inflammation and include nuchal rigidity and Kernig and Brudzinski signs. Kernig sign is present when pain and resistance are detected on attempted extension of the knee with the hip in 90° flexion. Brudzinski sign is present if passive flexion of the neck induces involuntary hip flexion. These signs may appear late in the young child with meningitis and are generally absent in comatose patients. In the infant signs of meningeal irritation may be minimal, but a bulging fontanelle and diastasis of the sutures (indicators of elevated intracranial pressure) are often observed. Evidence of meningeal inflammation may similarly be subtle in patients with either primary or secondary immunodeficiencies, and suspicion of meningitis in these susceptible children must therefore be high. Despite the frequency of increased intracranial pressure in this disease, papilledema is rarely noted and presence of this sign should raise concern about the possibilities of venous sinus thrombosis, subdural empyema, or brain abscess complicating meningitis. Careful neurologic examination will reveal some alteration of consciousness at the time of hospital admission in the great majority of patients. A variety of focal neurologic abnormalities may also be noted, including deafness, ataxia, limited extraocular movement, asymmetric facial expression, blindness, and motor deficits. Focal neurologic signs occur most commonly in infection due to *S. pneumoniae* and generally result from cortical vein thrombosis or occlusive arterial disease.

In addition to those physical findings directly referable to infection of the central nervous system, a number of other signs may also be present. Hypotension and tachycardia may occur secondary to vomiting and poor oral intake or from septicemia with resultant peripheral vasodilation. The most common skin rash observed is a purpuric or petechial eruption. This rash is observed most frequently with meningococcal infection but can be caused by any of the bacterial pathogens. Occasionally a diffuse maculopapular eruption may precede purpura and petechiae. Other signs may be present as a result of associated focal infection such as otitis media, sinusitis, buccal or periorbital cellulitis, arthritis, epiglottitis, pneumonia, or pericarditis. Recognition of these entities is important as they may influence management.

Laboratory Tests

Collection of CSF for analysis represents the most critical diagnostic step in the child with suspected meningitis. Any child who demonstrates any evidence of meningitis by history or physical examination should undergo lumbar puncture. Though such an approach will lead to a high number of negative lumbar punctures, it will also facilitate early diagnosis and hence allow more expeditious therapy of this serious disease. In the child who has a focal neurologic deficit or signs of elevated intracranial pressure such as papilledema, altered pupillary responses, or increased blood pressure with bradycardia, lumbar puncture should be delayed until a CT scan has been obtained to avoid the complication of cerebellar or uncal herniation. Other situations in which this procedure should be delayed or withheld include significant cardiorespiratory compromise in a neonate or infection in the area that the needle will traverse to obtain CSF. In all of these circumstances, blood cultures should be obtained and antibiotics should be administered immediately. Lumbar puncture should be performed later when the patient can safely tolerate the procedure. Though short-term antibiotic therapy will reduce the yield of CSF culture and to a lesser extent CSF gram stain, CSF morphologic and biochemical characteristics will remain unchanged for at least 2 or 3 days.

During lumbar puncture, the opening pressure should be determined whenever possible. This measurement is usually elevated in meningitis, with a mean value of 300 mm H_2O. When the pressure is very high, minimal amounts of fluid should be collected. CSF should be examined immediately, as WBCs begin to disintegrate after about 90 minutes. Analysis of CSF should include total WBC count and differential, protein concentration, glucose concentration relative to serum glucose, gram stain, and culture. Normal values for CSF in newborns, older infants, and children are shown in Table 60–2. In general in bacterial meningitis, the CSF WBC count is greater than $200/mm^3$, protein is greater than 100 mg/dL, glucose is less than 40 mg/dL with the ratio of CSF to serum glucose less than 0.5, and gram stain reveals bacteria. However, patients with meningitis do not always have abnormalities in all of these CSF parameters. Newborn infants may have normal CSF WBC counts as often as 30% of the time and also frequently have normal glucose concentrations and negative gram stains. In older children with early meningitis, CSF values may also be normal. It is therefore critical to perform a complete evaluation of CSF and await culture results in all cases.

Various immunoassays are available to detect bacterial antigens from group B streptococci, *H. influenzae* type b, *N. meningitidis*, and *S. pneumoniae* in CSF and other body fluids and may be especially helpful in establishing a causative agent in the child who has received antibiotic therapy prior to lumbar puncture. These techniques include counterimmunoelectrophoresis, latex agglutination and staphylococcal coagglutination tests, and enzyme immunoassay. Latex agglutination is the preferred test because of its simplicity, rapidity, and high sensitivity and specificity. Occasionally in patients with meningitis bacterial antigen is detected only in concentrated urine. Therefore, to optimize the yield of this technique, both CSF and concentrated urine should be assayed.

Other laboratory studies that should be obtained at the time of initial evaluation include blood cultures, serum glucose and electrolyte levels, blood urea nitrogen (BUN), serum creatinine, complete blood cell count (CBC), and possibly coagulation tests. As most infants and children with bacterial meningitis are initially bacteremic, blood cultures are especially important in the patient in whom lumbar puncture will be delayed until after the initiation of antibiotic treatment. The serum sodium concentration will provide information about the possibility of inappropriate secretion of antidiuretic hormone (ADH) and serve as a baseline level for future measurements. The combination of serum bicarbonate concentration, BUN, and serum creatinine will help in the assessment of the state of hydration and tissue perfusion. A CBC count provides a variety of valuable information. Though peripheral WBC counts are too variable and nonspecific to be useful in making or excluding a diagnosis of bac-

TABLE 60–2
Normal CSF Values

PARAMETER	PRETERM NEWBORN	TERM NEWBORN	INFANTS 1–3 MOS	>3 MOS THROUGH CHILDHOOD
WBC count (cells/mm^3)				
Mean	9.0	8.2	2.9	
Range	0–29	0–32	0–9	0–7
Polymorphonuclear cells (%)	57	61	0–5	0–4
Glucose (mg/dL)				
Mean	50	52	60	60
Range	24–63	34–119	40–80	40–80
CSF/Blood	0.74	0.81	0.5–0.65	0.5–0.65
Protein (mg/dL)				
Mean	115	90	40	20
Range	65–150	20–170	20–100	5–40

Values for preterm and term newborns adapted from Sarff et al: *J Pediatr* 1976; 88:473. Other values compiled from: Fishman R: *Cerebrospinal Fluid in Diseases of the Nervous System.* Philadelphia WB Saunders Co, 1980; Portnoy JM, Olson LC: Normal cerebrospinal fluid values in children: Another look. *Pediatrics* 1985; 75:484–487; Widell S: Protein content of CSF in normal children. Personal investigations. *Acta Paediatr* 1958; 47 (suppl 115):44–57.

terial meningitis, counts less than 3,000/mm ^{3} suggest severe disease and poor prognosis. Anemia has been best described in association with infection caused by *H. influenzae* type b, resulting from immune hemolysis of red blood cells that are coated with soluble bacterial antigens, but may occur with other pathogens as well. Thrombocytopenia may reflect disseminated intravascular coagulation, and measurement of platelet count in combination with coagulation studies (prothrombin time, PT; partial thromboplastin time, PTT; and possibly fibrinogen and fibrin split products) is of particular importance in the child with a petechial or purpuric rash.

MANAGEMENT

Treatment of bacterial meningitis should begin immediately after appropriate cultures are obtained. Initial antimicrobial therapy is based on the likely pathogens.

In newborn infants presenting with meningitis during the first week of life, initial empiric therapy should include a penicillin combined with an aminoglycoside. Ampicillin and gentamicin are generally used for the following reasons: ampicillin is effective against group B streptococci, *L. monocytogenes*, enterococci, and some gram-negative rods; and gentamicin provides broader coverage of the Enterobacteriaceae. For infants who present beyond the first week of life but before the age of 3 months, the preferred starting regimen is ampicillin and cefotaxime. This combination is superior to alternative regimens (e.g., ampicillin and gentamicin, ampicillin and chloramphenicol, or cefotaxime alone) because of the excellent coverage it provides against gram-negative bacilli, β-lactamase producing *H. influenzae*, and *Listeria* in addition to the other pathogens causing disease in this age group. In older infants (>3 months) and children, ampicillin in combination with chloramphenicol is the conventional drug regimen which has been used for many years and has been proven safe and effective. Several of the newer cephalosporins, specifically cefotaxime, ceftriaxone, and ceftazidime, represent acceptable alternative agents. These antibiotics may be especially useful against the rare isolate of *H. influenzae* resistant to both ampicillin and chloramphenicol. Other advantages include the lack of necessity for monitoring serum concentrations and their use as single agents administered between one and four times per day (depending on the drug), thereby potentially reducing the cost and hazard of multiple doses each day. These advantages should be weighed against the sparse data available on the effect of these drugs on long-term morbidity from meningitis.

After an organism has been isolated from culture, antibiotic therapy should be tailored according to the results of *in vitro* susceptibility testing. *L. monocytogenes* and enterococci can usually be treated with ampicillin alone, while group B streptococci can be satisfactorily treated with either ampicillin or penicillin. Some experts advise combination therapy with gentamicin for part or all of the course for meningitis caused by any of these pathogens. For neonatal meningitis caused by gram-negative enteric organisms, the synergistic regimen of ampicillin and an aminoglycoside remains the treatment of choice, but cefotaxime or ceftazidime may be necessary for resistant isolates. For *N. meningitidis* and most strains of *S. pneumoniae*, the prefered treatment is penicillin or ampicillin. Strains of pneumococci that are relatively resistant to penicillin are best treated with chloramphenicol or vancomycin. For *H. influenzae*, treatment is with ampicillin if the isolate is sensitive. For ampicillin-resistant strains, chloramphenicol or one of the above-mentioned cephalosporins should be used.

The duration of antimicrobial treatment for bacterial meningitis is determined by the organism causing disease and the clinical response to therapy. For uncomplicated meningitis due to group B streptococci or *L. monocytogenes*, treatment should extend for 14 days following sterilization of CSF. Infants with gram-negative meningitis require a minimum of 3 weeks of therapy, and in cases of delayed sterilization of CSF, 4 to 6 weeks may be necessary. In infants and children with meningitis caused by *N. meningitidis*, 7 days is considered satisfactory. Uncomplicated infection with *H. influenzae* should be treated for 7 to 10 days, while disease due to *S. pneumoniae* should be treated for at least 10 days. The preferred antibiotic and duration of therapy for infection with specific pathogens are summarized in Table 60–3. Dosage recommendations for these antibiotics and others commonly used in infants and children are shown in Table 60–4.

TABLE 60–3
Preferred Treatment for Common Causes of Bacterial Meningitis

ORGANISM	ANTIBIOTIC*	DURATION† (DAY)
Group B streptococci	Ampicillin or penicillin (± gentamicin)	Minimum 14
Listeria monocytogenes	Ampicillin (± gentamicin)	Minimum 14
Enterococci	Ampicillin (± gentamicin)	Minimum 14
Enterobacteriaceae	Ampicillin and aminoglycoside (cefotaxime or ceftazidime for resistant strains)	Minimum 21
Haemophilus influenzae	Ampicillin (chloramphenicol, cefotaxime, ceftriaxone, or ceftazidime for resistant strains)	7–10
Streptococcus pneumoniae	Penicillin (chloramphenicol or vancomycin for relatively resistant strains)	10
Neisseria meningitidis	Penicillin	7

*Ultimate choice of antibiotic must be guided by in vitro susceptibility testing.
†Duration of treatment is for uncomplicated infection.

During the course of treatment with aminoglycoside antibiotics or vancomycin, one should carefully monitor serum levels, especially in patients with impaired renal function, because of the toxicity of these drugs. Recommended peak serum levels are 4–8 μg/mL for gentamicin and tobramicin, 5 to 10 μg/mL for netilmicin, 15 to 25 μg/mL for kanamycin and amikacin, and 20 to 30 μg/mL for vancomycin. Trough serum levels should be less than 2 μg/mL for gentamicin, tobramycin, or netilmicin, less than 10 μg/mL for kanamycin and amikacin, and less than 12 μg/mL for vancomycin. Patients being treated with chloramphenicol should similarly have levels monitored, particularly neonates and children with hepatic dysfunction. In addition, one should note that concomitant therapy with phenobarbital, diphenylhydantoin, or rifampin will influence chloramphenicol metabolism and hence serum levels. The recommended peak serum level is 15 to 25 μg/mL.

PREVENTION

In an attempt to reduce the spread of invasive illness (secondary infection) due to *H. influenzae* type b and *N. meningitidis*, antibiotic prophylaxis is recommended under certain circumstances.

The risk of secondary *H. influenzae* disease among household contacts less than 4 years old is substantial, ranging from 2% to 6%. Spread of infection outside the family can also occur, particularly in daycare centers and nursery schools, but the precise frequency remains unclear. When a patient with *H. influenzae* meningitis has siblings younger than 4 years old, *all* household contacts should receive rifampin orally once daily for 4 days in a dose of 20 mg/kg (maximum 600 mg/dose). The treatment of daycare and nursery school contacts should be individualized; although the advisability of rifampin prophylaxis in daycare groups in which a single case of meningitis has occurred is controversial, most experts agree that rifampin should be administered to all children and supervisory personnel when two or more cases of invasive disease have occurred among attendees within 60 days. Since many patients younger than 2 years old do not develop protective antibody against *H. influenzae* type b and therefore are at risk for recurrent infection from exposure to colonized members of the household, some physicians advise prophylaxis of their families even if there is no sibling younger than 4 years old. In all of these circumstances the primary case should also receive rifampin to eradicate colonization which might persist despite parenteral antibiotics. Therapy should begin during hospitalization; for patients being treated with chloramphenicol, rifampin should be initiated just before discharge because of the effect on chloramphenicol metabolism. Prophylaxis should be administered to contacts within 7 days of diagnosis of the primary case and sooner if possible.

Secondary infection due to *N. meningitidis*

TABLE 60–4
Antibiotic Dosages for Infants and Children*

ANTIBIOTIC	AGE, WEIGHT	DOSE (MG/KG/DOSE)	INTERVAL (HR)
Amikacin	<4 wk	7.5 (loading dose 10)	q 12
	≥4 wk	10	q 8
Ampicillin	<1 wk	50	q 12
	≥1 wk	75	q 6
Carbenicillin	<1 wk, <2,000 g	75	q 8
	<1 wk, ≥2,000 g	75	q 6
	≥1 wk	125	q 6
Cefazolin	<1 wk	25	q 12
	≥1 wk	50	q 8
Cefotaxime	<1 wk	50	q 12
	1–4 wk	50	q 8
	>4 wk	45	q 6
Ceftazidime	<4 wk	30	q 12
	≥4 wk	50	q 8
Ceftriaxone	All ages	50	q 12
Chloramphenicol	<1 wk	25	q 24
	1–4 wk	25	q 12
	>4 wk	25	q 6–8
Clindamycin	<4 wk, <2,000 g	5	q 8
	<4 wk, ≥2,000 g	5	q 6
	≥4 wk	10	q 6
Gentamicin/ Netilmicin/ Tobramycin	<1 wk, <1,500 g	2.5	q 24
	<1 wk, 1,500–2,000 g	2.5	q 18
	<1 wk, >2,000 g	2.5	q 12
	1–3 wk, <1,500 g	2.5	q 12
	1–3 wk, >1,500 g	2.5	q 8
	3 wk–5 yr	2.5	q 8
	5–10 yr	2.0	q 8
	>10 yr	1.7	q 8
Kanamycin	<1 wk, <2000 g	7.5	q 12
	<1 wk, ≥2000 g	10	q 12
	1–4 wk, <2000 g	10	q 12
	1–4 wk, ≥2000 g	10	q 8
	>4 wk	10	q 8
Oxacillin	<1 wk, <2,000 g	25	q 12
	<1 wk, ≥2,000 g	50	q 12
	≥1 wk	75	q 6
Penicillin G	<4 wk	80,000 U	q 8
	≥4 wk	100,000 U	q 6
Piperacillin	<4 wk, <2,000 g	50	q 8
	<4 wk, ≥2,000 g	50	q 6
	≥4 wk	75	q 6
Ticarcillin	<4 wk, <2,000 g	75	q 8
	<4 wk, ≥2,000 g	75	q 6
	≥4 wk	80	q 4
Vancomycin	<1 wk, <1,000 g	10	q 24
	<1 wk, 1,000–2,000 g	10	q 18
	<1 wk, >2,000 g	10	q 12
	1–4 wk, <1,000 g	10	q 18
	1–4 wk, 1,000–2,000 g	10	q 12
	1–4 wk, >2,000 g	10	q 8
	4–8 wk	10	q 8
	>8 wk	10	q 6

occurs in 1% of family contacts and one per 1,000 daycare center contacts. Household, daycare center, and nursery school contacts of patients with meningococcal meningitis should receive antibiotic prophylaxis as soon as possible, preferably within 24 hours of presentation of the primary case. In most instances rifampin is the drug of choice in a dose of 10 mg/kg/dose (maximum 600 mg/dose) every 12 hours for 2 days. Some physicians recommend decreasing the dose for infants younger than 1 month to 5 mg/kg/dose. Occasionally an isolate of *N. meningitidis* will be sensitive to sulfonamides, in which case sulfisoxazole is an acceptable alternative. As with *H. influenzae*, patients may still harbor *N. meningitidis* despite parenteral antibiotics and thus should also receive rifampin or sulfisoxazole as appropriate before discharge home.

In an attempt to prevent primary cases of *H. influenzae* type b disease, routine immunization against this organism is recommended. There now is a "second generation" vaccine licensed for use which is a conjugate of *H. influenzae* type b capsular polysaccharide and diphtheria toxoid and is immunogenic in children 18 months or older. All children should receive a single dose of this vaccine at age 18 months. As 70% of invasive disease caused by *H. influenzae* type b occurs in children younger than 18 months, it is hoped that continued efforts in vaccine development will yield a vaccine that is immunogenic at younger ages as well.

For several years a quadrivalent meningococcal vaccine has been available in the United States that consists of purified bacterial capsular polysaccharide from serogroups A, C, Y, and W-135. Most endemic meningococcal disease in this country is caused by serogroup B, for which there is not yet an effective vaccine. Routine immunization of children against meningococcal infection is not recommended. However, the quadrivalent vaccine should be administered to children age 2 years and older in high risk groups (functional or anatomic asplenia, terminal complement deficiencies).

BIBLIOGRAPHY

Committee on Infectious Diseases, American Academy of Pediatrics: *Report of the Committee on Infectious Diseases, 1986 Red Book*. Elk Grove Village, Illinois, American Academy of Pediatrics, 1986.

Feigin RD: Bacterial meningitis beyond the neonatal period, in Feigin RD, Cherry JO (eds): *Textbook of Pediatric Infectious Diseaseus*, ed 2. Philadelphia, WB Saunders Co, 1987, pp 439–465.

Feigin RD: Prevention of infection with *Neisseria meningitidis* and *Haemophilus influenzae* Type b. *Pediatr Rev* 1985; 7:88–94.

Klein JO, Feigin RD, McCracken GH Jr: Report of the task force on diagnosis and management of meningitis. *Pediatrics* 1986; 78:959–982.

Klein JO, Marcy SM: Bacterial sepsis and meningitis, in Remington JS, Klein JO (eds): *Infectious Diseases of the Fetus and Newborn Infant*, ed 2. Philadelphia, WB Saunders Co, 1983, pp 679–735.

McCracken GH Jr, Nelson JD, Kaplan SL, et al: Consensus report: antimicrobial therapy for bacterial meningitis in infants and children. *Pediatr Infect Dis J* 1987; 6:501–505.

Nelson JD: Management problems in bacterial meningitis. *Pediatr Infect Dis* 1985; 4:S41–44.

Swartz MN, Dodge PR: Bacterial meningitis—A review of selected aspects. *N Engl J Med* 1965; 272:725–731, 779–787, 842–848, 898–902, 954–960, 1003–1010.

OTITIS MEDIA

Ralph F. Wetmore, M.D.

BACKGROUND

Acute otitis media is the occurrence of bacterial infection within the middle ear cavity. The presence of nonpurulent fluid within the middle ear cavity is termed otitis media with effusion. This fluid may be thin (serous) or thick (mucoid). This condition is alternatively known as serous otitis media, secretory otitis media, or glue ear.

Acute otitis media is the most common cause of bacterial infection in young children. As demonstrated in several studies, one-half of 1 year olds will have at least one episode of acute otitis media. By 3 years of age, one-third of children will have had three or more infections, and by age six, 90% will have had at least one infection. Otitis media with effusion is as common as infection in childhood. Increased recognition by the press and improved diagnosis, especially with new technology such as tympanometry, have made otitis media with effusion seem to increase in incidence. Some experts have suggested that there may be an increase in otitis media with effusion due to the treatment of acute otitis media with antibiotics.

The major pathogens of acute otitis media are *Streptococcus pneumoniae*, *Hemophilus influenza*, and group A β-*Streptococcus*. Other common organisms include *Branhamella* and *Staphylococcus*. Causative factors responsible for acute otitis media include eustachian tube dysfunction, upper respiratory infection, and allergy. Mechanical or functional obstruction of the eustachian tube allows egress of bacteria into the middle ear cavity. This anatomic problem is the major cause of recurrent acute otitis media in infants. Viral or bacterial upper respiratory infections may result in the spread of infection into the middle ear. Children with allergies are predisposed to upper respiratory illnesses and acute otitis media.

There are multiple factors involved in the pathogenesis of otitis media with effusion. As with acute otitis media, mechanical or functional problems with the eustachian tube is a major element in the development of otitis media with effusion. Tubal obstruction may be due to lymphoid tissue near the orifice of the eustachian tube or edema of the mucosa. In patients with cleft palate, inadequacy of the palatal muscles responsible for opening the eustachian tube leads to frequent problems with otitis media. Some authors think that vigorous sniffing by patients is responsible for the development of high negative middle ear pressure and is a causal factor for otitis media. Adenoid tissue is located in the region of the eustachian tube orifice; chronic adenoid problems including chronic adenoiditis or adenoid hypertrophy have been implicated in the development of otitis media with effusion. The role of allergy in the pathogenesis of otitis media with effusion remains unclear. Symptoms and laboratory evidence of allergy can be found in some patients; however, treatment of allergy has an inconsistent response in the long-term management of otitis media with effusion. Bacteria have been implicated in the pathogenesis of otitis media with effusion in many studies: approximately half of middle ear aspirates in untreated cases have positive results on bacterial cultures. This finding is the major reason for utilizing antibiotics in treatment. In at least one study, the duration of otitis media with effusion appeared to be much shorter in breast-fed infants than in bottle-fed children.

CLINICAL FINDINGS

History

The symptoms of both acute otitis media and otitis media with effusion are often dependent on the patient's age. In neonates and infants (up to 2 years of age), the most reliable symptom of otitis media is a change in behavior such as irritability or lethargy. Fever is an inconstant symptom. While many infants may tug at their ears, this finding may be seen in the presence of teething or may be just a habit. Decreased appetite, vomiting, or diarrhea may be the result of acute otitis media or its treatment with antibiotics.

Young children (2 to 4 years of age) may be able to verbalize complaints of ear pain. Otalgia may be seen with both acute otitis media and otitis media with effusion, although it is more severe with acute infection. Otalgia secondary to otitis media with effusion is often intermittent and often seems worse at night. Fever may be present with acute otitis media depending on the stage and severity of infection. Fever is typically not a symptom of otitis media with effusion. As with infants, young children frequently show behavioral changes with otitis media. These may range from lethargy to irritability with acute otitis media and from hyperactivity to indifference with otitis media with effusion. Young children with otitis media frequently complain of noises in their ears. While specific complaints of hearing loss are not verbalized by them, young children manifest hearing loss by saying "huh" or "what," ignoring directions, mispronouncing words, repeating the wrong words or turning up the television volume. Parents of these children may also complain of speech delay. As with infants, young children may have gastrointestinal symptoms as a result of either infection or treatment.

Children older than 4 years old will usually complain of ear pain with acute otitis media. This otalgia may be either mild or severe depending on the stage and severity of infection. Fever and change in personality may also be present with acute infection. Children in this age group with otitis media with effusion may also complain of otalgia that is intermittent in nature and seems worse at night. They may also complain of a variety of noises, popping sounds in the ear, or ear fullness. Some children may complain of hearing loss, although hearing loss may be discovered by schoolteachers or through screening audiometry. Indistinct speech will frequently accompany the mild hearing loss seen with otitis media with effusion.

Physical Examination

With acute otitis media, the earliest sign of infection is erythema of the tympanic membrane. This should not be confused with hyperemia over the malleus, which is a normal finding. With many viral syndromes there may be myringitis which is an inflammation of the tympanic membrane without true infection of the middle ear. This condition is difficult to distinguish from the early stages of acute otitis media and is a cause of misdiagnosis. Hyperemia of the tympanic membrane seen in a crying child may frequently be confused with acute otitis media. This hyperemia may be difficult to eliminate in an infant who cries everytime he is restrained or examined. Having the child held in a parent's arms or lap may permit an easier examination of the ears.

As a middle ear infection becomes more intense, physical examination reveals a loss of anatomic landmarks. Normally, the malleus is easily visualized, and in a patient with a translucent tympanic membrane, the incus can also be seen. In acute otitis media, these landmarks disappear as the tympanic membrane becomes opaque and bulges. As the tympanic membrane bulges with purulent fluid, pneumatic otoscopy will demonstrate diminished tympanic membrane mobility. The development of drainage in the external canal during an episode of acute otitis media is indicative of a spontaneous perforation of the tympanic membrane. Usually, these perforations are small and close spontaneously in a few days.

In otitis media with effusion, the color of the tympanic membrane varies according to the color of the fluid in the middle ear cavity. This may range from clear to amber to gray to blue. In contrast to what is seen in acute otitis media, the malleus, especially the short process, becomes more distinct as the tympanic membrane is retracted. The absence or reduction of tympanic membrane mobility is an essential finding in the diagnosis of otitis media with effusion; thus, pneumatic otoscopy is crucial to its diagnosis. Even in cases in which there is no obvious fluid behind the tympanic membrane, pneumatic otoscopy may indicate reduced compliance consistent with either fluid or severe eustachian tube dysfunction. In cases of prolonged otitis media with effusion there may be either small or large retraction pockets within the tympanic membrane. In severe cases the whole tympanic membrane will become draped over the medial wall of the middle ear.

Audiometric Studies

Middle ear immittance measures (tympanometry and acoustic reflexes) are an important tool in the diagnosis of otitis media. Immittance should not replace good physical examination, but rather should supplement it. The principle behind middle ear immittance measures includes the delivery of an acoustic signal to the tympanic membrane as the air pressure in the external meatus is systematically varied over a range from +200 to −300 mm H_2O pressure. The amount of the acoustic signal reflected from the tympanic membrane is measured under the various conditions of air pressure to derive a tympanometric curve of impedance as a function of pressure. Three general types of tympanometric functions are important to the diagnosis of otitis media that been labeled types A, B, and C (Fig 60–1). A normal, or A, curve is seen when the tympanometric function peaks in a range from +50 to −100 mm H_2O. A type C curve is seen in cases of eustachian tube dysfunction where the peak of the curve occurs anywhere from −150 to −400 mm H_2O. A flat, or type B, curve has no discernible amplitude peak and is seen in cases where the middle ear system is very stiff, such as found with otitis media with effusion. A flat curve will also be seen with other stiffening conditions, such as severe thickening of the drum. A perforation of the tympanic membrane will also produce a B curve; however, middle ear volume or static compliance measurements will help to distinguish this condition from otitis media with effusion.

Pure tone audiometry is a procedure that can be performed in the office setting as a screening tool for hearing loss. It has little practical value in the diagnosis of acute otitis media, although it may be abnormal. More importantly, it may confirm a mild hearing loss such as seen with otitis media with effusion. The typical hearing loss with otitis media with effusion is 20 dB to 40 dB. A normal hearing test in the office does not rule out otitis media with effusion. Hearing

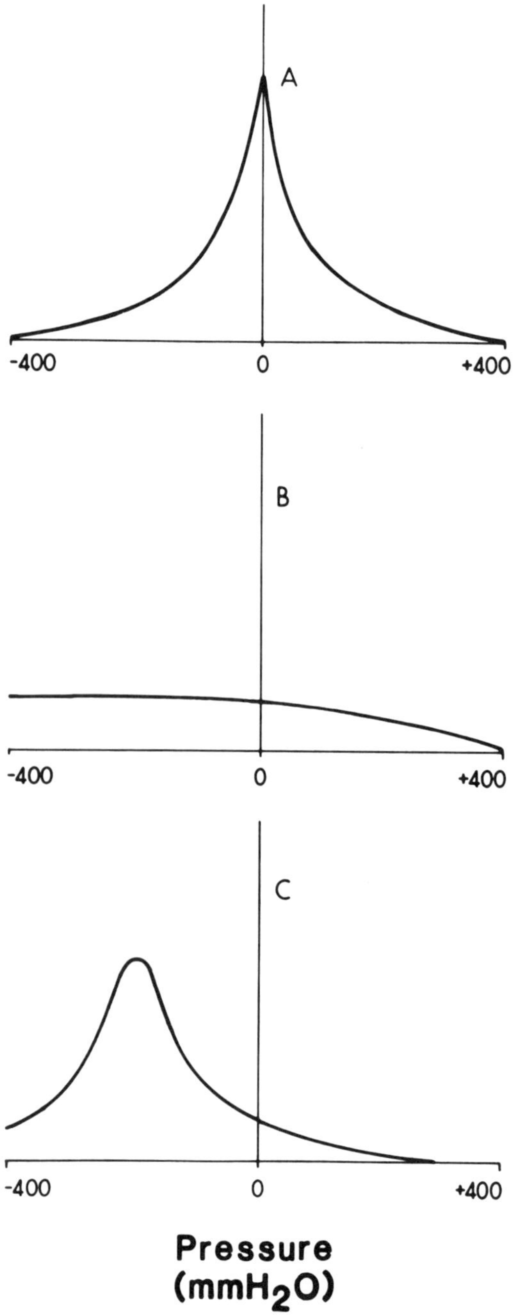

FIG 60–1
Types of tympanograms. *A,* normal curve. *B,* curve seen with middle ear effusion. *C,* curve seen with eustachian tube dysfunction.

loss greater than 40 dB is suggestive of other conditions, such as an ossicular discontinuity, or a sensorineural or a mixed hearing loss. If office audiometry fails to correlate with either the history or physical findings, a more complete audiometric assessment at a hearing center should be performed.

Tuning fork testing (Weber and Rinne) is important in the diagnosis of hearing loss in adults. Their reliability in children is age-dependent and variable. Normally, the Weber test will lateralize to the ear with a conductive hearing loss. Bone conduction will be greater than air conduction (negative Rinne test) in the presence of a conductive hearing loss, such as seen with otitis media with effusion.

Reflectometry is a newly developed screening device that has been used in the office. A signal is transmitted to the tympanic membrane and the amount of signal reflected can be translated into the degree of middle ear pathologic problems.

EARLY MANAGEMENT OF OTITIS MEDIA

Acute Otitis Media

While there is evidence that episodes of acute otitis media may be treated expectantly without antibiotics and with minimal sequlae, the current standard of care is oral antibiotic therapy for 10 to 14 days. There are a variety of oral antibiotics which are successful in the management of acute otitis media, and the choice of antibiotic depends on the preference of the physician, the cost, a history of drug allergy, and previous otologic history. Amoxicillin remains the antibiotic of choice in uncomplicated acute otitis media. Other antibiotics such as cefaclor, erythromycin and sulfisoxazole (Pediazole), trimethoprim and sulfamethoxazole (Bactrim), and amoxicillin/clavulanate (Augmentin), are popular in the treatment of otitis media, especially when resistant organisms are suspected. Antibiotic therapy should continue for 10 to 14 days; treatment courses of shorter duration may allow for the development of resistant organisms. Treatment failure as manifested by a continuation or worsening of pain, fever, irritability, or other symptoms is an indication to switch antibiotic therapy or consider referral to a specialist.

In the past, the use of either decongestants or

antihistamine-decongestant preparations was part of the standard care of acute otitis media. Several studies have shown them to have no proven benefit in the management of otitis media.

There are several forms of pain relief that are available to relieve the otalgia of acute otitis media. Analgesics such as acetominophen can be used in infants and young children, while codeine can be used in older children. Topical anesthetic drops (Auralgen) and the topical application of heat, such as a hot water bottle, may also provide relief. As noted, the failure of pain to resolve after instituting therapy is an indication to switch antibiotics or refer the patient to a specialist.

In the past, office myringotomy was widely practiced in the early treatment of acute otitis media. This has fallen out of practice today since the advent of successful antibiotic therapy. Injury to the tympanic membrane or the ossicles can occur in inexperienced hands, and emotional trauma related to the myringotomy can make subsequent examinations difficult. There are several conditions in which myringotomy or tympanocentesis should be considered. In neonates less than 1 month old or hospitalized neonates less than 3 months old, there may be infection with either gram-negative bacteria or *Staphylococcus*. Tympanocentesis should be part of the septic workup in such neonates when acute otitis media is suspected. Children undergoing chemotherapy or who are immunocompromised are often infected with unusual organisms, and tympanocentesis should be considered in these children during episodes of acute otitis media to identify the pathogen. Failure of several oral antibiotics to resolve acute infection or the development of a complication such as acute mastoiditis in an otherwise healthy child is also an indication for tympanocentesis to identify the offending organism and to provide a route of drainage.

Because of the possibility of persistent fluid or failure or complete resolution of infection, a follow-up examination should occur approximately 2 weeks after each episode of acute otitis media. Resolution of symptoms does not guarantee that either all infection or fluid has cleared, and physical examination is necessary to confirm that the ear has returned to normal.

Recurrent bouts of acute otitis media, especially over a short interval of time, are an indication for antibiotic prophylaxis. While there are no strict criteria for initiating antibiotic prophylaxis, three infections in 3 months or four infections in 6 months are the typical indications for prophylaxis. Sulfisoxazole was the first antibiotic used for recurrent acute otitis media, but other antibiotics such as amoxicillin have also been used.

Otitis Media with Effusion

The major thrust in the early treatment of otitis media with effusion should be antibiotic therapy. Several studies have shown the presence of bacteria in aspirates of middle ear effusions. Other studies have also shown the benefit of antibiotic therapy in the resolution of otitis media with effusion. In many children during the winter months, episodes of acute otitis media may coincide with the presence of otitis media with effusion, and antibiotic therapy is essential in the resolution of both. Antibiotic regimens, utilized in the treatment of otitis media with effusion, may include either therapeutic courses for 10 to 14 days or prophylactic regimens for 4 to 6 weeks. Amoxicillin, cefaclor, trimethoprim/sulfamethoxazole, erythromycin/sulfisoxazole, and amoxicillin/clavulanate, are usually utilized for therapeutic regimens, while sulfisoxazole and amoxicillin are used for prophylactic treatment. Initial treatment is followed by a repeat evaluation in 4 to 6 weeks.

In the past, decongestants and/or antihistamines were commonly used in the initial therapy of otitis media with effusion. Several studies have shown their ineffectiveness, and their use in otitis media with effusion is no longer essential. A short course of oral steroids has been shown to clear some middle ear effusions; this medication might be tried in children who have had minimal otitis media in the past. Since many children have chronic problems with otitis media with effusion, repeated use of oral steroids is not practical. Nasal steroids have been shown to be ineffective in the treatment of otitis media with effusion.

Older children or adolescents may be taught autoinflation of the eustachian tube. In this procedure, positive pressure is applied to the eustachian tube to attempt to clear negative middle ear pressure or fluid. While this may prove helpful for some older children, it is not practical in the management of otitis media with effusion in younger children.

Expectant therapy is a reasonable form of management of otitis media with effusion. This is especially true of children who are not having coinciding problems with acute otitis media. During the summer months, the incidence of otitis media with effusion diminishes; and observation of the patient without any medication may result in the resolution of fluid.

COMPLICATIONS OF OTITIS MEDIA

Otologic Complications

While complications of otitis media are uncommon, they are the major reason why chronic ear infections should be avoided. In the pre-antibiotic era, acute mastoiditis was a frequent complication of acute otitis media. Today it is seen rarely in infants and young children. These children present with fever, evidence of acute otitis media on physical examination and postauricular swelling. Mastoid radiographs show fluid in the mastoid air-cell system. Failure to respond to antibiotic therapy may result in coalescent mastoiditis, a destructive infection involving the ear and mastoid. Acute mastoiditis requires prompt and aggressive management including referral to an otologist for possible surgical drainage.

Hearing loss is a frequent symptom of both acute otitis media and otitis media with effusion. During an episode of acute otitis media, there is typically a temporary conductive hearing loss secondary to the purulent material in the middle ear cavity. As long as a middle ear effusion is present, there will also be a persistent hearing loss. In both acute otitis media and otitis media with effusion, the hearing loss will resolve after the purulent fluid or effusion has cleared. The effect of chronic hearing loss in the development of speech and language and in other areas of learning such as reading remains unclear. Significant sensorineural hearing loss clearly affects development; however, with a mild conductive hearing loss, such as that with otitis media, the effects are individual. Some children have no problems with speech development in the presence of chronic fluid, while others undergo significant delays with only intermittent fluid. Clearly, the individual needs of each child need to be recognized in the management of otitis media. Sensorineural hearing loss ranging from mild to profound may also be a rare complication of both acute otitis media and otitis media with effusion.

Both acute otitis media and otitis media with effusion can result in chronic perforation of the tympanic membrane. Most perforations with drainage during an episode of acute otitis media close spontaneously, but some may persist. Chronic otitis media with effusion can result in an atelectatic tympanic membrane which subsequently may form a chronic perforation. Small perforations may close without treatment, but large perforations result in hearing loss and require surgical repair.

Tympanosclerosis is hyalinization of the tympanic membrane, which is frequently the result of otitis media. These white plaques on the tympanic membrane are seen commonly. Typically they do not cause hearing loss, although complete hyalinization of the tympanic membrane may result in a conductive hearing loss.

Cholesteatoma results from keratinizing squamous epithelium being trapped medial to the tympanic membrane. Squamous debris from cholesteatoma continues to enlarge and subsequent infection results in destruction of normal structures, especially the ossicles and tympanic membrane. While cholesteatoma may be congenital, most cases are the result of chronic fluid or infection. The characteristic appearance of a cholesteatoma is a white lesion behind the tympanic membrane, although recognition may not always be obvious due to infection. Suspected cases of cholesteatoma should be referred for further evaluation.

Intracranial Complications

Intracranial complications of otitis media include meningitis, brain abscess, subdural empyema, and epidural abscess. In the pre-antibiotic era, intracranial complications as a result of acute otitis media were a common occurrence. Today these complications are more commonly a result of acute sinusitis.

The intracranial spread of infection from the ear and mastoid may be by one of several pathways: erosion of bone between the mastoid and the intracranial cavity; septic thrombophlebitis with spread of infection into the intracranial cavity; through preformed pathways between the ear and brain.

The development of an intracranial complication usually follows the onset of acute otitis media by several days. Symptoms of a severe headache or worsening otalgia, a change in sensorium, or the onset of nausea and vomiting signal the development of an intracranial complication. The institution of intravenous antibiotics and further evaluation including CT and lumbar puncture if indicated are the initial therapy. Otolaryngologic and neurosurgical consultations are also necessary.

SPECIALTY REFERRAL

Acute Otitis Media

After initiating antibiotic therapy for acute otitis media, there should be relief of pain within the next 24 to 48 hours. Failure of pain to subside is an indication to switch to a different antibiotic because of the possible presence of a resistant organism. Continued pain also signals the possible development of a complication, and an otologic referral should be made.

Drainage with an episode of acute otitis media indicates perforation of the tympanic membrane. Failure of the drainage to clear with antibiotic therapy is suggestive of an underlying problem such as a cholesteatoma. For this reason, an otologic referral should be made if drainage fails to clear with appropriate antibiotic therapy. A culture of the drainage may be helpful in guiding therapy.

The appearance of dizziness or vertigo during an episode of acute otitis media suggests the spread of infection into the cochlea. The resulting labyrinthitis can destroy both the vestibular and cochlear labyrinth, producing a profound sensorineural hearing loss and disturbance of balance. The appearance of this symptom necessitates an immediate referral.

In the management of recurrent acute otitis media, an infection while on a prophylactic regimen constitutes a breakthrough infection. Unless it can be demonstrated that poor patient compliance is the cause of the infection, one must assume that prophylaxis is not effective. A referral should be made for consideration of myringotomy with tube placement.

Some experts think that a prophylactic regimen for the treatment of recurrent acute otitis media should be used for 3 months. Resumption of infection following this 3-month regimen is an indication for referral to a specialist for consideration of myringtotomy with tube placement.

Otitis Media with Effusion

The persistence of middle ear effusion for approximately 6 weeks while on appropriate antibiotic therapy should signal referral to an otologist. This referral should be made on an individual basis depending on the time of year, previous otologic history, and current symptoms.

Recurrent bouts of fluid are also a cause for concern. The primary care physician can be mislead by the quick resolution of fluid; however, if the child has fluid with each upper respiratory infection, which occur frequently during the winter months, he most likely has recurrent otitis media. This produces long-term effects on speech and hearing equivalent to those of persistent fluid, and referral to a specialist should be made to evaluate the child. This is especially true in children who have an underlying sensorineural hearing loss or other developmental delays.

The persistence of a tympanic membrane perforation or the appearance of a white mass behind the tympanic membrane, suggestive of a cholesteatoma, are additional indications for referral to a specialist. A perforated tympanic membrane needs evaluation for damage to the ossicular chain and needs follow-up for possible surgical repair. Cholesteatoma has the potential for continued growth with destruction of the tympanic membrane and ossicles, damage to the cochlea and facial nerve or erosion into the intracranial cavity. For this reason, an expedient referral is necessary for prompt management.

BIBLIOGRAPHY

Brook I, Yocum P, Shah K, et al: Aerobic and anaerobic bacteriologic features of serous otitis media in children. *Am J Otolaryngol* 1983; 4:389–392.

Cantekin EI, Mandel EM, Bluestone CD, et al: Lack of efficacy of a decongestant-antihistamine combination for otitis media with effusion ("secretory" otitis media) in children. *N Engl J Med* 1983; 308:297–301.

Falk B: Sniff-induced negative middle ear pressure: Study of a consecutive series of children with otitis media with effusion. *Am J Otolaryngol* 1982; 3:155–162.

Gates GA, Avery CA, Prihoda TJ, et al: Effectiveness of adenoidectomy and tympanostomy tubes in the treatment of chronic otitis media with effusion. *N Engl J Med* 1987; 317:1444–1451.

Gates GA, Wachtendorf C, Holt GR, et al: Medical treatment of chronic otitis media with effusion (secretory otitis media). *Otolaryngol Head Neck Surg* 1986; 94:350–354.

Healy GB: Antimicrobial therapy of chronic otitis media with effusion. *Int J Pediatr Otorhinolaryngol* 1984; 8:13–17.

Smyth GDL: Management of otitis media with effusion: A review. *Am J Otol* 1984; 5:344–349.

Wallace IF, Gravel JS, McCarton CM, et al: Otitis media, auditory sensitivity, and language outcomes at one year. *Laryngoscope* 1988; 98:64–70.

UPPER RESPIRATORY TRACT INFECTIONS

Steven M. Selbst, M.D.

The most frequently seen patient in the pediatrician's or family practitioner's office is the child with fever, rhinorrhea, sore throat, and cough. Although the outcome of the upper respiratory tract infection (URI) is almost always excellent, it accounts for more sleepless nights, physician visits, and missed days of preschool, school, and work, than any other illness. What is a "common cold" to the patient may be more specifically defined by the physician. This chapter focuses on the diagnosis and management of some of the specific diagnostic entities within the category of URI, including pharyngitis, croup, and tracheitis. The section on croup also covers the differentiation between croup and epiglottitis, another important form of URI.

PHARYNGITIS

Pharyngitis (or tonsillitis, tonsillopharyngitis) is an inflammatory illness of the mucous membranes and structures of the throat. There are numerous causes of this infection, but consideration need only be given to a few. Adenovirus is the most common etiologic agent in young children, and other viruses such as influenza, parainfluenza, enterovirus, and the Epstein-Barr virus, also cause pharyngitis. Group A β-hemolytic *Streptococcus* is the most common and important bacterial organism, but this accounts for only a small part of the total number of cases of tonsillitis. Diphtheria is now a very rare cause of pharyngitis, and *Mycoplasma* is also an unusual agent in this infection. Gonococcal infections should be considered in sexually active teenagers. In about half of the children who present with sore throat, no pathogens (viral or bacterial) can be isolated.

Transmission of these infectious agents is by close-range airborne dissemination in most cases. In general, the bacterial infections are more common in the winter, and enteroviral infections are more common in the summer and fall. There is no sex predilection for pharyngitis. Children under the age of 3 years are unlikely to get streptococcal pharyngitis, whereas those aged 5 to 8 years are most likely to have "strep" throats.

Data Gathering

There is usually a sudden onset of fever and complaint of sore throat in children with pharyngitis. The parents may note that the child's throat is red and that the child's breath has a foul odor. Swollen lymph nodes of the neck may be noted and the child may complain of abdominal pain. In addition, the child may complain of headache, nausea, vomiting, anorexia, or pain in the back and extremities. Cough and rhinorrhea may accompany viral pharyngitis but not usually streptococcal infections.

On examination the child is usually febrile (38° to 40° C). However, some children with streptococcal pharyngitis may have little or no fever. In addition, cervical adenitis may be present along with erythema of the pharynx. Pharyngeal exudate and petechiae on the soft palate are also found and are especially associated with group A β-hemolytic *Streptococcus* and infectious mononucleosis. Furthermore, follicular lesions may be noted in the throat and are more characteristic of adenoviral infections, while ulcerative lesions may be noted with enteroviral infections.

Unfortunately, there is usually no way to make an etiologic diagnosis of pharyngitis on clinical findings alone, and a throat culture is imperative. A recent study in a private practice group found pediatricians to be only 76% accurate in correlating clinical features and cultures for group A β-hemolytic *Streptococcus*. In that study, fever, otitis media, and exudative pharyngitis occurred just as often in patients with a negative throat culture as in those with documented streptococcal infections. Palatal petechiae and cervical adenitis were more common in streptococcal pharyngitis. However, others have noted that only 50% of children with sore throat and adenitis actually have a culture that is positive for group A β-hemolytic *Streptococcus*. Cough, croup, and hoarseness are probably more commonly associated with viral pharyngitis. Therefore, because of the overlapping symptoms, without a throat culture one can only assume that pharyngitis is viral in origin if ulcerative lesions of herpangina are noted. Likewise, one can only assume that pharyngitis is due to group A β-hemolytic *Streptococcus* if the rash of scarlet fever is present.

Thus, in most cases of pharyngitis, the throat should be swabbed in an attempt to isolate group A β-hemolytic *Streptococcus*. A carefully obtained and accurately read throat culture has a dependability rate of 95% or better. Office culture kits are now available that are easy to use, relatively inexpensive, and provide results within 24 to 48 hours in most cases. Except in unusual situations, it is not necessary to culture for pathogens other than group A β-hemolytic *Streptococcus*.

It would be ideal to only selectively obtain cultures from children with sore throats. Some, therefore, recommend obtaining a throat culture only for children with a sore throat and a temperature greater than 99.1° F (taken orally), or for children with a temperature of 101° F or higher even in the absence of sore throat. While this routine would eliminate many unnecessary throat cultures, it also would result in failure to diagnose 12% of streptococcal infections. Recently, rapid test kits for group A *Streptococcus* have become available for office use. They have the advantage of being less expensive than throat cultures and they are highly specific for group A β-hemolytic *Streptococcus*. These kits may ultimately replace throat cultures in making a rapid (10-minute) diagnosis of streptococcal throat infection. However, recent studies have found them not highly sensitive.

Management

Throat lozenges, antiseptic mouthwashes, and decongestants have little, if any, value in treating pharyngitis. However, oral analgesics may be helpful in relieving symptoms of sore throat. Most importantly, all cases of streptococcal pharyngitis should be treated with antibiotics, whereas viral infections do not need such treatment. Whether antibiotic treatment will significantly shorten the duration of symptoms in streptococcal infections is still controversial. A classic study involving military recruits with streptococcal pharyngitis in the early 1950s implied that antibiotic treatment caused no significant clinical improvement. However, others think that prompt initiation of therapy in "classic" cases of streptococcal pharyngitis could afford relief and possibly prevent suppurative complications in some children, while cultures are pending. Recent studies show that pharyngeal injection and tender lymph nodes are significantly improved more quickly when patients were treated with antibiotics instead of placebo. Certainly, there is no justification in treating all children who complain of sore throat with antibiotics in hopes of achieving more rapid symptomatic improvement in those few who may have streptococcal infections. However, treatment should be considered in some ill or uncomfortable patients while results of culture are pending.

The primary goal in treating streptococcal pharyngitis is the prevention of rheumatic fever. Penicillin is the drug of choice. While intramuscular penicillin G benzathine in a dose of 25,000 to 50,000 U/kg, assures compliance, oral penicillin V is an alternative if given for a 10-day course. Ten days of erythromycin (40 mg/kg/day) is acceptable in cases of penicillin allergy. Finally, amoxicillin may be used to treat streptococcal infections, but its increased cost and broader spectrum does not justify its use instead of penicillin.

Once a child is treated for group A β-hemolytic streptococcal pharyngitis, it is not routine to obtain a culture of the throat after the antibiotic course is completed. Likewise, it is not cost effective to obtain throat cultures from or treat asymptomatic family members. Those who are symptomatic should have throat cultures and/or be treated with antibiotics if appropriate.

There is still considerable controversy about

performing tonsillectomies to prevent throat infections in children. While one recent controlled study showed that some children with multiple throat infections may benefit from surgery, the study had only a small number of patients, and the conclusions applied to only those few children with frequent significant infections.

Complications of pharyngitis are quite rare, with acute dehydration being the most common. Suppurative complications, such as parapharyngeal abscess and suppurative cervical adenitis occur in streptococcal infections, but they are quite unusual. These complications occur almost exclusively in untreated patients, but they should prompt the treating pediatrician to refer such a patient for hospital admission, intravenous antibiotics, and, possibly, surgical drainage.

Acute nephritis can also occur following upper respiratory tract infections with group A *Streptococcus*. Such a complication depends on the type of strain of the infecting group A *Streptococcus*. Antibiotic treatment of the preceding pharyngitis will not prevent glomerulonephritis if the patient is infected with the nephrogenic strain of *Streptococcus*.

Acute rheumatic fever remains an important complication of streptococcal pharyngitis. The incidence of rheumatic fever had been declining in the United States in the 1970s. However, there have been recent reports of increasing cases of this disease. This incidence rate varies slightly in different parts of the country and the world. It is likely that extensive efforts to diagnose and treat streptococcal pharyngitis are still needed.

CROUP

Croup, a viral infection that produces obstruction of the upper airway, is commonly caused by parainfluenza virus 1, 2, and 3, influenza virus A and B, and respiratory syncytial virus in children less than 5 years of age. *Mycoplasma pneumoniae* can cause croup in older children. These organisms narrow the airway below the true vocal cords by producing inflammation and edema. The obstruction that results may gradually progress to respiratory failure. Croup is a very common infection in children under 2 years of age, particularly in the winter. Croup must be differentiated from epiglottitis that is a bacterial infection (*H. influenzae* type B) which also produces upper airway obstruction (Table 60–5). Failure to make this distinction could be lethal for the patient since untreated epiglottitis is known to progress rapidly to complete airway obstruction. Croup should also be distinguished from a less common, but serious upper airway infection called bacterial tracheitis.

Data Gathering

The diagnosis of croup is often confirmed with a thorough history and complete physical examination. In general, croup has a gradual onset with URI symptoms often present for 2 or 3 days before medical attention is sought. This is quite different from the acute onset of epiglottitis and foreign body aspiration that also cause upper airway obstruction. It is important to learn what specific respiratory tract symptoms have been noted. Inspiratory noise, or stridor, is quite typical of croup and occurs in almost all patients. However, this symptom is also found usually with epiglottitis, foreign body aspiration, or other causes of upper airway obstruction. In contrast, a croupy cough (harsh, barking in quality) is characteristic for croup and is rarely noted in epiglottitis. In addition to these symptoms, children with croup often have a hoarse voice. Also, more than 80% of children with croup have fever, which may range from 38° to 40.5° C. Typically, the child

TABLE 60–5
Differentiating Croup From Epiglottitis

CROUP	EPIGLOTTITIS
Common infection	Uncommon
Young children (<3 yr)	Older children (usually)
Winter predominance	Not seasonal
Recurs in 5%	Rarely recurs
Viral etiology	Bacterial etiology
Subglottic edema	Supraglottic edema
Gradual onset	Rapidly progressive
Croupy cough	Cough is rare
Sternal retractions	Sternal retractions
Stridor characteristic	Stridor less consistent
Not toxic	Toxic appearing
Not drooling	Drooling occasionally
Low-moderate fever	High fever
No preferred position	Sitting quietly, leaning forward
Thin epiglottitis on lateral neck x-ray film	Round, large, epiglottis on lateral neck x-ray film

with croup has less fever than one with epiglottitis. Finally, it may be helpful to know if the child has had a similar episode in the past, since croup is known to be a recurrent illness, while epiglottitis is not.

Once the history is obtained, a brief, but careful physical examination is critical. It is important to determine if the patient has severe respiratory distress quickly so that prompt action may be taken if needed. Frequently, signs of moderate dyspnea are present. For instance, sternal retractions are quite common in children with croup and tachypnea, and nasal flaring is often seen as well. Uncommonly, the child with severe croup may be cyanotic. Drooling is also seen infrequently with croup, but it is more characteristic of epiglottitis, foreign body aspiration, or retropharyngeal abscess. In contrast, signs of dehydration may be noted in the child with croup. Although, most children with croup have fever at the time of the physical examination, they do not appear to be "toxic," as does the child with epiglottitis. They are also more often restless and "air hungry," than children with epiglottitis who are generally sitting up quietly. On chest examination the lungs are usually clear, with equal breath sounds, and inspiratory stridor is the outstanding noise that is heard. The findings of the remainder of the physical examination are usually normal in patients with croup.

If the diagnosis of croup is not obvious from the history and physical examination, the laboratory studies, particularly radiologic studies, may be quite helpful. For the majority of cases of croup, such x-ray films are not needed; but if epiglottitis is considered, a lateral neck x-ray film is invaluable. A lateral neck x-ray film that shows a thin epiglottis rules out epiglottitis as a cause of the stridor and makes croup far more likely if the signs and symptoms support this diagnosis. It is not necessary to obtain an anteroposterior (AP) view of the airway to confirm croup, though this would show the classic "steeple sign" or narrowed airway in the subglottic area. It is important to remember, that a child who is considered ill enough to require x-ray films to confirm the diagnosis should always be accompanied by a physician prepared to manage an obstructed airway if sudden problems were to arise.

The chest x-ray film is usually unremarkable in the child with croup, and further laboratory tests are rarely needed. A CBC count may suggest a viral illness, but this information is not critical. Finally, an arterial blood gas determination may provide useful information about oxygenation and CO_2 retention, but this is rarely needed for office management of croup.

Management

Once the diagnosis of croup is established, treatment is aimed at relieving airway obstruction. Humidity is the foundation of therapy for croup. There are several different ways to deliver humidified air to a child. An ultrasonic nebulizer, if available, is the preferred route. More practically, in an office setting, a child can be placed with his parent in a room with hot water running, so that the entire room fills with steam. The child may benefit from 10 to 15 minutes of exposure to this environment. At home, a simple room humidifier may be beneficial as well. Fever control is also important in reducing oxygen consumption and the work of breathing. Moreover, it is important to have the parents reassure the child since respiratory distress notably improves when the child is less agitated. Sedatives are not indicated in children with airway obstruction.

If humidity fails to relieve the respiratory distress, treatment with racemic epinephrine is warranted. A controlled double-blind study has shown that this drug is effective compared to normal saline in relieving airway obstruction. However, it must be administered by nebulized aerosol and requires the use of careful cardiac monitoring because of possible side effects such as tachyarrhythmias. Moreover, although the drug will promptly relieve symptoms of distress, the effects are known to be transient, and 2 hours after administration of racemic epinephrine, patients may be considerably worse. Thus, the drug is *not* recommended for outpatient management of croup. Likewise, since croup is usually a viral illness, antibiotics are not indicated in uncomplicated cases.

Finally, corticosteroids are of unproved value in treating croup. Several studies that have evaluated the efficacy of this treatment modality have been criticized for flaws in design or methods. While many recommend trying steroids for all hospitalized patients with croup, few would consider their use for common, mild cases treated as outpatients.

In outpatient management of croup, careful observation for signs of fatigue is crucial. Also, a child with croup must be encouraged (even forced) to maintain sufficient fluid intake at home. The work involved in excessive breathing with croup as well as accompanying fever make dehydration a real possibility. A child with croup should be referred for admission to the hospital if adequate fluid intake is not possible orally. Referral for admission is also recommended if the child is cyanotic or in severe distress when examined. Furthermore, the child with stridor at rest should be admitted, as should one who lives a great distance from medical care or who is unlikely to return for further care (i.e., inadequate supervision at home). A child who is otherwise compromised (previous airway disease) or who received racemic epinephrine treatment for prompt relief should also be referred for admission to the hospital.

TRACHEITIS

Bacterial tracheitis is an uncommon but distinct entity that has clinical features similar to both croup and epiglottitis. The entity has been known since the 1940s but has been referred to by many other confusing names such as acute laryngotracheobronchitis, acute laryngotracheitis, and membranous laryngotracheobronchitis. Most now agree that these infections all represent the same bacterial process that is an important cause of upper airway obstruction in young children.

Bacterial tracheitis is usually caused by *S. aureus*, but *H. influenzae* type B and *Streptococcus* have also been cultured from the thick tracheal secretions that are characteristic of this illness. The role of viruses in this illness is not clear since some physicians report parainfluenza virus type 1 was also isolated from tracheal secretions in some patients, whereas others could not isolate viruses. A recent report showed serologic evidence of viral infection in two patients with bacterial tracheitis, and it was concluded that viral infections of the upper respiratory tract contributed to invasion of bacteria in these patients.

Data Gathering

Bacterial tracheitis should be considered in young children with signs and symptoms of URI together with airway obstruction. Both sexes are at risk, and the age range has been reported as 1 month to 12 years old, with a mean age similar to that of patients with croup. The infection seems to be more common in the winter.

The child or infant with bacterial tracheitis will have a gradual onset of upper airway obstruction. This is more comparable to croup than epiglottitis. However, after a mild URI with barking cough, the child may develop a high fever and appear toxic, as would a child with epiglottitis. Inspiratory stridor is quite typical, but dysphagia and drooling are not usually found in bacterial tracheitis. The severe respiratory distress usually progresses and almost always requires emergency intervention to maintain the airway. When the airway is directly observed, there is marked subglottic narrowing, a normal epiglottis, and profuse thick tracheal secretions that are the hallmark of bacterial tracheitis. Occasionally, cardiorespiratory arrest results in children with bacterial tracheitis.

While the toxic appearance of a child with upper airway obstruction would lead one against making the diagnosis of croup, the laboratory evaluation of the illness of such a child will also help rule out epiglottitis. For instance, lateral and anteroposterior (AP) neck radiographs in children with bacterial tracheitis will show a normal-sized epiglottis and subglottic narrowing characteristic of croup. In addition, a chest x-ray film in those with bacterial tracheitis frequently shows pulmonary infiltrates. An elevated WBC count is not consistent, but there is often a left shift present to indicate that the tracheitis is due to a bacterial infection. Of course, culture of the purulent tracheal secretions would confirm the bacterial infection, but unlike epiglottitis, blood cultures are not positive in bacterial tracheitis. Also, a gram stain of the tracheal secretions may be helpful while cultures are pending. Furthermore, viral studies (culture, serologic analysis) may be useful in understanding the cause of the tracheitis infection, but they are not important in treating the patient. Finally, urine latex agglutination tests may be helpful in distinguishing bacterial tracheitis from viral croup infections, but this has not been well documented.

Management

Epiglottitis should be ruled out before therapy for tracheitis is begun. Standard therapy for croup such as hydration and humidity are rarely helpful in this particular infection. All patients who fail to respond to such treatment need immediate referral to the hospital for admission and probably intensive care. Nebulized racemic epinephrine should be tried next, but this is rarely helpful. Since bacterial tracheitis is a life-threatening illness, consultation for bronchoscopy and intubation should be sought quickly. Sometimes there is dramatic improvement after the thick purulent secretions are removed with bronchoscopy, but more often endotracheal intubation or tracheostomy is necessary. Continued vigorous suctioning of the artificial airway is then necessary. Furthermore, intravenous antibiotics play an important role in treatment, and oxacillin with chloramphenicol or cephalosporins are recommended. Studies have shown that hospitalization is considerably longer for bacterial tracheitis than one would expect for croup and epiglottitis, because of the persistent tracheal secretions. If treated appropriately, the prognosis for children with bacterial tracheitis is quite good.

BIBLIOGRAPHY

Otitis Media

Friedman AD, Fleisher GR, Henretig F, et al: Otitis media: Update on etiology and management. *Ann Emerg Med* 1982; 11:181–183.

Klein JO: Antimicrobial prophylaxis for recurrent acute otitis media. *Pediatr Ann* 1984; 13:398–403

Liston TE, Foshee WS, McCleskey FK: The bacteriology of recurrent otitis media and the effect of sulfasoxazole chemoprophylaxis. *Pediatr Infect Dis* 1984; 3:20–23.

Marchant CD, Shurin PA, Johnson CE, et al: A randomized controlled trial of amoxicillin plus clavulanate compared with cefaclor for treatment of acute otitis media. *J Pediatr* 1986; 109:891–896.

Papadeus VA, Fleisher GR: Otitis media in early infancy. *Am J Emerg Med* 2:251–253.

Pelton SI, Whitley P: Otitis media: Current concepts in diagnosis and management. *Pediatr Ann* 1983; 12:207–218.

Rowe DS: Acute suppurative otitis media. *Pediatrics* 1975; 56:285–294.

Schwartz RH, Puglise J, Rodrigues WJ: Sulfamethoxazole prophylaxis in the otitis-prone child. *Arch Dis Child* 1982; 57:590–593.

Teele DW, Klein JO, Rosner B, et al: Middle ear disease and the practice of pediatrics: Burden during the first five years of life. *JAMA* 1983; 249:1026–1029.

Pharyngitis

Hall CB, Breese BB: Does penicillin make Johnny's strep throat better? *Pediatr Infect Dis* 1984; 3:7–9.

Honikman LH, Massell BF: Guidelines for the selective use of throat cultures in the diagnosis of streptococcal respiratory infection. *Pediatrics* 1971; 48:573–582.

Hosier DM, Craenen JM, Teske DW, et al: Resurgence of acute rheumatic fever. *Am J Dis Child* 1987; 141:730–733.

Krober MS, Buss JW, Michels GN: Streptococcal pharyngitis: Placebo-controlled double blind evaluation of clinical response to penicillin therapy. *JAMA* 1985; 253:1271–1274.

Nelson JD: The effect of penicillin therapy on the symptoms and signs of streptococcal pharyngitis. *Pediatr Infect Dis* 1984; 3:10–13.

Paradise JL, Bluestone CD, et al: Efficacy of tonsillectomy for recurrent throat infection in severely affected children. *N Engl J Med* 1984; 310:674–683.

Peter G, Smith AL: Group A streptococcal infections of the skin and pharynx (part 2). *N Engl J Med* 1977; 297:365–370.

Randolph MF, Gerber MA, DeMeo KK, et al: Effect of antibiotic therapy on the clinical course of streptococcal pharyngitis. *Pediatrics* 1985; 106:870–875.

Rowe RT, Stone RT: Streptococcal pharyngitis in children: Difficulties in diagnosis on clinical grounds alone. *Clin Pediatr* 1977; 16:933–935.

Croup

Battaglia JD: Severe croup: The child with severe and upper airway obstruction. *Pediatr Rev* 1986; 7:227–233.

Cherry JD: The treatment of croup: Continued controversy due to failure of recognition of historic, ecologic, etiologic and clinical perspectives. *J Pediatr* 1979; 94:325–354.

Davis WH, Gartner JC, Galvis AG, et al: Acute upper airway obstruction: Croup and epiglottitis. *Pediatr Clin North Am* 1981; 28:859–880.

Denny FW, Murphy TF, Clyde WA Jr, et al: Croup: An 11 year study in a pediatric practice. *Pediatrics* 1983; 71:871–876.

Hen J: Current management of upper airway obstruction. *Pediatr Ann* 1986; 15:274–295.

Leipzig B, Oski FA, Cummings CW, et al: A prospec-

tive randomized study to determine the efficacy of steroids in the treatment of croup. *J Pediatr* 1979; 94:194–196.
Super DM, Castelli NA, Brooks LJ, et al: A prospective randomized double-blind study to evaluate the effect of dexamethasone in acute laryngotracheitis. *J Pediatr* 1989; 115:323–329.
Tunnessen WW, Feinstein AR: The steroid-croup controversy: An analytic review of methodologic problems. *J Pediatr* 1980; 96:751–756.
Westley CR, Cotton EK, Brooks JG: Nebulized racemic epinephrine by IPPB for the treatment of croup. *Am J Dis Child* 1978; 132:484–487.
Tracheitis
Campbell TP, Paris PM, Stewart RD: Tracheitis: The "other" cause of upper airway obstruction. *Ann Emerg Med* 1988; 17:66–68.
Denney JC, Handler SD: Membranous laryngotracheobronchitis. *Pediatrics* 1982; 70:705–707.
Edwards KM, Dundon MC, Altemeyer WA: Bacterial tracheitis as a complication of viral croup. *Pediatr Infect Dis* 1983; 2:390–391.
Jones R, Santos JI, Overall JC: Bacterial tracheitis. *JAMA* 1979; 242:721–726.
Liston SL, Gehrz RC, Siegel LG, et al: Bacterial tracheitis. *Am J Dis Child* 1983; 137:764–767.
Sofer S, Duncan P, Chernick V: Bacterial tracheitis: An old disease rediscovered. *Clin Pediatr* 1983; 22:407–411.

LOWER RESPIRATORY TRACT INFECTIONS

Paula Schweich, M.D.

Lower respiratory tract infections are a major cause of morbidity in children. The majority of these infections are self-limited and benign, but the clinician must be able to recognize and treat those situations that require specific treatment and aggressive support. This chapter will discuss the infectious lower respiratory tract diseases: bronchiolitis, pneumonia, afebrile pneumonitis, and tuberculosis.

BRONCHIOLITIS

Bronchiolitis is a clinical syndrome resulting from inflammation of the bronchioles. This disease is characterized by expiratory wheezing or inspiratory rales of acute onset following a viral upper respiratory tract infection (URI); it peaks in children 2 to 8 months of age, but may occur up to the age of 2 years. Bronchiolitis results in a spectrum of symptoms from mild to severe respiratory distress and is a major cause of hospitalization in young infants.

The causative agent in the majority of infants with bronchiolitis is the respiratory syncytial virus (RSV). The peak seasons for bronchiolitis are winter and spring, corresponding to the seasons for epidemics of RSV. Other viruses causing bronchiolitis include parainfluenza virus types I and III, adenovirus, enterovirus, influenza virus, and rhinovirus. *Mycoplasma pneumoniae* can also cause bronchiolitis.

The etiologic agent of bronchiolitis invades the epithelial cells of the lower respiratory tract, causing necrosis and sloughing of respiratory epithelium, increased mucus secretion, and edema of the airway wall. This process produces mechanically narrowed and obstructed peripheral airways in a nonuniform distribution throughout the lungs, with distal air trapping causing overdistention of the lungs and areas of atelectasis. The lung overdistention causes these infants to breathe rapidly with a high lung volume. Also, there may be areas in the lung that are perfused but poorly ventilated, resulting in hypoxemia and hypercarbia, often seen in the sicker infant with bronchiolitis. Young children tend to have more severe respiratory distress when they get bronchiolitis. The airways in these children are smaller and are more easily obstructed by the cellular debris, mucus, and edema.

Data Gathering

The diagnosis of bronchiolitis is suggested by the season, age of the child, and the clinical presentation. There is usually a prodrome of a URI including cough, rhinorrhea, and a low-grade fever. The child may have other symptoms of URI such as mild conjunctivitis, otitis media, or pharyngitis. The symptoms of URI are followed in 2 to 3 days by an increased respiratory rate of 60 to 80 breaths per minute, nasal flaring and chest retractions, wheezing, rales, and tachycardia. The wheezes or rales are usually bilateral and may be heard in different areas of the lung on repeated physical examinations. Infants with respiratory distress may feed poorly and have markedly decreased fluid intake, becoming irritable and dehydrated. In very mild cases, there may be no respiratory distress and breath sounds may be normal.

There are no routine laboratory tests for the diagnosis of bronchiolitis. The WBC count is usually normal, although it may be elevated with a left shift. Viral cultures from respiratory tract secretions are positive in up to 50% of infants with bronchiolitis, but are not available in time to be of help in diagnosis. Viral identification can be performed quickly in some centers with immunofluorescent techniques.

The chest radiograph is also nonspecific in bronchiolitis. Although the chest radiograph may be normal, there is usually diffuse hyperinflation with flattened diaphragms and often patchy or peribronchial infiltrates. There may be areas of atelectasis that are difficult to distinguish from pneumonia.

In infants with the acute onset of the first episode of wheezing and signs of a viral URI, there is no reliable way to distinguish a first asthmatic attack triggered by a viral infection from an episode of bronchiolitis. If, however, there is a strong family history of allergies or asthma, atopy in the patient, or a reversible component to the disease with bronchodilator therapy, the clinician should consider the diagnosis of asthma. These patients with asthma tend to improve more rapidly.

Other major diagnoses to be considered in the differential diagnosis are aspiration of foreign body, croup, obstruction by hypertrophied adenoids or retropharyngeal abscess, and congestive heart failure. A chest radiograph can be helpful to differentiate between these.

Management

The only specific therapy for bronchiolitis is the use of aerosolized ribavirin for suspected or proven RSV infection in high-risk or very ill infants. Otherwise, the management is supportive, as there is no proven specific therapy for either the airway obstruction or the viral infection. The child should be encouraged to drink clear fluids as often as possible, and antipyretics can be used for an increased temperature. A mist tent is not helpful, as the mist does not reach the lower respiratory tract to liquefy secretions. A subcutaneous injection of epinephrine (0.01 ml/kg of 1:1000), or a nebulized β-adrenergic agent may be helpful in older infants; if the child responds, there is a reversible bronchospastic component to the obstruction and treatment can be started with an oral bronchodilator such as metaproterenol syrup (2 mg/kg/day divided into three doses) or albuterol syrup (0.3 mg/kg/day divided into three doses) for 5 to 7 days. This is controversial treatment for children less than 18 months of age (some physicians feel that the smooth muscle on the small airways of infants is not responsive to bronchodilators); however, a trial of a bronchodilator should not harm the child. If the child does not respond to epinephrine or nebulized β-adrenergic agents, bronchodilators are generally not indicated.

Antibiotics are not indicated in the treatment of bronchiolitis. If the child's condition suddenly deteriorates and bacterial disease is suspected, tracheal secretions should be sent for gram stain and culture, blood cultures obtained, and ampicillin begun (150 mg/kg/day in four divided doses). Steroid treatment is not beneficial.

Children with bronchiolitis may have a worsening course for 24 to 72 hours, but then the majority improve quickly and are normal by 2 to 3 weeks. If there is concern about the infant's respiratory rate, fatigue, or ability to drink, the physician should check the infant frequently. It may be necessary to obtain an arterial blood gas determination to assess gas exchange. A minority of infants will have a severe enough abnormality of gas exchange to develop cyanosis.

The prognosis for children with bronchiolitis is generally excellent, and less than 5% of these children require hospitalization. If there is concern about dehydration, aspiration of fluids because the child is very young with a high respiratory rate, secondary bacterial pneumonia, or marked respiratory distress with impending respiratory failure, then hospitalization should be considered. Cyanosis, decreased inspiratory breath sounds, or lethargy may be indicative of impending respiratory failure. Complications such as persistent wheezing, superimposed bacterial pneumonia, lobar collapse, and apnea occur occasionally in the hospitalized patient.

Recent studies show that many children with bronchiolitis have increased airway reactivity when they become older children and their lung function studies may show peripheral airway obstruction of an extended period of time. There is a known strong association between bronchiolitis and later development of asthma.

It appears that those children with bronchiolitis who are atopic and have high IgE levels, family history of allergy, and nasal eosinophilia are more likely to develop asthma. It is not clear whether it is the bronchiolitis that predisposes these children to asthma, or whether there is another factor that predisposes these children to both diseases.

PNEUMONIA

Pneumonia is an infection that involves the terminal airways and alveoli of the lungs. Many children with URI also have a concurrent pneumonia. The incidence of pneumonia decreases with age, ranging from approximately 4% per year in young children, to 2% in children 5 to 9 years old, to less than 1% in children over 9 years old.

The normal airway is sterile from the trachea to the alveoli. Most pneumonias occur by aspiration, which spreads the organisms from the mouth or upper respiratory tract to the lower respiratory tract. Infection can occur because of virulence of the organism or susceptibility of the lower respiratory tract. Children with anatomic defects such as tracheoesophageal fistulae or abnormal palate, neurologic dysfunction (such as swallowing dysfunction or depressed cough reflex), foreign body aspiration, cystic fibrosis, or congestive heart failure have an increased incidence of pneumonia. Viruses may predispose to bacterial pneumonia by increasing secretions that are then aspirated, by decreasing motility of the cilia or effectiveness of the alveolar macrophages, or by altering the immune response. A less common cause of infection of the lung is by hematogenous spreading during bacteremia.

Table 60–6 shows the major causes of pneumonia in each age group. Viruses are a very common cause of pneumonia. RSV, parainfluenza viruses, and adenovirus are the most common viral agents causing pneumonia in children under 2 years old. The most common cause of pneumonia in infants and young children, RSV infections occur in yearly winter to spring epidemics of 6 to 8 weeks' duration, while parainfluenza virus infections may occur all year with superimposed epidemics. Adenovirus is noteworthy for its ability to cause a severe bilateral pneumonia with lobar infiltrates. Other viral causes of pneumonia in normal hosts include rhinovirus, enterovirus, and coronavirus. Generalized infections caused by varicella (chicken pox), rubeola (measles), and influenza may also be accompanied by pneumonia. Cytomegalovirus, herpes virus hominis, and rubella can cause pneumonia in neonates and immunocompromised hosts (see Acquired Immune Deficiency Syndrome, later in this chapter).

Table 60–7 presents the most common bacterial causes of pneumonia at each age. Bacteria are the major cause of pneumonia only in the first two weeks of life and account for less than 10% of pneumonia in normal children after that age. In the young infant, organisms from the maternal flora, such as group B *Streptococcus* and the enteric bacilli, may cause a fulminant respiratory tract infection that is difficult to distinguish from the respiratory distress syndrome. After the neonatal period, S. *pneumoniae* is the most frequent cause of bacterial pneumonia in all ages.

TABLE 60–6
Etiology of Pneumonia in Normal Children*

	AGE			
	LESS THAN 2 WK	2 WK–3 MO	3 MO–5 YR	6–18 YR
Common	Bacteria	Virus Chlamydia†	Virus	*Mycoplasma*
Less common	Virus	Bacteria	Bacteria	Virus
Occasional	Fungus		*Mycoplasma*	Bacteria

*Adapted from Long SS: *Pediatr Clin North Am* 1983; 30:297–321.
†Also consider other agents of afebrile pneumonitis syndrome.

TABLE 60–7
Organisms by Age in Bacterial Pneumonia

	LESS THAN 3 MO	3 MO–5 YR	6–18 YR
Common	Group B and D *Streptococcus* Enteric bacilli *Streptococcus pneumoniae*	*S. pneumoniae* *H. influenzae*	*S. pneumoniae*
Less common	*Staphylococcus aureus* *Hemophilus influenzae*	Group A *Streptococcus* Mouth flora *S. aureus*	*H. influenzae* Group A *Streptococcus* Mouth flora *S. aureus*

Data Gathering

Pneumonia in children is a clinical diagnosis. Most children with pneumonia will have an increased respiratory rate for their age, and many will have fever and a cough. Infants may feed poorly and be irritable, with no localized signs of infection, and require a full workup to rule out bacteremia, meningitis, pneumonia, and urinary tract infection. Older children may complain of chest pain, abdominal pain, or shortness of breath. More seriously ill children will present with cyanosis, nasal flaring, and retractions. On auscultation there may be normal or decreased breath sounds, rales, and/or wheezes. Transmitted breath sounds in a small chest may make the auscultatory findings difficult to interpret. Other findings associated with pneumonia include abdominal distention from partial ileus and meningismus.

The age of the child, history, and physical examination often suggest whether a child has viral, bacterial, mycoplasmal, or a more unusual pneumonia. Generally, bacterial pneumonia will have a more abrupt onset. The patient is more likely to have high fever frequently over 39° C, a wet-sounding or productive cough, and pleuritic chest pain. On physical examination, the patient may appear "toxic," and there may be decreased breath sounds and confined rales on auscultation. The progression tends to be more rapid than in viral pneumonia. Viral pneumonia is more likely to start with coryza, cough, and other upper respiratory tract symptoms. The fever usually is lower than that in bacterial pneumonia; the cough is nonproductive, and there may be other signs of viral illness such as headache, myalgias, pharyngitis, or rash. There are often other family members with a concurrent viral illness. On physical examination, an infant may be wheezing, and in many infants and children, the finding of rales and rhonchi are generally more diffuse than in bacterial disease. The findings on physical examination may be impressive compared to the general appearance of the child.

Mycoplasmal pneumonia is more similar in presentation to viral pneumonia, with low-grade fever and associated headaches and myalgias. There may be a history of exposure to others with a similar illness. There often is a gradually worsening, hacking paroxysmal cough. The auscultatory findings are usually unilateral, but not well localized.

The exact etiologic diagnosis is often difficult to determine because of the wide range and changing epidemiology of organisms, the difficulty of obtaining pulmonary secretions in children, and the invasiveness of a lung puncture. Laboratory studies and chest radiographs may be helpful as supportive data for the etiologic diagnosis, but are usually unnecessary unless there is a confusing clinical picture, a complication, or hospitalization is being considered.

Table 60–8 may help with differentiating the more common bacterial causes. The tests for bacterial disease include cultures and antigen detection. Cultures and gram stain can be obtained from secretions from the posterior pharynx or from the sputum in an older child who can cooperate. These are difficult to interpret, as many of the organisms that cause pneumonia are frequent colonizers of the throat in healthy children. More invasive procedures for obtaining a culture, such as thoracentesis for pleural fluid, transtracheal aspiration, and direct lung puncture are saved for the more se-

TABLE 60–8
Characteristics of Bacterial Pneumonias

	ONSET	PLEURAL FLUID	LABORATORY FINDINGS	CHEST X-RAY FILM	COMPLICATIONS	COMMENTS
Streptococcus pneumoniae	Subacute: preceded by URI, headache, malaise; acute: high, fever 103°–105° F with moderate to severe respiratory distress and chest pain	Rare	WBC left shift anemia	Lobar consolidation or patchy bronchopneumonia, atelectasis	Sepsis, meningitis, atelectasis	Lobar consolidation
Hemophilus influenzae	Subacute: insidious onset with prolonged cough; acute: as with *S. pneumoniae*	Common	WBC	Hilar nodes, lobar or bronchopneumonia, "shaggy" heart	Meningitis, soft-tissue; pericarditis	Concurrent otitis media in 50% of cases
Staphylococcus aureus	Acute: moderate to severe respiratory distress. Fulminating: especially in young infants	Common	WBC, Anemia	Hilar nodes, small focal lesions to consolidation	Sepsis, bone infection	Skin pustules and purulent conjunctivitis in young child; complicates viral infections
Group A *Streptococcus*	Subacute; acute	Less common	WBC	Same as *S. aureus*	Pericarditis, hyponatremia	Complicates viral infections

verely ill child. In a small number of patients, a positive culture of blood, pleural fluid, or the lung tissue will specifically identify the cause.

Antigen detection by counterimmunoelectrophoresis (CIE) or latex particle agglutination can be performed on serum, urine, pleural fluid, or CSF. These tests detect the capsular antigens of *S. pneumoniae* and *H. influenzae* type B. This test is available in some referral centers.

A 5-TU purified protein derivative skin test should be performed on any patient with pneumonia in which tuberculosis is a possibility.

Viruses can also be detected by culture and serologic techniques. A rapid test is the fluorescent antibody technique looking for RSV on smears of nasopharyngeal secretions. Sera obtained during the acute and convalescent stage can be used to detect antibody to any of the viruses and *Chlamydia*. All these organisms can also be cultured, although some with difficulty. Isolation of a respiratory virus from the nasopharynx is very strong evidence for its role in pneumonia, as these viruses are rarely carried asymptomatically.

It is not usually necessary to obtain a chest radiograph unless there is dullness to percussion, a recurring pneumonia, a toxic appearance of the child, or admission to the hospital. Chest radiographs alone are poor indicators of etiologic diagnosis, although certain appearances may be helpful along with the history and physical examination. The appearance of consolidation on a chest radiograph favors a bacterial cause. However, a radiograph showing hyperaeration with or without patchy infiltrates is also consistent with bacterial disease; complete lobar consolidation is less common in infants and children than in adults. The chest radiograph of a child with viral pneumonia often shows hyperaeration and may have perihilar or diffuse interstitial disease; however, there can also be an appearance of consolidation. Mycoplasmal pneumonia characteristically will have alveolar or interstitial patchy infiltrates in one or more lobes, and this pattern may migrate or progress.

The WBC count is another parameter that may be helpful along with the other data. In bacterial pneumonia the WBC count is usually over 15,000/mm^3, with a left shift. In viral and mycoplasmal pneumonias, the WBC count is usually less than 15,000/mm^3. The WBC count in viral pneumonia may have a lymphocyte predominance.

Management

If after considering all the data, the most likely diagnosis is viral pneumonia, there is no need for antibiotic treatment in most patients. Antibiotics will not shorten the course of disease nor prevent superinfection. However, treatment with antibiotics may be considered in a child who appears in a very toxic state, in a febrile child less than 3 months old, in an immunocompromised host, or if *M. pneumoniae* is a significant possibility. The treatment otherwise is supportive with antipyretics, fluids, and increased humidity. An antiviral agent (ribavirin) administered by continuous aerosol to infants for 3 to 6 days seems to cause more rapid improvement in signs and symptoms and also decreases viral shedding. In small infants with respiratory distress, monitoring is essential, and intravenous hydration and oxygen therapy may be necessary. The prognosis for an individual child with viral pneumonia is excellent.

Mycoplasma pneumoniae is very sensitive to erythromycin and the tetracyclines. The preferred drug of choice is erythromycin for 7 to 10 days, at a dose of 40 mg/kg/day divided into 6-hour intervals (maximum dose, 2 g/day). The treatment does not significantly improve the cough but may decrease the febrile course.

The initial antibiotic for bacterial pneumonia is chosen by knowing the most likely causative organisms for the patient's age, what antibiotics those organisms are usually sensitive to, and the current patterns of resistance. Broad-spectrum coverage is not recommended, as this may be less effective against the causative organism.

Oral therapy is appropriate for patients who are moderately ill with an uncomplicated pneumonia and who have no underlying diseases. Table 60–9 shows the drugs for initial treatment of uncomplicated pneumonia. A single initial dose of procaine penicillin given intramuscularly (IM) may be used to attain an early peak tissue concentration;* the usual oral

---

*Dose of IM penicillin procaine G should be determined as follows: child (15 kg), 300,000 U; child (15–30 kg), 600,000 U; child (30 kg), 1,200,000 U.

TABLE 60–9
Initial Antimicrobial Treatment*

AGE	ANTIBIOTIC (DOSE/KG), INTERVAL†
<3 mo	
Inpatient	Ampicillin (150 mg) q 6 hr and gentamicin (7.5 mg) q 8 hr; or ampicillin and cefotaxime (150 mg) q 6–8 hr.
3 mo–5 yr	
Outpatient	Amoxicillin (50 mg), q 8 hr; *alt*‡: erythromycin-sulfa (40 mg of erythromycin), q 8 hr; TMP-SMZ§ (10 mg of TMP), q 12 hr; amoxicillin plus potassium clavulanate (40 mg amoxicillin), q 8 hr; cefaclor (40 mg) q 8 hr. *Penicillin allergy:* erythromycin-sulfa (40 mg of erythromycin), q 8 hr.
Inpatient	Ampicillin (150 mg), q 6 hr; cefuroxime (100 mg) q 8 hr; *penicillin allergy:* chloramphenicol (50 mg), q 6 hr.
Comments	Use an *alt* outpatient drug if there is a high prevalence of β-lactamase producing *H. influenzae.*
6–18 yr	
Outpatient	Penicillin VK (50 mg), q 6 hr; *alt*‡: erythromycin (40 mg), q 6 hr; *penicillin alternative:* erythromycin (50 mg), q 8 hr.
Inpatient	Penicillin G (50,00 U), q 6 hr; nafcillin† (150 mg), q 4 hr; ampicillin† (150 mg), q 6 hr; *penicillin allergy:* chloramphenicol (50 mg), q 6 hr.
Comments	Some isolates of *S. pneumoniae* show "relative resistance" to penicillin; if *Mycoplasma* is suspected, use erythromycin.

*Adapted from Long SS: *Pediatr Clin North Am* 1983; 30:297–321.
†Parentheses suggest possible additional antibiotics.
‡Indicates alternate outpatient drug (see Comments).
§TMP-SMZ indicates trimethoprim-sulfamethoxazole.

antibiotic course is then started 24 hours later. Twenty percent to 50% of *H. influenzae* isolates are β-lactamase positive, and therefore resistant to amoxicillin. Therefore, amoxicillin with clavulanate, erythromycin-sulfa, trimethoprim-sulfamethoxazole or cefaclor may be a better choice.

The length of oral treatment for an uncomplicated pneumonia is 7 to 10 days, assuming there is a good clinical response. If the patient is severely ill, is an immunocompromised host, or has a complication, the patient will need parenteral therapy until there is clinical improvement.

If the specific cause is found by culture or other laboratory studies, or if the organism is found to be resistant to the antibiotic, the antibiotic therapy may need alteration. The pneumonia may be caused by a less common agent that was not covered in the initial therapy.

If there is a suspicion of penicillin allergy, usually from a history of urticaria or a pruritic rash after penicillin therapy, one should not use penicillin, its derivatives, or cephalosporins. Alternative drugs are included in Table 60–9.

In addition to antibiotic therapy, the moderately to severely ill child may require analgesia for chest pain. It is easier to follow the clinical course and detect complications if antipyretics are not used.

It is important to follow up all patients with pneumonia in the first few days for possible clinical deterioration. Most patients with uncomplicated bacterial pneumonia have their fever abate and improve clinically within 48 hours of appropriate treatment. Full recovery is often within 7 to 10 days. Another reevaluation in 2 to 3 weeks can assure the clinician that the patient has recovered. The chest radiograph does not need to be repeated unless there is suspected underlying disease or complication, the clinical course is unusually long, or the patient has repeated pneumonias. If the course is prolonged, complications should be sought with a careful physical examination, a chest radiograph, and any other necessary diagnostic tests.

Complications of viral pneumonia should be suspected if there is worsening respiratory distress after the peak of illness, an increasing WBC count, or a chest radiograph with consolidation or evidence of pleural effusion. Bacterial superinfection is more likely in older children with a systemic viral illness such as measles or varicella who have a severe viral pneumonia. It is rare following RSV or parainfluenza pneumonia. When there is a superimposed bacterial pneumonia, it may be fulminant and antibiotics covering all the common pneumonia-causing bacterial agents should be used.

Pleural effusions frequently complicate pneumonia caused by *H. influenzae* type b, *S. aureus,* and mouth flora. If an effusion is suspected clinically, lateral decubitus x-ray films, CT scans, or ultrasound (US) are useful studies for diagnosis. If an effusion is confirmed, the child should be referred for thoracentesis, both for diagnostic studies and therapeutic drainage. Lung abscesses are most common after aspiration of anaerobic mouth flora. Putrid breath and sputum and multiple organisms on gram stain are clues to this diagnosis. Other complications of bacterial pneumonia include atelectasis, meningitis, and the syndrome of inappropriate antidiuretic hormone.

Hospitalization is necessary in patients who are young infants, who appear toxic or in severe respiratory distress, who cannot take fluids well because of high respiratory rate or vomiting, or who fail to improve clinically while taking oral antibiotics. These patients as well as the patients who have complications or are immunocompromised need parenteral antibiotics. Initial parenteral antibiotic coverage is included in Table 60–9. If there is a possibility of hypoxia, an arterial blood gas level should be obtained, and oxygen therapy started if indicated.

The long-term prognosis for children with pneumonia is generally excellent. Some studies show that children who are hospitalized with lower respiratory tract disease, either pneumonia or bronchiolitis, have an increased incidence of respiratory tract symptoms than do controls. These children may have chronic impairment of lung function.

AFEBRILE PNEUMONITIS

Afebrile pneumonitis refers to a perinatally acquired pneumonia in young infants up to 4 months of age. It is caused by a heterogeneous group of infectious agents and is endemic throughout the year. It is theorized that the infant's nasopharynx or conjunctiva is colonized with bacteria from the mother's vaginal tract during birth. In some infants there is subsequent downward extension to the lungs. The organisms involved are *C. trachomatis, Pneumocystis carinii, Ureaplasma urealyticum, M. hominis,* and cytomegalovirus. Cytomegalovirus can also be transmitted through breast milk. The fact that the pneumonias caused by these organisms are indistinguishable from each other clinically and radiologically suggests that the host characteristics are more important than the offending agent.

Infants with lower respiratory tract disease may have an increased propensity to develop obstructive airway disease, often manifested by recurrent wheezing. Preliminary evidence suggests that infants with lower respiratory tract infection caused by *C. trachomatis* who are ill enough to require hospitalization may have more chronic sequelae than those infected with viral agents such as RSV.

TUBERCULOSIS

Tuberculosis continues to be an important health problem in the United States. It is primarily an urban disease, focused in certain minority groups and in the foreign born. Although overall the average annual incidence has decreased since the early 1960s, an increase has been observed during the past few years. This increase, mostly in urban areas, is most likely due to factors of poverty, overcrowding, immigration, and HIV seropositivity.

All ages of children are susceptible to tuberculosis, although infants and adolescents are at the highest risk. Each case in a child demonstrates recent transmission of *Mycobacterium tuberculosis* from another person, usually an adult, who is untreated. Children with active tuberculosis are rarely contagious because of small lesions and minimal coughing. The organism is transmitted by inhalation of tubercle bacilli which are aerosolized when a contagious person coughs, sneezes, or speaks. Once in the lung, the organisms multiply and spread through lymphatic channels and the bloodstream. They lodge in regional lymph nodes and distant organs. The child is asymptomatic during this period of spread. Over a period of weeks, specific immunity is acquired, and further spread is blocked.

After exposure, the time of maximum risk for active disease is the first 2 years. In most previously healthy hosts, the infection resolves spontaneously and never progresses to clinical disease.

Although much of childhood tuberculosis occurs in older children, the proportion of infected children with active disease is higher in children less than 3 years old. These children have primarily pulmonary or lymph node disease, with meningeal and miliary infection occurring rarely. Even with pulmonary disease, many children are asymptomatic or have nonspecific systemic symptoms. Progressive pulmonary disease when it occurs is more common in adolescents. Later clinical manifestations may include infection of the bones, joints, skin, ears, eyes, and kidneys.

Data Gathering

The diagnosis of tuberculosis is often based on the knowledge that a child has been exposed to an adult with clinical disease, or on a high index of suspicion for another reason. Infants exposed to disease are most likely to develop active disease and also suffer with more severe disease.

Initial diagnosis of infection is often based on a positive tuberculin test. Hypersensitivity develops and the tuberculin skin test becomes positive 2 to 10 weeks after infection. A reaction of at least 10 mm induration to 0.1 mL of 5 tuberculin units of purified protein derivative (PPD) administered by the intracutaneous route (Mantoux method) is the usual definition of a positive reaction.

A skin reaction between 5 and 10 mm is significant if the child has signs or symptoms of disease, or if he has had recent contact with an infectious case. If the skin reaction is equivocal, it should be repeated in 1 to 2 months. A negative reaction does not rule out the diagnosis if the child has signs and symptoms of tuberculosis.

If the tuberculin test is positive or equivocal, or a child has signs and symptoms compatible with tuberculosis, the history and physical examination should be followed by a chest radiograph. The physical examination, chest radiograph, and possibly results of cultures will determine whether the child has active disease, or if he is only a tuberculin reactor who needs preventive therapy.

The diagnosis of active disease is often based on detection of typical abnormalities on the chest radiograph. Radiographic abnormalities include lymphadenopathy of hilar, mediastinal or other lymph nodes, pulmonary involvement such as atelectasis, infiltration or consolidation, or pleural effusion.

Demonstration of the acid-fast bacilli by Ziehl-Neilsen stain of fluids or biopsy specimens is very helpful in diagnosis. Culture of *M. tuberculosis* is successful in approximately 25% of children with tuberculosis. The organism can be cultured from gastric washings, sputum, pleural fluid, CSF, urine and many tissues. Isolation may take 4 to 6 weeks, as the organism grows slowly. Attempts to culture the organism to determine drug susceptibility are particularly important when drug resistance is suspected.

When a child is found to be infected with *M. tuberculosis*, it is extremely important to identify the index case. This will help support the diagnosis, determine possible drug resistance from culture, and find and treat all infected individuals.

Management

Drugs for treatment of tuberculosis are shown in Table 60–10. Isoniazid and rifampin are bactericidal drugs that act on intracellular and extracellular organisms. Isoniazid is rapidly absorbed and diffuses well into all body fluids and tissues, including CSF. Hepatotoxicity is rare in children and if baseline liver function tests are normal, they do not need to be repeated unless there are clinical signs of toxicity. Pyrazinamide, streptomycin, and ethambutol are also bactericidal. Streptomycin is active against rapidly multiplying organisms and resistance is common. Ethambutol and ethionamide are only bacteriostatic. Although widely used in adults, ethambutol is not a good drug for young children since its principal side effect of optic neuritis cannot be well monitored.

The goal of treatment of tuberculosis is sterilization of the lesions in the shortest period of time. This will minimize development of resistant organisms and complications in the patient, and maximize patient compliance. Treatment of tuberculosis traditionally involved 12 to 24 months of continuous treatment, but recent data show that shorter treatment regimens are successful and there is rarely a need for retreatment. Medications can be given out at 2- to 4-week intervals, at which time the health care provider can determine compliance, and obtain any history of toxicity or complications. Physicians treating a patient with tuberculosis should work with the local health department.

The current recommendations of the American Academy of Pediatrics for treatment of un-

TABLE 60–10
Drugs Used for Treatment of Tuberculosis

DRUG	DAILY DOSE	TWICE WEEKLY DOSE	MAJOR ADVERSE REACTIONS
Isoniazid (INH)	10–20 mg/kg PO or IM (max 300 mg/day)	20–40 mg/kg* (max 900 mg)	Mild hepatic enzyme elevation (≤4%), peripheral neuropathy, hepatitis, hypersensitivity.
Rifampin (RIF)	10–15 mg/kg PO or IV	10–20 mg/kg* (max 600 mg)	Nausea, vomiting; orange discoloration of secretions and urine; hepatitis; febrile reaction; purpura (rare).
Pyrazinamide (PZA)	15–30 mg/kg PO (max 2 g/day)	50–70 mg/kg	Hepatotoxicity, hyperuricemia, arthralgias, skin rash, GI upset.
Streptomycin (SM)	20–40 mg/kg IM (max 1 g/day)	25–30 mg/kg	Ototoxicity, nephrotoxicity.
Ethambutol (EMB)	15–25 mg/kg PO (max 2.5 g/day)	50 mg/kg	Optic neuritis (retrobulbar neuritis), skin rash.
Ethionamide	15–20 mg/kg (max 1 g/day)	—	GI upset, hepatotoxicity, hypersensitivity.

*If INH and RIF are used in combination, use INH <10 mg/kg and RIF <15 mg/kg to decrease risk of hepatotoxicity.

complicated intrathoracic tuberculosis, including pulmonary disease, hilar and mediastinal lymphadenopathy, and pleural disease in children of all ages is a 9-month course of isoniazid and rifampin. These two drugs will eliminate the rapidly growing organisms. If drug resistance is suspected because the child is foreign born, had prior disease, or had a contact with drug-resistant disease, a third drug is added. The child must always be treated with at least two drugs to which the organism is likely to be susceptible. Treatment is daily for 4 to 8 weeks, and then can be continued two times a week. Extrapulmonary disease, such as that involving the bones, joints, genitourinary and GI tracts, is usually treated for 12 to 18 months; a third drug is added for the first 2 months. Tuberculous meningitis or disseminated disease, such as miliary tuberculosis, is treated with three or four drugs. Isoniazid, rifampin, pyrazinamide, and ethionamide all cross the blood-brain barrier in sufficient concentrations. The use of steroids for more severe disease is controversial.

The most important follow-up of these children is an ongoing clinical assessment. Although the standard duration of therapy is 9 months, this may be modified by the patient's clinical and radiographic response; treatment may be extended if the organism isolated from the patient or index case is resistant to the standard regimen. Children being treated for tuberculosis do not need routine laboratory studies. If the child had a positive sputum culture at the beginning of treatment, this can be rechecked. The chest radiograph can also be useful to follow up treatment response, although resolution of lesions may be very slow. If pulmonary infiltrates are identified at initial diagnosis, a chest radiograph can be obtained every 2 to 3 months. If initially there was only hilar adenopathy, a repeat chest radiograph is indicated in 6 to 12 months. Although follow-up radiographs should be obtained until the lesions have cleared, slow resolution is not a reason to extend treatment.

A large part of tuberculosis treatment involves prevention of disease in infected individuals. The American Academy of Pediatrics recommends testing of low-risk children at 12 to 15 months, at school entry, and in adolescence. Annual tuberculin testing is recommended only for children at high risk of infection. This would include children living in areas with a high prevalence of tuberculosis. The tuberculin test rather than the multiple puncture devices with dried or liquid tuberculin is used to evaluate suspected cases, contacts of tuberculosis patients, and testing of high-risk groups.

Children who are tuberculin reactive but healthy, with no evidence of clinical or radiographic disease, are treated with isoniazid for 1 year, daily for 1 month and then twice a week. This treatment prevents the development of active disease. Children who have been exposed to an active case of tuberculosis but who are tuberculin negative and healthy are treated with isoniazid for 3 months after contact is broken. At the end of 3 months, the tuberculin test is repeated, and if it has converted to positive, the child is treated for another 6 to 12 months.

BIBLIOGRAPHY

Bronchiolitis

Brooks LJ, Cropp GJ: Theophylline therapy in bronchiolitis. *Am J Dis Child* 1981; 135:934—936.

Carlsen K, Larsen S, Bjerve O, et al: Acute bronchiolitis: Predisposing factors and characterization of infants at risk. *Pediatr Pulmonology* 1987; 3:153–160.

Dunsky E: Bronchiolitis: Differentiation from infantile asthma. *Pediatr Ann* 1977; 6:45–55.

Hall CB, Hall WJ, Gala CL, et al: Long-term prospective study in children after respiratory synctial virus infection. *J Pediatr* 1984; 105:358.

Henderson FW, Clyde WA Jr, Collier AM, et al: The etiologic and epidemiologic spectrum of bronchiolitis in pediatric practice. *J Pediatr* 1979; 95:183–190.

Kendig EL, Chernick V: *Disorders of the Respiratory Tract in Children*. Philadelphia, W.B. Saunders Co, 1983.

McConnochie K: "Bronchiolitis, what's in the name?" *Am J Dis Child* 1983; 137:11–13.

Pneumonia and Afebrile Pneumonitis

Brasfield DM, Stagno S, Whitley RJ, et al: Infant pneumonitis associated with cytomegalovirus, *Chlamydia*, *Pneumocystis*, and *Ureaplasma*: Follow-up. *Pediatrics* 1987; 79:76–83.

Cohen GJ: Management of infections of the lower respiratory tract in children. *Pediatr Infect Dis J* 1987; 6:317–323.

Dworsky ME, Stagno S: Newer agents causing pneumonitis in early infancy. *Pediatr Infect Dis* 1982; 1:188–195.

Eichenwald MF: Pneumonia syndromes in children. *Hosp Prac* 1976; 89–96.

Gooch WM: Bronchitis and pneumonia in ambulatory patients. *Pediatr Infect Dis J* 1987; 6:137–140.

Hall CB, McBride JT, Walsh EE: Aerosolized ribavirin treatment of infants with respiratory synctial viral infection. *N Engl J Med* 1983; 308:1443–7.

Long S: Treatment of acute pneumonia in infants and children. *Pediatr Clin North Am* 1983; 30:297–321.

McCarthy PL, et al: Radiographic findings and etiologic diagnosis in ambulatory childhood pneumonias. *Clin Pediatr* 1981; 20:686–691.

Mok JYO, Simpson M: Outcome for acute bronchitis, bronchiolitis, and pneumonia in infancy. *Arch Dis Child* 1984; 59:306–309.

Morrison HR, Taussig LM, Fulginiti VA: *Chlamydia trachomatis* and chronic respiratory disease in childhood. *Pediatr Infect Dis* 1982; 1:29–33.

Paisley JW, Lauer BA, McIntosh K, et al: Pathogens associated with acute lower respiratory tract infection in young children. *Pediatr Infect Dis* 1984; 3:14–19.

Stagno S, Brasfield DM, Brown MB, et al: Infant pneumonitis associated with cytomegalovirus, *Chlamydia*, *Pneumocystis*, and *Ureaplasma*: A prospective study. *Pediatrics* 1981; 68:322–329.

Stickler GB, Hoffman AD, Taylor WF: Problems in the clinical and roentgenographic diagnosis of pneumonia in young children. *Clin Pediatr* 1984; 23:393–399.

Turner RB, Hayden FG, Hendley JO, et al: Counterimmunoelectropheresis of urine for diagnosis of bacterial pneumonia in pediatric outpatients. *Pediatrics* 1983; 71:780–783.

Wald ER: Management of pneumonia in outpatients. *Pediatrics Infect Dis* 1984; 3(suppl):21–23.

Tuberculosis

Jacobs RF, Abernathy RS: The treatment of tuberculosis in children. *Pediatr Infect Dis* 1985; 4:513–517.

Nemir RL, Krasinski K: Tuberculosis in children and adolescents in the 1980's. *Pediatr Infect Dis J* 1988; 7:375–379.

Report of the Committee on Infectious Diseases. American Academy of Pediatrics, ed 20, 1986.

Snider DE, Rieder HL, Combs D, et al: Tuberculosis in children. *Pediatr Infect Dis J* 1988; 7:271–278.

Woodring JH, Vandiviere HM, Fried AM, et al: Update: The radiographic features of pulmonary tuberculosis. *AJR* 1986; 146:497–506.

VIRAL HEPATITIS

John T. Boyle, M.D.

The term viral hepatitis is commonly used to describe infection with one of two viruses: hepatitis A (HAV) or hepatitis B (HBV). In recent years, this definition has been expanded to include non-A, non-B hepatitis and more recently delta hepatitis virus. Knowledge and understanding of viral hepatitis has grown tremendously in the past 10 to 15 years as an impressive array of sophisticated immunologic, biochemical, and biophysical techniques have been applied to further identify and characterize the disorder. For the primary physician, this knowledge has resulted in improved ability to diagnose hepatitis, to differentiate between acute and chronic infection, and, most importantly, to institute measures to prevent spread of the infection. Because there is no treatment for viral hepatitis, prevention of hepatitis is the primary goal of the primary care physician. Prevention demands (1) accurate diagnosis that depends on a high index of clinical suspicion since it is estimated that only 25% of cases are clinically apparent, and (2) knowledge of serologic markers that allow specific etiologic identification.

BACKGROUND

Hepatitis A

Hepatitis A virus is an RNA virus that has worldwide distribution. Since there is no known carrier state in humans, natural perpetuation of the virus is believed to occur outside the human host, most likely in fauna of contaminated water. Nevertheless, while human infection does occur from ingestion of contaminated shellfish, particularly clams and oysters, in the majority of cases transmission is human to human, with the most common mode being the fecal-to-oral route through such vehicles as contaminated food and water. It is interesting that the incidence of common-source outbreaks has decreased in the past 5 to 10 years. The previous fall-winter prevalence for school children is no longer observed. Common source outbreaks are still likely to be seen in daycare centers and facilities for the mentally retarded. The decrease in incidence of clinical HAV may reflect improved preventive immunoprophylactic measures, but it may also indicate an increased trend toward less severe, anicteric disease. Indeed recent epidemiologic studies suggest that 25% to 50% of the general population have antibody to HAV by 30 to 40 years of age, while only 3% to 5% of such individuals report an illness consistent with hepatitis. In one study, 20% of randomly selected asymptomatic urban adolescents had evidence of previous HAV infection, none of whom gave a past history of clinical hepatitis.

The exact method by which HAV gets from the intestine of infected individuals to the liver is unclear. The incubation period for HAV is 2 to 4 weeks. The HAV is cytotoxic to hepatocytes, with virus being shed into the blood as well as bile. Fecal shedding of virus antedates even prodromal symptoms, although peak shedding occurs during the clinical procedure. The severity of illness and the ensuing cellular destruction seem to depend on the intensity of viral replication. Most infections are anicteric and self-limited. Fecal viral shedding may continue for up to 14 days after appearance of jaundice or dark urine. There is no chronic fecal shedding.

Hepatitis B

HBV is a complex double-shelled DNA virus that has two antigenic components: a core component designated HBcAg and an outer surface component designated HBsAg. The component HBsAg is actually an outer protein envelope manufactured in excess to the core in the cytoplasm of infected hepatocytes. In addition, this unique virus contains a third antigenic component, HBeAg, that appears to be a reliable serologic index of HBV infectivity. Unlike HAV, HBV has an enormous human reservoir because acute infection may lead to a chronic viral carrier state in 5% to 10% of cases. Epidemiologic studies in the United States put the carrier rate in the general population at 0.1% to 0.5%.

Person-to-person spread is the most common, from the blood of carriers. While evidence of HBV virus has been found in all body secretions except feces and urine, a number of studies have shown that the virus is not infectious by the oral, nasal, or respiratory route. Most pediatric cases are acquired through close, intimate contact with an infectious individual by so-called inapparent parenteral spread, involving passage of virus through slight or insignificant breaks in the skin or mucous membrane barrier.

The incubation period for HBV may be as short as 6 days or as long as 6 months depending on the inoculum and the route of infection. Unlike HAV, replication and synthetic activity of HBV takes place with minimal or no cytopathogenic impact upon the hepatocytes. The hepatocellular injury is dependent on the nature and extent of the host's cell-mediated immune response to the HBV infection. In addition, evidence of immune complex disease with extrahepatic manifestations indistinguishable from serum sickness may be part of the prodrome in 5% to 10% of symptomatic HBV infections. Yet, as with HAV, the most frequent response to HBV exposure is an anicteric, asymptomatic, or self-limited infection. Development of a carrier state does not seem to be related to disease severity. For unknown reasons, infection seems to be ineffectively eliminated and persists without hepatocyte damage, or with histologic evidence of chronic persistent or chronic aggressive hepatitis.

Non-A, Non-B Hepatitis

Non-A, non-B is a cumbersome term that is used to identify a patient population that exhibits symptoms of viral hepatitis but who lack serologic markers for HAV and HBV, as well as other infectious agents known to produce a hepatitis-like illness. It is not known whether non-A, non-B represents only one or multiple infectious agents. Non-A, non-B shares many epidemiologic features of HBV and also is thought to be spread by the parenteral route. Non-A, non-B, the most common cause of post-transfusion hepatitis, accounts for well over 90% of cases. Acute infection is generally mild, but non-A, non-B has a disturbing tendency to progress to a chronic stage, perhaps even more frequently than HBV.

Delta Hepatitis Virus

Recently a new virus, the delta hepatitis virus (delta agent), has been described that seems to require the helper function of HBV to support its replication and expression. The delta agent has been described as a defective RNA viral genome that is dependent on HBsAg synthesis for its assembly, and thus can only infect patients with acute or chronic HBV infection. Some authorities believe that delta agent superinfection in patients with HBV may contribute to development of aggressive chronic active hepatitis or even fulminant hepatitis. Much remains to be learned about this newly discovered agent that can now only be diagnosed by detection of delta antigen by immunofluorescence of liver biopsy material.

DATA GATHERING

Symptoms

Most childhood cases of acute hepatitis produce minimal symptoms, are anicteric, and are usually confused with a gastrointestinal flu-like illness, particularly in the young child less than 10 years old. Symptoms of HAV and HBV overlap and are nonspecific. Today, with the availability of serologic markers, the concept of short-incubation (HAV) vs. long-incubation (HBV) hepatitis is not as important. Classically, clinical hepatitis consists of a prodrome of constitutional symptoms, followed by the acute onset of an icteric phase and then recovery. The prodrome consists of 5 to 7 days of low-grade fever, malaise, and easy fatigability, anorexia, nausea, vomiting, and epigastric or right upper quadrant abdominal pain. Pruritus and diarrhea are rare. Physical examination at this time may reveal tender hepatomegaly and occasional splenomegaly. The HBV may present with an atypical prodrome consisting of extrahepatic manifestations associated with immune complex disease such as rash, arthralgia, and arthritis. The rash is usually a papular acrodermatitis on the face, buttocks, and extensor surfaces of the arms and legs. When such a rash is associated with lymphadenitis and fever, it is termed the Gianotti-Crosti syndrome.

The icteric phase of viral hepatitis is characterized by the sudden onset of scleral icterus, jaundice, and passage of dark urine and light stools. In this stage, one finds tender hepatomegaly in all patients and splenomegaly in 10% to 15%. Although jaundice and laboratory parameters may increase for several days, the patient feels better. This divergence is classic for acute hepatitis and most often infers a good prognosis.

Differential Diagnosis

Agents capable of producing a viral hepatitis-like illness include Epstein-Barr virus (EBV; infectious mononucleosis), cytomegalovirus (CMV), herpesvirus, adenovirus, coxsackievirus, rheovirus, echovirus, rubella, arbovirus, leptospirosis, toxoplasmosis, and tuberculosis. Characteristically, these agents produce a predominantly systemic illness with multiorgan involvement. The illnesses caused by EBV and CMV most commonly mimic viral hepatitis. Both rarely produce jaundice, and high fever and diffuse adenopathy are more characteristic.

In teenage girls, *Neisseria gonorrhoeae* perihepatitis (Fitz-Hugh–Curtis syndrome) may occur as an extension of pelvic inflammatory disease. Symptoms and signs include fever, right upper quadrant abdominal pain, jaundice, and elevated levels of transaminases. Pelvic findings of acute salpingitis are present in most cases as well as a history of dysmenorrhea, menorrhagia, or vaginal discharge. Cervical culture may be negative in 15% to 20% of cases. *Chlamydia trachomatis* may also be a causative agent in Fitz-Hugh–Curtis syndrome.

Wilson disease is a treatable metabolic disorder of copper metabolism that may present with signs and symptoms indistinguishable from acute hepatitis.

All patients with suspected acute hepatitis should be questioned regarding recent medications ingested and environmental toxin exposure.

Diagnosis of Acute Hepatitis

Since most cases of acute hepatitis are mild, presenting only with nonspecific symptoms, it is important to perform a careful abdominal examination in all patients with viral prodromes, as tender hepatomegaly is often the only sign that suggests the correct diagnosis. A history of exposure to hepatitis is uncommon in the young child, more common in the adolescent. Obviously, knowledge of a recent outbreak of hepatitis in a patient's environment is most helpful.

General Laboratory Tests to Diagnose Acute Hepatitis

Biochemical laboratory tests in cases of suspected acute viral hepatitis include determination of serum transaminase values (aspartate aminotransferase [AST, SGOT] and alanine aminotransferase [ALT, SGPT]); alkaline phosphatase; bilirubin, direct and indirect; CBC count; PT; total protein, albumin, globulin; electrolytes, BUN, glucose; and ceruloplasmin (if no exposure to hepatitis).

In practice, this involves obtaining an automated CBC count and SMA-12 or Chemzyme screen analysis. The most sensitive indicators of ongoing hepatocellular injury are the serum transaminases, AST and ALT. At best, only a rough correlation exists between the structural alterations associated with hepatitis and the corresponding increase in values for transaminases. The absolute levels are not important, except when they exceed 3,000 U/L. Alkaline phosphatase level is usually normal or slightly increased. If levels are greater than two times the upper limit of normal for age, one should suspect either biliary tract disease, or EBV or CMV hepatitis. Direct-reacting hyperbilirubinemia (direct fraction greater than 30% of total) generally peaks 5 to 7 days after onset of jaundice. Hyperbilirubinemia may be present in the absence of scleral icterus or jaundice, as these signs usually cannot be appreciated until levels exceed 3 to 4 mg/dL. As with transaminases, the absolute level of serum bilirubin is unimportant unless it exceeds 20 mg/dL. Hemoglobin (Hb) level is usually normal. If Hb is decreased, consider G-6-PD deficiency, Wilson disease, or Coombs-positive anemia associated with chronic liver disease. The WBC count is also usually normal or slightly decreased, such that leukocytosis with WBC count greater than 25,000/mm^3 is considered a poor prognostic sign. An increased number of atypical lymphocytes may be noted in viral hepatitis as well as in infectious hepatitis. Prothrombin time is also normal in 95% of cases. Elevation of PT does correlate with disease severity and poor prognosis, especially if level does not correct following intramuscular (IM) injection of vitamin K. Total protein, albumin, and globulin levels are normal in acute hepatitis. Decreased albumin or increased globulin levels should suggest an acute flare of chronic liver disease. Baseline electrolytes and BUN are important because dehydration is one of the more common complications of anorexia and vomiting. Hypoglycemia is a major complication of severe hepatitis. Even in mild cases, levels of blood glucose in the range of 60 mg/dL are not uncommon and should not be cause for concern without other abnormal prognostic indicators.

Serum ceruloplasmin level as a screening test for Wilson disease should be drawn in all patients over 5 years of age with suspected hepatitis in whom a history of known exposure is lacking.

Serologic Diagnosis of Acute Hepatitis

Figures 60–2 and 60–3 contrast the sequence of clinical, serum biochemical, and serologic events in typical HAV and HBV infection. The serodiagnosis of acute hepatitis is best approached by testing first for anti-HAV IgM, HBsAg, and a Mono-spot or EBV serologic analysis. All these tests are now commercially available. The finding of serum IgM anti-HAV is diagnostic of HAV. The antibody is first present

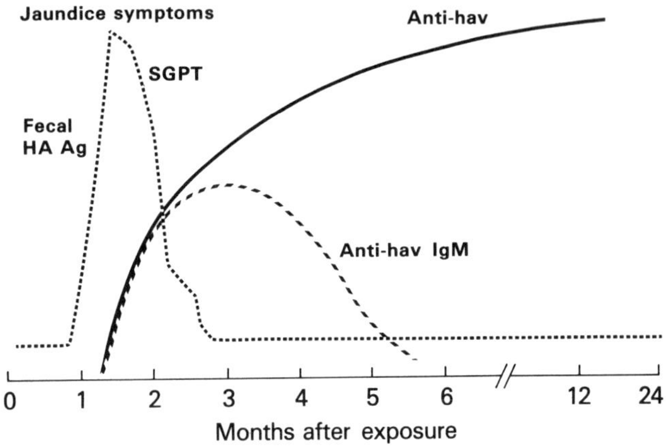

FIG 60–2
Time course of clinical, biochemical, and serologic events in typical case of acute type A hepatitis.

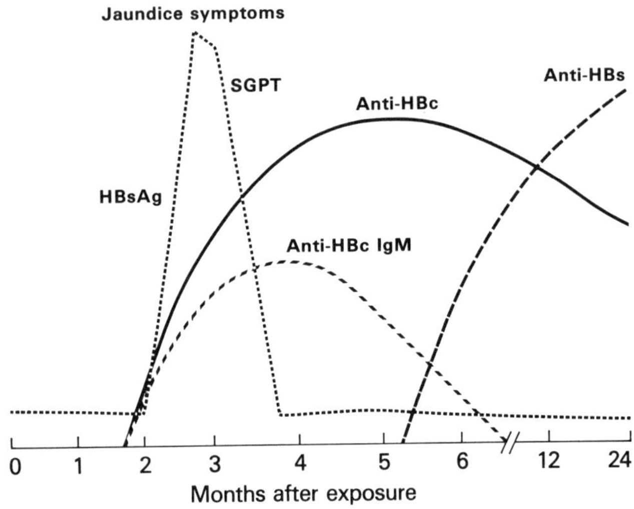

FIG 60–3
Time course of clinical, biochemical, and serologic events in typical case of acute type B hepatitis.

at the time of clinical symptoms. The component HBsAg, however, appears in the serum before the onset of clinical disease. A positive finding of HBsAg suggests the diagnosis of HBV in a symptomatic patient, but a negative finding does not rule it out, as HBsAg may rapidly be cleared from the serum within 1 week of onset of symptoms. If there is a strong suspicion, testing for anti-HBc (anti-HBcAg) is indicated to further exclude HBV, particularly if the disease is detected late. There are no specific tests for non-A, non-B hepatitis and ultimately this becomes a diagnosis of exclusion, particularly in patients with recent blood transfusion.

MANAGEMENT

Management of Acute Viral Hepatitis

There is no specific treatment for acute viral hepatitis. γ-Globulin has no influence on the course of the disease once symptoms occur. Today, the vast majority of patients can be treated at home. Traditionally, a low-fat, high-carbohydrate diet and bed rest have been recommended. Both are probably unnecessary, as neither influences the duration of the disease. Parents should be told to expect that their child's appetite will be poor. Small frequent feedings may be helpful. Ambulation and activity around the home should be allowed as tolerated. Drugs should be strictly avoided. The key for both the patient and household contacts is personal hygiene. Infants and small children should avoid contact with the infected child even after they have received immunoprophylaxis. Since shedding of virus may occur for up to 2 weeks after onset of jaundice, patients should be kept home and out of school for this time. After this, they may resume normal activity as tolerated, even if low-grade jaundice persists. Education of school authorities regarding such patients may be an important function of the primary care physician.

The indications for hospitalization of the patient with acute hepatitis are as follows:

1. Dehydration secondary to anorexia and vomiting.
2. Bilirubin level >20 mg/dL.
3. Abnormal prothrombin time.
4. WBC count >25,000/mm^3.
5. Level of transaminases >3,000 U/L.

Basically, hospitalization is required for dehydration, the most common complication of hepatitis, or for observation because of the presence of one or more of the factors considered to imply increased risk for fulminant hepatitis. The physician should also consider hospitalization for any patient for whom there is concern regarding poor home environment. While patients with acute hepatitis who are hospitalized should be isolated, it is not necessary for health care personnel to wear gowns, gloves, and masks when caring for these patients. Personal hygiene is essential.

Management of Fulminant Hepatitis

Fulminant hepatitis is a rare, catastrophic complication of viral hepatitis for which there is no specific therapy. Because a specific viral etiology is found in only 10% to 30% of patients, most cases are presumed to be non-A, non-B. Fulminant hepatitis is extremely rare following HAV. Two modes of presentation are seen. In the first, the child develops clinical hepatitis, but instead of improving, jaundice deepens, the level of transaminases starts to fall while the liver begins to shrink, the PT elongates, and progressive neurologic symptoms become apparent. In the second, a child manifesting a typical benign course of hepatitis suddenly relapses at a time when jaundice is decreasing. A course similar to the first mode of presentation then occurs. Fever, abdominal pain, and vomiting most often recur during the relapse.

At best, there is only a 20% survival from fulminant hepatitis. Prognosis is definitely related to level of intensive care management. These patients often develop significant cerebral edema and require intracranial pressure monitoring. Patients who have poor prognostic biochemical indicators and whose conditions continue to deteriorate clinically should be transferred to a pediatric tertiary care center equipped to provide the level of intensive care they require. Blood glucose level must be carefully monitored in such patients during transport.

Course and Follow-up of Acute Hepatitis

The jaundice of viral hepatitis gradually clears over 2 to 4 weeks. It may be 1 to 3 months before levels of transaminases return to normal. It is not unusual for a mild, short-lived relapse of both clinical symptoms and slight jaundice to occur in 10% to 15% of patients 8 to 12 weeks after the acute illness. This phenomenon has been called relapsing hepatitis and usually resolves in 2 to 3 weeks. Rarely, some patients develop a significant cholestatic form of acute hepatitis associated with high levels of direct-reacting hyperbilirubinemia and increased levels of alkaline phosphatase and cholesterol. Such patients usually complain of pruritus. Because of the concern of an extrahepatic biliary tract disorder in such patients, it is wise to perform an ultrasound to examine the gallbladder and bile ducts.

Because HAV infection does not lead to a chronic carrier state or chronic hepatitis, a patient who is positive for anti-HAV IgM can just be followed-up clinically without biochemical studies. Patients with HBV or non-A, non-B should have biweekly physical examination, as well as a check of serum bilirubin and either SGOT or SGPT (no apparent reason to measure both transaminases) until these parameters either return to normal or by continued abnormality fit the time criteria for a diagnosis of chronic hepatitis.

Chronic Type B Hepatitis

In patients with HBV, HBsAg should also be checked monthly. Persistence of HBsAg for 8 to 10 weeks indicates that the patient will probably not resolve the viral infection rapidly but will become a chronic carrier. Approximately 5% to 10% of adults with acute HBV become chronic carriers. The number is considerably greater in neonates infected by transmission from their mothers. Most chronic carriers are asymptomatic or have symptoms of mild fatigability or right upper quadrant pressure tenderness that can last 3 to 10 years. In the majority of individuals, levels of transaminases gradually fall to normal or near normal. Low-grade inflammation may lead to cirrhosis in some patients and a small percentage will die from liver failure. All chronic carriers should be followed up on a quarterly basis to determine infectivity status (positive HBeAg) and possible seroconversion to anti-HBe. In the latter case these individuals most likely will not develop severe chronic liver disease.

One of the major dilemmas for the primary care physician is the infectivity of HBsAg carriers. There has been one study that has demonstrated that classroom contact may at times be sufficient to allow for so-called inapparent parenteral spread of HBV. Chronic HBeAg-positive infants should not be placed in daycare centers or nursery schools, although school attendance in grade school should be allowed with precautions to maximize personal hygiene as best as possible. The dilemma of infectivity of HBV underscores the need to prevent this infection.

Chronic Hepatitis

Chronic hepatitis should be suspected in a patient who presents with (1) signs and symptoms of acute hepatitis but has markers of chronic illness such as decreased level of albumin or increased level of globulin, or (2) a patient with acute hepatitis who continues to have persistent hyperbilirubinemia or transaminemia with or without clinical symptoms for 6 to 8 weeks following initial presentation. The etiology is unknown but probably involves the host's immune response to hepatocellular injury. Clinical features include persistent jaundice, relapsing jaundice, extrahepatic complaints such as fever, arthritis, rash (particularly erythema nodosum), colitis, and, rarely, advanced features of liver failure including ascites and encephalopathy. Evidence of autoantibodies, particularly antinuclear antibodies (ANA) and anti-smooth muscle antibodies, is found in 60% of patients. Patients who fulfill the two criteria given above should be referred to a pediatric gastroenterologist for further evaluation. A diagnosis of chronic active hepatitis requires liver biopsy. The HBsAg-negative chronic active hepatitis is responsive to steroid therapy.

PREVENTION OF VIRAL HEPATITIS BY IMMUNOPROPHYLAXIS

Prevention of the spread of viral hepatitis should be one of the primary goals of the primary care physician.

Hepatitis A

Conventional immune serum globulin (ISG) confers passive protection against clinical HAV infection if given during the incubation period up until 6 days before onset of disease. In fact, 75% of those individuals receiving a dose of 0.02 mL/kg IM develop evidence of passive-active immunity with anti-HAV IgM. Postexposure immunoprophylaxis is suggested for (1) household contacts and close personal contacts, (2) institutionalized contacts, and (3) contacts within a daycare center. Contacts of an isolated case within a grade school classroom and routine play contacts do not require ISG. However, a second case within a class warrants immunoprophylaxis of the rest of the class. Immune serum globulin is protective for as long as 6 months. One potential method of determining who should receive ISG is to test susceptible contacts for anti-HAV IgG and to give ISG only to those who are negative. Preexposure prophylaxis is required for individuals traveling to areas where HAV is endemic. The dose is 0.02 mL/kg IM. If the stay is to be longer than 3 months, 0.06 mL/kg should be given every 4 to 6 months.

Hepatitis B

Postexposure immunoprophylaxis for HBV is recommended only for needle exposure, sexual contacts, and infants with an increased risk of neonatal hepatitis B. The best serologic marker for detecting susceptible contacts is anti-HBc. This antibody will detect individuals who have had both recent and past infection (Fig 60–3). Susceptible contacts with negative anti-HBc should receive HBV-hyperimmune γ-globulin (HBIG) in a dose of 0.06 mL/kg as soon after exposure as possible, and again 30 days after initial dose. Conventional immune serum globulin is not indicated for immunoprophylaxis of HBV. Today hepatitis B vaccine, prepared from formalin-inactivated highly purified HBsAg particles, is indicated as an adjunct to HBIG in high-risk susceptible contacts. Vaccination requires three IM doses (1.0 mL if the child is more than 10 years of age; 0.5 mL if less than 10 years); an initial dose, and boosters 1 month and 6 months later. Vaccination results in a high titer anti-HBS response in 95% of recipients. The vaccine has been found to be extremely safe, with soreness at the injection site being the major side effect.

Non-A, Non-B Hepatitis

Although there are no data regarding its effectiveness, conventional ISG (0.06 mL/kg) can be given to needle-stick or sexual contacts of patients with acute non-A, non-B hepatitis.

NEONATAL HEPATITIS B

Infants born to mothers who have had acute HBV infection during the third trimester, or chronic carriers of HBV (particularly HBeAg-positive carriers) are at risk to develop neonatal hepatitis B. In the United States where the carrier rate is less than 1%, neonatal acquisition of HBV from carrier mothers is said to be 5% to 10%. In contrast, in the Far East, where 40% to 50% of mothers are carriers, neonatal acquisition is close to 95%. Thus, it seems that the causes of acquisition are multifactorial. Infection seems to occur at birth by ingestion of virus from amniotic fluid, vaginal secretions, or placental or uterine blood, or through postpartum exposure by close contact, or via breast-feeding. Transplacental spread, if it occurs, is rare. The component HBsAg usually is first noted when the infant is 6 to 8 weeks of age. Neonatal HBV is usually an asymptomatic illness. However, a high percentage of the infants, particularly boys, become chronic carriers because of an ineffective immune response. The length of the carrier state is unknown. However, because of the dilemma of infectivity of such infants and children, prevention of neonatal HBV is essential. Whether all pregnant women in the United States should be routinely tested for HbsAg is debatable. The expected yield of one to five cases per 1,000 tests is higher than that seen in serologic monitoring for syphilis; however, HBsAg testing is much more expensive. For the present, HBsAg testing in pregnancy is recommended for the following high-risk patients: (1) refugees from the Far East or Africa, (2) patients with a history of acute or chronic hepatitis or those who have a household for sexual contact with such an individual, (3) patients with occupational exposure to blood, and (4) illicit drug users.

Infants at risk should receive hyperimmune HBV globulin (HBIG) 0.5 mL IM when in the delivery room, or not later than 48 hours postpartum. No special nursery precautions are indicated because at this point, the infant is not infective, although the carrier mother is infective. Mothers who are HBeAg-positive probably should avoid breast feeding. The initial dose of three HBV vaccine doses (0.5 mL) should be given in the first 24 hours of life and again at 1 month and 6 months of age. Because these infants with carrier mothers will have continued exposure, serologic evaluation when they are 1 year of age should include anti-HBc and anti-HBs. If both are positive, passive-active immunity has occurred and the infant probably has lifelong immunity. If anti-HBs titer alone is positive, it is probably the result of vaccination and the infant should be followed up yearly with anti-HBs titer until further experience with the vaccine determines that no further booster will be required.

BIBLIOGRAPHY

Chin J: Prevention of chronic hepatitis B infection from mother to infants in the United States. *Pediatrics* 1983; 71:289.

Dienstag JL: Non-A, non-B Hepatitis: I. Recognition, epidemiology, and clinical features. *Gastroenterology* 1983; 85:439.

Jacobson IM, Dienstag JL: The delta hepatitis agent: Viral hepatitis, type D. *Gastroenterology* 1984; 86:1614.

Koff RS: *Viral hepatitis*. New York, John Wiley & Sons, 1978.

Krugman S: The newly licensed hepatitis B vaccine: Characteristics and indications for use. *JAMA* 1982; 247:2012.

Roy CC, Silverman A, Cozzetto FJ: Acute liver disease, in Silverman A, Roy CC (eds): *Pediatric Clinical Gastroenterology*, ed 2. St Louis, CV Mosby Co, 1983, p 576.

Roy CC, Silverman A, Cozzetto FJ: Chronic liver disease, in Silverman A, Roy CC (eds): *Pediatric Clinical Gastroenterology*, ed 2. St Louis, CV Mosby Co, 1983, p 675.

Schafer DF, Hoofnagle JH: Serological diagnosis of viral hepatitis. *Viewpoints Dig Dis* 1982; 14:5.

Seeff LB, Hoofnagle JH: Immunoprophylaxis of viral hepatitis. *Gastroenterology* 1982; 77:161.

Tabor E, Jones R, Gerety RJ, et al: Asymptomatic viral hepatitis Types A and B in an adolescent population. *Pediatrics* 1978; 62:1026–1030.

SEXUALLY TRANSMITTED DISEASES

Donald Schwarz, M.D.

In addition to the classic sexually transmitted diseases (gonorrhea, syphilis, chancroid, lymphogranuloma venereum, granuloma inguinale), more recently described entities with newly understood frequency include genital papillomas, herpes, candidiasis, nonspecific vaginitis, trichomoniasis, lice, scabies, hepatitis, and HIV-associated disease. These disease entities and their underlying pathogens are becoming increasingly recognized in pediatric practice.

Unlike other infectious diseases, these processes, which are spread through sexual contact, often carry with them both physical and important psychosocial problems. The clinician must be both comfortable with the physical diagnosis and management of the disease entity and sensitive to the associated social issues.

THE PREPUBERTAL CHILD

In the prepubertal child, a sexually transmitted disease must be considered a marker for sexual abuse until proven otherwise. The clinician must remain vigilant for signs and symptoms of child abuse.

In prepubertal girls, vaginitis may occasionally be caused by a sexually transmitted disease. Symptoms of vaginitis include odor, dysuria, frequency, and discomfort. Information from the history, physical examination, and laboratory evaluation help distinguish causes of vaginitis. Common causes of vaginitis that are not related to sexually transmitted diseases include foreign bodies (frequently beads, small toys, or retained tissue; often associated with a particularly foul odor), pinworms, scabies, varicella lesions, streptococcal or staphylococcal disease, and irritative vaginitis (caused by reaction to powders, creams, bubble bath, or poor hygiene). *Gardnerella* vaginitis or *Candida* vaginitis may be acquired through venereal or nonvenereal contact. Further investigation is needed in these cases. Papillomas, trichomonal, herpes simplex, gonococcal, or chlamydial disease must carry a high suspicion for sexual transmission. Infectious causes of vaginitis require appropriate antibiotic treatment.

Any pharyngeal or anal infection with a pathogen that is sexually transmitted (including *Gonococcus, Chlamydia,* herpesvirus, syphilis, or human papillomavirus) must be assumed to be secondary to abuse. In young children with anal symptoms in particular, a directed history and careful physical examination are essential. Diagnostic testing for *Neisseria gonorrhoeae, Chlamydia trachomatis, Treponema pallidum,* and herpes simplex virus should be performed.

Pelvic inflammatory disease (PID), presenting with lower abdominal pain, while reported in young girls, is exceedingly rare. All other causes of abdominal pain must be ruled out before PID is assumed to be present. In cases of lice, scabies, or papillomas of the genital area, the clinician should be careful to inquire about sleeping patterns and shared use of clothing and towels.

For nonvenereal causes of vaginitis, sitz baths and local irrigation with saline solution usually suffice. Occasionally systemic antibiotics are required (for streptococcal infections).

ADOLESCENT WOMEN

Routine screening for sexually transmitted diseases should be performed on all adolescent women who are sexually active, those who are pregnant, those being evaluated for sexual abuse, rape, or incest, and those with a history of sexual activity in the past. In addition, the differential diagnosis for recurrent urinary tract infection should include sexually transmitted disease. Screening tests should be performed at least annually in women who are sexually active; and in women who have multiple sexual partners, an examination should be performed at least every 6 months.

Diagnosis

An evaluation of a patient for a sexually transmitted disease begins with a sexual history. This history should review the age of onset of menses and last menstrual period, pregnancy history, history of previous sexually transmitted diseases, recent use of antibiotics, time of last pelvic examination, symptoms since last examination, number and frequency of partners and their symptoms, and use of contraceptives. Any history of lesions of the genitalia, pain on intercourse, vaginal discharge, pruritis, unexplained rash, joint complaints, urinary discomfort, or infection in a partner should raise the question of a sexually transmitted disease.

After obtaining a history, a complete physical examination is done. Particular attention should be paid to unexplained fever, rash, mucous membrane findings, new murmurs, abdominal symptoms, joint findings, and lesions around the anus. A complete pelvic examination should be performed.

Ulcerating Lesions

The pelvic examination should begin with inspection of the external genitalia. An ulcerating lesion anywhere in the genital area should be considered secondary to syphilis until proven otherwise (see below). The classic chancre of syphilis is a nonpainful, indurated, usually single ulcer of several millimeters to slightly over a centimeter in size. It is usually accompanied by firm, nonfluctuant, painless local lymph nodes. It is highly infectious. The chancre of syphilis must be differentiated from the usually multiple and smaller ulcerative lesions of herpes simplex disease. These lesions are frequently clustered and confluent. Herpes may also present with clustered vesicles. These lesions are usually painful, may be pruritic, and progress from vesicle to ulcers to crusted lesions over a number of days. They frequently leave hyper- or hypopigmented areas after the acute lesions have healed (see below).

A third cause of an ulcerative lesion is chancroid. Chancroid is the result of infection with *Hemophilus ducreyi* (a gram-negative bacillus). Chancroid is an acute, localized infection that presents with single or multiple papules which progress to painful necrotizing ulcers at the site of infection. Regional adenopathy with painful suppurative lymph nodes is also frequently present. Extragenital lesions do occur. Diagnosis of chancroid is made by culture from the ulcer, or from pus from a suppurating lymph node. Chancroid is treated with ceftriaxone, 250 mg IM for one dose, or trimethoprim/sulfamethoxazole, one double-strength tablet (80 mg trimethoprim and 400 mg sulfamethoxazole) twice a day for 7 days.

Granuloma inguinale is caused by *Calymmatobacterium granulomatis*, which causes subcutaneous nodules, vesicles, or papules in the genital area that extend and often ulcerate. The lesions are quite destructive and may be associated with squamous cell carcinoma. Diagnosis is made by punch biopsy or by giemsa stain of granulation tissue taken directly from lesions. Granuloma inguinale is treated with doxycycline 100 mg twice daily for 21 days.

Rash

External erythemetous rash around the genital area which may be accompanied by discharge can be caused by candidal infection. Generalized disorders in which genital lesions may occur include erythema multiforme, varicella, aphthous ulcerations of Behçet disease or Crohn disease, and Kawasaki syndrome. A crusted pruritic rash in the genital area may be caused by scabies. Scabitic lesions of the genital area resemble those on other parts of the body with a classic linear pattern. Scabies should be treated with lindane or a preparation of pyrethins and piperonyl butoxide. Erythemetous, intensely pruritic areas within the pubic hair may be the result of lice infestation (*Pediculosis pubis*). Treatment should be a lindane preparation (Kwell, Scabene) or pyrethins with piperonyl butoxide.

The rash of secondary syphilis may be generalized and accompanied by mild constitutional symptoms. It is described in detail below.

Other Lesions

Inspection of the genital area is not complete without examining the introitus for abscesses of Bartholin glands. Bartholin gland abscesses are caused in the great majority of cases by *N. gonorrhoeae*. Treatment is not complete without incision and drainage of the lesions.

Classic wart-like lesions around the genital area are caused by either human papillomavirus (venereal warts) or *T. pallidum* (condyloma lata of syphilis). The two lesions may occasionally be differentiated by the drier, more cornified appearance of common papillomavirus lesions. Condyloma lata are classically moist with a broad base. They are extremely infectious. Definitive diagnosis requires syphilis serologic testing.

Molluscum contagiosum may be transmitted through any intimate contact. Between one and twenty white, translucent, or flesh-colored lesions that are 3 to 7 mm in diameter with central umbilication may be present. They may be accompanied by pruritis or mild irritation. Biopsy is diagnostic.

Adenopathy

After genital inspection, the inguinal lymph nodes are palpated. Diseases that frequently cause regional inguinal adenopathy include syphilis, candida, chancroid, lymphogranuloma venereum, and granuloma inguinale. Lymphogranuloma venereum (LGV) is caused by *Chlamydia trachomatis* types L-1, L-2, or L-3. It is a systemic lymphatic infection beginning often with small, painless, papular or nodular lesions at the portal of entry. This is followed by subacute regional lymphadenitis. Other symptoms include chills, fever, headache, abdominal and joint pain, and anorexia. Diagnosis is made by culture from lymph node drainage or serum complement fixation tests. LGV is treated with doxycycline 100 mg orally twice daily for 21 days or until lymphadenopathy has resolved.

Internal Examination

After completing inspection and palpation of inguinal lymph nodes, an internal examination is performed with a speculum lubricated only with warm water. On speculum examination, if discharge is present a sample should be taken for wet preparation with saline solution and with 10% solution of potassium hydroxide. The characteristics of the discharge and the presence or absence of vaginitis, foreign body, and any evidence of vaginal trauma including abrasion and focal vaginitis should be noted. The cervix should be inspected for its transition zone, and any lesions noted. Table 60–11 provides a differential diagnosis of vaginal discharge.

Vaginitis

Herpes simplex vaginitis classically gives a thin, copious, non-foul-smelling discharge. It may be associated with inguinal adenopathy, pruritis, dysuria, labial edema, and pain on intercourse. Diagnosis is made by culture with special viral medium or Tzanck preparation (Wright staining of smears from lesions which reveal multinucleated giant cells and cytoplasmic vacuoles). Serologic tests for herpes simplex virus antibodies are confirmatory but not diagnostic. Treatment is with acyclovir 200 mg orally five times per day for 10 days for initial attacks and for 5 days for recurrence. Suppressive therapy is discussed below.

The discharge associated with *Trichomonas vaginalis* infection is typically thick, frothy, copious, yellow-green, and foul smelling. It is associated with vaginitis and classically causes a strawberry cervix (areas of punctate hemorrhage). Diagnosis of *Trichomonas* is made either by direct visualization of motile organisms on wet preparation with saline (75% sensitive), Papanicolaou smear (80% sensitive), or culture (85% sensitive). Appropriate treatment for *Trichomonas* vaginititis is with metronidazole either 2 g given once by mouth or 500 mg by mouth twice daily for a week.

Gardnerella vaginalis infection leads to a thick, copious, foul-smelling, white-yellow discharge. It is associated with pruritis and vaginitis, and is frequently found in women with *Trichomonas* infection. Diagnosis is made by wet preparation in which clue cells are seen. These cells are large epithelial cells covered with small, hairlike bacteria. The "whiff test" (application of 10% potassium hydroxide to a sample of vaginal pool discharge yields a fishy smell from amines produced by *Gardnerella* bacteria) is quite specific but not highly sensitive. Cul-

TABLE 60–11
Differential Diagnosis of Vaginal Discharge

ORGANISM	DISCHARGE	DIAGNOSIS	TREATMENT
Herpes	Thin, copious not foul smelling	Culture (special medium)	Acyclovir, oral or topical
Trichomonas	Thick, copious, yellow-green, foul smelling	Wet prep (75% sensitivity), Papanicolaou smear (80% sensitivity), culture (85% sensitivity)	Metronidazole 2 g PO × 1
Gardnerella	Slightly thick, copious, foul smelling, white-yellow	Wet prep: clue cells. 10% KOH: whiff test. Culture: send swab.	Metronidazole 500 mg PO BID for 7 days
Candida	Cottage cheese–like	10% KOH (heat), culture: send swab	Clotrimazole 100 mg intravaginally. Miconazole 2% cream or nystatin cream or tablets
Chlamydia	Any discharge	Culture (special medium) and monoclonal antibodies (rapid-slide). Gram stain (look for 10 or more WBC/hpf).	Doxycycline 100 mg PO BID for 7–10 days
Gonococcus	Any discharge	Culture (both Martin-Lewis and chocolate agar).	Ceftriaxone 250 mg IM

REMEMBER: Treat both *Gonococcus* and *Chlamydia* in symptomatic women.

ture of the vaginal pool will also lead to diagnosis of *Gardnerella*. *Gardnerella* vaginitis is treated with metronidazole 500 mg orally twice daily for 7 days.

Candida albicans (monilial) vaginitis, often associated with intense pruritis, produces a cottage cheese–like discharge. Predisposing factors to monilial infection include diabetes mellitus, pregnancy, use of broad-spectrum antibiotics, and oral contraceptive use. Diagnosis is made by applying a 10% solution of potassium hydroxide to a sample of the vaginal pool on a slide and then heating gently. Filamentous hyphae and budding yeast forms may be seen when potassium hydroxide dissolves cell walls. *Candida* forms are occasionally seen on Gram stain as well. *Candida* can be cultured in many laboratories. Simple transport medium is required. Treatments for *Candida* vaginitis include clotrimazole 100 mg applied intravaginally at bedtime for 1 week or miconazole 100 mg intravaginally at bedtime for 1 week or 200 mg for 3 days. They are equally effective.

Of note, partners of patients with *Trichomonas* vaginitis must be treated to prevent reinfection in women with vaginitis. No treatment is necessary, though, for partners of patients with *Gardnerella*- or *Candida*-induced vaginitis. These are never eradicated from the vaginal pool, and treatment of partners makes no difference to rates of recurrence.

Vaginal discharge in the absence of vaginitis should suggest chlamydial or gonococcal disease. *C. trachomatis* leads to a cervicitis with resulting discharge. Diagnosis is made by culture with special transport medium or with direct fluorescent antibody or monoclonal antibody testing. Chlamydial infection is treated with doxycycline 100 mg orally twice daily for 7 to 10 days.

N. gonorrhoeae also leads to cervicitis without vaginitis. Discharge may be creamy to green-white. Diagnosis is made by culture of endocervical discharge. To maximize the chances of a positive result on culture, pharynx and rectum should also be cultured for *N. gonorrhoeae* in symptomatic individuals. If culture is done, both a restrictive medium such as Martin-Lewis or Thayer-Martin medium *and* chocolate agar are preferrable, as about 10% of *N. gonorrhoeae* will not grow on restrictive media. Plates should be placed in a CO_2-enhanced environment. Transgrow, a modified restrictive medium, contains CO_2 and is suitable for transport for longer than 2 hours. Treatment in areas with low prevalence of penicillinase-producing gonorrheal organisms can be with amoxicillin 3 g orally once, taken 30 minutes after 1 g of probenicid. If penicillinase-producing organisms are prevalent, recommended treatment is ceftriaxone, 250 mg intramuscularly, given once. Alternatively in penicillin-allergic patients, spectinomycin 2 g intramuscularly given once can be used. Ceftriaxone will also eradicate rectal and pharyngeal disease.

To diagnose sexually transmitted diseases appropriately on pelvic examination, the following order should be used for collection of specimens: (1) samples of the vaginal pool for wet preparation and potassium hydroxide preparation; (2) vaginal culture for *Gardnerella, Candida,* and *Trichomonas* (if appropriate); (3) endocervical specimen for culture for *N. gonorrhoeae*, with a specimen plated on both restrictive and on chocolate agar; (4) a Papanicolaou smear (annually) in all sexually active adolescents; (5) a cervical specimen for *Chlamydia* testing. If available, *Chlamydia* culture is the most sensitive test for infection. It should be the screening test of choice. However, growth of *Chlamydia* in culture is inhibited by the presence of other organisms and pus. As a result, in some centers both *Chlamydia* culture and a rapid diagnostic procedure should be performed.

After completing speculum examination, bimanual examination is performed. Any tenderness on cervical motion, tenderness of the adnexa, or mass should be noted and appropriately handled. In young adolescents, tenderness of the cervix and adnexal structures may be confirmed, after regloving, through a rectal-bimanual examination.

Pelvic Inflammatory Disease

The presenting complaint in patients with PID may range from vague abdominal discomfort to florid signs and symptoms of acute abdomen.

In addition to the classic symptoms of abdominal pain, nausea, vomiting, and fever, the patient may have increased vaginal discharge, menorrhagia, metorrhagia, dysuria, urgency, or urinary frequency. Right upper quadrant pain, pleuritic in quality or referred to the right shoulder and back, suggests Fitz-Hugh–Curtis syndrome, a perihepatitis reported with both gonococcal and chlamydial infections. Physical examination may reveal a mildly to severely ill patient with abdominal or adnexal tenderness; signs of peritoneal inflammation are not uncommon. Adnexal fullness or an adnexal mass suggests tubo-ovarian abscess; right upper quadrant tenderness or an audible friction rub suggests Fitz-Hugh–Curtis syndrome.

Evaluation should focus primarily on excluding other causes of an acute abdomen that would necessitate prompt surgical intervention. In particular, acute appendicitis and ruptured ectopic pregnancy should be ruled out. Endometriosis or corpus luteum hemorrhage should be distinguished from PID. Fever and laboratory evidence of acute inflammation are not typically a feature of those two disorders.

Toxic shock syndrome, while quite uncommon, should be considered in any severely ill young woman who is menstruating, especially if she uses tampons. Fever, rash, and hypotension are the hallmarks of the disorder, and multisystem involvement is the rule. Abdominal pain, vomiting, and diarrhea are commonly seen.

In patients with symptoms suggestive of urinary tract infection, urinalysis and culture should be performed. In those with abdominal pain and right upper quadrant tenderness hepatitis secondary to hepatitis virus A or B or non-A, non-B, cytomegalovirus, and Epstein-Barr virus should be considered. Acute cholecystitis, perforated peptic ulcer, subphrenic or perinephric abscess, acute pyelonephritis, nephrolithiasis, and pneumonia (especially right lower lobe) should be ruled out. Fitz-Hugh–Curtis syndrome is a perihepatitis rather than a parenchymal disease, and for that reason liver function test results are usually normal. On cholecystography, the gallbladder may not be seen early, but subsequent studies will be normal. Like PID, Fitz-Hugh–Curtis syndrome is largely a clinical diagnosis.

In a toxic-appearing patient, particularly a patient in septic shock, the clinician should consider postabortal PID with organisms such as *Clostridium perfringens*.

Several laboratory tests have been used in the initial evaluation of patients suspected of having PID, but none is very sensitive or specific. Less than 25% of patients are estimated to have leukocytosis, and approximately 40% each are estimated to have mild or moderate elevation of erythrocyte sedimentation rate. Organisms isolated from patients with PID include: *N. gonorrhoeae, C. trachomatis,* and mixed anaerobic flora, thus initial therapy while awaiting culture results should include broad-spectrum antibiotics (see below). Endocervical, rectal, and pharyngeal cultures for gonococcus isolation should be performed. Cervical cultures or rapid diagnostic testing for *Chlamydia* should be obtained. Pregnancy testing should be performed for all patients with suspected or proved PID. US may be helpful in the evaluation of patients with adnexal fullness or mass to visualize the occasional tubo-ovarian abscess (TOA), a complication of PID. Gynecologic consultation should be obtained for patients with TOA.

The diagnosis of PID is often clinical and frequently unclear. As 15% of women have been shown to be infertile after only one episode of PID, the clinician who evaluates a sexually active adolescent woman with abdominal pain must have a high index of suspicion for PID. Treatment should be initiated as early as possible to reduce the risk of complications.

Patients with uncomplicated PID are often adequately treated as outpatients. Outpatient therapy includes doxycycline, 100 mg by mouth, twice a day for 10 days and ceftriaxone, 250 mg intramuscularly once. Ampicillin and penicillin treatment is not recommended because of the high rate of penicillinase-producing *N. gonorrhoeae* in the United States. For those patients treated in an ambulatory setting, reevaluation within 72 hours of initiation of therapy is essential. At that time, symptoms should have resolved and fever should have abated.

The Centers for Disease Control (CDC) recommend hospitalization for patients with PID in the following situations:

1. If the diagnosis is uncertain.
2. If a surgical emergency, particularly appendicitis and ectopic pregnancy, cannot be excluded.
3. If a pelvic abscess is suspected.
4. If severe illness precludes outpatient management.
5. If the patient is pregnant.
6. If the patient is unable to follow or tolerate an outpatient regimen.
7. If the patient fails to respond to outpatient therapy.
8. If clinical follow-up 48 to 72 hours following the initiation of antibiotic treatment cannot be arranged.

Not mentioned by the CDC, but routinely accepted in many centers, is the policy that all young adolescents (14 years of age and younger) with suspected PID should be hospitalized to assure adequate treatment and education.

Inpatient therapy for PID may include any of the following:

1. Doxycycline 100 mg IV bid and cefoxitin 2.0 g IV qid
2. Clindamycin 600 mg IV qid and gentamycin (or tobramycin) 2.0 mg/kg IV followed by 1.5 mg/kg IV qid
3. Doxycycline 100 mg IV bid and metronidazole 1.0 mg IV bid

ADOLESCENT MEN

All adolescent men who are sexually active, those suspected of being victims of sexual abuse, and those who have a history of previous sexual contact should be considered at risk for sexually transmitted diseases. For sexually active adolescent men, annual screening should be done and should include cultures for gonorrhea and *Chlamydia*, urinalysis, and a serologic test for syphilis.

The visit begins with a sexual history. In boys it is important to determine the time since the last physical examination, the number and frequency of sexual partners, any history of homosexual encounters, any symptoms since the last examination, any history of sexually transmitted diseases, any history of symptoms of disease in partners, recent use of antibiotics, and use of condoms. A complete physical examination should be performed to look for similar systemic symptoms as in adolescent women. The genitalia should be inspected for findings characteristic of syphilis, herpes, *Candida*, scabies, lice, papillomas, lymphogranuloma venereum, chancroid, and granuloma inguinale, as for women. In uncircumcised men, the foreskin must be retracted and inspected for lesions. Any penile discharge should be noted and appropriate cultures obtained.

The physical examination includes palpation of the scrotal contents for tenderness and stripping of the penis for discharge.

Urethritis

Discharge in men should be sent for routine culture for *N. gonorrhoeae*, and either culture or rapid diagnostic testing for *C. trachomatis*. An appropriate sample is obtained with either a swab or wire loop, and samples for *N. gonor-*

rhoeae should be plated on both restrictive medium and chocolate agar or on an appropriate transport medium. Gram staining of urethral discharge from men, when appropriately done, is 95% sensitive and 97% specific for *N. gonorrhoeae*. Culture is confirmatory. *Chlamydia* culture is 99% sensitive and specific in men. Indications of urethritis can be found with a screening urinalysis. If a spun urine specimen has greater than 10 WBCs per high power field, one can be 93% certain that infection is present.

It must be remembered that 45% of men with gonococcal urethritis will also carry *Chlamydia*. The presence of overgrowth of gonococcal organisms and pus inhibit the growth of *Chlamydia* in culture. In men with gonococcal urethritis, the clinician must remember to obtain pharyngeal and rectal cultures. Treatment for gonococcal disease is outlined above for women as is treatment for chlamydial infection. In men with urethritis resistant to these treatments, *Trichomonas* infections should be considered, especially if partners have symptoms of infection. Treatment with metronidazole should be given to men with unresponsive urethral symptoms.

Other less frequent causes of urethritis include herpes simplex disease (external lesions are usually present), urethral trauma, such as that caused by accidental insertion or self-insertion of catheters or other instruments (hematuria is frequently present), and Reiter syndrome (usual triad for Reiter syndrome includes urethritis, anterior uveitis or conjunctivitis, and arthritis of lower extremity large joints). In cases of urethritis resistant to antimicrobial therapy, the clinician should consider referral to a urologist for evaluation of urethral stricture, intraurethral ulceration, condyloma acuminatum, or foreign body not readily palpated. Urethrographic or urethroscopic study may be indicated. All men with urethritis should be examined for tenderness and inflammation of the prostate gland.

Epididymo-orchitis

Epididymo-orchitis may be caused by sexually transmitted organisms. It must be differentiated from surgical conditions such as torsion of the testis or appendix testis and incarcerated inguinal hernia. *N. gonorrhoeae, C. trachomatis,* infections, and rarely syphilis cause sexually transmitted epididymitis. Gonococcal infection and chlamydial disease will be diagnosed with cultures, rapid diagnostic, and Gram-stain techniques. Syphilis is diagnosed with serologic testing. Other causes of epididymitis include common pathogenic bacteria such as *Staphylococcus, Streptococcus,* or coliforms extending from a nearby genitourinary focus. Tuberculosis is a rare cause of epididymitis. A positive result of a urine culture in a patient with epididymitis should suggest an underlining genitourinary tract anomaly.

Orchitis is most frequently caused by mumps, Coxsackievirus, Echovirus, or Adenovirus and may be difficult to diagnose. Mumps orchitis is likely in the patient with a history of parotitis 4 to 6 days preceding testicular involvement. Serum amylase values may occasionally be elevated, but often they will have returned to normal by the time testicular swelling has developed.

Scrotum trauma and tortion of the testis, as well as incarcerated inguinal hernia, must always be considered when tenderness is found within the scrotal sac.

SPECIFIC DISEASE ENTITIES

Syphilis

After many years of decreasing frequency, the number of syphilis cases is again increasing. The reported number of cases of congenital syphilis increased by more than 21% in the United States in the second half of 1987.

The natural history of syphilis can be broken down into three stages. Primary syphilis occurs 3 to 4 weeks (range, 10 days to 10 weeks) after initial infection with *T. pallidum*. Primary syphilis is a local infection. Symptoms include large local lymph nodes (draining the portal of entry) and a chancre (non-painful ulcerating lesion at the portal of entry, which involutes 4 to 6 weeks after initial symptoms). A chancre is more commonly seen in men than in women.

Secondary syphilis, marked by rash and/or condyloma lata, occurs 3 weeks after the onset of primary symptoms or 6 weeks to 6 months into the course of the disease. Secondary syphilis is a systemic infection and may be accompanied by mild, generalized symptoms. Rash is a common symptom of secondary syphilis.

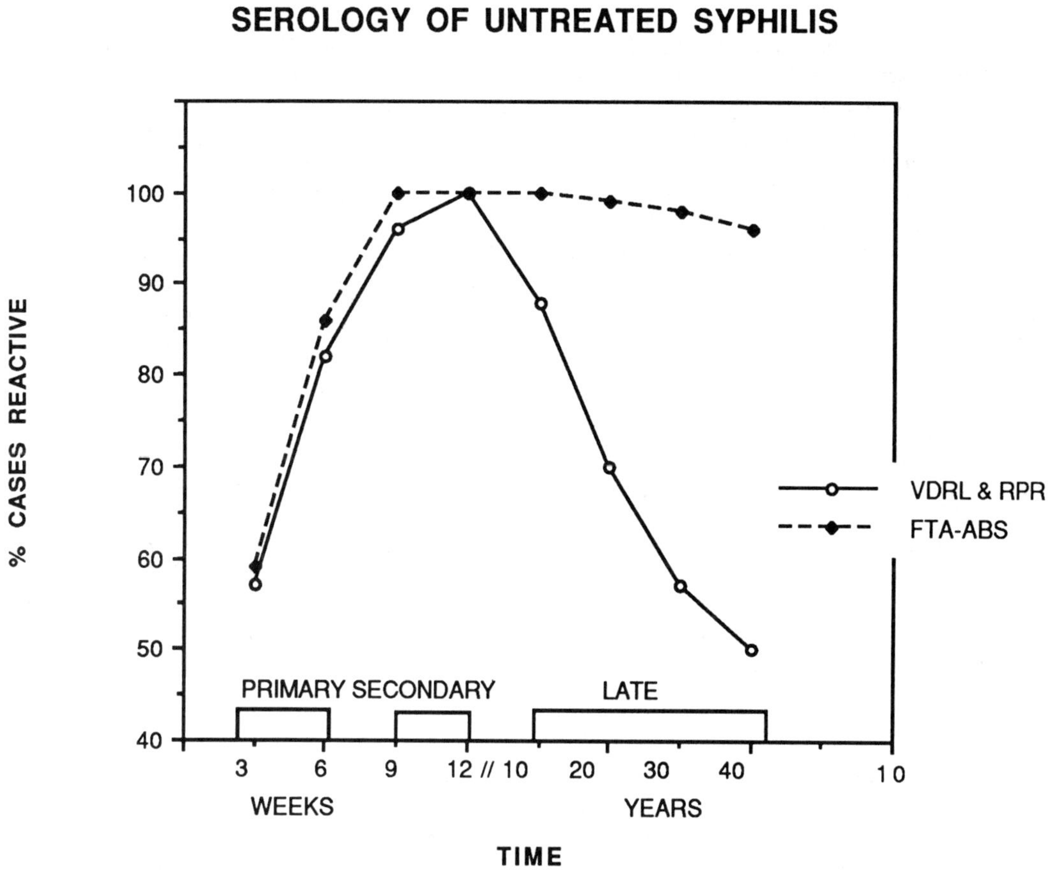

FIG 60–4
Serology of untreated syphilis.

This rash may last weeks to months. It is usually macular, non-pruritic, and located on the extensor surfaces of the extremities and on the chest. It may occur on palms, soles, or mucous membranes. It may be petechial, papular, or even vesicular.

Condyloma lata are moist, warty lesions that usually occur near the portal of entry. They may be found on the vulva, perineum, thighs, or buttocks. Condyloma lata resemble venereal warts caused by human papilloma virus. They can occasionally be differentiated by the wider base and less cornified appearance of lesions due to syphilis. Their surface may be grayish and necrotic.

After symptoms of secondary syphilis abate, a period of latency may occur. This may happen at any time after primary syphilis. During this time, patients may have recurrent eruptions and lesions on mucosa, skin, eyes, viscera, and bone. One need not progress through primary syphilis to secondary syphilis to latency. It is not unusual to have no primary or no secondary lesions.

Tertiary syphilis, which affects neurologic, cardiovascular, rheumatologic, and integumentary systems should not be seen in pediatric patients as it has a latency period of about 20 years.

Testing for syphilis is done with rapid antibody screening of blood samples. In patients with rapid test results that are positive, a titer is performed. As with other diseases, positive syphilis serology is not diagnostic of current infection in the face of recent treatment with appropriate antibiotics. As shown in Figure 60–4, stages of syphilis, serologic results may be negative at the time of primary lesion. As a result, any suspect lesion in a patient with a history of sexual activity should be appropriately treated at the time of the visit unless follow-up and abstinence can be assured. In patients with normal serologic results and a primary lesion, a second serologic test should be done 4 to 6 weeks after the initial visit. If serologic test results are positive, treatment should be initiated. Treatment for early primary syphilis includes either benzathine penicillin, 2.4 million units once, or tetracycline, 500 mg orally four times a day for 15 days. For syphilis of more than 1 year's duration, treatment must include benzathine penicillin G, 2.4 million units weekly for 3 weeks, or tetracycline, 500 mg orally four times a day for a month. Treatment for congenital syphilis is penicillin G, 25,000 U/kg IM or IV twice a day for at least 10 days, or procaine penicillin G, 50,000 U/kg IM daily for at least 10 days. Cure of syphilis is only suggested when titers begin to decrease.

Human Papillomavirus

Human papillomavirus (HPV) infection leads to condyloma accuminata or venereal warts. One to two percent of all Papanicolaou smears in the United States show cytologic signs of HPV. Papillomas may occur in the lower genital tract of women, on the penis, in the urethra of men and women, and on oropharyngeal mucosa. Papillomas may be totally invisible to the naked eye (flat warts). They can be seen only through close inspection with a hand lens or culposcopy after application of 3% acetic acid. Prevalence of HPV infection appears to have been rising since the 1960s when registries began. It is estimated that 2% of women in middle-class communities, and 10% in indigent populations are infected with HPV.

The virology of papilloma infection is complex. Types 6 and 11 cause exophytic (that is, visible) lesions, which may be associated with itching, burning, and pain. Virotypes 16, 18, 31, and 35 are more likely to cause flat lesions, which are tiny and difficult to see. These may occur on the cervix or external genitalia. They are easier to treat than the more visible lesions but more difficult to diagnose. More than one type of papilloma virus may exist in the same patient at a given time. All serotypes have oncogenic potential but types 16, 18, 31, and 35 have a stronger association with neoplasia than types 6 and 11. Cervical HPV increases the relative risk of cervical cancer by 2,000 times. In a 6-year follow-up study of 846 patients with human papilloma virus on Papanicolaou smear in 1979, 30 had carcinoma in situ by 1985. Of note, the adolescent cervix is particularly vulnerable to dysplasia because of squamous metaplasia occurring as the squamocolumnar junction migates outward in adolescence.

External lesions of papillomavirus may have a typical cauliflower-like appearance on the genitalia. These are easily identified. It is important to check the perianal area and the crural folds in patients who have visible lesions on the external genitalia. Cervical condylomas appear as leukoplakia (white spots on the cervix). The presence of HPV is confirmed with Papanicolaou smear; however, the false-negative rate is 20%. In patients with confirmed evidence of HPV on Papanicolaou smear, the smear should be repeated every 3 months. Colposcopy and direct biopsy are usually needed for diagnosis. These should be performed by an experienced gynecologist.

Treatment

Treatments for external lesions include (1) podophyllin, although the long-term cure rate is only 20% and podophyllin is known to be mutagenic, and (2) trichloroacetic acid, which is used successfully in many centers in strengths of either 25% or 85%. Eighty-five percent solutions should be used only by experienced practitioners. If cervical lesions or dysplasia is present, treatment is needed. Treatments include cryocautery, cone biopsy, and laser vaporization of lesions.

Visible HPV lesions of the internal vaginal area in women should be treated with laser vaporization. These treatments are best handled by experienced gynecologists.

In men with HPV lesions, or in partners of women with know papilloma virus infections, diagnosis of flat warts may be made by swathing the genitalia in gauze soaked in 3% acetic acid solution. With a hand lens, lesions will appear as white spots after 5 minutes of soaking. Treatment is generally performed in a urologist's office, as inspection of the distal 1 to 2 cm of the urethra is necessary for complete treatment of HPV lesions in men.

Herpes Simplex

Herpes simplex is a chronic viral infection marked by latency and repeated, recurrent localized lesions. The primary episode of infection is more severe and prolonged than recurrent attacks. The primary attack lasts up to 3 weeks, with initial symptoms beginning 5 to 7 days after infection (range, 1 to 45 days). Lesions are often multiple, bilateral, and coalescent. Lymphadenopathy is commonly found in primary disease. Half of patients will have systemic symptoms with primary disease, including fever, headache, and malaise. Local symptoms include dysuria, pain, itch, and vaginal or urethral discharge. Pain generally lasts 1 to 2 weeks. Ulcers last 4 to 14 days before crusting. All symptoms are more common in women than men. Extragenital lesions occur in as many as one-third of patients.

Overall, 60% of patients will have a recurrence. Herpesvirus lives in dorsal root ganglia between attacks. The first recurrence usually occurs within 4 to 6 months of primary symptoms. Recurrent episodes are shorter and milder than primary ones. Only 5% to 10% of patients will have systemic symptoms during recurrent attacks. Lesions in recurrent attacks usually last about 10 days. Many patients will have a prodrome 1 to 2 days before an attack. Recurrence is more likely with Herpes simplex type 2 infection than with type 1 infection. The average patient will have three to five recurrences per year. Stress, fever, menses, heat, sexual activity, and depression may all bring on a recurrence.

Diagnostic tests for herpes include the Tzanck preparation, in which a scraping is smeared on a slide and Wright stained. The Tzanck preparation is 30% to 50% sensitive for herpesvirus infection. Papanicolaou smears will result in diagnosis in 40% of cases, because of the virus' predilection for the cervix. Available from most large diagnostic centers, herpesvirus culture is between 94% (for vesicular stage) and 27% (for crusting lesions) sensitive. Appropriate diagnostic material from herpes lesions is obtained by unroofing lesions or removing crusts before swabbing for a sample.

Transmission of the virus is through direct contact, although the agent can live on inanimate objects. True asymptomatic shedding does occur in women (from the cervix), though the period of shedding is short (generally 1 to 5 days), and the virus titer is lower than in symptomatic shedding. Virus has been identified in saliva, vaginal fluid, and in semen.

The most feared complications of herpesvirus infection are neonatal acquisition of herpes and cervical carcinoma. Herpesvirus has been isolated from cervical samples obtained from patients with carcinoma in situ of the cervix.

Herpesvirus lesions are treated with acyclovir. Acyclovir inhibits viral DNA polymerase through substitution for a nucleoside base. The drug is available in oral, topical, and intravenous form. Topical acyclovir reduces the duration of viral shedding by 3 to 4 days during a primary outbreak. Ointment is applied four times a day for 7 days. It has little effect on symptoms. In recurrent episodes, ointment may reduce shedding by about 1 day.

Oral acyclovir is more effective than the topical form during primary outbreaks. Dosage for oral acyclovir is 200 mg five times a day for 10 days. Oral acyclovir reduces pain and other symptoms. Oral acyclovir is also effective in treating recurrent infection. To be maximally effective, it must be administered within the first 48 hours of an outbreak.

Oral acyclovir can be used for prophylaxis for recurrent attacks of herpes. Continuous prophylaxis may be helpful in the patient who experiences frequent recurrences, but has no effect on long-term prognosis. Prophylaxis does not prevent asymptomatic shedding.

BIBLIOGRAPHY

Adger H, Shafer MA, et al: Screening for *Chlamydia trachomatis* and *Neisseria gonorrhea* in adolescent males: Values of first-catch urine examination. *Lancet* 1984; 2:944.

Benenson AS, ed: *Control of Communicable Diseases in Man*, ed 13. Washington DC, American Public Health Association 1985.

Brunham RC: Therapy for acute pelvic inflammatory disease: A critique of recent treatment trials. *Am J Obstet Gynecol* 1984; 148:235.

Centers for Disease Control: 1985 STD Treatment Guidelines, U.S. Atlanta, 1985.

Corey L, Adama HG, Brown ZA, et al: Genital herpes simplex virus infections: Clinical manifestations, course, and complications, *Ann Intern Med* 1983; 98:973.

Eschenbach DA: Epidemiology and diagnosis of acute

pelvic inflammatory disease. *Obstet Gynecol* 1982; 55:142S.
Farmer MY, Hook EW, Heald FP: Laboratory evaluation of sexually transmitted diseases. *Pediatr Ann* 1986; 15(10):715.
Fouts AC, Kraus SJ: *Trichomonas vaginalis*: Reevaluation of its clinical presentation and laboratory diagnosis. *J Infect Dis* 1980; 141:137.
Guinan ME: Oral acyclovir for treatment and suppression of genital herpes simplex virus infection. *JAMA* 1986; 255:1747.
Hermansen MC, Chusid MJ, Sky JR: Bacterial epididymo-orchitis in children and adolescents. *Clin Pediatr* 1980; 19:812.
Mertz GJ, Schmidt O, Jourden JL, et al: Frequency of acquisition of first-episode genital infection with herpes simplex virus from symptomatic and asymptomatic source contacts. *Sex Transm Dis* 1985; 12:33.
Murphy MD: Office laboratory diagnosis of sexually transmitted diseases. *Pediatr Infect Dis J* 1983; 2:146.
Reid R, Laverty CR, Coppleson M, et al: Noncondylomatous cervical wart virus infection. *Obstet Gynecol* 1980; 55:476.
Rice RJ, Thompson SE: Treatment of uncomplicated infections due to *Neisseria gonorrhoeae*. *JAMA* 1986; 255:1739.
Rosemberg SK, Reid R: Sexually transmitted papillomaviral infections in the male. I. Anatomic distribution and clinical features. *Urology* 1987; 29:488.
Sanders LL, Harrison HR, Washington AE: Treatment of sexually transmitted chlamydial infections. *JAMA* 1986; 255:1750.
Sanfilippo JS: Adolescent girls with vaginal discharge. *Pediatr Ann* 1986; 15:509.
Stamm WE, Wagner KF, Amsel R, et al: Causes of the acute urethral syndrome in women. *N Engl J Med* 1980; 303:409.
Stone KM, Grimes DA, Magder LS: Primary prevention of sexually transmitted diseases. *JAMA* 1986; 255:1763.
Swinker ML: Clinical aspects of genital herpes. *Am Fam Physician* 1986; 34:127.

GENITOURINARY INFECTION

Margaret Delaney, M.D.

Urinary tract infections are a significant cause of morbidity in children. They can present as minor problems or as life-threatening episodes which may be the first sign that a patient has or is at risk for developing serious renal disease. Since renal damage is irreversible once it is present, it is essential to identify early those patients at risk, with the aim of preventing further injury to the growing kidney. Patients with urinary tract infections often require long-term bacteriologic and clinical follow-up and in some cases long-term therapy.

Criteria for Diagnosis

The definitive diagnosis of a urinary tract infection rests on the urine culture. The criteria for bacteriuria is greater than or equal to 10^5 organisms per milliliter of urine of a single species. This number generally represents growth caused by organisms in the urine and not by contamination from the collection vessels or from bacteria in the periurethral, urethral, anal, or vaginal areas. Bacterial counts of 10^3 to 10^5 organisms per milliliter are suspicious, while bacteria counts less than 10^3 per milliliter suggest contamination. Urine cultures yielding small numbers of bacteria must be repeated and consideration given to factors contributing to equivocal counts such as: increased urine excretory rates due to excess fluid intake, dilute urine, acid urine having a pH less than 5, and the presence of fastidious organisms or bacteriostatic agents in the urine.

Terminology

The term "urinary tract infection" refers to a group of conditions that have in common the presence of significant numbers of bacteria in the urine. Cystitis and pyelonephritis refer to the level of infection and may be defined in clinical, radiologic, or histopathologic terms. Cystitis refers to inflammation of the bladder and is clinically manifested by symptoms of suprapubic pain, dysuria, frequency, and dribbling. The patients are usually afebrile and hematuria may or may not be present. It is often associated with proximal urethritis.

Pyelonephritis refers to inflammation of the renal parenchyma, calyces, and pelvis. The symptom complex of acute pyelonephritis, a well-defined clinical entity, includes malaise, chills, and high fevers accompanied by flank pain, costovertebral angle tenderness, and, often, vomiting. In radiologic terms, pyelonephritis refers to abnormalities above the ureterovesicle junction. The term "chronic pyelonephritis" has multiple definitions and thus can be misleading. It may refer to the chronic stages or end result of bacterial infection of renal parenchyma characterized by a decrease in renal size or scarring. It can also refer to certain histologic lesions of the renal parenchyma or to specific radiologic findings that include papillary shrinkage or a defect in the renal outline. Finally, it may refer to the continuous excretion of bacteria or to frequent recurrences.

Distinguishing between upper and lower urinary tract disease is important because of the differences in therapeutic response, prognosis, recurrence patterns, and methods for follow-up. In clinical practice, however, the distinction is often academic and a definitive diagnosis based on histopathologic or radiologic findings is seldom made. In children especially, symptoms are often not classic and may even be absent. Furthermore, there is a larger amount of overlap in the clinical presentations. Exact methods to localize the site of involvement in children are often unreliable and not widely available.

The terms acute pyelonephritis and cystitis can be viewed as clinical entities representing ends of the spectrum of urinary tract infections in children, in whom the differentiation is often impossible on clinical grounds and impractical by laboratory investigations.

Epidemiology

In newborns screened for urinary tract infection, there is a 0.7% to 1% occurrence rate, being more common in boys. In infancy, boys and girls are equally affected, but beyond 6 months of age there is a preponderance in girls. The risk of having a symptomatic urinary tract infection during childhood is 3% for girls and 1% for boys. In preschool and school-aged children, the prevalence of urinary tract infections is 1% to 2% in girls, and 0.03% in boys. Most infants and young children with symptomatic urinary tract infections outgrow their susceptibility, girls at a later age than boys.

Pathogenesis

It is assumed but not proved that urinary tract infections occur via the ascending route except in neonates, in whom most infections are hematogenous in origin. The reservoir for bacteria is the gastrointestinal tract. In men, underlying renal tract abnormalities are more common.

The body has certain defense mechanisms to prevent the continuing multiplication and colonization of organisms that may ascend into the bladder. The mechanisms by which the bladder cleans bacteria are incompletely understood and the precise role of any one mechanism remains unclear. Clues to their nature have come from individuals lacking the specific mechanism and are more inferential than proved. Local factors suggested as being important include urinary bactericidal substances, urinary pH, urine osmolality, and the local and systemic immune response. Structurally, complete bladder emptying provides a wash-out mechanism for organisms that do ascend.

Conversely, any residual urine from a mechanical or functional obstruction to flow that inhibits complete emptying of the bladder predisposes to infection. Meatal stenosis, an anatomical narrowing of the terminal urethus, usually does not impede the flow of urine and does not cause infection in most cases.

Clinical observations have suggested other factors that may encourage bacterial invasion of the bladder. These include fecal soiling; chronic constipations; the shorter urethra in women; local irritation from worms, chemicals, or bubble bath; increased vaginal pH; and decreased cervicovaginal antibody production. The exact significance of these factors, however, remains subject to debate.

Individual susceptibility may influence one's tendency to develop an infection. In girls prone to urinary tract infections, a high concentration of gram-negative bacteria has been found in the periurethral flora. Such colonization is rarely found in healthy children over 4 to 5 years of age. It is noted that their propensity to infection may parallel a defect in some mechanisms that normally clears the periurethral area of gram-negative flora. Uroepithelial cells bind *Escherichia coli* more avidly in infection-prone women. An epithelial receptor that binds most pyelonephritic *E. coli* has been identified and is associated with a glycosphingolipid of the P blood group. Winberg postulates that differences in susceptibility in humans may be attributed in part to the density and availability of these receptors. Another area of investigation centers on strains of bacteria having certain virulence factors that enable them to infect the host. Much, however, remains unknown and further clarification of the factors involved in the pathogenesis of urinary tract infections is the subject of ongoing research.

It is also important to note factors that determine the degree of renal damage. These include age at diagnosis, presence of earlier unrecognized infection, therapeutic delay, obstruction, and bacterial virulence.

The relationship between infection and ureteral reflux is incompletely understood and the management of reflux is controversial. As Winberg notes "there have been few unbiased studies analyzing the impact of vesicoureteral reflex on the course and prognosis of urinary tract infections and fewer on the benefits and hazards of such procedures to correct reflux." Reflux, found as an accompanying feature in up to 50% of urinary tract infections, appears related to age. There is spontaneous resolution of reflux in 85% of nondilated ureters and in 41% of dilated ureters. There appears to be a familial occurrence, although the modes of inheritance have not been established.

While it remains unproved that reflux, by preventing complete emptying of the bladder, increases susceptibility to recurrent infection, it is accepted that the combination of reflux and infection by transporting bacteria from the bladder to the renal parenchyma predisposes to scar formation. The relationship between gross reflux and scarring has been demonstrated in many patients, while the effect of minor degrees of reflux remains under investigation. Because of the potential risks for patients with reflux and the complexities of the issues surrounding their management, it is recommended that they be referred to a specialist for consultation (see Chapter 99).

Bacteriology

E. coli is the causative organism in greater than 80% of noncomplicated first infections and in more than 75% of recurrences. Other organisms including *Proteus*, Enterobacteriaceae, *Klebsiella*, and *Staphylococcus* are more likely seen in complicated infections. The pathogens that usually come from the gastrointestinal tract are often found to be the dominant organism in the fecal flora. In patients with underlying renal abnormalities and in the debilitated host, *Pseudomonas*, fungal, and anerobic infections occur commonly.

Data Gathering

Clinical Features.—The clinical presentation depends on such factors as age, sex, pattern of previous infections, and the presence of anatomic defects. Symptoms tend to be fewer the greater the number of previous infections and the closer the recurrence. Infections with enterococcus, *Proteus*, *Pseudomonas*, or *Staphylococcus* may cause fewer symptoms than those with *E. coli*. Symptoms are often vague, nonspecific, or even absent. Infants and toddlers may present with fever; gastrointestinal complaints, such as anorexia, weight loss, failure to thrive, vomiting, ileus, abdominal pain, and diarrhea; skin manifestations, such as pale gray coloration or hypersensitivity of the skin to touch; CNS findings, including lethargy, irritability, and meningismus; and respiratory distress. Older children are more likely to have the classic symptoms although they are not a constant finding at any age. Symptoms of cystitis include dribbling, enuresis, dysuria, urgency, frequency, and abdominal or suprapubic pain. Fever, pyuria, and hematuria may or may not be present. Other symptoms of urinary tract infection in older children are vaginal discharge, abdominal tenderness, anorexia, and vomiting.

The history and physical examination are always important and may give clues to the presence of an underlying abnormality. In addition to delineating the presenting symptoms, the history should elicit information on previous fevers, urinary tract infections, and the recent use of antibiotics. One should note any history of trauma, sexual activity, urethritis, or use of foreign bodies and establish patterns of drinking, micturition, and defecation. Any family history of renal disease, hypertension, or urinary tract infection should be ascertained.

The physical examination should include measurements of height, weight, and blood pressure. In particular, one should look for findings that may suggest obstruction such as the presence of an abdominal mass or palpable bladder. The genitalia and rectum should be examined and in men it is helpful to evaluate the urinary stream. In examining the back, one should note any skin abnormalities in the lumbar area that may suggest dysraphism.

Laboratory Diagnosis.—To accurately diagnose infection, the urine sample must be properly collected and stored. Suprapubic aspiration of urine has generally been underutilized but is the method associated with the least ambiguity. Any growth from a correctly performed suprapubic aspiration is significant. In patients less than 1 year old in whom the bladder is an abdominal organ, suprapubic aspiration is easily performed and is the preferred method of collection. Other patients for whom suprapubic aspiration is indicated are young children with diarrhea, incontinence, or poor hygiene; any seriously ill patient in whom an accurate diagnosis is necessary before beginning therapy; patients for whom previous cultures have shown mixed organisms of questionable significance; and patients with bladder or urethral outflow obstruction. Complications of this technique include hematoma formation and puncture of abdominal viscera. They are, however, rare. Catheterization is an alternative to suprapubic aspiration in children older than 1 year. There is a small chance of contamination by the urethral or perineal flora, but with proper sterile technique, there is little danger of introducing organisms into the urinary tract.

When voided specimens are used in cooperative patients, they should be midstream clean-catch urine specimens. After spreading the labia in females and retracting the foreskin in males, the external genitalia should be cleansed with povidone-iodine (Betadine) and then rinsed. The specimen should then be collected in a sterile container. If the specimen is not obtained by a nurse, the patient or parent must be given instructions on the proper method of collection. With the clean-catch method, two positive specimens showing growth of greater than 10^5 organisms of a single species are considered significant. While one positive midstream urine culture carries an accuracy of 80%, two positive cultures are 95% accurate. Three positive cultures carry on accuracy of almost 100%. Since some contamination may be unavoidable despite precautions, clean-catch urine cultures are helpful only when negative. If positive, other methods of collection should be used to confirm the diagnosis. Bagged urine specimens should be used solely as a screening method and never for diagnosis if treatment is to be instituted before the result of the culture is available. To correctly obtain a bagged urine specimen, the bag is attached after the perineal area has been cleansed and is left on no more than 3 hours. Once the patient has voided, the bag should be detached within 15 minutes. Even when obtained correctly, there is a high risk of false-positive results. Ideally the patient should not have taken antibiotics for 72 hours before the culture since even at low concentrations in the blood, antibiotics may be in active form in high concentration in the urine.

The Uricult is an accurate method of demonstrating significant bacteriuria. This consists of a glass slide with blood agar on one side and clear agar on the other, the latter inhibiting the growth of gram-positive organisms. After the slide has been dipped into a urine sample or placed in the urinary stream, the excess urine is allowed to run off and it is incubated at room temperature or 37° C. The bacterial count is quantitated by comparison with a standardized chart. If growth is present, the organisms can be identified in a microbiology laboratory.

There are a number of chemical tests commercially available for use in screening for bacteriuria that are based on the principle of detecting in the urine some product of bacterial metabolism. These tests aim to obviate the special preparation of the patient necessary for a urine culture and to obtain immediate information. While useful in mass surveys of screening of asymptomatic patients for research purposes, they are not useful in clinical practice.

A routine urinalysis is of little use in diagnosing an infection. Bacteria or pyuria in the sediment serve only to suggest the need for urine culture. There is debate over the best method for performing urine microscopy, i.e., whether it is better to examine centrifuged or uncentrifuged and stained or unstained urine for bacteria and WBCs. A Gram stain of an uncentrifuged urine demonstrating bacteria correlates with bacteria in more than 95% of cases. The hemocytometer counting chamber enables one to examine fresh unspun, unstained urine in a standardized manner. Urine containing more than 5 bacteria/mm^3 or more than 10 WBCs/mm^3 has a high correlation with bacteriuria. Pyuria, however, can be absent or may be present in conditions other than urinary tract infection such as trauma, severe dehydration, febrile illnesses, chemical inflammation, and genital infections. Thus bacteria or WBCs seen in the unspun urine are helpful only in making a tentative diagnosis before the definitive result of the culture is available.

It is difficult to anatomically localize the site of a urinary tract infection on a clinical basis. Methods of localization include measurement of renal concentrating capacity, antibody-coated bacteria, erythrocyte sedimentation rate, C-reactive protein, urinary lactic dehydrogenase (LDH) isoenzymes, and *E. coli* antibody titers as well as bladder wash-out techniques and ureteral catheterization. Technical complexities, lack of availability, and unreliability, however, make individual methods of localization impractical in the routine diagnosis of childhood infections. Despite considerable research, individual tests that can be applied on a broad clinical basis are not available.

Radiologic investigations are used to assess the effects of the previous infection, to identify those at risk for progressive renal damage, and to detect anomalies that, in the presence of infection, could lead to further damage unless recognized and corrected. Recommendations concerning the patients to be evaluated, timing, and the specific investigations to be performed vary. Most agree, however, that all children undergo some form of imaging approximately 2 to 4 weeks after the first documented UTI to look for vesicoureteral reflux, scarring, and/or structural abnormalities. Earlier evaluation is indicated for patients who are severely ill or toxic appearing, those who fail to respond clinically, those with severe hypertension, and those with new onset of renal insufficiency.

There is no definitive schema for imaging following the first UTI. Advances in US and nuclear medicine have brought into question the traditional evaluation of voiding cystourethrography (VCUG) and intravenous pyelography (IVP). VCUG remains the definitive method of evaluating the lower urinary tract, providing detailed images of the collecting system, bladder, and urethra as well as an accurate grading of reflux. Direct radioisotope cystography has the advantage of a lower radiation dose and allows continuous monitoring, which is less likely to miss transitory reflux. Because it does not provide the essential anatomic detail of the vesicoureteral junction and bladder outlet, it is not recommended as the initial evaluation. Renal US is a noninvasive means of delineating anatomic and structural abnormalities. The sensitivity, however, is related to the skill of the examiner. US is particularly useful in acutely ill patients, where obstruction or abscess is suspected, and in situations in which renal function may not permit adequate visualization of the kidneys, such as in the neonatal period or in the presence of renal insufficiency. IVP remains the best method for visualizing detailed anatomy of the renal parenchyma and pelvicalyceal system and is useful for assessing renal growth. It is not helpful in the neonatal period when the kidneys are poorly visualized despite normal renal function and is contraindicated in situations in which an osmotic load may aggravate dehydration or renal failure, in severe hypertension, and in patients with a history of allergic reaction. Dynamic radioisotope scans such as the DTPA (^{99m}Tc-diaminotetraethylpentacetic acid) scan allow evaluation of differential renal function and provide information about possible urinary obstruction. The DMSA (^{99m}Tc-dimercaptosuccinic acid) scan is a static radioisotope scan and gives information about cortical mass. It is the most sensitive means of detecting scars and areas of inflammation before atrophy and scarring occur. The renal radiation dose, however, is ten times higher than that of IVP or a DTPA scan.

Investigations following up the first UTI should include a VCUG and renal US. If these studies are normal, further evaluation can be deferred pending a recurrence. If reflux is present, IVP or a DMSA scan should be obtained. It must be emphasized that radiologic investigation of the urinary tract is a dynamic field and the choice of the appropriate studies should be made in consultation with an experienced radiologist. It is also essential that all radiologic investigations be performed and interpreted by persons experienced with children to obtain the maximal amount of information with the least amount of exposure to the patient.

MANAGEMENT

The goals in management are: eradicating the acute infection, preventing further infection, recognizing those at risk for developing renal disease while removing, where possible, any contributing factors, and preventing the development of progressive renal damage with its consequences (including hypertension and problems associated with pregnancy). The physician should always look for evidence of obstruction that may require immediate surgical intervention. Findings suggestive of obstruction include bladder distention, a flank mass, hypertension, impaired renal function, failure to eradicate the infection, and an unusual causative organism.

Ideally, the diagnosis should be confirmed before treatment is begun. In the majority of patients seen in offices or clinics, one is able to wait for the culture results, while in hospitalized patients it is often necessary to institute antibiotic therapy before the results of the culture are available. In these patients, it is imperative that specimens for culture have been properly obtained.

As the most likely organism in uncomplicated lower urinary tract infections is *E. coli* with broad susceptibility, the usual choices for treatment in this situation are a short-acting sulfonamide, ampicillin, nitrofurantoin (Macrodantin), or trimethoprim-sulfamethoxazole (Table 60–12). All are readily absorbed from the gastrointestinal tract, concentrated well in the urine, and have low toxicity. Parenteral antibiotics are indicated for all patients with pyelonephritis or signs of systemic illness, neonates, and those who are unable to tolerate oral fluids or medications because of vomiting or severe flank or abdominal pain. The general recommendation for duration of therapy is 10 days to 2 weeks, which is adequate to eradicate infection regardless of whether there is renal parenchymal involvement. The merits of single-dose therapy, which has been advocated in adults with uncomplicated lower urinary tract infections, are being investigated in children. The indiscriminate use of single-dose therapy, however, is hazardous and because differentiation between upper and lower tract disease is often unreliable and impractical, single-dose therapy is not recommended.

In addition to antibiotics, various supportive measures can be employed. These include encouraging fluids to ensure an adequate diuresis and frequent urination to allow complete bladder emptying. A bladder analgesic such as pyridium, 7 to 10 mg/kg/day, or urine acidification with ascorbic acid, 250 to 500 mg three times per day, may provide symptomatic relief. Good hygiene with avoidance of chemical irritants and bubble baths should be emphasized. Vomiting and dehydration should be treated when present. Patients who require hospitalization include patients who require intravenous therapy, those with renal insufficiency, those with high fevers who appear "toxic," and those in whom poor compliance is suspected.

FOLLOW-UP

The immediate purpose of follow-up is to assess the patients' response to therapy both clinically and bacteriologically. Long-term aims of follow-up are the prevention of further infection and the removal of any underlying condition that may predispose to infection. In such cases surgery may be indicated for lesions causing obstruction or stasis.

The response to treatment should be prompt. Within 24 to 48 hours of starting therapy, the urine culture should be negative and symptoms should be controlled. The patient's clinical

TABLE 60–12
Antibiotics for Use in Uncomplicated Lower Tract Infections

DRUG	DOSE (MG/KG/DAY)	NO. OF DAILY DOSES	COMMENTS
Sulfisoxazole (Gantrisin)	120–150	4	Not with neonatal jaundice
Nitrofurantoin (Macrodantin)	5–7	4	Not for use in first month of life; GI side effects—best given with food or milk; no controlled studies on efficiency in treating acute febrile pyelonephritis; not effective with glomerular filtration rate <50% of normal
Ampicillin (Amoxicillin)	75–150 (25–50)	4 (3)	
Trimethoprim-sulfamethoxazole	5–7/25–35	3–4	Not to be used in children <2 mo old

condition should be reviewed 2 to 3 days after diagnosis. While a repeated urine culture is not always indicated at this time, a urine culture should be obtained approximately 3 days after completion of therapy.

Recurrences, which occur in the majority of females with uncomplicated infections, may be asymptomatic. Follow-up cultures should, therefore, be obtained at periodic intervals for a period of time. Since most recurrences take place within 2 years, an example schedule for obtaining follow-up cultures would be: 3 days after completion of therapy, monthly for 3 months, every 3 months for 9 months, and then twice yearly for 1 year. Longer follow-up is warranted in patients with pyelonephritis in whom there is a 30% to 40% recurrence rate for children without renal tract abnormalities. Although most recur within the first 6 months, 1% may have recurrences up to 6 years from the initial infection.

Recurrences of infection may be due to relapse or reinfection, the latter being more common. A relapse may be due to an unresolved infection secondary to drug resistance or due to obstruction of adequate drainage. Relapses can also result from the persistence of bacteria in a focus not amenable to therapy. Most recurrences occur within the first few months. In women, 80% of recurrences are due to infection with a new organism, while in men most are due to reemergence of an organism that has been partially suppressed. In women without obstruction, the risk of recurrence is 30% within 1 year and approximately 50% within 5 years of the initial infection. The risk of reinfection is much greater than the risk of a first infection and increases with the number of previous infections. The clinical presentation often is less severe.

Recurrences within the first few months are caused by resistant organisms and follow the use of sulfonamides and ampicillin but not nitrofurantoin. The initial course of antibiotics induces changes in the sensitivity of organisms in the gastrointestinal tract and periurethral area. Nitrofurantoin, which is absorbed in the upper small intestine, does not alter colony flora and therefore does not induce antibiotic resistance. In recurrent infections it is best to wait for the sensitivity pattern before instituting treatment. In situations in which immediate therapy is needed, a drug different from that initially used should be employed.

Recurrent infection and issues relating to antibiotic prophylaxis such as patient selection, duration of treatment, radiologic follow-up, bacteriologic surveillance, and compliance are best managed with the assistance of a specialized team that includes a pediatric nephrologist, urologist, and radiologist. Nonetheless, the long-term implications of recurrent urinary tract infections are important to physicians since there may be an association with otherwise unexplained pyelonephritis, hypertension, and problems related to pregnancy (toxemia, perinatal morbidity, prematurity) that develop in adulthood. The purposes of prophylaxis are to prevent recurrent infections after the existing infection has been eradicated, to maintain a symptom-free state in the patient, and to prevent progressive renal damage. Recommendations for those who should receive prophylaxis vary, but generally include patients with closely spaced episodes of recurrent infections and infants and toddlers with reflux.

BIBLIOGRAPHY

Burns MW, Burns JL, Krieger JN: Pediatric urinary tract infection: Diagnosis, classification and significance. *Pediatr Clin North Am* 1987; 34: 1111–1120.

Corman LI: Simplified urinary microscopy to detect significant bacteriuria. *Pediatrics* 1982; 70: 133–135.

Gordon I: Imaging the urinary tract, in Holliday MA, Barratt TM, Vernier RL (eds): *Pediatric Nephrology*. Philadelphia, Williams & Wilkins, 1987; pp 300–329.

Kunin CM: Urinary tract infections in children. *Hosp Pract* 1976; 11:91–98.

Lerner GR, Fleischmann LE, Perlmutter AD: Reflux nephropathy. *Pediatr Clin North Am* 1987; 34: 747–770.

Stamm WE: Measurement of pyuria and its relation to bacteriuria. *Am J Med* 1983; 28:53–57.

Winberg J: Clinical aspects of urinary tract infection, in Holliday MA, Barratt TM, Vernier RL (eds): *Pediatric Nephrology*. Philadelphia, Williams & Wilkins, 1987; pp 626–646.

Winberg J, Bollgren I, Källenius G, et al: Clinical pyelonephritis and focal renal scarring: A selected review of pathogenesis, prevention, and prognosis. *Pediatr Clin North Am* 1982; 29:801–814.

VULVOVAGINITIS, URETHRITIS, EPIDIDYMITIS, AND BALANITIS

Margaret Delaney, M.D.

VULVOVAGINITIS

The term vulvovaginitis refers to inflammation of varying degrees of the vulva and vagina. Symptoms include perineal and vulvar discomfort, described variously as pain, burning, or itching. Dysuria may occur due to irritation caused by urine coming in contact with inflamed areas. A variable amount of discharge is usually present. The first signs in nonverbal children may be irritability, scratching of the perineal area, and pain with defecation or voiding.

Data Gathering

Although the history may or may not be helpful in establishing the cause, it should include questions pertaining to specific causes of vulvovaginitis.

CAUSES OF VULVOVAGINITIS

Bacterial
Nonspecific (mixed infections secondary to poor hygiene)
Specific
Gonococcus
Gardnerella vaginalis (Hemophilus vaginalis or Corynebacterium vaginale)
Shigella
Streptococcus
Secondary to infections elsewhere (eg., skin, nasopharynx, ear, gastrointestinal tract, urinary tract)
Nonbacterial
Candida
Trichomonas
Herpesvirus
Chlamydia
Mycoplasma
Pinworms
Foreign body
Contact reactions due to allergy or irritation (with nylon or rayon underclothing, medications, soaps or detergents, bubble baths, vulvar sprays)
Systemic illnesses with vaginal manifestations (with bullous impetigo, *Shigella*, chicken pox, diphtheria, scarlet fever, histiocytosis X, acrodermatitis enteropathica, draining pelvic abscess)
Vulvar skin diseases (seborrheic dermatitis, psoriasis, lichen sclerosus, condyloma acuminatum, molluscum contagiosum)
Neoplasia
Granulomatous diseases (syphilis)

While certain etiologic agents may cause a specific type of discharge, the cause is seldom established by its nature. In the acute phases of infection the discharge is often thick and profuse; while in the chronic phases, it tends to become scanty. A malodorous discharge is suggestive of a foreign body.

In obtaining the history, it is important to note infections elsewhere, current antibiotic therapy, and use of other medications. One should ask about trauma and the child's hygiene including toilet habits, methods of wiping, and the use of deodorants, bubble baths, perfumes, or sprays. Tight-fitting pants or leotards and dyed underwear may be contributing factors. Finally, the history should include questions about sexual activity or possible sexual abuse.

The general examination should include a rectal examination, which may be helpful in eliciting the vaginal discharge and in palpating a foreign body or tumor. Vaginoscopy enables the physician to define the extent of the infection and should be carried out in cases of vaginal bleeding and where suspicion of a foreign body, neoplasm, or congenital anomaly exists. It is essential that the procedure be performed by experienced personnel to minimize trauma to the patient.

The age of the patient is an important factor in establishing the differential diagnosis. Differing etiologic patterns in premenarchal and postmenarchal patients are due to differences in the host environment and the factor of sexual activity in postmenarchal patients (see Sexually Transmitted Diseases, in this chapter). Because the vaginal mucosa in premenarchal children lacks estrogenic stimulation, it is thin, atrophic, and easily traumatized. The neutral pH and absence of glycogen and lactobacilli make it a good culture medium. Other factors that predispose young girls to vulvovaginitis are the proximity of the vulva and vagina to the anus and the lack of thick labia and pubic hair, which normally constitute a protective environment. Contributing hygienic factors include wiping from back to front after defecation or voiding, and sliding off the toilet seat.

Rising estrogen levels and sebaceous gland activity in postmenarchal patients induces thickening of the vaginal wall, the development of rugae, and cornification of the superficial cell layers. Lactobacilli, which metabolize glycogen, become prevalent and the vaginal pH drops from 7 to 5. These changes allow different organisms to become more common as pathogens. The leading causes of vaginal discharge in postmenarchal patients are *Gardnerella vaginalis* vaginitis; endocervicitis due to *Chlamydia*, gonococcus, or *Trichomonas;* herpetic ulcers; candidal vaginitis; *trichomonas vaginitis; and mucus from endocervical erosions seen with the use of oral contraceptives.*

There are several causes of physiologic discharge in children. Newborn infants may have a transient gray-white discharge consisting of desquamated vaginal mucosal and cervical epithelial cells that hypertrophied as a result of prenatal hormonal stimulation. Estrogen withdrawal may also cause a bloody vaginal discharge in infants and rarely, drainage from an ectopic ureter can present as a vaginal discharge. Physiologic leukorrhea occurs several months prior to the onset of menses. This white discharge is composed of desquamated vaginal epithelial cells, WBCs, and endocervical mucus. It is bothersome, but baths and frequent changes of underwear can alleviate symptoms. Reassurance, however, is all that is necessary in most cases.

Management

The most common type of vulvovaginitis occurring in premenarchal girls is a nonspecific vulvovaginitis resulting from poor hygiene. It is caused by nongonococcal pyogenic bacteria unrelated to specific diseases and produces a primary vulvitis with secondary vaginitis. As this is a diagnosis of exclusion, it should be made only after the physical examination is performed and appropriate cultures are obtained. The mainstay of treatment for nonspecific vulvovaginitis is personal cleanliness. The mother must be instructed on the importance of such measures as having the child wipe from front to back, using toilet tissue free of dyes and perfumes, and bathing often with frequent changes of underwear. Loose-fitting white cotton panties should be used and leotards or pants that prevent the circulation of air and allow the buildup of moisture and heat should be avoided. In the acute phase, in which weeping lesions and a vesicular dermatitis are present, compresses with Burow's solution (1:40) or plain water are helpful. Tepid sitz baths with plain water, colloidal oatmeal, baking soda, or starch also provide relief. Soap, which may irritate the area, should be avoided. In the presence of denuded, excoriated skin, topical medications should not be used since they may be systemically absorbed and could cause either an allergic reaction or dermatitis secondary to the medicine itself or its vehicle. After the acute phase has subsided, the area can be washed twice a day with a bland nonmedicated soap, rinsed, and blotted dry. Antipruritic lotions or hydrocortisone cream or lotion may be used, but pastes and ointments that can cause occlusion of the skin should be avoided.

Most children will respond to the above measures. For those who do not, intravaginal medications such as Sultrin vaginal cream (containing sulfathiazole, sulfacetamide, and sulfabenzamide) may be used. Approximately 1 mL is inserted into the child's vagina nightly for 1 week; the mother must be instructed on proper technique. Vaginal suppositories containing aminoacridine hydrochloride are effective with anaerobes, gram-positive bacilli, and *Proteus.* Topical estrogens are no better than the above methods and sexual precocity may result from prolonged administration. In cases in which vulvovaginitis remains refractory to all modes of therapy, one should consider the possibility that a foreign body or pinworms are present or that proper hygiene is not being practiced. After 1 month, 15% to 20% of children will have recurrences, which are usually due to poor perineal hygiene. Systemic antibiotics are rarely indicated in the treatment of nonspecific vulvovaginitis, but may be used in cases in which an infection is resistant to other therapies.

(For discussion of gonorrhea and other specific causes of vulvovaginitis see the earlier section on sexually transmitted disease.)

URETHRITIS

Inflammation of the urethra occurs in both men and women. There are infectious and noninfectious etiologies that vary with age, sexual activity, and hygiene.

CAUSES OF URETHRITIS

Infectious
Gonococcal
Nongonococcal
  Chlamydia
  Ureaplasma
  Trichomonas
  Candida
  Herpes simplex type 2
  Syphilis
Fecal contamination
Allergy
Pinworms
Chemical irritants
  Bubble bath
  Soap
Trauma
  Mechanical
  Masturbation
Foreign body
Systemic illness
  Stevens-Johnson syndrome
  Reiter syndrome

The most common causes in preschool children are fecal contamination and physical or chemical irritation, whereas gonorrhea and nongonococcal urethritis account for most cases in adolescents. Dysuria, the main symptom, may be accompanied by hematuria and pyuria. Meatal tenderness and pruritus may be present, and in cases in which inflammation is marked, the urinary stream may be diminished. Discharge is an inconstant finding and can vary from clear mucus to a copious purulent exudate. Systemic symptoms are usually absent. After delineating the nature of the complaint, one should establish whether there has been trauma, use of irritants, or use of foreign bodies as well as ascertaining any history of sexual contact. Physical examination reveals meatal erythema and tenderness. A discharge, if not obvious, can sometimes be elicited by manual stripping of the urethra.

In addition to urethritis, gonococcus causes prostatitis, epididymitis, and balanitis in men; whereas in women leukorrhea is usually more prominent. The organism, which has an incubation period of 2 to 8 days, may be transmitted by sexual or nonvenereal means such as close contact with an infected object or person. While patients may be asymptomatic, there is often a sudden onset of a thick profuse discharge with the absence of fever. In men and prepubertal girls, a Gram stain showing a leukocytic exudate with the presence of gram-negative intracellular diplococci is presumptive evidence for gonococcal infection. In sexually active women, a culture is necessary to make the diagnosis. When gonococcal infections occur in prepubescent children, one must look into the home and social environment and consider the possibility of sexual abuse.

The incidence of nongonococcal urethritis (NGU) depends on the population studied. In college men, it accounts for 80% to 90% of urethritis. *Chlamydia* is responsible for 30% to 50% of NGU; *U. urealyticum*, a genital *Mycoplasma*, is causative in some cases, while in others the cause is unknown. In sexually active patients, it may occur sequentially or together with gonococcus presenting as a persistent discharge in a patient initially treated for gonococcal infection. Because the incubation period is longer than that of gonorrhea, there is usually a longer period between sexual contacts. The exudate, which is less profuse, may be intermittent.

Cultures for *Chlamydia* and *Ureaplasma* are now available. While cultures are the most accurate means of identifying an organism, a rapid microimmunofluorescent test is also available for identification of *Chlamydia*. Untreated, the symptoms of chlamydial urethritis will often resolve. Although spontaneous clearance of the infection can occur, in most cases the organism persists.

Chlamydia is suspect as one of the causes of the acute urethral syndrome in women. This syndrome consists of the acute onset of dysuria, urinary frequency, and pyuria. Hematuria is absent and urine cultures are negative. Suprapubic tenderness is often present.

Less common infectious causes of urethritis are *Trichomonas*, *Candida*, and herpes simplex. *Trichomonas* infections cause intense urethral burning and a white frothy discharge. The meatus appears red and irritated. *Candida* causes a sore, reddened balanitis and a white curd-like discharge. Urethritis due to herpes is usually associated with herpetic penile lesions and tender inguinal adenopathy.

Noninfectious causes of urethritis include foreign bodies that may cause dysuria, frequency, and hematuria. In some instances, they may be visible on radiographs. Trauma due to mechanical causes of masturbation may result in pain, dysuria, and bleeding. In these cases, fever is usually absent, although secondary infection may occur. Fecal contamination or pinworm infestation produce pyuria, hematuria, and dysuria. Chemical irritants, which include bubble baths, soaps, and detergents, usually cause transient dysuria and no systemic signs.

To establish the diagnosis, urethral discharge may be obtained by gently squeezing or manually stripping the distal urethra or by inserting a moist cotton swab into the meatus. Wet mounts and a Gram stain should be performed. An average of four or more WBCs per high-power field (×1,000) in three to five fields on Gram stain indicates urethritis. Routine cultures as well as those for *Candida*, gonococcus, and *Chlamydia* should be obtained.

Men and prepubertal girls in whom the Gram stain of the urethral exudate shows gram-negative intracellular diplococci are presumed to have a gonococcal infection. Culture and sensitivity testing are important to identify resistant organisms and to assess response to therapy. In the absence of gonococcus, patients are presumed to have NGU. Although in the adolescent clinical syndromes can frequently establish the diagnosis, cultures for *Chlamydia* should always be obtained. General measures employed in treating patients with urethritis include instruction on good hygiene, fluids, rest, and avoidance of sexual intercourse. Hot baths and heat applied locally may help to alleviate local irritative symptoms.

The treatment of patients with urethritis caused by sexual contact is similar to that of sexually active patients with vulvovaginitis. Twenty percent to 50% of sexually active patients with gonococcal urethritis also have NGU. Many are due to simultaneous acquisition of both organisms, because the 2- to 3-week incubation period is longer than for gonococcus. Thus, one may see a therapeutic response during the incubation period followed by the reappearance of urethritis. In this situation, a 1-week trial of tetracycline is recommended. Lack of response may be due to tetracycline-resistant *Ureaplasma* or urethritis caused by *Trichomonas* or *Candida*.

EPIDIDYMITIS

Acute epididymitis is uncommon in children. It is usually caused by the spread of organisms from the urethra or bladder; the coliform organisms that cause bacteriuria being the most common cause in children.

Symptoms of epididymitis include variable degrees of enlargement and tenderness of the epididymis; in the chronic state the symptoms may be mild. On examination there is localized painful swelling of the epididymis, which remains in the normal posterolateral position. A urethral discharge, pyuria, and erythema may be present and some patients are febrile. The main diagnostic difficulty is differentiation from testicular torsion, which is a surgical emergency. This should be definitively excluded by Doppler flow studies, radionuclide scan, or surgical exploration.

The treatment of epididymitis includes rest, scrotal support with elevation, and ice packs or cold compresses. Patients should be observed for the development of abscess formation. Antibiotics when given empirically usually do not produce a dramatic response. If a specific organism is isolated, specific therapy is indicated.

BALANITIS

Inflammation of the penis and foreskin is often related to the presence of the foreskin, which if phimotic or redundant may predispose to infection, especially if hygiene is poor. The condition occurs commonly in infancy, when the penis may be irritated by wet, soiled diapers and, with poor hygiene, becomes secondarily infected.

Symptoms include difficulty voiding, a narrowed stream, dysuria, and urinary retention. Erythema and swelling are usually present and when secondary infection exists, there may be cellulitis of the penile skin and regional adenopathy. Causative organisms include gram-negative cocci, *Candida*, and gonococcus. The possibility of syphilis should be excluded. The cause is established by a Gram stain and cultures of the area. Specific antibiotic therapy depends on the organism isolated. In all cases the importance of good hygiene must be stressed.

This involves cleansing the glans and foreskin and keeping the area dry. If phimosis is present, circumcision or a dorsal slit may be performed to allow drainage.

BIBLIOGRAPHY

Altchek A: Vulvovaginitis, vulvar skin disease, and PID. *Pediatr Clin North Am* 1981; 28:397–432.

Berger RE: Sexually transmitted diseases, in Walsh PG, Gittes RF, Perlmutter AD, et al (eds): *Campbell's Urology*. Philadelphia, WB Saunders, 1986; pp 909–912.

Fleisher GR: Genitourinary infections, in Fleisher G, Ludwig S (eds): *Textbook of Pediatric Emergency Medicine*. Baltimore, Williams & Wilkins, 1988; pp 458–461.

Govan DE, Kessler R: Urologic problems in the adolescent male. *Pediatr Clin North Am* 1980; 27:109.

Huffman JW: Gynecologic infections in childhood and adolescence, in Feigin RD, Cherry JD (eds): *Textbook of Pediatric Infectious Disease*. Philadelphia, WB Saunders Co, 1987, pp 555–565.

Marks M: Urethritis, in Feigin RD, Cherry JD: *Textbook of Pediatric Infectious Diseases*. Philadelphia, WB Saunders Co, 1987, pp 517–520.

Paradise JE, Campos JM, Friedman HM, et al: Vulvovaginitis in premenarchal girls: Clinical features and diagnostic evaluation. *Pediatrics* 1982; 70: 193–198.

Paradise JE: Pediatric and adolescent gynecology, in Fleisher G, Ludwig S (eds): *Textbook of Pediatric Emergency Medicine*. Baltimore, Williams & Wilkins, 1988, pp 721–729.

ACQUIRED IMMUNE DEFICIENCY SYNDROME

Gary S. Marshall, M.D.

In the summer and fall of 1981, the medical community was first alerted to a syndrome of cellular immunodeficiency, opportunistic infection, and Kaposi sarcoma occurring in young, urban, homosexual men. One could not have then foreseen that at this writing, only 7 years later, recognizing and treating related syndromes caused by the same transmissible agent would be a major concern of the primary care physician. The possibility of a pediatric acquired immune deficiency syndrome (AIDS) might have been anticipated when early epidemiologic studies identified close sexual contact and blood or blood product exposure as risk factors for disease transmission. This possibility became reality in December 1982 with the report from Los Angeles of a 20-month-old former premature, multiply transfused infant with organomegaly, hematologic abnormalities, dysgammaglobulinemia, cellular immune dysfunction, and opportunistic infections. Similarly affected infants were simultaneously recognized in other urban centers of California, New York, and Miami, most of whom had been born to mothers with or at high risk for AIDS. By 1983, pediatric AIDS was generally recognized as a distinct clinical entity.

What has occurred since these initial events is unprecedented in the history of medicine in general and in the care of infants and children in particular. Two years after the epidemic was uncovered, the causative agent, a virus called human immunodeficiency virus (HIV, formerly referred to as HTLV-III or LAV), was identified by scientists in Paris and in Bethesda, Maryland. The molecular biology of this virus, its routes of transmission, and its effects on the host immune system were quickly delineated. Despite early efforts aimed at risk behavior modification and the institution of serologic screening of donor blood 3 years ago, the total number of reported cases has increased exponentially, owing in part to the long latent period between infection and disease and to transmission by virus carriers prior to the onset of clinical illness. As of October 31, 1988, there were 76,932 total cases reported to the Centers for Disease Control (CDC, Atlanta) with 43,177 deaths. The rise in pediatric cases has paralleled that in adults in a delayed fashion, so that at present, 1,218 cases have been reported from 43 states, the Virgin Islands, and Puerto Rico; this directly reflects the spread of HIV from its earlier confines in relatively closed populations to women of childbearing age through intravenous drug abuse and heterosexual contact.

The spectrum of illness recognized as due to HIV has broadened steadily. The emphasis has shifted somewhat from AIDS itself, which is only the tip of the iceberg, to the protracted but relentless immune dysfunction and consequent predictable clinical syndromes that follow infection with the virus. The identification of new HIV-related syndromes in children has necessitated several revisions of the CDC case definition, which at first closely paralleled that in adults. The current classification system for pediatric AIDS takes into account this broad spectrum of illness and includes some syndromes that appear to be unique to children.

More has been learned about HIV infection in a shorter period of time than about any other disease entity in history. Cofactors in disease progression are being pursued and a serologically distinct but related virus, HIV-2, has been discovered. Antiviral therapies are being investigated, and in the case of zidovudine (formerly called azidothymidine; AZT), instituted; vaccine development is under way, and supportive treatments are improving. In the coming years of the pandemic, it can be expected that most pediatricians will face HIV-infected patients at some point in their careers. This section will discuss HIV and its epidemiology with respect to children, and will attempt to provide guidelines by which the infected child can be recognized and diagnosed.

BACKGROUND

HIV, a retrovirus, reproduces by reversing the classic flow of genetic information, transcribing its RNA genome into DNA which integrates into the genetic material of the infected cell. Once there, this "proviral" DNA can lie dormant and be passed down (much like other genes) to daughter cells through the normal process of mitosis, or it can serve as a template from which progeny virus RNA and protein are made. This lytic cycle can result in cell death. Although the viral genome is relatively small, it has evolved an elaborate set of regulatory genes, allowing it to lie dormant in the cell, sequestered from the immune system, or, when appropriate, to rapidly replicate and spread.

The major virion envelope glycoprotein, gp120, has been shown to bind a cellular antigen called CD4, initiating the infectious cycle. Infection of several nonlymphocytic cell types has been demonstrated; some undoubtedly play a major role in pathogenesis, such as infected monocytes or macrophages, which probably serve as reservoirs of virus in the body. However, it is the universal presence of CD4 on T cells of the helper (T4) phenotype that directly accounts for the devastating immunosuppression seen in AIDS. T4 cells play a central role in initiating and coordinating the immune response to invading microorganisms. They first interact in a specific fashion with scavenger antigen-presenting cells, proliferate, and secrete soluble factors (cytokines), that stimulate B cells into antibody secretion and activate cytotoxic T cells that are capable of killing virus-infected cells. It is the selective depletion of T4 cells in AIDS patients that results in such profound humoral and cellular immunologic derangement. An absolute decrease in T4 cell numbers in the peripheral blood is probably the single most important factor determining the clinical course of HIV infection, since it paves the way for opportunistic organisms. HIV probably has direct effects as well, most notably in the CNS, that contribute to the diversity of clinical syndromes seen in AIDS.

Only three routes of transmission are known to be involved in the spread of HIV: inoculation of blood through transfusion, needle sharing, or by accident; homosexual or heterosexual contact; and perinatal exposure. Several facts regarding transmission are particularly relevant to pediatric HIV infection:

1. The virus is inefficiently transmitted, so that repeated exposures or large inocula appear to be necessary. Transmission by casual contact has never been documented.
2. Transmission by blood products, responsible for a larger proportion of current childhood cases than adult cases, has been almost eliminated by voluntary donor exclusion, the screening of donor blood for HIV antibody since April 1985, and heat treatment of clotting factor concentrates.
3. Although most sexually acquired disease in the United States is seen in homosexual men, the number of cases among heterosexuals is increasing (this mode of transmission is the leading one worldwide). Since 29% of women with AIDS appear to have been infected through heterosexual contact, this form of transmission may indirectly result in a large number of infected children.
4. Intravenous drug abusers occupy a key position in the AIDS epidemic, since they are the principle bridge to other adult populations via heterosexual contact. Intravenous drug abuse is also a prominent factor in childhood infection,

since the largest proportion of infected women of childbearing age are drug abusers or the sexual partners of men who abuse drugs.

5. Given the link between pediatric AIDS and intravenous drug abuse, it is not surprising that most cases have occurred among poor, urban, black and Hispanic populations.

6. Transmission from an infected woman (who may be asymptomatic) to her offspring may occur in utero, at the time of birth, or postnatally by breast feeding. The rate of transmission by seropositive women is variable, but is estimated to be 25% to 50%.

Epidemiologic features of AIDS in adults and children are summarized in Table 60–13. The majority of adult cases have occurred among non-drug abusing men who are homosexuals or bisexuals, heterosexual intravenous drug abusers, or persons with both of these risk factors. Blood product administration accounts for 4% of adult and 19% of childhood cases; these numbers can be expected to decrease in the future. The vast majority of pediatric cases, 78%, occur in the children of women with AIDS or at risk for AIDS.

Table 60–14 provides some information about rates of infection in various population groups in the United States. Clearly, seroprevalence rates vary widely by location and risk factor. Of interest, rates among unselected women of childbearing age may be higher than 2% in some areas.

TABLE 60–13
Epidemiology of AIDS in the United States*

RISK FACTOR	ADULTS (%)	CHILDREN (%)
Homosexual contact	62	0
Intravenous drug abuse	20	48 (mother)
Homosexual contact and intravenous drug abuse	7	0
Heterosexual contact	4	28 (mother)
Blood products (includes patients with hemophilia)	4	19 (child)
Undetermined	3	3 (mother) 2 (child)
Race		
White	58	23
Black	26	53
Hispanic	15	23
Other	1	1
Sex		
Male	92	55
Female	8	45

*Data from Rogers MF, Thomas PA, Starcher ET, et al: *Pediatrics* 1987; 79:1008–1014; and AIDS Weekly Surveillance Report (October 31, 1988) Centers for Disease Control, Atlanta.

WHEN TO CONSIDER HIV INFECTION

No doubt HIV infection will find its way into the differential diagnosis of an increasing variety of disease states in children. The currently identified clinical manifestations can be broadly categorized as follows: (1) effects thought to be more or less direct consequences

TABLE 60–14
HIV Seroprevalence Rates in Selected United States Populations*

	ANTIBODY POSITIVE (%)					
GROUP	HIGH	LOCATION	YEAR	LOW	LOCATION	YEAR
Homosexual, bisexual men	70	San Francisco	1978–1987	0	Pittsburgh	1984
Intravenous drug abusers	65	Brooklyn	1986	0	Tampa	1986
Patients with hemophilia†						
Type A	100	Los Angeles	1983–1984	33	Albuquerque	1984–1985
Type B	69	Worcester, Mass.	1984	0	Hershey, Pa.	1982–1984
Women partners of infected men	46	New York	1987	0	Arkansas	1987
Women prostitutes	45	New Jersey	1986–1987	0	Memphis	1985–1986
Unselected women (prenatal or delivery)	2.3	New York	1986–1987	0.0	Wisconsin	1986
Massachusetts newborns‡	0.80	Inner city	1986–1987	0.09	Suburban/rural	1986–1987

*Data from Centers for Disease Control: *MMWR* 1987; 36(Suppl 6):1–48.
†Differences in prevalence are due to more benign nature of hemophilia B, necessitating fewer clotting factor treatments.
‡Filter-paper blood specimens obtained by needle stick for metabolic screening, tested for HIV antibody; reflects seroprevalence rate among women bearing live infants.

of retrovirus infection, such as lymphadenopathy, progressive encephalopathy, lymphoid interstitial pneumonitis, cardiopathy, or the proposed AIDS embryopathy; (2) effects that are related to immunosuppression, including opportunistic infections such as *Pneumocystis carinii* pneumonia or disseminated cytomegalovirus (CMV), as well as opportunistic malignancies such as non-Hodgkin lymphoma; and (3) more generalized conditions that result from a combination of the above processes, such as failure to thrive or "wasting syndrome."

Whereas recognition of symptomatic infection in the appropriate epidemiologic context is not difficult, the clues to asymptomatic infection are more subtle. Recognition of asymptomatic children is imperative, however, since it appears that the majority will develop AIDS. Furthermore, it may be just this group that is targeted for research into new antiviral therapies. To recognize the HIV-infected child, one must maintain a high degree of suspicion and a current state of knowledge regarding epidemiologic risk factors and clinical presentations.

SUSPECTING HIV ON EPIDEMIOLOGIC GROUNDS

Children Born to Mothers With or at Risk for HIV Infection.—For the 244 children with perinatal AIDS diagnosed prior to December 31, 1985, 61% of their mothers were intravenous drug abusers, 18% were Haitian (HIV is endemic in Haiti and presumably heterosexually transmitted), 14% were the sexual partners of drug abusers, and 5% were the sexual partners of other infected men. Mothers at risk for transmission might also include those who received blood transfusions prior to mid-1985, or those who recently emigrated from other endemic areas, such as sub-Saharan Africa. The importance of an extensive social history, with specific inquiry into parental illicit drug use and sexual practices, is underscored by these statistics. One must always keep in mind that these issues are sensitive and difficult, but no less vital, to address; a concerned, straightforward, nonjudgmental approach is mandatory. Testing an asymptomatic mother for HIV antibody can provide persuasive, albeit indirect, evidence for or against infection in her child. All too often, an affected child is the first indication of an infected mother.

Children at Risk From Blood or Blood Product Transfusion.—It is now recommended that anyone receiving blood products (whole blood, cellular components, plasma, or clotting factors) prior to April 1985, be tested for HIV antibody. Products such as immunoglobulin, albumin, plasma protein fraction, and hepatitis B vaccine have carried no risk of transmission and the current risk from screened donor units is extremely small. Children in this group include hemophiliacs, who account for 6% of pediatric AIDS cases, as well as some former premature infants and children surviving life-threatening medical illnesses or major trauma or surgery who are now more than 3½ years old. The risk was higher from regional products, like whole blood, in cities such as New York, Miami, Newark, and San Francisco, whereas the risk from pooled products, like clotting factors, was unrelated to geographic location. The importance of a thorough medical history cannot be overemphasized.

Children Engaged in "Adult-Type" Risk Behaviors.—Some older children and adolescents engage in activities linked to HIV transmission, including homosexual intercourse, heterosexual promiscuity, prostitution, and intravenous drug abuse. Although few cases to date can be related to these activities, as the virus continues to spread in drug-abusing and heterosexual populations, this issue will increase in importance. HIV infection in a child whose mother is uninfected and who has never received a blood transfusion should raise the possibility of sexual abuse. For the pediatrician caring for adolescent patients, a detailed personal sexual and drug-use history is essential.

• • •

The above epidemiologic risk categories for children point directly to interventions that might prevent some childhood infections. On the societal level, effective treatment programs for intravenous drug abuse are needed, as are strategies to discourage young people from drug use. National education programs regarding the dangers of promiscuous, anonymous sex and the benefits of condoms and spermicide (which is also viracidal) use have already begun. High-risk women should be screened for antibody, and if positive should be counseled regarding birth control; if already pregnant, they should know the approximate 25% to 50% risk of having an infected baby and be offered the option of abortion. There is no current recommendation for cesarean section in pregnant HIV-infected women, although blood and other fluids present at delivery are presumptively infectious and should be treated as such. Infected women in the United States and other developed countries who complete pregnancies should be advised to bottle feed, since breast milk has been implicated as a vehicle for transmission in a few cases. Intravenous drug users who are under the care of the pediatrician should be referred for treatment (at best) or counseled on needle sterilization with diluted household bleach (at worst). All adolescents should receive factual age- and culture-appropriate guidance regarding safe sexual practices; this is particularly true for the adolescent man who is homosexual.

SUSPECTING HIV ON CLINICAL GROUNDS

Immunodeficiency

Pediatricians are accustomed to suspecting and working-up immunodeficiency disorders, since prior to the AIDS epidemic, most such conditions became evident during the first few years of life. The hallmarks of immunodeficiency in childhood include constitutional signs such as failure to thrive, unexplained fever, and chronic malabsorptive diarrhea, as well as susceptibility to infection, manifest as either unusually severe, persistent, or recurrent experiences with commonly infecting organisms or infections caused by organisms that rarely infect normal children. Examples of these infection patterns seen in children with AIDS are listed in Table 60–15. The types of opportunistic infections encountered in children with AIDS differ somewhat from those seen in adults (Table 60–16).

In any child with opportunistic infections, congenital disorders such as severe combined immunodeficiency, DiGeorge syndrome, agammaglobulinemia, or Wiskott-Aldrich syndrome should be considered, but HIV testing should also be done, regardless of the epidemiologic circumstances (some pediatric AIDS patients cannot be unequivocally placed into known risk categories). Most children with perinatally acquired disease present with opportunistic infections within the first few years of life, but other signs of HIV infection usually present earlier, typically in the second half of the first year. Recent data suggest that children with perinatal infection can be divided into two risk populations: those with very short incubation periods (median, 4.1 months) and those with an incubation period comparable to that in adults (median, 6.1 years). Accordingly, some children can remain asymptomatic for many years prior to the diagnosis of AIDS. The devel-

TABLE 60–15
Examples of Opportunistic Infections in Children with AIDS

INFECTIONS	CLINICAL FEATURES	DIAGNOSIS
Common agents		
Oral *Candida* (thrush)	Mucosal white patches	KOH wet mount
Esophageal *Candida*	Dysphagia, retrosternal pain	Endoscopy with biopsy
Disseminated CMV	Retinitis, enteritis, pneumonitis, hepatitis	Culture and histopathologic studies
Salmonella	Diarrhea, sepsis	Stool and blood cultures
H. influenzae, Pneumococcus	Recurrent sepsis, pneumonia	Blood culture, chest radiograph
Opportunistic agents		
Pneumocystis carinii (pneumonia)	Fever, tachypnea	Chest radiograph, bronchoalveolar lavage with silver stain
Cryptosporidia	Diarrhea	Acid-fast stool smear
Disseminated *Mycobacterium avium-intracellulare*	Fever, enteritis	Blood culture
Cryptococcus (meningitis)	Headache, altered mental status	CSF antigen test, culture

KOH = potassium hydroxide, CMV = cytomegalovirus.

TABLE 60–16
Differences Between Adult and Pediatric HIV Infection in the United States

FEATURE	ADULT	PEDIATRIC
Time from infection to symptoms	5–7 yr	4 mo to 6 yrs*
Mononucleosis syndrome accompanying seroconversion	Common	Rare
Embryopathy	—	Suggested
Kaposi sarcoma	Common	Rare
Lymphoid interstitial pneumonitis, parotid swelling	Rare	Common
Progressive neurologic disease	Common	Pronounced
Lymphopenia	Common	Unusual
Opportunistic infections		
Recurrent bacterial sepsis	Unusual	Common
Cryptococcal meningitis	Common	Unusual
Cerebral toxoplasmosis	Common	Unusual
Oral hairy leukoplakia	Common	Unusual

*Data from Auger I, Thomas P, DeGruttola V, et al: *Nature* 1988; 336:575–577.

opment of opportunistic infections before the first birthday is an ominous sign. The median survival time from diagnosis in such patients is 6.5 months, compared with 19.7 months in those diagnosed after 1 year of age. These figures derive from the first few years of the epidemic and reflect only those children with the most severe manifestations of HIV infection.

Laboratory investigation of patients with signs of immunodeficiency can provide corroborative evidence of HIV infection, although the derangements seen can be numerous and diverse (Table 60–17). The majority of children with symptomatic HIV infection (i.e., opportunistic infections) show evidence of T4 lymphocyte depletion, manifest as either an inverted ratio of T4 cells to T8 cells (i.e., ratio less than 1.0) or more accurately, T4 cell numbers less than 400/mm^3. Absolute lymphopenia, or a decrease in total lymphocyte count below 1,500/mm^3, is strikingly rare when compared with adult patients. The majority of children develop polyclonal hypergammaglobulinemia, either in response to the direct activation of B cells by HIV or impaired T cell regulation of immunoglobulin synthesis; patients with hypogammaglobulinemia have also been described. At some point in almost all cases there is evidence of impaired functional antibody synthesis, and this has important implications for HIV tests based on the detection of HIV-specific antibody. Compromised cellular immune responses can be

TABLE 60–17
Immunologic Features of Pediatric HIV Infection

ABNORMALITY	TEST
Normal or decreased lymphocyte count	CBC count differential
Decreased number of T4 cells	Lymphocyte subsets
Decreased T4/T8 cell ratio	Lymphocyte subsets
Depressed in vitro cellular response	Lymphocyte stimulation response to antigens and mitogens
Cutaneous anergy	*Candida;* tetanus, mumps skin tests (if previously immunized)
Dysgammaglobulinemia	IgG, IgA, IgM levels
Decreased functional antibody response	Tetanus, diphtheria antibody levels (if previously immunized)

demonstrated by poor reactivity to skin test antigens and diminished in-vitro lymphocyte stimulation responses to antigens and mitogens. Indeed, absence of skin test reactivity is predictive of a poor outcome. Other immunologic abnormalities that are less clinically useful are seen, including impaired cytokine production, decreased thymic hormone levels, and increased circulating immune complexes.

HIV-Associated Syndromes

Opportunistic infections are usually the final common, often lethal, pathway of HIV infection. However, a number of other clinical syndromes may predate or accompany this manifestation of HIV disease, some of which were included in the now less preferred term AIDS-related complex (or condition; ARC). Their recognition is imperative since they may be the only clues to the presence of HIV in some patients.

These syndromes vary in their expression between adults and children. Some are common to both, such as persistent generalized lymphadenopathy or immune thrombocytopenic purpura (ITP); others are almost unique to children, such as lymphoid interstitial pneumonitis (LIP) and chronic parotid gland swelling, or unique to adults, such as the mononucleosis-like syndrome accompanying seroconversion (including fever, rash, lymphadenopathy, pharyngitis, malaise, myalgias, headache, and arthralgias). As further examples, Kaposi sarcoma is much more common in adults than children, but CNS deterioration is probably more pronounced in children. Some of the major differences between adult and pediatric HIV infection are listed in Table 60–16; those HIV-associated syndromes most commonly seen in children are discussed below.

Embryopathy.—There is good evidence that HIV can infect the fetus in utero, but there is considerable disagreement over whether such infection can have generalized effects on the developing fetus resulting in recognizable dysmorphic features. This possibility was suggested by workers in New York who noted the following characteristics in children with perinatal AIDS: growth failure, microcephaly, hypertelorism, prominent boxlike forehead, flattened nasal bridge, long palpebral fissures, blue sclerae, oblique eyes, short nose with flattened columella, prominent philtrum, and patulous lips. This putative embryopathy has been challenged, however, on several grounds: the subjective nature of many of the above findings; the lack of strictly blinded observations; failure to compare morphologic features with racially appropriate norms; the existence of alternate explanations for some features, such as growth failure; and the presence of confounding variables such as maternal drug exposure during pregnancy. In fact, recent controlled data fail to substantiate a craniofacial dysmorphism in perinatally infected infants.

Persistent Generalized Lymphadenopathy, Hepatosplenomegaly, and Parotid Gland Enlargement.—In retrospect, the first signs of the impending AIDS epidemic were probably present in 1979, when physicians in California and New York noticed a syndrome of persistent generalized lymphadenopathy in homosexual men. Many of those originally diagnosed with AIDS in 1981 had had persistent generalized lymphadenopathy for several years, and by 1983 persistent generalized lymphadenopathy was recognized as a definitive pre-AIDS syndrome. This chronic lymphadenopathy typically lasts for 3 to 5 years in adults, during which time the patient may be otherwise asymptomatic or suffer constitutional signs like fever, fatigue, and night sweats as the number of T4 cells continues to decline. Histologically, the lymph nodes appear to progress from follicular and paracortical hyperplasia to atrophy of germinal centers and fibrosis with lymphocyte depletion.

The vast majority of infected children also develop chronic adenopathy along with hepatosplenomegaly. A minority, probably less than 15%, develop nontender, nonfluctuant, salivary gland enlargement; if present, this finding is quite characteristic of HIV infection. The lymph nodes are usually nontender, mobile, and are present at noncontiguous sites. Hepatic transaminase levels may or may not be elevated. Biopsy is advised only if other treatable conditions, like leukemia or lymphoma, are serious considerations. Infections with *M. tuberculosis*, Epstein-Barr virus (EBV), and *Toxoplasma* can cause similar findings, and it should be noted that these infections can also occur with HIV infection.

Lymphoid Interstitial Pneumonitis (Pulmonary Lymphoid Hyperplasia).—Approximately 50% of children with AIDS develop this slowly progressive, chronic pneumonitis characterized clinically by cough and mild respiratory difficulty with superimposed episodes of acute respiratory insufficiency and, in some cases, the insidious onset of digital clubbing and oxygen dependency. LIP is differentiated from *Pneumocystis* pneumonia by its indolent course and the typical absence of fever and adventitial sounds, although secondary bacterial pneumonias do occur. Patients with LIP tend to be older at the time of diagnosis (mean age, 18 months) than those who present with opportunistic pneumonias (mean age, 6 months), more commonly exhibit persistent generalized lymphadenopathy and salivary gland enlargement, and appear to have a better long-term prognosis.

Radiologically, a diffuse, symmetric, reticulonodular pattern is seen throughout the lung, and hilar and upper mediastinal adenopathy is not uncommon (Figure 60–5). In contrast, *Pneumocystis* appears as a diffuse mixed alveolar and interstitial infiltrate with air bronchograms that progresses rapidly to opacification (Figure 60–6). The diagnosis of lymphoid pneumonitis can be confirmed with results of open lung biopsy, which shows infiltration of lymphocytes and plasma cells into the alveolar septa and peribronchial areas, in the absence of demonstrable infectious agents. This disease is not a malignancy per se, but rather an opportunistic lymphoproliferation, the etiology of which may involve polyclonal activation of lymphocytes by HIV or persistent EBV infection (EBV DNA can be detected in biopsy tissue and elevated serum EBV antibody titers are seen in some patients with LIP). Steroids have been advocated in treating this disorder, but controlled trials are lacking.

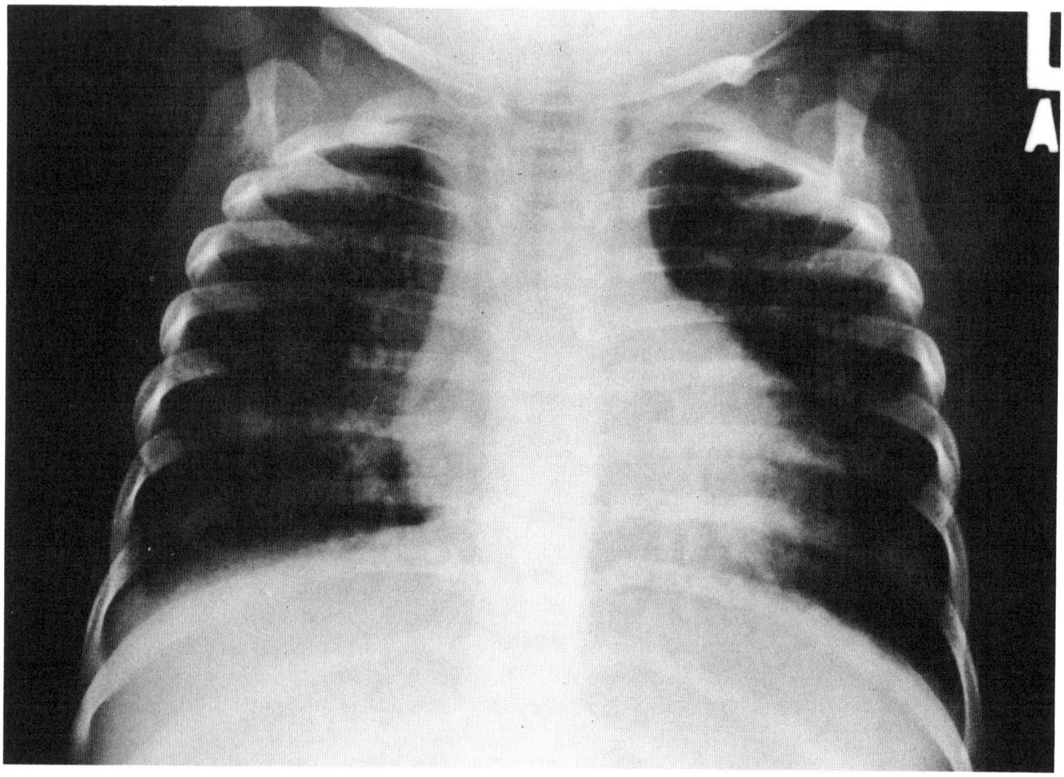

FIG 60–5
Posteroanterior chest radiograph in a 1-year-old HIV-positive girl with chronic cough. A diffuse reticulonodular interstitial infiltrate is evident throughout, including the periphery and bases, and prominent hilar adenopathy is seen on the left. These findings are typical of lymphoid interstitial pneumonitis.

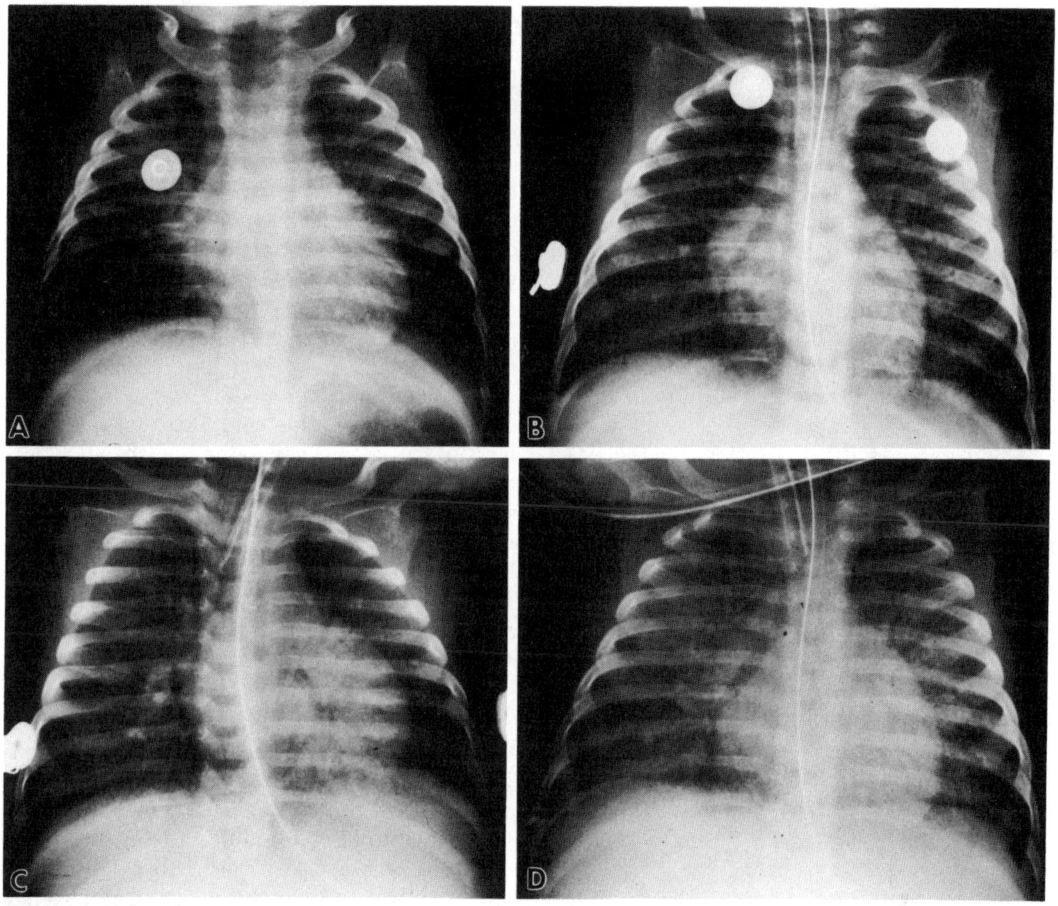

FIG 60–6

Chest radiographs in a 4-month-old baby born to a mother who was an intravenous drug abuser. **A,** at admission the infant had fever, cough, and tachypnea. **B,** by the second hospital day intubation for artificial ventilation was necessary, and a symmetric, diffuse parenchymal density was evident. **C,** air bronchograms and worsening infiltrate were noted on the fourth day. **D,** relative opacification was noted 5 days after admission. Silver-stained material from a bronchoscopic bronchoalveolar lavage revealed the presence of *Pneumocystis carinii.* The patient died on the seventh hospital day.

Encephalopathy.—CNS syndromes in AIDS can be due to opportunistic infections (e.g., toxoplasmosis, progressive multifocal leukoencephalopathy, cryptococcal meningitis) or malignancies (e.g., lymphoma). In addition, HIV itself is thought to have direct CNS effects, constituting a major feature of natural infection. Studies in adults have shown a high frequency of asymptomatic leptomeningeal involvement as well as encephalitis and aseptic meningitis during early HIV infection. Similarly, the AIDS dementia complex, characterized by cognitive, motor, and behavioral dysfunction, eventually affects the majority of adult patients and may be present prior to the development of, or to the exclusion of, opportunistic infections. Primary CNS infection probably involves more than 50% of children with HIV. Common features of this encephalopathy include developmental delay or loss of developmental milestones, intellectual deterioration, impaired brain growth (secondary microcephaly), and generalized weakness with pyramidal tract signs. Pathologic reflexes may be present, as well as hypotonia, pseudobulbar signs, ataxia, and isolated seizures. These findings are progressive in a majority of patients, particularly in those with AIDS, although this progressive form can be seen in patients who have not yet had opportunistic infections. In other patients, for unknown reasons, the neurologic signs appear to be relatively static, at least for a while. Neurologic symptoms have been noted as early as 2 months of age and as late as 5 years in perinatal infection. Progressive encephalopathy is highly correlated with fatal outcome, the time interval between onset to death averaging about 8 months. Encouragingly, improvement in cognitive function has recently been demonstrated in children treated with AZT.

CT scans in children with HIV encephalopathy generally show cerebral atrophy with enlargement of subarachnoid spaces and ventricles and occasional calcifications in the basal ganglia and periventricular white matter. The CSF is usually normal, but can show mild lymphocytic pleocytosis and protein elevation. Intra–blood-brain barrier synthesis of HIV antibody can be demonstrated in many patients by comparison of CSF and serum antibody levels. At least in adults, HIV can be isolated from and HIV antigens detected in CSF directly. At autopsy, histopathologic studies show inflammatory cell infiltrates, multinucleated giant cells, and perivascular inflammation, and HIV has been detected in the brain tissue of some children.

Wasting Syndrome.—In 1985, a wasting syndrome, locally referred to as "slim disease," was reported among seropositive African adults. The distinguishing features of this disease were extreme weight loss and intractable, non-bloody diarrhea, often leading to death and occurring in the absence of other clinical criteria for AIDS. In children, slim disease translates loosely into failure to thrive, which is evident in the majority of patients and can predate the onset of opportunistic infections. Diarrhea can be recurrent or protracted, necessitating hospitalization and parenteral nutrition; specific pathogens may not be identified. True protein-calorie malnutrition documented by anthropometric measurements, low serum albumin, elevated serum cholesterol, and anemia may be present. The pathogenesis of failure to thrive in children with AIDS is likely to be multifactorial, involving HIV encephalopathy and enteritis, and perhaps psychosocial factors as well.

Immune Thrombocytopenic Purpura.—In 1982, it was noted that some homosexual men presenting with ITP had immunologic derangements similar to men experiencing opportunistic infection; longitudinal follow-up studies showed rates of progression to AIDS similar to those in asymptomatic HIV carriers. The same entity was recognized as a presenting feature of childhood HIV infection in 1986. It is distinguished from the more common ITP by its early age of onset (8 or 9 months, compared with greater than 1 year) and the association with other stigmata of HIV infection. The mechanism of thrombocytopenia may involve the deposition of immune complexes on the platelet surface or the generation of specific antiplatelet antibodies followed by sequestration and destruction in the spleen. Anecdotal experience suggests a beneficial effect of steroids, but watchful waiting may be in order. HIV testing should be done on any child less than 1 year of age who presents with petechiae, ecchymoses, and isolated thrombocytopenia.

Malignancy.—Kaposi sarcoma, a previously rare tumor of endothelial origin, occurs in epidemic proportions among homosexual men with AIDS. It presents as painless, non-pruritic, blue-violet to brown nodules arising on the extremities or mucosal surfaces that can aggressively spread to involve the lymphatic system and viscera. Kaposi sarcoma was noted to occur in 4% of the first 307 reported children with AIDS; almost all of these children were born to Haitian parents. The reasons behind its low incidence in children are unclear but may relate to the absence of cofactors, or perhaps even a second transmissible agent that is present in homosexual populations. A role for decreased immune surveillance is suggested by the occurrence of this tumor in immunocompromised patients without AIDS.

Non-Hodgkin lymphomas, particularly B cell–derived tumors, are known to be associated with HIV. They occur in approximately 6% of adult AIDS patients and exhibit unusually aggressive phenotypes, with frequent extranodal involvement. In fact, the brain is the primary site of involvement in almost one quarter of patients. Primary lymphoma of the brain occurs in as many as 3% of HIV-infected children, representing the most common lymphoid malignancy and the most common cause of CNS mass lesions. Histologically, these tumors are similar to those seen in adults. The presentation is often one of focal neurologic deficits (hemiparesis, cranial nerve deficits, visual disturbance) and seizures developing above the background of diffuse encephalopathy. The CT scan shows multicentric enhancing hyperdense mass lesions, but occasional hypodense ring lesions occur and must be differentiated from focal infectious processes. Brain biopsy is thus mandatory to confirm the diagnosis and determine therapy.

Other Organ System Disease.—Some investigators have noted organ system involvement in AIDS that appears to be unrelated to known causal agents.

Hepatitis has been described, manifest as hepatomegaly with elevated transaminase levels in the absence of infection with known hepatotropic viruses such as hepatitis A, hepatitis B, EBV, and CMV, or bacteria such as *M. tuberculosis*. Results of biopsy show a form of chronic hepatitis, with lobular and portal lymphocytic infiltration, hepatocellular and ductal destruction, sinusoidal cell hyperplasia, and endothelialitis; giant cell hepatitis has also been described. Progression to jaundice and liver failure can occur.

A cardiopathy similar to that seen in adults has also been reported. Patients present with signs of congestive heart failure and exhibit radiologic and electrocardiographic stigmata of cardiomegaly with global ventricular dysfunction. Echocardiography may document the development of valvular abnormalities. Enteroviral infection and other concurrent viral or bacterial infections should be ruled out in this setting.

Several types of renal disease are known to accompany AIDS in adults, most notably a disorder characterized by proteinuria, azotemia, and focal and segmental glomerulosclerosis that rapidly progresses to end-stage renal disease. Investigators caring for large numbers of pediatric AIDS patients have noted frequent subclinical renal abnormalities, and in some patients severe progressive renal disease.

The expanded spectrum of clinical manifestations of HIV infection prompted the CDC to develop a new classification system for HIV infection in children. This system, as published in April 1987, is outlined in Table 60–18.

DEFINING HIV INFECTION

The mainstay of defining infection with HIV is the detection of antibodies that arise and persist after exposure to the virus. Such antibodies are usually screened for with an enzyme-linked immunosorbent assay (ELISA) that uses whole virus antigen ("first generation" tests) or recombinantly expressed subunit antigens ("second generation" tests). Sera that are repeatedly reactive on ELISA are then confirmed to be positive by Western blot (immunoblot), wherein antibodies to individual virion components can be visualized. Both tests are required for definitive diagnosis. Other tests for antibody have also been used, such as the immunofluorescent test, which detects antibody to antigens expressed in infected cells. It should be mentioned that some states require informed consent before

TABLE 60–18
CDC Classification System for Pediatric HIV Infection*

Class P-0 (indeterminate infection): antibody positive perinatally exposed infants who do not meet CDC definition of infection
Class P-1 (asymptomatic infection)
- Subclass A: normal immune function
- Subclass B: abnormal immune function (e.g., hypergammaglobulinemia, T4 lymphopenia)
- Subclass C: immune function not tested

Class P-2 (symptomatic infection)
- Subclass A: nonspecific findings (e.g., fever, failure to thrive, persistent generalized lymphadenopathy)
- Subclass B: progressive neurologic disease
- Subclass C: lymphoid interstitial pneumonitis
- Subclass D: secondary infectious diseases
  - Category D-1: infections fitting surveillance definition (e.g., *Pneumocystis*, cryptosporidiosis)
  - Category D-2: recurrent bacterial infections
  - Category D-3: other infections
- Subclass E: secondary malignancies
  - Category E-1: cancers fitting surveillance definition (e.g., Kaposi sarcoma, B cell lymphoma)
  - Category E-2: other cancers
- Subclass F: other diseases (e.g., cardiopathy, hepatitis)

*Adapted from Centers for Disease Control: *MMWR* 1987; 36:225–230, 235.

HIV testing can be done, and in all cases, the confidentiality of test results must be safeguarded.

Antibody testing, however, is not without pitfalls, particularly in children. First, symptomatically and asymptomatically infected adults and children who have no detectable HIV antibody have been reported. It is not known whether this represents failure of the detection methods used or specific defects in antibody synthesis by the host. Second, in a well-known phenomenon, patients with AIDS can revert to seronegative status as the disease progresses, presumably due to "burn out" of the antibody-synthesizing machinery. Studies have shown that as many as 10% of infected children and 25% of children with AIDS may not be identified by ELISA screening alone; the Western blot may detect some of these false negative results.

Third, false-positive antibody tests occur in children due to the persistence of transplacentally acquired maternal antibody. For this reason, the CDC now classifies any perinatally exposed child less than 15 months of age (the theoretical limit of maternal antibody persistence) with HIV antibody but without immunologic abnormalities, symptoms, and culturable virus as indeterminately infected (Table 60–19). Antibody that is detectable after 15 months of age almost certainly implies definitive infection in perinatally-exposed as well as parenterally- or sexually-exposed children. The utility of testing for IgM antibody to HIV, which does not cross the placenta and therefore would indicate de novo synthesis by the infected baby, is as yet unclear. One experimental test that may be useful someday has a similar basis: measurement of HIV antibody synthesis by the baby's B cells in vitro. These latter two assays may be available in some research laboratories.

There are additional tests available to the clinician evaluating antibody-positive children with indeterminate infection and antibody-negative children with suspected infection. One is virus culture, which is generally done from blood and is now commercially available. While culture represents a gold standard of infection, it may not be positive in all children with AIDS. Similarly, there are ELISA-based "antigen capture" assays that can detect the presence of viral antigen in body fluids; the utility of this test in infants is currently under investigation. Several new experimental tests for HIV may be the key to newborn diagnosis in the future. These include in situ hybridization, wherein HIV nucleic acid is detected directly in the mononuclear cells of the baby, and the polymerase chain reaction, whereby HIV-related DNA sequences are amplified in vitro and detected by standard hybridization methods. The latter technique can detect previously undetectable amounts of HIV genetic material.

TABLE 60–19
CDC Definition of HIV Infection in Children*

Perinatal infection, age less than 15 mo:
Virus culture positive
Antibody positive with evidence of cellular and humoral immunodeficiency and class P-2 symptoms
Symptoms meeting CDC surveillance definition of AIDS
Perinatal infection, age greater than 15 mo, or other modes of transmission:
Virus culture positive
Antibody positive
Symptoms meeting surveillance definition

*Adapted from Centers for Disease Control: *MMWR* 1987; 36:225–230, 235.

FINAL COMMENT

HIV infection represents a formidable challenge to the physician. Recognition of the infected child requires extensive knowledge of the epidemiology of HIV transmission and the increasing variety of clinical and immunologic manifestations. Meticulously obtained historical information, careful clinical assessment, and longitudinal evaluation are required. Definition of infection can be a problem; for this and for assistance in management, infectious disease or immunology subspecialists may be helpful resources.

It is not enough to recognize that AIDS victims in this country are irreversibly stigmatized and feared. The physician caring for children with AIDS must also be sensitive to the fact that these children are almost always victimized twice. All of them are terminally ill. Most of them are also the estranged components of broken, underprivileged homes; the majority have sick, dying, or dead parents. The remainder of pediatric AIDS patients are survivors of life-threatening conditions such as extreme prematurity or have ongoing diseases such as hemophilia. Compassion is the first step in the fulfillment of our medical mission.

BIBLIOGRAPHY

Ammann AJ: The acquired immunodeficiency syndrome in infants and children. *Ann Intern Med* 1985; 103:734–737.

Ammann AJ, Levy J: Laboratory investigation of pediatric acquired immunodeficiency syndrome. *Clin Immunol Immunopathol* 1986; 40:122–127.

Auger I, Thomas P, DeGruttola V, et al: Incubation periods for pediatric AIDS patients. *Nature* 1988; 336:575–577.

Belman AL, Diamond G, Dickson D, et al: Pediatric acquired immunodeficiency syndrome: neurologic syndromes. *Am J Dis Child* 1988; 142:29–35.

Blanche S, LeDeist F, Fischer A, et al: Longitudinal study of 18 children with perinatal LAV/HTLV III infection: Attempt at prognostic evaluation. *J Pediatr* 1986; 109:965–970.

Borkowsky W, Krasinski K, Paul D, et al: Human immunodeficiency virus infections in infants negative for anti-HIV by enzyme-linked immunoassay. *Lancet* 1987; 1:1168–1171.

Centers for Disease Control: Classification system for human immunodeficiency virus (HIV) infection in children under 13 years of age. *MMWR* 1987; 36:225–230, 235.

Centers for Disease Control: Human immunodeficiency virus infection in the United States: A review of current knowledge. *MMWR* 1987; 36: 1–48.

Connor E, Grupta S, Joshi V, et al: Acquired immunodeficiency syndrome–associated renal disease in children. *J Pediatr* 1988; 113:39–44.

Curran JW, Jaffe HW, Hardy AM, et al: Epidemiology of HIV infection and AIDS in the United States. *Science* 1988; 239:610–616.

Desposito, F, McSherry GD, Oleske JM: Blood product acquired HIV infection in children. *Pediatr Ann* 1988; 17:341–345.

Duffy LF, Daum F, Kahn E, et al: Hepatitis in children with acquired immune deficiency syndrome: Histopathologic and immunocytologic features. *Gastroenterology* 1986; 90:173–181.

Epstein LG, Sharer LR, Oleske JM, et al: Neurologic manifestations of human immunodeficiency virus infection in children. *Pediatrics* 1986; 78:678–687.

Epstein LG, DiCarlo FJ Jr, Joshi VV, et al: Primary lymphoma of the central nervous system in children with acquired immunodeficiency syndrome. *Pediatrics* 1988; 82:355–363.

Falloon J, Eddy J, Wiener L, et al: Human immunodeficiency virus infection in children. *J Pediatr* 1989; 114:1–30.

Fauci AS: The human immunodeficiency virus: Infectivity and mechanisms of pathogenesis. *Science* 1988; 239:617–622.

Friedland GH, Klein RS: Transmission of the human immunodeficiency virus. *N Engl J Med* 1987; 317:1125–1135.

Jason JM, Stehr-Green J, Holman RC, et al: Human immunodeficiency virus infection in hemophilic children. *Pediatrics* 1988; 82:565–570.

Marion RW, Wiznia AA, Hutcheon G, et al: Human T-cell lymphotropic virus type III (HTLV-III) embryopathy: A new dysmorphic syndrome associated with intrauterine HTLV-III infection. *Am J Dis Child* 1986; 140:638–640.

Minnefor A, Oleske J, Connor E, et al: Pediatric AIDS. *Antibiot Chemother* 1987; 38:52–58.

Pahwa S, Kaplan M, Fikrig S, et al: Spectrum of human T-cell lymphotropic virus type III infection in children: Recognition of symptomatic, asymptomatic, and seronegative patients. *JAMA* 1986; 255:2299–2305.

Qazi QH, Sheikh TM, Fikrig S, et al: Lack of evidence for craniofacial dysmorphism in perinatal human immunodeficiency virus infection. *J Pediatr* 1988; 112:7–11.

Rogers MF, Thomas PA, Starcher ET, et al: Acquired immunodeficiency syndrome in children: Report of the Centers for Disease Control national surveillance, 1982 to 1985. *Pediatrics* 1987; 79:1008–1014.

Rubinstein A, Sicklick M, Gupta A, et al: Acquired immunodeficiency with reversed T4/T8 ratios in infants born to promiscuous and drug-addicted mothers. *JAMA* 1983; 249:2350–2356.

Rubinstein, A, Bernstein L: The epidemiology of pediatric acquired immunodeficiency syndrome. *Clin Immunol Immunopathol* 1986; 40:115–121.

Rubinstein A, Morecki R, Silverman B, et al: Pulmonary disease in children with acquired immune deficiency syndrome and AIDS-related complex. *J Pediatr* 1986; 108:498–503.

Saulsbury FT, Boyle RJ, Wykoff RF, et al: Thrombocytopenia as the presenting manifestation of human T-lymphotropic virus type III infection in infants. *J Pediatr* 1986; 109:30–34.

The AIDS Issue. *Sci Am*, Oct, 1988.

Serwadda D, Mugerwa RD, Sewankambo NK, et al: Slim disease: A new disease in Uganda and its association with HTLV-III infection. *Lancet* 1985; 2:849–852.

Silverman BK, Waddell A (eds): *The Surgeon General's Workshop on Children with HIV Infection and Their Families.* Rockville, Md, US Department of Health and Human Services, DHHS Publication No HRS-D-MC 87-1.

Steinherz LJ, Brochstein JA, Robins J: Cardiac involvement in congenital acquired immunodeficiency syndrome. *Am J Dis Child* 1986; 140:1241–1244.

RECURRENT INFECTIONS

Mary Ellen Conley, M.D.

Every physician who cares for children repeatedly faces the issue of what to do with the child with recurrent infections. Some children seem to be sick all of the time. The mother says she feels as if she lives in the doctor's office. The grandmother says something must be wrong. The physician pages through the chart. The child has had many infections, but too many? And, if too many, what can and should be done?

HOW MANY IS TOO MANY?

In a study done of 246 full-term, first-born children, Hoekelman found that although 36% of the children had no infections at all in the first year of life, 13% of the children had four or more infections in the same period. When it is recognized that the children included in this study are in the lowest-risk group and that children who are born prematurely, who have older siblings, or who are in a daycare facility have infection rates that are two to three times greater than these low-risk patients, we estimate that normal children may have up to eight to ten infections a year in the first few years of life. If these infections are upper respiratory tract infections, otitis, or gastroenteritis, if the child is well between infections, if the screening tests described at the end of the chapter are normal, and particularly if the child is growing normally, there is no need to worry. That is not to say the infections are not a nuisance to the family, but they should not be a cause of worry or considered a harbinger of worse things.

WHEN TO WORRY?

There are certain signs that indicate that a physician should look further into the causes of multiple infections. These signs do not indicate that the patient has an immunodeficiency. Immunodeficiencies are rare and other causes of recurrent infection are more common. These signs include:

1. Two or more life-threatening infections (requiring hospitalization and intravenous therapy) within 5 years or less.
2. Prolonged infections or infections that are unresponsive to typical therapy.
3. Infections with unusual organisms.
4. Infections interfering with normal growth.
5. Infections in a child with a family history of similar infections, childhood death, or immunodeficiency.

RECURRENT INFECTIONS NOT DUE TO IMMUNODEFICIENCY

The cause of recurrent infections may not be due to a defect in the child at all. Sometimes recurrent infections are caused by a failure to completely eradicate a particularly resistant organism. A child whose otitis media is due to an organism that is resistant to the antibiotic being used may seem to have recurrent ear infections. Another example is the child with recurrent pyoderma. Some staphylococci are unusually virulent. The *Staphylococcus* may be carried by several family members but only one or two are afflicted with the pyoderma. As soon as the patient completes a course of therapy for the pyoderma, he becomes reinfected by the asymptomatic carrier. Several circumstances that should increase the physician's suspicion that this is occurring are: (1) recurrent skin infections in an individual who was completely well and without infections for several years prior to the onset of the staphylococcal infections; (2) a chronic skin condition such as eczema or psoriasis in a family member; or (3) employment of a family member in a health care facility or microbiology laboratory.

Recurrent infections may be due to increased environmental exposure to contagious agents. Not only the children who go to daycare centers, but the younger siblings of children in daycare centers or kindergarten may have repeated mild infections. Medical students who are doing a rotation in a pediatric walk-in clinic and military recruits who work and sleep in close contact with many individuals are also more subject to infections.

If a child has recurrent infections but only at

a single anatomic site, such as the middle ear or the lungs, then a localized defect should be sought. Recurrent pneumonias may be due to cystic fibrosis, α-l-antitrypsin deficiency, foreign body, recurrent aspiration, tracheoesophageal fistula, or other anatomic defects. Asthma with intermittent atelectasis also masquerades as recurrent pneumonia. Asthma and atelectasis should be suspected if the infection is associated with what seems to be a viral upper respiratory tract infection, the "pneumonia" resolves quickly, and the child has a history that suggests an allergic predisposition. Occasionally, a child who has had recurrent meningitis can be found on careful examination to have an abnormal communication between the skin and the CSF, most often a dural sinus. In these cases, the organisms that cause the meningitis are usually *Staphylococcus* or enteric organisms.

Children with certain systemic defects also have an increased incidence of infection. Worldwide, malnutrition is the most common cause of persistent or recurrent infection. During certain infections (most notably, measles, but also other systemic viral infections), the individual is more susceptible to bacterial infections. Some metabolic diseases, such as diabetes, may be associated with frequent infections. Patients who have had a surgical or a physiologic splenectomy also have a higher incidence of bacterial sepsis.

IMMUNE DEFICIENCIES

In considering the possibility that a child might have an immune deficiency, it is helpful to recognize that defects in each limb of the immune system present with typical clinical findings. The four limbs of the immune system: (1) B cells or antibody production, (2) T cells or cell-mediated immunity, (3) phagocytes, and (4) complement, have overlapping functions to provide maximum protection for the individual but defects in each limb tend to be associated with particular kinds of infection.

B Cell Defects

Defects in antibody production are the most common of the immune defects, the easiest to diagnose and often the most amenable to treatment. There are many causes of antibody deficiency including failure of B cell precursors to mature into B cells, failure of B cells to further differentiate into plasma cells, failure of plasma cells to secrete the immunoglobulin they have synthesized, and loss of immunoglobulin. Some patients have normal serum concentration of immunoglobulins (proteins with certain biochemical properties), but they fail to make specific antibodies (proteins that bind to specific antigens like tetanus toxoid or pneumococcus). Antibody deficiency for any of these reasons tends to result in infections with encapsulated pathogenic bacteria, particularly pneumonococcus and *H. influenzae*. Congenital agammaglobulinemia usually presents in children between 6 and 18 months of age, after maternally derived antibody has decayed. Presentation is sometimes dramatic, with rapidly progressive sepsis, meningitis, or pneumonia. Otitis, sinusitis, and pneumonia are the most common infections in antibody deficiencies even in children treated with replacement γ-globulin. Children with antibody deficiencies whose conditions are diagnosed early, before they have developed chronic pulmonary scarring or damage at some other site, and who are treated appropriately with γ-globulin replacement and aggressive antibiotic treatment usually do not require repeated hospitalization for acute infections.

T Cell Defects

T cell deficiencies, no matter what the cause, tend to present with viral, fungal, or parasitic infections of insidious onset. The infant develops a cold, rhinorrhea, and tachypnea that does not resolve; thrush recurs when therapy is stopped; diarrhea is common and persistent. There may be rashes. Complete congenital T cell deficiencies usually present as severe combined immune deficiency because normal antibody production requires T cell help. Babies with severe combined immune deficiency usually come to medical attention between 3 and 6 months of age because of persistent pneumonitis, diarrhea, and failure to thrive. On initial examination they may be found to be infected with as many as four or five different viruses.

The child with DiGeorge syndrome, congenital absence, or hypoplasia of the thymus and parathyroids, most often presents not with recurrent infections but with the associated defects of DiGeorge syndrome, cardiac defects, or hypocalcemia. The infections that these children acquire may be as much related to the cardiac defects as to the T cell immune deficiency.

Phagocytic Defects

For normal phagocytic function to occur, there must be a sufficient number of phagocytes, polymorphonuclear leukocytes, and monocytes in the peripheral circulation. Chemotactic function must be normal; that is, the phagocytes must reach their target. The phagocytes must ingest the foreign particle or substance. Finally, the phagocyte must be able to kill or degrade the invader. If there is a defect anywhere along this pathway, the patient is likely to have infections at the body surfaces, particularly the skin, the oral cavity, the conjunctiva, and the lungs. *Staphylococcus*, enteric bacteria, and fungi, especially *Candida* and *Aspergillus*, are most commonly involved. Some patients may also have intermittent, spontaneously resolving fevers.

Complement Defects

Defects in the complement pathway result in more varied clinical problems than defects in the other limbs of the immune system. Early complement component defects, C1, C2, and C4 deficiencies, may be associated with lupus-like syndromes, or occasionally with recurrent infections due to pathogenic encapsulated bacteria. Defects in the late complement components, C5, C6, C7, and C8, make the patient unusually susceptible to infections with *Neisseria*, both gonococcus and meningococcus. Patients are usually completely well between infections and may not come to medical attention until adolescence or adulthood. Any patient with a systemic neisserial infection who has a past history of severe neisserial infection or a family history of systemic meningococcal or gonococcal diseases should be evaluated for a complement defect.

DATA GATHERING

If a child has had recurrent infections, there are several simple laboratory tests that can be done to help evaluate the possibility of an immune deficiency. These include a CBC count, quantitative serum immunoglobulins, including serum IgE, functional antibody titers, and a total hemolytic complement (CH_{50}). In a CBC count, special attention should be given to the absolute number and appearance of the neutrophils. If a child is neutropenic but does not have an acute bacterial infection and has been previously well, the neutrophil count should be repeated and the child should be followed up carefully but the physician need not be alarmed. Acute viral suppression is the most common cause of neutropenia in childhood. If the neutropenia persists beyond 3 weeks, the child should be referred to an immunologist or a hematologist. The absolute lymphocyte count should also be noted. Infants with T cell deficiencies are frequently lymphopenic. Quantitative serum immunoglobulins should always be done rather than a protein electrophoresis or immunoelectrophoresis. The latter two tests are less sensitive and less specific than quantitative serum IgM, IgG, IgA, and IgE. The results of quantitative serum immunoglobulins should always be compared to age-appropriate standards. Children with agammaglobulinemia or hypogammaglobulinemia usually have serum concentrations of IgM, IgG, and IgA that are much less than 2 standard deviations below the norm. Because serum concentrations of IgA do not reach adult levels until the second decade of life. It is not unusual for children to have a delay in production of IgA so we usually do not make the diagnosis of IgA deficiency before the child is 3 years of age. The quality of antibody production can also be evaluated. Isohemagglutinins or anti–blood group substances are measured in every hospital blood bank and, except in the patient who is blood type AB, can provide good evidence of functional antibody production. In children who have received their measles-mumps-rubella vaccine, an antirubella titer can also be obtained. This test is usually readily available because it is used in obstetrics. The total hemolytic complement assay, or CH_{50}, is a functional assay that gives a normal result only if each of the complement components is present in adequate concentrations.

MANAGEMENT

There are certain management pitfalls that the physician should try to avoid. Sometimes a small child or infant with recurrent upper respiratory tract infections is found to have an IgG concentration at the low range of normal. The physician may be tempted to treat the patient with γ-globulin, but this should be avoided as it can suppress the child's own antibody production and make later diagnostic studies more difficult, and it labels the baby as a fragile, sick child. If the serum IgM level is in the normal range and the child has not had documented systemic bacterial infections, serum immunoglobulin levels should be repeated in 4 to 6 months and the parents should be reassured. Another vexing situation is the 8- to 18-year-old child who has persistent malaise, low-grade temperatures, and headaches or coughs. Findings of all laboratory studies and physical examination are completely normal and the child is appropriate in height and weight. The parents and the child should be carefully questioned about school attendance under these circumstances. School avoidance frequently presents as persistent undocumented infections. Specific management of school refusal is discussed in Chapter 90.

When a child has had many mild infections, it is sometimes difficult to reassure the mother that the child does not have a significant problem. It can be helpful to point out all the good signs if they are present: normal growth and development, no life-threatening infections, and normal laboratory tests. It is very helpful to point out that each infection has a beginning and an end, rather than it being one prolonged infection. If there is suspicion that the child does have recurrent infection on an immunologic basis, then consultation with an immunologist should be sought.

BIBLIOGRAPHY

Ammann AJ, Wara DW: Evaluation of infants and children with recurrent infections. *Curr Probl Pediatr* 1975; 5:11.

Hoekelman RA: Infectious illness during the first year of life. *Pediatrics* 1977; 59:119–121.

Johnston RB: Recurrent bacterial infections in children. *N Engl J Med* 1984; 310:1237–1243.

Stiehm ER (ed): *Immunologic Disorders in Infants and Children.* Philadelphia, WB Saunders, 1989.

61 INFLAMMATORY BOWEL DISEASE

John T. Boyle, M.D.

Once considered rare in pediatric practice, chronic inflammatory bowel disease (IBD) is now being recognized with increasing frequency in older children and adolescents. Inflammatory bowel disease is a general term used to denote two specific entities: ulcerative colitis and Crohn disease. Ulcerative colitis is characterized by inflammation and ulceration confined to the colonic mucosa. Crohn disease is a transmural inflammatory process that involves all layers of the bowel wall. The inflamed bowel contains noncaseating granuloma in greater than 50% of cases. Twenty years ago it was thought that Crohn disease only affected the small bowel. Today we know that in 60% of cases, both the small and large bowel are involved.

BACKGROUND

Fifteen percent to 20% of all IBD occurs in the pediatric age group, and 50% to 60% of all cases in this age group are Crohn disease. The cause of both conditions is unknown. Because there is no known cause, there is no specific treatment except for ulcerative colitis, which can be cured with surgical resection of the entire colon. Nevertheless, medical therapy is effective in controlling symptoms and preventing complications. Because early diagnosis makes therapeutic choices more rational, an important role of the primary care physician is early diagnosis and recognition of potential complications. Since there are no specific markers of disease activity, the condition of each patient must be managed according to his or her own specific needs. Thus, experience in dealing with numbers of these patients is essential in deciding the best medical therapy for these patients. Accordingly, they should be referred to the care of a pediatric gastroenterologist. The primary care physician by continuing to administer general pediatric care develops a unique role as patient advocate and, as such, can collaborate with the subspecialist to provide necessary input in making important management decisions in this chronic illness.

PATHOPHYSIOLOGY

There is no evidence that IBD seen in children is a different disease than that seen in adults. Theories concerning etiology have variously emphasized psychosomatic, allergic, genetic, microbiologic, and immunologic factors. Emotions and personality do not cause this disease but may alter clinical manifestations when the disease is active. Similarly, no specific dietary constituent has been implicated in the pathogenesis of the disease. There is no simple mendelian genetic mechanism at work in transmission of IBD, yet multiple familial occurrences are well documented in 15% to 20% of patients with IBD. Since no specific infectious agent has been identified, one hypothesis states that IBD results from the establishment of a state of hypersensitivity to a number of bacterial or viral antigens normally present in the gastrointestinal (GI) tract. The theory assumes a genetic predisposition and a breakdown in the normal GI mucosal barrier. The theory also assumes that ulcerative colitis and Crohn disease represent polar extremes of the single pathologic process.

DATA GATHERING

The usual presenting symptoms of crampy pain in the lower quadrant of the abdomen, diarrhea with or without rectal bleeding, weakness, fatigability, and weight loss are common to ulcerative colitis and Crohn disease. The onset of Crohn disease is usually more insidious. A careful history will evoke a positive history of some blood in the bowel movements in both diseases when colonic involvement is present. Inflammatory bowel disease is always a likely diagnosis in any patient with bloody diarrhea of greater than 3 weeks' duration. Often, however, extraintestinal manifestations or complications of IBD may be the major initial complaint and overshadow the GI manifestations. Presentations that should make one think of IBD are summarized below. It is important to remember that in ulcerative colitis, extraintestinal symptoms are almost always seen concurrently with gastrointestinal symptoms, whereas in Crohn disease extraintestinal symptoms are more likely to overshadow or actually antedate gastrointestinal symptoms.

CLINICAL PRESENTATIONS ASSOCIATED WITH IBD

- Nocturnal diarrhea or abdominal pain
- Weight loss in excess of 10% of weight when well
- Perianal fistula
- Fever of unknown origin (rare)
- Growth retardation
- Delayed puberty, primary amenorrhea
- Ankylosing spondylitis and sacroiliitis
- Migrating polyarthritis involving large joints
- Erythema nodosum and/or pyoderma gangrenosum
- Chronic active hepatitis and/or pericholangitis

Severe growth failure occurs in 30% to 40% of patients under the age of 21 years with Crohn disease and in 10% of patients with ulcerative colitis. Typically, children with growth failure have cessation of linear growth associated with poor weight gain, loss of subcutaneous fat, and marked delay in sexual maturation. Most physicians use standard linear growth curves to assess the growing child. Under normal circumstances, the growth of a child is a very regular process. Serial measurements of stature when taken by the same observer show a remarkably smooth, consistent progression from year to year. It is important not to define growth retardation as a height less than the third percentile. In fact, growth retardation is a deceleration in height gain—usually manifested by crossing height percentiles. Thus, a patient whose normal growth channel is the 90th percentile for age and whose growth decelerates, crossing percentiles to the 50th percentile, has growth retardation.

A growth velocity curve is the most sensitive indicator of growth deceleration because significant changes may be appreciated before crossing of major percentile lines is observed on standard linear growth curves. In IBD, it is not uncommon to find growth failure preceding the clinical onset of bowel disease, often by years. Growth failure does not correlate with severity of symptoms. While the etiology of growth failure appears to be multifactorial, dietary insufficiency is the primary factor in most cases. Often despite denying GI symptoms, these patients have low caloric intake even for their height age (age at which their actual height would be 50% on a standard growth chart).

DIAGNOSIS

Preliminary workup of suspected IBD should be performed by the primary physician. The importance of the history cannot be overemphasized. History of recent antibiotic intake and family history are important and often overlooked. Abdominal examination is often nonspecific although a fullness or mass in the right lower quadrant may indicate Crohn disease. Rectal examination is important in detecting perianal disease such as fissures or fistula as well as appraising stool guaiac (Hemoccult). Laboratory data are also nonspecific. The complete blood count may reveal evidence of hypochromic, microcytic anemia. The sedimentation rate is elevated in 90% of patients with Crohn disease. Certainly a normal sedimentation rate should not deter further workup in a suspicious case.

The differential diagnosis of infectious disease of the GI tract mimicking IBD is described below. Possible infective organisms or diseases are as follows:

CAUSATIVE ORGANISMS

Salmonella species
Shigella species
Campylobacter species
Yersinia enterocolitica
Aeromonas hydrophila
Neisseria gonorrhoeae
Clostridium difficile
Tuberculosis
Entamoeba histolytica
Lymphogranuloma venereum

Since IBD is primarily a diagnosis of exclusion, the primary care physician should rule out known infectious causes before referring the patient to a pediatric gastroenterologist. Most microbiology laboratories have the special techniques available to culture *Campylobacter*, *Yersinia*, and *Aeromonas*. *Clostridium difficile* is an anaerobe that is the causative agent of pseudomembranous enterocolitis, a complication of antibiotic therapy. Indeed, pseudomembranous enterocolitis has now been described following treatment with almost all routine antibiotics used in pediatric practice, including penicillin, ampicillin, amoxicillin, erythromycin, and trimethoprim-sulfamethoxazole. While most laboratories are capable of culturing *C. difficile*, only specialized labs are usually able to demonstrate the enterotoxin produced by this organism that produces the inflammatory disorder. Rectal cultures for gonorrhea should be obtained particularly for adolescent females. This organism extends to the rectum in 20% to 50% of females with gonorrhea, although development of symptomatic acute colitis is rare (2% to 5%). Practically speaking, amebiasis is the only parasitic infection in the United States that may mimic IBD. This organism is best diagnosed with specific serologic tests that are positive at the time of acute colitis in 90% of patients. Lymphogranuloma venereum is another sexually transmitted disorder that should be ruled out by appropriate serologic testing if inguinal adenopathy is a finding on physical examination.

Once infectious causes have been ruled out, it is best for the primary care physician to refer the patient to the pediatric gastroenterologist for further diagnostic evaluation. The next diagnostic study should be flexible colonoscopy (usually left side of the colon only) with colonic biopsies. An air-contrast barium enema can be performed on the same day as the endoscopy since small punch biopsies performed through a flexible endoscope do not increase the risk for complications during contrast radiography. An air-contrast upper GI tract radiologic series with small bowel follow-up studies is then performed on a separate day to complete the diagnostic workup. Double air-contrast radiography is the state-of-the-art technique for determining anatomic sites and extent of mucosal inflammation in the small and large bowel. Endoscopy is still needed since it may reveal inflammation even with negative findings of a double-contrast barium enema, and it is a method to obtain multiple biopsies that can often distinguish Crohn disease from ulcerative colitis by the presence of noncaseating granuloma.

It is not necessary to admit most patients with presumed IBD to the hospital for diagnostic workup. Nevertheless, the ability to educate the patient and family regarding the disorder and evaluate nutritional parameters will often lead the gastroenterologist to utilize a short admission for the diagnostic workup.

MANAGEMENT

While the primary care physician should not assume direct care of this disorder, for reasons stated above, he or she should have some understanding of the philosophy of treatment. The general goals of treatment are: (1) to attain the best possible clinical and laboratory control of the inflammatory disease with the least possible side effects from medication; (2) to promote growth through adequate nutrition; and (3) to permit the patient to function as normally as possible, i.e., school attendance, sports. Not all of these goals are always attainable. Sulfasalazine and steroids remain the mainstay of therapy for both ulcerative colitis and Crohn disease. Indications for steroid therapy include: (1) poor response to sulfasalazine therapy; (2) severe colitis (defined as one or more of the following five conditions: grossly bloody diarrhea occurring five times a day, oral temperature of 100° F; resting pulse rate of 100 beats per minute; hematocrit level of 30% or serum albumin value of 3.0 gm/dl; or toxic megacolon); and (3) extraintestinal manifestations such as arthritis. The fact remains that many gastroenterologists are willing to tolerate mild-to-moderate active disease or treat with only sulfasalazine and symptomatic medication if they believe that the dose of steroids required for complete disease suppression will result in undesirable side effects, especially growth suppression.

As far as patients with growth retardation, a dramatic reversal of malnutrition and a change in growth velocity can be expected in all children treated with adequate nutrition in conjunction with medical therapy to adequately control symptoms of inflammatory bowel disease. Improvement in nutritional status may be accomplished by a variety of methods. Occasionally, with heightened awareness of the nutritional needs, patients will be compliant for oral supplemental alimentation with any one of a number of high-caloric formulas. When oral supplementation fails, other means of providing nutritional support include: overnight continuous nasogastric feeding, intravenous parenteral alimentation in the hospital, or, in select patients, intravenous parenteral alimentation in the home. Whether or not a patient can achieve true catch-up growth with nutritional support is still controversial. Catch-up growth means that the patient returns to his or her normal growth channel. Factors that affect the ability for catch-up growth include duration of malnutrition, onset of puberty, disease activity, and steroid therapy. The importance of disease activity is brought out by the experience with surgery to treat growth retardation. Patients have shown catch-up growth following surgery if the inflammatory process remains in remission. However, rough figures for recurrence of active disease following an operation for Crohn disease are 20% after 2 years and 40% after 3 to 3½ years. The risk of recurrence is much higher in ileocolitis than in ileal disease alone.

The current indications for surgery in IBD are as follows:

INDICATIONS FOR SURGERY

Uncontrollable massive bleeding
Perforation or imminent perforation (toxic megacolon)
Acute fulminant disease not responding within 1 month to intensive medical management
Continuous incapacitating disease despite 1 year of adequate medical management
Chronic intermittent course with recurrent severe attack or long periods of disability
Retardation of growth and sexual maturation
Duration of more than 10 years and dysplasia of rectal mucosa

Because of the age of pediatric patients, surgery has always been viewed as a last resort, even when the patients were very ill. In recent years, attitudes of pediatric gastroenterologists are changing, certainly in regard to patients presenting with acute severe colitis. About 10% of patients with ulcerative colitis and a considerably smaller percentage of patients with Crohn disease present with criteria for severe colitis as listed above. All are now treated initially with bowel rest, blood transfusion, high-dose intravenous corticosteroids, intravenous antibiotics, and intravenous hyperalimentation. It is now generally accepted that patients who do not respond dramatically to this aggressive medical management within 3 to 4 weeks should undergo surgery.

It is important to realize that total proctocolectomy will cure ulcerative colitis. In recent years, the development of several endorectal pull-through procedures, similar to those performed to treat Hirschsprung disease or imperforate anus, have been used to treat ulcerative colitis. Not only are such procedures sphincter-saving, therefore allowing continued bowel continuity, but the complication of impotence is avoided. This latter complication of the standard proctocolectomy and permanent ileostomy, the procedure that has been the mainstay of surgical treatment of ulcerative colitis, can now be avoided in young patients.

BIBLIOGRAPHY

Brown R, Tedesco FJ: Differential diagnosis of infectious disease of the gastrointestinal tract mimicking inflammatory bowel disease. *Intern Med for Specialist* 1984; 5:140.

Fonkalsrud EW: Inflammatory bowel disease in children. *Surg Clin North Am* 1981; 61:1125.

Kelts DG, Grand RJ: Inflammatory bowel disease in children and adolescents. *Curr Prob Pediatr*, vol 10, 1981.

Kelts DG, Grand RJ, Shen G, et al: Nutritional basis of growth failure in children and adolescents with Crohn's disease. *Gastroenterology* 1979; 76:720.

Kirsner JB, Shorter RG: Recent developments in "nonspecific" inflammatory bowel disease. *N Engl J Med* 1982; 306:775, 837.

Kirschner BS, Klick JR, Kalman SS, et al: Reversal of growth retardation in Crohn's disease with therapy emphasizing oral restitution. *Gastroenterology* 1981; 80:10.

Kirscher BS, Voinchet O, Rosenberg IH: Growth retardation in inflammatory bowel disease. *Gastroenterology* 1978; 75:504.

Werlin SL, Grand RJ: Severe colitis in children and adolescents: Diagnosis, course, and treatment. *Gastroenterology* 1977; 73:828.

62 LUMPS AND BUMPS

Moritz M. Ziegler, M.D.

Superficial visible masses, commonly detected by parents, require prompt recognition and appropriate treatment and disposition. The major task for the primary care physician is to decide how serious the problem is and how quickly evaluation and treatment should be initiated. Fortunately, malignancy is not a common cause of visible lumps and not all lesions need to be removed. The following discussion is based on the location of the mass and is written to help the physician make the appropriate diagnosis and initiate the proper treatment.

HEAD AND FACE MASSES

Sebaceous cysts are soft masses usually found on the scalp, face, or back. These cysts are often called epidermoid or pilar cysts. Epidermoid cysts vary from 0.2 to 5 cm, are nontender, and may be mobile. The contents are thick and cheesy epithelial debris. These cysts may become infected, requiring excision or drainage. Pilar cysts occur on the scalp and are similar in appearance to epidermoid cysts.

Inclusion or dermoid cysts, located either in the midline of the face, scalp, or over the lateral aspect of the eyebrow, are subcutaneous, vary in diameter from several millimeters to more than a centimeter, and are mobile and nontender. These lesions should be removed to establish a diagnosis and to prevent erosion of the skull. Rarely they are characterized by dumbbell extension through the tables of the skull. They do not recur.

Preauricular lesions may be classified as a simple pit with a cutaneous orifice, a sinus tract with an associated subcutaneous cyst, a tract extending to the auditory canal or to the base of the skull, or as a cutaneous tag with or without a cartilaginous component. Unilateral or bilateral, they are quite common in the population at large. Cutaneous tags themselves can be removed for cosmetic purposes, while the sinus and cysts do not require treatment unless there is a history of infection or if there is a palpable cystic component in the subcutaneous tissue lying below the sinus.

NECK MASSES

MIDLINE NECK LESIONS

These lesions include submental lymph nodes in the upper midline of the neck. These lymph nodes, which are normally present, may become enlarged following an infection in the floor of the mouth or the perioral area. Dermoid cysts, located anywhere within the midline of the neck from the mandible to the supraclavicular fossa, most commonly are nontender, mobile, and in the subcutaneous tissue. A thyroglossal duct cyst originates from the normal descent of the thyroid gland and occurs anywhere along the tract from the base of the tongue down the midline (though they may be eccentric) of the neck to just above the thyroid cartilage. The lesions, usually painless, move with swallowing and protrusion of the tongue.

If a patient consults a physician because of the discovery of an undiagnosed but asymptomatic mass on the neck, then referral for elective surgery is appropriate. A patient who has tenderness and redness of the neck should be treated with antibiotics. A limited incision and drainage is appropriate for an acute abscess; but with the diagnosis of an infected thyroglossal duct cyst, such an incision should be followed up with a delayed definitive operation after clearing of the infection to remove the cyst and its associated tract that penetrates the central portion of the hyoid bone after the infection has cleared. This removal will prevent recurrent infections and will prevent the rare occurrence of carcinoma in cyst remnants in adults.

Lesions of the thyroid gland include goiters due to hyperthyroidism (toxic goiters) or hypothyroidism (nontoxic goiters), or solitary or multiple nodules. Thyroid neoplasms usually are solitary, nonfunctioning nodules, while thyroiditis may produce nodules, diffuse enlargement, or no change in thyroid size.

LATERAL NECK LESIONS

Cervical lymphadenitis, the most common neck lesion, is characterized by the onset of swelling and tenderness in the neck followed by heat and redness of the overlying area, a sequence that often follows an episode of pharyngitis or otitis. If these lymph nodes have a hard texture and are in the location of a known lymph node group, a course of antistaphylococcal antibiotic therapy is indicated. With progression of the infection and suppuration, the inflamed lymph nodes demonstrate central softening as abscess formation occurs. Such suppurative lymphadenitis is best treated with drainage in addition to the antistaphylococcal antibiotics. Needle aspiration with Gram stain and culture of the aspirate will help in the choice of antibiotics. Aspiration plus antibiotics is often the only treatment necessary for controlling suppurative lymphadenitis. If repeated aspiration is necessary or if systemic toxicity exists, then surgical drainage and parenteral antibiotics are the preferred method of treatment.

Tuberculosis lymphadenitis (scrofula), a chronic lymphadenopathy with tenderness and enlargement suggesting an inflammatory process, is best evaluated with a diagnostic chest x-ray and tuberculin skin test, though a negative skin test may occur with an infection by an atypical mycobacterium. The rubbery, woody lymph nodes are treated best with surgical excision (with culture and histologic examination), since fistulae may result from needle aspiration or simple incision and drainage.

Malignant neoplasms of the neck include a lymph node affected by leukemia or lymphoma or a lymph node enlarged from metastatic disease. The most common solid tumor in childhood that causes lymph node metastases is neuroblastoma. Definitive histologic diagnoses of neoplastic involvement of cervical lymph nodes require an excisional biopsy, proper specimen handling for touch preparation and lymphocyte markers, histologic studies, and proper staining and culturing for bacteria, fungi, and acid-fast organisms. Only needle aspiration is safe in the realm of the primary care physician, while formal excisional biopsies and drainage procedures require the skills of a surgeon.

Salivary glands most commonly are affected by a stricture of the duct system, collagen diseases, sarcoidosis, or vascular lesions such as hemangioendotheliomas. Salivary gland infection in the lateral neck induces inflammation of the submandibular gland or parotid gland with or without secondary abscess formation. These processes are unusual, result in systemic symptoms of infection and sepsis, and require prompt antibiotic therapy and/or operative drainage.

Branchial cleft cysts and sinus tracts in the lateral neck occur either along the anterior border of the sternocleidomastoid muscle from the upper to the lower neck (branchial pouch II cysts and sinus tracts), or they occur in the submandibular triangle up onto the anterior face (branchial pouch I cleft deformities). Such lesions range from a pore in the skin, to a subcutaneous cyst associated with that pore, to a proximally ascending sinus tract. Additionally, there may be only a subcutaneous cystic component or a subcutaneous cartilaginous remnant.

Elective surgical referral for branchial cleft lesions is done to establish the histologic diagnosis of a subcutaneous nodule, to excise a skin-communicating cystic mass that would be prone to infectious problems requiring interval drainage and subsequent excision, or to prevent the statistically increased likelihood of an in situ carcinoma forming in a branchial cleft remnant.

Lymphangiomas are congenital aberrant lymphatic system tumors varying from a single cyst to a cluster of grapes multicystic lesion due to a abnormal continuity in or dilatation of lymphatic channels. Such lymphangiomas or cystic hygromas are most commonly located in the neck, although they can be found throughout the child's body especially on the chest wall, axilla, and the extremities. These spongy, soft-tissue tumors are variable in size and filled with clear yellow or hemorrhagic fluid. Aspiration of fluid from the mass will usually confirm the diagnosis. Lymphangiomas are not characterized by spontaneous regression, but they do demonstrate a gradual coalescence with restriction of their boundaries and better definition of their margins. Patients with lymphangiomas frequently have a history of recurrent lymphangitis with associated acute swelling, tenderness, and erythema of the overlying skin; these lesions require broad-spectrum antibiotic therapy. Hospital admission is indicated if the acute inflammatory swelling might compromise the airway or if there is evidence of a proximal lymphangitis or systemic infection. Surgical referral is indicated electively or urgently depending on the clinical spectrum displayed.

VASCULAR MALFORMATIONS

These lesions range from mild skin discoloration to large soft tissue masses. There are three general types: port-wine stain, strawberry hemangioma, and cavernous hemangioma. The port-wine stain (nevus flammeus) is a purplish discoloration usually found around the face and neck. These lesions, consisting of mature capillaries, may need cosmetic coverage since conventional surgery or sclerosing therapy is less effective. Laser therapy has been used effectively. Capillary hemangiomas (nevus vasculosus), a raised reddish lesion, is also known as a strawberry hemangioma. After an initial proliferative phase (the peak of the growth period occurring when the child is 1½ to 3 years old), these lesions spontaneously regress. As regression begins, the central portion begins to undergo an ischemic change. This is followed by the development of an irregular surface with a whitish sheen, and then there may be occasional ulceration and crust formation. During this involution, the hemangioma may become infected. Hemangioendotheliomas are characterized by a discolored cutaneous involvement associated with a soft-tissue swelling beneath the surface of the skin. If untreated, these lesions will regress. Large hemangiomatous lesions may cause complications that include platelet trapping with a secondary bleeding diathesis or cardiac failure. Cavernous hemangiomas consist of large lakes of vascular channels and they are not characterized by spontaneous regression. Many lesions are true mixed hemangiomas with capillary, port-wine, and cavernous components, and the treatment needs to be individualized. Venous lakes, in the head and neck area, especially in the supraclavicular fossa, are most visible when children increase their intrathoracic pressure. During a Valsalva maneuver, a bulge anterior to the sternocleidomastoid muscle or in the supraclavicular space may appear representing a venous lake of the jugular system.

THORACIC MASSES

BREAST

Breast lesions that require emergency treatment are infectious in nature and include a breast abscess in a neonate or an older child. These swellings, usually secondary to staphylcocci, are tender, red, and warm. If antibiotic therapy does not clear the lesion or if central fluctuation develops, careful drainage is necessary, avoiding injury to the underlying breast bud.

Gynecomastia, or breast enlargement in boys, may be unilateral or bilateral and frequently presents as a tender breast enlargement with a palpable subareolar nodule. Enlargement may persist for up to 2 years before regression occurs. Only in the face of unusual signs or symptoms, excessive size change, or with chronicity is surgical referral indicated.

Breast tumors are usually benign in adolescents and carcinoma of the breast in a young girl is very rare. Most breast tumors in girls are fibroadenomas characterized by a discrete, firm, nontender nodule. Such palpable fibroadenomas may vary in size with menstruation and they may be especially sensitive to growth hormones. A breast tumor associated with a nipple discharge most commonly will be an intraductal papilloma. Adolescents may also develop breast lesions that are secondary to true fibrocystic disease.

The rapidity with which one proceeds to surgery for a breast mass should be tempered in the young girl. A dominant nodule is ideally managed with serial examinations over one or two menstrual cycles to confirm the persistent presence of the mass before proceeding to biopsy. In a child less than 5 years old, an inappropriately performed biopsy may damage the breast bud and subsequently limit breast development; therefore, biopsies should rarely be performed in that age group.

CHEST WALL

Chest wall deformities either protrude as a pigeon chest (pectus carinatum) or retract as a funnel chest (pectus excavatum). Other costochondral and sternocostal abnormalities exist including the absence of the second, third, and fourth ribs along with the overlying pectoralis muscle (Poland syndrome) or even the absence of a part of the sternum with the exposure of the underlying heart or its surrounding membranes (ectopia cordis). These lesion produce cosmetic abnormalities and may produce functional limitations as well, and elective surgery is indicated.

ABDOMINAL MASSES

Abdominal wall lesions may occur in the midline, the lateral abdominal wall, and in the inguinoscrotal region.

MIDLINE ABDOMINAL WALL LESIONS

These lesions may be localized to the area around the umbilicus or above and below that region. A weeping umbilicus may be due either to a granuloma at the site of the previous umbilical cord attachment, a patent urachus secondary to a persistence of the urachal remnant connected to the dome of the bladder, or a patent omphalomesenteric duct, an epithelialized remnant extending from the antemesenteric border of the distal ileum to the umbilicus. A granuloma is best treated with topical cauterization with silver nitrate and usually no further difficulties occur. A patent urachus requires surgery after a study for the presence of bladder neck or posterior urethral valve distal urinary tract obstruction. A patent omphalomesenteric duct represents an extension of the area of the ileum from a Meckel diverticulum and requires formal laparotomy with excision of the bowel with the draining sinus.

Umbilical hernias are an extremely common developmental anomaly. Such hernias represent a failure of closure of the abdominal wall at the body stalk or umbilical cord. Umbilical hernias are characterized by a fascial defect through which a true peritoneal sac bulges. The more common course of a neonatal umbilical hernia is gradual contracture of the fascial ring with spontaneous closure of the defect after months to several years. Elective surgery is deferred in boys until the age of 4 or 5 years and in girls until the age of 2 or 3 years. Strangulation of the hernia or skin rupture with evisceration is rare. Supraumbilical hernias, fascial defects located just above the umbilicus with associated protrusion of intra-abdominal contents, are not characterized by spontaneous regression, and the detection of a supraumbilical hernia is an indication for elective surgery. A midline fascial attenuation extending from the umbilicus to the xiphoid process of the sternum with prominent rectus muscle margins on either side is a normal anatomic variant termed diastasis recti. This finding is best demonstrated by a Valsalva maneuver or by having the patient lie supine with subsequent lifting of the head to tense the abdominal wall musculature. A midline 1.0-cm to 1.5-cm subcutaneous abdominal wall nodule between the xiphoid process and umbilicus most likely represents an epiplocele. An epiplocele, in contrast to a true ventral hernia, is a protrusion of preperitoneal fat through a small midline fascial defect. Epiploceles may present as an acute abdomen because of incarceration and strangulation of the fat, and in that circumstance the patient requires a prompt surgical evaluation. Most often epiploceles present as an undiagnosed soft-tissue nodule; for those lesions that are symptomatic or that seem to be enlarging, we recommend elective surgical excision with closure of the fascial defect.

LATERAL ABDOMINAL WALL LESIONS

Lateral abdominal wall protrusions include the very rare lumbar hernia located in the posterior lateral lumbar triangle. A spigelian hernia is similarly rare and occurs along the lateral border of the rectus abdominus muscle where it interdigitates with the oblique musculature. Both lumbar and spigelian hernias may require elective and, rarely, urgent surgical repair of the fascial weakness; but their major interest is their very infrequent occurrence and peculiar presentation.

Inguinal hernia represents failure of closure of the processus vaginalis, an obliteration that occurs in the last trimester of pregnancy, and appears later on the patient's right side. Patency of the processus vaginalis may result in a physiologic hydrocele in which case the proximal processus has been obliterated, but fluid has been trapped in the distal scrotum; it may produce a hydrocele of the spermatic cord in which there is a loculation of fluid in the mid-processus vaginalis with a proximal patency; or it may produce a frank communicating or hernia-hydrocele in which the entire processus is patent and is filled either with fluid from the abdominal cavity or with other intra-abdominal contents, depending on the diameter of the neck of the hydrocele sac. A physiologic hydrocele is characterized by a mild scrotal swelling that had been present since birth, and there is neither a history of a suprapubic bulging nor of intermittent scrotal size change. A hydrocele of the spermatic cord is represented by a swelling confined to the midinguinal canal with an empty space in the area of the deep inguinal ring. It is at times impossible to make a distinction between this lesion and an incarcerated inguinal hernia. If an ancillary rectal examination or cross table radiograph does not exclude an incarcerated inguinal hernia, then prompt surgical review and surgical exploration are indicated. A communicating hydrocele may also be noted in the newborn period but it is characterized by an intermittent scrotal size change. It is more appropriate to designate these lesions as an indirect inguinal hernia when the diameter of the neck of the patent processus vaginalis is large enough to accommodate other intra-abdominal contents such as omentum, the intestine, or an ovary. Inguinal hernias are more common in the premature child, on the right side, in boys, and in children with a family history of such hernias. An inguinal hernia should be electively repaired to prevent the potential complications of incarceration and strangulation. Though this complication is not common, occurring in only 5% to 10% of children, it is a devastating event that complicates the operative safety and repair of such a hernia.

The differential diagnosis of an inguinal canal swelling in the presence of a normally placed scrotal testis includes the following: an inguinal hernia, a hydrocele of the spermatic cord, or ilioinguinal lymphadenopathy, the latter being suggested especially in the presence of an infected distal extremity lesion. If the swelling is sudden in onset, if the child seems irritable with signs and symptoms of a partial bowel obstruction, and if the mass is tubular in nature extending out of the area of the deep inguinal ring, then an incarcerated inguinal hernia is the likely diagnosis. Emergency hernia reduction is best accomplished by the examiner applying simultaneous V-shaped distal traction with the upper hand at the area of the deep inguinal ring, while performing a distal-to-proximal transscrotal compression of the hernia contents with the lower hand. After reducing such an incarcerated hernia, hospital admission may be necessary and early elective surgical repair is indicated; but if the hernia cannot be reduced, then prompt surgical exploration is necessary to avoid strangulation of the contents of the hernia.

PERINEAL MASSES

SCROTUM

Undescended testis may arrest in descent anywhere within the abdomen, the inguinal canal, the medial-to-lateral thigh, or most commonly, the suprapubic pouch. It is also possible that the empty scrotum represents agenesis of the testis. The diagnosis of an undescended testicle requires a clear understanding of embryology and a relaxed child examined in a comfortable and warm environment. Undescended testicles most commonly need to be differentiated from the retractile testis in which the gonad can be identified, grasped, and pulled to the bottom of the scrotum. True undescended testes require elective surgical evaluation. However, the child presenting with pain and an acutely tender groin mass with the absence of a palpable testis in the scrotum on that side should be suspected of having either incarceration of a hernia associated with that undescended testis or torsion of the undescended testis. Testicular torsion itself is an uncommon event, but torsion of an undescended testis is statistically more likely. Such a diagnosis represents a true surgical emergency and testicular salvage is possible only by rapid surgical intervention.

Testicular torsion may also occur in the intrascrotal testis in which the gonad is twisted either extravaginally or intravaginally; and the twisted and foreshortened spermatic cord pulls the testis to the top of the scrotum. These suddenly tender scrotal masses usually are associated with pain, nausea, and vomiting and are absolute surgical emergencies requiring rapid differential diagnosis by physical examination, urinalysis, and use of Doppler ultrasound or nuclear medicine scanning to evaluate testicular blood flow. The differential diagnosis of a painful scrotal mass includes an incarcerated hernia, testicular torsion, acute epididymitis, and torsion of the appendix testis. The latter diagnosis is made by localizing a discrete tender spot on the spermatic cord-testis surface in a patient in whom scrotal pain is not severe. At times it is possible to visualize the infarcted tissue as a blue dot beneath the scrotal skin. Epididymitis may produce abnormal results on a urinalysis and it will produce an increased vascularity by either ultrasound or flow scanning techniques. Still another cause of the acutely tender scrotum is acute hemorrhage into a testicular tumor.

ANORECTUM

Anal fissures most often occur secondary to local anal canal trauma secondary to constipation. Fissures are the most common cause of bright red rectal bleeding in childhood and are best diagnosed by either direct physical inspection or by the use of limited proctoscopy with a proctoscope. Acute fissures are best treated by stool softeners, sitz baths, and rectal lubricants such as glycerin suppositories. Chronic fissures require elective surgery. Perianal abscesses require drainage and adequate decompression, a procedure best performed in the operating room. Drainage of a small abscess in an infant in the emergency room is also appropriate. Sitz baths help treat the acute inflammatory response and keep the area clean. A late appearing anal fistula extending from the crypts of the rectal glands through perianal soft tissue to the skin requires elective surgery. Perianal fistulae, fissures, and abscesses in older children may herald the presence of underlying inflammatory bowel disease.

Rectal prolapse may be without apparent cause or it may be associated with underlying chronic constipation, cystic fibrosis, or hookworm infestation. Usually the prolapsed rectum can be reduced with gentle compression. Efforts should be made to soften the stool, add a lubricant to the diet, and limit the time a child spends on the toilet. Surgery is rarely necessary.

Pilonidal dimples are common congenital variations in children. Such dimples may present only as a skin lesion over the sacrococcygeal area, or there might also be a subcutaneous sinus leading to a cyst beneath the skin. The acute pilonidal abscess may require incision and drainage, and elective surgical removal of such chronically infected areas is then indicated. For the shallow broad-based noninfected dimple, surgical referral or prophylactic excision is not indicated.

MASSES ON THE EXTREMITIES

CYSTS

A wrist ganglion, which is a synovial sheath cyst, is a common cystic lesion of the extremities. These are usually located on the dorsum of the wrist though they can be located in any joint or tendon synovial sheath area. These tense, spongy subcutaneous masses may produce discomfort that is treated best by splinting or joint rest, and a surgical referral can then be made to decide whether or not aspiration or excision is indicated. A Baker cyst represents a ganglionic type of synovial sheath cyst located in the popliteal space. These lesions may produce a mass as well as discomfort, and elective surgery is indicated.

VASCULAR MALFORMATIONS

Enlarged extremities (whether they be an arm or a leg) may occur over an entire half of the body or it may involve but one extremity. Such enlargement may be due to hemihypertrophy or to other vascular or lymphatic anomalies of the extremities. Hemihypertrophy should raise the suspicion of possible associated problems including a higher incidence of Wilms' tumor; and such children with diagnosed hemihypertrophy should be screened with serial renal ultrasound. Vascular extremity anomalies represent a tremendous challenge in treatment and usually they represent hemangioendotheliomas or mixed lymph-hemangiomas. Arteriovenous malformations may also be a part of such vascular hamartomas. Such vascular extremity lesions carry the same complications as vascular lesions elsewhere in the body (platelet trapping, high-output cardiac failure, bleeding following traumatic injury). An additional problem unique to the extremity vascular malformation is overgrowth of the hyperemic limb. All of these lesions require elective surgical review.

Lymphangiomas of the extremities are characterized by recurrent episodes of lymphangitis and cellulitis secondary to bacterial trapping in aberrant lymphatic channels. These lesions require repeated courses of antibiotic therapy; and there may be some benefit in utilizing chronic prophylactic antibiotics to suppress such infections. Lymphatic anomalies also include congenital lymphedema (Milroy disease) or traumatic lymphedema. Such abnormalities characterized by an intact arterial and venous system on examination require elective referral.

SKIN LESIONS

Integumentary lesions seen on the extremities of children include viral warts or verruca vulgaris producing local pain and discomfort or cosmetic problems only. Symptomatic plantar warts on the ventral surface of the feet can cause significant discomfort; and such children are best referred for elective treatment by the topical application of epidermal exfoliatives, electrodessication, or cryotherapy.

Nevi are classified as raised or flat, pigmented or nonpigmented, and are hair-bearing or hair-free. Spider nevi or spider angiomas represent true vascular hamartomas and are not true nevi. Nevi that are congenital do have a documented increased incidence of malignant degeneration, and such patients should be referred for either prolonged follow-up or for surgical excision. The presence of irritation and erythema, bleeding, growth, or darkening are all warning signs that biopsy and surgical excision should be considered. The location of a nevus on the plantar surface of the foot, the palm of the hand, or the genitalia are, per se, not indications to consider surgery.

BIBLIOGRAPHY

Koop CE: *Visible and Palpable Lesions in Children.* New York, Grune & Stratton, 1976.

63 MALIGNANT DISEASE

Steven A. Shapiro, D.O.

Malignant tumors that occur in children differ in many ways from those that occur in adults. Approximately half of all pediatric malignancies are not solid tumors, but are leukemia or its related lesions. When solid tumors do occur, they are sarcomas (tumors arising in connective tissue) that may grow to a considerable size or even metastasize before producing symptoms. Even the few adult tumor forms (such as epithelial tumors or carcinomas) seem to occur in solid viscera (adrenal, liver) rather than in hollow structures when they occur in childhood.

There are no efficient screening tests for cancer in children. Procedures such as a Papanicolaou smear or proctoscopic examinations are useless as screening modalities during childhood. A careful physical examination remains the technique yielding the greatest results. Physical findings may change rapidly as an examination may be negative for an abdominal mass one day and positive the next because of hemorrhage into the lesion or tumor growth lifting it out of a fossa. The primary care specialist who treats children must maintain an awareness that cancer does occur in childhood, and, therefore, any illness that presents as more than the typical transient childhood malady should have the possibility of malignancy included in its differential diagnosis.

Malignant disease may be recognized by three pathophysiologic mechanisms: (1) a mass lesion may be noted, (2) there may be unusual signs and symptoms, or (3) chronic vague symptoms may be persistent. In the first group, those patients whose presenting complaint is the tumor itself, the diagnosis can usually be made promptly. The advice to watch a lesion, with the expectancy and hope that it will disappear, should never be given. Except for an inflammatory lymph node or a hemangioma, mass lesions in children should not be expected to disappear. Any mass that is not diagnosed by characteristics of location (e.g., thyroglossal duct cyst) or specific cause (e.g., specific trauma) should be considered malignant until proved otherwise, and thus will require excisional biopsy of the entire mass.

In those patients who have unusual symptoms that are directly referrable to the tumor, the physician will be able to make the diagnosis if there is a high index of suspicion for cancer. These signs and symptoms include problems such as unusual bleeding from the gums or rectum in leukemia, girdle pain or limb dysfunction with a spinal cord tumor, repetitive morning vomiting or staggering ataxic gait with a brain tumor, and hematuria from a Wilms tumor. If cancer is not routinely considered as a diagnostic possibility, then these patients will not be able to receive therapy while the disease is still manageable.

The third group are those children with no symptoms at all, or with symptoms so nonspecific that they resemble the vague complaints of any number of more likely diagnoses. These forms of cancer are most often diagnosed late. In some patients, nonspecific symptoms are misconstrued as behavior problems. In others the tumor produces low-grade fevers, fretfulness, and failure to thrive. Again, the only way such a clinical picture can lead to the correct diagnosis is by having a high index of suspicion for cancer. In working with pediatric patients, there is a psychological barrier to overcome as no one likes to entertain a diagnosis as unpleasant as cancer. The physician must remain alert that signs and symptoms produced by a malignant tumor are not misdiagnosed because they mimic other more acceptable diagnoses.

A caring and devoted primary care physician guided by the results of several key evaluations can reasonably be the major force in easing the family's shock and profound grief when the diagnosis of cancer in the child becomes a reality. However, before any discussion of the disease takes place, it is essential that the diagnosis is not in doubt. It is unwise to base the conversation on preliminary tests to avoid subsequent qualifications or retractions.

In the remaining portions of this chapter, the most common childhood malignancies will be reviewed, with emphasis on their presenting signs and symptoms. An approach toward making the diagnosis by the primary care physician in the local setting will also be recommended (see related Chapters 15, 38, 39, 41, 43, and 62).

ACUTE LEUKEMIA

Less than a generation ago, there was no effective therapy for acute lymphocytic leukemia (ALL) of childhood. Spontaneous remissions are rare in ALL, and at the time of diagnosis the average patient could have been expected to survive only a few months. Today, remission can be induced in 90% of patients, and 5-year leukemia-free survival rates can be expected in at least 60%. It is the most common malignancy of childhood occurring in nearly 4/100,000 children under the age of 14 years.

DATA GATHERING

The patient may present with a myriad of apparently disconnected symptoms suggesting renal, neurologic, or even cardiac disease. Table 63–1 summarizes the most common presenting complaints among children along with their frequency. Carefully question parents about fever, infections that persist and pains in the

TABLE 63–1
Frequency of the More Common Presenting Complaints Among Children

FINDING	PERCENT
Fever	61
Pallor	55
Hemorrhage	52
Anorexia	33
Fatigue	30
Bone pain	23
Abdominal pain	19
Joint pain	15
Lymphadenopathy	15
Weight loss	13

From Sutow WW, Vietti TJ, Fernbach DC: *Clinical Pediatric Oncology*, ed 3. St Louis, CV Mosby Co, 1980. Used by permission.

TABLE 63–2
Presenting Characteristics of 1,024 Patients With Acute Leukemia as Reported by The Southwest Oncology Group

CHARACTERISTIC	PERCENT
Age (yr)	
<2	14
2–5	47
6–10	24
>11	15
White blood cell count (1,000/cu mm)	
<10	34
10–24	25
25–49	22
>50	19
Hemoglobin (gm/100 ml)	
<7	44
7–11	43
>11	14
Sex (male)	57
Race (white)	85
Hemorrhage (yes)	48
Blasts (%)	
<65	25
65–84	22
85–94	28
≥95	25
Platelets (1,000/cu mm)	
20	29
20–49	23
50–99	20
≥100	29
Liver enlarged	79
Spleen enlarged	69
Cervical nodes enlarged	62
Inguinal nodes enlarged	54
Axillary nodes enlarged	47

From Sutow WW, Vietti TJ, Fernbach DC: *Clinical Pediatric Oncology*, ed 3, St Louis, CV Mosby Co, 1980. Used by permission.

chest, bones, joints, and back. This pain may not be severe and can take many forms. Determine if there has been an increase in the frequency of nosebleeds or easy bruising; ask about lumps or masses. Finally, verify abdominal enlargement, which may suggest hepatosplenomegaly, by asking how the child's clothing has fit recently.

On physical examination, the child with acute leukemia may have a slightly elevated temperature (101° to 102° F). The conjunctival membrane in the eye and the nailbeds may be pale or there may be boggy or bleeding gums. Lymph nodes may be palpated in the neck, groin, and axilla, or there may be splenomegaly and hepatomegaly. In boys, the testes should be carefully palpated for enlargement or change in consistency. Infiltration with leukemic cells is the most likely causative factor if this is noted.

Several basic laboratory tests are all that are needed to initially indicate the diagnosis of leukemia. A complete blood cell (CBC) count, with differential cell, platelet, and reticulocyte counts, along with a serum chemistry profile including urea nitrogen, creatinine, uric acid, calcium, and liver function studies are usually sufficient. Table 63–2 summarizes the presenting characteristics of leukemia in one large pediatric cancer study group. Further classification as to cell type, morphologic characteristics, and leukemia cell surface markers should be performed at the facility where treatment is to be started. With careful guidance by the primary care physician, this transition to the referral center can be accomplished with expediency and with thoughtful concern toward the emotional support of the family.

NON-HODGKIN LYMPHOMA

Non-Hodgkin lymphomas (NHL) are malignant tumors that originate in lymphatic tissues (e.g., lymph nodes, mesentery, Peyer patches, appendix, and, rarely, spleen). Extralymphatic sites of origin include bone, ovaries, and skin. In contrast to the adult forms in which the disease can remain indolent and localized for years, childhood NHL has a tendency to proliferate rapidly and spread outside the primary site in weeks to months. Metastasis occurs to the bone marrow and central nervous system (CNS). If extensive marrow involvement occurs, the distinction between NHL and acute leukemia may be extremely difficult. The types of lymphomas seen in children are almost always poorly differentiated and diffuse, and they entirely efface the architecture of the tissue of origin.

Classification of NHL is controversial. Histologic, cytologic, and immunologic studies are readily employed, and the tumors are also classified according to stage that reflects the degree of tumor burden. The staging system described in the section on Data Gathering is best suited to pediatric NHL that often presents as Stage III or IV disease.

Non-Hodgkin lymphomas usually occur before puberty or in early adolescence. The childhood incidence is 0.5 cases/100,000 children under 15 years. Patients with any form of immunodeficiency state, either inherited or acquired, have an exceptionally high incidence of NHL. Those patients having undergone renal or cardiac transplant, patients receiving chronic immunosuppressive therapy, and patients with Hodgkin disease treated with radiation therapy and chemotherapy have an unusually high incidence of NHL.

DATA GATHERING

About 25% of NHL in childhood presents as a stage I or II disease; Murphy's clinical staging classification suited for children with NHL is presented below. The presentations can include localized swelling in the cervical or inguinal nodes, nasopharyngeal masses, mediastinal masses, bone pain, and an "acute" abdomen.

MURPHY'S CLASSIFICATION

Stage I

Single nodal or extranodal tumor with the exclusion of mediastinum or abdomen

Stage II

Single extranodal tumor with regional involvement of the lymph nodes or two or more lymph node areas on the same side of the diaphragm

Resectable primary gastrointestinal tract tumor (usually ileocecal), with or without involvement of mesenteric lymph nodes

Stage III

Intrathoracic tumors

Extensive unresectable intra-abdominal disease

Paraspinal or epidural tumors.

Two single tumors on opposite sides of the diaphragm

Stage IV

Any of the above with involvement of CNS, bone marrow, or both

While African Burkitt lymphoma, a form of NHL, arises in the jaw in over half of the patients, this is an uncommon finding in American patients, in whom only 20% of lesions occur in the jaw and about 15% arise in cervical lymph nodes. American Burkitt lymphoma usually causes generalized abdominal enlargement, pain, nausea, vomiting, constipation, and, in half of the cases, malignant ascites. The above symptoms can also suggest a primary tumor arising in the ovaries or in retroperitoneal lymph nodes, but kidney and bowel are sometimes involved. Burkitt tumor cells proliferate exceedingly rapidly, which allows the tumor to extend locally over a period of days to weeks. This usually leads to ascites, pleural effusion, and renal failure. Extension of the disease to the meninges and bone marrow is common. If untreated, the tumor is rapidly fatal, usually due to renal failure. Even when treated, the disease tends to recur within a few months either in the abdomen or as leukemia.

Mediastinal NHL occurs commonly in boys during late childhood or early adolescence. If untreated, metastasis to bone marrow, CNS, and testes is quite common. Presenting signs and symptoms include the presence of a bulky thoracic tumor in the anterior mediastinum, which may be associated with cardiovascular or circulatory (superior vena cava syndrome) compromise.

MANAGEMENT

When localized NHL is suspected, a biopsy of the lymph node or mass should be obtained promptly. Prior to this, chest radiographs and CBC counts are essential to make certain that there is neither a mediastinal mass nor any evident leukemic process. Once the primary care physician has ascertained a suggestion of the type of process involved, expedient referral for definitive therapy should be accomplished.

Combination therapy with surgery and chemotherapy, with or without radiation therapy, can make the prognosis for local NHL excellent.

HODGKIN DISEASE

Like NHL, Hodgkin disease is a malignancy of the lymph nodes. Usually it begins in a cervical lymph node and spreads in a predictable and orderly sequence from one lymph node region to the next. If left untreated, it progresses to involve organs outside the lymph nodes. In contrast to NHL, spread to the bone marrow and CNS is rare. The malignant cell in Hodgkin disease is the Reed-Sternberg cell, which is thought to originate from either a B-lymphocyte or a histiocyte precursor.

Hodgkin disease is classified according to the extent of disease at presentation and the histologic composition of the involved lymph node. As a general rule, the greater the number of lymphocytes and the fewer the Reed-Sternberg cells, the better the prognosis.

The incidence of Hodgkin disease is similar to that of NHL; 0.6 cases per 100,000 children under 15 years. Although Hodgkin disease has been reported in infants, it is rare in children under 5 years of age. In the United States Hodgkin disease tends to occur in the higher socioeconomic classes. There has been much literature about a possible viral etiology of Hodgkin disease, but these studies have been difficult to confirm. However, it has been established that Hodgkin disease patients have higher antibody titers than other children to the Epstein-Barr virus.

DATA GATHERING

Hodgkin disease most often manifests as a mass in the neck; about 4% of the cases present as masses in the groin. The mass may have been present for days, months, or years. Some patients initially complain of adenopathy localized to a few lymph node regions; others notice generalized adenopathy. Anterior mediastinal masses occur in one half of the patients. Nonetheless, large mediastinal Hodgkin tumors can present with the same cardiovascular or respiratory symptoms as mediastinal NHL. Most patients with Hodgkin disease are well, but 30% will present with fever and involuntary weight loss. At the time of diagnosis, the fever may be low grade or high grade. The typical Pel-Ebstein fever, a high debilitating fever followed by a drenching sweat, is usually a sign of very advanced disease.

MANAGEMENT

In the past, the majority of patients in the United States underwent staging laparotomy and splenectomy. Treatment with large-field radiation therapy and with multiagent chemotherapy has made it apparent that most patients with Hodgkin disease can be cured. However, it has been shown that splenectomy carries a high risk of hyperacute pneumococcal infection in children. Furthermore, radiation causes major growth disturbances in children under 18 years. On the other hand, chemotherapy and large-field irradiation predisposes to the development of leukemia and NHL in approximately 5% of patients. In view of the above, many pediatric oncology centers are beginning to investigate staging procedures without laparotomy and to use different combinations of chemotherapy in association with lower doses and smaller fields of radiation therapy to attain long-term disease control. Thus, it is important for the primary care physician to begin the process of defining the extent of disease from the moment it is recognized. A CBC count with sedimentation rate and chest radiograph are minimal procedures to ascertain the full extent of the disease. Furthermore, lymph node biopsy can be attempted if tissue is easily accessible. Once histologically confirmed, the child should be referred to a physician with special expertise in handling childhood Hodgkin disease for the purpose of planning the therapeutic approach.

HISTIOCYTOSIS

Histiocytic diseases include a heterogenous group of benign and malignant disorders in which the cell of origin, the histiocyte (tissue macrophage), appears to be the predominant cell type. It is invariably difficult to determine whether the histiocytes are benign or malignant. They may appear histologically benign and metastasize, and conversely they can appear histologically malignant and behave with relatively benignity.

DATA GATHERING

Recent studies have brought order into the classification of histiocytic diseases by grouping them pathophysiologically into three groups: (1) lipid storage diseases; (2) reactive diseases, including what was formerly called histiocytosis X and familial erythrophagocytic lymphohistiocytosis; and (3) neoplastic diseases, which include histiocytic medullary reticulosis and acute monocytic leukemia. The distinction between these diseases is often impossible to clarify.

The spectrum of eosinophilic granuloma syndromes includes solitary eosinophilic granulomas in bone, multiple eosinophilic granulomas of bone, and disseminated eosinophilic granuloma (Letterer-Siwe disease). A solitary eosinophilic granuloma presents as a painless or mildly painful swelling in the skull, long bones, ribs, pelvis, or vertebrae. Radiologically the lesion is lytic with well-defined borders.

When there are multiple eosinophilic granulomas arising over an extended period in long bones or the skull, changes in the skull can occur that cause proptosis, diabetes insipidus, cholesteatoma, or loss of teeth (Hand-Schüller-Christian disease). Occasionally, paraplegia has resulted from this process.

When widespread eosinophilic granulomas in bone and soft tissue occur in an infant, Letterer-Siwe disease is the usual cause. Typical signs and symptoms include failure to thrive, chronic seborrhea, chronic otitis media, purpuric rash, generalized adenopathy, and hepatosplenomegaly. Chest radiographs may demonstrate interstitial pneumonitis. The CBC count may be normal, but bone marrow involvement or splenomegaly may lead to pancytopenia.

MANAGEMENT

The primary physician should consider histiocytic diseases in those infants with constitutional signs and symptoms of failure to thrive and in young children who present with bone lesions unassociated with any other signs of a neoplastic process.

BRAIN TUMORS

Children with tumors of the CNS present a difficult problem for any pediatric practitioner's care. They are the most common solid tumors in children, with an incidence second only to the leukemias. In the United States, approximately 1,200 new cases of primary childhood CNS tumors are diagnosed yearly. The past two decades of clinical research have seen the advent of newer diagnostic techniques along with improvements in anesthesia, surgery, radiation therapy, and hormonal replacement therapy. With these newer modalities, a note of cautious optimism with respect to brain tumor therapy and the resultant quality of life may be offered to the family.

The precise etiology of brain tumors is not known, but hereditary and environmental factors are contributing causes. Hereditary diseases such as neurocutaneous syndromes are associated with intracranial neoplasms. Approximately 15% of children with neurofibromatosis will develop intracranial tumors, which are usually cerebral, hypothalamic, or optic gliomas. Children with tuberous sclerosis develop intracranial lesions as well. These are usually subcortical hamartomas and subependymal low-grade astrocytomas. Von Hippel-Lindau disease is seen in association with retinal angiomatosis and cerebellar hemangioblastoma. Families have been reported in which several siblings have developed brain tumors. A less common occurrence is the association of medulloblastoma with the autosomal dominant basal cell nevus syndrome.

Environmental factors that have been implicated in the etiology of brain tumors include ionizing radiation, presumed infectious agents in animals, and industrial toxic exposure. There are intriguing reports of the increased incidence of brain tumors among children of parents who are employed in the chemical or aircraft industry.

DATA GATHERING

The inherent nature of the child is to persist at as normal a level of activity for as long as possible. This is all too often the case when discussing tumors of the CNS. Symptoms are usually determined by the location of the tumor in association with age of the child. In Table 63–3, the location and relative frequency of occurrence is defined. Tumor histologic composition and relative frequency of occurrence are organized in Table 63–4.

Most childhood tumors are in the posterior fossa and cause their first symptoms by com-

TABLE 63–3
Location of Pediatric Brain Tumors*

LOCATION	PERCENT
Posterior fossa	60
Supratentorial	40
Midline region	15
Cerebral hemispheres	25

*From Walker RW, Allen JC: Pediatric brain tumors. *Pediatr Ann* 1983; 12:383.

TABLE 63–4
Incidence of Brain Tumors by Tumor Histology*

TYPE OF TUMOR	PERCENT
Medulloblastoma	20
Astrocytoma (cerebellar)	17
Astrocytoma (other)	16
Glioblastoma	5
Ependymoma	9
Craniopharyngioma	8
Optic nerve glioma	5
Meningioma	2
Pineal (germinoma)	2
Other†	16

*From Bell WE, McCormick WF: Increased intracranial pressure in children. Philadelphia, WB Saunders Co, 1978.
†These included sarcomas, pituitary adenomas, oligodendrogliomas, and primitive neuroectodermal tumors.

pression of the fourth ventricle, leading to increased intracranial pressure and hydrocephalus. In one series, 86% of almost 300 children with the diagnosis of brain tumors presented with signs of increased intracranial pressure, manifested as headache, vomiting, and episodic "gray-out" of vision. These findings are often associated with signs of cerebellar dysfunction such as gait disturbance (ataxia), hemiparesis, behavioral changes, dementia, diplopia, vertigo, and visual difficulties. Table 63–5 summarizes the most common presenting symptoms and their frequency.

The most common presentation usually begins with a bifrontal or diffuse headache that often occurs in early morning just after awakening, and remits within 1 or 2 hours. Its pathogenesis is unknown. Occasionally, the headache is abrupt in onset, short-lived, and is associated with exercise, change in position, or transient increases in thoracic pressure. These headaches, associated with the maneuvers

TABLE 63–5
Common Presenting Symptoms of Brain Tumors*

SYMPTOM	PERCENT
Raised intracranial pressure	85
Headache	70
Vomiting	75
Episodic blindness	10
Disturbance of gait	40
Mental symptoms	35
Diplopia	25
Vertigo	25
Hemiparesis	15
Seizures	10
Head tilt	10

*From Gjerris F: Clinical aspects and long-term prognosis of intracranial tumors in infancy and childhood. *Dev Med Child Neurol* 1976; 18:145–159. Used by permission.

listed, are due to a sudden rise in intracranial pressure and are called *plateau waves.* These tend to last 10 to 20 minutes.

Cerebellar signs depend on the location within the cerebellum. Medulloblastoma and ependymomas are usually midline lesions arising in the region of the fourth ventricle. Lesions in this area will produce truncal ataxia and result in a broad-based gait. Cerebellar astrocytomas are most often confined to one hemisphere and produce an ipsilateral ataxia in the limbs and loss of fine motor coordination. Nystagmus is another frequent sign of cerebellar tumors. While head tilt is an uncommon finding, the physician evaluating the condition of the child with this complaint should make a careful neurologic assessment, looking specifically for asymmetry. The child will hold his neck flexed toward the side of the lesion and will invariably resist attempts at passive movement.

Gliomas involving the brain stem generally infiltrate the region without causing ventricular obstruction. They will more often show various cranial nerve abnormalities and long-tract signs such as spastic gait, hemiparesis, and up-going toes (Babinski sign).

Supratentorial lesions have various clinical presentations. A rapidly growing cerebral glioma will produce focal neurologic deficits, seizures, or both. These are caused by pressure from the tumor and its surrounding edema on contiguous structures.

Temporal lobe lesions often are responsible for visual field defects, while frontal lesions can cause hemiparesis.

Despite the multiplicity of presentations with CNS disease, the diagnosis of an intracranial neoplasm can, in the majority of cases, be made on the basis of a history and careful neurologic examination. In the younger child, the skull should be checked for local tenderness, a "cracked-pot sound" (Macewen sign) with gentle percussion, bossing of the frontal or parietal bones, venous congestion, and exophthalmos. Computed tomography (CT) scans and magnetic resonance (MR) imaging have revolutionized the diagnostic evaluation of the child suspected of having an intracranial neoplasm. When a positive scan is obtained, angiography gives further information about blood supply to the tumor and degree of vascularity, as well as further definition as to location. These combined modalities in association with the operating microscope have given the neurosurgeons the most advantageous position ever in contemplating a surgical approach, with the greatest likelihood for as complete a resection as clinically possible.

TABLE 63–6
Tumors in Upper Abdomen*

BENIGN	MALIGNANT
Renal	
Hydronephrosis	Wilms tumor
Polycystic kidney	Adenocarcinoma
Benign neoplasms	
Renal hypertrophy	
Adrenal	
Adrenal hyperplasia	Neuroblastoma
Benign neoplasms	Ganglioneuroblastoma
	Adenocarcinoma
	Pheochromocytoma
Liver	
Hepatosplenomegaly	Hepatoblastoma
Benign neoplasms	Hepatocellular carcinoma
Benign hyperplasia	Metastatic tumor

*From Jones PG, Campbell PE: *Tumors of Infancy and Childhood.* Oxford, England, Blackwell Scientific Publications Inc, 1976. Used by permission.

ABDOMINAL, GENITOURINARY, AND RETROPERITONEAL TUMORS

The discovery of an abdominal mass requires an immediate orderly investigation to determine its precise nature. As is the case with many signs and symptoms in pediatrics, the etiology of the masses differs among infants and children of various ages. The spectrum of intra-abdominal and pelvic tumors is summarized in Tables 63–6 and 63–7.

DATA GATHERING

Wilms tumor and neuroblastoma are the most common intra-abdominal neoplasms of young children. Wilms tumor presents as a large flank mass in a well child; abdominal neuroblastoma, outside of infancy, presents as a midline or flank mass in an ill child. Hepatic tumors are sometimes associated with systemic illness. Tumors arising in the pelvis, regardless of cause, may first cause neurologic deficits or abdominal pain.

For most of these tumors, staging usually depends on the amount of tumor that has been removed surgically. Stage I tumors are usually those that are completely removed. If there is microscopic or gross residual or if there is spread to regional lymph nodes, the tumor is considered stage II or III. Tumors presenting with wide-spread distant metastasis to other organ systems are considered stage IV. Histologic classification is apparent for each tumor category and has gained in significance only recently as survival has improved.

WILMS TUMOR

Wilms tumor (nephroblastoma), the most common intrarenal neoplasm of childhood, is an embryonal neoplasm of mixed histologic composition. About 5% of all Wilms tumor occurs bilaterally. Wilms tumor occurs in approximately 8 in 1,000,000 children under 15 years of age; 65% of children presenting with Wilms tumor are under 5 years. There is a significant association between Wilms tumor and congenital anomalies, including aniridia, hemihypertrophy, genitourinary anomalies, hemangiomas, hamartomas, and cardiac anomalies. There are several case reports of familial Wilms tumor as well as reports of families in which some of the members had the congenital anomalies listed above, while other members had Wilms tumor.

TABLE 63–7
Tumors of Lower Abdomen and Genitalia*

BENIGN	MALIGNANT
Retroperitoneum	
Presacral teratoma	Soft-tissue sarcoma
Anterior meningomyelocele	Bone sarcoma
	Lymphoma
Ganglioneuroma	Neuroblastoma
Lipoma	Teratoma
Bladder and urethra	
Abscess	Rhabdomyosarcoma
Ureterocele	Leiomyosarcoma
Polyp	
Neurogenic bladder	
Bowel	
Appendicitis	Lymphoma
Feces	Adenocarcinoma
Duplication cyst	Carcinoid
Carcinoid	
Female genitalia	
Vagina	
Cysts	Rhabdomyosarcoma
Hydrocolpos	Clear-cell sarcoma
Hematocolpos	Endodermal sinus
Adenoma	
Neurofibroma	
Uterus and fallopian tubes	
Abscess	Rhabdomyosarcoma
Papilloma	Adenocarcinoma
	Embryonal carcinoma
Ovary	
Teratoma	Teratoma
Cyst	Dysgerminoma
Granulosa theca cell	Arrhenoblastoma
Fibroma	Adenocarcinoma
Hemangioma	Choriocarcinoma
	Metastatic tumor
Male genitalia	
Prostate gland	
Abscess	Rhabdomyosarcoma
Testis	
Hydrocele	Rhabdomyosarcoma
Testicular torsion	Embryonal carcinoma
Orchitis	Seminoma
Teratoma	Leukemia
Leydig or Sertoli cell tumor	
Spermatic Cord	
Hydrocele	Rhabdomyosarcoma
Hernia	Leukemia
Inflammation	
Adrenal rest	
Benign tumors of connective tissue	

*From Jones PG, Campbell PE: *Tumors of Infancy and Childhood.* Oxford, England, Blackwell Scientific Publications Inc, 1976. Used by permission.

DATA GATHERING

The majority of children with Wilms tumor have an abdominal mass discovered accidentally by their parents while bathing or clothing the child or by the physician on routine physical examination. The mass is solitary and deep in the flank and can be either firm or soft. Abdominal pain, fever, anorexia, malaise, vomiting, and weight loss are rare presenting complaints. Gross hematuria occurs in less than 25% of the cases and usually indicates invasion of the renal pelvis with tumor. Hypertension, seen in a small number of patients, is thought to be the result of excessive renin secretion secondary to renal artery compression. By a related mechanism, polycythemia occasionally occurs. More often, anemia results from bleeding into the tumor.

In performing the physical examination, the physician should note the size of the liver and spleen, the site and size of the mass, blood pressure, and the presence of any of the congenital abnormalities listed above. Laboratory evaluation should include determination of CBC count, BUN, and creatinine. Radiographs of the abdomen (kidneys, ureters, bladder [KUB]) may disclose a mass-displacing bowel. Intravenous pyelography (IVP) usually demonstrates the intrarenal mass that distorts the calyces (Fig 63–1). In those cases in which the kidney is not visualized, ultrasound can usually demonstrate the mass.

At this point, children with a presumed Wilms tumor should be referred to a (pediatric) surgeon experienced in the diagnosis and treatment of this tumor. Wilms tumor exemplifies the advances of multimodal therapy in the pediatric oncology center; disease-free survival rates now approach 90%. Even patients with metastatic disease or bilateral tumors can be treated successfully.

NEUROBLASTOMA

Neuroblastoma is a malignant tumor arising from sympathetic tissue in the adrenal medulla, or in the sympathetic chain along the craniospinal axis in the neck, posterior mediastinum, the pelvis, or intra-abdominally. This tumor commonly metastasizes to bone, bone marrow, skin, liver, and lymph nodes.

After CNS tumors, neuroblastoma is the most

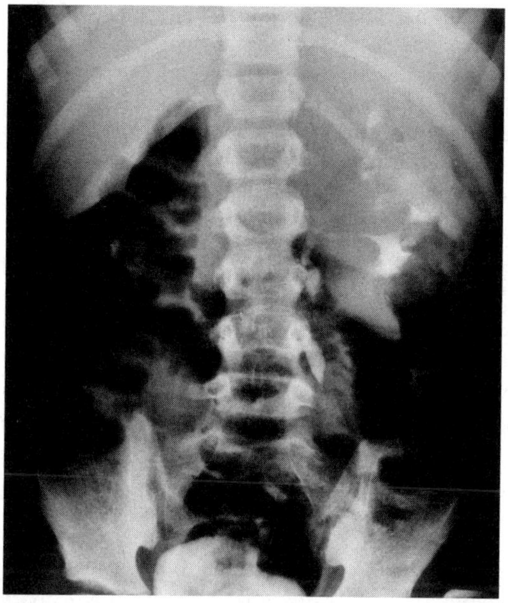

FIG 63–1
Wilms tumor. Displacement of collecting system can be seen on left.

common solid tumor of childhood. Approximately 50% occur in children before the age of 2 years and 80% are found in children under 5 years. Neuroblastoma occurs in approximately 1/100,000 children under 16 years.

DATA GATHERING

Approximately two thirds of patients present with widespread metastases. Signs and symptoms include irritability, anorexia, weight loss, pallor, and subcutaneous lumps. Adrenal neuroblastoma, as well as nonadrenal intra-abdominal tumors, can cause a palpable abdominal mass. When the cervical sympathetic ganglia are involved, Horner syndrome (ptosis, miosis, anhidrosis) can be seen on the affected side, or hoarseness arising from recurrent laryngeal nerve compression can occur. Spinal cord compression syndrome can occur when neuroblastoma arising in sympathetic ganglia extend into and out of the intervertebral foramina. This is often referred to as a "dumbbell tumor." Thus, rapidly occurring paraplegia in a child under 5 years old should be considered neuroblastoma unless another cause has been proved. Skeletal lesions lead to bone pain or pathologic fractures. When periorbital metastasis occurs, proptosis and periorbital ecchymosis or "black eyes" are noted. The physician should not confuse these black eyes for those associated with battered children. Rarer presentations include opsomyoclonus ("dancing eyes-dancing feet"), hypertension, tachycardia, skin flushing, and chronic diarrhea all manifested as a result of excessive catecholamine secretion from the tumor itself.

Patients with a rare characteristic of neuroblastoma (noted as stage IV-S) demonstrate the ability of the tumor to undergo spontaneous regression or mature to a more benign lesion. These children present in the first few months of life with gross hepatomegaly or skin nodules. The primary tumor may not be obvious. When the primary physician encounters massive hepatomegaly in an otherwise healthy-appearing child, the diagnosis of stage IV-S neuroblastoma should be considered.

Once neuroblastoma is suspected, the evaluation should include a CBC count, IVP, chest radiograph, skeletal survey, bone scan, and bone marrow aspiration and biopsy. The latter two procedures are best performed by those physicians prepared to treat the tumor. All patients should have quantitative evaluation of urinary catecholamine levels, including vanillylmandelic acid (VMA) and homovanillic acid (HVA), along with other serologic markers available to assess the aggressiveness of the tumor.

Even though the majority of these tumors respond initially to therapy, most will become refractory to treatment and the disease is invariably fatal.

SOFT TISSUE SARCOMAS

These tumors are derived from mesenchymal tissue: muscle, tendon, nerve, fat, and endothelium. Less common are fibrosarcoma, neurofibrosarcoma, synovial sarcoma, mesenchymoma, malignant fibrous histiocytoma, and leiomyosarcoma. Rhabdomyosarcoma arises from striated muscle and is the most common soft-tissue sarcoma of children under 15 years, accounting for 6% of all pediatric malignancies. The annual incidence of this tumor is 8.4 in 1,000,000 white children and 3.9 in 1,000,000 black children. Approximately 70% of cases present before the child is 10 years old. The peak incidence is between 2 to 6 years of age (median age, 5 years).

Soft tissue sarcomas are classified according to their apparent tissue of origin as can be seen from the various less common varieties mentioned above. Rhabdomyosarcoma is further subdivided according to histologic subtypes (embryonal, alveolar, or pleomorphic) and with respect to the extent of disease after surgery.

DATA GATHERING

Sarcomas usually occur as a lump in soft tissues. This may be painless or painful and specific symptoms may depend on the location of the tumor. Orbital tumors cause rapidly developing unilateral proptosis. Nasopharyngeal tumors can present with recurrent epistaxis, chronic sinusitis, chronic nasal obstruction, or dysphagia. Middle ear rhabdomyosarcoma can cause chronic otitis media, ear pain, and cranial nerve palsies. Neck tumors can cause dysphagia, hoarseness, or simply a painless lump in the posterior cervical triangle. Urinary tract obstruction or constipation is usually produced when rhabdomyosarcoma arises in the bladder or the prostate. In girls, sarcoma botryoides of the vagina or uterus may present as protrusion of hemorrhagic polyps from the introitus. In a paratesticular region, the tumor presents as an expanding nontender mass in the scrotum, usually located above and separate from the testis; this mass may be confused with a hernia and may be associated with a hydrocele. In the extremities or trunk, a painless mass is the most frequent presentation. Metastasis commonly occurs to the lungs, CNS, bones, liver, bone marrow, and regional lymph nodes. Head and neck tumors usually extend to the base of the skull.

All children with this histologic diagnosis proven with biopsy should have a CBC count and bone marrow evaluation. Radiography of the primary tumor site, the lungs, and a skeletal survey should be performed. Additionally, bone and liver scans should be obtained. All patients with head and neck tumors should undergo tomography of the base of the skull and/or whole-brain CT. Other tests, such as examination of cerebrospinal fluid, IVP, MR imaging, cystography, lymphangiography, and gallium scanning may be indicated depending on the primary site of the tumor.

The primary care physician, when confronted with a soft-tissue mass in a child, should consider cancer in the differential diagnosis and promptly begin the evaluation and biopsy of the mass, or refer the child to a physician or surgeon trained in the care and treatment of the disease. No therapy should be instituted until the final outcome of the staging procedures listed above are available.

BONE TUMORS

Malignant tumors of bone are sarcomas that arise from the cells of cortical or cancellous bone (osteogenic sarcoma), cartilaginous bone (chondrosarcoma), periosteum (periosteal sarcoma), or reticuloendothelial cells of the marrow (Ewing's tumor). For practical purposes, osteosarcoma and Ewing's tumor are the only malignant bone tumors with which the primary care physician should be familiar.

Osteosarcoma and Ewing's tumor are most common during adolescence, with 50% of the cases diagnosed in the second decade. Approximately 300 cases are diagnosed in the United States each year, giving an incidence of approximately 3 in 1,000,000 children under the age of 15 years. Sixty percent of all osteosarcomas occur just above or below the knee. While osteosarcoma shows no racial predilection, Ewing's tumor is an exceedingly rare tumor in blacks. Despite the well-documented association of osteosarcoma with ionizing radiation, most adolescent patients with osteosarcoma have had no excessive exposure to sources of radiation. Likewise, the cause of Ewing's tumor is largely unknown.

DATA GATHERING

All patients with malignant bone tumors complain of pain or a painful lump that frequently is realized after a notable episode of trauma. This may occasionally be associated with hemorrhage into the tumor. The pain is usually at night and may awaken the patient. While most patients with osteosarcoma are well, approximately one-third of those with Ewing's tumor will have some constitutional symptoms such as fever, weight loss, anorexia, and malaise.

When the tumor occurs in an extremity, examination may reveal a hard, tender swelling.

Larger tumors may feel warm, owing to increased vascularity. Trunk lesions, especially those arising in the pelvis, are difficult to diagnose. Since the mass is buried deep in gluteal tissue, neither radiography nor physical examination may offer any clues. Meticulous neurologic tests, having the patient walk on the heels and toes, stand on either leg, and flex and abduct the hips in concert with superficial and deep-tendon reflex symmetry, may provide findings of some abnormalities.

Bone tumors usually require radiographs and a biopsy of the lesion for confirmation. Plain radiographs will reveal changes associated with a destructive process in bone. "Codman's triangle" created from periosteal elevation and the typical "sunburst" appearance produced by tumor blood vessels growing perpendicularly into extracortical tumor tissue are seen. Later, one may see an "onion skin" periosteal reaction caused by repetitive episodes of the lesion pushing out the periosteum and the periosteum responding by producing calcium.

A bone scan or MR image will be especially useful in diagnosing Ewing's tumor if the history and physical examination suggest that trauma alone cannot account for the pain. Other studies including determinations of CBC count, sedimentation rate, serum lactic dehydrogenase in Ewing's tumor, and serum alkaline phosphatase in osteogenic sarcoma are often useful. A chest radiograph should be obtained to determine whether there are obvious metastases. This can be correlated further with chest CT.

Once any infectious process has been ruled out, a biopsy is indicated. This should be performed by an orthopedic surgeon who has expertise in the total management of neoplastic bone lesions. The clinical course of osteosarcoma is that of a highly malignant neoplasm. The tumor rapidly disseminates hematogenously, with pulmonary metastases generally being the first site of recurrent disease. Prior to recent advances in therapy, metastatic disease occurred within 6 to 9 months from the time of diagnosis, with death ensuing 6 months later. Following the development of pulmonary metastases, dissemination to other bones and visceral organs frequently occurs. With more effective chemotherapy, the incidence of metastases has decreased and those patients who still do develop pulmonary metastases tend to have fewer with a later onset.

THE CONCEPT OF CURE

Defining "cure" for a child with cancer is not simple. Terms such as "long-term disease-free survival" or "no evident disease" are more likely expressions of our own clinical inadequacies. An equally important problem is that the disease and its treatment are frequently associated with sequelae that prevent complete restoration to normal health or that alter subsequent growth and development.

The primary care clinician should realize that the diagnosis and treatment of cancer, albeit far superior to any prior science and technology thus seen in modern medicine, must still resolve several difficult issues. The construction of medical treatment regimens that minimize acute and late effects and the design of intervention strategies to reduce the psychological and social impact of the disease on children and families must be further researched.

Society must also undergo some degree of modification of attitudes so that as the number of survivors increase, more acceptance in the community is realized.

BIBLIOGRAPHY

D'Angio GJ: Neuroblastoma Overview—1986. *Med Pediatr Oncol* 1987; 15:159–162.

Hakami N, Monzon CM: Acute non-lymphocytic leukemia in children, in Jellinger K (ed): *Therapy of Malignant Tumors*. New York, Springer-Verlag, 1987, pp 567–575.

Jacobi G, Kornhuber B: Malignant brain tumors in children, in Jellinger K (ed): *Therapy of Malignant Brain Tumors*. New York, Springer-Verlag, 1987; pp 363–493.

Jones PG, Campbell PE: *Tumors of Infancy and Childhood*. Oxford, Blackwell Scientific Publications, Inc, 1976.

Magrath IT: Malignant non-Hodgkin's lymphomas in children. *Hematol Oncol Clin North Am* 1987; 1:577–602.

Mauer AM: The concept of cure in pediatric oncology, altered realities. *Am J Pediatr Hematol Oncol* 1987; 9:58–61.

Meyers PA: Malignant bone tumors in children: Ewing's sarcoma, in Jellinger K (ed): *Therapy of Ma-*

lignant Tumors. New York, Springer-Verlag, 1987, pp 667–673.

Meyers PA: Malignant bone tumors in children: Osteosarcoma. *Hematol Oncol Clin North Am* 1987; 1:655–665.

Murphy SB: Childhood non-Hodgkin's lymphoma. *N Engl J Med* 1978; 299:1446–1448.

Ruymann FB: Rhabdomyosarcoma in children and adolescents, a review. *Hematol Oncol Clin North Am* 1987; 1:621–654.

Steinherz PG: Acute lymphoblastic leukemia of childhood. *Hematol Oncol Clin North Am* 1987; 1:549–566.

Sullivan MP: Hodgkin's disease in children. *Hematol Oncol Clin North Am* 1987; 1:603–620.

Sutow WW, Vietti TJ, Fernbach DC: *Clinical Pediatric Oncology*, ed 3. St Louis, CV Mosby Co, 1980.

64 NEPHROSIS

Thomas L. Kennedy III, M.D.

As every physician in training learns, nephrotic syndrome consists of heavy proteinuria, hypoalbuminemia, edema, and hyperlipidemia. To the nephrologist, the nephrotic syndrome is defined by proteinuria in excess of 40 mg/sq m/hr (approximately 50 mg/kg/day), since the other components are all the consequences of this primary abnormality. To the child and his family, however, the nephrotic syndrome is the severe, generalized edema, which can be both frightening and debilitating.

BACKGROUND

ETIOLOGY AND EPIDEMIOLOGY

The nephrotic syndrome is an uncommon condition in childhood. The exact incidence is unknown, but several studies suggest a yearly incidence of two to seven cases per 100,000 children less than 15 years of age. Although the nephrotic syndrome has occurred in families and some immunogenetic markers are more common in patients with nephrotic syndrome, there is no recognizable genetic pattern and the vast majority of cases are sporadic. Male patients predominate, with a ratio of about 2:1.

The nephrotic syndrome is not a single entity and the heavy proteinuria that characterizes it may occur in association with virtually any glomerular disease. In childhood, however, one form comprises 80% of all cases of nephrotic syndrome. This entity has gone by several names, including lipoid nephrosis, nil disease, minimal lesion nephrotic syndrome, and the idiopathic nephrotic syndrome of childhood, but minimal change nephrotic syndrome (MCNS) is the term with widest current acceptance. The name originates from the observation that histologic examination of the kidney reveals only slight abnormalities. On light and immunofluorescent microscopy, there are usually no pathologic abnormalities. On electron microscopy, there is "fusion" of the foot processes of glomerular epithelial cells.

The etiology of MCNS is unknown. The observation has frequently been made that the onset and relapses occur in temporal relationship to an infection or an allergic episode. However, such a precipitating event is not always present and cause and effect cannot be proved. Furthermore, speculation and anecdotal evidence implicating diet and food additives in the nephrotic syndrome have no convincing support. Although minimal change disease may occur at any age, it is most common between ages 2 and 5 years and accounts for more than 90% of cases of nephrotic syndrome in this age group.

PATHOPHYSIOLOGY

A persuasive body of evidence has developed that strongly implicates an immunopathogenesis in minimal change disease. Some of this evidence includes clinical observations and some is derived from in vitro experiments using serum and white blood cells (WBCs) from patients with the condition. Observations exist, however, that cause doubt on a primary immunologic dysfunction. It is possible that the immune abnormalities are secondary to the low serum proteins and the hyperlipoproteinemia.

There is further uncertainty regarding the etiologic role of the immunologic dysfunction and the pathophysiology of the nephrotic syndrome as it is currently understood. The renal glomerulus possesses a filtration barrier that retards the loss of certain substances from the blood on the basis of molecular size, configuration, and charge. The barrier normally possesses a net negative charge that prevents the filtration of anionic molecules such as albumin. In the nephrotic syndrome, the glomerular negative charge is lost and albumin—and, to a more variable extent, other serum proteins—becomes filterable. It is not known how or why the negative charge disappears.

As the kidney loses protein, serum levels begin to decline. The body unsuccessfully attempts to compensate by increasing the hepatic synthesis of albumin. The hypoproteinemia that develops causes a concomitant fall in plasma oncotic pressure and plasma water begins to move from the intravascular to the interstitial space. The serum protein level at which edema develops varies among children but generally is less than 2.4 g/dL.

The elevated levels of cholesterol and lipids are not totally understood but are due, in part, to the nonspecific increase in hepatic synthetic pathways. Also contributing to the hyperlipidemia is the urinary loss of lipoprotein lipases that are important in the metabolism of lipoproteins.

DATA GATHERING

CLINICAL MANIFESTATIONS

The child with nephrotic syndrome almost invariably presents with edema. The onset may be dramatic or insidious, but it is usually rapid enough that discovery of heavy proteinuria on a routine screening urinalysis is uncommon. Generally, the swelling is first recognized in the periorbital area, is intermittent, and frequently is attributed to allergic symptoms. As the edema becomes generalized, renal disease is suspected and proteinuria is documented.

The child with nephrotic syndrome should be evaluated for the possibility of associated renal disease. In addition, detailed information and education should be provided to the family. This latter aspect cannot be overemphasized because it is extremely important that the family appreciates the recurrent nature of what is usually a chronic condition and the stress such an illness can place on them. They should understand the pathophysiology of the edema so they see the value of restricting salt intake, but not fluids, during relapses. They must know how to detect proteinuria and be committed to routine urine testing and to keeping a diary. They should appreciate the role of infection in precipitating relapses, the danger of infection in the child on high-dose steroids, and the expected and untoward effects of prednisone. Hospitalization may be necessary in children with severe anasarca, abdominal symptoms, or infection.

HISTORY

In evaluating the child with nephrotic syndrome, important history includes questions that would suggest the presence of preexisting renal disease including previous episodes of nephritis, abnormalities on screening urinalyses, and a history of hypertension or urinary tract infections. Also important is an inquiry regarding a family history of renal disease. Questions must be asked regarding possible infections, since infections not only frequently precede the onset of nephrotic syndrome, but also occur more often in the hypoproteinemic, edematous child and may be life threatening. A history of oliguria is usually obtained and may be misleading to the extent that it may suggest acute renal failure. Renal failure, however, occurs only rarely in MCNS. More frequently, the oliguria is appropriate and reflects the kidney's response to intravascular volume depletion caused by the hypoproteinemia.

PHYSICAL EXAMINATION

The physical examination can help document intravascular volume depletion when significant postural changes in blood pressure exist. A fall in systolic blood pressure of 10 mm Hg or more when the patient changes from the supine to the erect position is of concern. Hypertension should make one suspect significant renal disease. After obtaining the patient's height and weight, it is important to determine the ideal weight for height to estimate the amount of edema and to calculate medication doses on the basis of "dry" weight or surface area. Great care must be taken on physical examination to exclude the presence of infection, including those that may not be obvious (e.g., sinusitis, perianal abscess, or urinary tract infection) or those that may appear trivial (e.g., paronychia, dental or gingival infection). The edema, which tends to be pitting and dependent, may be obvious or may occur as mild ascites and/or pleural effusion. Scrotal and labial edema are of concern not only because of the discomfort they cause but also because an overlying cellulitis may develop. The presence of abdominal discomfort associated with anorexia and diarrhea is often attributable to bowel wall edema, but this discomfort makes careful abdominal and rectal examination essential to assess the possibility of peritonitis. An interesting but clinically insignificant and unexplained finding in the child with nephrotic syndrome is softening of the cartilage in the ear.

LABORATORY

Laboratory tests are directed at confirming the presence of nephrotic syndrome, determining whether it is MCNS or part of some other renal disease and excluding the possibility of infection. Laboratory evaluation of the child with nephrotic syndrome is summarized below.

LABORATORY EVALUATION

Confirm the diagnosis of nephrotic syndrome

- Urine dipstick for protein (usually 3+ to 4+) or urine protein/creatinine >1.0
- 24-hour urine protein (>40 mg/sq m/hr)
- Determination of serum total protein and protein electrophoresis
- Determination of serum cholesterol and triglyceride levels (not essential)

Rule out other renal disease (not all tests are necessary in every child)

- Determination of blood urea nitrogen (BUN) creatinine
- Glomerular filtration rate (creatinine clearance)
- Urinalysis (sediment examination for cellular casts)
- C3, CH50 determinations
- Other serologic tests: antinuclear antibody, antistreptolysin O titers, hepatitis B surface antigen, circulating immune complexes, cryoglobulins
- Renal ultrasound

Rule out infection

- Complete blood cell (CBC) count
- Cultures (as indicated, including paracentesis for abdominal tenderness)
- X-ray films (as indicated, including chest, abdomen, sinus)
- Tuberculin skin test (before starting steroids)

The CBC count is helpful in several respects. An elevated hematocrit level may indicate intravascular volume depletion. On the other hand, anemia may occur in long-standing nephrotic syndrome secondary to loss of transferrin in the urine or may indicate the presence of renal insufficiency. The WBC count is a useful guide to the presence of possible infection until steroids are begun. Because of increased levels of fibrinogen, cholesterol, and α-globulins, the sedimentation rate is elevated and, therefore, not a reliable indicator of infection in the child with nephrotic syndrome.

Serum protein concentrations show marked reduction in albumin concentrations (frequently in the range of 1.0 g/dL), increases in α_2-globulin fraction, and variable changes in the γ-fraction.

Although a 24-hour urine is helpful to quantitate the protein loss, the urine protein-creatinine ratio on random specimens recently has been shown to accurately reflect the nephrotic state.

The use of urine protein electrophoresis and comparison of the renal clearance of different-sized proteins, the so-called protein selectivity index, is not specific enough to be of help in evaluating the condition of an individual with nephrotic syndrome.

The BUN and creatinine levels will indicate or exclude renal insufficiency. The level of BUN may be elevated disproportionately to that of creatinine (prerenal azotemia) as a manifestation of the intravascular volume depletion. A creatinine clearance should be obtained, with the urine collected for protein quantitation for more precise determination of glomerular filtration rate. Although the creatinine clearance is generally normal in MCNS, a reduction at the time of diagnosis usually reflects decreased renal blood flow rather than glomerular disease.

The urinalysis may be helpful in differentiating MCNS from other causes of nephrotic syndrome. Microscopic hematuria may be present in up to one-quarter of children with MCNS but the presence of an "active" sediment, that is the presence of mixed cell types and cellular casts, suggests other renal disease.

Complement proteins are rarely reduced in the child with MCNS and suggest other renal lesions, including acute poststreptococcal, membranoproliferative, or lupus glomerulonephritis.

Other laboratory studies are not routinely indicated for every child. Rather, they should be considered in the child with signs and symptoms of other diseases or with atypical presentation of the nephrotic syndrome.

The renal biopsy remains the definitive diagnostic test, but may be reserved for certain circumstances. These include: (1) the child older than 12 years at diagnosis; (2) the child whose presentation and prior evaluation strongly suggest renal disease other than minimal-change disease; (3) the child who is steroid resistant; and (4) the child who is a candidate for immunosuppressive therapy. Most children with nephrotic syndrome do not require a biopsy and the diagnosis of MCNS is generally presumed rather than documented anatomically.

DIFFERENTIAL DIAGNOSIS

The differential diagnosis of nephrotic syndrome is lengthy and may be considered as broad groupings that include the nephrotic syndrome that occurs as the primary manifestation of a glomerulopathy and the one that occurs secondary to a systemic disease or toxic injury. The following classification of the nephrotic syndrome is not exhaustive. Only a very few of the conditions listed occur frequently enough in the pediatric age range to deserve mention in this discussion.

DIFFERENTIAL DIAGNOSIS OF NEPHROTIC SYNDROME

Primary renal disease

- Without glomerulonephritis
  - Minimal change nephrotic syndrome
  - Focal segmental glomerulosclerosis
  - Congenital nephrotic syndrome
- Associated with glomerulonephritis
  - Mesangial proliferative
  - Membranoproliferative
  - Membranous

Occurrence with systemic disease

- Infections
  - Viral (hepatitis B, HIV, Epstein-Barr virus, cytomegalovirus, etc.)
  - Bacterial (acute poststreptococcal glomerulonephritis, subacute bacterial endocarditis, shunt nephritis, etc.)
  - Parasitic (malaria, schistosomiasis, etc.)
  - Congenital syphilis
- Malignant disease
  - Lymphoma (e.g., MCNS in Hodgkin disease) and leukemia
  - Solid tumors (Wilms tumor, carcinomas)
- Metabolic disease
  - Diabetic nephropathy
  - Hypothyroidism
- Inflammatory disease
  - Systemic lupus erythematosus
  - Henoch-Schönlein purpura
  - Systemic vasculitides (e.g., polyarteritis)
- Miscellaneous diseases
  - Sickle cell disease
  - Hemolytic-uremic syndrome
  - Renal venous thrombosis

Associated with exogenous agents

- Allergens
  - Pollens, inhalants
  - Venoms (e.g., bee, snakes)

Immunizations
Toxins
  Heavy metals
  Heroin
Medications
  Captopril
  Penicillamine
  Nonsteroidal anti-inflammatory agents

Focal segmental glomerulosclerosis (FGS) comprises about 5% to 10% of cases of childhood nephrotic syndrome. It may mimic minimal change disease in its presentation although a more insidious onset, hematuria, hypertension, and azotemia are all more common. It is generally unresponsive to steroid and immunosuppressive therapy and leads to slowly progressive renal insufficiency. Focal segmental glomerulosclerosis has been reported with increased frequency in children with vesicoureteral reflux, in children with one kidney, and in some families. There are some nephrologists who believe that it may be a transition form of minimal change disease, although this is controversial.

Mesangial proliferative glomerulonephritis also accounts for about 5% to 10% of cases of childhood nephrotic syndrome. Its presentation is much like MCNS. Initially, it often responds to steroid therapy, although children with this condition have more frequent relapses and more commonly become steroid resistant. The outlook for this condition is more uncertain than that for MCNS or FGS. As with the other forms of nephrotic syndrome, definitive diagnosis depends on tissue histologic studies obtained by renal biopsy.

Membranoproliferative glomerulonephritis (MPGN; formerly called mesangiocapillary glomerulonephritis) comprises about 5% of cases of childhood nephrotic syndrome. Membranoproliferative glomerulonephritis may be divided into three types and is frequently characterized by persistent hypocomplementemia. Although the outlook for patients with MPGN has traditionally been considered unfavorable, chronic drug therapy with prednisone given on alternate days and most recently antiplatelet therapy with aspirin has improved the prognosis.

Membranous nephropathy is noted because it is so infrequent in children while it is the most common form of nephrotic syndrome in adults. There is no adequate therapy, although the course in children may be marked by spontaneous remissions.

The congenital nephrotic syndrome (also called Finnish-type or microcystic disease) is inherited as an autosomal recessive disorder presenting at birth or shortly thereafter and characterized by resistance to any form of therapy. The massive protein loss leads to growth failure, malnutrition, and fatal infection unless aggressive management, such as parenteral alimentation and eventual renal transplantation, is instituted.

MANAGEMENT

It is important to realize that of all the laboratory tests that may help to diagnose MCNS, the best predictor of MCNS short of a renal biopsy is the response to steroid therapy.

Of children with MCNS, 90% respond to glucocorticoids with complete, albeit usually temporary, resolution of proteinuria. The drug with the widest use is prednisone, begun at a dose of 60 mg/m^2/day (or 2 mg/kg/day, maximum 80 mg) in two to three divided doses. The drug should be given in this manner for a maximum of 1 month or at least 2 weeks after the urine has been protein free. The average time from the onset of therapy until onset of remission is about 10 to 14 days. During this interval, it is frequently very difficult for both parents and physicians to stand by and watch the child become more edematous. Measures such as aggressive diuretic therapy are generally ill-advised and potentially dangerous (see supportive therapy). Patience is the most important attribute during this period. Depending on the amount of edema, remission may be associated with a dramatic and marked diuresis that can lead to electrolyte disturbances, including hyponatremia and hypokalemia. After the diuresis, the child will frequently feel fatigued and appear tired with dark discoloration around his eyes.

When remission is attained, the prednisone is given on alternate days as a single morning dose with breakfast. The initial alternate-day dose and tapering schedule may vary somewhat among nephrologists, but the majority favor a slow decrease over a 2- to 3-month period. The alternate-day schedule is effective and minimizes steroid toxicity.

Children who have persistent proteinuria after receiving 4 weeks of daily steroids require special treatment or a renal biopsy and therefore require consultation with a pediatric nephrologist.

MCNS can be classified as follows:

1. Steroid sensitive: Patients respond to steroids and can stay protein-free without treatment for various lengths of times.
2. Steroid dependent: Patients respond to steroids but require continuous treatment with low-dose steroids.
3. Steroid resistant: Patients do not respond to steroid treatment.

The child with MCNS who responds to prednisone may follow several patterns. First, the nephrotic syndrome may resolve and never recur. This ideal outcome accounts for only about 20% of cases. Second, there may be infrequent relapses (e.g., less than two per year) occurring for several years, responding each time to steroids and eventually resolving. This category accounts for about 30% of cases. Third, 40% of children have frequent relapses of heavy proteinuria, requiring repeated and often prolonged courses of steroids. These children are at risk of developing steroid toxicity. When such toxicity becomes intolerable, the child should be considered to receive immunosuppressive drugs capable of inducing long-term remissions in both steroid-dependent and steroid-resistant MCNS. The difficulty is deciding when the myriad of steroid side effects becomes intolerable, since the potential toxicities of the alternative alkylating agents are significant.

Steroid side effects such as growth failure, hypertension, aseptic necrosis of bone, steroid-induced psychosis or severe myopathy are clearly unacceptable. Of these, problems with growth are most common and growth rates must be followed closely.

The impact of other side effects are more variable. For example, the cushingoid changes, acne, and hirsutism may be totally unacceptable and lead to noncompliance in an adolescent woman, so the decision to use alternatives to prednisone must be individualized.

IMMUNOSUPPRESSIVE THERAPY

Only about 10% of children with MCNS require immunosuppressive therapy. The drugs that are effective are cyclophosphamide (Cytoxan) and chlorambucil (Leukeran). Each has its proponents but neither has been shown to be superior to the other. The drugs are given at a lower dose and for a shorter period of time than when used to treat malignant disease (for cyclophosphamide, 2 mg/kg for 8 weeks; for chlorambucil, 0.2 mg/kg/day for a total dose of 12 mg/kg). For this reason, their potential toxicities are less common when used in children with MCNS. By convention, they are given in conjunction with prednisone (generally 2 mg/kg/day in divided doses for 14 days, then every other day), even when the child is steroid resistant. Short-term side effects of both are leukopenia, and weekly WBC counts should be obtained. Administration is temporarily interrupted for total WBC counts less than 4,000/mm^3 or for total granulocyte counts less than 1,500/mm^3. Other potential short-term effects include anorexia, mild hair loss, hemorrhagic cystitis with cyclophosphamide (good oral hydration must be emphasized), and focal seizures with chlorambucil. All of these are uncommon. Long-term effects include infertility, the possibility of sustained immunologic dysfunction, and the occurrence of malignant disease. Unfortunately, the exact risk is unknown, but it appears to be small. The remissions obtained are frequently prolonged or permanent, but, if not, will sometimes appear to decrease the frequency of relapses. Cases of children who convert from a state of steroid resistance to steroid responsiveness following immunosuppressive therapy are well documented.

LONG-TERM FOLLOW-UP

Relapses

Recurrence of proteinuria may develop at any time in the child with nephrotic syndrome. The most common triggering event is infection, although many times transient proteinuria may occur in association with an infection and disappear when the illness resolves. For this reason, it is wise not to start steroids or increase the dose in a child who develops infection-associated proteinuria until it is clear the protein loss is persistent after the child is well. Likewise, once the decision is made to use steroids, they should be given in full doses (i.e., 2 mg/kg/day) and not reinstituted in half-doses or other nonsystematic fashion that can lead to prolonged courses and steroid toxicity. Remission is defined as 5 consecutive days of protein-free urine (dipstick reading negative or trace) and the transition to alternate-day therapy can be made at that time.

Patterns may become apparent for the occurrence of relapse in certain children and, if recognized, the timetable for decreasing steroids can be tailored for that individual. For example, some children may require a more gradual transition from daily to alternate-day steroids, while others appear to relapse only when their dose is reduced below some critical level. At any rate, it is good practice to pay close attention to the child on a tapering dose of prednisone and to avoid reducing the dose at the time of an intercurrent illness.

The use of chronic, low-dose, daily (2.5 mg of prednisone) or alternate-day steroid therapy has been advocated to prevent proteinuria in children with frequent relapses. The efficacy of such therapy remains to be fully established.

Supportive Therapy

Dietary measures may be used to aid in the management of MCNS. The diet should include optimal amounts (1.5 to 2.0 g/kg/day) of high biologic value protein, but there is no reason to increase intake above this level since the body will not utilize the excess protein ingested. Moderate salt restriction will help reduce the rate of edema formation, but should not be so severe that it will affect the palatability of the diet. Fluid restriction should not be instituted, since thirst in the child with nephrosis frequently indicates intravascular volume depletion.

For the same reason, diuretic therapy should be undertaken with caution. In a child with MCNS who is incapacitated by anasarca, who has respiratory distress because of pleural effusions, or who has abdominal discomfort and anorexia because of ascites, the use of intravenous infusions of 25% albumin (1 g/kg/dose given over 60 to 90 minutes and followed by 1 mg/kg of furosemide) may be used. These infusions may provide significant, temporary relief through the diuresis they evoke. Because the hyperoncotic albumin temporarily increases the intravascular volume through movement of edema from the interstitium, hypertension may develop and the blood pressure must be monitored closely. Routine oral diuretic therapy becomes very useful in chronic forms of nephrotic syndrome, in which the blood volume is not contracted and edema can be minimized.

Other supportive measures include attention to the prevention and prompt treatment of infectious disease. In the child who has had a relapse of MCNS, peritonitis remains a threat. The most common organism is *Streptococcus pneumoniae* but *Hemophilus influenzae*, and *Escherichia coli* have also been reported and antibiotic therapy must be chosen appropriately.

It is important to remember that the nephrotic syndrome is a hypercoagulable state and venipuncture in deep veins (e.g., the femoral vein) should be avoided.

Although its efficacy in children with MCNS is unknown, the pneumococcal vaccine should be considered. If the vaccine is administered, it should be given preferably when the child is in remission and off steroids.

Despite reports of immunizations precipitating relapses in children with MCNS, such cases are uncommon and the routine schedule of immunizations may be followed at the physician's discretion.

Outcome

The "statistically average" child with MCNS will have approximately five relapses over a 5-year period and then permanently go into remission. However, such prognostication is unreliable for any individual, since some children have no relapses and some children have many relapses extending well into adulthood.

The ultimate outlook for permanent remission and preservation of normal renal function is good for steroid-sensitive patients with MCNS. Of greatest concern is therapy-related morbidity that includes steroid-induced growth retardation and obesity and the long-term dangers of the alkylating agents. The morbidity, if any, related to the hyperlipidemia of MCNS is unknown.

The risk of MCNS transforming into another glomerulopathy such as focal glomerulosclerosis or mesangial proliferative glomerulonephritis is also unknown and, as mentioned earlier, is controversial. If such transformation occurs, however, it is quite uncommon. The physician, therefore, may remain very optimistic when counseling the family of a child with MCNS regarding outcome.

Use of Consultants

The pediatric nephrologist need not provide total care for the child with MCNS. Consultation at the time of diagnosis may provide useful suggestions with regard to the evaluation and initial therapy. The nephrologist can also provide the necessary information the family will need to know to adequately care for their child and realistically deal with the future course. Later, the nephrologist can be helpful in the management of children with frequent relapses who may require many changes in their steroid regimen. The nephrologist must assume responsibility for the child who requires a renal biopsy or the use of immunosuppressive medication and should play an active role in the care of children with nephrotic syndrome other than MCNS.

BIBLIOGRAPHY

Berns JS, Gaudio KM, Krassner LS, et al: Steroid-responsive nephrotic syndrome in childhood: A long-term study of clinical course, histopathology, efficacy of cyclosphosphamide therapy and effects on growth. *Am J Kidney Dis* 1987; 9:108.

Brenner BM, Stein JH (ed): Nephrotic syndrome. *Contemp Issues Nephrol* 1982; 9.

McVicar M, Chandra M: Pathogenic mechanisms in the nephrotic syndrome of childhood. *Adv Pediatr* 1985; 32:269.

Strauss J, Zilleruelo G, Freundlich M, et al: Less commonly recognized features of childhood nephrotic syndrome. *Pediatr Clin North Am* 1987; 34:591.

65 THE POISONED PATIENT

Gary C. Cupit, Pharm.D.

Accidental poisoning remains one of the leading causes of death in children below 5 years of age. While the incidence of accidental poisoning remains high, the decline in mortality can be attributed to factors such as safety closures on containers, improved medical training of physicians, consumer awareness, the voluntary efforts of industry in regard to packaging and the quantity of medication in containers, and the development of a system of regional poison control centers.

In many situations, the poison that a pediatric patient ingests is readily known since it is an accidental ingestion and is rapidly discovered by a parent or babysitter. However, it is not unusual for the diagnosis to be made as an afterthought when a child has been evaluated for an involved metabolic problem or even after death. Poisoning should always be suspected in the following situations: (1) a trauma victim; (2) a comatose patient for whom the etiology is unknown; (3) a pediatric patient with a life-threatening arrhythmia or an arrhythmia of unknown etiology; (4) patients with severe metabolic acidosis or anion gap, and (5) patients rescued from a fire. In each of these situations, there needs to be a systematic approach to the poisoned patient. It is the intent of this chapter to provide such a framework.

DATA GATHERING

CLINICAL EVALUATION AND HISTORY

Identification of the poisonous agent is one of the most important aspects of the history. Prior medical history, current medications, and allergies should be determined from parents, siblings, or relatives. History taken for a toxic ingestion requires that much information be gathered not only about the patient but also about the circumstances by which the poisoning occurred and the agent responsible for the ingestion. A collection of selected questions to be asked during the history is provided below:

1. Who is giving history (parent, babysitter, etc)?
2. Was there an exposure?
3. What was the toxic agent (exact nature or name of each item)?
4. What were the circumstances of the exposure?
5. To how much was the victim exposed?
6. What was the route of exposure?
7. When was the exposure?
8. What is the age, weight, sex, and name of the victim?
9. What was the condition of the victim prior to the exposure?
10. What is the present condition of the victim?
11. When did symptoms, if any, begin?
12. Can you describe the symptoms?
13. Are the symptoms getting worse?

When a patient is poisoned, it is critical to determine whether the patient has developed symptoms from the poisoning. Symptoms usually occur within 2 to 4 hours after an ingestion of most poisons. Nontoxic amounts generally do not result in any symptoms. In a small number of poisons, symptoms may be delayed from several hours to several days. The degree of the severity of the symptoms is related to the amount and toxicity of the substance ingested.

When combining the clinical presentation of a patient with the history of the compound that is thought to have been ingested (or even in those situations where the compound is unknown), the formulation of a *symptom complex* is most helpful. For example, if a patient is comatose and has constricted pupils (miosis), a diagnosis of narcotic overdose is likely. If a patient also has depressed respirations, it would most likely be a narcotic overdose. The combination of the recognition of symptom complexes and a good history are the keys to making a diagnosis in poisoned patients. While these components are being analyzed, the patient must have the "ABCs" evaluated and treated if necessary. That is, his airway must be protected and assured, breathing must be adequate, and cardiovascular systems must be sufficient to maintain good circulatory perfusion. Once basic life support measures have been instituted and while other management procedures are being performed, specimens of blood, urine, saliva, sweat, or other appropriate body fluids should be obtained for qualitative and quantitative toxicologic screens.

MANAGEMENT

BASIC POISONING MANAGEMENT

There are a number of procedures that may be utilized to terminate a patient's exposure to toxic substance or to reduce its harmful effects. The most frequent routes of entry for a poisonous substance is either by inhalation, ocular exposure, cutaneous exposure, or ingestion. Each of these routes requires separate treatments to reduce toxicity.

Inhalation.—Individuals who have inhaled toxic gases or chemicals should be removed from the presence of the toxic environment as rapidly as possible. Rescuers should be aware of the dangers of these fumes and take precautions against inhaling any toxic compounds. Protection may include the use of protective breathing devices for rescuers if adequate ventilation cannot be assured. Where appropriate, the administration of oxygen should be instituted immediately.

Ocular Exposures.—The exposure of the eyes to a corrosive or dangerously toxic compound requires immediate irrigation with tepid water, isotonic saline, Ringer's lactate, or an ophthalmic irrigating solution. A gentle, continuous stream should be used for at least 5 to 10 minutes. For corrosive products, the irrigation should be continued for at least 15 to 30 minutes. All eyes exposed to toxic compounds should receive a complete ophthalmologic examination.

Cutaneous.—When a toxic compound is splashed on the skin or the skin is immersed in the substance, immediate flushing with water and then soap and water should be instituted. When clothing covers the skin, the area should be irrigated with water immediately prior to removal of the clothing to ensure a prompt dilution of the toxic substance. Clothing should then be removed to further irrigate the involved area. Care should be taken by hospital personnel in handling clothes and shoes.

Ingestion.—After oral ingestion, the principal treatment should focus on gastrointestinal decontamination. The oral administration of water is often recommended for the initial management of the poisoned patient. This is based on the impression that this will dilute and further delay gastrointestinal absorption of a poison. There are several studies, however, indicating that the administration of a large volume of water may actually enhance the absorption of an ingested poison. It is now recommended that the dilution of poisons ingested orally be avoided. It is suggested, however, that dilution with water may be useful, with the demulcents, in the management of corrosive ingestions.

Induced Emesis.—The induction of emesis by stimulation of the posterior pharynx by a tongue blade, catheter, finger, or inverted tablespoon is often recommended. Hazards of these procedures include laceration of the posterior pharynx and trauma to the oral cavity with the introduction of a blunt object in resistant patients. More importantly, this approach is not always effective. These results, when compared with those of other studies, indicate that mechanical stimulation is much less effective than administering a pharmacologic emetic such as ipecac. Only when an appropriate chemical emetic or other procedure such as gastric lavage is unable to be instituted should mechanical emesis ever be considered. Chemically induced emesis is most frequently recommended and agents include sodium chloride, copper sulfate, and soaps.

Sodium chloride or salt water solutions for the induction of emesis has been advocated for many years but are not safe and should not be used.

Copper sulfate used as an emetic has been known for many years. This agent has been previously administered in a dose of 150 to 250 mg, dissolved in 30 to 60 mL of water. While this agent is efficacious, concerns about its use are based on the potential toxicities that may exist. Elevations in serum copper concentrations, increased urinary excretion of copper, and proteinuria as well as frank renal and hepatic damage, are all reported complications. These reasons argue against its routine use as an emetic.

Soaps and detergents have been known to cause emesis in patients who have ingested these compounds for some time now. There has been a reported study utilizing liquid dishwashing detergents as a means of inducing emesis. Doses of three tablespoonfuls of liquid dishwashing detergent diluted in 8 oz of water were given. After administration, emesis occurred in an average of 7 minutes and was successful in 91% of patients drinking the solution. While not as equally effective as ipecac, this approach may offer an alternative when ipecac is not readily available.

Pharmacologic Emesis.—The two agents that are most frequently used in the pharmacologic category are syrup of ipecac and apomorphine. Both agents act by stimulating the chemoreceptor trigger zone in the medulla, plus ipecac acts as a local gastric irritant. Syrup of ipecac is the most popular and widely available emetic for the induction of emesis. After the administration of ipecac syrup, emesis occurs within 30 minutes in over 90% of patients. The dose of ipecac syrup that is most frequently recommended is as follows: infants under 1 year of age, 10 mL; children 1 to 2 years of age, 15 mL; and patients more than 12 years of age, 30 mL.

Administration of ipecac is to be followed by the administration of 5 to 7 mL of liquid per kilogram of body weight in children or 8 to 12 oz of liquid in adults. If emesis does not occur within 20 to 30 minutes, the dose of syrup of ipecac may be repeated. If the emesis still does not occur, gastric lavage should be instituted. The administration of liquids following the dose of syrup of ipecac appears to improve its success. Clear fluids should be used and liquids such as milk avoided since they may reduce the onset of emesis. It should be remembered that only modest amounts of fluid should be administered prior to the administration of ipecac, single large volumes may increase passage of the toxin into the small intestine, thereby enhancing absorption. Other variables that had previously thought to influence the efficacy of syrup of ipecac have been evaluated. For example, many clinicians thought that ipecac-induced emesis may be influenced by medications that have antiemetic properties, e.g., anticholinergics, phenothiazines, and tricyclic antidepressants. The time to onset of emesis after administration of ipecac syrup was similar in those patients who had ingested antiemetic agents and those who had not. Ambulation of patients after administration of syrup of ipecac has been thought to improve the time of onset and the overall response rate of an emesis. Recent studies, however, have questioned the benefit of ambulation and have shown that in both pediatric and adult patients, having the patient walk about the office or bouncing the child on one's knee does not alter either the rate of onset or the efficacy of the procedure.

To maximize the benefits of ipecac-induced emesis, many clinicians have advocated the storage of ipecac at home for use in case of accidental poisoning. Many studies have shown that when syrup of ipecac is available in the home and is used only after contacting a poison control center or physician, safe and effective emesis can be performed at home. Other clinicians have emphasized that when syrup of ipecac is available in the home, complications may result if it is administered without consultation with a health professional or a poison control center.

The major concern about ipecac toxicity is that of cardiotoxicity. Several well-controlled studies have documented, however, that there is no increase in cardiac problems in patients given ipecac syrup. Reports of cardiotoxicity with ipecac-induced emesis have been either from the administration of ipecac fluid extract or the long-term use of ipecac syrup as a means of weight control.

Apomorphine is available for parenteral use only, whereas syrup of ipecac is available as an oral preparation. Apomorphine is administered in a dose of 0.07 to 0.10 mg/kg, administered subcutaneously. Emesis usually begins within 4 to 6 minutes and may persist for as long as 45 minutes. Apomorphine is 85% to 100% effective in inducing emesis after administration. While apomorphine has been shown to be a rapid-acting emetic, there are some serious disadvantages to its use.

Apomorphine is a narcotic derivative, available by prescription only and is a 6-mg hypodermic tablet that must be dissolved in water for injection prior to its use. Another major concern is that when apomorphine is used, its narcotic activity may produce both central nervous system and respiratory depression. This sedative side effect makes emergency management difficult and interpretation of the effects of some ingested poisons confusing. The sedation is reversible by the administration of naloxone, but this makes its use more complicated. The protracted vomiting that occurs with the use of apomorphine is considered to also be an undesirable and unnecessary side effect.

Gastric Lavage.—The role of gastric lavage in the management of poisoning is an item of controversy even today. Of concern is that gastric aspiration and lavage can be performed only under the direction of medical personnel, resulting in a significant delay of the onset of treatment while the patient is being transported to a health care facility. The procedure itself requires a minimum of 20 to 30 minutes. Then if complications do not intervene (such as laryngeal spasm, cyanosis, or aspiration), there remains the question of effectiveness of lavage when compared to induced emesis.

Proponents of gastric lavage suggest that in many studies, lavage is not correctly performed. This criticism is based on the incorrect use of nasogastric tubes as opposed to large-bore gastric lavage tubes specifically designed for this procedure. Also, insufficient amounts of lavage fluid are often used. Other clinicians express concern that when evaluations of gastric lavage are performed, the position of the subject being lavaged is extremely important and must be considered. By using a modified Sim position with the patient on the left side, it is possible to achieve an excellent return rate of many compounds during lavage.

Other factors known to influence the efficacy of lavage are the temperature of the fluid used in lavage, the properties of the drug ingested and the frequencies of lavage. A comparison of various temperatures of water used in lavage solutions have shown that tepid water appears to be the most preferable. Tepid water has been shown to result in a delay of gastric emptying time when compared with colder solutions.

Dosage form or pharmacologic properties may influence lavage efficacy. Medications that are enteric-coated may be lavaged more effectively using an alkaline solution to dissolve the coating to enhance removal of the medication. Medications that have anticholinergic properties and delayed gastric emptying have a greater recovery rate on initial lavage and on repeat lavage than do other medications. When gastric lavage is considered, it must be remembered that the patient's airway must be protected at all times with the use of an artificial airway, preferably a cuffed endotracheal tube.

Adsorption Therapy.—The oral administration of compounds to bind ingested poisons in the gastrointestinal tract and, thus, decrease their absorption is a method used with great frequency in the treatment of the poisoned patient. This is rapidly becoming the method of choice for eliminating many toxins. At the current time, activated charcoal is the standard for all comparisons of adsorption of drugs in the gastrointestinal tract. To date, it is the most effective orally administered adsorbent (toxins that are known to be adsorbed by activated charcoal are listed below).

Acetaminophen	Nicotine
Amphetamine	Parathion
Arsenic	Phenothiazines
Atropine	Phenylbutazone
Barbiturates	Phenylpropanolamine
Carbamazepine	Phenytoin
Diazepam	Propoxyphene
Digitalis	Salicylates
Ethanol	Silver
Ipecac	Strychnine
Malathion	Sulfonamides
Morphine	

Activated charcoal powder is administered orally as a suspension in water or by nasogastric tube. Charcoal tablets or universal antidote are not recommended. Newer preparations of activated charcoal suspended in sorbitol or propylene glycol are currently being marketed. The optimal ratio of activated charcoal to ingested drug on a weight basis is usually 10:1. When the exact amount of drug ingested is unknown, the recommended dosages are 1 g/kg for a minimum of 20 to 25 g in a child and a minimum of 50 to 100 g in an adult.

The palatability of charcoal slurries has been a recurring problem in poison treatment. As a result, several charcoal preparations that contain sweeteners, flavors, or other agents have been tried. Agents that should be avoided when administering activated charcoal are milk, ice cream, or flavoring agents such as chocolate. Cherry flavoring does not appear to adversely affect charcoal adsorbency.

Maximum prevention of drug absorption occurs when a sufficient amount of charcoal is administered when the time interval between drug ingestion and administration of charcoal is brief. Repetitive dosing of activated charcoal may further decrease drug absorption if the drug undergoes enterogastric or enterohepatic circulation. Reductions of 20% to 30% have been reported for phenobarbital, digoxin, amitriptyline, carbamazepine, and phenylbutazone. This method of enhancing gastrointestinal clearance by activated charcoal has been termed "gastrointestinal dialysis," since the use of charcoal for this purpose is analogous to the use of albumin in peritoneal dialysis. The renewed enthusiasm for activated charcoal has prompted many investigators to compare the efficacy of ipecac-induced emesis with the administration of activated charcoal alone. Present studies have shown that acetaminophen, tetracycline, aminophylline, and acetysalicylic acid achieve lower plasma concentrations after ingestion with activated charcoal than with coadministration of ipecac. A previous study has shown that apomorphine-induced emesis and administration of activated charcoal have an equivalent benefit in reducing salicylate absorption, with a combination of apomorphine and activated charcoal having an even greater benefit. Conventional induction of emesis by ipecac followed by the administration of activated charcoal has not been studied in this manner. It appears that a combined approach may be superior to either agent when used alone.

Cathartics.—The administration of saline cathartics such as sodium sulfate, magnesium sulfate, or magnesium citrate is commonly recommended for reducing gastrointestinal absorption of acutely ingested poisons. Acting as an osmotic agent, the presence of a large volume of fluid leads to increased peristaltic activity and a decrease in gastrointestinal transit time causing defecation. Data supporting the efficacy of catharsis as a means of decreasing absorption of these compounds is inconclusive at this time. The main reason for instituting cathartic agents is that activated charcoal administration is associated with constipation. Saline cathartics may minimize this side effect. For the adult, the oral dose of sodium or magnesium sulfate is 15 to 20 g administered as a 10% or 20% oral solution; the pediatric dose is 250 mg/kg.

Antidotal Therapy.—Those antidotes that should be available for immediate administration include: atropine (cholinesterase inhibitor, insecticides), methylene blue (methemoglobinemic agents), oxygen (carbon monoxide), and naloxone (narcotic respiratory risk). Other antidotes usually do not require urgent administration and may be given subsequent to initiation of other management modalities. Antidotes do not diminish the need for good supportive care or other therapy. The overall number of ingestions for which a specific antidote is necessary or available is small. Indiscriminate use of antidotes without other forms of management should be discouraged. Table 65–1 summarizes a list of commonly used antidotes, suggested doses, and their indications for use.

Enhanced Elimination of an Absorbed Poison.—The procedures available for enhancing the elimination of an absorbed poison are diuresis, dialysis, and hemoperfusion. Since these procedures provide great risk and are often beyond the scope of office practice, it is unlikely that these procedures would be per-

TABLE 65–1
Selected Local and Systemic Antidotes

POISON	LOCAL ANTIDOTE	SYSTEMIC ANTIDOTE
Acetaminophen	Activated charcoal (not to be used if *N*-acetyl-L-cysteine is to be given)	*N*-acetyl-L-cysteine (Mucomyst), initial dose of 140 mg/kg PO in Coke, Pepsi, Fresca, grapefruit juice, or water; then, 70 mg/kg every 4 hr for 68 hr (17 doses)
Acids, corrosive	Dilute with water or milk, then administer antacid	
Alkali, caustic	Dilute with water or milk, then give demulcent	
Amphetamines	Activated charcoal	Chlorpromazine, 1 mg/kg IM or IV; administer slowly if given IV; may repeat in 15 min; reduce to 0.5 mg/kg if other CNS depressants involved.
Anticholinergics	Activated charcoal	Physostigmine (adult dose, 2 mg; child, 0.5 mg) may be given IV, IM, or SC; may repeat in 15 min until desired effect is achieved; subsequent doses may be given every 2–3 hr as needed
Anticholinesterases Organophosphates	Activated charcoal	Atropine, 1–2 mg (for children under 2 yr, 1 mg or 0.05 mg/kg) IM or IV, repeated every 10–15 min until atropinization is evident; then give pralidoxime chloride 25–50 mg/kg (1 g in adults) IV, repeat in 8–12 hr as needed
Carbamates		Atropine as above, but *do not* use pralidoxime

TABLE 65–1
Selected Local and Systemic Antidotes *(continued)*

POISON	LOCAL ANTIDOTE	SYSTEMIC ANTIDOTE
Antihistamines	See Anticholinergics	
Belladonna alkaloids	See Anticholinergics	
Carbon monoxide		100% oxygen inhalation for no more than 2 hr, followed by inhalation of room air
Cholinergic compounds	See Anticholinesterases	
Cyanide		Adult: amyl nitrite inhalation (inhale for 15–30 sec every 60 sec) pending administration of 300 mg sodium nitrate (10 mL of 3% solution) IV slowly (over 2–4 min); follow immediately with 12.5 g sodium thiosulfate (2.5–5 mL/min of 25% solution) IV slowly (over 10 min); for children, sodium nitrate should not exceed recommended dose, because fatal methemoglobinemia may result*
Detergents, cationic	Ordinary soap solution	
Ethylene glycol	See Methanol	
Fluoride	Calcium gluconate or lactate, 150 mg/kg, or milk	Calcium gluconate, 10 mL of 10% solution, given slowly IV until symptoms abate; may be repeated as needed
Heavy metals	Milk or egg whites Usual chelates used:	Dimercaprol (BAL) 3–5 mg/kg dose, deep IM every 4 hr for 2 days, then every 4–12 hr for up to 7 additional days; edetic acid (EDTA) 75 mg/kg every 24 hr, deep IM or slow IV infusion, given in 3–6 divided doses for up to 5 days; may be repeated for a second course after a minimum of 2 days; each course should not exceed a total of 500 mg/kg of body weight; penicillamine 100 mg/kg/day (maximum 1 g) taken PO in divided doses for up to 5 days; for long-term therapy do not exceed 40 mg/kg/day
Arsenic	Dimercaprol	
Cadmium	Satisfactory use not demonstrated	
Copper	Dimercaprol, penicillamine	
Gold	Dimercaprol	
Lead	Dimercaprol, EDTA, penicillamine	
Mercury	Dimercaprol, penicillamine	
Silver	Satisfactory use not demonstrated	
Thallium	Satisfactory use not demonstrated	
Hypochlorites	See Alkali, caustic	
Iodine	Starch solution, 3%–10%	
Iron	Sodium bicarbonate, 1%–5% solution, preferably by lavage	Deferoxamine, 20–40 mg/kg IV, given as slow drip over 4–hr, not to exceed 15 mg/kg/hr; followed by 20 mg/kg every 4–8 hr until urine color normal or iron level normal (can give 20 mg/kg IM every 4–11 hr if no IV sites available)

*Dosages of sodium nitrate and sodium thiosulfate are as follows:

HEMOGLOBIN	SODIUM NITRATE IV (INITIAL DOSE, 3%)	SODIUM THIOSULFATE IV (INITIAL DOSE, 25%)
8 g	0.22 mL (6.6 mg)/kg	1.10 mL/kg
10 g	0.27 mL (8.7 mg)/kg	1.35 mL/kg
12 g (nl)	0.33 mL (10.0 mg)/kg	1.65 mL/kg
14 g	0.39 mL (11.6 mg)/kg	1.95 mL/kg

TABLE 65–1
Selected Local and Systemic Antidotes *(continued)*

POISON	LOCAL ANTIDOTE	SYSTEMIC ANTIDOTE
Isoniazid	Activated charcoal	Pyridoxine (vitamin B_6) 1 mg/g of Isoniazid (INH) ingested in divided doses, given slowly IV (5 mg/50 mL each bolus); if seizures present, initially give 5 mg IV over 3–5 min; may repeat dose at intervals of 5–15 min until seizures stop or consciousness regained
Methanol		Ethanol, loading dose to achieve blood level of 100 mg/dL; adult: 0.6 gm/kg body weight + 7–10 g to be infused IV over 1 hr; child: 0.6 g/kg body weight + 4–5 g to be infused IV over 1 hr; maintenance doses should approximate 10 g/hr in adults to 5 g/hr in children, to be adjusted according to measured blood ethanol levels.
Methemoglobinemic agents (nitrates, chlorates, nitrobenzene)		Methylene blue, 1–2 mg (0.1–0.2 ml/kg) of a 1% solution given IV slowly over 5–10 min if cyanosis is severe (or methemoglobin level greater than 40%)
Narcotics	Activated charcoal	Naloxone, 0.005–0.01 mL/kg (adult 0.4 mg) given IV at intervals of 2–3-min as needed (second choice of agents includes levallorphan, 0.2 mg/kg or nalorphine 0.1 mg/kg, given as above)
Oxalate	Dilute with water or milk, then give calcium gluconate or lactate 150	Calcium gluconate, 10 mL of 10% solution, given slowly IV until symptoms abate; may be repeated as needed
Phenol	Dilute with water or milk, then give activated charcoal, castor oil, vegetable oil	
Phenothiazines (neuromuscular reaction only)		Diphenhydramine, 0.5–1.0 mg/kg, given IM or IV; or benztropine, 2 mg, IM or IV
Physostigmine	See Anticholinesterases	
Quaternary ammonium compounds	See Detergents, cationic	
Thallium	Activated charcoal; may be given continuously to remove metal, excreted via enterohepatic circulation	See Heavy metals
Tricyclic antidepressants	See Anticholinergics	
Warfarin		Vitamin K_1, 0.5–1.0 mg/kg, given IM or IV; adults, 10 mg IM or IV; children, 1–5 mg IM or IV

formed at the time of initial evaluation; rather this is a situation in which the patient should be prepared for transport to a health care facility after initial stabilization and assessment. The value of these procedures may be determined by consultation with a regional poison control center.

SUMMARY

Acute and chronic poisonings present a significant challenge to the practicing pediatrician. While the toxic ingestion may not be known, the route of exposure and resulting symptoms should be easily determined. It is imperative that as the diagnosis of the toxin to which the victim has been exposed becomes apparent, basic first aid and life support be initiated. With laboratory confirmation of ingestions requiring a minimum of 1 to 2 hours, pertinent history and symptoms can be invaluable in establishing a course of treatment.

Termination of a toxic oral exposure may consist of dilution, emesis, lavage, or the administration of activated charcoal. At this point, if further treatment is required, consideration should be given to transportation of the patient to an appropriate health care facility. While antidotal therapy may be instituted or enhancement of certain bodily functions, e.g., forced alkaline diuresis, may increase the elimination of toxins, these procedures are normally performed in an emergency room environment. It is hoped that with increased awareness of the dangers of poisons, prevention of deaths caused by poisoning will become an integral part of the practicing pediatrician's expertise. It is important to develop and maintain a good working relationship with the regional poison control center.

BIBLIOGRAPHY

Aronow R (ed): *Handbook of Common Poisonings in Children*, ed 2. Evanston, Ill, American Academy of Pediatrics, 1983.

Haddad LM, Winchester JF (eds): *Clinical Management of Poisoning and Drug Overdose*. Philadelphia, WB Saunders Co, 1983.

Hanson W (ed): *Toxic Emergencies*. New York, Churchill Livingstone, 1984.

Henretig FM, Cupit GC, Temple AR: Toxicologic emergencies, in Fleisher G, Ludwig S (eds): *Textbook of Pediatric Emergency Medicine*, ed 2. Baltimore, Williams & Wilkins Co, 1988 pp 548–599.

Temple AR (guest ed): Symposium on medical toxicology. *Emerg Med Clin North Am* 1984; 2:3–197.

66 SEIZURE DISORDERS

Robert Ryan Clancy, M.D.

Recurrent epileptic seizures are a common pediatric neurologic disorder affecting approximately 0.5% of children. The majority of affected individuals can have the epilepsy successfully diagnosed, evaluated, and managed by a knowledgeable primary care physician. This chapter will review recent developments in the medical and neurologic approach to children with epilepsy in the setting of an office practice. Neonatal seizures, status epilepticus, and seizures complicating acute medical or neurologic illnesses will not be addressed.

BACKGROUND

The key to the successful management of a seizure disorder is an initial accurate diagnosis of epilepsy and the correct classification of the type of seizure. Children are vulnerable to a wide variety of nonepileptic medical or neurologic disorders that abruptly "seize" them, provoking sudden attacks of disordered consciousness, behavior, involuntary movements, disturbed body tone, posture, or sensation. These nonepileptic abnormal events (e.g., migraine, gastroesophageal reflux, and breath-holding attacks) may mimic genuine epilepsy and lead to an initial incorrect diagnosis and inappropriate or unnecessary evaluation and treatment.[1]

The term "seizure" means literally to "grab hold of." For example, it would be correct to state "a child was *seized* with a fit of laughter" without any connotation of epilepsy. Similarly, the term "convulsion" implies any forceful involuntary contraction of the voluntary muscles. It would, therefore, also be correct to state that "a child coughed *convulsively*," with no implication of an epileptic mechanism. Epilepsy, however, is a sign of a neurologic disorder characterized by *recurrent* attacks of abnormal brain function (the seizures themselves) arising from abrupt, uncontrolled, repetitive electrical discharges of cortical neurons. Convulsive epileptic seizures (e.g., grand mal) display prominent motor signs. Nonconvulsive epileptic seizures (e.g., simple petit mal) lack these motor features.

The classification of seizures (Table 66–1) has recently undergone another revision reflecting an increased understanding of the correlation between epileptic clinical and EEG phenomena.[2] The new classification broadly divides all seizures into partial or focal onset (arising from a limited area of cortex of one hemisphere) or generalized onset seizures (arising simultaneously from both cerebral hemispheres).

Simple partial seizures are focal onset seizures that do not impair consciousness (consciousness implies full awareness of self and the environment and a normal ability to react to external stimuli) but rather manifest as a restricted disturbance in muscle control (e.g., isolated twitching of facial muscles), general sensation (e.g., warmth or tingling of an extremity) or special sensation (e.g., unformed visual hallucinations). Some simple focal seizures may gradually evolve into a complex partial seizure, signified by an altered consciousness. Either may culminate in a grand mal convulsion. Complex partial seizures are focal onset seizures that disturb or impair consciousness. The older terms (temporal lobe, psychomotor, or limbic lobe seizures) have been largely abandoned because partial seizures that disturb consciousness can arise from any lobe of the brain.

Generalized seizures appear simultaneously and symmetrically in both cerebral hemi-

TABLE 66–1
Revised Classification of Seizures

Partial seizures	
Simple: Preserved consciousness	*Complex:* Loss or clouding of consciousness
Simple or complex partial seizures may display motor signs (e.g., clonic jerking, distorted posture), somatosensory symptoms (e.g., simple tingling, warmth), special sensory symptoms (e.g., simple distortions of smell, taste, vision), autonomic signs (e.g., sweating, pallor, piloerection), or psychic symptoms (e.g., fear, anger, complex hallucinations). Psychic symptoms are far more common with complex partial seizures than with simple partial seizures.	
Generalized seizures	
Nonconvulsive	*Convulsive*
Typical absence seizure: true petit mal with three cps spike wave discharges on EEG	Tonic (abrupt increase of muscle tone)
Atypical absence seizure: EEG shows "slow" spike slow wave discharges at one to two cps; onset and termination of absence seizure may be gradual rather than abrupt	Atonic (abrupt decrease of muscle tone)
	Clonic (repetitive muscle jerking)
	Tonic-clonic (the classic grand mal seizures)
	Myoclonic (brief, shocklike muscle contractions)

spheres. Consciousness is disturbed immediately and motor manifestations, if any, are bilateral. The commonly recognized grand mal seizure exemplifies a generalized convulsive seizure composed of a predictable sequence of loss of consciousness, tonic stiffening of the trunk and limb musculature followed by a series of coarse clonic jerking of the extremities. The familiar petit mal seizure typifies a generalized nonconvulsive seizure producing partial or complete mental arrest or "absence" but lacking forceful muscle contractions.

Clinical observations alone may sometimes be insufficient to correctly discriminate between some of the classified types of seizures, and information gathered from the electroencephalogram (EEG) and other ancillary tests may assist the correct classification of seizures. For example, it is now recognized that automatisms (involuntary, semicoordinated purposeless integrated motor activities that appear during or after the clouded consciousness of a seizure) may accompany petit mal and are not pathognomonic for complex partial seizures. This distinction is more than of academic interest because it provides the basis for selecting the preferred anticonvulsant regimen. Ethosuximide (Zarontin) is highly effective in controlling petit mal absence but has little value in controlling the mental lapses of complex partial seizures. Conversely, carbamazepine (Tegretol) may completely abort absence due to complex partial seizures but will not eliminate petit mal attacks.

DATA GATHERING

The initial medical and neurologic examination of the child with suspected seizures seeks to: 1) provide a precisely detailed description of the sequence of events that comprised the attack, including the presence of a warning or aura, loss or preservation of consciousness, presence or absence of unilateral or bilateral motor signs and postictal signs and symptoms; 2) clarify the medical context in which the seizures arose; 3) define the past and present neurologic health of the patient, including a detailed physical and neurologic examination; and 4) provide specific therapy to remove the cause of the seizures or to treat the seizures themselves with appropriately selected anticonvulsants. The history should also inquire about unusual circumstances of the seizures (for example, extreme sleep deprivation) or the possibility of an environmental factor responsible for triggering the attack. The latter might include flickering lights (television, discotheques), reading, tactile stimulation, sound, or musical passages.

The medical and neurologic etiologies of seizures are legion. It is not feasible or desirable to devise a single rigid diagnostic formula that can successfully evaluate all children with seizures. The patient's age, prior medical and neurologic health, type of seizure, and the medical context in which the seizures arose should be thoughtfully integrated to provide a reasonable framework to tailor the patient's evaluation. For example, a thorough toxicology screen is necessary to adequately evaluate the condition of a teenage boy whose first seizure arose during a party. On the other hand, a lumbar puncture is usually performed to fully assess the condition of an ill-appearing infant after the first febrile seizure.

THE EEG IN EPILEPSY

The EEG remains the most commonly used tool to complement the history and physical examination of patients with suspected epilepsy. The EEG provides unique information to help confirm the diagnosis of epilepsy, classify the type of seizures, assist in discriminating focal onset from generalized seizures, raise the suspicion of an underlying structural CNS abnormality, suggest the preferred drug treatment, and sometimes formulate a neurologic prognosis.

The EEG cannot substitute for clinical judgment in establishing the diagnosis of epilepsy. A normal interictal EEG does not refute the diagnosis of epilepsy, nor does an "epileptically" abnormal EEG confirm it unless a seizure is clinically recognized. All EEG studies of epileptic patients report a sizable number of patients with normal interictal EEGs.[3] The yield of epileptically abnormal EEGs can be increased by recording the EEG within 1 week of a clinical seizure, obtaining serial tracings, and by enhancing or activating procedures. These include recording a portion of the tracing during sleep, prior all-night sleep deprivation, hyperventilation, photic stimulation, and sometimes the use of special recording electrodes such as nasopharyngeal leads. In general, the yield of abnormal EEGs is not materially influenced by the patient's consumption of anticonvulsants except for petit mal epilepsy. The administration of ethosuximide or valproic acid can normalize the EEG in petit mal.[4] Certain historical facts can be ascertained to increase the likelihood of recording an epileptically abnormal EEG. For example, some patients' seizures are clustered in the early morning. Scheduling the tracing for the early morning, therefore, might show an abnormality that may not be present if recorded later in the day.

A small number of healthy, nonepileptic children may display incidental focal or generalized epileptiform abnormalities on their records obtained for evaluating nonepileptic phenomena, such as headaches or learning disabilities.[5] The results of the EEG examination should be carefully correlated with the patient's clinical complaints in all instances. At times, it is necessary to discard the epileptic EEG abnormality as irrelevant to the clinical complaints at hand rather than assuming that epilepsy is the basis for the problem.

Many patients with epilepsy will continue to manifest abnormal EEGs despite good clinical control of their seizures. The often repeated advice of treating the patient rather than the EEG is particularly relevant in this circumstance. Routinely repeating the EEG examination on an arbitrary annual basis contributes little to the patient's neurologic care. It is unnecessary to automatically repeat EEGs at regular intervals if the clinical attacks or seizures are under good control. Repeating the EEG is indicated if there is a poor response to treatment, if a new type of seizure appears, if pseudoepileptic seizures are suspected, and when the physician contemplates discontinuation of treatment after a suitable period of seizure-free existence.

NEURORADIOLOGY FOR THE EPILEPTIC CHILD

It is recognized that a variety of structural CNS abnormalities are responsible for provoking seizures in some epileptic children. Cerebral hemorrhage, localized infection, contusion, tumor, stroke, calcification, porencephaly, vascular anomalies, and CNS malformations may announce their presence with a focal onset or generalized seizure. The clinician often desires an image of the intracranial contents to exclude a structural cause for epilepsy.

The yield of clinically useful information obtained from routine plain skull x-ray films is surprisingly low in children with chronic epilepsy. Its greatest application presently is to detect linear or depressed skull fractures immediately after head trauma. Computed tomographic (CT) scanning has largely supplanted the routine skull x-ray film in the evaluation of epilepsy in children.

Several studies have examined the utility of CT scanning in epileptic children. The incidence of any CT scan abnormality in children with normal intelligence and neurologic examinations who have generalized seizures is about

5%. Children with focal onset seizures have a much higher rate of abnormal CT scans, but most of the findings are nonspecific focal or generalized abnormalities, such as cerebral atrophy, cortical "scars," porencephalic cysts, and other conditions that have no therapeutic import. The yield of therapeutically significant clinical information, such as the demonstration of a resectable tumor or vascular anomaly, is less than 2% in CT scans obtained from children with focal seizures.

One common variety of partial epilepsy does not necessitate routine CT scans: so-called benign focal epilepsy of childhood (rolandic epilepsy, central-temporal epilepsy, sylvian seizures).[6] This inherited form of partial seizures usually begins at 4 or 5 years of age. The clinical seizure may be confined to sleep or may arise diurnally. A witnessed attack is usually heralded by focal twitching of the facial muscles, speech arrest, and salivation and may culminate in a grand mal convulsion. The EEG reveals a characteristic pattern of sharp waves in the central-temporal (sylvian) regions. A family history of similar seizures is present in about 30% of cases. This form of epilepsy is considered benign in spite of its focal nature, because it is not associated with any underlying structural CNS abnormality. Furthermore, seizure control is typically achieved easily and the disorder generally remits during later adolescence.

A single CT scan performed during the initial evaluation of the epileptic child is generally sufficient in most cases. Repeating the CT scan annually or on a routine basis is usually not necessary. The appearance of new signs or symptoms, such as headaches or hemiparesis, is a clear indication for repeating the CT scan, even if the original study was entirely normal. Some low-grade gliomas are not radiologically apparent early in their course, but may appear months or years after the onset of seizures. Children with neurofibromatosis and tuberous sclerosis are especially vulnerable to develop intracranial tumors so a high index of suspicion should be exercised for these individuals.

The introduction of magnetic resonance (MR) imaging can identify structural abnormalities previously undisclosed by routine CT scans, especially in those with complex partial seizures.[7] The superior resolution of this imaging modality allows small hamartomas, tumors, arteriovenous malformations, and focal scars to be more readily identified. However, calcifications may be missed with MR imaging and are best identified with CT. In some individuals, both CT and MR imaging examinations will be necessary for the full radiographic evaluation of possible structural abnormalities.

MANAGEMENT

THE SINGLE, UNPROVOKED SEIZURE

The term epilepsy implies the presence of *recurrent* seizures. However, a single, unprovoked seizure may arise as a solitary experience that interrupts the lives of otherwise healthy individuals. The risk of additional seizures and, therefore, epilepsy, following an initial isolated seizure is estimated at between 27% and 43% in adolescents and adults.[8] In young children the risk is higher. Individuals who have suffered a single seizure require the same careful medical and neurologic evaluation as those who have suffered repeated attacks, but neurologists disagree whether all such patients must be treated with anticonvulsants. Many prefer to await the second seizure before embarking on a commitment to chronic use of anticonvulsants.

FEBRILE SEIZURES

Approximately 4% of children between the ages of 6 months and 5 years will experience one or more febrile seizures. The clinical characteristics of the seizure, past medical and family histories, physical and neurologic examinations supplemented by the results of the EEG examination will permit most cases to be classified as either simple or complex febrile seizures (Table 66–2).

Children with simple febrile seizures have approximately the same risk of later life (nonfebrile) seizures as their healthy counterparts.[9] This condition is considered an age-dependent CNS response to fever and is distinguished from genuine epilepsy. Although the risk of later nonfebrile seizures is acceptably low, affected children may experience repeated febrile seizures until they have sufficiently matured. The risk of repeated febrile seizures is greatest in infants whose first febrile seizure appeared before 1 year of age. The goal of treatment of

TABLE 66–2
Simple and Complex Febrile Seizures

CHARACTERISTICS	SIMPLE FEBRILE SEIZURES	COMPLEX FEBRILE SEIZURES
Description of seizure	Generalized tonic, clonic, or tonic-clonic; sometimes atonic (limp)	Focal motor
Duration of seizure	≤15 min	>15 min
Repetition	One seizure within 24 hr	Clusters within 24 hr
Previous health	Normal	Suspected or definite neurologic abnormality
Family history	Negative for epilepsy; may be positive for febrile seizures	Positive for idiopathic or genetic non-febrile epilepsy
EEG	Nonspecific background slowing in the immediate postictal period; usually normal if recorded 7–10 days after the febrile seizure	Frank focal or generalized epileptiform abnormality
Risk for future nonfebrile seizures (epilepsy)	Approximately equal to the general population	≤10%

simple febrile seizures is, therefore, the prevention of recurrent *febrile* seizures. There is no evidence that treatment reduces the risk of future (nonfebrile) epilepsy. The daily prophylactic administration of phenobarbital to achieve a minimum blood level of 15 μg/mL substantially reduces the risk of recurrent febrile seizures. Phenytoin (Dilantin) is not efficacious as a prophylactic drug. Carbamazepine (Tegretol) is not useful in cases of phenobarbital failure. Sodium valproate (Depakene) does protect against recurrences; however, the risk of serious or fatal adverse side effects in children under 2 years of age[10] precludes its widespread use for this generally benign and self-limited condition. Anticonvulsants are usually administered for at least 2 years and discontinued 1 year after the last febrile seizure.

Children with complicated febrile seizures, with preexisting neurologic abnormalities or a family history of idiopathic or genetic nonfebrile seizures face up to a 10% risk of future epilepsy. Prophylactic anticonvulsant treatment is usually prescribed for these children.

RECURRENT NONFEBRILE SEIZURES

The goal of treatment of recurrent nonfebrile seizures is the complete elimination of further attacks without exposing the patient to significant systemic, cognitive, or behavioral adverse side effects. The key to the successful management is an accurate initial diagnosis of epilepsy (by carefully considering and excluding nonepileptic events that may mimic true seizures), the identification and removal of the possible cause of the seizures, the correct classification of the type of seizure disorder, and the selection of the appropriate type and dosage of anticonvulsant.

Ideally, the smallest dose of a single anticonvulsant that empirically controls the seizures is the "correct" amount of medication. If low doses of a single drug are unsuccessful, the dosage is gradually increased until seizure control is achieved or dose-related drug side effects appear. When clinical toxicity appears before acceptable seizure control, a second drug is introduced and gradually substituted in place of the initial ineffective drug. After trials of single anticonvulsants have been exhausted, two-drug combinations can be tried.

The selection of the particular anticonvulsant is largely determined by the classified type of seizure. Table 66–3 lists specific anticonvulsants that are considered generally useful for various types of seizures.[11] Maintenance dosages and pharmacokinetic properties are outlined in Table 66–4. For many medications, a lower dose is introduced initially and gradually increased until a maintenance level is achieved.

TABLE 66–3
Anticonvulsants Useful for Different Types of Seizures

Tonic-clonic	Classic petit mal	Atypical petit mal
Carbamazepine	Ethosuximide	Valproate
Valproate	Valproate	Clonazepam
Phenytoin	Clonazepam	Diazepam
Phenobarbital	Methsuximide	Clorazepate
Primidone	Trimethadione	Adrenocorticotrophic hormone
Mephenytoin	Acetazolamide	Ketogenic diet
Myoclonic	**Atonic**	**Focal**
Valproate	Valproate	Carbamazepine
Ethosuximide	Clonazepam	Phenytoin
Clonazepam	Ketogenic diet	Phenobarbital
Diazepam		Primidone
Clorazepate		Valproate
Adrenocorticotrophic hormone		Clorazepate
Primidone		Methsuximide
Ketogenic diet		Mephenytoin
		Ethotoin

TABLE 66–4
Dosages, Pharmacokinetics, and Therapeutic Blood Levels of Commonly Prescribed Anticonvulsants

ANTICONVULSANT						
GENERIC NAME	TRADE NAME	APPROXIMATE TOTAL DAILY DOSE (MG/KG) (CHILDREN)	DOSAGE INTERVAL (DOSES/DAY)	SERUM ELIMINATION HALF-LIFE (HR)	TIME TO REACH STEADY STATE (DAYS)	THERAPEUTIC BLOOD RANGE
Phenobarbital	Luminal	3–6	1–2	46–136	14–21	15–40 μg/ml
Phenytoin	Dilantin	3–8	2	10–34	7–8	10–20 μg/ml
Carbamazepine	Tegretol	20–30	3	12–25	3–6	6–12 μg/ml
Primidone	Mysoline	5–20	3	5–16	2–3	5–12 μg/ml
Ethosuximide	Zarontin	20–50	2	20–60	5–11	40–100 μg/ml
Valproate	Depakene	15–60	3–4	6–15	1–2	50–100 μg/ml
Methsuximide*	Celontin	5–20	1–2	70	15	10–40 μg/ml
Diazepam	Valium	0.1 to 2.0	3	24–53	5–8	200–600 ng/ml
Clorazepate	Tranxene	0.1 to 1.0	1–2	48	10	15–40 ng/ml
Clonazepam	Klonopin	0.1 to 0.35	2–3	18–50	4–9	10–70 ng/ml
Trimethadione	Tridione	20–40	3–4	10	2	20–40 μg/ml

*Methsuximide is rapidly converted to its active metabolite, *N*-desmethylmethsuximide. Figures reflect the pharmacokinetic properties of this metabolite.

DETERMINATION OF SERUM DRUG LEVELS

Many clinical laboratories offer the clinician direct measurements of serum levels of anticonvulsants that are available for delivery to the nervous system. Therapeutic blood levels of anticonvulsants are usually reported as a range of values. For example, the therapeutic range of phenobarbital is often cited as 15 μg/mL to 40 μg/mL. This implies that many, but not all, patients will require a minimum blood level of 15 μg/mL to achieve seizure control and that many, but not all, patients will experience dose-related side effects at blood levels exceeding 40 μg/mL. These therapeutic range values should be regarded as approximate guidelines rather than absolute barriers to be blindly ob-

TABLE 66–5
Anticonvulsant Serum Levels

TIMING OF SERUM LEVEL DETERMINATIONS
After introducing a new drug and establishing a maintenance dose
After changing the dose of a drug that has been chronically administered
After adding a new medication that effects the metabolism of the first
To adjust the dose in growing children with changing drug requirements
To ensure a maintenance level above the minimum therapeutic range in patients with infrequent seizures in whom treatment response cannot easily be titrated against the administered dose
To determine which of several administered drugs is responsible for clinical toxicity
To adjust the dose in patients with concurrent renal or hepatic disease

served. Therefore, it would be allowable to exceed the upper therapeutic range if the patient has experienced a definite, but incomplete, response with a lower dose of medication and remains free from drug-related side effects. Similarly, it would be unwarranted to increase the dose of an anticonvulsant if the patient already experiences side effects despite a blood level that strictly falls within the therapeutic range.

The determination of blood levels of anticonvulsants can only materially benefit the patient if the information is thoughtfully integrated with the entire clinical picture.[12] The routine determination of blood levels without a specific question or goal in mind will probably not benefit the patient. Tables 66–5 and 66–6 outline some practical guidelines to suggest the timing and interpretation of anticonvulsant blood level determinations.

POLYPHARMACY

Some epileptic patients do not achieve acceptable seizure control when receiving standard doses of one or two anticonvulsants. It is then tempting for the physician to prescribe a complex regimen of high doses of multiple anticonvulsants in an attempt to completely prevent more seizures. There is little evidence that this practice of polypharmacy substantially improves seizure control. Moreover, considerable evidence has suggested that high doses of single or multiple anticonvulsants can produce subtle but measurable disturbances of mental functions including intelligence, mood, perception, short-term memory, attention, concentration, and speed of problem solving.[13]

The effects of anticonvulsants on mental function in children have received abundant attention recently. Most physicians are aware that phenobarbital frequently provokes unwanted behavior (moodiness, hyperactivity, and sleep disturbances) in treated children.[12] However, there is not a similar broad awareness of and sensitivity to the mental side effects of commonly prescribed anticonvulsants.[13] Moreover, the presence of cognitive side effects

TABLE 66–6
Anticonvulsant Serum Levels

INTERPRETATION OF SERUM LEVELS	
LOW DRUG LEVELS DESPITE A CORRECTLY PRESCRIBED DOSE	HIGH DRUG LEVELS DESPITE A CORRECTLY PRESCRIBED DOSE
Noncompliance; incorrect dose or wrong drug	Patient accidentally or deliberately taking more than prescribed dose
Determination of blood level before steady-state is achieved (about five elimination half-lives: 5 × T½)	Reduced metabolism or excretion due to drug interaction
Reduced gastrointestinal (GI) absorption	Unique, individual variation in GI absorption and/or metabolism
Pregnancy	Hepatic or renal disease
Increased metabolism due to drug interaction	Laboratory error
Increased metabolism due to unique, individual biochemical variations (uncommon)	
Laboratory error	

may not be discernable with the customary clinical observation in the physician's office or via the traditional neurologic examination. Rather, the impairment of cognitive function requires specific, sensitive neuropsychological evaluations.[14]

A few practical conclusions can be drawn on the basis of the investigations presently available: some anticonvulsants expose patients to fewer mental side effects than others.[15] Valproate and carbamazepine have a more favorable profile of cognitive side effects than the traditional agents such as phenobarbital, primidone, and phenytoin. For all anticonvulsants, mental side effects are more likely to appear at higher dosages and drug levels than at lower ones. The coadministration of two or more drugs (polytherapy) may have additive mental side effects.

The practice of polypharmacy is often ineffective and may be frankly detrimental to the patient. The clinician must, therefore, carefully weigh the benefits of marginal improvement in seizure control against the risk of impaired mentation due to drug toxicity. For some individuals, total seizure control at the expense of chronic intoxication may be undesirable, and the patient may have to be willing to accept occasional seizures.

MEDICALLY REFRACTORY SEIZURES

Despite the best efforts of the primary care physician, some children's seizures persist with sufficient severity or abundance that they interfere substantially with their intellectual, academic, personal, and social development. Patients with medically refractory seizures deserve referral to a neurologist who is knowledgeable in epilepsy or to a regional comprehensive epilepsy center. Many programs provide facilities for intensive monitoring of the EEG and anticonvulsant blood levels and expert manipulation of the patients' medications. Patients may enjoy substantial benefits by exposing an incorrect diagnosis or classification of epilepsy, determining the presence of unsuspected pseudoepileptic seizures, or obtaining the safe reduction or elimination of polypharmacy. Some children with intractable epilepsy may be selected as suitable candidates for "seizures surgery." If their habitual focal seizures consistently arise from a single expendable brain region, a sharp reduction or total cessation of seizures can be achieved by excising the offending area. Similarly, children with refractory generalized epilepsy may benefit from surgical transection of the corpus callosum that prevents the free transmission of epileptic discharges between the cerebral hemispheres.[16]

RESTRICTIONS ON THE EPILEPTIC CHILD

Young people with epilepsy must be urged to explore the same activities and aspire to the same goals that challenge all children. They should not be sheltered from the hard work, struggles, discipline, failures, and disappointments that are healthy experiences during normal growth and development. Maturity, performance, independence, and self-confidence will remain dormant if the epileptic child is denied the opportunity to meet a challenge, prove his or her competency, and claim responsibility for both success and failure.

Reasonable limitations are imposed by all parents on their children. Parents of epileptic children should be equally expected to exercise their authority and discipline. Either capricious restrictions or overindulgence may harm their children. However, some special restrictions do apply to the epileptic child. Water submersion accidents represent a genuine threat to the life of the epileptic child. Swimming and boating must be meticulously supervised by an accompanying adult. Scuba diving cannot be sanctioned. Similarly, climbing at high elevations along narrow ledges or bicycling along the edge of a road could prove fatal if a seizure caused the child to lose control.

Society also places restrictions on epileptic individuals. Driving privileges are not extended to epileptics unless they have been seizure-free for a predetermined period of time. Epileptics may not be inducted into the armed forces, and some employers have public hiring policies excluding epileptics. Whether or not these restrictions are fair or necessary, they nevertheless exist. Part of the clinician's obligation to his epileptic patients is to advise them regarding these restrictions so that educational and career planning are realistic.

PSYCHOSOCIAL ASPECTS OF EPILEPSY

The majority of children with epilepsy are otherwise intelligent, well-adjusted, healthy individuals. Still it is recognized that educational, behavioral, psychiatric, and socialization disorders are over-represented among the epileptic population. The relative contributions of biologic factors (the epilepsy itself, possible underlying brain injury, anticonvulsant side effects) and environmental influences vary among individuals. The intrusion of this unwanted, socially embarrassing illness amid the normal turmoil of childhood and adolescence can precipitate unwanted behavior or a frank psychiatric disturbance that can be more disabling than the seizures themselves. In some cases, the anticonvulsant (particularly barbiturates[17]) may incite the untoward behavior, and reduction of dose or substitution with another drug can ameliorate the symptoms. If this simple maneuver fails, the clinician should not resign the child to this unhappy state. Skilled psychological or psychiatric intervention can be and often is effective in helping the child and family cope with this facet of the illness.

BIBLIOGRAPHY

1. Pedley TA: Differential diagnosis of episodic symptoms. *Epilepsia* 1983; 24:S31–S44.
2. The Commission on Classification and Terminology of the International League Against Epilepsy: Proposal for revised clinical and electroencephalographic classification of epileptic seizures. *Epilepsia* 1981; 22:489–501.
3. Marsan CA, Zivin LS: Factors related to the occurrence of typical paroxysmal abnormalities in the EEG records of epileptic patients. *Epilepsia* 1979; 11:361–381.
4. Callaghan N, O'Hare J, O'Driscoll D, et al: Comparative study of ethosuximide and sodium valproate in the treatment of typical absence seizures (petit mal). *Dev Med Child Neurol* 1982; 24:830–836.
5. Cavazzuti GB, Cappella L, Nalin A: Longitudinal study of epileptiform EEG patterns in normal children. *Epilepsia* 1980; 21:43–55.
6. Beaussart M, Faou R: Evolution of epilepsy with rolandic paroxysmal foci: A study of 324 cases. *Epilepsia* 1978; 19:337–342.
7. Riela AR, Penry JK, Laster DW, et al: Magnetic resonance imaging and complex partial seizures, in Ellington RJ, Murray NF, Halliday AM (eds): *The London Symposium (EEG Suppl 39)*. London, Elsevier Science Publishers, 1987; pp 161–173.
8. Hauser WA, Anderson VE, Lolwensen RB, et al: Seizure recurrence after a first unprovoked seizure. *N Engl J Med* 1982; 307:522–528.
9. Nelson KB, Ellenberg JH: Prognosis in children with febrile seizures. *Pediatrics* 1978; 61:720–727.
10. Dreifuss FE, Santilli N, Langer DH, et al: Valproic acid hepatic fatalities: A retrospective review. *Neurology* 1987; 37:379–385.
11. Clancy RR: New anticonvulsants in pediatrics: carbamazepine and valproate. *Curr Prob Pediatr* 1987; 17:133–209.
12. Stores G: Behavioral effects of antiepileptic drugs. *Dev Med Child Neurol* 1975; 17:647–658.
13. American Academy of Pediatrics Committee on Drugs: Behavioral and cognitive effects of anticonvulsant therapy. *Pediatrics* 1985; 76:644–647.
14. Vining EPG, Mellits ED, Dorsen MM, et al: Psychologic and behavioral effects of antiepileptic drugs in children: A double-blind comparison between phenobarbital and valproic acid. *Pediatrics* 1987; 80:165–174.
15. Mattson RH, Cramer JA, Collins JF, et al: Comparison of carbamazepine, phenobarbital, phenytoin and primidone in partial and secondarily generalized tonic-clonic seizures. *N Engl J Med* 1985; 313:145–151.
16. Wyllie E: Corpus callostomy for intractable generalized epilepsy. *J Pediatr* 1988; 113:255–261.
17. Brent DA, Crumrine PK, Varma RR, et al: Phenobarbital treatment and major depressive disorder in children with epilepsy. *Pediatrics* 1987; 80:909–917.

67 TRAUMA

LACERATIONS AND BURNS

John M. Templeton, Jr., M.D.

In recent decades, emergency departments in hospitals throughout the United States have been burdened with a number of acute, minor problems that used to be handled in the physician's office. In the case of lacerations and burns, it is understandable that an anxious parent would seek help in an emergency department. However, many simple lacerations and burns could be handled in the office setting. The following is a discussion of office management of these problems.

Lacerations are of three main types. The first and most common type is a simple laceration, which usually is linear or somewhat curved and penetrates the skin and subcutaneous tissue in a plane that is relatively perpendicular to the surface of the skin. The second type of laceration is a tangential or flap laceration in which the skin, subcutaneous tissue, and other structures are cut in an oblique fashion. Such flap lacerations can be curved or may be angled similar to the apex of a triangle. The final type of laceration is a complex laceration. This type involves three or more cuts in the injured surface radiating in different directions, emanating from a single common wound. Such complex lacerations are the result of a forceful blunt injury or a jagged tear. When complex lacerations have the appearance of a star they are referred to as stellate. All three types of lacerations can involve deeper structures such as fascia, muscle, tendons, vessels, and nerves.

PRINCIPLES OF WOUND MANAGEMENT

1. *Remove all foreign bodies,* such as gravel, grass, and dirt. When sutures are required, use a suture strong enough to do the job but not so big as to leave unnecessary foreign material in the wound.

2. *Debride devitalized tissue.* Lacerations due to blunt trauma are particularly likely to be associated with crush injury to the skin and deeper structures. This crush tissue usually incurs both necrosis due to the trauma itself, and infarction due to thrombosis of the vascular supply to the traumatized area. In the case of some tangential flap-type lacerations, the apex of the flap may be so pointed that it may no longer have adequate blood supply to support it. All such devitalized areas should be debrided back to a point at which one achieves fine capillary bleeding.

3. *Avoid secondary injury to the wound.* If a fresh wound is left open and unprotected for more than a few minutes the edges become dessicated, resulting in further cellular death and compromised circulation. Except during periods of assessment, cleaning, and repair, the wound should be protected by a sterile saline dressing. Also, any antiseptic solutions normally used for cleansing the skin are cytotoxic to unprotected tissue such as fat and muscle. If one is soaking a wound to cleanse it, a mild or dilute antiseptic solution should be used. Then, prior to closing the wound, all of the antiseptic solution should be thoroughly lavaged from the wound with saline.

4. *Maximize the blood supply to the wound.* In general, avoid epinephrine-containing solutions, especially in regard to distal organ situations such as the fingers, nose, and ears. Avoid using tourniquets on the digits and avoid the use of excessive pressure dressings.

5. *Minimize the final bacterial count* in the wound by means of vigorous saline lavage prior to closing the wound. Use sterile gloves whenever the wound is examined.

6. *Avoid leaving a dead space* in the depth

of the wound. Inadequate repair of muscle fascia and subcutaneous tissue will result in a dead space that will fill with serum and may become an ideal culture medium for infection. Even in the absence of secondary infection the seroma will cause an increased inflammatory response.

When one can be assured of compliance with the above principles of wound management, closure of the wound per primum or "by first intention" is the optimal form of management. The majority of well-handled wounds closed primarily should be completely sterile within 12 to 24 hours after primary closure.

Some wounds, however, are associated with much more severe tissue damage, and/or contamination with bacteria and foreign material. In such cases, all of the principles of wound management cannot be achieved. The patient is better served by not closing the wound initially and instead letting it heal "by secondary intention" or by delayed primary closure. In healing by secondary intention, the healing occurs by exaggerated fibrocapillary proliferation, scar formation, and finally wound contracture. Healing by delayed primary closure refers to the practice of allowing the lesion to develop healthy granulation tissue and then approximating the wound edges resulting in faster healing and less scar.

DATA GATHERING

What To Do When the Parent Calls

When a parent calls and says that her child has just incurred a laceration, the following first-aid advice should be given. Initially, anything clean, such as a cloth, towel, or washcloth, may be applied to the wound with modest pressure. The child should be placed in a supine position and should be comforted and reassured. If the child is excited he is less likely to remain still and more likely to raise his blood pressure, resulting in an increased tendency toward bleeding. Thus, it is important to make sure that the child is kept warm and comfortable.

Assessing the Injured Child

Once the child arrives in the office, an accurate history of the nature of the injury or surgical problem should be taken. It is important to determine what the environment was, where the child was injured, and what the apparent injuring item was (e.g., glass, corner of a table). An injury that occurs outdoors or in a trash heap may raise more concerns about a potentially contaminated wound or the presence of a foreign body. It is very important to make sure that the injury correlates with the history given to make sure that no intentional injury was involved and to make sure that there is no potential for other more serious occult injuries. One should determine the child's immunization status and his history of allergies (including allergies to drugs, antiseptics, iodine, and tape). Take vital signs including pulse and blood pressure, first in a supine and then upright position. Make sure that the child's neurologic status is normal and that peripheral circulation is intact, particularly distal to the site of injury.

When to Refer to the Hospital

As noted previously, the patient and family are usually best served if management of minor acute problems and follow-up care is done in the office. However, after initial assessment of the wound, there are several important findings that may lead the office physician to recommend care in a hospital setting: (1) serious injuries to deeper structures (including neurologic injury, excessive blood loss, tendon injury, closed-compartment injury, and underlying fracture); (2) need for more specialized care or equipment; (3) need for intravenous antibiotics; (4) concern for social environment; or (5) legal consideration.

MANAGEMENT

Once the assessment is complete and there is no need to refer the child, the management phase begins. If one has carefully planned and provided for appropriate supplies (Table 67–1), the total time to take care of most minor lacerations should range between 15 and 30 minutes. It is usually necessary for the physician to have a nurse or helper to facilitate treatment of the wound. Preferably the assessment of the child and complete treatment of the wound can all be done in one location. A separate area that has all the necessary supplies, in a quiet part of the office, usually serves best.

TABLE 67–1
Suture Materials

SUTURE MATERIAL AND NEEDLE TYPE	NEEDLE SIZES ETHICON	NEEDLE SIZES DAVIS & GECK
Chromic catgut		
Tapered needle	5–0, RB-1	5–0, T-31
Polyglycolate (Ethicon: Vicryl; Davis & Geck: Dexon Plus)	4–0, RB-1	5–0, T-31
Tapered needle	5–0, TF	5–0, T-30
	4–0, RB-1	5–0, T-31
	3–0, RB-1	3–0, T-31
Cutting needle	5–0, PC-1	5–0, SBE-2
Black monofilament nylon		
Cutting needle	5–0, P-3	5–0, PRE-2
	4–0, PS-2	4–0, PRE-4
	3–0, PS-1	3–0, PRE-6

Calm the Child and Family

Explain to the parent or guardian the nature of the child's problem, the treatment you plan to give, and the follow-up care required. Explain to the child that the wound needs to be repaired and that mother or father will be with him to help the doctor make him all better. Honestly explain that there may be a little pain initially but that you will then take the pain away by making his sore "go to sleep." When a child or guardian is willing, it is a great asset to have a calm, supportive parent who is willing to stay by the side of the child and to hold his or her hand, and to provide verbal reassurance that he or she is going to be made all better and will be able to go home very soon. A helpful parent may, in fact, know things of a diverting nature, such as talking about another sibling who also had to have a laceration "fixed up," and can thereby engage the attention and cooperation of the child. If the parent indicates that she would rather not be present, a sympathetic nurse can often fulfill this same function of reassurance. In this way the child and parent or nurse can go through the process together of getting "fixed up."

Initial Preparation of the Wound

Gently remove the bloody dressings from the wound while wearing sterile gloves and a mask. Have a sterile field prepared and, using gauze and a mild antiseptic solution in a basin, clean the wound. Often, bleeding will have stopped by the time the patient arrives in the office. If so, it is best to concentrate on gently cleaning the skin surrounding the wound. Vigorous rubbing of the wound itself restimulates further bleeding and should not be done until one is ready for a final lavage with saline preparatory to closing the wound. When the wound area has been cleaned, the wound should be thoroughly lavaged with sterile saline. This is most easily done by using a 30- or 50-mL syringe with which saline can be sprayed into the wound to remove any loose debris and remaining antiseptic solution.

Nonanesthetic Care of the Wound

Because the instillation of local anesthesia is usually somewhat painful, it may be the most upsetting part of wound repair. Fortunately, many minor lacerations are short and have edges that already lie comfortably coapted together. So long as the wound has been palpated to make sure there are no retained foreign bodies, the skin surrounding the wound can be prepared with a light layer of povidone-iodine (Betadine) solution (make sure not to get any of the antiseptic into the wound). When this has dried, or has been wiped away, a small amount of benzoin should be applied on each side of the wound and the wound edges closed with surgical tape strips. Most children like the idea that their "sore" can be healed with a "Band-Aid." An additional dressing should be applied over the wound so as to prevent contamination of the as yet unhealed wound.

In the case of patients who present late with contaminated wounds (more than 12 hours after injury) or wounds that are already infected, one may elect not to close the wound at all. Once again, one should make sure that there is no foreign body or devitalized tissue in the wound. If debridement is required, then local anesthetic is indicated. If no debridement is required, a light sterile fine mesh packing or wick may be placed in the wound and a bulky dressing applied (see section below on wounds left open).

Preparation of the Surgical Field

Sterile drapes may be used to isolate the injured area from the surrounding clothes and other nonsterile items. It is important to have at least a foot of sterile field all around the wound so that the end of the suture can lie on the sterile drape while the suture is being placed. If the laceration is in the head or neck area, placement of the drapes may represent a sudden threat to the child because of loss of visual contact with either a supporting parent or with the physician. It is important, therefore, to tell the child that the drapes are there to keep everything clean and that the parent or supporting nurse will still be there. Alternatively, a clear plastic drape may be used. Then the skin surrounding the wound should be cleaned once again with an antiseptic solution such as Betadine solution, making sure that none of the solution gets into the wound. Any excess solution can be wiped away.

Anesthetic Preparation

Most lacerations require one or more sutures. Although instilling local anesthetic may be almost as painful as putting in a single suture, it is usually best to use some local anesthesia. It is helpful to enlist the child's help as a participant by asking him to tell you if he feels any pain. Explain that if he feels pain you will quickly make the pain go away. In general, pain following instillation of an anesthetic will last for 10 to 15 seconds followed by fairly effective anesthesia. The child who is 6 years old or older will often be able to understand well what you tell him and may be able to cooperate to a considerable degree if you do not violate the trust relationship.

Most wounds that are to be closed per primum are considered clean. For this reason the anesthetic solution may be instilled through the edge of the wound, which is already somewhat more anesthetized than the surrounding skin. Lidocaine (Xylocaine) 1% without epinephrine is usually the best choice for local anesthetic. The total dose of lidocaine 1% should not exceed 5 mg (0.5 mL)/kg. If one needs to use a larger volume, dilute the lidocaine in a 1:1 ratio with sterile saline solution. Lidocaine 0.5% is an effective anesthetic agent, but it takes a bit more time to take effect. After explaining to the child that he may now feel some pain, one can begin to instill the anesthetic material just under the dermis using a fine 25-gauge needle for a distance of about 1.0 to 1.5 cm around the periphery of the wound. It is less painful to do this if the lidocaine is instilled slowly and then the needle is advanced into the area that has just received the lidocaine, after a few seconds' delay. More and more anesthetic solution can then be slowly instilled until the wound is thoroughly anesthetized. After injecting anesthetic, it is best to wait 60 seconds to make sure that the anesthetic has taken effect. Test the skin margins with a needle, again asking the child to report any pain sensation so that you can "make it go away."

Final Assessment and Preparation of the Wound

With the wound edges now anesthetized, the wound should be inspected once again to make sure that there are no foreign bodies or devitalized tissue present and that there are no unexpected major structures injured. Sometimes fine particulate foreign-body material is densely stuck to the ragged edges of the wound. Such areas should be debrided with scissors. If any devitalized tissue is noted it should also be debrided. If a specific bleeding point, such as a vein, is identified, it may be clamped and tied with a 4–0 chromic tie. If the edges of the wound appear to be unduly contused and blue or purple, it is likely that this margin of tissue will not survive. Using a scalpel, 2 to 3 mm of the wound edges can be excised to remove devitalized tissue (Fig 67–1).

Management of the Deep Portion of the Wound

If the superficial fascia and muscle has been divided but no other injuries are apparent, 4–0 or 3–0 polyglycolate suture may be used to close the opening in the fascia. Usually the sutures do not need to be closer than 5 to 8 mm. If the subcutaneous tissue is fairly widely separated, it can be approximated by using 4–0 chromic sutures, placing them approximately 1 cm apart. Once there is complete closure of the depths of the wound, thereby eliminating dead space, the skin edges can be closed.

Closure of the Skin

Optimal closure of the skin edges involves simple interrupted sutures using monofilament nylon placed in such a fashion that the wound

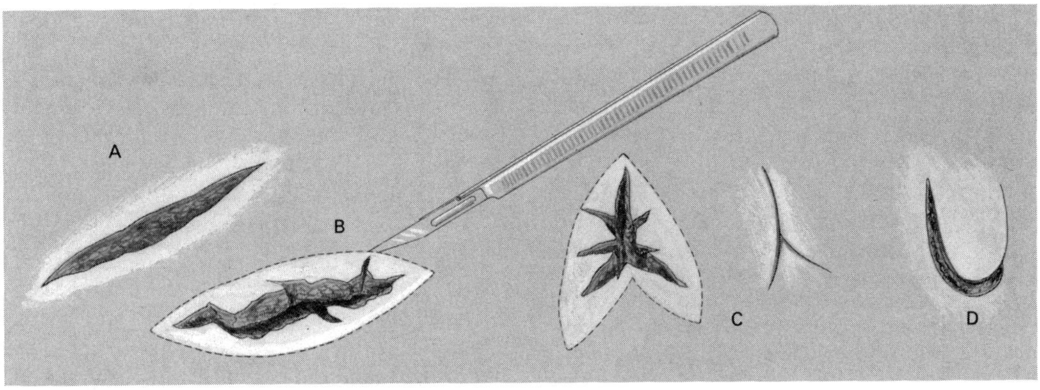

FIG 67–1
Preparation of wound edges to allow optimal closure by removal of jagged edges. *A,* simple; *B,* elliptical; *C,* stellate wound repair by excision; *D,* flap repair.

edges are slightly everted. It is very important to incorporate the same amount of skin and subcutaneous tissue on both sides of the wound so that there will be balanced tension on the edges of the wound. Closure of the skin edges should be gentle enough so that the edges just barely touch together (Fig 67–2). If one is not careful, the suture may become inadvertently tight, producing a garotting effect on the encircled skin and tissue. The result of placing skin sutures too tightly is that they begin to cut through the skin, resulting in more prominent cross-hatching marks ("railroad tracks"). Furthermore, because such sutures cut into the tissues, they are painful and difficult to remove. An improved cosmetic result can be obtained by placing surgical tape strips between each of the specific sutures and removing the nylon sutures 1 or 2 days earlier.

There are additional ways to protect the tissue from unnecessary trauma. First, in grasping each particular tissue layer, use the forceps as gently as possible and only for a few moments. Second, a suture should be selected that will

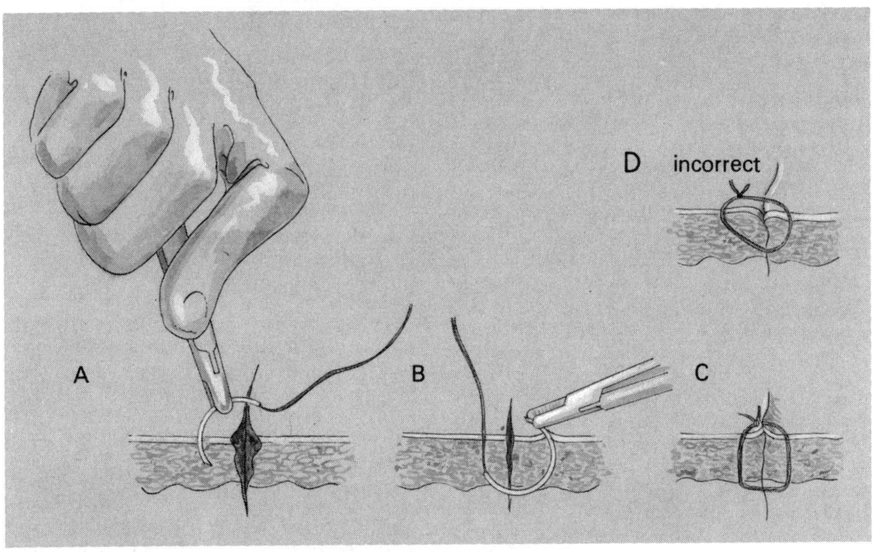

FIG 67–2
Technique for simple suture. **A,** placement of needle perpendicular to skin surface. **B,** follow through the curve of the needle. **C,** symmetrical correctly placed suture. **D,** incorrect placement of suture.

have adequate strength but that will result in as little inflammation of the tissue and skin as possible. Using an unnecessarily heavy suture results in an increased inflammatory response. Third, in longer wounds, or ones that have a curved or tangential shape, it is especially important to place the center suture for each layer first so that proper realignment of the wound edges is assured. Subsequent sutures can then be placed lateral to the midpoint.

Management of Special Wound Situations

Flap Wounds.—Tangential or flap wounds can exist in a simple, curved or an angle-type wound, or can occur as multiple flaps in a stellate wound. When the apex of a flap is a sharp angle, realignment of the wound edges is more difficult. The use of a few interrupted subcuticular sutures in the dermis near the tip (but not at the tip) is adequate for realigning the skin. The blood supply to these acutely angled tangential flaps is often not good, and placement of the sutures through the tip may result in its final loss of viability. A Steri-Strip to align the tip results in better healing. After securing the center point or apex of a tangential flap, one can place interrupted sutures along the lateral margins of the remaining wound to provide further support. When repairing a flap-type wound it is important to place the needle through the flap edge first. The edges of the mobile flap can then be moved back and forth until it is properly aligned with the skin on the opposite side.

Eyebrow Lacerations.—Because of the bony prominence of the orbit under the eyebrows, children frequently get eyebrow lacerations from striking their head against a hard object. The physician should avoid shaving the eyebrow off because in a few patients the eyebrows will not grow back well. Also, one loses helpful landmarks in returning the tissue to its preinjury location. Following the same general principles in closing the wound, one can usually close such lacerations with a few interrupted loop knot-type sutures. Be sure individual hairs are free of the sutures.

Lip Lacerations.—In all areas of the body it is helpful to try to realign the edges of the laceration so that the natural skin lines are reapproximated. This is particularly important in the lip when the vermilion border has been divided. Such repairs may be done in an office setting, but usually require careful reconstruction of the deeper layers of the lip if they have been divided as well. Sutures of 5–0 chromic catgut are usually adequate for these deeper layers. Then for the skin itself fine nylon sutures of a 6–0 or 5–0 size should be used.

The Scalp.—Lacerations of the scalp are different in several ways from lacerations in other areas. Because of the rich collateral blood supply of the scalp and because skin of the scalp is under more tension than skin in most other locations, bleeding from the scalp can be prodigious. Without effective tamponading of a vigorously bleeding scalp wound, a child can readily lose 10% to 15% of his total blood volume.

On arrival in the office the child should be taken to the treatment area but the wound should not be examined until all the supplies and equipment are ready. Additional sterile bandages should be available in case the wound must be quickly redressed to tamponade recurring bleeding points. One should have 10 mL of lidocaine, 1%, with epinephrine ready for use. The maximum dose one should give is 7 mg (0.7 mL)/kg. Because major bleeding from the scalp occurs from both small and larger vessels and because it occurs so rapidly, it is often difficult to see where the specific, large bleeding vessels are. Rapidly instilling lidocaine with epinephrine around the periphery of the wound for a distance of 1 cm and then retamponading the wound for 1 or 2 minutes will usually allow effective vasoconstriction of the arterioles. Then the specific larger bleeding vessels that usually do not respond to infiltration of epinephrine can be clamped with a hemostat and selectively ligated. A figure-of-eight suture with 3–0 chromic catgut around both sides of the clamped bleeding vessel is usually required to obtain specific hemostasis. This is because these vessels tend to retract and are not controlled by simple ligation.

Once the anesthetic has taken effect and bleeding has been controlled, one can further prepare the wound for primary repair. Shaving the hair back for a distance of 1 to 2 cm provides a margin of unimpeded skin to be used in repairing the wound. This limited shaving also facilitates examination of the wound edges to make sure that they are still viable and to provide room for debridement of any devitalized tissue. However, one should not overly debride the margins of the scalp wound unless they are clearly devitalized. There is not much laxity in the scalp and it may be difficult to close the wound primarily if there is excessive skin loss. Once the shaving is complete, the wound should be thoroughly lavaged with 300 to 500 mL of saline to remove any hair particles or other foreign debris. Any foreign material that remains stuck to the wound, or any remaining devitalized tissue should be carefully and thoroughly debrided.

If the galea has been violated, interrupted sutures approximately 1 cm apart using 3–0 or 2–0 Vicryl sutures or chromic sutures can be used for reapproximation. If the dermis of the scalp is fairly thick, the deep portion of the dermis can be reapproximated with interrupted sutures of 4–0 or 3–0 Vicryl. The skin can be reapproximated with an interrupted or running suture of 3–0 nylon. Often, obtaining adequate apposition of the skin edges in a scalp wound requires more tension than is true for skin lacerations elsewhere in the body. It is important, however, not to tie down the skin sutures any more tightly than necessary to achieve gentle apposition of the wound edges. In the hair-bearing area of the scalp, cosmetic effect will not be as important a consideration as elsewhere in the body, but it is important to remember that wound healing will be impeded if excessively tight sutures are used.

Once the wound has been closed it is better to apply a dressing to the wound that can be removed fairly easily and not result in the sticking of the dressing to the skin, sutures, or hair. A piece of Telfa, cut to fit the shaved area of the scalp, can be applied over the wound after coating the skin edges with benzoin and allowing it to dry. In the case of an older cooperative child, a light layer of benzoin can be put on top of the Telfa and one or two more layers of Telfa applied in a similar fashion to provide a cushion for the dressing. An alternative is to apply a piece of adhesive-backed plastic (Op-Site or Tegaderm) cut to size, on top of the initial layer of Telfa. In the case of younger children it is better to apply several bulky layers of sterile dressing over the initial layer of Telfa and then to use a roll of gauze to wrap around the head and secure the bandage to the wound.

Wound Dressings

The role of a dressing is to prevent secondary contamination and infection of the wound, to protect the wound from accidental secondary trauma before it is healed, and to facilitate optimal healing with minimal scar formation. In the case of a young child, the dressing is also intended to keep probing or scratching fingers out of the wound.

In the days following repair of the wound the fibrocapillary tissue laid down at each layer of the wound is delicate. If the wound is kept immobilized there are less likely to be shearing forces tearing apart or separating these early fibrocapillary proliferation layers. Whenever such shearing or tearing does occur, additional fibrocapillary proliferation is required resulting in enhanced scar formation.

To provide optimal comfort and healing of the wound the following guidelines are suggested:

1. Apply a Telfa dressing directly over the wound and sutures so that undue sticking to the dressing does not occur.
2. Apply at least two or three layers of sterile gauze over the Telfa to provide padded protection.
3. Where appropriate, as on the extremities, use a roll-type gauze bandage to hold the dressing in place. Tape may be used to secure the edges of the roll of gauze, including to the adjacent skin, to keep the rolled gauze from slipping up or down.
4. In general, where tape is used on the skin, it is best to use paper tape.
5. Where the injury involves particularly active areas, such as the hand or other joint areas, one should apply a large amount of loose, bulky dressings secured with a roll of gauze, taped to keep the dressing secure and thereby providing a splinting effect. Such a dressing will minimize any motion along the wound interface.

Tetanus Management

If the patient is known to the treating physician, or if the parent can give reliable evidence of the child's immunization status, one can follow the following simple guidelines in regard to a booster shot for tetanus toxoid. A fully immunized patient does not require a tetanus booster more frequently than every 10 years.

Most physicians, however, tend to give a booster if there has been more than an interval of 5 years. Clearly, the older standard of a booster every 1 or more years after the last shot is not necessary.

If the wound has a high potential for tetanus infection, as would be the case in a major destructive injury that occurred in a barnyard or a garbage dump, the patient is probably better treated in a hospital setting with antibiotics and careful wound management. If the wound is simple and if the family cannot provide reliable evidence of adequate immunization, the child should be started on an immunization program.

Suture Removal

Two factors determine how soon one can consider removing the skin sutures: the blood supply of the area involved, and the tension on the wound interface. In general, the blood supply is greatest in the head and neck area resulting in more rapid and effective fibrocapillary proliferation. As one descends toward the lower extremities the blood supply diminishes somewhat. In some areas of the body, skin wounds are under increased tension due to underlying bone, as in the scalp, or due to muscle activity, as in the face or hand. Although the neck does not have quite as good blood supply as the face or scalp, the tensions on the skin edges of the neck wound are not as great. The sutures, therefore, can be removed in the neck somewhat sooner than they can be in the face and scalp. Suggested times for suture removal are as follows: neck, 3 to 4 days; face and scalp, 5 days; eyelids, 3 days; trunk and upper extremities, 7 days; and lower extremities, 8 to 10 days.

Office Management of Wounds Electively Left Open

A wound that is not closed primarily must either heal by secondary intention or by a delayed primary closure several days after the wound has occurred. The main purpose in leaving a wound open in such a manner is to minimize the potential for proliferation of bacteria and the development of a wound infection. Wound infections are not only a hazard in regard to reseparation of the wound edges, but are a nidus of infection of previously uninvolved tissue with the potential for local tissue necrosis, elaboration of toxic substances, and systemic sepsis.

More serious wounds and injuries are likely to be handled in a hospital setting. Nevertheless, the same principles for avoiding secondary wound infection apply in the cases of smaller more limited wounds. In general, one should consider leaving the wound at least partially open when (1) the laceration was due to an animal bite, especially a human bite; (2) the laceration occurred in a contaminated locale such as a garbage dump or barnyard; (3) the laceration occurred many hours before the patient was brought for medical attention; and (4) the laceration was of a puncture type, such as in the hand or foot, when playing outdoors.

The tissue layer most susceptible to secondary infection is the subcutaneous tissue because it has the least adequate blood supply. For this reason this layer is the most important one to leave open. If a contaminated wound is relatively fresh, and if one can visualize all layers of the wound fairly well, one may consider debriding any compromised muscle and fascia and closing these layers in the expectation that satisfactory wound healing may occur. The skin and subcutaneous layer would be packed loosely and left open. If the wound margins cannot be well seen, or if there are signs of early infection, debridement may be employed as indicated but none of the wound should be closed. In such a situation one should clean and debride the wound and then apply a saline-soaked, sterile fine mesh gauze to the entire wound surface followed by a light bandage of absorbable gauze. Alternatively, Betadine-soaked fine mesh gauze may be used. The Betadine may play little role in local antisepsis, but since it is somewhat cytotoxic it may elicit a more prominent inflammatory response, leading to better local blood supply and bacterial control. If the wound is relatively clean when it is first dressed, a change of dressing is not required for two or three days. Then the wound should be redressed at least once a day in the same manner until fresh, healthy granulation tissue is obtained. Such tissue is characterized by a bright red irregular surface that readily bleeds when wiped with a gauze. If the wound is already infected or badly contaminated, more intensive open wound treatment is required.

The dressings should be soaked off every 8 to 12 hours and the wound cleaned and redressed. These dressing changes should continue twice or three times a day until good granulation tissue develops.

In most wounds that are appropriately cleaned and debrided initially there will be adequate granulation tissue by 3 to 5 days after the injury. Then the wound field can be prepared as for a primary wound closure, anesthetized, and closed in appropriate layers, including closure of the skin. Some wounds treated by the open technique may be deeper than they are wide. If the granulation tissue appears to be healthy and if the skin edges appear to lie comfortably together, a physician can elect simply to tape the edges together and protect the wound with a bulky dressing until healing is complete.

There are some situations in which one may decide to close a wound that normally would be left open. In the case of an animal bite of the face, for example, the cosmetic result is such an important consideration that one might elect to repair a small clean wound primarily to minimize scar formation. The use of tape strips for the skin still allows potential for drainage should any infection develop. When infection in the face occurs it is associated with a considerable amount of cellulitis, which may then progress to periorbital cellulitis with the potentially fatal hazard of cavernous sinus thrombosis. For these reasons children with animal bites of the face are probably most safely managed by admission to a hospital, repair of the laceration in an operating room, and coverage with intravenous antibiotics.

The other circumstance in which one might individualize management of a wound is when medical attention is sought many hours after the original injury. The usual guideline is to not close such a wound if the interval has been greater than 12 hours. One might, however, elect to treat a 6-hour-old badly contaminated crush wound in an open fashion. By contrast, an 18-hour-old clean knife wound laceration may be closed safely.

BURNS

Burns are a quite common form of injury in children. In many cases the burns are mild enough to be treated in an office setting. The four usual causes of burn injuries are ultraviolet light from the sun, or from thermal, chemical, or electrical sources. Assessment of a burn injury involves a determination of the apparent depth of injury and the percent of the patient's total body surface area that is involved. First-degree burn injuries involve the epithelium only, and as such are quite superficial. The dermis, nerve endings, and skin appendages such as sweat glands are intact. Usually, skin with a first-degree burn can continue to provide an effective barrier to the penetration of bacteria and the evaporative loss of water. In first-degree burns the patient presents with various degrees of erythema, edema, pain, and tenderness to touch.

Second-degree burns represent partial thickness injury to the skin. There is injury into but not through the dermal layer. Deep second-degree burns can result in loss of most of the dermis with preservation only of sweat glands and hair follicles. Because the deeper layers of the dermis are still viable in second-degree burns, the site of injury is characterized by erythema, pain, and blanching on palpation. When a second-degree burn is relatively superficial, blisters are usually present. Third-degree burns represent full-thickness injury of the skin into or even beyond the subcutaneous tissue. The entire skin has been killed, and therefore presents as a tough brownish leathery surface that has no pain or blanching.

It often is not possible to distinguish between third-degree burns and deep second-degree burns. In different parts of the same burn there can be all gradations from first-degree through third-degree injury. Physiologically, the severity of the burn injury is determined by the percent of the total body surface area that is involved with both second-degree and third-degree burns. For children, any second-degree burn involving 10% or more of the body surface area or any third-degree burn involving more than 2% of the body surface area should be managed in an emergency department or burn center. Such children usually require admission to the hospital. In addition, patients with second- or third-degree burns of the hand or perineum should also be admitted for inpatient care. Finally, any child who incurred his burn as a result of a fire in a closed space should be admitted because of the risk of smoke inhalation injury.

Sunburn

In spite of these stipulations, many burns are suitable for management in an outpatient setting. Sunburn is a common problem in children because their skin is thinner than that of an adult, and the child is often unaware of the dangers of sunburn. The sunburn usually presents a bright red erythema of the skin with various degrees of edema. Pain may present acutely within 2 to 4 hours following excessive exposure. The pain is usually proportional to the amount of associated edema. Therefore, the first line of treatment should involve cool compresses with or without ice, which may be applied intermittently for periods of 10 to 15 minutes. One may also use baths of tepid water to which starch or Aveeno powder has been added. If pain and discomfort is still a major problem, emollients such as cold cream or cocoa butter, or creams and lotions such as Eucerin or calamine lotion may be applied to the involved areas. If edema is a prominent feature, 0.5% to 1.0% corticosteroid sprays or lotions may be used.

Pain and discomfort will usually peak and begin to resolve within 24 hours. Children with a more severe case of sunburn may have greater prolongation of symptoms or may develop systemic toxic effects such as fever, chills, malaise, delirium, or prostration. Any child with significant systemic symptoms should be admitted to the hospital for more extensive treatment.

Thermal Burns

In children with thermal burns that are mild enough to be treated on an outpatient basis, the usual causes are being scalded or touching a hot stove or cooking utensil. If a parent calls immediately to tell you about the burn, the single most effective immediate treatment is to immerse the burned area in cool or cold water. Quick use of cold water will immediately stop any further thermal injury.

In the office the child's burn should be cleansed with sterile saline solution at room temperature. If blisters are intact they should not be opened for at least 24 hours. An intact blister will lessen discomfort to the patient and will provide temporary protection against infection. Usually within 24 to 48 hours after a second-degree burn is incurred, the blister begins to lose its integrity. It should then be debrided at that point for more effective cleansing of the involved skin. The main problem with second-degree or third-degree burns is secondary bacterial invasion. In the case of a relatively deep second-degree burn, secondary bacterial invasion can result in additional tissue destruction, and thereby convert a second-degree injury to a third-degree injury. For this reason a topical antiseptic should be used. For all areas except the face the burns should be lightly washed twice a day and a layer of 1% silver sulfadiazene (Silvadene) cream applied to the wound. Because silver sulfadiazene quickly runs off a weeping burn surface, sterile gauze should be applied over the wound to keep it in contact with the burn, and held in place with a loose rolled gauze dressing. For small second-degree burns of the face, it is best to cleanse the wound and apply Polysporin ointment three times a day.

Superficial second-degree burns will usually successfully reepithelialize within 7 to 10 days. Deeper second-degree burns may take up to 20 days. Follow-up in the office can usually be done at 2 days, 5 days, and 10 days following injury. The parents, however, should be warned to watch for increasing redness or discoloration of the normal tissue around the burn site or for the presence of odor or inappropriate pain from the burn area itself. Such findings are suggestive of secondary infection (such as streptococci). If secondary infection does develop the patient should be admitted to the hospital for more intensive management.

Chemical Burns

Chemical burns can occur from a variety of substances. Fortunately, children are not generally involved with chemical burns because most of the acids or bases that produce these burns are not widely available in the home. If a child gains access to a garage or workshop where strong chemicals are kept, however, a spill on the skin may occur. The strong chemicals may be acid or base. In the majority of situations the appropriate treatment is to lavage the area of chemical burn thoroughly with water. This has the effect of diluting the concentration of the chemical and washing the material away. Two types of chemicals, however, should not be treated with water. Strong acids such as sulfuric acid or nitric acid should be neutralized with lime water or soap. Also, a burn from sodium metal should be neutralized with a weak acid such as acetic acid. The appropriate sequence in handling a child with a chemical burn to the skin is to first identify the chemical agent. This may require sending a family member back to the garage or workshop to find out what the chemical was. Except for the above-mentioned exceptions, the chemical burn should be lavaged with water following which any loose debris or tissue such as blister fragments may be removed. Then a bismuth-tribromophenate in petrolatum (Xeroform) gauze with bulky absorbent gauze on the outside may be applied loosely with a rolled gauze to the burned area. Finally, once the chemical agent is known, a burn center or poison control center should be called for further advice and recommendations.

Electrical Burns

Electrical burn injuries usually involve a point of entry and exit in the body. Such injuries can be highly deceptive in that these two sites may appear to have only a small area of damaged tissue. Because of the conductivity of certain tissues such as blood vessels, however, much greater internal tissue damage may occur. In children, the most common type of electrical burn is a labial burn, which is the result of the child chewing on an electrical cord. In such burns the tissue damage is confined usually to one corner of the mouth. There are signs of full-thickness injury in that the area may be relatively nonpainful and have an area of dry, leathery tissue. Local conservative wound care involves washing the involved area four to five times a day with benzalkonium chloride (Zephiran), allowing the area to dry, and applying a thin layer of antibiotic ointment. The child should be fed with a cleft lip feeder. Arm splints should be used to keep the child's hands away from the wound.

Traditionally, such injuries have been treated on an outpatient basis with careful warnings given to the parents that major bleeding from a labial artery may occur 1 to 3 weeks after the initial burn. In such cases the bleeding is best controlled with pressure and application of sponges wet with epinephrine. In contrast to conservative or expectant care some plastic surgeons have stressed the benefit of oral stents to minimize subsequent scar formation and wound contracture. To be effective, such treatment needs to be started early. If such treatment is available in the patient's locale, then immediate referral for further therapy is warranted.

BIBLIOGRAPHY

Caravajal HF, Parks DH: *Burns in Children*. Chicago, Year Book Medical Publishers, 1988.

Eather KF: Regional anesthesia for infants and children. *Int Anesth Clin* 1975; 13:19–48.

Edgerton MT: *The Art of Surgical Technique*. Baltimore, Williams & Wilkins, 1988.

Fleisher GR, Ludwig S: *Textbook of Pediatric Emergency Medicine*, ed 2. Baltimore, Williams & Wilkins, 1988.

McGregor IA: *Fundamental Techniques of Plastic Surgery*, ed 7. New York, Churchill-Livingstone, 1980.

Schwartz SI (ed): *Principles of Surgery*, ed 5. New York, McGraw-Hill, 1989.

Wind GG, Rich NM: *Principles of Surgical Technique*, ed 2. Baltimore, Urban & Schwarzenberg, 1989.

HEAD TRAUMA

Frederick Tecklenburg, M.D.

Head injury is one of the most common childhood accidents confronting the primary care physician. Each year approximately 5 million children present to medical attention for evaluation of head trauma. Since the majority of these injuries may be managed on an outpatient basis, the physician's office will frequently be the site of assessment and disposition. Alternatively, roughly 200,000 children will be hospitalized, primarily for careful and serial neurologic observation. Fifteen thousand patients suffer more severe craniocerebral trauma requiring prolonged hospitalization and an additional 3,000 to 4,000 pediatric patients die. An untold number of children sustain permanent neurologic sequelae. The key to appropriate management of head injuries is early recognition of potential complications, coupled with the rapid and orderly initiation of therapy.

Brain injury due to head trauma has been conceptualized as primary and secondary injuries (Fig 67–3). Primary injuries are the direct biomechanical damage to the head incurred at the moment of trauma. Fractures, cerebral contusions and lacerations, and the initial neuronal and vascular damage that occur at traumatic impact are examples of primary injuries that unfortunately are seldom amenable to therapy. Secondary brain injuries are the result of reactive central nervous system (CNS) lesions such as brain swelling, intracranial hemorrhages, and seizures, or the result of systemic pathologic conditions, including hypoxia, hypercarbia, hypotension, anemia, hyperthermia, and electrolyte imbalance. If a child deteriorates after the traumatic event, a secondary factor is responsible. These multiple secondary factors are treatable, but if left unchecked, they will ultimately lead to additional brain insults via hypoxemia, ischemia, or increased intracranial pressure. Thus, the goal of the primary care physician is to sort out those patients with minor head trauma and to recognize and refer those patients who may need management of secondary head injury factors.

ANATOMIC CONSIDERATIONS

The infant and young child's head occupies proportionately more of the total body mass than the adult. The brain weight and head circumference of the newborn are, respectively, 25% and 60% of adult values; by 2 years of age, these dimensions are 75% and 87% of adult average values. This relative cephalic preponderance, coupled with the child's inquisitive nature and lack of judgment, creates a predisposition to head injury.

Scalp

The scalp consists of several layers, easily remembered by the acronym: skin, connective tissue, aponeurosis, loose areolar tissue, periosteum.

The connective tissue is a very vascular subcutaneous layer that anchors the skin to the aponeurosis (galea) via fibrous septa. The minimal adhesiveness of the aponeurosis to the per-

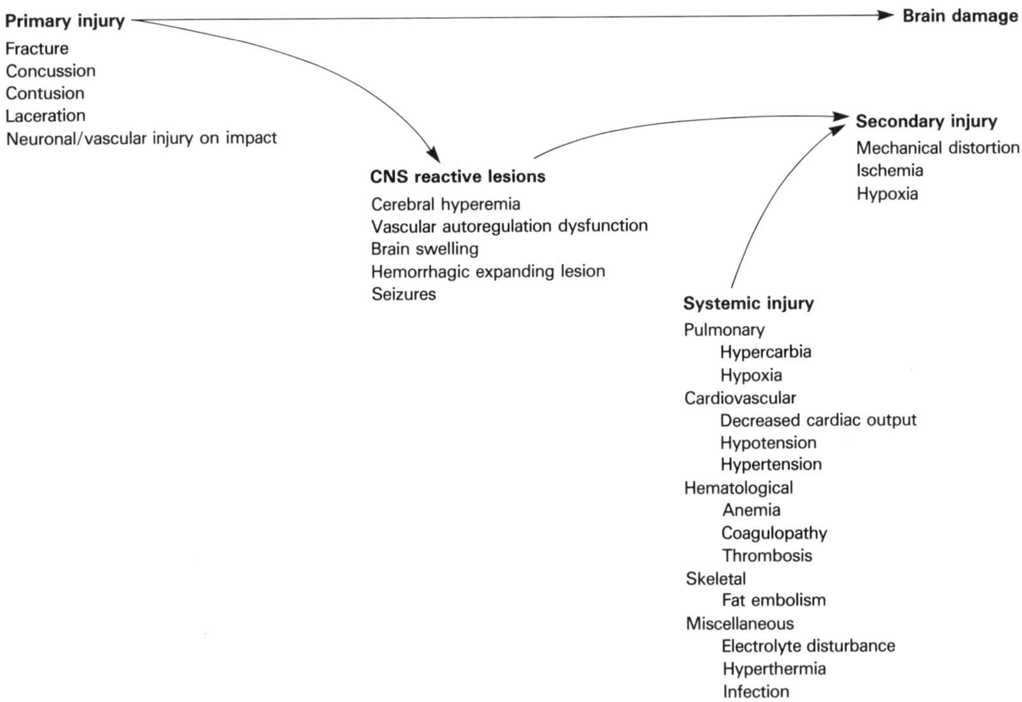

FIG 67–3
Pathophysiology of head trauma. Factors in primary injury and CNS systemic factors that lead to brain damage.

icranium accounts for the large flaps, "scalping" injuries, and gaping wounds that occur when the galea is lacerated. Underneath this layer is a clinically significant potential space consisting of loose areolar tissue and the emissary veins. A subgaleal hematoma results from hemorrhage into this space, and in the infant it may be sufficiently expansive to induce anemia and, occasionally, shock. The periosteum is the outermost covering of the individual cranial bones.

The Skull

The infant's skull is more flexible than the adult's because of the intrinsic nature of young bone, the flexible sutural ligaments, and the fontanelles. This resiliency has a protective effect by absorbing some of the local traumatic impact forces. But the calvarial elasticity may also allow more detrimental movement of the brain during acceleration and deceleration of the head.

The base of the skull contains the anterior, middle, and posterior cranial fossae. By early childhood these surfaces become more irregular and sharply defined, predisposing the brain to parenchymal damage by sudden accelerative forces. The ridged orbital roofs and cribriform plate of the ethmoid form the floor of the anterior fossa, a potentially injurious surface to the inferior portions of the frontal lobes. The middle cranial fossa's anterior anatomic boundary, the lesser wings of the sphenoid, presents a damaging obstacle to any anterior motion of the temporal lobes. The multiple foramina and air sinuses traversing through bones of the middle cranial fossa make this portion of the base especially prone to fracture. Fractures into these spaces have obvious clinical implications as discussed below.

The Meninges

The meninges envelop the CNS and are integral to the intracranial vascular system. Vessels superficial to the meninges include the middle meningeal arteries that are the most common source of epidural hemorrhages. The dura mater, the outermost meningeal covering, consists of two layers: an endosteal layer tightly adherent to the inner table of the skull, and a meningeal layer surrounding the brain parenchyma. The latter separates from the outer layer to penetrate certain crevices of the brain creating the falx cerebri, tentorium cerebilli, falx cerebelli, and diaphragma sella. These anatomic septa limit the amount of brain rotary movement, and fold upon themselves to form the major venous sinuses. The tentorium cerebelli separates the posterior fossa from the occipital lobes of the cerebrum and is clinically most important. Anteriorly, this membrane opens to form the tentorial incisura, an aperture for the midbrain, posterior cerebral artery, and oculomotor nerves. Pressure differentials at this membrane may lead to brain herniation through the tentorial opening and compression of the structures traversing it.

Interior to the dura is the arachnoid mater, a thin impermeable membrane that contains the cerebrospinal fluid (CSF) in the subarachnoid space. The CSF cushions the brain from trauma and easily exits into the spinal subarachnoid space to dissipate increasing intracranial pressure. The subarachnoid space also contains the cerebral vasculature, which branches from the internal carotid and vertebral arteries. Disruption of these cerebral arteries and veins produces bloody spinal fluid and the clinical stigmata of subarachnoid hemorrhage. The pia mater is the innermost meningeal membrane, closely adhering to the brain surface.

The Brain

Consciousness requires a state of alertness and cognitive function or, on a neuroanatomic basis, an intact ascending reticular activating system (ARAS) and cerebral cortex. Numerous mechanical and/or biochemical factors can affect these anatomic sites and, thus, the level of consciousness.

DATA GATHERING

History

The initial history should include the details of the traumatic event, the patient's neurologic status before and after the accident, the suspected presence of associated injuries, and any care administered prior to the patient's presentation. Questions should address the presence or absence of loss of consciousness, tonic-clonic movements, somnolence, irritability, ab-

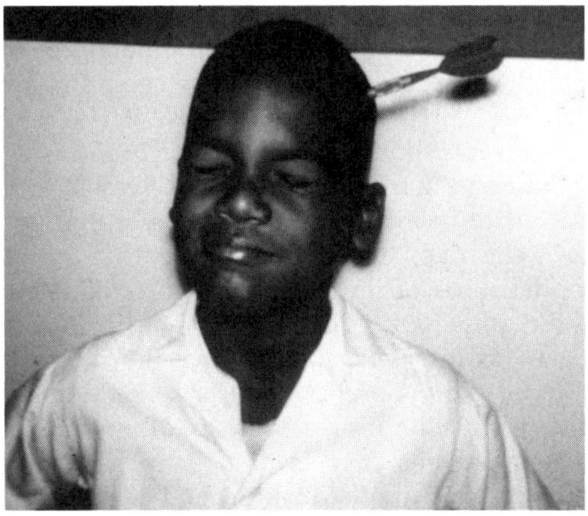

FIG 67–4
Missile injury to the head that fortunately missed injuring the brain.

normal behavior or verbalizations, emesis, ataxia, or weakness. Knowledge of the patient's mental status before and after the accident and, more importantly, any progression of neurologic signs or symptoms is crucial to patient management. If the patient is verbally responsive, the examiner should elicit any complaints of head or neck pain, visual changes, paresthesias, or amnesia.

It is important to ascertain the height of fall, the quality of impact surfaces, and the shape and velocity of striking objects (Fig 67–4). The mechanism of injury will influence the clinician's diagnostic and management plans. For example, a two-story fall necessitates a careful search for associated injuries and a longer period of observation. A diving injury immediately dictates that a cervical spine fracture be ruled out.

Finally, the history may reveal discrepancies or unlikely events that could suggest a diagnosis of child abuse. Routine, yet essential, information regarding allergies, chronic illness, and current medications should be known.

Physical Examination

The physical examination of the alert and conscious patient may proceed in a routine, thorough manner, with emphasis placed on the head, neck, and neurologic examinations. Examination of the head includes careful palpation of the calvarium, fontanelles, and facial bones; inspection of scalp wounds for underlying fractures; and the search for signs of any oral or mandibular trauma. If there are no complaints of neck pain or evident neck spasm, cervical range of motion and palpation of the cervical spine should be tested. A complete neurologic examination should include evaluation of mental status, cranial nerves, cerebellar function, sensation, deep-tendon reflexes, and muscular tone and strength. Nonspecific but important signs to recognize in the infant include irritability, pallor, high-pitched crying, "ocular apathy," or poor social interaction. Notation of the vital signs, especially pulse and blood pressure, is essential information for a complete neurologic assessment.

The patient with moderate or severe head trauma often requires simultaneous physical examination and therapy, which should always follow the sequence in the acronym: *A*irway, *B*reathing, *C*irculation, *D*isability. After assuring an adequate airway, ventilation, circulation, the physician must rapidly assess the neurologic *d*isability. The remainder of the physical examination may then be completed, emphasizing repeated A,B,C,D evaluation to optimize the care of the patient with a head injury.

A neurologic flow sheet facilitates an objective and serial recording of the patient's neurologic status. The descriptive terms of consciousness (alert, lethargic, obtunded, stuporous, comatose) should be replaced with the Glasgow Coma Scale (GCS). This scale is reliable in the hands of multiple observers, and the score itself has management and prognostic implications. The scale consists of scores for three responses: eye opening, verbal, and best upper limb movement (Table 67–2). The eye-opening response to speech does not require a command to open the eyes, and the response to painful stimuli should not include facial stimuli. A note should be made if the eyes are open but not blinking or if they are occluded by periorbital edema. The verbal response score for nonverbal patients (infants and young children) has not been standardized. The painful stimulus for the best upper limb response should be nailbed or supraorbital pressure. Raising the hand above the chin in response to supraorbital pressure is a localizing response. An abnormal flexion and extensor response are decorticate and decerebrate posturing, respectively. The

TABLE 67–2
Glasgow Coma Scale

Eye opening	
Spontaneous	4
To speech	3
To pain	2
None	1
Verbal response	
Oriented	5
Confused	4
Inappropriate	3
Incomprehensible	2
None	1
Best upper limb response	
Obeys	6
Localizes	5
Withdraws	4
Abnormal flexion	3
Abnormal extension	2
None	1

GCS ranges from 3 to 15; morbidity and mortality rise sharply with scores from 7 to 3.

Radiology

Skull series have no place in the evaluation of the unstable patient with closed head trauma. Computed tomography (CT) of the head is the procedure of choice in the patient with a persistently altered or deteriorating level of consciousness, or the patient with focal neurologic findings.

Criteria for skull x-ray films in the stable child with a history of head trauma include the following: (1) clinical signs of basilar or depressed skull fractures; (2) history of loss of consciousness greater than 5 minutes; (3) missile or open injuries; and (4) age less than 12 months, with a history of significant traumatic force, e.g., a fall greater than 2 ft. The location and extent of fractures are more important variables regarding management. Fractures overlying the middle meningeal groove, deep venous sinuses, or the rim of the foramen magnum, have potential intracranial vascular complications and warrant careful patient observation. Skull radiographs should include a stereolateral pair (one upright to rule out a sinus air-fluid level), posteroanterior and Towne views. Alternatively, in the patient who must remain supine and immobile, the lateral views may be obtained with a horizontal beam; the other views, with anteroposterior beams. If facial fractures are suspected, a Waters view may be indicated. Other views can be obtained if a fracture is detected in the initial series.

MANAGEMENT

After the initial assessment of the stable head-injury patient, serial observation is a mainstay of management. Any deterioration must be recognized and addressed promptly to reduce the potential morbidity of craniocerebral trauma. In the alert and responsive child, this continued observation may be carried out by reliable caretakers. The decision for home disposition should meet several criteria: absence of a life-threatening mechanism of injury, no neurologic symptoms other than a resolved momentarily altered consciousness, dependable parents, and a normal neurologic examination. Instructions to parents should include obvious signs and symptoms of deterioration or complications as summarized below.

Contact your physician if any of the following exist:

1. A fall greater than your child's height
2. Sleepiness, or difficulty arousing from usual sleep time
3. Vomiting or pallor
4. Severe headache
5. Weakness or dizziness
6. Complaints of visual disturbance
7. Fluid draining from ear or nose
8. Stiff or painful neck

Seek emergency care if:

1. Child is unresponsive
2. Seizures develop

The decision to hospitalize a child for observation after minimal head trauma is based on several considerations:

1. History of loss of consciousness
2. Amnesia
3. Vomiting
4. Skin fracture
5. Age of patient; infant or neonate
6. Associated injuries
7. Mechanism of injury
8. Social issues
9. Systemic disease

10. Seizures
11. Change in level of consciousness

Most authorities on head trauma recommend hospitalized observation if a history of loss of consciousness for more than 5 minutes is obtained. This recommendation must be tempered with parents' ability to estimate time elapsed in an emergency setting. Although retrograde amnesia is common in uncomplicated concussion syndromes, anterograde amnesia is indicative of a more severe injury and warrants further observation until cleared. One or two episodes of emesis within the first couple hours of trauma is often associated with mild head injury, but emesis associated with somnolence or persistent vomiting requires a longer period of medical surveillance. The clinical significance of isolated linear fractures that do not cross underlying vasculature is debatable. There is no question, however, that open, basilar, or depressed fractures mandate immediate neurosurgical attention. The physician's threshold for admission should be lowered in the infant or neonate with any symptoms or signs. The mechanism of injury is another consideration in the decision regarding hospitalization. A child who was struck by a moving vehicle or fell a significant distance often requires prolonged observation for head and other associated internal injuries. Social issues include a parent's ability to observe the child and the suspicion of child abuse. Chronic conditions or diseases such as coagulopathies, osteogenesis imperfecta, or ventricular shunts, may predispose to intracranial hemorrhages or fractures. A history of a brief seizure on impact or within several hours of head trauma should prompt admission for closer observation, although the stable patient does not require anticonvulsant therapy. Finally, any symptom or sign suggesting a change for the worse in the level of consciousness will necessitate longer periods of observation.

Specific Clinical Situations

Scalp Lacerations.—When scalp lacerations are extensive, local hemostasis is a management priority. If direct pressure does not control the hemorrhage, hemostat application and sutural ligation of the severed arterial branches are indicated. Under sterile conditions, the wound should be inspected for debris, and the skull palpated for fractures. Evidence of bone fragments or open or depressed fractures dictates neurosurgical evaluation prior to closure. The galea must be sutured first to achieve normal healing, and the more superficial scalp sutures may be ligated slightly tighter than usual to achieve further hemostasis. A pressure dressing also helps stem continued bleeding.

Subgaleal Hematoma.—The subgaleal hematoma is a common scalp lesion that presents as a localized or diffuse fluctuant swelling. Bloody fluid accumulates in the potential space between the galea and periosteum, dissecting the two layers. A clinically significant hemorrhage may occur into this space in the young child or infant, but surgical treatment is rarely, if ever, indicated. These lesions do not transilluminate and may require several weeks for resolution.

Subgaleal Hygroma.—A subgaleal hygroma is an uncommon scalp accumulation of CSF usually occurring secondary to a laceration of the dura and arachnoid membranes by a skull fracture. Clinically they resemble a subgaleal hematoma, but a positive transillumination and skull fracture suggest the diagnosis. Neurosurgical referral is indicated.

Cephalohematoma.—A cephalohematoma is a subperiosteal hematoma of an individual cranial bone. It most commonly affects the parietal bone after parturition and on palpation is firm with a central depression (due to its organized perimeter). It does not cross the suture line and does not transilluminate. Calcification of the elevated periosteal layer not uncommonly occurs, and resolution may require 2 weeks to 3 months. No therapy is required; aspiration is contraindicated.

Skull Fractures.—Skull fractures indicate a significant traumatic force occurrence, but the fracture per se does not necessarily correlate with the presence or absence of intracranial pathologic conditions. The linear fracture is the most common fracture and has little serious clinical implication unless it overlies a vascular channel or penetrates an air sinus. On radiographs, the linear fracture usually appears relatively straight and nonbranching; it rarely crosses sutures. Occasionally, a linear fracture is diastatic in which case the clinician should beware of an underlying contusion or laceration. In addition, diastatic sutural fractures occur with trauma in young children and have significant intracranial hemorrhage potential. The lambdoid suture that overlies the transverse venous sinus is most commonly affected. Increased intracranial pressure at a young age can also lead to generalized split sutures before the sutural ligaments calcify.

A late and rare complication of linear fractures is a "growing" fracture. Growing fractures are thought to arise because the meninges have been lacerated on initial injury and a pulsating arachnoid cyst forms that erodes the fracture margin. The reshaped fracture widens into an irregular bony defect and a leptomeningeal cyst develops. These scalp masses become evident several months to years after the initial fracture and may pulsate and transilluminate. Neurosurgery is usually required.

Depressed fractures often result from significant traumatic forces acting on a small cross-sectional area (e.g., a blow from a hammer) and have obvious implications for underlying brain tissue. Unless seen in a tangential view on radiographs, these fractures often appear as an increased sclerotic density because of overlapping bone surfaces. Occasionally, these fractures are open (a compound fracture) or comminuted, and, thus, require neurosurgical debridement and inspection for parenchymal injury. Most neurosurgeons would consider surgical elevation of the bone edges if the depression is either greater than the thickness of the skull or 5 mm.

Basilar skull fractures are in the basal portion of the skull—specifically the frontal, ethmoid, sphenoid, temporal, and occipital bones. Clinical indicators of these fractures include periorbital subcutaneous hemorrhages ("raccoon eyes"), CSF rhinorrhea or otorrhea, cranial nerve palsies, hemotympanum, or postauricular ecchymosis (Battle sign). In the young child, the dura closely adheres to the basilar skull accounting for the associated meningeal tears in basilar fractures. These skull fractures are often difficult to demonstrate on routine radiographs, though sphenoid and frontal sinus air-fluid levels or opacification and pneumocephaly may suggest their presence.

CSF rhinorrhea implies a fracture near the cribriform plate of the ethmoid and may require tomography or CSF radionuclide studies to identify it. Fractures of the temporal bone's petrous ridge causing otorrhea or hemotympanum can be equally hard to demonstrate radiologically. The CSF leaks often increase with coughing or head-down position, and on filter paper the leaks display a "water-ring" if bloody. Infectious complications, primarily pneumococcal or *Hemophilus influenzae* meningitis, are the main reason for clinical concern. There is no clear consensus on the use of prophylactic antibiotics. Fortunately, in many cases the CSF leaks close within a week.

Concussion.—Concussion is a mild closed head injury, with an associated brief impairment of consciousness. Although an organic lesion is not consistently demonstrable, the ascending reticular activating system (ARAS) and cerebral cortex are the probable sites of this temporary neuronal dysfunction. Clinically, the child exhibits variable degrees of impaired consciousness, from coma to lethargy, and often has associated anorexia, vomiting, or pallor. Sleepiness, confusion, or abnormal behavior may continue for several hours. The older child or adult often reports amnesia for the events leading to the accident (retrograde amnesia). A posttraumatic or anterograde amnesia reflects a temporary difficulty forming new memories after the injury. The length of the posttraumatic amnesia correlates with the severity of the head injury. There is usually an uneventful recovery in concussions.

An alternate presentation of concussion especially in infants and younger children is the pediatric concussion syndrome. A delayed deterioration of consciousness occurs minutes to several hours after seemingly minimal head trauma. The change in mental status is usually heralded by pallor, vomiting, and irritability. The patient may be mildly ataxic and often becomes somnolent. There are no focal findings, and the syndrome resolves in several hours. The differential diagnosis of delayed deterioration of consciousness also includes posttraumatic seizure manifestations, brain swelling, and intracranial hemorrhage. Neurosurgical consultation and CT scan are warranted in this setting.

Cerebral Contusion or Laceration.—Contusions are hemorrhagic bruises of the brain demonstrable on CT scan and are often associated with local swelling. The sites of contusions tend to be in the cerebral cortex adjacent to significant focal skull impacts or in areas of the brain anatomically predisposed to accelerative forces (the anterior and orbital surfaces of the frontal lobes, anterior temporal lobes, and areas adjacent to free falx edges). A cerebral contusion does not necessarily cause unconsciousness, though prolonged impairment of consciousness is common. The neurologic signs depend on the site of the contusion and are often focal.

Lacerations are tears in the brain substance that occur at similar sites. In addition, the unmyelinated state of nerve fibers in young infants predisposes their white matter to tears on rotational accelerative forces. The major morbidity of lacerations is related to the site and extent of the tear itself and secondary vascular complications (i.e., intracranial hemorrhages).

Intracranial Hemorrhage.—*Epidural Hemorrhage.*—Epidural hematomas are relatively rare (less than 3%) in pediatric severe head trauma, but early recognition and prompt treatment will improve outcome. They occur more frequently in older children and have a mortality rate of 10% to 20%. The majority of epidural hematomas originate from a hemorrhaging middle meningeal artery that quickly separates the meningeal dura layer from the inner table of the skull. In children, however, a substantial minority of epidural hematomas are due to meningeal and diploic vein hemorrhage. These hematomas may occasionally occur in the posterior cranial fossa secondary to a bleeding deep venous sinus. Another crucial anatomic difference in young children is the dura mater's tight adherence to the skull. These factors are probably responsible for the variable and occasionally subacute presentation of pediatric patients with epidural hemorrhage.

Patients with an epidural hematoma often present with a rapid and focal neurologic deterioration without regaining consciousness. This type of injury often has an arterial source of bleeding and associated brain lesions. Not unexpectedly mortality is higher with an earlier presentation. Some patients will present with the classic triad of concussion, intervening lucent phase, and then neurologic deterioration. The period of "lucency" is usually not a totally asymptomatic interval but simply an improvement in the level of consciousness. Over a variable period of time, the child progressively develops neurologic signs of increased intracranial pressure and impending transtentorial herniation. In supratentorial epidural hematomas, the CT scan reveals a biconvex increased density with varying amounts of "midline shift." The incidence of cranial fractures is at least 50% in pediatric epidural hemorrhages, and approaches 100% in adults. In the pediatric patient epidural hemorrhage may also occur in the posterior cranial fossa after occipital trauma, and commonly causes nuchal rigidity, cerebellar signs, vomiting, and continued impaired consciousness. An occipital fracture is usually present.

Subdural Hemorrhages.—Posttraumatic subdural hemorrhages are an important source of neurologic morbidity in pediatric patients. Subdural hematomas occur five to ten times more frequently than bleeding in the epidural space and tend to affect infants more often than older children. The subdural hemorrhage is almost exclusively venous in origin, most frequently from cerebral vein disruption at the sagittal sinus. These anastomoses are very sensitive to the shearing forces generated by rotational acceleration.

In the young infant, the onset of symptoms may be relatively slow because of the venous source of bleeding and the increased calvarial compliance. Nonspecific symptoms such as vomiting, irritability, and low-grade temperature may develop. Some infants, however, will not present until the subacute or chronic phase of subdural collection. In the subacute phase, the subdural blood organizes into a hemorrhagic cyst over several weeks and expands in size via the osmotic pressure of red blood cell (RBC) breakdown products. Regardless of time course, the majority of patients with subdural hemorrhage will eventually have a focal or generalized seizure. Physical examination often reveals an irritable or lethargic baby with a bulging fontanelle, "sunsetting" eyes, retinal and preretinal hemorrhages, and hypertonicity. Only a minority of these patients have an associated skull fracture. The CT scan will commonly demonstrate bilateral crescentic-shaped subdural collections. If the subdural hemorrhage is older than 1 week, the collection may appear isodense on CT, necessitating contrast medium to establish the diagnosis. The mortality seen in patients with subdural hematomas is lower than in patients with epidural hemorrhage, but the morbidity is higher due to underlying brain damage. Older children with subdural bleeding tend to present in a more acute state, with symptoms and signs of increasing intracranial pressure and impending transtentorial herniation.

Subarachnoid Hemorrhage.—Subarachnoid hemorrhage is a common finding on CT scans of pediatric patients with severe head trauma. Although the major cerebral vessels traverse the subarachnoid space, the more fragile and smaller leptomeningeal vessels are often the source of hemorrhage. The clinical course is usually dominated by associated brain injuries, although headache, nuchal rigidity, and low-grade fever may occasionally be attributed to subarachnoid blood. Rarely, a communicating hydrocephalus develops due to hemorrhagic debris blocking the CSF circulation. On CT scan, a linear increased density is commonly seen in the interhemispheric fissure.

Intraparenchymal Hemorrhage.— Acute intracranial hemorrhage is a common finding in fatal head injuries. Clinically this lesion is indistinguishable from other severe intracranial mass lesions. The hemorrhages predominate in the frontal and temporal lobes and may have associated focal neurologic findings.

Brain Swelling.—Acute brain swelling is a common occurrence in the pediatric patient with severe head trauma. A child with a deteriorating neurologic status after a period of "lucency" is more likely to have generalized cerebral swelling rather than an intracranial hemorrhage. The initial basic pathophysiology is increased cerebral blood volume or cerebral hyperemia. The increased cerebral blood flow early in the posttraumatic course has therapeutic implications regarding hyperosmolar agents. The CT scan reveals a small ventricular system and decreased subarachnoid cisternal spaces. Within 1 to 2 days after trauma, a "vasogenic" cerebral edema may develop. This is primarily white matter edema due to disruption of the blood-brain barrier. This form of brain edema can dramatically increase the intracranial pressure.

Seizures.—Seizures develop in approximately 10% of children hospitalized for head trauma. Posttraumatic seizures can be temporally divided into immediate, early, and late seizures. An "immediate" seizure manifests within seconds of impact and probably represents a traumatic depolarization of the cortex. It may occur with mild trauma, is brief, and probably has no prognostic significance.

"Early" seizures account for about half of the posttraumatic fits and take place within the first week of the traumatic event. They are usually due to focal injury by contusion, laceration, ischemia, or edema. Young children seem more susceptible to development of early posttraumatic seizures. The majority of affected patients present in the first 24 hours after the trauma. Roughly equivalent numbers of patients have generalized or focal seizures, and 10% to 20% will develop status epilepticus. Approximately one fourth of patients with early seizures will continue to have seizures after the first week (i.e., posttraumatic epilepsy).

Late posttraumatic seizures that occur 1 week or longer after trauma probably reflect cortical scarring. The severity of head injury, dural laceration, and intracranial hemorrhage are all factors in this form of seizure. Close to 5% of hospitalized head trauma patients have late posttraumatic fits. The long-term prognosis is more guarded; as many as three-fourths of these patients will develop epilepsy.

BIBLIOGRAPHY

Bruce DA, Schut L, Bruno LA, et al: Outcome following severe head injuries in children. *J Neurosurg* 1978; 48:707.

Harwood-Nash DC, Hendrick EB, Hudson AR: The significance of skull fractures in children. *Radiology* 1971; 101:151.

Ivan LP, Choo SH, Ventureyra EC: Head injuries in childhood: A two-year survey. *Can Med Assoc J* 1983; 128:281.

Leonidas JC, Ting W, Binkiewicz A, et al: Mild head trauma in children: When is a roentgenogram necessary? *Pediatrics* 1982; 69:139.

Raimondi AJ, Hirschauer J: Head injury in the infant and toddler. *Child's Brain* 1984; 11:12.
Raphaely RC, Swedlow DB, Downes JJ, et al: Management of severe pediatric head trauma. *Pediatr Clin North Am* 1980; 26:707.
Rosman NP, Oppenheimer EY: Posttraumatic epilepsy. *Pediatr Rev* 1982; 3:221.
Snoek JW, Minderhoud JM, Wilmink JT: Delayed deterioration following mild head injury in children. *Brain* 1984; 107:15.
Young B, Rapp RP, Norton JA, et al: Failure of prophylactically administered phenytoin to prevent early posttraumatic seizures. *J Neurosurg* 1983; 58:231.

FACIAL TRAUMA

Dee Hodge III, M.D.

Almost every child experiences facial trauma several times in his life. Some children, due to their level of activity or type of play, experience it several times a day. Most facial trauma is minor and does not require the attention of a physician. In other instances, because the face is the site of the vital sensory organs, facial trauma is more of a concern and the child is brought to the pediatrician or family practitioner.

In this chapter the more common forms of facial injuries will be discussed in regard to their evaluation, diagnosis, treatment, and conditions for referral.

EYE

In evaluating injuries to the eye, it is important to have a general approach to the examination and a few useful tools. Minimal equipment needed by the physician includes: eye chart for evaluation of visual acuity, adequate light and magnification, topical anesthetic (e.g., proparacaine hydrochloride (0.5%), fluorescein dye, and dilating or cycloplegic drops (e.g., tropicamide 1%). Lid retractors and a slit lamp are useful but not essential in the office setting. A good history is most important in determining what happened, when, where, and how the child is doing now. Having a standard approach will aid in the evaluation of the injured eye; for example:

1. Evaluate visual acuity.
2. Check extraocular movement.
3. Check face and periorbital area for asymmetry ecchymosis, eyelid laceration.
4. Examine conjunctiva and fornices including eversion of upper lid.
5. Evaluate cornea including examination with use of fluorescein.
6. Examine anterior chamber and compare with other side.
7. Note pupil size and shape.
8. Examine lens and posterior chamber.
9. Conclude with funduscopic examination.

Chemical burns and occlusion of the central retinal artery are the only true ocular emergencies. These should be referred immediately as minutes count as far as survival of the eye. Medical attention within hours is needed for the other injuries noted here. They are divided into nonpenetrating and penetrating injuries of the eye.

Nonpenetrating Injuries of the Eye

Abrasions.—Abrasions of the lid can be treated in the same manner as any abrasion to the skin. Special care should be taken to clean the abrasion of any imbedded foreign material to prevent long-term retention of the foreign body or tattooing.

Corneal abrasions are the most common injuries to the eyes of children. Presenting signs and symptoms include uncomfortable sensation, blurred vision, red eyes, tearing, and photophobia. The examination is facilitated by the use of topical anesthesia followed by fluorescein dye to demarcate the abrasion. Most abrasions can be treated in the office. Antibiotic drops or ointment with follow-up in 24 hours is the treatment of choice. The use of patching is controversial and is often not needed. Follow-up is extremely important at 24- or 36-hour follow-up visit, and any large abrasion that has persisted should be referred to an ophthalmologist.

Contusion.—Contusion of the eyelid or "black eye" results from blunt trauma to the orbit and surrounding structures. A careful examination is needed to rule out any associated injury to the globe or bone structures. If the injury is isolated to the eyelid, then cold compresses and analgesics are the only treatment needed. Often these injuries will look worse on the day after the injury and parents should be prepared for this progression.

A contusion to the globe usually results in subconjunctival hemorrhage. This type of hemorrhage may also occur spontaneously or in association with nose blowing or forceful vomiting. After complete examination, if there is no suspicion of a bleeding tendency or child abuse, assurance may be given to the parents that it will resolve in a few weeks with no need for further follow-up.

Hyphema.—Hyphema is defined as accumulation of free blood in the anterior chamber. The most common cause is blunt trauma resulting in rupture of iris or ciliary body blood vessels. Spontaneous hyphemas are known to occur, most often in diseases that include purpuric skin lesions, sickle cell disease, ocular tumors, and congenital and acquired coagulation factor deficiencies. Most fill less than 30% of the anterior chamber and last from 5 to 7 days. Loss of full visual acuity due to the hyphema may produce drowsiness, but the physician must be careful not to overlook concomitant neurologic trauma.

The diagnosis is made by examining the eye and finding blood in the anterior chamber. This is easily seen when a light source is placed lateral to the eye and shone across the anterior chamber. A slit lamp will show even microscopic amounts of blood. Hyphemas have been graded based on the amount of blood occupying the anterior chamber: in grade I, one-fourth of the chamber is filled; grade II, one-half; grade III, three-fourths; grade IV, the entire chamber is filled with blood, or "black ball" hyphema.

Management of hyphema, the responsibility of the ophthalmologist, includes hospitalization for daily observation and bed rest. All patients without history of trauma should have determination of prothrombin time and partial thromboplastin time and a sickle preparation done. Complications include rebleeding that may occur on the fourth to fifth day, elevation in intraocular pressure, and corneal staining.

Corneal and Conjunctival Foreign Body.—Foreign bodies are also a common problem in the pediatric patient population. A foreign body may be the cause of a corneal abrasion and, indeed, the signs and symptoms are the same. Visual acuity is normal. The sensation of a foreign body is useful in locating the foreign body, and, therefore, the use of anesthetic drops should be avoided in this situation. Fluorescein also may be useful in locating the offending object. Most of the objects can be removed by lavage or by lifting the object with a cotton swab. More resistant objects may need to be removed with the aid of a slit lamp and magnification by the ophthalmologist.

Penetration of the globe by a foreign body is a true emergency and must be ruled out. If the history and the physical examination are compatible with a high velocity foreign body or vision is decreased, or if the eye is more inflamed or softer than expected the patient should be promptly referred to an ophthalmologist.

Chemical Burns.—Chemical burns are one of the true ophthalmologic emergencies. Alkali burns are more devastating than acid burns. Acids precipitate tissue protein so the injury is more superficial and slower to penetrate into the tissues of the eye. Alkali, on the other hand, allow rapid deep penetration into the tissues of the eye because of saponification of fat and destruction of cells.

Initial treatment by parents at home is essential and consists of irrigation with water for 20 minutes before transport to the office. There should be continued irrigation in the office with 2 L of fluid or until the pH level of the conjunctival sac is between 7.3 and 7.7. Immediate referral to an ophthalmologist is indicated.

Rupture of Eyeball.—Rupture of the eyeball may result from a number of different types of injuries but most commonly is caused by blunt trauma. The most common site is along the limbus though rupture may occur occasionally around the optic nerve. If rupture is suspected, do not try to force the eye open but refer the patient immediately to an ophthalmologist.

Penetrating Injuries of Eye

Any suspected penetrating injury, as mentioned earlier, needs prompt treatment by an ophthalmologist. Every lacerated eyelid should be considered to have a penetrating wound to the globe. Other signs and symptoms of penetration are: decreased vision on physical examination, lacerated cornea or conjunctiva, localized scleral swelling, shallow anterior chamber, distorted or peaked pupil, external presentation of the iris or other intraocular contents, or a white pupil. If penetration of the globe is suspected, vigorous examination should be avoided at all cost since the increased pressure on the globe may cause extrusion of the intraocular contents. If intraocular foreign bodies are suspected, x-ray films of the orbit and ultrasound (US) are useful in locating the foreign body. It is again stressed that all patients with suspected penetrating injury must be referred.

Lid Lacerations.—Lacerations to the lid comprise the majority of lid injuries after contusion and abrasions. Lacerations that do not involve the lid margins may be sutured in the usual manner using 5–0 or 6–0 nylon after instilling topical anesthetic without epinephrine. Lacerations near the inner canthus frequently involve the canaliculi and should be evaluated by the ophthalmologist. Any through-and-through laceration should raise the suspicion of injury to the globe and should also be referred for examination by an ophthalmologist.

Periorbital Trauma.—Blunt trauma to the orbit causes a sudden increase in intraorbital pressure. The medial wall and orbital floor are the weakest bones of the orbit, thus giving way. Orbital floor fractures may result in entrapment of orbital fat, inferior rectus muscle, inferior oblique muscle, or a combination of the above. Examination may reveal proptosis or an inability of upward gaze. X-ray film of the orbit may show entrapment of the inferior rectus, the so-called "teardrop sign." If no intraocular injury is found, then conservative treatment is advocated. This includes ice, to reduce swelling during the first 24 hours, followed by heat. Oral antibiotics are considered helpful by some to reduce the chance of infection across the violated sinus. All children should be referred to an ophthalmologist.

NASAL TRAUMA

Epistaxis

Bleeding from the interior of the nose may be caused by injuries, infections, septal perforations, tumors, and blood dyscrasias; however, most nosebleeds are not associated with any of these conditions. Drying of the mucosa and trauma from nose-picking are the most common cause of bleeding from the area of Kesselbach plexus in the anterior nasal septum.

Bleeding from the anterior septum often stops with simple measures. Pinching the nostrils for a full 10 minutes will stop the bleeding in most instances. If bleeding continues, identifying the exact source of bleeding is necessary. The anterior nasal chamber can often be adequately visualized through a surgical head otoscope fitted with a nasal speculum. If no active bleeding is seen, more equipment is needed including optimal illumination and exposure with a head mirror, nasal speculum, and suction tip. If the bleeding point is identified, dry the area and cauterize it with a silver nitrate stick or touch the area with cotton dampened with 2% tetracaine and 3% ephedrine.

Exact sites of bleeding deep within the nose can rarely be identified. Usual sites include the posterior ethmoid, a branch of the external carotid, or septal branch of the sphenopalatine artery. Posterior nasal hemorrhage usually requires sedation, postnasal packing, and hospitalization. The need for posterior packing used in conjunction with anterior packing is very rare in children.

Without a history of recurrent epistaxis, workup of bleeding disorders is unwarranted. Recurrent epistaxis is defined as greater than ten nosebleeds per year without history of nasal trauma or nasal allergy (see Chapter 39 for more details).

Nasal Fractures and Septal Hematoma

For many children with nasal trauma, medical attention is not sought unless the injury is severe enough to cause swelling, cosmetic deformity, airway obstruction, or epistaxis. The child's nose does not respond in the same way as an adult's because of differences in structure. Because of more cartilage, incomplete fracture is more often seen, and with less likelihood of mobility and crepitus. Nasal fractures fall into four categories: (1) *greenstick*—an incomplete fracture that is never compounded by tearing of the underlying mucosa. The diagnosis cannot be made with conventional radiography. The diagnosis can be made clinically by the finding of point tenderness, but it is impossible to make the diagnosis in the presence of edema; (2) *linear fracture*—a simple fracture without displacement or comminution; (3) *lateral fracture*—the most common type of fracture found in children. There is an inward fracture of the traumatized nasal bone and an outward fracture of the opposite nasal bone. Findings of x-ray film are often positive; (4) *frontal fracture*—caused by a straight-ahead blow to nose.

The primary diagnosis of fracture may be difficult. Signs in order of frequency include: epistaxis, swelling of nasal dorsum, ecchymosis of the eyes, tenderness of the nasal dorsum, obvious nasal deformity, and crepitus of the nasal bones. Any change in appearance of the nose since injury may be helpful. Any deviation is pertinent, but seeming absence of deviation may be misleading because of edema. If edema is present, delay definitive palpation until it subsides in 3 to 4 days. Crepitus, if present, is considered diagnostic. Internal examination of the nose is important. Any deviation of the nasal septum increases likelihood of later abnormality. X-ray film examination is diagnostic in only 50% of the cases.

A septal hematoma may also result from nasal trauma and occurs more frequently in children because the septal cartilage tends to buckle more easily. Small hematomas must be searched for and treated if present. Evacuation of the hematoma is necessary to prevent the possibility of avascular necrosis of the septal cartilage and septal abscess. Consultation with an otorhinolaryngologist is advised.

Foreign Bodies of the Nose

Many times children will present with the complaint of a foreign body in the nose, but more often than not the complaint is of a unilateral foul-smelling discharge. Foreign bodies are often visible in the anterior antrum with a nasal speculum. Foreign bodies include paper, toys, beads, etc., and, thus, the majority are radiolucent. The physician may try to remove the foreign body if it is in the nasal vestibule and can be grasped easily with forceps. The child must be well restrained. The mucosa may be sprayed with a topical vasoconstrictor such as phenylephrine (Neo-Synephrine) to decrease edema and bleeding. The object should never be pushed posteriorly or irrigated because of the danger of aspiration. Once the object is removed, the patient should be treated with amoxicillin, 25 to 50 mg/kg/day for 10 days. If removal is impossible, referral is indicated.

Maxillary and Mandibular Fractures

Problems in diagnosis and treatment of these fractures are often secondary to difficulty in examination, small size of the structure, and lack of development of paranasal sinus. Fortunately, these injuries are rare as a lack of pneumatization, the flexibility of developing bone, and mixed dentition produce more stable structures, and therefore a greater force is needed to cause these fractures. When mandibular or maxillary fractures are present they may be associated with intracranial and cervical spine injuries. Rapid evaluation for other injuries is necessary. Management of the airway and treatment of shock, as always, is of first priority. Facial bones heal rapidly, therefore, stabilization is required within 5 days of injury lest malalignment occur.

Fractures of the maxilla are secondary to excessive force directed at a small area. Fractures to the maxilla are frequently associated with nasal injury, soft-tissue trauma, and involvement of the orbit. Examination of any suspected bone facial injury should follow these sequential steps: First, the supraorbital ridges are palpated. Next, the infraorbital ridges are palpated using the examiner's first three fingers to determine symmetry or fracture. The zygomatic arches are then palpated. The infraorbital rims, zygomatic bodies, and maxilla are inspected from the top of the head and then palpated to determine depressions and/or displaced fractures. Next, the nasal bones and maxilla are examined for stability, and the nose is examined intranasally to determine septal placement. Occlusion is observed to determine dental relations. Finally, the mandible is palpated, then distracted to determine sites of discomfort and possible mandibular fracture. If a fracture is suspected or confirmed by x-ray film, then referral of the patient is in order.

Fractures of the mandible are most often caused by direct blow. Fracture is unusual in children but, when seen, most commonly occurs at the subcondyle. Other fracture sites include the angle of the jaw, symphyseal, and body of the mandible. Diagnosis is based on change in occlusion and pain or difficulty opening the mouth. If a fracture is suspected, refer the child to an otorhinolaryngologist or dental surgeon.

EAR

External Trauma

External trauma to the ears includes laceration, blunt injury, and thermal injury. Lacerations are common and may be treated in the same manner as lacerations in other areas of the body. Special care and consultation may be needed if there is extensive damage to the auricular cartilage. Blunt injury is typified by ecchymosis and hematoma. Ecchymosis is treated conservatively, but hematomas must be evacuated immediately because of the likelihood of damage to the cartilage. Treatment of burns and frostbite is described in the section on environmental trauma.

Foreign Bodies

Foreign bodies in the external canal are extremely common and include stones, beads, paper, erasers, and, frequently, insects. Objects may be rolled out with an ear curet or grasped and removed with forceps. Irrigation of the ear with body temperature water is another useful method of removing these objects, provided that the object, such as a dry pea, will not absorb water and become more impacted. It must be noted that insects must be killed with alcohol or mineral oil before removal is attempted. Once the object is removed, the external canal should be treated with antibacterial otic suspension.

Trauma to Middle Ear

Trauma that results in injury to the tympanic membrane or structures of the middle ear must be referred to the otorhinolaryngologist. Minor abrasions along the external auditory canal may be cleansed by irrigation and treated with antibacterial otic suspension for 3 to 5 days.

BIBLIOGRAPHY

Collet BI, Traumatic hyphema: A review. *Ann Ophthalmol* 1982; 14:52.

Ervin-Mulvey LD, Nelson LB, Freeley DA: Pediatric eye trauma. *Pediatr Clin North Am* 1983; 30:1167.

Fortunato MA, Fielding AF, Guernsey LH: Facial bone fractures in children. *Oral Surg* 1982; 53:225.

Frey T: Pediatric eye trauma. *Pediatr Ann* 1983; 12:487.

Gussack GS, Luterman A, Rodgers K, et al: Pediatric maxillofacial trauma: unique features in diagnosis and treatment. *Laryngoscope* 1987; 97:925–930.

Kiley V, Stuart JJ, Johnson CA: Coagulation studies in children with isolated recurrent epistaxis. *J Pediatr* 1982; 100:579.

Kirchner JA: Epistaxis. *N Engl J Med* 1982; 307:1126.

Moran WB Jr: Nasal trauma in children. *Otolaryngol Clin North Am* 1977; 10:95.

Potsic WP, Handler SD: Otorhinolaryngology emergencies, in Fleisher G, Ludwig S (eds): *Textbook of Pediatric Emergency Medicine.* Baltimore, Williams & Wilkins Co, 1983.

Yarington CT Jr: Maxillofacial trauma in children. *Otolaryngol Clin North Am* 1977; 10:25.

Yarington CT Jr: The initial evaluation in maxillofacial trauma. *Otolaryngol Clin North Am* 1979; 12:293.

DENTAL TRAUMA

Linda P. Nelson, D.M.D., M.ScD.
Edward Sweeney, D.M.D.

Since teeth have an important cosmetic function as well as aiding in communication and mastication, one of the most worrisome events occurs when the child sustains trauma to the oral-facial structures. Such injuries are frequently associated with pain and bleeding, as there may be lacerations, tooth fractures, or even loss of teeth. No two dental emergencies are ever alike; the physician will often be the parents' first contact; therefore, this chapter will attempt to organize the clinical findings so that the physician can logically assess the need for and the type of dental referral.

EPIDEMIOLOGY OF ORAL-FACIAL TRAUMA

During the first year of life, dental injuries are usually both infrequent and minor and usually result from falls from cribs or carriages. With increased efforts in ambulation during the second year of life, the frequency of dental injuries increases. The position of the head and angulation of the teeth at the time of the fall often dictate the type and severity of the dental injury. For example, a young child who falls face down on the floor will rarely "knock out a tooth," but the child who falls on his chin and then onto his nose will often fracture or totally loosen a primary tooth. The frequency of injuries in the primary (deciduous) dentition peaks between the ages of 15 months to 3 years. As the child reaches school age and adolescence, playground accidents become more frequent. Many of these injuries are not related to falls but rather to contact sports, especially football, baseball, soccer, and hockey. The typical sports-related injury involves a fracture of the crown of the maxillary anterior tooth as it is contacted by either a fist, an elbow, or a baseball bat. Falls from bicycles are also a significant source of dental injury. Facial and dental injuries resulting from automobile accidents are often multiple, with soft-tissue injuries to the lower lip and chin as well as dental crown fractures caused by hitting the dashboard.

Fighting injuries occur in the older adolescent. Typically there is a luxation injury of maxillary anterior teeth, as well as root fractures and injury to supporting bone. Multiple bone fractures are a frequent finding, especially in the mandible, where developing molars predispose the angle to fracture.

The prevalence of dental injuries varies from 4% to 30% depending on the study cited. The majority of dental injuries involve a single maxillary anterior tooth. Various studies indicate that many children are accident prone and sustain repeated trauma to their teeth, probably as a result of the unfavorable anterior malocclusion described as "buck teeth."

DATA GATHERING

Oral-facial injuries always require that the health care provider complete an adequate medical history and assessment. Airway management and control of acute bleeding problems are paramount. A neurologic assessment should be made in all cases of head and neck trauma and proper disposition made as indicated. In addition to the medical assessment, certain dental questions may help clarify the nature of the problem.

1. *Ask general questions.* A medical history must include questions on congenital heart defects, bleeding disorders, and other systemic illnesses that might necessitate antibiotic prophylaxis or other types of medication.

2. *When did the injury occur?* If the nerve (pulp) of the tooth is exposed, the treatment and prognosis may be influenced by a prompt (less than 45 minutes from the time of injury) referral. If a tooth is avulsed (exarticulated), the time interval between initial avulsion and reimplantation is critically significant in determining the prognosis of the tooth.

3. *Where did the injury occur?* The place of the traumatic incident may necessitate inquiring as to whether tetanus immunizations are up to date.

4. *How did the injury occur?* Although the exact mechanisms of most dental injuries are unknown, the type of trauma can provide clues as to the type of dental injury to suspect. A direct traumatic blow to a tooth often results in a fracture to the crown of a maxillary anterior tooth. This direct blow is usually against a piece of furniture such as a coffee table or a fist or elbow. An indirect traumatic injury would be a blow to the chin in a fall. In indirect trauma, due to the archery bow shape of the mandible, the condyles may be forced against the articular disc, which may result in a condylar fracture and/or symphyseal fracture.

5. *Emergency dental treatment rendered elsewhere?* It is important to know whether an avulsed tooth was reimplanted into the socket or was stored in milk, water, or allowed to dry. If a tooth is discolored and has been for some time, it is probably the result of a previous injury, and thus requires no emergency treatment at this time.

6. *Is there spontaneous pain from the teeth?* The positive finding of spontaneous pain from traumatically injured teeth may indicate an exposed nerve (pulp) or damage to the tooth-supporting structures such as hemorrhage into the periodontal ligament. Crown-root fractures may also give rise to spontaneous pain. These types

of injuries require immediate referral to a dentist.

7. *Is there any pain during mastication and do the teeth "bite together" as they did prior to the injury?* If the occlusion has been altered so that the "bite" shifts, this may indicate a jaw fracture or luxated tooth. Immediate referral to a dentist or oral surgeon is indicated for a detailed evaluation.

MANAGEMENT

Injuries to Teeth

In the sections that follow, injuries to (1) teeth, (2) bone, and (3) soft tissue will be reviewed with regard to the identification and management of specific injuries.

The part of the tooth that can be seen on visual inspection is the crown. The part buried in the alveolar bone is the root that is anchored to the bone by collagenous fibers (periodontal ligament).

Enamel, which covers the crown, is the hardest substance in the body. Unlike the reparative qualities of bone, enamel—once injured—cannot be repaired. The major function of enamel is to resist impact. Mastication alone may exert 50 to 100 lb/in^2 of pressure between anterior teeth and 150 to 200 lb between posterior teeth. Simple fractures involving only enamel usually require no emergency treatment unless the fracture line causes a sharp edge, which can be smoothed by simple polishing.

Dentin is the yellowish bonelike material underlying the enamel; composed of basically the same materials as enamel, it has a greater protein content and surrounds the pulp chamber. A fracture that exposes dentin must be treated as soon as possible to insulate and prevent any communication between the dentin and the pulp. Dentinal fractures usually will result in sensitivity to cold and hot liquids or even to cold air. The degree of sensitivity to temperature is usually indicative of the closeness of the line of fracture to the pulp. That is, the closer the fracture line is to the pulp, the greater the sensitivity, and, therefore, the greater the need for an immediate referral to a dentist for pulp protection and an esthetic tooth-colored acrylic restoration. If the physician suspects a simple dentin fracture (that is, one with no bleeding from the central core of the tooth and minimal sensitivity), referral to a dentist should be made as soon as convenient or within 48 hours of the accident.

The dental *pulp* is the soft-tissue component of the tooth that fills the central core or pulp chamber and root canal of the tooth. This soft tissue contains fibroblasts, inferior alveolar nerve fibers, blood vessels, and lymphatics. Any overstimulation of the pulp will result in a pulpitis or inflammation. A pulpitis that is minor in duration and severity is often self-limiting or reversible. Therefore, any dental trauma must be clinically examined by gently wiping the tooth with a moist gauze to ascertain if there is bleeding from the "root canal." If a pink hue emanates from the central core, the pulp may be exposed even though there is no active capillary bleeding. Timing is critical to the successful treatment of pulp exposures. If bleeding is noted from the central core, it is imperative that the patient be referred to a dental office as soon as possible. If the exposure is relatively small (1 mm in diameter) and the exposure has been present less than 45 minutes, the dentist can apply a calcium hydroxide covering and probably retain the vitality of the tooth. Any tooth with a pulp exposure should be referred for immediate treatment even if the exposure time is greater than 45 minutes.

Cementum is the enamel analogue that covers the root and is very similar to bone. It is not as hard as enamel nor is it as resistant to abrasion. The periodontal ligaments anchor the cementum and, thus, the root of the tooth to the alveolar bone. It is the periodontal ligament that is necessary for the viability of the tooth within the alveolar socket, if a tooth is luxated due to trauma or avulsed. Irreversible damage to the periodontal ligament can cause ankylosis of the root to the alveolar bone and/or inflammatory external resorption of the root and subsequent loss of the tooth.

A *crown-root fracture* is defined as a fracture involving enamel, dentin, cementum, and, usually, the pulp. Crown root fractures in the anterior teeth are usually caused by direct trauma from a fall or fist. They may be longitudinal or horizontal in direction, causing either a portion of the crown or the entire crown to be mobile without mobility of the root. The pain will often be intense from such an injury and immediate dental referral will often lead to pulp removal or, in some severe cases, extraction.

Sometimes displacement of fragments in crown-root fractures may be so minimal that they are overlooked for several days until there is necrosis of the pulp with the accompanying pain of infection.

If the injury is severe enough to cause a fractured tooth, there is often an accompanying soft-tissue laceration. For example, lower lip lacerations are often associated with maxillary anterior fractures. It is important for the examining physician to remember that tooth fragments can easily become lodged deep in the soft-tissue wound. Sutures should not be placed until oral radiographs confirm the absence of hard-tissue debris.

Luxation Injuries.—For purposes of prognosis and therapy, five different types of luxation injuries are recognized. They are concussion, subluxation (loosening), intrusion, extrusion, and avulsion (or exarticulation). The teeth most frequently injured through luxation are the maxillary anterior incisors. Due to the resiliency of maxillary alveolar bone in the young child, primary teeth tend to be intruded or extruded as a result of injury, whereas permanent teeth tend to sustain tooth-related fractures more readily. Without the aid of intraoral radiographs, the physician must diagnose luxation injuries based on clinical findings and history alone.

Concussive Injuries.—These injuries produce no increased loosening of the teeth, as there is only minor trauma to the periodontal ligaments. The patient will complain of "sore teeth," especially if they are percussed with a metal instrument. No dental referral is necessary unless there is increased sensitivity in the subsequent 48 hours.

Subluxated Teeth.—This term denotes teeth with either increased mobility or a lateral shift in position. There is often associated gingival crevice bleeding present, indicating damage to the periodontal ligaments. Lateral displacements are often associated with fractures of the alveolar socket. Displaced teeth are evident by visual inspection, but increased mobility is a more elusive clinical finding as anterior teeth normally have some degree of mobility owing to the elasticity of the periodontal fibers. It is, therefore, necessary to check contralateral teeth in the same or opposing arch to determine what a normal mobility pattern is for that child. Hypermobile teeth or displaced teeth usually require immediate reduction and splinting; therefore, a referral to a dentist should be made as soon as possible consistent with the medical needs of the patient. With prompt referral, the prognosis for subluxated teeth is excellent.

Extruded Teeth.—These teeth appear elongated and often have a marked lingual deviation of the crown. There is always gingival bleeding since the periodontal ligaments have been disrupted. If a primary tooth is extruded and so loose that there is fear of aspiration, have the child bite into gauze and transport the child to a dentist as soon as possible. It is recommended that extruded primary teeth *not* be replaced into the alveolar socket by the physician since reimplantation could traumatize the nearby calcifying permanent tooth. Permanent teeth that are extruded can be gently teased back into the alveolar socket as the child bites into gauze. There should be immediate referral of the child to a dental office for splinting.

Intruded Teeth.—These are teeth that have been driven into the alveolar bone. These injuries may mimic either a tooth fracture, since only part of the crown may be visible, or an exarticulated (avulsed) tooth, because the entire crown may be within the alveolar bone. The history of the traumatic injury will often lead to the correct diagnosis that can be confirmed radiologically. Intruded teeth generally have a poor prognosis as compared to other luxation injuries, because of the severity of the compression of the blood and nerve supply to the tooth. Generally, the more deeply intruded the tooth, the greater the compression of the pulp, and the worse the prognosis. Whereas, intrusions of less than 4 mm generally require no treatment and the teeth reerupt without sequelae, teeth intruded more than 4 mm generally do not reerupt and usually abscess. Any intrusion should be evaluated by a dentist at the time of injury. Even if no treatment is indicated, the dentist will obtain important baseline radiographs. Deeply intruded primary teeth are often extracted to prevent subsequent damage to the developing permanent tooth due to abscess formation.

Exarticulations or Avulsions.—This term applies to teeth totally "knocked" out of the alveolar socket. The maxillary anterior teeth are those most often affected. Avulsion of permanent teeth occurs predominantly between the ages of 7 and 9 years when the roots are still not fully formed. These injuries tend to be seasonally associated with bicycle or sledding accidents. The amount of time the tooth is out of the alveolus is critical. If the initial contact is made by telephone, the parent or adult should be instructed to reimplant the tooth, thereby reducing the extra-alveolar time and improving the prognosis.

In reimplantation, the tooth should be held by the crown so as not to disrupt further the delicate periodontal fibers that remain on the surface of the root. If the tooth appears dirty, it may be held under gently running temperate tap water. As exarticulated teeth are conical and slippery, they are easily lost when wet; therefore, instruct the parent to place a stop over the drain. Immediately replace the tooth back into the socket. Local anesthesia is usually not necessary, nor is it necessary to remove any blood clots as these will be forced out during reimplantation. Immediate referral to a dentist is necessary so the tooth can be splinted. During transport the child should bite into gauze or use finger pressure to retain the tooth in the socket. If the reimplantation *cannot* be performed at the scene of the injury, at home, or in the physician's office, then the tooth should be transported in milk, saline, or the buccal vestibule of an adult and brought along with the child to a dental office as soon as possible for reimplantation and splinting. Antibiotic coverage is often indicated.

Timing is critical, with teeth that have an extra-alveolar period of less than 30 minutes yielding the best prognosis. Teeth that have extra-alveolar periods of more than two hours, especially in a dry environment, usually develop necrotic periodontal ligaments and are eventually lost due to root resorption. However, even if the time out of the alveolar bone exceeds 2 hours, the tooth should still be reimplanted since the week or months that the tooth will remain can be used to prepare the child for its eventual loss and to allow the dentist to prepare a suitable prosthetic device to replace the tooth when it eventually is lost. Most dentists recommend that a primary tooth should *not* be reimplanted, thus eliminating further potential trauma to the permanent tooth developing apically to the primary.

Injuries to Bone

Bone injuries are usually the result of automobile accidents or fights. Clinically, fractures of the alveolar process are easily diagnosed by displacements or mobility in several teeth. When the mobility of a single tooth is measured by digital pressure, several proximal teeth will also move. The maxillary anterior region is often involved. An immediate referral to a dentist is indicated. The dentist will take intraoral and extraoral radiographs to rule out mandibular or maxillary fractures and, if the injury is limited only to the alveolar bone, treatment will usually consist of reducing the fragment and splinting the mobile teeth to adjacent sound teeth.

Jaw fractures in children usually occur to the mandibular condyles or to tooth-supporting areas and are usually of the "greenstick" nondisplaced variety. Clinically, a child with condylar fracture will have pain upon mouth opening and, therefore, some degree of trismus. As well, there may be deviation of the mandible toward the affected side. Fractures on tooth-supporting areas occasionally exhibit displaced fragments and disturbances in segments of the arch. Palpation along the alveolar process will often reveal a discontinuity or "step" at the site of the fracture. Gingival laceration is often an accompanying feature.

If immediate referral to a dentist is impossible due to other medical considerations, treatment of jaw fractures can be delayed for 24 to 48 hours without any adverse effect on the prognosis. The child should be placed on a soft diet and encouraged not to open his or her mouth unless absolutely necessary.

Soft-Tissue Injuries

Gingival lacerations are often associated with fractured or luxated teeth or alveolar bone in children. Although there is often an inclination on the part of the referring physician to suture these lacerations prior to transport to a dentist, this should be discouraged. If the tooth has been luxated or there is an alveolar bone fracture and repositioning is indicated, it is more difficult to digitally manipulate the tooth back into proper position if the gingiva has been sutured. Usually, suturing of the gingiva is the last procedure to be done in supporting the repositioned tooth. Fragments of fractured teeth are sometimes lodged in these open wounds and, therefore, must be removed prior to suturing.

Most tongue and mucosal lacerations heal without suturing. Suturing is indicated when the free border of the laceration results in a large flap or there is a through-and-through laceration. Tongue and mucosal lacerations bleed profusely, owing to the high vascularity of the tissues. Due to the excessive muscular movements of the tongue, the sutures are placed much deeper than elsewhere in the body. Most tongue lacerations are sutured with 3–0 chromic resorbable suture in deeper muscle and 2–0 chromic resorbable suture in superficial areas. Mucosal lacerations that result in a flap are often sutured with 3–0 chromic catgut if deep, and 3–0 or 4–0 silk if superficial. The decision to administer antibiotics is difficult as the wound is by definition contaminated by the oral flora of the mouth. Antibiotic therapy is at the discretion of the physician or dentist and is based upon the severity and history of the wound.

Many of the dental or oral-facial injuries associated with contact sports can be reduced or eliminated by proper use of custom-fitted mouth guards. To prevent many oral injuries, the dentist may take impressions of the child's mouth and closely adapt soft-plastic trays that are more effective than those that are not custom-made.

BIBLIOGRAPHY

Andraeson JO: *Traumatic Injuries of the Teeth.* St Louis, CV Mosby Co, 1981.

Berkowitz R, Ludwig S, Johnson R: Dental trauma in children and adolescents. *Clin Pediatr* 1980; 19:3.

Josell SD, Abrams RG: Symposium on oral health. *Pediatr Clin North Am* 1982; 29:3.

Nelson LP, Neff JH: Dental emergencies, in Fleisher G, Ludwig S (eds): *Textbook of Pediatric Emergency Medicine.* Baltimore, Williams & Wilkins Co, 1988.

Pinkham JR: *Pediatric Dentistry: Infancy through Adolescence.* Philadelphia, WB Saunders Co, 1988.

Stewart RE, Barber TK, Troutman KC, et al: *Pediatric Dentistry: Scientific Foundations and Clinical Practice.* St Louis, CV Mosby Co, 1982.

ENVIRONMENTAL TRAUMA

Dee Hodge III, M.D.

Environmental trauma refers to those environmental conditions that may injure the child because they are so extreme. These include: (1) heat illness; (2) sunburn; (3) cold exposure; and (4) frostbite.

HEAT ILLNESS

Heat-related illnesses encompass three distinct syndromes: (1) heat cramps or involuntary cramping of muscles; (2) heat exhaustion, which is characterized by hypotension and weakness secondary to acute depletion of the extracellular fluid space by sweating; and (3) heatstroke, which is an acute medical emergency related to the failure of thermoregulatory control. There is a common pathophysiologic mechanism to all of these syndromes.

Heat transfer between the environment and the skin is effected by conduction, convection, radiation, and evaporative cooling. The rate of net heat loss is dependent on the balance of heat production and heat loss. Although each mechanism of heat transfer plays a part, it is evaporative cooling that is the principal avenue of heat loss. When the atmospheric temperature is equal to, or in excess of, that of the skin temperature, sweat loss becomes the principal means of dissipating heat. The higher the humidity, the less sweat evaporates and, therefore, little cooling occurs. High humidity and high ambient temperature are the adverse environmental conditions setting the stage for heat-related illnesses.

Children do not adapt to extremes of temperature as effectively as adults when exposed to high temperature levels. This is true for several reasons including: (1) Children have a greater surface-area-mass ratio than adults, which induces a greater heat transfer between the environment and the body. (2) Children produce more metabolic heat per unit mass with even minimal exercise. (3) Sweating capacity is not as great in children as in adults. (4) The capacity to convey heat by blood from the body core to the skin is reduced in the exercising child. Obesity, febrile state, cystic fibrosis, gastrointestinal tract infection, diabetes insipidus, diabetes mellitus, chronic heart failure, caloric malnutrition, anorexia nervosa, sweating insufficiency syndrome, and mental deficiency all potentiate the risk of heat stress.

Data Gathering

Heat cramps occur acutely during or after intense physical exercise. The physiologic basis for heat cramps is related to the acute loss of sodium through sweating. Water replacement may be sufficient but does not compensate for the electrolyte loss. The ensuing alteration in the sodium-potassium balance in the muscle membrane results in involuntary painful contraction of the muscle.

Heat exhaustion is the most common of the heat stress injuries. There are two identifiable subsyndromes: heat exhaustion due to water depletion and heat exhaustion due to salt depletion. In heat exhaustion due to water loss, the individual is usually sweating. The body temperature may be mildly elevated to 38° C to 39.5° C (100° F to 103° F), but not to the levels encountered in acute heatstroke. Postural or frank hypotension is present. This form of heat exhaustion may progress to heatstroke. In heat exhaustion due to salt depletion, water replacement is adequate, but sodium intake fails to meet sodium losses incurred by intense sweating. Body temperature is normal, thirst is unusual, and muscle cramps may be present, but hypotension and increased heart rate are common.

Heatstroke is classically defined by the triad of hyperpyrexia, neurologic symptoms, and anhydrosis. Temperature is in excess of 41° C (106° F). Multiple organ systems may be involved, resulting in hepatic abnormalities, electrocardiogram (ECG) changes, renal abnormalities as a result of either hypotension, myoglobinuria, or thermal injury, and hematologic abnormalities.

Management

As in any injury, prevention is better than treatment. Intense exercise should be banned under environmental conditions that are conducive to heat stress. The American Academy of Pediatrics Committee on Sports Medicine has outlined criteria for acclimatization and curtailing exercise.

In heat-related illness the following guidelines are suggested for treatment:

Heat Cramps.—Oral salt replacement (or occasionally intravenous [IV] salt replacement) is an important measure. Massage of the affected muscles should be carried out.

Heat Exhaustion.—Remove the patient to a cool environment to avoid further sweat loss. Obtain blood pressure and rectal temperature. If the patient is hypotensive, IV fluid challenge with 10 to 20 mL/kg of normal saline over one hour is recommended. If the patient is normotensive, oral administration of an electrolyte preparation is all that is necessary. Appropriate fluids that contain sodium and potassium include Sportsade, Gatorade, and Pedialyte.

Heatstroke.—The most urgent treatment is rapid lowering of the body temperature. Direct cooling with use of ice packs can be accomplished in the office or at the scene, while awaiting ambulance transfer to the hospital. If IV fluids are available, these should be started to support blood volume. The remainder of the treatment should occur in the hospital where continuous hemodynamic monitoring can be accomplished.

SUNBURN

Sunburn is the result of exposure to sunlight in excess of its beneficial aspects. Ultraviolet solar radiation (UVR) in the 290- to 320-nm range is responsible for sunburn and is referred to as the "burn band" (UVB). Factors that increase the exposure and intensity of UVB, and thereby the risk of sunburn include high altitude, latitudes close to the equator, spring and summer months in the northern hemisphere between 10:00 A.M. and 2:00 P.M., and wide-open spaces of sand or snow that reflect UVR.

There is no single accepted theory for the pathogenesis of sunburn. The minimal erythema dose is defined as the least amount of radiation capable of inducing barely perceptible redness. The erythema is due to vasodilation of blood vessels in the dermis. There is also increased vascular permeability, which results in edema of the dermis. Prostaglandins also seem to play a role in pathogenesis, though it is not understood at this time.

Data Gathering

After the exposure to the minimal erythema dose, there is an immediate erythema that appears and then fades. This is followed by delayed erythema that appears about 4 to 6 hours later, becomes maximal at 15 to 24 hours, and lasts up to 3 days. Maximal tanning appears at about 3 to 5 days. With sunburn there is erythema and edema of the dermis associated with itching and tenderness. Severe overexposure results in fever, vomiting, delirium, and shock. Severe cases with greater than 70% surface-area burn have a similar clinical picture to that of extensive first- and second-degree thermal burns. Healing occurs with desquamation of the skin.

The condition of the sunburned patient is usually easily assessed by history together with the clinical signs. Marked photosensitivity may be due to drugs or systemic disease. Drugs causing phototoxic reaction include: psoralins, tetracyclines, sulfonamides, thiazides, and retinoic acids. Drugs causing photoallergic reactions include: phenothiazines, sulfonamides, para-aminobenzoic acid esters, and halogenated salicylamides. Systemic disorders associated with photosensitivity include polymorphous light eruption, erythropoietic protoporphyria, and systemic lupus erythematosus.

Management

Prevention is the most effective management. Other than protective clothing, sunscreens offer the best protection for susceptible individuals. There are two types of available sunscreens: chemical screens that filter and reduce the intensity of UVR reaching the cells of the skin, and physical screens that are opaque and reflect and scatter light.

Treatment of mild sunburn includes application of cool tap water or compresses with 1:10 dilution of Burow solution for 15 minutes, four or more times a day. Emollients or plain emulsifying ointments are used to soothe and relieve dryness. Aspirin is effective for pain relief. Local anesthetics do not appear to have a major effect and topical steroids have been shown to be noneffective in relief of many of the symptoms of sunburn. In moderate-to-severe sunburn, the treatment is the same as in mild sunburn but, in addition, hospitalization and the administration of IV fluids may be indicated (see Chapter 49).

COLD EXPOSURE

Hypothermia is defined as a core temperature of less than 35° C (95° F). While more common in the adult population due to old age, lack of adequate housing, alcohol and drug ingestions, endocrine disorders, and CNS disorders, in children the condition may be due to prolonged exposure after automobile accidents, cold water immersion, or becoming wet and exhausted during winter sports activities.

Maintenance of body temperature involves a balance between heat production and heat loss. In response to cold exposure, the thermoregulatory center in the hypothalamus sets in motion a coordinated response including increased thyroid and adrenal output via the pituitary (nonshivering thermogenesis), sympathetic nervous system output leading to peripheral vasoconstriction and increased heart rate, and shivering of skeletal muscles leading to increased heat production. Accidental hypothermia occurs when these mechanisms cannot compensate for exposure to low ambient temperatures.

Data Gathering

The clinical signs of hypothermia are related to the decrease in the core temperature. Mental confusion, impaired gait, lethargy, and combativeness are all early signs. Shivering is a useful sign, but patients whose temperature has fallen below 33.3° C (92° F) may not shiver or even feel cold.

"Paradoxical undressing," described in adults, is believed to be due to the failure of peripheral vasoconstriction at low body temperatures, apparently causing a sensation of heat, leading some confused hypothermic patients to take their clothes off.

Acidosis may be respiratory, secondary to ventilatory failure, or metabolic, secondary to circulatory collapse and increased lactic acid production. Urine flow is increased, resulting in a "cold diuresis." Increased urine output combined with extracellular fluid shifts can lead to significant volume depletion.

Cold insult to the cardiovascular system causes decreased cardiac output and hypotension. Cold-induced myocardial irritability leads to conduction disturbances, with ventricular fibrillation. Other ECG changes include sinus bradycardia, T-wave inversion, prolonged intervals, atrial fibrillation, and the characteristic Osborne "J" wave. A useful staging guide to hypothermia has been developed for adults but has not been correlated for pediatric patients: *Mild hypothermia (35° C to 32° C)* is usually benign. Ataxia, slight clumsiness, slowed response to stimuli, and dysarthria are common. Shivering starts at this stage. In *moderate hypothermia (32° C to 25° C)*, shivering stops and is replaced by muscular rigidity. Delirium, stupor, and coma may be present. The patient is often arousable and can be conversant. Temperatures below 30° C are particularly dangerous. Basal metabolic rate is less than 50% of normal. In *severe hypothermia* (less than 25° C) death may ensue if hypothermia is present for more than 2 hours. Patient is unresponsive, purposeful movements and reflexes are absent. The pupils are unreactive. Vigorous cardiopulmonary resuscitation may be required.

Patients who appear dead after prolonged exposure to cold temperatures should not be considered dead until they have a near-normal core temperature and are still unresponsive to cardiopulmonary resuscitation.

Management

Therapy may be divided into two categories: general supportive measures and specific rewarming techniques. Recognition of cold injury is the key. In the field, wet clothing should be removed and further heat loss prevented by blankets, body heat, and, if available, administration of heated humidified oxygen. If possible, warmed IV solutions without potassium should be administered. Hospitalization and intensive monitoring is required by all but the mildly hypothermic patient. Minimal and artful handling is needed because of the ease of precipitation of ventricular fibrillation in the cold heart. Specific rewarming techniques should not be used in the field or in the office situation.

FROSTBITE

Extreme cold injury is uncommon in civilian life, but the number of cases has continued to increase during recent years as the number of participants in outdoor winter sports has increased. The incidence in children is unclear, but those most likely to be injured are those who become wet or exhausted.

The precise mechanism of tissue injury is still unclear, but the extent of injury is determined by the duration of exposure, humidity, wind speed, contact with water or metal, immobility, and dependency of a part. Frostbite is a thermal injury and the tissue damage is similar to a burn in many respects. High-altitude frostbite is produced by rapid freezing. This type of injury is seen in extremely cold temperatures (−40° C to −52° C), with vasoconstriction and deposition of ice crystals in tissue. Slow freezing is most commonly seen. The initial response is vasoconstriction of the exposed part. With continued exposure, there is decreased blood flow, with stasis and, ultimately, occlusion of the vessels.

Data Gathering

Traditional classification describes four degrees. *First-degree* frostbite is characterized by erythema of the skin and edema of the involved part without blister formation; *second-degree* frostbite, by blister and bleb formation; *third-degree* frostbite, by necrosis of the thick layers of the skin and subcutaneous tissues without loss of a part; and *fourth-degree* frostbite, the most severe, by complete necrosis with gangrene and loss of the affected part. Many now advocate a simplified classification: superficial and deep.

Initially the frozen tissue exhibits pallor. As early as 1 hour after freezing, subcutaneous edema becomes manifest as the part thaws. A line of demarcation between frozen and unfrozen tissue, a hyperemic zone owing to reactive vasodilatation, may be seen. Edema becomes maximal approximately 48 to 72 hours after thawing and gradually subsides. It may take as long as 60 to 90 days before a final line of demarcation between viable and nonviable tissue becomes obvious.

Management

Superficial Frostbite.—"Frost nip" is the only type of frostbite that can be treated satisfactorily in the field. Adequate rewarming can be accomplished by the removal of clothing from the affected part and placing the part into the axilla or against the torso of a partner or parent. Rubbing the frostbitten part with snow or exercising it in an attempt to hasten rewarming will cause further damage.

Deep Frostbite.—Rewarming should not be attempted until adequate facilities are at hand. Once the rewarming process has begun, refreezing or weight-bearing on the affected part will result in additional injury. Rewarming should be accomplished via water bath maintained at 40° C to 42° C (104° F to 108° F). Rewarming should be continued until a flush has returned to the most distal tip of the thawed part, approximately 20 to 30 minutes. After rewarming, thawed parts, like burned tissue, are extremely sensitive to trauma and susceptible to infection. The patient should be kept warm. Dependent position of the affected part should be avoided, and blisters should be left intact. Tetanus toxoid is recommended, and extreme care should be taken to prevent infection and avoid abrasion or other trauma. Whirlpool baths are recommended once or twice daily until healing is complete. Conservative surgical management is recommended.

BIBLIOGRAPHY

Heat Illness

Clowes GHA, O'Donnell TF: Heat stroke. *N Engl J Med* 1974; 291:564–66.

Committee on Sports Medicine, American Academy of Pediatrics: Climatic heat stress and the exercising child. *Pediatrics* 1982; 69:808–809.

O'Donnell TF: Management of heat stress injuries in the athelete. *Orthop Clin North Am* 1980; 11:841–855.

Wadlington WB: Heat stroke in infancy. *Am J Dis Child* 1976; 130:1250–51.

Sunburn

Lane-Brown M: New concepts in prevention and treatment of sunburn. *Drugs* 1977; 13:366–372.

Leach J: Sunburn: Effects and management. *Pediatr Rev* 1983; 5:13–17.

Pathak MA: Sunscreens: Topical and systemic approaches for protection of human skin against harmful effects of solar radiation. *Am Acad Derm* 1982; 7:285–312.

Russo PM, Schneiderman LJ: Effect of topical corticosteroids on symptoms of clinical sunburn. *J Fam Pract* 1978; 7:1129–1132.

Frostbite

Espainosa GA: Management of frostbite injuries. *J Natl Med Assoc* 1981; 73:1125–1130.

Lapp NL, Juergens JL: Frostbite. *Mayo Clin Proc* 1965; 40:932–948.

Hypothermia

Grace TG: Cold exposure injuries and the winter athelete. *Clin Orthop* 1987; 216:55–63.

Martyn JW: Diagnosing and treating hypothermia. *Can Med Assoc J* 1981; 125:1089–1096.

Reuler JB: Hypothermia: Pathophysiology, clinical settings, and management. *Ann Intern Med* 1978; 89:519–527.

Welton DE, Mattox KL, Miller RR, et al: Treatment of profound hypothermia. *JAMA* 1978; 240:2291–2292.

ORTHOPEDIC TRAUMA

Henry H. Sherk, M.D.

Children with a complaint of musculoskeletal pain and a history of injury comprise a large group of patients brought to the office of the primary care physician. Because of the frequency with which such patients are seen and the commonness of the diagnoses with which they present, there is a tendency to label such patients as "routine" and proceed rather quickly and automatically along a line of investigation and treatment. However, such children require not only a full awareness of the diagnostic possibilities on the part of the physician but also a careful diagnostic evaluation. Without an organized approach to the assessment of an injured child, one can either miss important injuries or order unnecessary studies, prolong the evaluation, and possibly overtreat.

The child with physical findings that are suggestive of injury and confirmatory findings with radiography requires treatment, not decision-making. If, however, the child has no physical findings, the physician must decide whether the complaint and severity of injury justify radiography, whether symptomatic treatment should be given, and whether additional evaluation is indicated should the symptoms persist. If the patient has positive physical findings and radiographs reveal no musculoskeletal injury, the physician must make similar decisions regarding symptomatic treatment and the need for additional evaluation. A child with musculoskeletal pain and no history of injury requires an assessment that may lead to a wide variety of diagnostic considerations. In such an individual, examination and radiography can very quickly establish the diagnosis of an occult fracture or a dislocation. If, however, there are no abnormal physical findings and if radiographs reveal no musculoskeletal injury, one must be alert to the possibility of developmental abnormalities such as the osteochondroses or more serious diseases such as an infection or tumor.

This chapter deals with the common minor fractures, dislocations, sprains, and benign developmental conditions seen in office practice. In each section specific entities (i.e., upper limb, lower limb) are reviewed with regard to data gathering and management.

FRACTURES OF THE CLAVICLE

One of the most common injuries in children is a fracture of the clavicle. In older children the diagnosis is usually unmistakable on clinical examination, but in infants and very young children it may be less obvious. Overriding of bone fragments, severe swelling, ecchymosis, local tenderness, crepitus, and drooping of the shoulder on the affected side lead the physician to the diagnosis. At times, this symptom complex allows the child and parent to make the diagnosis before they bring the injured patient to the physician for treatment of the "broken collar bone." However, in greenstick fractures the findings are more subtle, as there may be no deformity and very little swelling. The patient may permit passive motion, but more often is fretful and has a pseudoparalysis due to pain when mobilization of the shoulder is attempted. Radiographs, of course, establish the diagnosis in doubtful cases and confirm it in more obvious situations.

Treatment is gratifying in almost every case. Children under 6 or 7 years of age require no reduction even if the fracture is displaced. Symptoms resolve quickly over a period of 2 weeks, with a clavicle strap or a posterior figure-of-8 bandage (Fig 67–5). In infants, even this degree of support may be unnecessary, particularly if there is minimal displacement of the fracture. One can expect rapid union of the fragments and obliteration of the deformity noted on radiography as remodeling and remolding take place with further growth. Older children may require a longer period of support with the bandage until discomfort subsides and union occurs. Reduction is rarely necessary and it is difficult to maintain, so that even strikingly comminuted displaced clavicle fractures can be expected to heal well.

Congenital pseudoarthrosis of the clavicle is probably not related to trauma and rarely causes enough deformity, functional impairment, or discomfort to justify surgery. Patients most often request surgery for cosmetic reasons but the postoperative scarring and frequent recurrence rate make cosmesis an inadequate indication for surgical treatment.

An interesting, though unusual, variant of a clavicle fracture is an epiphyseal separation at the proximal end of the clavicle at the sternoclavicular joint. It is recognizable clinically as swelling and tenderness at the medial end of the clavicle after an injury. Because of the late ossification of the proximal clavicular epiphysis (at the age of 17 years), the diagnosis is difficult to make with radiographs. Treatment should be as conservative as possible with local adhesive strapping and a posterior figure-of-8 bandage for support.

FRACTURES OF THE PROXIMAL HUMERUS

Some dislocations of the shoulder are rare in young children. The patient under 7 years old with swelling and pain about the shoulder probably has a transverse fracture of the proximal humerus just below the lesser tuberosity. From the age of 7 years to adolescence, shoulder injuries are usually epiphyseal separations, and after adolescence patients usually sustain shoulder dislocations or acromioclavicular sep-

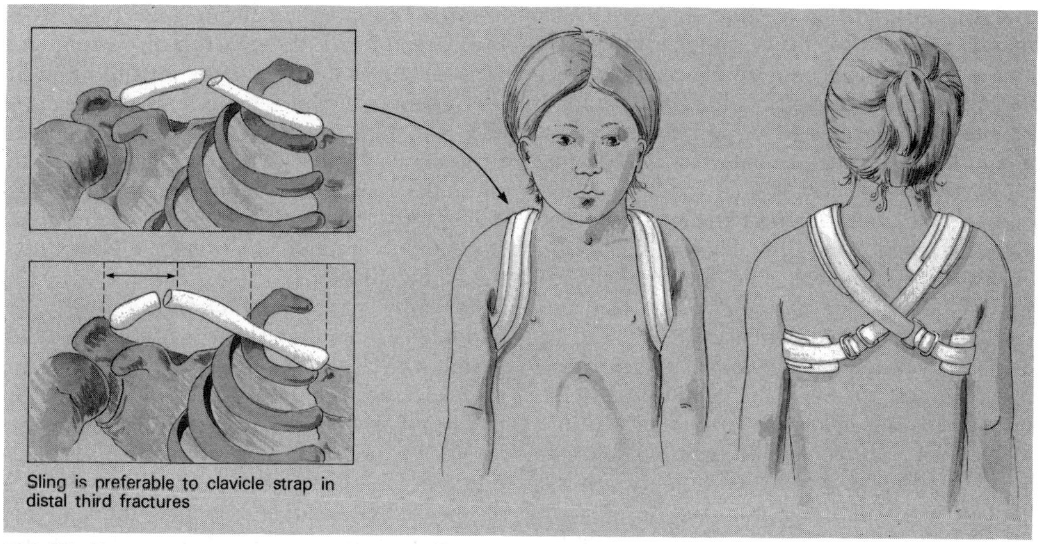

FIG 67–5
Method for applying figure-of-8 bandage to fractured clavicle.

arations. Fractures of the proximal humerus in very young children have a propensity to unite quickly, even in the face of bayonet apposition or even a moderate degree of angulation. In an office setting, it is possible to treat such patients with a Velpeau dressing or sugar-tong plaster splints with an excellent chance of satisfactory healing. The bone deformity can be expected to remodel well over a period of several months.

Displaced epiphyseal fractures in older children, on the other hand, probably require more aggressive treatment than can be provided on an outpatient basis. Such patients may require anesthesia for reduction, plaster support in the "salute position," or overhead traction to maintain alignment. Rarely, a patient with this type of injury may need open reduction to disengage the biceps tendon when it is trapped between the fragments. In patients who have minimal deformity, however, the outpatient setting may suffice and a Velpeau dressing or shoulder spica cast can secure sufficient immobilization to permit uncomplicated healing. Malunion of this type of fracture results in anterior angulation of the humerus just below the humeral head. Patients with this type of residual deformity have limited shoulder flexion and if outpatient treatment seems suitable for a given individual, adequate follow-up radiographs must be taken frequently enough in the early stages of treatment to prevent this complication.

SHOULDER DISLOCATIONS

Shoulder dislocations occur infrequently in young children and are uncommon until adolescence. Nevertheless, in an outpatient practice youthful athletes often present with this type of injury and may benefit from prompt treatment by the primary care physician. Recognition of the injury is not difficult. Patients have severe pain with an acute shoulder dislocation and the appearance of the affected shoulder is obviously different even to the untrained eye. The acromion is very prominent. Often the head of the humerus is visible and palpable beneath the corocoid process and the shoulder has a square appearance, lacking the normal roundness of the deltoid muscle.

Before undertaking treatment, a radiograph is essential. If the radiograph reveals no fracture, the primary physician can often treat the patient's severe shoulder pain by reducing the dislocation promptly. Some sedation may be necessary in heavy muscular adolescents, but longitudinal traction against the countertraction of a sheet passed under the axilla can very often achieve reduction without resorting to general anesthesia. If manipulation does fail, anesthesia may be necessary to permit the reduction.

Following a first episode of shoulder dislocation, in adolescent patients recurrent dislocation of the shoulder is a frequent complication.

Prolonged support in a sling and swath or shoulder immobilizer may minimize the possibility of a recurrence, and young patients with this injury should be restricted in this way for 4 to 6 weeks. The external support should allow the anterior ligaments, capsule, and subscapularis muscle to heal such that these anatomic structures will be competent enough to prevent another episode. Before the external support is withdrawn completely, the patient should carry out a program of range of motion and muscle-strengthening exercises. It should be noted that adult patients do not require prolonged support after an initial shoulder dislocation because the older age groups have a low incidence of recurrence but a high incidence of shoulder stiffness after this type of injury. Older patients can begin the exercise program immediately, using a sling only for comfort for a few days.

FRACTURES OF THE SHAFT OF THE HUMERUS

Fractures of the shaft of the humerus in newborns may be the result of a difficult delivery, but in infants and young children the presence of this type of fracture suggests parental abuse or at least a direct blow to the upper arm. Falls in young patients usually result in fractures of the wrist, forearm, or shoulder, and not the shaft of the humerus.

Fractures of the humeral shaft have an excellent prognosis and heal promptly with the Velpeau wrap-around dressing in infants or with a sugar-tong splint in older children.

INJURIES ABOUT THE ELBOW

The most serious bony injury of the upper limb is a supracondylar fracture of the humerus. This fracture is not generally suitable for office treatment and, in general, most patients with this injury should be admitted to the hospital. Patients with displaced supracondylar fractures have intense discomfort, severe swelling, and obvious vascular compromise so that there is usually little debate over the need for prompt emergency treatment in a hospital setting.

Other types of elbow injuries, however, may also have major potential for causing long-range impairment but may present much less dramatically. Hence, they may receive less attention and possibly go unrecognized and untreated. The most significant injury in this regard is a fracture through the capitellum. It is well known that this fracture fails to unite unless open reduction and pin fixation achieve and maintain a virtually perfect alignment. Even minor degrees of displacement permit the capitellar fragment to migrate and fail to heal. Nonunion of the capitellum causes the distal fragment to migrate proximally and, in turn, the elbow develops a valgus deformity traction neuropathy, with stretching of the ulnar nerve and late degenerative arthritis of the elbow. Patients with fractures through the capitellum, therefore, require recognition by the primary physician and referral for definitive treatment.

Other elbow injuries seen commonly in patients in ambulatory care settings are fractures of the radial head and medial humeral epicondylar fractures. Treatment of these injuries should be as conservative as possible. Radial neck fractures can be permitted up to 30° of angulation before requiring open reduction (never an excision, as in adults) and medial humeral epicondylar fractures need open reduction only if they are displaced into the elbow joint or if they are so displaced as to compromise the ulnar nerve as it passes posteriorly behind the medial humerus. In general, both of these fractures—radial neck and medial humeral epicondyle—can be treated with splinting for 4 weeks before permitting active motion. If in doubt, however, the primary care physician should refer the child for consultation and discussion of the possible need for open reduction.

Elbow dislocation may occur without fracture but before manipulating the injury, radiographs must be obtained to rule out the presence of a complicating bone injury. If one thereby establishes the fact that the patient's pain, deformity, swelling, and ecchymosis are solely related to dislocation of the elbow joint, the primary care physician might consider reduction with traction with the elbow at a right angle. Reduction of a dislocated elbow in a child is usually easily done, and only in older patients might anesthesia be required. After reduction the physician should protect the elbow in a splint for 3 to 4 weeks before removing support and permitting active use of the elbow joint.

Pure dislocations of the elbow, however, are rare in children and one should be on the lookout for associated fractures of the medial epicondyle, radial neck, capitellum, and olecranon. In general, complex elbow injuries require specialized care and should be referred from the primary care setting.

NURSEMAID'S ELBOW

A common minor elbow injury in children is the pulled elbow, nursemaid's elbow, or radial head subluxation. The lesion is usually present in young children and results from pulling the child vigorously by the wrist or hand. The mechanism of the injury is longitudinal traction applied while the arm is in pronation. This action pulls the radial head part way out of the encircling annular ligament. Part of the annular ligament thus is caught between the radial head and the capitellum. When traction is released, the annular ligament remains in that location and prevents the forearm from returning to a supinated and fully extended position. The child refuses to move the arm and complains of pain in the elbow. Radiographs are normal. One can reduce the subluxation usually by supinating the forearm and extending the elbow slightly. Occasionally one can feel a click or snap as this is done. Young children cry loudly when the elbow is reduced, so that it may be wise to carry out the procedure after warning an apprehensive parent about what will happen. When the reduction is achieved, the pain disappears quickly and the child will begin moving the arm rather freely. Recurrence of the subluxation is not unusual, but, despite this, support with a sling for a week seems all that is required in the way of postreduction treatment. Most young children will not conform to the sling once the reduction is achieved. After the second or third recurrence, the child may require immobilization in a long arm cast. Nursemaid's elbow is not seen in children over 4 or 5 years of age.

FOREARM AND WRIST INJURIES

The primary care physician can and should be involved in the treatment of forearm and wrist injuries. As some injuries are more complex, the physician should have a working knowledge of the types of injuries encountered and realize which injuries will need more aggressive treatment than is possible to provide in an office setting.

In a primary care setting minimally displaced fractures can often be treated successfully simply by immobilization. The physician should have adequate skill in applying the cast, remembering to apply plaster smoothly and evenly over adequate padding and making sure it is well molded over bony prominences. Casts should not be circular or tubular but should be contoured to follow the cross-sectional configuration of a limb. Patients should have adequate checks after the cast has been applied for evaluation of neurovascular status, and they should have careful follow-up with serial radiography to rule out late displacement. In general, patients with displaced forearm and wrist fractures should be considered for referral since reduction may require anesthesia.

CLASSIFICATION OF FOREARM AND WRIST FRACTURES

- Distal third fractures of the radius or ulna
  - Greenstick
  - Displaced
- Shaft fractures of the radius or ulna
  - Greenstick
  - Displaced
- Epiphyseal fractures of the distal radius, with or without involvement of the distal ulna
- Fracture dislocations
  - Monteggia
  - Galeazzi

Fractures of the Distal Third of the Forearm

Angulation of the distal end of a bone readily self-corrects with growth in young children and up to 30 degrees of deformity is acceptable in children under 6 years of age. In these injuries the treating physician would be justified in applying a long arm cast without manipulation. In undisplaced fractures and "buckle fractures" a short arm cast will suffice.

In patients with severely angulated greenstick fractures or displaced fractures of the distal third of the radius and/or ulna, reduction is considered necessary. Remodeling and remolding might eliminate deformity with time in young children but angulation of 30 degrees or more might result in a permanent deformity, and thus should be corrected if possible. A gentle manipulation (with the patient under sedation or with local anesthesia injected into the hematoma) might be attempted in greenstick fractures but displaced fractures of the distal third of the forearm are more difficult to reduce and often require more vigorous treatment. This type of treatment usually requires general anesthesia. The fracture should be immobilized after manipulation in pronation and slight flexion.

Shaft Fractures of the Forearm

Greenstick fractures develop progressive deformity and angulate rather markedly if not treated correctly. One must break through the intact cortex on the side of the bone away from the fracture and then reduce the malalignment prior to casting. It is possible to engage in this type of treatment in a primary care setting but usually results are better and the entire situation less stressful for the patient if the manipulation is done under general anesthesia.

Complete and displaced fractures of the forearm also require suitable analgesia and adequate reduction to avoid permanent deformity and for these reasons are best splinted by the primary care physician and referred for definitive treatment.

Epiphyseal Fractures

Epiphyseal separations to the distal radius can occur above or in conjunction with a fracture of the distal ulna. Minimal displacement requires no reduction but patients should be immobilized in a long arm cast for 5 or 6 weeks (Fig 67–6). Patients with displaced epiphyseal separations present more serious problems. Vigorous manipulation or delayed manipulation may so damage the epiphyseal plate that growth arrest occurs and patients may develop a significant radial shortening. Therefore, patients with this type of injury are, in general, not good candidates for treatment in a primary care setting.

Fracture Dislocations

Fracture dislocations of the forearm are complex injuries that usually involve a fracture of a shaft of one bone and dislocation of the radial head or distal ulna. In the Monteggia fracture and its variants, the radial head is dislocated and the ulna fractured. In the Galeazzi fracture the distal radioulnar joint is separated and the distal radius is fractured. In general, these fractures may present more difficulty in treatment than the primary care physician would want to accept. It is essential, however, that one make the diagnosis, a requirement that mandates radiographs with views of the ends of the bones as well as their midshafts. In addition, one should suspect a diagnosis of a dislocation in a fracture of a single bone of the forearm.

HAND INJURIES

Hand injuries in children usually consist of finger fractures and fingertip injuries, although teenagers occasionally present with fractures of the carpal navicular. The severe industrial cases—the cornpicker injuries and crush injuries with clothes wringers—are now much less common in small children. Most minor hand injuries are suitable for care in the primary setting, provided that the physician recognizes several common pitfalls.

For example, fractures of the proximal phalanx at or just distal to the epiphyseal plate occur very frequently and usually are minimally displaced. Such fractures can be treated by

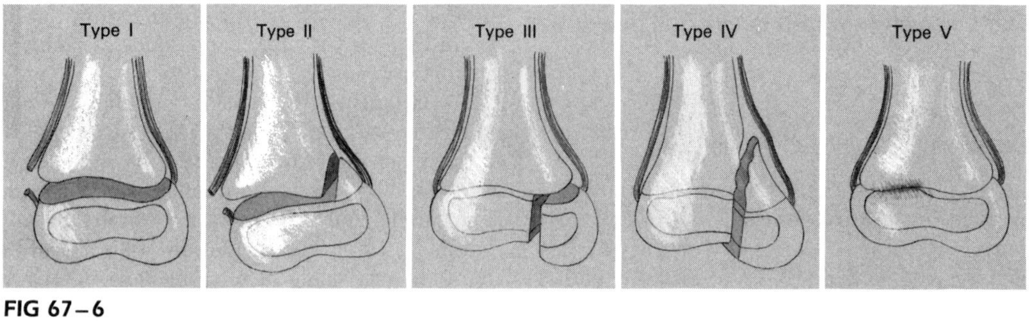

FIG 67–6
Salter Harris classification of epiphyseal fractures.

"buddy taping" or strapping with adhesive the injured finger to an adjacent digit. The same type of treatment is also suitable for undisplaced fractures of the shaft of a phalanx. In treating fractures of the phalanges, one should remember not to immobilize only one digit and one should avoid rotational malalignment. Ask the patient to flex all four fingers while looking at the hand from the volar direction. All four fingertips should come together to point to the proximal part of the carpal navicular. If rotational malalignment is not corrected, the involved finger will not do this and will overlap an adjacent finger.

Fractures of the fifth metacarpal usually result from fighting. They merit only very conservative treatment; even if the child or young adolescent maintains a considerable degree of angulation at the fracture site, the functional result will be good. These injuries should be treated with volar splints for 3 or 4 weeks until union is sufficient to permit normal activities.

Fractures of the condylar parts of the phalanges and fractures of the distal phalanx of a digit may not be amenable to treatment in the primary care setting. Displaced condylar fractures can leave the child with permanently angulated fingers unless the fracture is openly reduced and pinned. Fractures of the tendinous insertions of the extensor digitorum communis on the base of the distal phalanx can leave the child with a permanent mallet finger unless splinted in hyperextension. Such fractures may also require pin fixation to prevent deformity but usually splinting in extension is sufficient. In young children a mallet finger deformity is usually caused by an epiphyseal separation. In adolescents the deformity results from a fracture through the epiphysis into the growth plate.

Dislocation of the metacarpal-phalangeal joint may not permit reduction by closed means since the joint capsule and flexor tendon can become interposed between the distal end of the metacarpal and proximal part of the proximal phalanx (Fig 67–7). If one or two gentle attempts do not achieve reduction of this type of injury, open surgical reduction should be carried out as soon as possible. This is accomplished by splitting the interposed volar plate and retrieving the displaced tendon.

Tendon lacerations and open fractures should be referred from the primary setting for definitive treatment in a hospital.

LOWER LIMB INJURIES

Fractures of the pelvis, hip fractures, femoral shaft fractures, and epiphyseal separations about the knee are all major injuries that probably would not involve the primary care physician. These injuries require hospitalization and prolonged care in a hospital setting. Some undisplaced tibial shaft fractures in young children may be treatable with splinting or cast fixation in the office, but, in general, patients with significant long bone fractures in the lower limb require hospitalization.

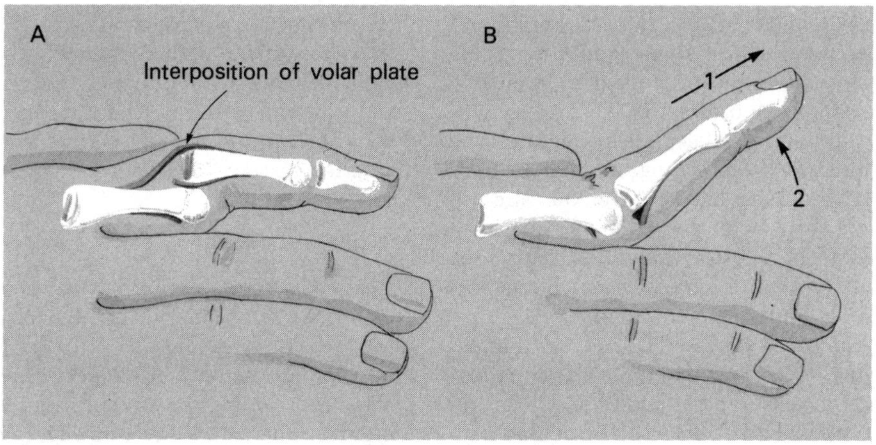

FIG 67–7
Technique for repositioning of dislocated finger.

AVULSION FRACTURES OF THE PELVIS

Major fractures of the pelvic ring usually result from severe injury but the primary care physician may be called on to treat avulsion fractures of the pelvis. These occur in immature adolescents who with vigorous muscle contraction avulse a muscle origin. The anterior superior and anterior inferior iliac spines are common sites of injury, with avulsion of the origins of the sartorius and rectus femorus, respectively. The hamstring muscles, in addition, avulse the ischial tuberosity. The patients usually have a good deal of swelling, ecchymosis, and pain, and there is little chance that the physician will not order a radiograph to establish the diagnosis since the patients have such an acute clinical picture. Treatment with bed rest, analgesics, and an ice bag usually suffices. These patients can most often be treated at home after the diagnosis has been made. It usually takes 2 months for the fractures to heal sufficiently to permit a return to regular activities.

KNEE INJURIES

Knee injuries in children are generally different from those seen in adult patients. The torn menisci and ruptured cruciate and collateral ligaments of the adolescent and older athlete are much less common in young patients. The bone-cartilage interface of the epiphyseal plate is the weakest component of the knee in children. In young adults the epiphyseal plates have closed and the bone is young and very strong. In children, therefore, a major stress on the knee will most likely cause an epiphyseal separation, while in a young adult the same step will produce a ligamentous tear. In elderly patients with osteoporosis, the same injury will probably produce a tibial plateau fracture. The implications of the foregoing are that in children internal derangements of the knee are unusual and a child suspected of having one more likely has an epiphyseal separation. This type of injury may require more aggressive diagnostic measures and treatment than can be provided in the office setting. The injuries that occur in such cases are fractures of the tibial spines, epiphyseal separations of the distal femur or proximal tibia, and intraarticular fractures of the femoral condyles.

Patellar fractures and dislocations, however, may not require more specialized care than is available in the outpatient setting. Acute dislocations of the patella can be reduced and immobilized by the primary care physician. If adequate radiographs including tangential views have established the fact that no osteochondral fracture fragments are loose in the joint, then support in plaster for a few weeks should let the soft tissues heal satisfactorily. Patients should, of course, restore quadriceps and hamstring strength with an exercise program before resuming athletics. If an osteochondral fragment is loose in the joint, it should be removed.

Recurrent subluxations and dislocations may require surgical correction. Fractures of the patella do not occur very often in children and it is easy to mistake a bipartite patella (a congenital lesion) for an injury. Fractures of the patella in children may require open reduction and should probably be referred for consideration of that possibility.

TIBIAL STRESS FRACTURES

Stress fractures of the tibia are often not recognized as such, and as a diagnostic problem, they may prove troublesome. They usually cause pain in the lower leg that is associated with a good deal of local tenderness. Patients often have negative findings on radiographs at first. With passing time, a radiograph will reveal hazy callus forming external to the tibia at the level of a transverse radiolucent line. The appearance of the radiograph may also suggest a tumor of bone or an early infection. A bone scan is positive in all three conditions so that the true diagnosis occasionally can only be inferred. Treatment with reduction of activities, weight bearing with crutches, and analgesics usually permits healing to occur with minimal discomfort. An occasional patient may require a long leg cast.

ANKLE FRACTURES

Some ankle fractures can be treated quite successfully by the primary care physician. Undisplaced fractures of the distal fibula, for example, respond well to 3 or 4 weeks of support in plaster and can be treated quite successfully in the office. The caveat here, however, is the recognition of the fact that children—especially young children—do not often "sprain" their ankles, and swelling and pain of the lateral ankle in this age group is probably a minimally displaced fracture of the distal fibula through the epiphyseal plate.

The pitfalls to be avoided in treating ankle injuries in children are related to the Tillaux, triplane, and medial malleolar fractures. The primary care physician's responsibility in the management of this type of case is recognition, since these injuries may require open reduction for the best result. The Tillaux fracture occurs through the lateral part of the distal tibula epiphysis and the lateral half of the epiphysis is displaced for various degrees from its normal position. If a Tillaux fracture is associated with a complete distal tibial separation with a retained metaphyseal spike (Salter II) (see Fig 67–6), the injury is a triplane fracture. With such severe damage to the epiphyseal cartilage, growth arrest can occur and adequate reduction with internal fixation is necessary to minimize that complication. Medial malleolus fractures in children also have the potential for causing growth arrest, with subsequent varus deformity and shortening. This type of injury also probably requires at least consideration of open reduction and is best referred.

FOOT INJURIES

Injuries of the hindfoot are uncommon except for cases with major crushing injury. In children with a painful swollen ankle and a "normal" radiograph, however, one should be sure to look for an osteochondral fracture of the talus. This lesion is recognizable as a small fragment of bone at the edge of the superior surface of the talus, where it articulates with either the medial or lateral malleolus. Under most circumstances the fracture can be expected to heal with support in a non-weight-bearing short leg cast. Occasionally, however, the fragment may separate itself from the talus and become a loose body in the joint. Under these circumstances, the patient will require an arthrotomy of the joint for its removal.

Fractures of the os calcis in children are very unusual. They require only a compression dressing and elevation under most circumstances. Unless potential skin necrosis complicates the fracture, the primary care physician should be able to treat this patient on an outpatient basis.

Most of the children with foot injuries who present in an office setting have metatarsal fractures or phalangeal injuries. The fracture most often seen is at the base of the fifth metatarsal and is not to be confused with normal ossification of the epiphysis in that location. One can recognize the difference with no trouble since in younger children the epiphyseal plate is disposed longitudinally. Fractures of the fifth metatarsal, however, are transverse. Metatarsal fractures in children heal promptly with a compression dressing or short leg cast for 3 or 4 weeks. Older athletic adolescents may fracture the base of the fifth metatarsal repeatedly, however, and eventually develop nonunions. Surgical treatment may be necessary in established nonunions and one should protect such individuals with casts for longer periods.

Fractures of the phalanges of the toes usually require little formal treatment. When undisplaced or minimally displaced, they can be supported with adhesive strips securing the toe to an adjacent digit. Angulated broken toes should be reduced by passive manipulation before taping the digit.

OSTEOCHONDROSES OF THE LOWER LIMB

The term osteochondroses refers to a group of conditions that occur during the juvenile period and are characterized by similar radiologic findings of increased density and fragmentation of an epiphyseal or apophyseal center. The epiphysis, which is located at the metaphyseal ends of long bones, is where bony growth is occurring, and the apophysis is the name given to the location where muscle or tendon attaches to the bone. Historically, the cause of the bone fragmentation has been attributed to avascular necrosis.

However, recent evidence indicates that many of these lesions—especially the apophyseal lesions—are actually due to abnormalities of enchondral ossification, possibly due to mechanical factors related to traction on the bone via the muscular attachment. Therefore, the osteochondroses are a radiologic classification and not an etiologic classification. There are very classic locations where this phenomenon occurs and each is identified by its own eponym. A brief description of each syndrome will follow.

In general, the patient presents with a history

of progressive pain in a particular location. There is usually no history of a definite traumatic episode. Some patients may make reference to some minor traumatic event or date the onset of symptoms, but a good etiologic correlation or explanation is usually not confirmed. The pain generally is exacerbated with activities and subsides with rest. The management, which for the most part is always conservative, consists of various forms of immobilization, rest, and anti-inflammatory medications.

Freiberg Infarction (Osteochondrosis of the Metatarsal Head)

This lesion represents true avascular necrosis of a metatarsal head. It usually involves the second metatarsal head but occasionally involves one of the more lateral metatarsals and, rarely, the first metatarsal. On radiographs, there is the appearance of a crushed and fragmented distal metatarsal head. It more commonly occurs in individuals in whom the first metatarsal is shorter than the second and increased stress from repetitive weight bearing has been implicated as an etiologic factor.

The typical patient is an adolescent who presents with localized pain and swelling of the involved metatarsal head. On physical examination, swelling and limitation of motion of the involved metatarsal pharyngeal joint are noted. As stated previously, the findings on radiography are characteristic.

Treatment in the adolescent should initially always be conservative and nonoperative. Initial management should consist of recommending that the patient wear a low-heel shoe with a metatarsal bar or pad to redistribute the weight bearing away from the involved metatarsal and prescribing anti-inflammatory medication depending on the severity of symptoms. If the pain is severe or persists, then a short leg walking cast is used for 3 to 4 weeks. If this fails, a brief period of non-weight bearing with the aid of crutches is instituted until the symptoms resolve. If symptoms were to arise in a patient who is skeletally mature, then the treatment would be resection of the involved metatarsal head.

Köhler Disease (Osteochondrosis of the Tarsal Navicular)

This is also a true avascular necrosis of the tarsal navicular. It is believed that repetitive compressive forces lead to fragmentation and loss of blood supply. The navicular bone occupies the apex of the longitudinal arch of the foot and is subjected to constant stress during weight bearing. It is also the last tarsal bone to ossify. The combination of late ossification and constant stress is felt to be the reason as to why the tarsal navicular is at risk for this particular problem. This theory is supported by the fact that Köhler disease is more common if tarsal navicular ossification is delayed. It is more common in boys since their navicular ossifies later than that of girls.

Typically, the patient presents with a history of progressive pain and swelling around the medial aspect of the midfoot in the region of the tarsal navicular. The average age of onset for this phenomenon is 4 years in girls and 5 years in boys. Physical examination reveals pain and swelling of the tarsal navicular. Two variations on radiography should be noted: the tarsal navicular may either appear as a thin wafer of bone with patchy increased density suggestive of collapse or may appear normal in size and shape with minimal fragmentation but definite uniform increase in density compared with surrounding tarsal bones.

Treatment is again symptomatic. First, treatment with an arch support and restriction of activities is instituted. If the pain persists, a short leg walking cast is applied and usually the pain subsides within 4 weeks. Refractory cases can be treated with guarded weight bearing with either a pediatric walker or crutches, depending on the age of the child. Short courses of anti-inflammatory medicines such as aspirin are often a good adjuvant. This is usually a self-limited problem with normal ossification within two years of presentation.

Sever Disease (Calcaneal Apophysitis)

This is not a true avascular necrosis but merely represents a self-limited traction apophysitis of the calcaneus at the insertion of the Achilles tendon. This condition is more common in boys, possibly reflecting their type of athletic activity. Age of presentation is usually between 6 and 10 years. The typical patient presents with pain and tenderness over the posterior aspect of the calcaneus. The patient complains of an insidious onset of pain that is aggravated by activity (especially running and jumping activities) and is relieved by rest. Physical examination may reveal pain, tenderness, and mild swelling around the insertion of the Achilles tendon. The pain is exacerbated by resisted plantar flexion and passive hyperdorsiflexion of the foot. The appearance on radiographs is classic, showing increased density and fragmentation of the posterior calcaneal apophysis.

The treatment again is conservative and consists of a mild restriction of activities (mainly running and jumping) and a 1-in. heel pad to elevate the heel and decrease the tension of the Achilles insertion. In severe cases a short leg walking cast may be required for 3 to 4 weeks. Aspirin for a short course is helpful. Once the symptoms have resolved heel-cord stretching exercises should be instituted to prevent any recurrence.

Osgood-Schlatter Disease (Traction Apophysitis of Tibial Tubercle)

This disease is quite similar to Sever disease but occurs at the anterior tibial tubercle where the patellar tendon inserts onto the tibial tubercle. It is a traction apophysitis similar to Sever disease, but anatomically the tibial tubercle is located right at the proximal tibial epiphysis and some investigators refer to this entity as traumatic or traction epiphysitis. Regardless of the name, it is basically an inflammation of the tibial tubercle at the insertion of the patellar tendon. The typical patient is an adolescent boy, aged 11 to 15 years, who is active in sports. The patient presents with pain and local swelling around the tibial tubercle. The pain is exacerbated by running activities, stair climbing, bicycling, or any other activity that involves active contraction of the quadriceps mechanism. Physical examination reveals local pain and swelling around the tibial tubercle. In addition, resistive knee extensions and passive hyperflexion cause increased pain around the tibial tubercle.

On radiographs, Osgood-Schlatter disease in younger patients reveals soft-tissue swelling anterior to the tibial tubercle and occasionally thickening of the patellar tendon. Bone changes are usually seen in older adolescents and appear as prominent irregular tibial tuberosities or fragmented, often with one large fragment located anterior and superior to the tibial tubercle. This is often referred to as an ossicle or unresolved lesion. Osgood-Schlatter disease is usually self-limited and subsides when the tibial tubercle fuses when the patient is about 15 years of age.

Treatment for Osgood-Schlatter disease is symptomatic. If the symptoms are severe enough to interfere with a patient's activities, then a mere decrease in activity level usually suffices. It is most important to cease the aforementioned activities of running, bicycling, and stair climbing. Anti-inflammatory drugs such as aspirin and a knee immobilizer are adjuvants. The knee immobilizer is worn during symptomatic episodes and serves the purpose of keeping the knee in full extension, thereby resting the quadriceps and decreasing the tension on the tibial tubercle. For refractory cases, a plaster cylinder cast can be applied for 4 to 8 weeks. Surgery is reserved for patients with refractory symptoms in whom a definite, separate large fragment or ossicle is identified on a radiograph and could thus be excised surgically. Full return to function without residual impairment is the usual outcome.

BIBLIOGRAPHY

Alpar EK, Thompson K, Owen R, et al: Mid shaft fractures of forearm bones in children. *Injury* 1981; 13:153.

Blount WP: *Fractures in Children.* Baltimore, Williams & Wilkins Co, 1955.

Canale TS: Fractures and dislocations in children in Crenshaw AH (ed): *Campbell's Operative Orthopedics.* St Louis, CV Mosby, 1987, 1983–2013.

Chapcahal G (ed): *Fractures in Children.* New York, Thieme-Stratton, 1981.

Green DP: Hand injuries in children. *Pediatr Clin North Am* 1977; 24:903.

Kennedy JC (ed): *The Injured Adolescent Knee.* Baltimore, Williams & Wilkins, 1979.

Peiro A, Aracil J, Martos F, et al: Triplane distal tibial epiphyseal fractures. *Clin Orthop Related Res* 1981; 160:196.

Pollen AG: *Fractures and Dislocations in Children*. Edinburgh, Churchill Livingstone Inc, 1973.

Rang M: *Children's Fractures*, ed 2. Philadelphia, JB Lippincott, 1983.

Rockwood CA Jr, Wilkins KE, King RE (eds): *Fractures in Children*. Philadelphia, JB Lippincott, 1984.

Sharrar W: *Pediatric Orthopaedics and Fractures*. Philadelphia, JB Lippincott Co, 1971.

Slater RB, Harris WR: Injuries involving the epiphyseal plate. *J Bone Jt Surg (Am)* 1963; 45:587.

Tachdjian MO: *Pediatric Orthopedics*. Philadelphia, WB Saunders Co, 1972.

Weber BG, Brunner C, Freuler F (eds): *Treatment of Fractures in Children and Adolescents*. New York, Springer-Verlag, 1980.

OFFICE MANAGEMENT OF MINOR SURGICAL PROBLEMS

John M. Templeton, Jr., M.D.

Minor surgical problems in children have the following characteristics: (1) the disorder is relatively superficial and can be diagnosed by simple inspection and palpation and (2) procedures required for treatment can be performed within 15 minutes using local anesthesia. These procedures can be easily handled in an office setting with a relatively low investment in equipment and expense. Performing the procedures in the office is cost saving for the parent and may be less anxiety provoking for the patient.

The main drawback in performing minor surgical procedures in the office is the limitation in time for the busy primary care physician. Nevertheless, if one takes the time to instruct office staff, the receptionist or office nurse will usually identify which patient needs a procedure and prepare the child in a designated, well-equipped treatment room. The nurse can initiate local cleansing and soaks if indicated. If local anesthesia is required, the primary care physician can instill local anesthesia and then see another patient while waiting 15 minutes for the local anesthetic to take full effect.

The only other drawback to the primary care physician performing minor surgical procedures in his office is a medical-legal one. If the procedure is not minor and if a qualified surgical consultant is readily available, the physician may be advised to refer the patient. However, if surgical help is not readily available and the physician feels comfortable in managing the problem, the patients and their families will be grateful for having the procedure done by a physician they know and trust.

ABSCESSES

An abscess is an area of local pyogenic infection that has produced tissue breakdown with the development of pus within this area. An abscess can occur anywhere in the body. When they occur deep to fascial and muscle planes, they are best thought of as complex. Patients with such abscesses often require admission to the hospital for the purposes of general anesthesia to facilitate adequate drainage and the use of intravenous antibiotics. Fortunately in children, most abscesses are superficial. Because of the child's size, such abscesses tend to point earlier and lend themselves to easy incision and drainage. The infective organisms generally reflect the bacteriologic composition of adjacent body compartments. The bacteria grown from a perianal abscess, therefore, are likely to be different from those obtained from a cervical abscess.

In taking a history, one may discover a predisposing basis for the abscess. Examples of this include: a puncture wound or insect bite, or the presence of a preexisting cystic mass or superficial sinus tract. Most abscesses slowly evolve from an area of apparent cellulitis with erythema, swelling, and tenderness. Over the course of 1 to 3 days, the surrounding erythema becomes brighter red; blanching on palpation becomes more prominent; and the skin begins to take on a shiny quality beneath which there is a somewhat distinct mass that is quite tender. By palpating the mass between one's two index fingers, one often can appreciate fluctuance indicating that frank accumulation of pus has occurred and that incision and drainage is indicated. If these features are not present, one may be dealing with a cellulitis rather than a mature abscess. Since many cases of cellulitis can be treated adequately with frequent warm soaks and antibiotics and never develop an abscess, an incision and drainage in an area of cellulitis is not likely to be helpful. If it is unclear whether a local infection represents cellulitis or an abscess, needle aspiration can be used to help in the assessment. Attaching a 22-gauge needle to a 5-mL syringe that contains 0.5 mL of nonbacteriostatic sterile water, and after thorough prepping of the involved area, one can insert the needle for a distance of 1 to 2 cm while applying back suction. If no purulent material is obtained, the nonbacteriostatic water can be injected into the tissue and then aspirated to provide enough material for culture and sensitivity. If, on the other hand, purulent material is obtained, the needle can be detached from the skin and left in place to serve as a guide for incision and drainage. The purulent material in the syringe can be sent for culture and sensitivity.

Whether or not a needle has been used for initial assessment, the tissue around the suspected abscess site should be thoroughly cleansed and prepared. The final preparation should be with a strong topical antiseptic such as povidone-iodine (Betadine). The field should be draped to isolate the area and to prevent spread of purulent material from beyond the immediate area of drainage. Next, an attempt should be made to identify natural skin lines in the area of the abscess. In most cases, the incision should be planned in a line parallel to natural skin lines to minimize any subsequent scar formation (Fig 67–8).

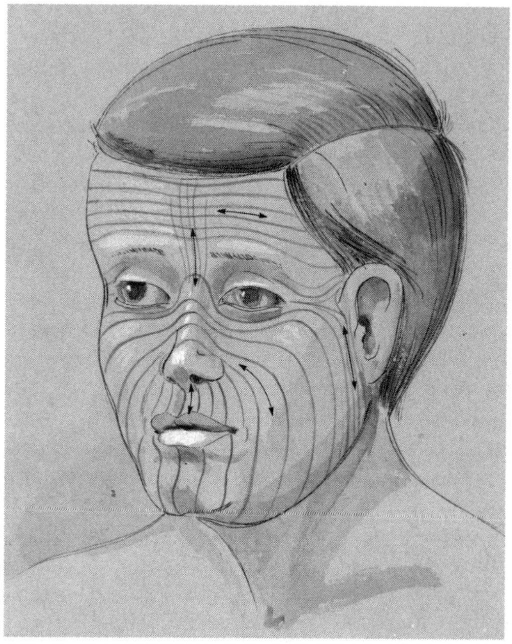

FIG 67–8
Natural skin lines of the face. Incisions of the face as elsewhere should be made in lines parallel to these lines.

The instillation of local anesthesia such as 1% lidocaine (Xylocaine) is often useful because it eliminates the initial pain when the incision is made. The physician must confirm that the patient is not allergic to the anesthetic. At a minimum, an area at least 1.5 cm long should be anesthetized. This is because an incision for drainage of an abscess that is less than 1 cm may often prove to be inadequate. If an assistant is present, he can spray ethyl chloride on the planned site of incision and drainage a second before the incision is made. In using ethyl chloride, it is important to make sure that none of it sprays into the face of the patient. In addition, enough spray is needed to make a prominent white area develop before adequate anesthesia is achieved. Even in the presence of an intense local white reaction, the local anesthetic effect wears off within 5 to 10 seconds. It is difficult, therefore, for a single person both to "freeze" the abscess area and then to perform the incision.

In spite of adequate anesthesia to the skin, the second stage of the procedure is always somewhat painful. Once the incision has penetrated the center of the abscess, a blunt hemostat should be inserted and spread widely in order to break any internal loculations and to assure adequate drainage. One should have a means of collecting some of the pus for culture. Even though most abscesses are due to a coagulase-positive *Staphylococcus,* the organism should be identified in case the patient does not respond properly to treatment.

Once the abscess has been evacuated, it is helpful to place some packing within the center of the abscess. This is usually best accomplished by lightly inserting 0.25- or 0.5-in. width iodoform gauze to the point that a small portion is left protruding from the skin incision. Although there initially appears to be bleeding with the incision and drainage, gentle pressure on the wound margin for 3 to 5 minutes will usually result in complete hemostasis. A bulky sterile dressing should then be applied over the drainage area. In some cases it is advisable to start the patient on a 5-day regimen of oral antibiotics such as cephalexin (Keflex) or dicloxacillin.

Follow-up instructions should include the following: (1) 24 hours after drainage ceases, the dressing and the underlying packing should be removed. Removal of this packing results in some additional debridement effect. Unless the cavity is quite deep or the length of the incision is inadequate, further packing of the wound is not needed. (2) Whether or not further packing is used, the abscess area should receive warm soaks three times a day. These soaks may be done by using local compresses or preferably by immersing the involved area under water. With each soak, the prior dressings and any remaining packing should be removed. At the end of the soak, a sterile dressing should be reapplied. (3) When the wound has closed successfully by secondary intention, soaks and protective dressings may be discontinued. (4) One can arrange to see the child in 3 to 7 days following the procedure. The family should be instructed to bring the child back sooner should there be progressive inflammation and tenderness in the area surrounding the site or if the child shows persistent fevers or signs of toxic effects.

Contraindications to drainage of an abscess in the office include: (1) a known preexisting medical problem such as a bleeding disorder, an immunologic deficiency, or diabetes mellitus. Complications often occur in such patients and they should, therefore, be treated in a hospital setting. (2) A child who already has evidence of systemic toxicity, including a high fever and poor appetite. (3) A child who is less than 6 months of age and has a large abscess in the head and neck area.

There are a number of specific types of superficial abscesses that may be encountered in children.

Lymphadenitis

Any area in which there is a concentration of lymph nodes such as the neck, inguinal area, or axillae may develop lymphadenitis and subsequent abscess. If the child has little or no systemic symptoms, and if the child is older than 6 months of age, the majority of these may be drained in the office. Most children with lymph node abscesses will have them in the cervical area. While it is possible to treat some of these abscesses with repeated needle aspiration, success in this approach generally requires continuous intravenous antibiotics because of the incomplete drainage obtained from needle aspiration alone. Although incision and drainage may result in residual scar, the child will have more rapid relief of symptoms. From the viewpoint of cost, patient benefit, and time expended, formal incision and drainage is still the standard of care for managing most abscesses.

Perianal Abscess

The origin of perianal abscess, in most cases, is an inflammation in the depth of one of the anal crypts. If this local cryptitis breaks through the epithelium of the anal canal, infection extends through the superficial fibers of the adjacent external sphincter muscle until the skin is reached. The child may have one or two days of fretfulness and pain on passing stool before the infection becomes obvious. Most abscesses in this area appear in the skin just lateral to the anocutaneous junction. They are rarely larger than 1 cm, are usually bright red, and are tender when palpated locally. When one examines the rectum, but is careful not to touch the abscess, there is usually no other evidence of tenderness or disease around the rectum. The purpose of the rectal examination prior to performing drainage of an apparent perianal abscess is to make sure there is not a larger area of induration and tenderness extending more deeply into the pelvis alongside the rectum. In such cases the infection has broken through the deep portion of the external sphincter mechanism and has now entered easily dissected planes in the ischiorectal space. These deep infections can be quite extensive and life-threatening. When there is any doubt about the possibility of a more deeply extending infection, the patient should be admitted to the hospital and should undergo incision and drainage under general anesthesia so that the physician can adequately break up any loculated pockets of pus within the abscess cavity.

Most children with perianal abscess are less than 1 year of age. Perianal abscess in the neonatal period may indicate immune deficiency. A perianal abscess in an older child should raise the concern of a possible underlying inflammatory bowel condition. In general, the typical perianal abscess is rounded, superficial, and quite discrete. It, therefore, lends itself readily to a localized incision and drainage in the office. It is hard to keep packing inside these superficial abscesses. It is, therefore, better to start the child on frequent sitz baths in the tub, starting 4 to 6 hours after the incision. In most cases the abscess cavity will appear to have healed by secondary intention within 1 week. Parents should be cautioned, however, that one in three children with an episode of perianal abscess will develop recurring local infections. These infections often will drain spontaneously and finally evolve into a fistula in ano. Once a fistula in ano is well established and mature, an elective operative procedure will be required to excise the fistula.

Secondary Abscess in Congenital Cysts

There are a number of cysts or sinus tracts that can be present in children on a congenital basis. In the head and neck area, two of the most common types of superficial congenital malformations are a thyroglossal duct cyst and branchial cleft cysts, with or without a sinus tract. A thyroglossal duct cyst occurs in or quite near to the midline anterior neck in the region of the hyoid bone. It tends to move prominently when the child swallows. Prior to secondary complications such as infection, it is usually smooth, fairly discrete, and slightly mobile. Because these cysts often maintain a sinus tract communication with the foramen cecum, they are susceptible to infection.

The origin of branchial cleft sinus tracts or cysts is the result of failure of complete fusion between each of the branchial arches during fetal development. These cysts or sinus tracts often retain some potential communication with the pharynx or skin rendering them susceptible to secondary infection. Every child with a preexisting lump or cyst in these areas should be referred to a pediatric surgeon for elective removal because of the increased likelihood of developing secondary infection. When infection does develop, the definitive management of these lesions is complicated. Initially, a formal incision and drainage are required because the preexisting cystic cavity has become an abscess. Then the infection in the congenital cyst will need to heal completely before it is safe to proceed with definitive surgical resection. Some of the branchial cleft sinus tracts, especially those of the second branchial cleft variety, are associated with a small but visible pore entering the skin along the medial margin of the sternocleidomastoid muscle. Patients who are found to have such a skin pore, especially if there is intermittent mucus drainage from the pore, should be referred for evaluation by a pediatric surgeon. The sinus tracts are also susceptible to secondary infection. Their management is, therefore, much easier if they can be handled on an elective basis before an abscess occurs.

One other type of congenital cyst that frequently is associated with a skin pore is a dermoid cyst or sebaceous cyst. The visible pore in the skin in such cases immediately overlies the cyst. Because such lesions have a potential for the entry of bacteria, a secondary abscess will often develop. When an abscess in a dermoid cyst does develop, it requires initial incision and drainage and complete healing before one can proceed with definitive treatment.

Pilonidal Sinus Abscess

Some young children may be noted to have a dimple in the midline in the interbuttocks groove in the region of the coccyx. If the opening of the dimple is wide enough to allow viewing of the base of the dimple, secondary infections are unlikely. On the other hand, some pilonidal sinuses have a very narrow tract. With the onset of puberty, increased growth of hair may occur in this area. Often one or several strands of hair may extend along this small sinus tract impeding normal drainage and resulting in the development of an abscess. The patient and the family may not be aware of any abnormalities in this area until progressive pain and tenderness is noted overlying the coccyx. Within a few days a frank abscess may present. The usual organisms involved are *Staphylococcus* or *Escherichia coli*. Once an abscess is clearly established, a formal incision and drainage will be required. In addition to evacuation of the purulent material, one should look for and remove any hairs that are seen extending down along the sinus tract. Because the abscess cavities are often fairly large by the time the patient presents for treatment, the family should be instructed in how to provide local hot soaks followed by repacking with new iodoform gauze two to three times a day. These abscess cavities may take 2 to 3 weeks before they close entirely. One to 2 months after infection has fully resolved, the patient should then undergo an elective excision of the still present pilonidal cyst.

MINOR SURGICAL PROBLEMS OF THE HAND

For a number of reasons, the hand is often a site for infections and trauma. Younger children are often unaware of dangers in the environment. When they fall, the hand often takes the brunt of the injury. Likewise fingers may be caught in narrow spaces or crushed in a car door. Many children have the propensity to chew or suck on their fingers, giving rise to infections.

While many hand problems, if recognized early, can be treated on an outpatient basis, what may appear initially to be a minor problem may within 24 hours turn into a major problem. Because the hand is so important in human development and function no hand problem should ever be taken lightly. Warning signs and symptoms that a more serious process is involved include: generalized swelling of the palm or dorsum of the hand, evidence of dissemination of infection such as lymphangitic streaking, generalized pain on moving the finger joints, or inability to perform simple tasks such as pinching or curling and uncurling of fingers. The presence of any one of these signs makes it mandatory that the patient be referred for care by a hand specialist in the hospital setting.

Nevertheless, there are a number of localized and early problems involving the hand that are appropriate for care in the office. The following are examples of such localized problems:

Felon

An infection in the pulp of the distal digit is called a felon. If the felon occurred as a result of a discernible puncture of the overlying skin, an abscess in the skin at the puncture site may develop. This abscess may be treated with incision and drainage followed by frequent soaks and antibiotic ointment dressings. Often, however, a felon will not show signs of pointing. This undrained infection within the pulp of the fingertip can produce serious complications. Excessive pressure in the pulp's base may lead to ischemic necrosis of soft tissue. Since most felons are the result of infections from coagulase-positive staphylococci, fat between the septa is often destroyed. Dissemination of infection may extend to the underlying phalanx, with extension along the flexor tendon sheath. In this manner the whole finger and even the hand may be jeopardized.

On examination the fingertip is painful, red, and tense. Even slight pressure worsens the pain. Frank fluctuance is rarely present. Early drainage is mandatory. Anesthesia for fingertip problems is best achieved by a digital nerve block. The hand should first be thoroughly cleansed with surgical antiseptic soap and then prepped with antiseptic solution such as povidone-iodine. After the hand has been draped and isolated, 1% lidocaine can be used to infiltrate the proximal digital dorsal and volar nerves on each side. It is important to make sure that there is no epinephrine in the lidocaine solution. Epinephrine instilled around the digital arteries may produce such sustained vascular occlusion that necrosis of a portion of the finger may occur.

As shown in Fig 67–9, the needle can be inserted on the side of the flexor aspect of the finger near the web space and then advanced down to the proximal phalanx. When the periosteum is hit with the needle, the needle can be drawn back 1 or 2 mm. The syringe is aspirated to make sure that blood is not obtained and then an initial 0.5 to 1.0 mL of anesthetic can be instilled. Next, the needle can be drawn back part way and then advanced toward the extensor surface of the finger, near to the phalanx. Additional anesthetic can be instilled. Usually 1 to 2 mL is sufficient to provide block of the two digital nerves within 10 minutes. The same procedure should be done to block the dorsal and volar digital nerves on the opposite side of the phalanx.

As shown in Figure 67–10, an incision should be made close to and parallel to the edge of the nail. An incision at this point will minimize potential damage to digital nerves and avoid troublesome scar formation. A curved mosquito hemostat can be advanced first to the side of the phalanx, and then further advanced along the anterior surface of the bone. A similar counterincision on the opposite side can then be made, and the mosquito hemostat tip can be advanced out through this counterincision. A small piece of Penrose drain or sterile rubber band can be pulled through this

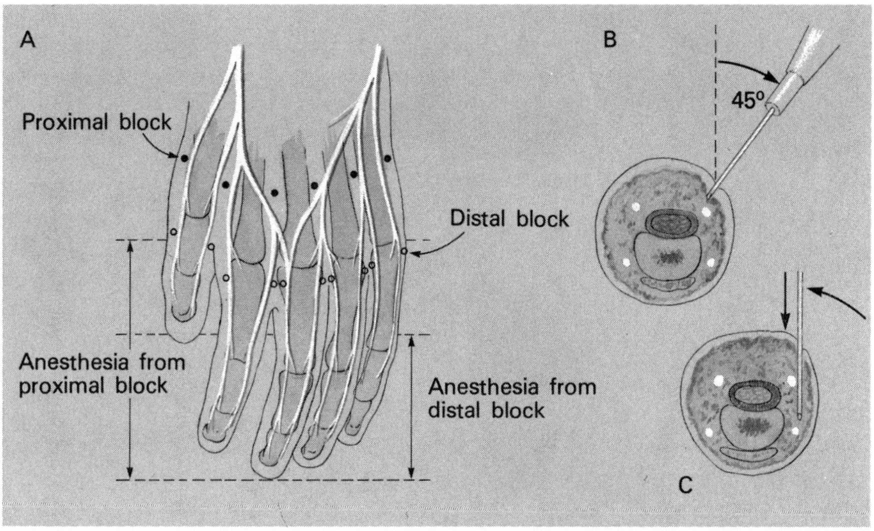

FIG 67–9
A, nerves supplying the hand with sites for proximal block *(black dots)* and distal block *(white dots)* with corresponding areas of anesthesia. For most distal lesions of the digits, a distal block is preferred. **B,** insert needle at 45-degree angle until periosteum is reached, then retract 1 to 2 mm in, aspirate, and then inject 0.5 to 1 mL of anesthesia. **C,** then advance the needle toward the extensor surface, aspirate, and then inject 1 to 2 mL of anesthesia.

space and left in place. Dicloxacillin therapy should be started and the patient should be seen again within 24 hours to make sure that the infection is responding appropriately. If the patient is doing well, the drain may be removed after 48 hours and the patient may start frequent warm soaks.

Paronychia

At the base of the fingernail is a flap of thin epidermis called the eponychium (cuticle). This area is vulnerable to trauma, including that which occurs as a result of biting or sucking of the fingers. As a result bacterial invasion may occur, leading to a local cellulitis overlying the base of the nail. When the infection is fairly early and localized, it can be managed by local hygiene and maneuvers to foster spontaneous drainage. Three times a day the entire hand should be washed with warm soap and water for 20 minutes. Then a loose-fitting finger cot that is partially filled with povidone-iodine or polymyxin β-bacitracin-neomycin (Neosporin) ointment can be applied over the finger so that maceration of the inflamed skin occurs. With maceration, spontaneous drainage usually follows. Usually 2 to 3 days with such treatment is sufficient. It is important to make sure that the finger cot is loose enough so that it does not produce a tourniquet effect at the base of the finger.

If the infection is more advanced, the entire base of the nail may be involved. There will often be a collection of pus that is visible under the skin. As shown in Figure 67–11, local incision and occasionally debridement of the skin overlying the abscess is usually necessary. A digital nerve block should be utilized in such cases before undertaking such drainage.

If the paronychia is far advanced, the proximal base of the fingernail may serve as a foreign body and thereby perpetuate the infection. In such cases one must first excise the overlying eponychium and then excise the involved portion of proximal nail that frequently is surrounded by pus on all sides. When formal drainage of a superficial or deep paronychia is required, therapy should be started with dicloxacillin or cephalexin until the specific culture report is returned. Hot soaks three times a day followed by the application of sterile loose dressing is important until healing is complete.

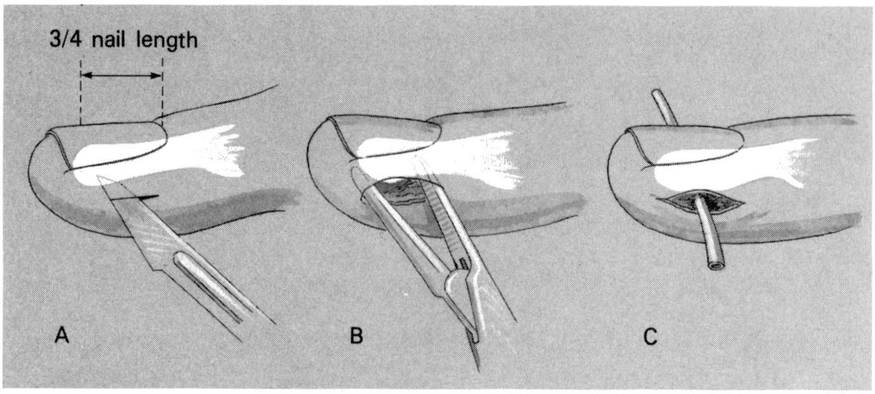

FIG 67–10
Drainage of felon. **A,** incision of felon parallel to edge of nail. **B,** hemostat advanced along anterior surface of bone. **C,** small drain is placed.

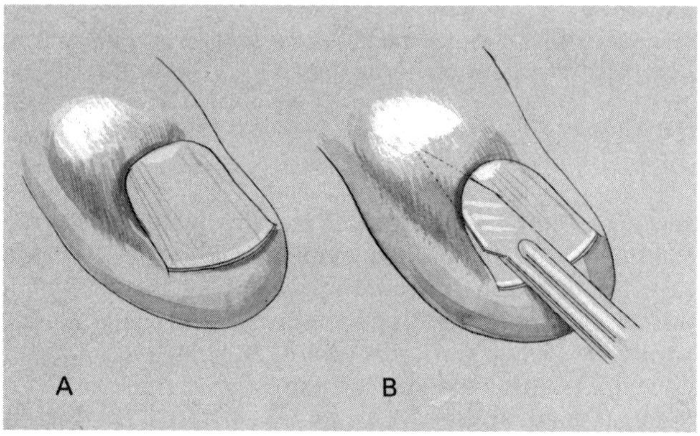

FIG 67–11
A, paronychia involving base of nail. **B,** after digital nerve block, local incision of abscess along the surface of the nail will provide drainage. If the overlying skin is necrotic, it should be debrided as well.

Subungual Hematoma

A direct blow to the fingernail, as with a hammer, often will cause bleeding between the nail bed and the nail. This bleeding will result in a hematoma that slowly expands over several hours leading to persistent and often throbbing-type pain. At this point one will usually notice a blue-black zone under the nail at the site of the hematoma. Drainage of the hematoma will provide immediate relief of pain and will minimize any potential for secondary pressure effects. If the hematoma extends almost to the tip of the nail, then the nail can be separated from the end of the nail bed resulting in drainage. Usually, however, the hematoma is under the proximal portion of the nail. The easiest maneuver to achieve drainage is to heat a straightened portion of a paper clip with a burning match until it is red-hot and then apply it with slight pressure to the nail over the center of the hematoma. Doing this two or three times will slowly burn a hole through the nail until there is a sudden extrusion of dark watery blood. One can also use a no. 11 scalpel blade to cut through the nail overlying the hematoma (Fig 67–12). This is done in a rotary fashion until a hole is cut through the nail down to the hematoma. This requires a moderate amount of pressure, however, and will add to the patient's pain and discomfort unless one has initially utilized a digital nerve block. After the blood has been drained, one should soak the finger two to three times a day and then keep a light dressing over the area until the dead space has closed in completely.

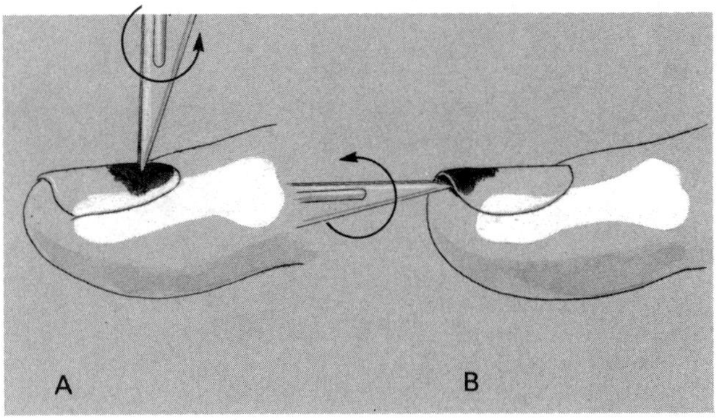

FIG 67–12
Drainage of subungual hematoma. **A,** proximal hematoma drained through nail. **B,** distal hematoma drained directly.

Subungual Splinter

While playing, children occasionally catch a splinter under the finger nail. Usually the splinter is wood, but other items such as a sliver of metal or plastic can produce the same injury. Because it is a penetrating injury, bacteria are often present. The presence of bacteria and a foreign body may lead to local infection and complications. Removal of the splinter is, therefore, important for both comfort and treatment. If the splinter is not totally embedded, it is better not to pick at the wooden splinter, as it may cause it to break into fragments making removal of the deeper portion more difficult. Instead the edge of the nail should be trimmed back as closely as possible to the tip of the finger. Then after thorough cleansing of the hand, the object can often be caught against the under surface of the nail with a needle or a scalpel tip and gently stroked out of its pocket. If the splinter has broken off and is embedded under the nail, direct exposure of the splinter can be obtained by scraping a portion of the overlying nail away as shown in Figure 67–13. Once the splinter is exposed, it can be removed and local cleansing can be done. The hand should be soaked three times a day, after which an antibacterial ointment dressing should be applied. As with all wounds involving foreign bodies, one should make sure that the patient has adequate protection against tetanus.

Fingertip Amputations

Children are prone to crush injuries or amputation injuries of the tip of the finger. In most cases such injuries involve only the distal half of the distal phalanx. They usually involve part or all of the nail bed. In many cases, the bone of the tip of the phalanx is partially exposed or amputated. In contrast to the treatment for adults, it is very important when treating children to avoid at all costs debriding back bone or the nail bed to obtain a primary closure. After placement of a digital nerve block, any frankly necrotic tissue should be gently debrided. After thorough cleansing with the use of dilute antiseptic surgical soap followed by saline lavage, the fingertip should be dressed with a sterile petrolatum gauze and bulky absorbent gauze to immobilize and protect the finger. Such relatively minor fingertip injuries will usually heal spontaneously in a few weeks with a quite acceptable cosmetic and functional result. In cases of a more severe or proximal injury or the development of secondary infection, the patient should be referred immediately to a hand specialist.

Entrapped Rings

Children have a fascination for rings and will often put more than one on a hand. Sizing of rings for children is often not accurate, especially if one child borrows another child's ring to try it on. This leads to the ring becoming trapped proximal to the proximal interphalangeal (PIP) joint. Very often the mother or child will have attempted to pull the ring off by using soapy water or mineral oil. In such cases prolonged attempts at pulling on the ring may have resulted in edema of the distal portion of the finger, making removal even more difficult.

Commercial ring cutters are available. When the ring is an inexpensive one or is thin, removal of a ring in this fashion is quite easy. A

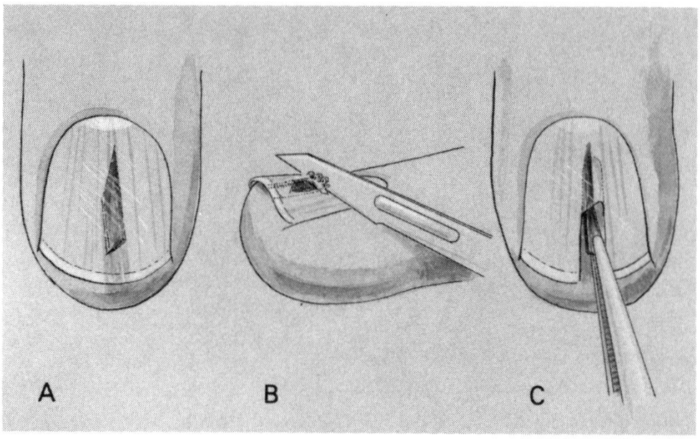

FIG 67–13
Removal of splinter. **A,** splinter embedded under the nail too deep to reach by distal approach. **B,** shaving a portion of overlying nail to expose splinter. **C,** removal of splinter with hemostat.

thick ring may take more time and effort. An alternative to using a ring cutter is to attempt to milk the edema and swelling out of the distal finger so that the ring may be slid over the PIP joint. A No. 1 silk suture works well in such cases. One end of the silk is used to wrap the soft tissues of the finger tightly, beginning at the distal end and slowly wrapping the silk more and more proximally, thereby squeezing any edema back toward the hand. The wrapping is continued all the way down to the ring, at which point the proximal portion of the silk is passed underneath the ring. Then this end of the silk is lifted outward at right angles to the axis of the finger and unraveled in the reverse direction. This maneuver, thereby, coaxes the ring up and over the blockage at the PIP joint. This maneuver is greatly assisted by having the patient's hand and involved finger kept in an elevated position over the head for 10 to 15 minutes before attempting the ring removal.

Hair Strangulation of a Digit

Young children, particularly those in the first year of life, often grab their mother's hair or loose threads. Occasionally a single strand of hair or thread may completely encircle a finger or toe, leading to constriction of the digit. Distal to the constricting band, the digit becomes swollen and red. One can usually identify a clear line of demarcation between the normal proximal tissue and the edematous distal tissue.

On examination the constricting material may not be immediately discernible because it has cut so deeply into the skin. This is particularly true in the case of a strand of hair if the hair was wet when it became wrapped around the finger. Subsequent drying will lead to further shrinkage and constriction of the digit. Retraction of the skin surrounding the indentation will finally reveal the constricting object. It is imperative to remove this band as soon as it is identified. It is helpful to use a magnifying lens to see and remove all of the material producing the constricting band. In most cases the band can be grasped with the tip of a fine mosquito hemostat. The portion that has been grasped with the hemostat can then be cut with a no. 11 scalpel blade. If one is sure that the constricting band is a hair fiber, one may also use a depilatory agent (e.g., Nair) to dissolve the hair. After removal of the band, the hand should be placed in an elevated position to allow further resolution of edema in the distal digit. If the digit has not been irreversibly compromised, it should return to normal within 48 to 72 hours.

OTHER MINOR SURGICAL PROBLEMS

Foreign Bodies

Because of their general level of activity and their occasional lack of attention to safety measures, children are prone to soft tissue injuries that result in the embedding of foreign bodies. Falls in an area where bits of rough gravel or cut glass are present often result in small lacerating injuries that may not suggest the presence of a foreign body. Carrying sharp items or not paying attention to where one steps or sits may result in the embedding of a broken pencil tip or penetration of the foot or buttocks by pins or other sharp objects.

It is very important for the physician to obtain an accurate history as to the location and circumstances in which a child may have incurred a small puncture-type injury. If there is any reason to suspect entry of a foreign body a radiograph should be obtained. Metallic items and glass will be seen on a radiograph, whereas organic material such as wood splinters is usually not radiopaque. If a foreign body is seen on a radiograph, it is usually removed before complications develop. The presence of organic material in the tissue, however, may go unrecognized and is, therefore, more often associated with complications. Moreover, such material is likely to elicit a greater inflammatory response than is a smooth-surfaced object such as glass. Because of the concomitant presence of bacteria, this enhanced inflammatory response results in a purulent reaction that soon evolves into a localized abscess. The abscess is helpful in that it tends to enhance the body's attempt to extrude the foreign material and points the way for the physician who is called on to treat the problem. Such a localized abscess should be prepared and opened as described above. Exposure of the abscess cavity will usually result in extrusion of the foreign object. Subsequent treatment should be the same as with any abscess.

Foreign objects that are appropriate for removal in an office setting are those that are in the subcutaneous tissue and/or are readily palpable. The end of the needle, for example, may be palpated just under the surface of the skin, although the tip of the needle may extend more deeply. When a foreign body cannot be felt and radiographs show that the foreign body is deep to superficial fascia, the patient should be referred to an appropriate surgical specialist for assessment and probably removal of the object. This is particularly true in the case of penetrating objects in the foot and buttocks because much time and effort can be saved by removal of the foreign body under fluoroscopy. As with all penetrating injuries, it is very important to make sure that the patient is immunized for tetanus.

Fishhook Injuries

Fishhook injuries can occur in almost any part of the body, usually as a result of misadventures with casting. Often, attempts to remove the fishhook at the scene of the injury result in the fishhook becoming more deeply embedded.

Occasionally, when the fishhook has punctured a slender structure such as a finger or an auricle the bared end of the hook will be seen to have partially exited on the side opposite to the point of entry. In such cases the tip of the fishhook may be grasped with a hemostat. Next, the shank of the fishhook is cut flush with the skin at the entry site. Then the distal fragment can be drawn out with little or no discomfort.

In most cases, however, the fishhook is deeply embedded in the patient's soft tissues. Any attempts to remove the fishhook should be designed to neutralize the effect of the barb at the end of the hook. Most techniques involve some manipulation of the fishhook that may be a bit painful and frightening to the child. Therefore, after local cleansing with surgical soap and antiseptic solution, one should instill 1 or 2 mL of local anesthetic around the entry site and around the embedded portion of the fishhook. The most commonly used technique to neutralize or disengage the barb is to place a piece of heavy silk around the exposed curve of the fishhook and to loop this silk two or three times around the index and ring fingers of one hand. With the other hand, one should grasp the straight shank of the fishhook with a thumb and middle finger and use the index finger to press the curve of the shank downward, thereby disengaging the barb from the tissue within. Holding this downward pressure with one hand, one can then use the other hand to pull on the silk suture steadily outward in a line that is parallel to the straight shaft of the fishhook. This will have the effect of straightening the curve of the hook slightly enough to allow extraction of the fishhook.

Insect Bites

There are a number of insects that have the ability to penetrate the skin for sucking, as in the case of mosquitoes, or to puncture the skin, often accompanied by the release of an irritating or toxic material. The more serious forms of insect bites include those of poisonous spiders. Because the effect of their envenomation can lead to serious local and systemic symptoms, children with such bites should be referred to a hospital. Much more common than spider bites are stings from insects of the Hymenoptera order. Honeybees, wasps, yellow jackets, and hornets can live and thrive in environments close to man. For certain susceptible individuals, stings from these insects can be life-threatening. It is estimated that 40 to 50 people die each year in the United States as a result of anaphylactic reactions following a sting from one of these insects. Immediate treatment with subcutaneous epinephrine 1:1,000 (0.1 mL to 0.3 mL) and a tourniquet above the site of the sting may help to lessen the life-threatening effects of an anaphylactic reaction. Even in individuals who are not so sensitive, a systemic toxic reaction can occur when ten or more stings have occurred. Such systemic symptoms may include vomiting, diarrhea, muscle cramps, headaches, and dizziness. Rarely, convulsions may occur. If such symptoms are pronounced or protracted, the patient should be taken to a hospital. If these symptoms pass quickly, however, one may then proceed with local care and treatment of each sting site. One should first cleanse the area with soap and water. Then, using a knife blade held at a right angle to the surface of the skin, the stinger can be scraped out of the skin. Cold compresses may provide local symptomatic relief. One can then apply a solution of one fourth of a teaspoon of meat tenderizer (chymopapain) and 1 teaspoon of tap water to the sting site. In addition one can give the patient diphenhydramine (Benadryl) 5 mg/kg/24 hr in four divided doses by any route. This medication may particularly help to reduce any associated systemic signs and symptoms (see Chapter 51).

Zipper Injury to the Penis

On occasion a young boy who is in a hurry to get back to playing after urinating will zip up the fly of his trousers so quickly that the skin of the shaft of the penis is caught in the zipper. If the portion of skin that is caught is small and appears to be caught by only one of the small zipper teeth, one can quickly pull the zipper back, detaching the skin. This will be painful for a moment but then the problem will be resolved.

If the skin is tightly entrapped involving several of the small teeth of the zipper, it is more effective to infiltrate the skin of the shaft of the penis with 1% lidocaine around the involved area. Because of the partially closed nature of the zipper, one will not be able to see the entire circumference of the shaft. Instead, the anesthesia can be instilled subcutaneously down for a distance of 1 cm beyond where one can see. With effective anesthesia the child can be reassured that he will have no more pain and discomfort. It may then be possible to thrust the zipper handle quickly downward to try and disengage the zipper from the skin. If this is not feasible because of the secondary development of edema, it is better to take a pair of heavy scissors and cut the involved portion of zipper off of the pants. With the patient's pants removed, one can better see the entrapped area. Then the teeth with their attachment to the cloth of the zipper can be individually pulled and cut away until the entrapped skin is released.

After removal of the zipper, the involved area of skin should be thoroughly washed and cleansed and dressed with polymyxin β-bacitracin ointment (Polysporin) and a light, fluffy dressing. It is a good idea for the child to lie down for the rest of the day to help to resolve any local edema. Starting the next day the child should take sitz baths two or three times a day, after which a local polymyxin β-bacitracin ointment dressing should be applied until the area has healed satisfactorily.

BIBLIOGRAPHY

Barkin RM (ed): *Emergency Pediatrics*. St Louis, CV Mosby Co, 1984.

Fleisher GR, Ludwig S (eds): *Textbook of Pediatric Emergency Medicine*, ed 2. Baltimore, Williams & Wilkins Co, 1988.

Pascoe D, Grossman M (eds): *Quick Reference to Pediatric Emergencies*, ed 3. Philadelphia, JB Lippincott Co, 1984.

Reece, RM (ed): *Manual of Emergency Pediatrics*, ed 2. Philadelphia, WB Saunders Co, 1978.

Welch KJ, Randolph JG (eds): *Pediatric Surgery*, ed 4. Chicago, Year Book Medical Publishers, 1986.

section iv

Developmental Disabilities

Developmental disabilities represent a major portion of childhood chronic illnesses. Most of these disabilities have multiple associated problems that result in intellectual, physical, and emotional or behavioral handicaps. Although these multiple problems often require diagnostic and therapeutic input from multiple and diverse health care professionals, the primary care physician has the responsibility of integrating and coordinating the overall health care for these children within their local community and home setting. Frequently, the success of a family's ability to cope with their child's disability is dependent on the medical and emotional support they receive from their primary care physician. The following section discusses several of the more common and/or severe developmental disabilities, including mental retardation, cerebral palsy, spina bifida, speech and language delays, hearing impairment, learning disability, hyperactivity, autism, cleft lip and palate, and chromosomal disorders, with a focus on the identification, assessment, and management of the disorders. There are also separate chapters that specifically address office screening or assessment of developmental disabilities, the educational and legal rights of the developmentally disabled child, and the impact of a developmentally handicapped newborn, toddler, and child on family functioning.

68 MYELOMENINGOCELE

Edward B. Charney, M.D.

Spina bifida with myelomeningocele is one of the most significant handicapping conditions of childhood. It is a birth defect that may adversely effect the motor, sensory, psychosocial, emotional, and cognitive development of the child, and may produce tremendous psychological and economic stress on the entire family. By the nature of its multisystem involvement, many children with this disorder receive specialized care from a multidisciplinary team that often consists of a developmental pediatrician, neurosurgeon, orthopedist, urologist, nurse, social worker, and physical or occupational therapist. The primary care physician, however, may be the one to whom both the family and team of specialists turn for day-to-day medical management, assistance in locating community resources, and provision of ongoing emotional support. Familiarity with the nature of the birth defect, its functional implications, and management issues can be valuable in the physician's fulfillment of this role.

NATURE OF THE BIRTH DEFECT

Spina bifida describes the separation or nonfusion of the vertebral spinal arches whereas myelomeningocele describes the cystic dilatation of the meninges around a malformed neural tube (Fig 68–1). Neural tube defects including myelomeningocele, meningocele (cystic dilatation of meninges around a normal spinal cord without neurologic deficits), anencephaly, and encephalocele result from incomplete neural tube closure at around 28 days' gestation. It occurs in approximately 0.7 to 1.0 per 1,000 live births in the United States.

Although many theories for etiology have been proposed, the cause remains unknown. There is, however, a well-documented higher incidence in affected families with estimated recurrence rates 50 times higher than the general population; increased frequency of other congenital malformations (i.e., cleft palate/lip, congenital heart disease) among both the affected child and family members; and a higher incidence in Ireland (4 per 1,000 live births) with lower, but still increased incidence among Irish descendants living elsewhere. On the basis of these observations and other epidemiologic data, it has been suggested that a predisposition with polygenic mode of inheritance exists and, possibly, that certain environmental factors play a contributory etiologic role. Maternal periconceptual dietary deficiencies in folic acid and/or other vitamins are presently being investigated as one such environmental factor.

Prenatal diagnosis may be established through amniocentesis at 16 to 18 weeks of pregnancy. Fetuses with open neural tube defects will have an increased amniotic fluid level of α-fetoprotein, an α-globulin synthesized by normal embryonal yolk sac, liver cells, and gastrointestinal tract. Ultrasonography (US) and amniotic fluid levels of acetylcholinesterase can significantly enhance prenatal diagnosis.

The level in the spinal cord at which neural tube closure was incomplete, determines the degree of motor paralysis and sensory loss of the child (Fig 68–2). Sensation is either totally or partially absent in the skin over the paralyzed muscle groups. Musculoskeletal deformities develop primarily around those joints that are either totally or partially paralyzed. Deformities may develop on a dynamic basis with imbalanced muscle strength about the joint, or on a positional basis where effects of gravity and/or position lead to contractures about a to-

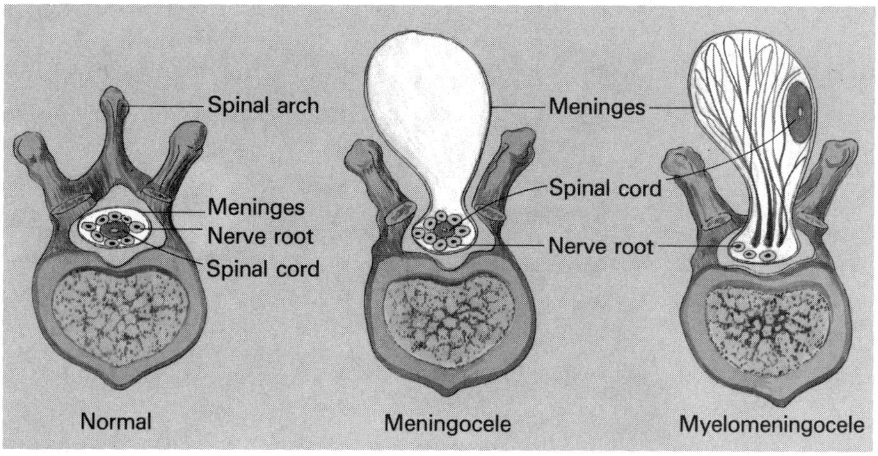

FIG 68–1
Nomenclature of neural tube defects.

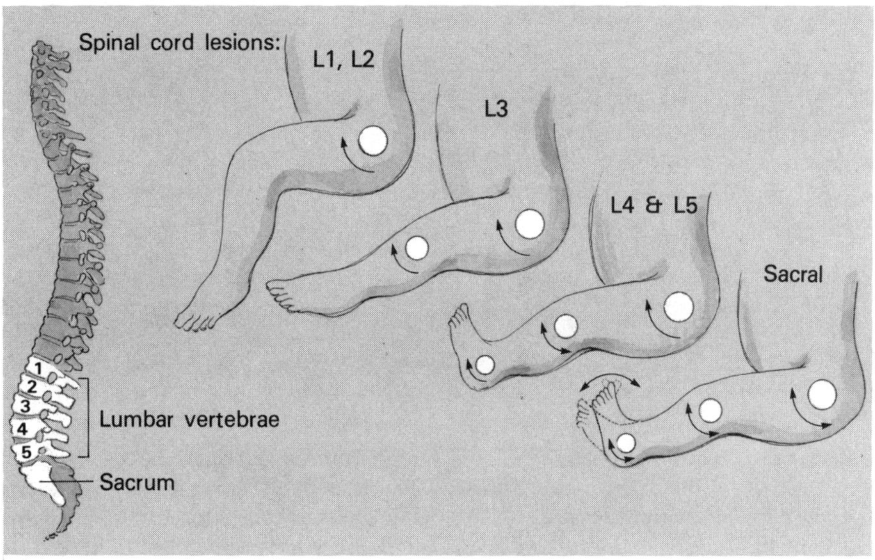

FIG 68–2
Motor activity and level of spinal cord lesion. Lesions at L-1, L-2 allow only hip flexion, while lesions at L-3 allow extension of knee. Patients with lesions at L-4 and L-5 dorsiflex flex ankles and those with sacral lesions can also plantarflex ankles and move toes (see Table 68–1).

tally paralyzed joint. Spinal deformities of scoliosis or kyphosis may be associated with congenital anomalies of the spine and rib cage, such as hemivertebrae or fused ribs.

Often there is not just an isolated birth defect of the spinal cord and spine, but rather there commonly are associated congenital malformations of the brain. Ninety percent have an Arnold-Chiari type II malformation of the hindbrain, where there is downward displacement of the medulla and posterior cerebellum into the cervical vertebral canal (Fig 68–3). Hydrocephalus develops in 60% to 95% as CSF flow and absorption are compromised from the Arnold-Chiari malformation as well as from the frequently accompanying aqueductal stenosis or occlusion. Additional clinical complications of this malformation include cranial nerve pal-

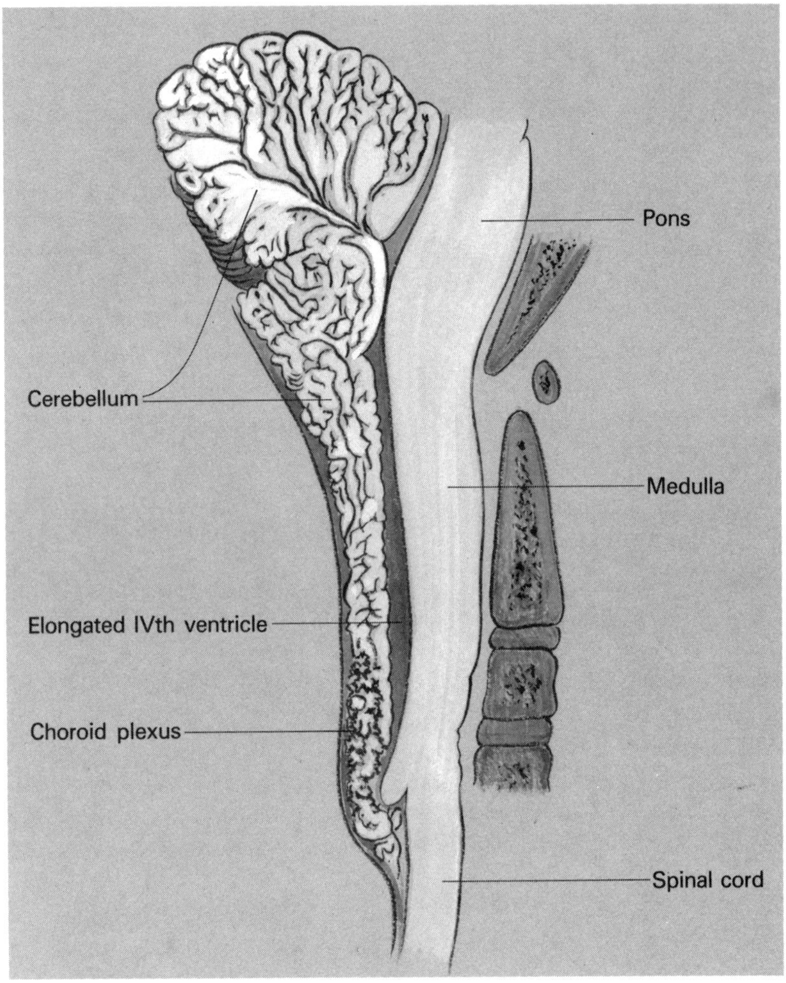

FIG 68–3
Arnold-Chiari malformation.

sies with strabismus, vocal cord paralysis with stridor, swallowing difficulties, and apnea. Other less well-defined anatomic lesions in the brain may contribute to seizure disorder in 15%, mental retardation in 35%, and visual perceptual problems in 80%.

FUNCTIONAL IMPLICATION

Infants and children with thoracic lesions have flaccid paralysis of both lower extremities with variable weakness in abdominal and trunk musculature. Those children with high lumbar lesions (L-1, L-2) have voluntary hip flexion and adduction but flaccid paralysis of the knees, ankles, and feet (see Fig 68–2). Ninety percent to 95% of children with thoracic or high lumbar paralysis have associated hydrocephalus. They also are particularly prone to musculoskeletal deformities of the spine, hips, and entire lower extremity. These children may be capable of walking; however, they require extensive bracing and crutches for independence (Table 68–1).

Children with midlumbar (L-3) paralysis have strong hip flexion and adduction and fair knee extension, but paralyzed ankles and toes (see Fig 68-2). Approximately 85% have associated hydrocephalus. Musculoskeletal deformities of the lower extremities may be common and independent ambulation can be accomplished with either extensive, moderate (Fig 68–4), or minimal bracing.

Children with low lumbar lesions (L-4, L-5) have strong hip flexion and adduction, knee ex-

TABLE 68–1
Degree of Paralysis and Functional Implications

PARALYSIS	HYDROCEPHALUS (%)	AMBULATION	BOWEL/BLADDER INCONTINENCE (%)
Thoracic or high lumbar (L-1, L-2)	95	"May" walk with extensive braces and crutches	>90
Midlumbar (L-3)	85	"Can" walk with either extensive, moderate or minimal braces, and usually with crutches	>90
Low lumbar (L-4, L-5)	70	"Will" walk with moderate, minimal, or no bracing with or without crutches	>90
Sacral (S-1 to S-4)	60	"Will" walk with minimal or no braces and usually without crutches	>90

tension, and ankle dorsiflexion with often weak or absent ankle plantar flexion, toe extension/flexion, and hip extension (see Fig 68-2). Seventy percent have associated hydrocephalus. They are particularly prone to deformities of the ankles or feet and often need moderate, minimal, or no bracing for independent ambulation.

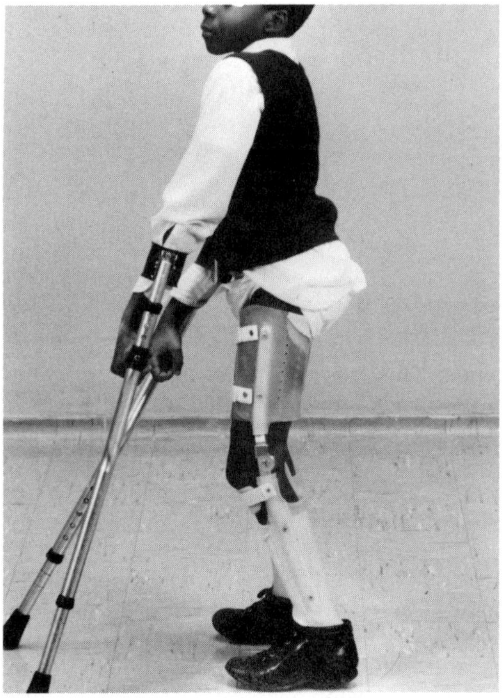

FIG 68–4
Knee-ankle-foot orthosis (KAFO) or long leg bracing with Lofstrand (forearm) crutches.

Children with sacral lesions usually only have mild weakness of the ankles and/or toes (see Fig 68-2). Approximately 60% have associated hydrocephalus. Musculoskeletal deformities are usually of the feet, and the vast majority will walk independently with only minimal or no bracing.

Bladder and bowel problems are present in at least 90% of children, irrespective of their degree of lower-extremity paralysis. Motor and sensory innervation of both organs are normally mediated through the S2-4 level of the spinal cord and therefore, incomplete neural tube closure of this area results in a neurogenic bladder and bowel. In general, there are two major types of neurogenic bladder, one that fails to empty adequately or one that fails to store adequately (Fig 68–5). Failure in emptying is usually associated with paralysis or ineffective bladder detrusor contractility and/or ineffective urethral relaxation. Infants and children with this type of bladder are at risk for urinary tract infections associated with urinary stasis, hydronephrosis (when abnormally increased bladder pressure and vesicoureteral reflux are present) (see Fig 68–5, *E*), and overflow incontinence. Failure to adequately store urine is often a result of either uninhibited bladder detrusor contractility and/or ineffective urethral resistance. Although urinary tract infections and hydronephrosis are relatively uncommon complications of this bladder type, urinary incontinence is usually present.

Problems in bowel control are primarily related to either ineffective involuntary relaxation or contraction of the internal anal sphinc-

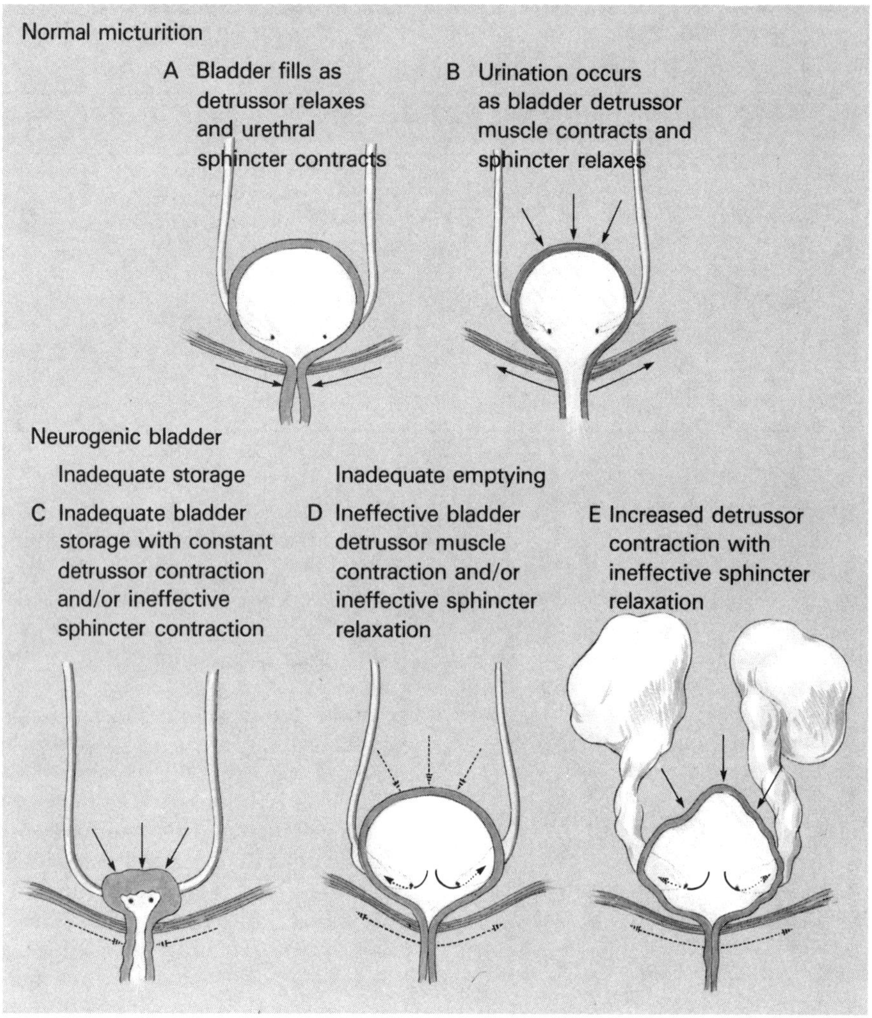

FIG 68–5
Normal functioning bladder (**A** and **B**) vs. neurogenic bladder (**C, D,** and **E**).

ter (Fig 68–6). The inability to establish relaxation results in constipation with a full rectum that is unable to completely empty its fecal contents through a tight sphincter. Unless the rectum is emptied regularly, constipation will produce a hugely dilated colon with "overflow" or "bypass" diarrhea interspaced with infrequent passage of hard stools. Inability to maintain some normal contraction of the internal sphincter, on the other hand, usually results in frequent diarrhea and a tendency for rectal prolapse. Irrespective of the status of the internal sphincter, almost all children with myelomeningocele have no anal or perianal somatic sensation. This, along with an inability to voluntarily control their external sphincter, make them unable to sense or control stool passage.

MANAGEMENT

Treatment of children with myelomeningocele should be individualized according to the needs of both child and family. There is also considerable variation of these needs with the different developmental stages of the child. When reviewing management issues it is best, therefore, to examine separately the child with

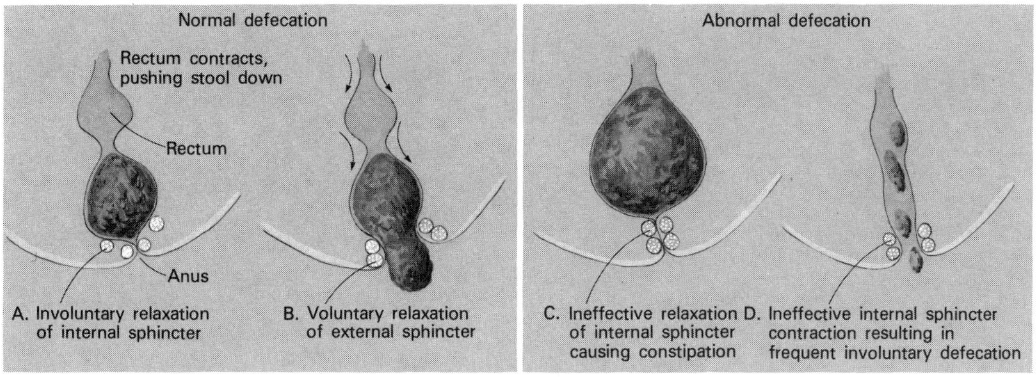

FIG 68–6
Normal functioning bowel (**A** and **B**) vs. neurogenic bowel (**C** and **D**).

myelomeningocele as a newborn, infant, preschooler, school-aged child, and adolescent. Recognition of the importance of developmental stages in management affords the clinician a somewhat easier task when formulating a whole-child total care plan.

NEWBORN

Controversial issues in the newborn management of myelomeningocele have included both the selection process and optimal time for surgical intervention. During the 1950s and 1960s, early surgical back closure was performed on most infants, irrespective of their clinical severity, as advances in surgical technique were made and the ventricular shunt was improved. The enhanced survival of these infants, however, was observed to be associated with an increased number of more severely disabled children. Retrospective and prospective studies in the 1970s identified a number of "adverse criteria" at birth that were associated with severe disabilities later in life. These "adverse criteria" included: thoracolumbar lesions with paralysis of the legs below the knees, congenital hydrocephalus with head circumference greater than the 95th percentile, congenital kyphoscoliosis, birth anoxia, and other severe birth defects. A selection process was then advocated and practiced whereby infants with one or more of these criteria did not receive surgical intervention. Although survival rates diminished, as approximately 90% of those without surgery died during the first year, the number of severely impaired survivors decreased among those selected for surgical intervention.

Consideration of withholding life-prolonging measures for any handicapped newborn is an ethical and moral dilemma for both physician and parents. Resolution of this dilemma often necessitates a decision-making process over a period of time. Until very recently, it had been cited that time was not available for such a process in management of the newborn with myelomeningocele. It was believed that delay in surgery beyond 48 hours was associated with increased morbidity. Recent data, however, suggest that there may be no increase in mortality or morbidity if surgery is delayed 1 or 2 weeks. This additional time may afford both the physician and parents a period to seek additional consultation and emotional support before establishing a treatment plan for the newborn.

When surgical intervention is decided on, the infant will usually first have surgical closure of the myelomeningocele defect. Evaluation for development of hydrocephalus may then be done by head circumference measurements and brain US or computed tomography (CT). Management of the hydrocephalus usually involves a shunting procedure whereby cerebrospinal fluid (CSF) from the ventricular system is internally diverted to another place in the body for better absorption. A ventriculoperitoneal (VP) shunt is commonly utilized; however, a ventriculoatrial (VA) shunt may be used when peritoneal absorption is poor (Fig 68–7). Additional routine diagnostic studies performed during the initial hospitalization include intravenous pyelography (IVP) and/or re-

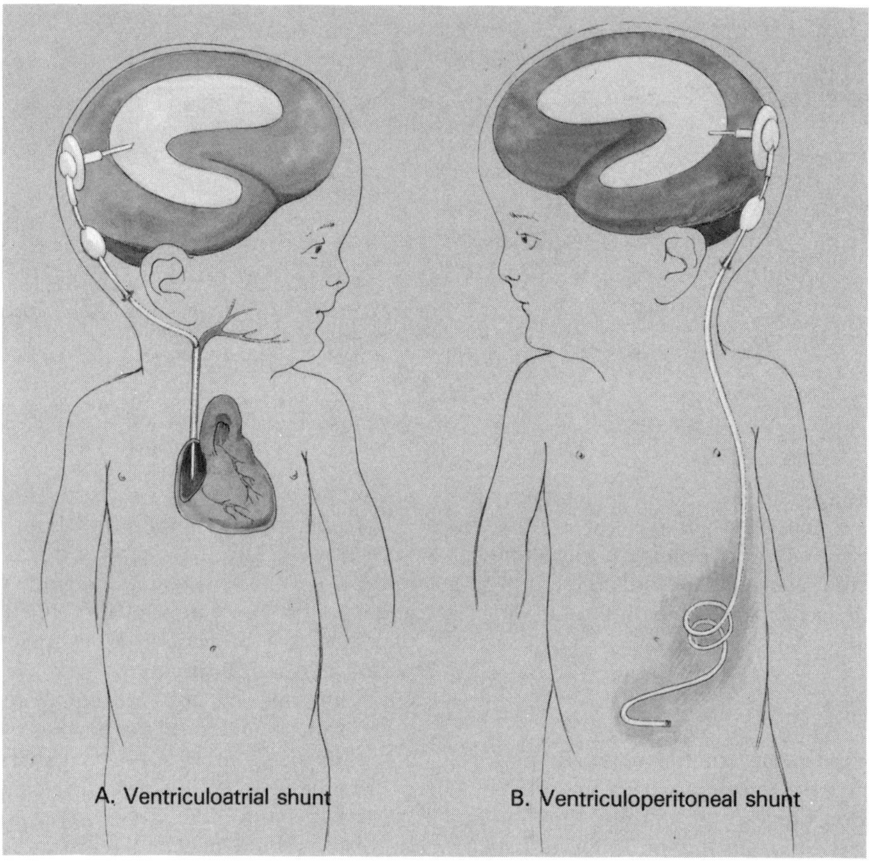

FIG 68–7
Ventricular shunting procedure for hydrocephalus. **A,** ventriculoatrial shunt. **B,** ventriculoperitoneal shunt.

nal US. The presence of hydronephrosis should be investigated with voiding cystography (VCUG). Poor bladder emptying may require a vesicostomy or intermittent catheterization of the bladder. A vesicostomy (Fig 68–8) usually results in decompression of the bladder and upper tracts by permitting complete emptying. The infant's care is simpler than with intermittent catheterization as only a diaper is required.

INFANT

During the infant's first few months at home, most parents will have considerable concern over whether or not their child's shunt is working. Approximately 50% of all infants with shunts will require at least one revision during the first year of life. Mechanical shunt malfunction without infection is far more common than shunt infection alone as a cause of shunt revision. Signs and symptoms of shunt malfunction may be insidious or acute. Often, the earliest sign in the younger infant may be an increased velocity in head growth accompanied by a fullness or bulging in the anterior fontanelle. Lethargy, vomiting, and irritability are particularly common symptoms of the older infant with shunt dysfunction. If these signs and symptoms are reflective of increased intracranial pressure alone, then the clinical signs of common childhood febrile or afebrile illnesses including otitis media, diarrhea, or upper respiratory illness are usually absent. Although shunt infections may also present with lethargy, irritability, and vomiting, they often have an otherwise unexplained fever and commonly occur within a shunting postoperative period of several weeks to months. Other signs of increased intracranial pressure in the infant may include an acute onset of a sixth nerve palsy with abduction pare-

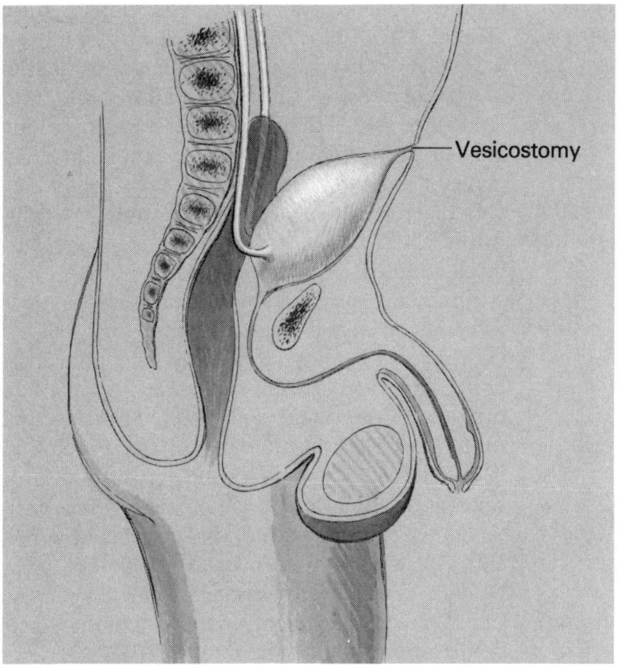

FIG 68–8
Vesicostomy with dome of bladder brought out to skin.

sis or vocal cord paralysis and stridor. A croupy cough and stridor in an infant with myelomeningocele is often more likely associated with shunt malfunction than it is with an infectious respiratory process such as tracheolaryngobronchitis. Diagnostic studies for assessing the functional status of a shunt often include brain CT or US for ventricular size; plain radiographs of head, neck, chest, and abdomen for continuity of shunt tubing; and sterile collection of ventricular fluid through the shunt system for chemical and bacteriologic analysis.

Motor paralysis or weakness may contribute to both the development of musculoskeletal deformities and delays in gross motor skills during the first year. Parental instruction in proper positioning and passive stretching exercises for the child can often minimize the development of these deformities. Some infants, however, such as those with rigid equinovarus deformities (club feet), will require casting and/or surgical correction during this time. Delays in gross motor skills including head and trunk control and independent sitting, crawling, and standing are common, particularly among those with significant motor paralysis. The valuable developmental experience of independent environmental exploration may be compromised by these delays. Individualized therapy plans are therefore developed so as to enhance gross motor as well as other developmental skills in these young children.

Management of the neurogenic bladder during infancy is directed at ensuring adequate emptying, preserving normal upper tracts, and preventing urinary tract infection. Although the Credé maneuver with suprapubic pressure has previously been recommended for bladder emptying, recent evidence has been accumulating that suggests it may often be unnecessary and, at times, harmful. Surveillance to ensure adequate bladder emptying and prevention of hydronephrosis therefore utilizes repeat IVP and/or renal US, often at 6 months and 1 year of age. The prevention or control of urinary tract infections often is dependent on regular collections, either by midstream or urethral catheterization, of urine specimens for culture. In general, during infancy even asymptomatic bacteria is treated with a course of oral antibiotic therapy. The indication and efficacy of daily low-dose prophylactic antibiotic therapy remains controversial.

Bowel difficulties generally require no more intervention than the routine well-baby dietary counseling. If after such counseling constipation persists, a trial of a daily mild rectal suppository (i.e., glycerin) may be employed to avoid the complications of a persistent distended rectum. Dietary counseling is also important in avoiding obesity, since many of these infants have decreased caloric requirements on account of decreased motor activity. Obesity later in childhood can significantly compound and complicate an existent motor and/or psychosocial disability.

Anticipatory guidance for parents of these young infants is a critical part of their routine well-baby care. Parents often need repeated explanations of their child's birth defect, including its effect on the infant's overall development, what to expect as potential complications or management interventions, and the emotional effect of such a disability on both parents and siblings. A process of better appreciation and understanding of these issues on the part of parents often affords them a somewhat easier time in coping with a child's problem later in life. The primary care physician has the unique opportunity of seeing these infants and parents on a regular basis and may thereby be instrumental in establishing both the medical and emotional support necessary for this process.

PRESCHOOL

One of several major goals of management during these years is independence in mobility. Sometime between 12 months and 5 years of age a child with myelomeningocele may learn to walk, depending on the level of paralysis, with or without the assistance of braces and/or crutches. Motor strength in the legs alone, however, does not ensure success in walking. Rather, a developmental readiness in both cognitive skills and motivation must be complemented by a therapeutic program before many of these children learn to walk. For some, musculoskeletal deformities of the hips, knees, or feet may interfere with functional standing or walking. Surgical management of these deformities during these years may then become necessary. Postoperative care may include casting of an immobilized joint for several weeks. It is not uncommon for these children to sustain fractures soon after cast removal, as their slender and osteoporotic bones fracture easily with minimal trauma. Painless swelling and redness of the involved leg usually develops within several days. Most lower-extremity fractures will heal with only temporary discontinuation of weight bearing while maintaining the child in braces, rather than casts. Sores to anesthetic skin often become problematic as the child becomes mobile, and anticipatory guidance should be directed at avoiding sunburn, tight-fitting shoes or braces, crawling on rough surfaces, and excessively hot baths.

Another major goal of management at this time is the achievement of fecal and urinary continence. Success in this area may afford the child an enhanced self-esteem while enabling him to remain clean and free of soiling and odor. Between 2 and 3 years of age, the family is encouraged to sit the child on the potty for several minutes after every meal. Often with the benefit of the postprandial gastrocolic reflex and gentle abdominal pressure or the Valsalva maneuver, the child may learn to have a regular timed bowel movement, thereby avoiding accidents other times of the day. If by 3 or 4 years of age this method of timed evacuation has not produced continence, then the families are instructed in the use of a nightly rectal suppository (i.e., glycerin or bisacodyl) to stimulate regular emptying. Constant soiling or frequent loose bowel movements may be a sign of constipation with "bypass" diarrhea. More complete bowel emptying can then be accomplished with intermittent use of an enema. If modification of stool consistency is necessary for continence, then dietary manipulation is generally utilized rather than oral medications.

Attempts at achieving urinary continence are generally introduced after bowel continence has been achieved. This usually involves a clean intermittent catheterization (CIC) program wherein parents and child are instructed in the clean, but not sterile, insertion of a catheter through the urethra about four times a day. If parents and child are compliant and there is complete bladder emptying without uninhibited detrusor contractions or diminished urethral resistance, continence may be achieved. In those children with bladders that cannot store urine adequately, a pharmocologic intervention may be necessary, consisting of either anticholinergic agents (e.g., propantheline bromide, oxybutynin chloride) to diminish uninhibited detrusor contractions or adrenergic agents (e.g., imipramine hydrochloride) to increase urethral resistance. Once adequate storage is accomplished, continence may be achieved with regular bladder emptying by CIC. Complications of CIC including epididymitis or urethral injury are rare. Asymptomatic bacteria is common. Courses of oral antibiotic therapy are utilized primarily in those with vesicoureteral reflux, upper tract damage, or symptomatic infections (i.e., incontinence, fever). Urinary tract surveillance continues during these years with regular IVP or renal US. Development of vesicoureteral reflux with hydronephrosis may be managed initially with either a trial of CIC or vesicostomy for minimizing bladder pressure and enhancing emptying (see Fig 68–8).

Although shunt malfunctions are most common during the first year, they can occur at any age. The older the child is, the more likely he or she will complain of headache as a manifestation of the increased intracranial pressure. Nausea, vomiting, lethargy, and/or strabismus are also frequently associated with malfunctioning shunt systems in the older child.

Assessment of the child's motor, language, and psychosocial development is another important aspect of overall treatment in these young children. Early intervention programs or other community educational resources may be extremely helpful for both the child with developmental delays and his or her family. When the child reaches the age to enter either kindergarten or first grade, psychological evaluation for school readiness may be available through the local community school system. Ideally, decisions regarding appropriate school or classroom setting should be based primarily on the child's cognitive and emotional development, rather than just on the degree of physical disability.

SCHOOL AGE

Throughout the school-age years, emphasis in management must be directed at establishing and/or maintaining independence in self-care skills and self-respect. The latter is usually dependent on independence in mobility, toilet needs, avoidance of obesity, and success in school. Socialization among both disabled and nondisabled peers must also be developed for all the extensive medical and surgical intervention to be of value in producing a successful long-term functional outcome.

In general, the vast majority of children who can walk both at home and in their local community with braces and crutches will have achieved this skill by 6 years of age. For those children who are unable to walk on the basis of either severe paralysis, mental retardation, obesity, poor motivation, or severe musculoskeletal deformities, independent mobility in a wheelchair is encouraged. Progressive spinal deformities of scoliosis or kyphosis may interfere with functional sitting, standing, or walking during this time. In extreme situations, these deformities may also result in restrictive lung disease and cor pulmonale later in life. Although initial management of these deformities might include a plastic body jacket for trunk support, some may progress in severity and necessitate surgical fusion of the spine.

When CIC was successful in establishment of urinary continence, the child is encouraged to be an active participant in his or her toilet needs by performing self-catheterization, being responsible for the care of catheters, and regulating timing of the procedure. When continence has not been achieved, surgical intervention may be considered in a well-motivated youngster with urodynamic study evidence of a dysfunctional bladder that is unresponsive to pharmocologic measures. There are several surgical procedures for incontinence, including insertion of an artificial urinary sphincter (Fig 68–9) or bladder augmentation with an intestinal patch (Fig 68–10) that can enhance low-pressure bladder storage capacity and thereby afford the child an opportunity to be continent. Surveillance of the upper tracts is continued throughout these years with IVP or renal US and routine blood pressure measurement is utilized for identification of the unusual, but still possible, complication of hypertension secondary to renal damage.

The visual perceptual motor deficits that are frequently present in children with hydrocephalus commonly result in poor school performance. Unfortunately, the child's inability to attain the academic level of his or her classmates may be misinterpreted as either laziness, immaturity, or mental retardation, when in fact it may be symptomatic of a specific learning disability. Recognition and appreciation of this potential complication on the part of the school

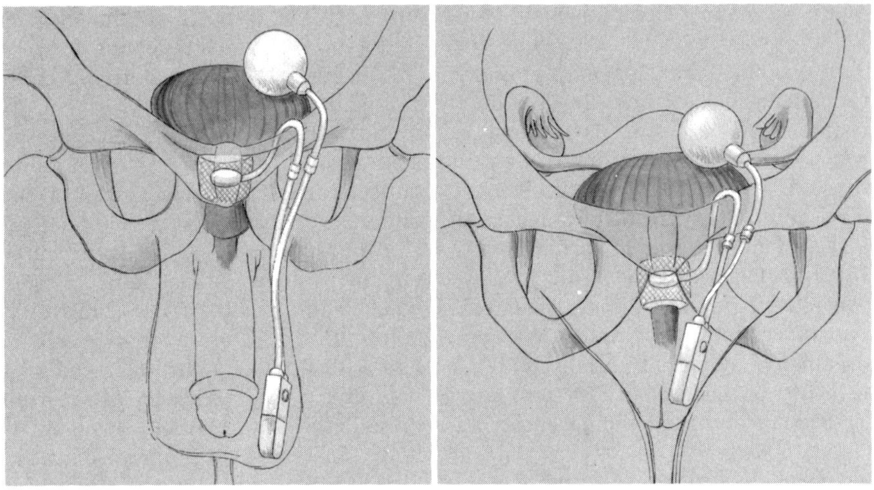

FIG 68–9

Artificial genitourinary sphincter (Scott-American Medical Systems). Pressure in cuff around bladder neck-urethra maintains continence. When pump in scrotum or labia is activated, fluid is transferred from the cuff to the retroperitoneal balloon, permitting bladder emptying. After several minutes the cuff automatically refills, restoring continence.

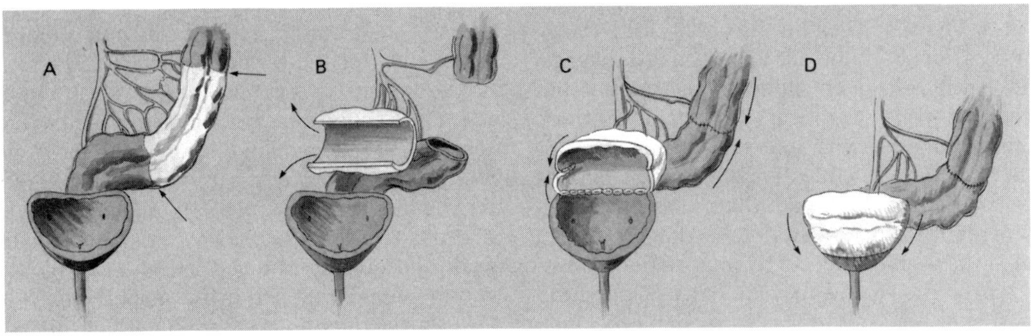

FIG 68–10

Augmentation sigmoid cystoplasty. **A,** segment of sigmoid to be used for augmentation is outlined and bladder has been widely opened. **B,** sigmoid segment converted into a patch in order to eliminate effective peristaltic contraction. **C,** bowel continuity restored by intestinal anastomosis. Sigmoid patch being sutured to bladder. **D,** augmentation sigmoid cystoplasty completed.

system can lead to early identification of the problem through appropriate psychometric testing. Remedial help may then be arranged with resource room or full-time specialized educational classroom settings. A successful experience in school, both in academic achievement and social acceptance by peers, can then contribute significantly to the establishment of an enhanced self-respect that is critical for a smoother emotional transition into adolescence.

ADOLESCENCE

Although a significant part of adolescent treatment is directed toward establishing emotional well-being, appropriate schooling and realistic planning for the future, there are still some physical problems requiring attention. As some adolescents, particularly those with high paralysis, become more dependent on wheelchairs for mobility, they are prone to development of pressure decubitus ulcers of their anesthetic buttocks. Local wound care and avoidance of additional pressure or trauma is the major mode of therapy. Prevention of these sores may be accomplished by reminding the adolescent of the need for frequent positional changes while in the wheelchair and for maintaining adequate seating adaptations.

Sexual counseling is particularly important during the adolescent years. Abnormal sexual function is associated with a neurogenic bowel and bladder, since organ innervation is similar through the sacral portions of the spinal cord. For men, penile erection may be partial or not sustained, ejaculation may be absent or retrograde, and orgasm may not be precipitated by direct genital stimulation. Surgical management with artificial penile implants may be beneficial and orgasm can be attained through stimulation of nonanesthetic erotic areas of the body. Women are generally fertile and can undergo normal labor and delivery. Both men and women have a 1 in 10 risk of parenting an infant with a neural tube defect.

It is not surprising that many of these children, by the nature of their disability, have significant problems in adolescent adjustment. Achievement of self-identity and independence is often difficult and depression with social isolation is not uncommon. Although anticipation of these problems with appropriate intervention plans throughout childhood may be effective, additional support systems are often necessary during the adolescent years. Professional counseling may need to supplement guidance counseling through the school and social groups in the community. Parents of these teenagers and other family members can also benefit from additional emotional support and guidance.

CONCLUSION

With recent advances in medical, surgical, and diagnostic technology, the majority of children with myelomeningocele now have the opportunity to live a normal life span. The quality of this life, however, is dependent to a considerable degree on supportive services available to them on both a national and local level. Emphasis must be placed, therefore, on the responsibility that society has to these disabled individuals if they are not only to survive, but also to become functional and productive citizens in the world.

BIBLIOGRAPHY

Brocklehurst G (ed): *Spina Bifida for the Clinician,* Clinics in Developmental Medicine, no 59. London, Spastics International Medical Publications, 1976.

Charney EB, Weller S, Sutton LN, et al: Myelomeningocele newborn management: Time for a decision making process. *Pediatrics* 1985; 75:58–64.

Charney EB, Weller SC, Sutton LN, et al: Management of Chiari II complications in infants with myelomeningocele. *J Pediatr* 1987; 111:364–371.

Freeman J: *Practical Management of Meningomyelocele.* Baltimore, University Park Press, 1974.

Shurtleff DB: Myelodysplasia: Management and treatment. *Curr Probl Pediatr* 1980; 10:1–90.

Shurtleff DB: *Myelodysplasias and Extrophris: Significance, Prevention, and Treatment.* New York, Grune & Stratton, 1986.

Liptak GS, Bloss JW, Briskin H, et al: The management of children with spinal dysraphism. *J Child Neurol* 1988; 3:3–20.

69 CEREBRAL PALSY

Edward B. Charney, M.D.
Helen M. Horstmann, M.D.

Cerebral palsy is a disorder of movement and/or posture that results from nonprogressive damage to a developing brain. Although the lesion or site of damage may be static, there is a progression of multiple associated complications over time. Medical attention to these disabling complications is enhanced by physician familiarity with some basic background knowledge of the disorder, methods for early identification, techniques for assessment, and modes of management. This chapter examines these issues as they pertain to delivery of health care in a primary care physician's office.

BACKGROUND INFORMATION

ETIOLOGY

The damage to the developing brain may occur prenatally (e.g., infection, chromosomal anomaly, maternal drug abuse), perinatally (e.g., prematurity, asphyxia, sepsis), or postnatally (e.g., head trauma, meningoencephalitis). Close to 50% of children with cerebral palsy, however, may have no clearly evident identifiable cause.

CLASSIFICATION

The location and/or extent of brain damage may be correlated with a classification system that defines the two major types of cerebral palsy as being spastic and nonspastic (Fig 69–1).

Spastic cerebral palsy, the most commonly encountered type, is associated with various degrees of damage to the motor cortex. The clinical signs of spasticity, which are hypertonicity with exaggerated stretch and deep tendon reflexes, may be present in one or more extremity. If the brain damage is diffuse with bilateral involvement, there may be *spastic quadriplegia* with total body involvement and spasticity of all four extremities. When only one side of the motor cortex has been damaged, there may be *spastic hemiplegia* with involvement of the contralateral arm and leg. In some children, there is bilateral damage that results in spasticity of all four extremities with subtle or mild involvement of both upper extremities and significant functional impairment in both lower extremities. These children, who often have a history of prematurity, are described as having *spastic diplegia.*

Nonspastic cerebral palsy is associated with damage to portions of the brain involved in movement other than the motor cortex. *Dyskinetic cerebral palsy* is correlated with damage to the basal ganglia of the brain. Chorea, athetosis, and dystonia, the major types of dyskinetic cerebral palsy, are clinically marked by involuntary body movements that interfere with function. *Ataxic cerebral palsy* is associated with cerebellar damage and is clinically apparent by the presence of imbalanced and incoordinated voluntary movements of the trunk and extremities. Some children have brain damage involving several portions of the brain and have a mixed type of cerebral palsy with various features such as spasticity, dyskinesia, and/or ataxia.

ASSOCIATED DISABILITIES

The numerous associated disabilities of cerebral palsy result from either the ramifications of the movement disorder itself or from additional sequelae of the brain damage (Table 69–1). The

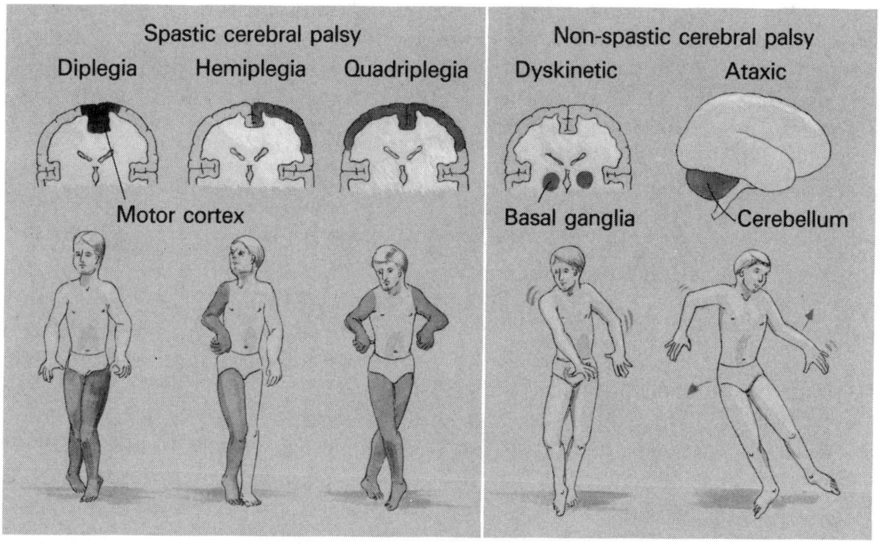

FIG 69–1
Classification of cerebral palsy.

TABLE 69–1
Associated Disabilities

Movement disorders
Head
Ocular
Strabismus
Oropharynx
Feeding
Speech
Drooling
Congestion
Trunk/extremities
Mobility
Gross/fine motor delays
Activities of daily living
Constipation
Obesity
Musculoskeletal deformities
Additional complications of brain damage
Mental retardation
Seizures
Learning disability
Hyperactivity
Hearing impairment
Language disorder
Secondary handicaps
Emotional/psychological
Educational
Peer socialization

more severely motor-involved infants and children often have movement disorders of the head that include the ocular and oropharyngeal areas. Strabismus is quite common and there are often problems with feeding, speech production, excessive drooling, and upper airway congestion. Movement disorder of the trunk and extremities will often compromise mobility and cause significant delays in attaining both fine and gross motor milestones of infancy and early childhood. As the child gets older, independence in many of the routine activities of daily living such as self-feeding, bathing, dressing, and self-grooming, may be limited by these movement problems. Immobility and difficulty with feeding in the more severely involved youngster is often associated with constipation. Decreased mobility in some children with cerebral palsy may contribute to obesity. Also, the inability to have normally balanced motion about certain joints can result in various musculoskeletal deformities such as equinus feet, hip dislocation, scoliosis, and wrist flexion, which may further compromise mobility and other activities of daily living.

Beside their disorders of movement and posture, children with cerebral palsy may have additional sequelae of brain damage, which include mental retardation, seizures, learning disability, hyperactivity, hearing impairment, and language disorders. Mental retardation is more commonly seen in children with total body motor involvement. Seizures are particularly common among children with either spastic hemiplegia or quadriplegia. The specific learning disability seen in children with cerebral palsy and normal intellect is primarily related to an attention deficit disorder as well as defects in visual or auditory perceptual processing. Hearing impairment or deafness is most commonly encountered in those children in whom brain damage resulted from congenital rubella or kernicterus.

Any of the aforementioned problems, either alone or in combination, may lead to secondary handicaps. These include disturbances in the child's emotional and psychological well-being, educational achievement, peer socialization, and employment opportunities as an adult, as well as his economic and emotional stability within the family. Early identification, comprehensive assessment, and coordinated treatment of the child with cerebral palsy may minimize or alleviate some of these most significant secondary handicaps.

IDENTIFICATION

Delay in attaining motor developmental milestones during the first year of life is often the first clinical sign of cerebral palsy. Abnormal muscle tone when present during this time is usually hypotonic in nature and signs of spasticity may not develop until about 1 year of age. Although motor problems with poor head control and feeding difficulties may be the earliest sign during infancy, many will present with delays in sitting, crawling, standing, and walking. Some infants, particularly those with more severe and extensive brain damage, will also have persistence of primitive reflexes (Fig 69–2) beyond the age at which they should normally disappear. Infants with spastic hemiplegia may not have significant delay in motor development, but rather will have an asymmetric crawl or abnormal early establishment of hand preference before 18 to 24 months of age.

A definitive diagnosis of cerebral palsy is often difficult during the first year of life, especially in the premature infant in whom motor delays may reflect maturational age in central nervous system (CNS) development. Nevertheless, it is important for the physician to identify those infants "at risk" (with abnormal development) and monitor their progress closely over time. It is hoped that with close surveillance of this "at risk population," early identification can in turn lead to early referrals for early intervention.

ASSESSMENT AND MANAGEMENT

Office assessment of infant and toddler development can be accomplished by parental report of developmental milestones achieved and through tests such as the Denver Developmental Screening Test (see Chapter 78). Developmental progress in the older child may be assessed by obtaining history and records of school performance. Early assessment of cognitive skills in many children with cerebral palsy is often difficult. Some may have normal cognitive ability, yet their speech is unintelligible due to associated dysarthria. Also, their fine motor impairment may interfere with successful achievement of problem-solving tasks on tests requiring motor coordination. The primary care physician, however, can play a major role in assessing the cognitive skills by listening to parental concerns, observing the child in the office, and then making referrals to medical or educational programs that are experienced and skilled in cognitive evaluations of these youngsters. Some children with higher cognitive abilities than their expressive language or motor skills would suggest, may gain social and educational benefits from the newer bioengineered nonverbal communication devices.

Aspects of the physical examination that deserve particular attention include assessment of vision and hearing. Use of the Hirschberg light test or cover and cross-cover test can help in evaluating the presence of strabismus. Otoscopic examination should detect serous otitis media associated with chronic upper-airway congestion. Tests for hearing can be initiated in the office by evaluating language development and, most importantly, by listening to parental concerns about a child's hearing ability. Referral for consultation with the ophthalmologist, otolaryngologist, or audiologist may then be arranged as necessary.

Assessment of overall nutritional status and dietary counseling are important responsibilities of the primary care physician. Since feeding difficulties may be encountered as early as

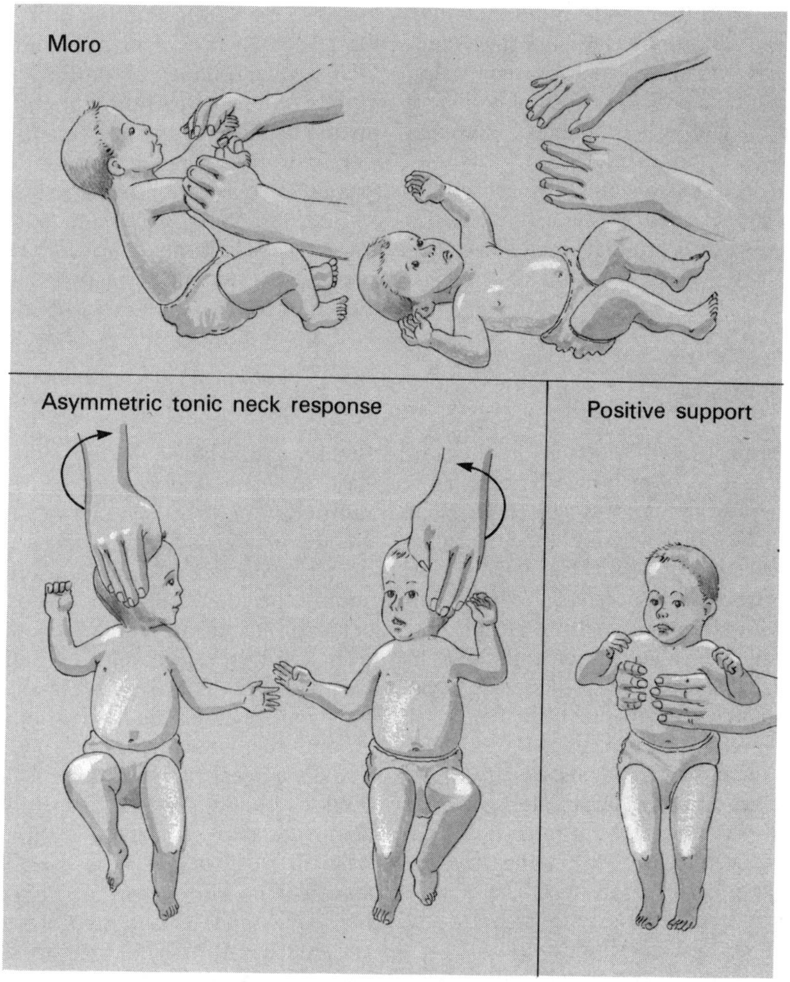

FIG 69–2

Primitive reflexes. *Moro reflex:* with sudden extension of the head there is rapid symmetrical abduction and upward movements of the arms followed by gradual adduction and flexion. Response usually normally disappears by 4 months of age. *Asymmetric tonic neck reflex,* or "fencer" position: with head rotation there is extension of the "chin side" upper extremity and flexion of the contralateral or "occiput side" extremity. Obligatory or persistence (more than 30 seconds) of this response is abnormal. *Positive support reflex:* with stimulation of the hallucal area on a hard surface, there is prolonged (more than 30 seconds) equinus or plantar flexion positioning of the feet. This response is often suggestive of future spasticity.

the first month of life, parents should be made aware of feeding techniques that may minimize or alleviate the infant's problem in sucking, chewing, or swallowing. Speech and language pathologists working with programs caring for children with cerebral palsy can often assist in teaching parents the use of these techniques. Dietary counseling for the school-aged and adolescent child is a critical part of the management plan to prevent obesity. It is not uncommon for teenagers with cerebral palsy to lose the ability to walk independently, as their musculoskeletal deformities can no longer accommodate or carry their excessive weight. Diets of 600 to 1,200 calories daily and regular exercise programs should be prescribed for these youngsters.

Another area of functional assessment that requires attention by the primary care physician is that of the child's bowel elimination pattern. Constipation, associated with immobility and inadequate dietary fiber, is often seen in those children with total body motor involvement and feeding difficulties. Recommendations for dietary changes, such as decreasing dairy product intake and adding stool softeners or occasional laxatives and enemas, may be necessary in individual cases.

Assessment and management of associated learning problems, seizures, behavioral problems, and family stress are discussed elsewhere in the text.

MUSCULOSKELETAL ASSESSMENT AND MANAGEMENT

The concept of positional influence on adjacent joints forms the basis of orthopedic assessment and management of the musculoskeletal system of the child with cerebral palsy. Most muscles cross at least one joint and frequently they cross two joints. Tightness or spasticity of one of these muscles alters the position of not only these joints but of the adjacent joint. In order to maintain a balanced, erect position, the head must be centered over the feet in stance. If there are any fixed contractures, this must be compensated for at various levels. For instance, if the hamstrings are tight and cause a flexor stance through the knees, there must be ankle dorsiflexion or weight-bearing on the toes for the child to stand on the ground. The hip or trunk must also compensate with flexion, pelvic tilt, or lumbar lordosis (Fig 69–3).

The child should be in a functional upright position for assessment by the primary care physician; the child should be walking, if possible. The position at each joint should be noted. Examination in both supine and prone positions should be done when the child is relaxed. The amount of contracture at each joint should be recorded, as should the amount of voluntary control. Particular attention should be directed at those muscles that often produce joint deformities by causing adduction through the hips, flexion through the hips and knees, equinus at the ankles, and varus or valgus through the feet. A quick assessment of possible ambulation prognosis can be related to the presence or absence of postural reflex activity at 1 year of age. The presence of either the asymmetric tonic neck, Moro, extensor thrust (Fig 69–2), symmetric tonic neck, or neck-righting reflex, or the absence of the foot placement or parachute reaction do not carry a good prognosis for independent ambulation.

The management of musculoskeletal deformities often requires the direction of an orthopedist experienced in the care of children with cerebral palsy. Plans in management should focus on increasing function and comfort for the child. Functional gains may be in areas such as walking, sitting, hand use, or general hygiene care. Achievement of these general goals may utilize modes of therapy that include bracing, casting, or surgery.

BRACING

Bracing has changed rather markedly over the past 20 years. Most major centers now use a minimum of bracing, and usually use lightweight plastic orthoses. Braces cannot be expected to correct a fixed deformity, but instead should be used to hold a position already achieved or to inhibit an overactive muscle from creating a dynamic deformity. The most frequent type of brace used is an ankle-foot orthosis made of molded polyethylene to control an equinus deformity and to prevent foot-drop due to a weak anterior tibialis. Occasionally, long-leg braces are used to control the position achieved after hamstring lengthening. In the past, long-leg braces were used to counteract spastic hamstrings, especially after contractures had developed. This is no longer thought to be an appropriate use of bracing. Since bracing has been particularly ineffective in controlling adduction and flexion at the hip, surgery should be considered for this problem.

CASTING

Casts have long been used to stretch out a tight joint. This can be achieved over 2 or 3 weeks with a cast that allows ambulation. Most frequently, casts are used to stretch out the triceps surae and thereby allow a toe walker to develop a heel-toe gait. If the child is preambulatory, frequently the use of a cast is preferred by therapists, particularly those trained in neurodevelopmental techniques. The flat-based cast with a toe extension (Fig 69–4) provides a stable base for standing and helps relax other muscles more proximally, probably since the stable base frees the more proximal muscles from being used to help achieve balance.

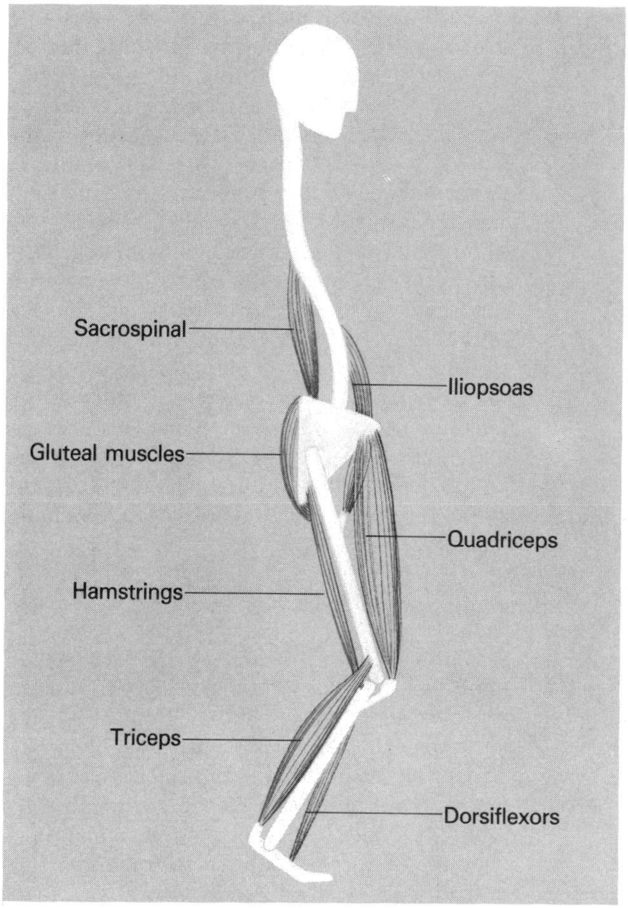

FIG 69–3
Primary deforming muscles of lower extremity.

SURGERY

Most surgery in children with cerebral palsy should be undertaken after the child has achieved neuromaturation, usually after the age of 2 years. It should be part of the overall program for the child, in conjunction with therapy, schooling, and social considerations. Prior to surgery, an orthopedic surgeon should evaluate the child more than once to get an accurate impression of the child's tone and function.

The purpose of the surgery is to avoid fixed deformities, including muscle contractures, particularly before this has evolved into a bone deformity, especially around the hip. When possible, immobilization should be minimized so that the child will begin a therapeutic program within a few days after surgery. This greatly decreases the amount of rehabilitation time and minimizes the amount of time a child must miss from usual activities. While too little surgery is better than too much surgery, several procedures should be done simultaneously by an orthopedic surgeon who is experienced in the care of children with cerebral palsy in an effort to minimize hospitalization. Frequently, surgery is done at several joint levels, all during one period of anesthesia.

Hip

The spastic iliopsoas causes flexion at the hip and is thought to be a contributor to hip subluxation. When the child's hip contracture results in crouching at the hip and there is hip subluxation on radiography (Fig 69–5), an iliopsoas recession in combination with an adductor tenotomy can be helpful. If tightness of the adductor results in hygiene problems or

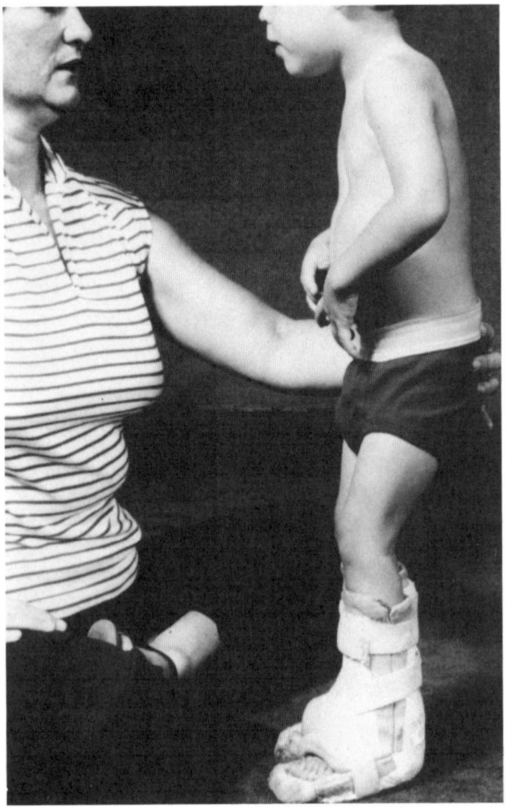

FIG 69–4
"Inhibitive"-type cast, which assists upright stance.

scissoring while walking (Fig 69–6), transfer or release of the adductors should be considered. Frequently the combination of tight hip adduction, flexion, and femoral anteversion results in hip subluxation and later hip dislocation as the hip pulls out of the joint. Hip dislocation can occur at any age. In a significant percentage of children the subluxated or dislocated hip becomes painful and is associated with degenerative joint changes. Once the degenerative changes have set in, pain relief is difficult. Because of this, there is a feeling that orthopedic surgical intervention is helpful when a hip is subluxating, even in a severely retarded child. The soft tissue procedures alone, such as adductor tenotomy or iliopsoas recession, often do not maintain the hip in the joint and a varus derotation osteotomy (Fig 69–7) is frequently indicated.

Knee

Flexion at the knee is usually due to a relative imbalance between the hamstring and quadricep muscles with the hamstring muscles being more spastic or more contracted (see Fig 69–3). Hamstring lengthening is indicated when knee flexion contracture exceeds 10° or there is flexion of the knees throughout the stance phase of walking. Children should begin weight-bearing and ambulating within a few days after surgery for optimum results.

FIG 69–5
Bilateral subluxated hips with mild uncovering and lateral migration of femoral heads out of the acetabulum.

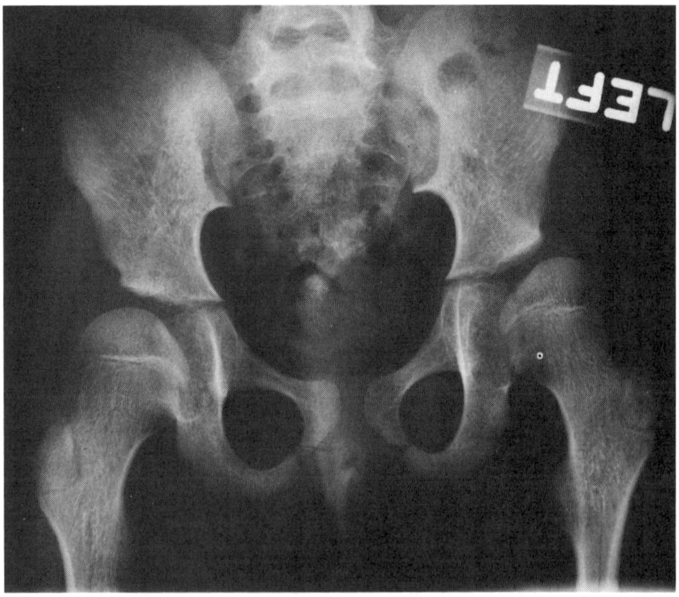

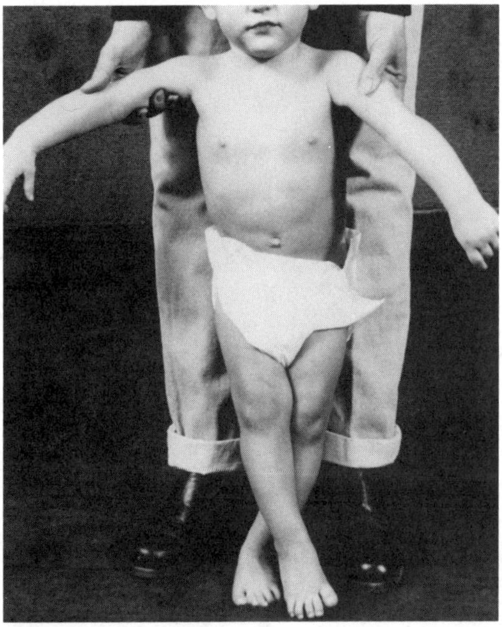

FIG 69–6
Scissoring posture with adduction spasticity and one lower extremity crossing over the other during assisted walking.

Foot

Although a child with cerebral palsy is frequently born with normal-looking feet, foot deformities are common in these children as they get older (Fig 69–8). The deformities become more fixed as the child becomes more spastic, and the muscle imbalance stronger. The aim in the management of these feet is to avoid structural deformity. Most deformities can initially be managed with the use of appropriate orthoses, but if the problems persist, surgery to balance the deforming forces is necessary.

The foot can be in an equinus position with the child on his toes or a calcaneous position where there is excessive dorsiflexion. Talipes equinus results from an overactive gastrosoleus complex. If bracing fails to relieve talipes equinus, Achilles tendon lengthening is appropriate. When done with minimal dissection, children can get up and walk the next week in a short-leg cast.

With medial or lateral imbalance, the foot can be in either valgus with pronation or in varus with supination. A valgus or pronated foot is a flat foot with prominence of the talus medially. This can be due to a muscle imbalance with overactivity of the peroneal muscles, or it can be associated with hypotonia and ligamentous laxity where the ligaments are sufficiently lax that the medial longitudinal arch is flattened. If this problem is neglected, not infrequently a fixed bony deformity results, which is cosmetically unappealing and difficult to correct surgically. When there is a valgus deformity in combination with an equinus deformity, there is frequently breaking through of the midfoot, with a rocker bottom deformity resulting. A varus or supinated deformity of the midfoot and hindfoot is most commonly seen in a hemiplegic child and is due to a spastic

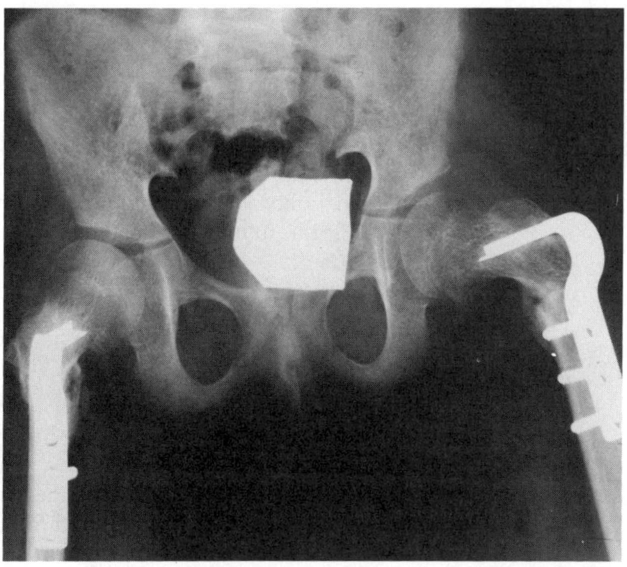

FIG 69–7
Bilateral varus derotation osteotomy to redirect the femoral heads into the acetabulum. This is fixed with metal plate and screws.

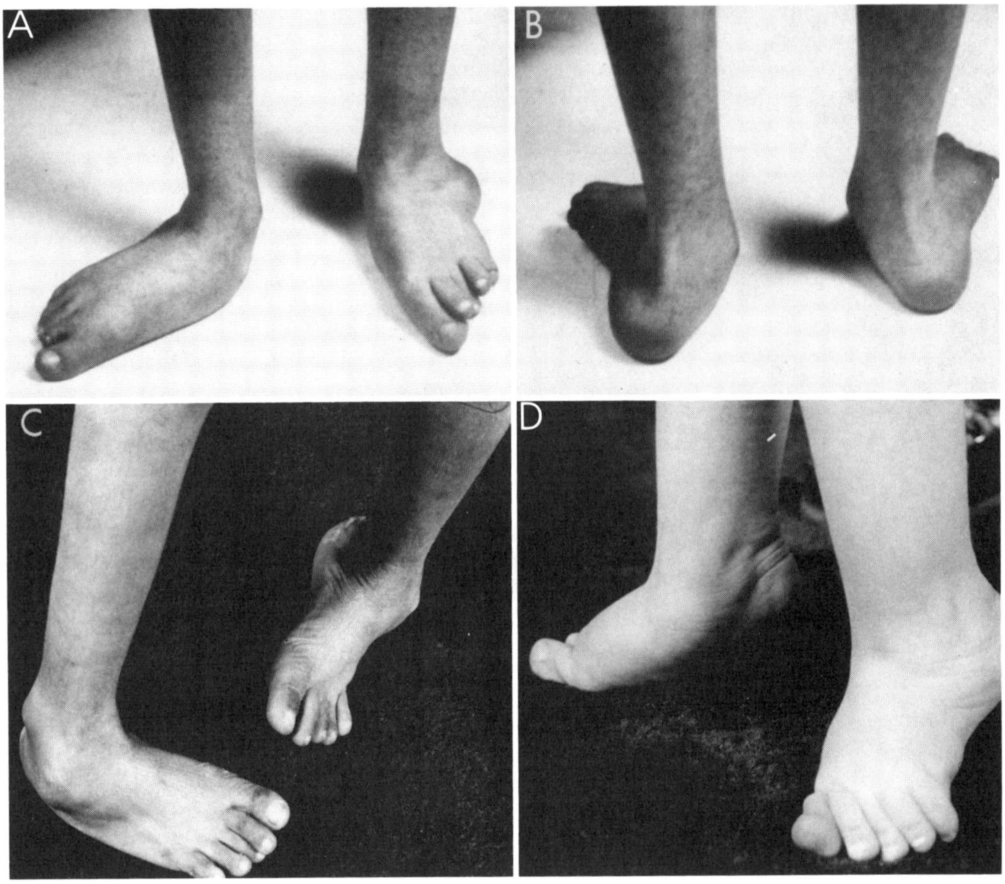

FIG 69–8
Valgus feet with hindfoot and midfoot in flat foot **(A)** or pronated **(B)** positioning. **C,** equinovarus feet with overactive posterior tibialis causing midfoot supination. **D,** equinovalgus feet with tight heel cords causing plantar flexion and tight peroneals causing collapse or pronation of the midfoot.

posterior tibialis muscle, often with contribution from the anterior tibialis muscle. Bracing seldom relieves the problem while surgery to balance the overpull results in dramatic improvement.

Spine

When scoliosis develops, it commonly occurs sometime after the child is 10 years of age. The physical examination is the most reliable way of checking for scoliosis as children with cerebral palsy tend to lack trunk control and can be postured with a curved pattern with lateral flexion through their spines. A structural scoliosis has trunk rotation of one side more than the other (Fig 69–9). Postural kyphosis is frequent with lack of trunk control and should not be considered a structural problem if the child has flexibility in the spine. Bracing treatment (Fig 69–10) is helpful in the control of scoliosis in cerebral palsy, but not as successful as in idiopathic scoliosis because of difficulties holding spastic children in a brace. Posterior spinal fusion is frequently necessary and should be considered when the child's curve approaches 60°.

Upper Extremity

The entire upper extremity tends to be involved in children with cerebral palsy. The typical deformity involves shoulder abduction, flexion through the elbow, pronation through

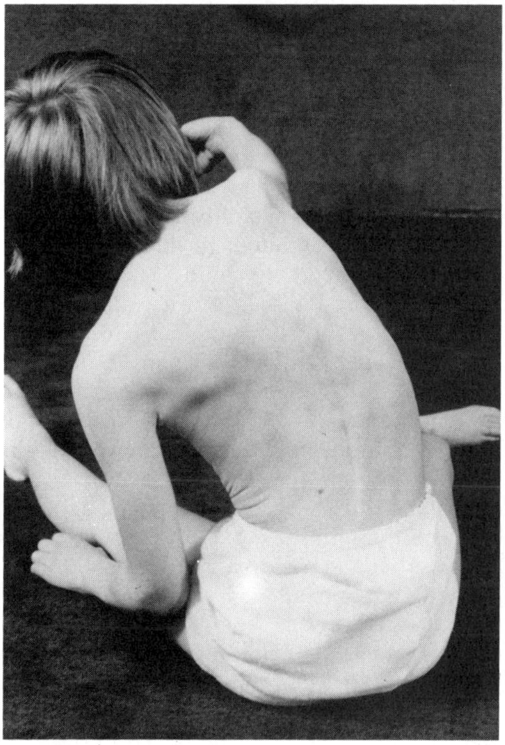

FIG 69–9
A typical scoliosis seen in cerebral palsy with a right thoracolumbar convexity.

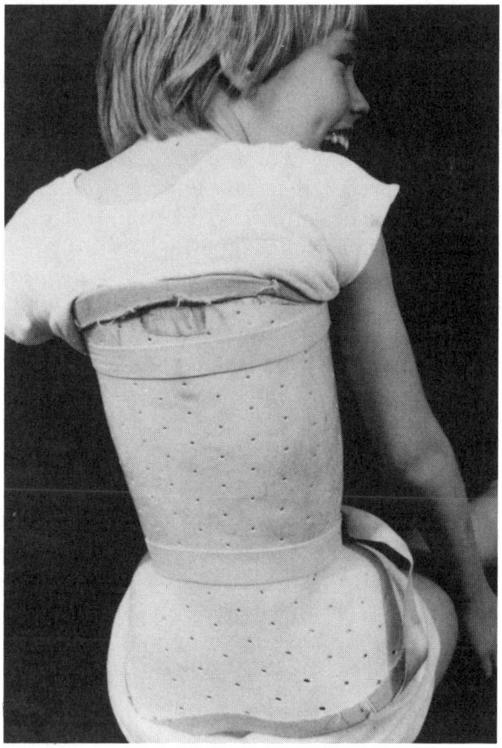

FIG 69–10
Underarm thoracolumbar sacral orthosis, which improves sitting balance and contains the scoliosis.

the forearm, flexion through the wrist, thumb-in-palm deformity with an unstable metacarpophalangeal joint, and hyperextended metacarpophalangeal joints or tight finger flexors (Fig 69–11). The child frequently has a tenodesis grasp and release. The hemiplegic child tends to have more involvement of his upper extremities than his lower extremities, while the diplegic child tends to have relatively better use of the upper extremities. The total body involved child can have severe lack of control of the upper extremities, which precludes effective use of hands for any but the most gross movements. Most upper extremity deformities in cerebral palsy should be operated on after age 4 years, when the mature pattern can be assessed and the child can cooperate with the postoperative management. A normal hand is never achieved due to decreased stereognosis and proprioception. Splinting should be used initially and surgery only after adequate assessment has been done.

Elbow flexion contractures are frequent and

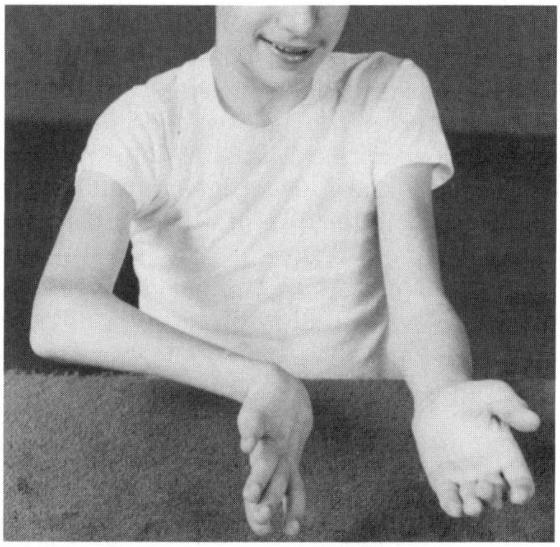

FIG 69–11
Spastic right hemiplegic upper extremity.

do not respond well to splinting. Occasionally the problem is sufficent that the child does better with a lengthening of the biceps brachialis. Wrist flexion deformity is common. If there is good voluntary motion of the flexi carpi ulnaris, it can be transferred to the extensor carpi radialis or brevis. In considering wrist procedures, it is important to consider the grasp activity of the fingers. Frequently a child uses a tenodesis grasp for voluntary control. When the child flexes the wrist the fingers extend, and when the child extends the wrist the fingers flex. A tenodesis grasp is therefore a contraindication to a wrist fusion. To correct a persistent thumb-in-palm deformity the adductor pollicis is partially released and the first dorsal interosseous is partially released at its origin. Weak thumb extension and abduction can be improved by a muscle transfer with rerouting of the extensor pollicis longus tendon.

THERAPEUTIC GOALS

Both physical and occupational therapy are helpful in overall management of children with cerebral palsy. The understanding of therapeutic goals is integral to efficient use of a therapist's time and to optimize the outcome for a child. A good therapy program is like a good coaching program, and it can help bring the child to his or her fullest potential. It cannot, however, go beyond the limits of the child's potential. A disabled child will continue to have deficits in spite of the best of therapy, surgery, and other environmental input, just as all the tennis lessons in the world cannot make most of us world class tennis players. Early developmental programs have been established for handicapped and developmentally disabled children to help them obtain the optimum result.

At the infant level, an effort should be made to stimulate the child with sensory input as well as motor input. A child's environmental stimulation should include input with sensory stimulation to all the senses including tactile, visual, and auditory. Adequate positioning of the trunk can allow the child's hands to be used for play activity and exploration, whereas, without adequate positioning, the hands may need to be used for balance. The child at the preschool age needs mobility to interact with his peers. While optimum posture and movement must be sought, it should not be achieved at the expense of limiting mobility, if the child is mentally capable. Ambulation can often be achieved through crutches or a walker. If this is not possible, a self-propelled wheelchair is the solution. Optimally, a child should be able to achieve mobility similar to that achieved by his peers. If necessary, the use of an electric wheelchair by a child with at least a mental age of 3 or 4 years is appropriate.

By the time the children are in school, more time will be concentrated on specific educational needs. By this time, contractures and bracing should be minimized. Throughout childhood, an effort should be made to combine fun with therapy. If adaptive sports programs are needed, these should be utilized to augment the child's mobility and balance. There are increasing numbers of programs available for these children including swimming programs, skiing programs, horseback riding, wheelchair games, and wheelchair athletics, all of which help in the interfacing of motor, cognitive, and social development.

BIBLIOGRAPHY

Bleck E: *Orthopedic Management in Cerebral Palsy*. Philadelphia, JB Lippincott, 1987.

Rang MR, Silver R, DelaGarza J: Cerebral palsy, in Lovell WW, Winter RB (eds): *Paediatric Orthopedics*. Philadelphia, JB Lippincott, 1986; pp 345–396.

Taft L (ed): Cerebral palsy. *Pediatr Ann* 1986; 15. March 1986.

70 GENETIC DISORDERS

Richard I. Kelley, M.D., Ph.D.

At least three of 100 infants are born with a congenital defect or genetic disorder, many of which are associated with a degree of developmental disability. Moreover, of children coming to medical attention because of problems in development, approximately half have a genetically determined disorder. Genetic disorders and congenital malformations are often classified according to the presumed mechanism of disease, as summarized in Table 70–1.

Despite the variety and variability of inherited diseases, a useful, systematic approach to the evaluation of a child suspected to have a genetic disorder can be followed by the primary care physician. This chapter will present an approach to the diagnosis of some of the more common genetic developmental disabilities using basic information obtained from the patient's history, physical examination, and laboratory studies. Specific diagnostic and management problems of the genetic developmental disorders most often encountered by the primary care physician will then be discussed in more detail.

EVALUATION OF A GENETIC DISORDER

HISTORY

When taking the medical history of a child with a birth defect or developmental disability, an attempt should be made to identify the problem as prenatal, perinatal, or postnatal in onset. Special emphasis should be placed on the prenatal history, specifically addressing: the possibility of congenital infection; maternal exposure to radiation, anticonvulsants, alcohol, medications, and other possible teratogens; maternal diseases, such as diabetes, phenylketonuria (PKU), and other endocrinologic or metabolic disorders. Because most organogenesis is complete by the 12th week of gestation, precise dating of a prenatal event or exposure more often than not will exclude its role in causing a particular abnormality and thereby relieve much parental guilt.

The importance of obtaining all measurements at birth and regularly thereafter, especially head circumferences, cannot be overemphasized. A disproportionately small head circumference at birth is often the only clue to the prenatal onset of a disease affecting the central nervous system (CNS). Moreover, poor growth, especially when associated with feeding-related complaints, such as vomiting, irritability, tachypnea, or lethargy, is common to many genetic disorders, especially those caused by defects of intermediary or energy metabolism. Unusual urinary or body odors reported by the parents should be evaluated carefully. Classic metabolic odors such as "maple syrup" or "sweaty feet" are usually described by parents only as "bad" or "foul." The diet dependency of some metabolic disorders should also be recognized. Not infrequently, the diagnosis of galactosemia and many organic acidurias and urea cycle defects will be preceded by a diagnosis of milk intolerance or other food allergy and a history of multiple formula changes.

A carefully developed family history, working stepwise back through three generations, should always be taken. A developmental disability or birth defect of any nature should be explored, keeping in mind the marked variability of some syndromes. Information about miscarriage, stillbirth, and children dying in infancy should be sought and notation made of parental ages at the time. Ethnic origins, con-

TABLE 70–1
Classification of Genetic Disorders and Other Birth Defects

CATEGORY	EXAMPLES
Chromosomal abnormalities	
Autosomal trisomies and monosomies	Down (trisomy 21) syndrome
Minor deletions and duplications	Prader-Willi, aniridia-Wilms syndromes
Sex chromosome disorders	Turner, Klinefelter syndromes
Mendelian (single gene) disorders	
Autosomal dominant	Neurofibromatosis, tuberous sclerosis
Autosomal recessive	Homocystinuria, Zellweger syndrome
Sex-linked recessive or dominant	Fragile X syndrome, aqueductal stenosis, incontinentia pigmenti
Idiopathic multiple congenital anomalies	Rubinstein-Taybi, William syndromes Noonan, CHARGE syndromes
Multifactorial defects	Neural tube defects, hydrocephalus, isolated mental retardation
Environmentally determined defects	Congenital infections, teratogens (alcohol, anticonvulsants), maternal metabolic disease

sanguinity, or membership in religious sects with relatively closed genetic pools (e.g., Amish, Hutterite) can be important clues to the diagnosis of an autosomal recessive disorder.

PHYSICAL EXAMINATION

For many genetic disorders, retarded somatic as well as mental development is common. Microcephaly, defined as a head circumference more than three standard deviations below the mean for age or more than two standard deviations below that predicted by the skeletal size, is an important finding, especially when there is no evidence of perinatal or postnatal injury. In addition, asymmetries or other abnormalities of the cranial contour often reflect underlying brain defects. Similarly, because the forebrain has an inductive effect on the early development of the face, infants with abnormal frontal lobe development (e.g., holoprosencephaly, Zellweger syndrome) commonly have abnormal midfacial structures: low nasal bridge, epicanthal folds, hypo/hypertelorism, shallow supraorbital ridges, anteverted nares, flattened philtrum, and capillary hemangiomas. Careful attention should also be given to the eye examination. Detecting colobomas, Brushfield spots, epibulbar dermoids, corneal clouding, cataracts, optic nerve hypoplasia or atrophy, cherry-red spots, and pigmentary retinopathy can be critical for the diagnosis of a genetic CNS abnormality, storage disease, or congenital infection.

A high-arched, narrow palate or one with prominent lateral palatine ridges may reflect abnormal shaping of the palate because of deficient or abnormal tongue movements and are important early objective signs of neurologic disease in the newborn or young infant. In the child with developmental delay, otherwise typical clefts of the lip or palate are more likely to be part of a malformation syndrome than simple multifactorial defects. Similarly, common heart defects such as septal defects or pulmonic stenosis may have syndromic, diagnostic significance in the retarded child. The presence or absence of hepatic or splenic enlargement should be carefully noted at each examination. Visceromegaly may be an early clue to the diagnosis of a storage disorder, such as one of the mucopolysaccharidoses or sphingolipidoses, but may also be a late or subtle finding.

Abnormalities of the genitalia such as hypospadias or cryptorchidism can be important diagnostic findings in genetic syndromes but are particularly significant when associated with midfacial defects because of the possibility of a related hypothalamic (i.e., hypogonadotropic) disturbance, as in the septo-optic dysplasia malformation sequence. While gross malformations of the extremities usually lead to an immediate genetic evaluation at birth, more subtle skeletal abnormalities may gain importance later as indicators of a prenatal developmental disturbance; for example, clinodactyly (incurvature of the finger), simian creases, partial cutaneous syndactyly, brachydactyly (short fingers), and contractures are frequent findings. Some abnormalities of the hands can be relatively specific, such as broad thumbs and toes in the Rubinstein-Taybi syndrome or unequal metacarpal length in Turner syndrome and Albright hereditary osteodystrophy.

A detailed examination of the skin is especially important because of the collective relatively high prevalence and variability of the neuroectodermal syndromes (Table 70–2). Neurofibromatosis, with an incidence of one in 3,000 births, is the most prevalent neuroectodermal disorder and one of the most prevalent genetic diseases. Although most affected individuals have normal intelligence, mild-to-moderate retardation in neurofibromatosis is common. Also noteworthy is the significant proportion (10%) of children with infantile spasms who have tuberous sclerosis, a disorder characterized by multiple hypopigmented skin lesions that are often poorly distinguished and easily overlooked in infancy. In neurofibromatosis and tuberous sclerosis, children who have seizures, multiple skin lesions, and severe developmental delay may have inherited the disorder from an undiagnosed parent who, in the absence of a detailed skin examination, seems to be completely normal. Other important dermatologic abnormalities that should be noted are the thickened hair and skin of most mucopolysaccharidoses, abnormal hair patterning, which may indicate a prenatal abnormality of brain formation, and cutaneous hemangiomas and telangiectasia, particularly those on the face or head, which may be associated with underlying vascular malformations of the brain.

Relatively few neurologic abnormalities have much diagnostic specificity for genetic disorders. Particularly severe hypotonia in infancy is an important feature of Down, Zellweger, Prader-Willi, and Lowe syndromes, and myotonic dystrophy; dystonia in an infant boy may be the only sign of X-linked Lesch-Nyhan syndrome. Ataxia is a prominent characteristic of several genetic syndromes, for example, ataxia-telangiectasia and Cockayne and Menkes syndromes; progressive or episodic choreoathetosis can be an important sign of glutaric aciduria and several other inborn errors of organic acid metabolism.

Abnormalities found on physical examination should always be interpreted in relation to other family members. The parents' observation that their retarded child resembles no one in the family is significant, as is the finding that a specific malformation is present in family members without retardation. Family photographs can be especially helpful in such matters. The extreme variability of some genetic syndromes, such as the neuroectodermal syn-

TABLE 70–2
Neuroectodermal Disorders

SYNDROME	INHERITANCE	SKIN FINDINGS
Tuberous sclerosis	Autosomal dominant	Hypopigmented macules, adenoma sebaceum, shagreen patches
Neurofibromatosis	Autosomal dominant	Café au lait spots, subcutaneous neurofibromas, Lisch nodules (iris)
Sturge-Weber disease	Sporadic	Port-wine nevus in trigeminal area
Focal dermal hypoplasia	X-linked dominant	Focal dermal atrophy, lipomatous nodules, irregular pigmentation
Nevus sebaceous syndrome	Unknown	Linear, yellow-orange lesions of forehead or midface area
Incontinentia pigmenti	X-linked dominant	Blistering at birth, with later whorled hyperpigmentation
Hypomelanosis of Ito	Unknown (?X-linked)	Streaked or whorled areas of hypopigmentation on limbs or trunk

dromes, also requires the physician to examine or question parents about specific physical findings in them, for example café au lait spots or hypopigmented macules. Furthermore, in some families, milder degrees of mental retardation may follow a dominant inheritance pattern, sometimes in association with subtle physical abnormalities such as borderline microcephaly. Tactful questioning about the parents' schooling and employment experiences and measurement of head circumferences can be revealing. This is particularly relevant to X-linked recessive disorders, such as fragile X syndrome, in which the heterozygote mother not infrequently manifests a mild form of the disorder.

LABORATORY AND SPECIAL STUDIES

Chromosome Studies

Karyotyping of peripheral blood lymphocytes is now offered by many medical centers and commercial laboratories. For confirmation of a clinical diagnosis of Down syndrome, Turner syndrome, or other whole trisomy or monosomy, conventional analysis, which provides a simple chromosome count and detection of only large chromosomal deletions or duplications, is adequate. For the recently identified fragile-X syndrome, more sophisticated analytical methods, available usually only in major genetic centers, are necessary. An important caveat when ordering chromosomal studies is to be certain that an adequate number of metaphases is examined, at least 20, to rule out mixed (mosaic) populations of normal and abnormal cells. In cases of partial deletions or duplications, parental karyotypes should also be examined to determine if the abnormal chromosome was derived from a balanced translocation in one of the parents. In special circumstances, karyotyping can be done on skin fibroblast cultures or, for an emergent diagnosis of trisomy 13, 18, or 21, on a bone marrow aspirate.

With increasing sophistication of high-resolution chromosome banding techniques, a number of formerly idiopathic malforma-tion/mental retardation syndromes have been found to be caused by minute chromosomal deletions or by chromosome breaks occurring at very specific loci. Examples include Prader-Willi syndrome (15q), aniridia-Wilms syndrome (11q), bilateral retinoblastoma (13q), Miller-Dieker lissencephaly (11p), and Di George syndrome (22q). In addition, a substantial proportion of patients with certain X-linked disorders, such as glycerol kinase deficiency, have been found to have microscopically resolvable deletions or rearrangements of the X chromosome. As a result, almost any child with multiple congenital malformations or unexplained developmental disability should undergo high-resolution karyotyping, even when the diagnosis of a classic nonchromosomal syndrome seems clear.

Metabolic Testing

In recent years, techniques for identifying inborn errors of metabolism as causes for developmental delay have rapidly advanced beyond the traditional spot tests for galactosuria, mucopolysaccharidoses, and phenylketonuria, but many are available only in a few major pediatric centers. In general, unless the family history or clinical findings strongly suggest a specific diagnosis, the broadest possible metabolic evaluation should be ordered and should include, at a minimum, the tests listed in Table 7–3.

This battery of tests can be done on only 10 mL of a 24-hour urine collection. Storage disorders, except for many of the mucopolysaccharidoses, cannot be detected with screening tests but instead require specific enzymatic assays or biopsies for histologic and chemical analysis. A number of metabolic diseases can be diagnosed with common laboratory tests, such as uric acid for Lesch-Nyhan syndrome (high uric acid) or defects of molybdenum metabolism (low uric acid). Because screening tests are expected to have false-positive results, more detailed follow-up studies are often required. Unfortunately, most "metabolic screens," even at major medical centers, are inadequate, especially for detecting many newly discovered organic acidurias. Furthermore, state neonatal screening programs only test for the most common, treatable metabolic diseases, such as phenylketonuria and hypothyroidism, and should never be assumed to be either complete or infallible. Follow-up or duplicate studies are often required.

TABLE 70–3
Screening Tests for Inborn Errors of Metabolism

TEST	MAJOR DISORDERS DETECTED
Urine	
Ferric chloride	Phenylketonuria, tyrosinemia, histidinemia, alkaptonuria
Acetest	Ketosis (acetone, acetoacetate)
Reducing substances	Galactosemia, hereditary fructose intolerance
Mucopolysaccharide (Berry)	Mucopolysaccharidoses
2,4-dinitrophenylhydrazine	Tyrosinemia, maple syrup urine disease, phenylketonuria
p-Nitroaniline	Methylmalonic, ethylmalonic aciduria
Nitroprusside	Cystinuria, homocystinuria
Nitrosonaphthol	Tyrosinemia, malabsorption syndromes
Amino acid chromatography	Numerous aminoacidopathies, renal transport defects (generalized and specific)
Organic acid–gas chromatography	Numerous organic acidurias, lactic acidoses
Plasma	
Lactic acid	Lactic acidoses, Leigh disease, biotinidase deficiency, other organic acid abnormalities
Ammonia	Urea cycle defects, organic acidemias associated with hyperammonemia

Anatomic Defects

Because, for many genetic syndromes, there are often clinically unsuspected abnormalities in several different organ systems, special investigations, such as ultrasound and computed tomography (CT), are often required to look for silent anatomic defects, either for diagnostic clues or for complete definition of an already established diagnosis. A skeletal survey, for example, may provide a valuable clue to a diagnosis, such as early dysostosis multiplex in a mucopolysaccharidosis, while CT or magnetic resonance imaging may demonstrate subtle brain malformations or unsuspected hydrocephalus.

DIAGNOSTIC AND MANAGEMENT ISSUES

CHROMOSOME DISORDERS

Abnormalities of the number (aneuploidy) or structure of the 22 pairs of autosomes and two sex chromosomes are generally divided into complete chromosome monosomies and trisomies and partial monosomies and trisomies, including ring chromosomes, duplications, deletions, and other chromosome rearrangements. Although collectively chromosome abnormalities are common, occurring in about one in every 160 births, only half of these are likely to come to medical attention in early childhood. This is because some of the sex chromosomal abnormalities are infrequently ascertained before puberty, and because approximately one-third of chromosomal defects are balanced rearrangements without phenotypic abnormalities. Of the remainder, Down syndrome (trisomy 21, mongolism), with an overall incidence of approximately one in every 1,000 births, is the most common defect seen by the primary care physician.

Except for the sex chromosome aneuploidies, most of which have relatively mild physical and mental abnormalities (if any), chromosome disorders are in general characterized by multisystem malformations and relatively severe mental retardation. However, there are no special or pathognomonic findings in the physical examination that should lead one to consider a chromosome disorder over other causes of multiple congenital anomalies and developmental delay. Rather chromosomal analysis should now be a routine part of the diagnostic evaluation of unexplained malformations or developmental delay.

Down Syndrome

Down syndrome is the most common major genetic disorder encountered by physicians and is associated with significant morbidity and mortality in the first few years of life. Because the diagnosis of Down syndrome is now rarely missed at birth, the role of the primary care physician in caring for a child with Down syndrome usually begins at birth with parental counseling and guidance and screening for medical problems associated with Down syndrome. Thereafter, the primary care physician must regularly review the special educational and medical needs of the child with Down syndrome and help formulate the goals and program for each child.

Intelligence and Education.—Although the intelligence quotients (IQs) of most children and adults with Down syndrome fall between 25 and 60, the individual child with Down syndrome usually experiences an average decline in IQ of 20 to 25 points from infancy to adulthood. This decline occurs partly because of the increasing weight with age of cognitive factors in the measurement of IQ and partly because of a true degeneration of skills, especially in the adult years. Nevertheless, children with Down syndrome usually progress and socialize well throughout childhood. Most are described as good-natured, friendly, eager to please, and usually function in the trainable retarded range. On a statistical basis, children with mosaic Down syndrome, that is, a mixture of normal cells and trisomy 21 cells, develop somewhat better than those with complete trisomy 21 and occasionally have IQs in the 70s. However, without exception, adults with Down syndrome lack the basic cognitive skills required for independent living. Rather, most remain at home or live in community shelters. Children with Down syndrome are usually enrolled in an infant stimulation program in the first 6 months and later continue in equivalent programs run by local school systems or organizations for the handicapped. Some are able to attend normal classes in the lower grades.

Despite the conclusions of a number of studies that early intervention programs fail to improve the basic intellectual performance of children with Down syndrome, other studies have found that a well-structured, intensive program may limit the expected fall in IQ. Equally important, however, is that early intervention programs usually provide a valuable source of emotional and technical support for parents coping with raising a retarded child and facilitate the integration of a child with Down syndrome into the family and other social routines. In contrast, there is little that is encouraging about the many different dietary and pharmacologic treatments for Down syndrome that have been promoted over the years. Major controlled studies on the effects of thyroxine, trace minerals, multivitamins, and 5-hydroxytryptophan on psychomotor development in Down syndrome have failed to demonstrate any convincing benefits. Careful attention to nutrition of the retarded child is important, but it is doubtful that nutritional or pharmacologic therapy of Down syndrome will substantially alter ultimate performance.

Medical Problems.—In the first few years, congenital heart disease, frequent infections, and seizures are the major medical problems that confront the physician caring for a child with Down syndrome. Congenital heart disease occurs in about 50% of children with Down syndrome and is the major cause of morbidity and mortality in the first year. Half of the defects can be classified as endocardial cushion defects, while septal defects, tetralogy of Fallot, and patent ductus arteriosus constitute most of the other half. Pulmonary hypertension and congestive heart failure from inoperable cardiac lesions are the most common causes of death. Because of the high risk and initially silent nature of some heart defects, all children with Down syndrome should have a detailed cardiac evaluation including echocardiography at birth. Other congenital malformations, particularly those of the gastrointestinal tract, may be appreciated at birth or become symptomatic in later months. Duodenal atresia or stenosis, pyloric stenosis, diaphragmatic hernias, and Hirschsprung's disease are all more common in Down syndrome than in normal children. Cryptorchidism is also common and clinical hypogonadism essentially universal in the adult man with Down syndrome. Adult women also are frequently hypogonadal, but regular menstruation is common and fertility not unknown.

Chronic upper or lower airway infections are more common in Down syndrome but require only standard therapy. However, chronic or recurrent wheezing not infrequently is a sign of reflux and recurrent aspiration and should be evaluated appropriately. Visual and auditory problems (strabismus, cataracts, severe refractive errors, and hearing disorders [mostly conductive]) are common in Down syndrome and require prompt attention to allow maximal developmental achievement. Seizures occur in about 5% of children with Down syndrome and include a high proportion of infantile spasms. Those who develop infantile spasms have a particularly poor prognosis for development.

A disease of particular concern in Down syndrome is acute leukemia, which has a remarkably high incidence of about 1%. This high rate is for true leukemia and does not include the even more common, leukemia-like but self-limiting leukemoid reaction in newborns with Down syndrome. Another life-threatening complication in the older Down syndrome patient is atlantoaxial instability. Although fatal dislocations are uncommon, up to 30% of children with Down syndrome have sufficient cervical instability that activities that could result in neck injury, such as tumbling, should be avoided. Finally, hypothyroidism, once thought to be the primary cause of Down syndrome, is indeed more common in Down syndrome, and at least one measurement of thyroid function during childhood years is probably warranted.

Apart from these areas of increased risk, the medical care of the child with Down syndrome is usually relatively routine. Standards for the reduced rate of growth in Down syndrome are available for the first 3 years, which facilitates the recognition of chronic disease in Down syndrome. In most communities, support services, education, and training are well-established for the management of Down syndrome from infancy to adulthood. And, whereas the majority of children with Down syndrome in the past were institutionalized, today most remain at home or enter sheltered workshops.

Other Autosomal Abnormalities

Individually, autosomal abnormalities other than Down syndrome are rare, but collectively constitute a major cause of more severe degrees of retardation, especially when there are coexisting multiple congenital anomalies. There are no special guidelines for the management of these children but, more often than in Down syndrome, the physician is faced with the care of a chronically ill and disabled child who has severe, sometimes hopeless, developmental problems. Death in the first year of life from heart disease, apnea, aspiration, or infections is common. Although children with minor chromosomal deletions or duplications may as a group fare relatively better than children with larger chromosomal defects, individual congenital malformations and mental retardation can be as severe as in whole chromosomal aneuploidies such as trisomy 13 or trisomy 18.

Sex Chromosome Abnormalities

Aneuploidies of the sex chromosomes, principally Turner syndrome (45,XO), Klinefelter syndrome (47,XXY), 47,XXX, and 47,XYY, are common karyotypic abnormalities, each with an incidence between 0.3 and 1.0 per 1,000 births. Except for Turner syndrome, with both short stature and characteristic dysmorphic features, most patients with aneuploidies of the sex chromosomes manifest few distinguishing physical or developmental characteristics before puberty. If not diagnosed in infancy, women with Turner syndrome often first come to medical attention because of delayed sexual maturation. In contrast, men with Klinefelter syndrome are infrequently diagnosed before puberty and usually have normal masculinization, but may then be diagnosed because of infertility or other clinical characteristics of hypogonadism.

There is controversy about the frequency or degree of developmental disability associated with the common sex chromosome disorders. Statistically, individuals with Turner syndrome have slightly lower than average full-scale IQs, which usually reflect relatively normal verbal skills but weaknesses in space-form perception and generally lower performance IQ components. From a functional standpoint, however, intellectual deficits in Turner syndrome are uncommon. In Klinefelter syndrome, mild deficits of verbal skills, and, in some studies, an increased incidence of behavior and adjustment problems are commonly reported. On the other hand, there are many individuals with either Turner syndrome or Klinefelter syndrome who have superior intelligence. Because of major biases of ascertainment for these disorders, the true incidence of disability is uncertain. Similar uncertainty about developmental disability also exists for two other common sex chromosome abnormalities, 47,XXX and 47,XYY, which are much less frequently identified because of their usually normal phenotypes. Statistically, both 47,XXX and 47,XYY appear to be associated with mild intellectual deficits, but, again, substantial overlap with normals occurs. Women with triple X syndrome (47,XXX) may also come to medical attention because of fertility problems, while a proportion of men with 47,XYY syndrome have been identified because of juvenile delinquency or defiant and aggressive personalities. Because these observations are likewise complicated by biases of ascertainment, the true incidences of such complications are not known.

MENDELIAN DISORDERS AND IDIOPATHIC SYNDROMES

There are several hundred mendelian disorders that feature some degree of developmental disability. To these can be added a large number of idiopathic syndromes and syndromes with as yet uncertain heritability. Most of these syndromes are rare, overlap phenotypically, and are difficult to diagnose without the help of an experienced geneticist. For obvious reasons, dominantly inherited mendelian disorders associated with substantial developmental disability are uncommon except within highly variable syndromes such as the neuroectodermal disorders, neurofibromatosis, and tuberous sclerosis. A positive family history outside of the patient's sibship is uncommon for autosomal recessive genetic disorders, except within genetic isolates where the prevalence of the gene is high. On the other hand, affected individuals in other generations and sibships are common in X-linked recessive disorders, but easily overlooked without taking a family history. Typically, for X-linked recessive disorders, affected men of heterozygote women manifest the complete syndrome while heterozygote females may have a milder form of the disorder or may be normal.

FRAGILE X SYNDROME

Fragile-X syndrome is a recently delineated form of sex-linked mental retardation associated, under specific lymphocyte culture conditions, with a fragile site on the X chromosome (Xq27). Despite the presence of a distinct chromosome abnormality in this disorder, fragile X syndrome segregates and expresses itself in most respects as a true X-linked mendelian disorder and is not classified as a chromosome disorder per se. The average man with fragile X syndrome functions in the moderately-to-severely retarded range (IQ usually 30 to 60) but often has particularly severe deficits in speech and language. Pronounced behavioral abnormalities, including hyperactivity, autism, and even frank psychosis, are common. In addition, men with fragile X syndrome typically have macro-orchidism, mild macrocephaly, prominent ears, prognathism, and joint laxity, but others may appear phenotypically normal. Seizures may occur in up to 20% of affected men.

The incidence of fragile X syndrome is surprisingly high: approximately one per 1,000 male births and up to 5% of moderately-to-severely retarded men. After Down syndrome, it is the most common genetic cause of significant developmental disability. Furthermore, as in other X-linked genetic disorders, women who are heterozygous for fragile-X syndrome are variably affected. They may have entirely normal or only dull normal intelligence, but rarely severe mental retardation. Mentally normal men with the fragile-X chromosome marker have been ascertained as part of extended family studies, but they are rare.

The diagnosis of fragile X syndrome with special cytogenetic studies is now available in many genetic centers, but must be specifically requested. The often subtle physical abnormalities of men with fragile X syndrome behooves the practitioner to include the fragile X test in the routine evaluation of the phenotypically normal, retarded man. Demonstration of the marker X chromosome in heterozygote women is less reliable and false-negative results for obligate heterozygotes are common.

MULTIFACTORIAL DISORDERS

Children with developmental disabilities who come to medical attention usually do so because of frank physical or mental defects or because they deviate significantly from their family's norm. However, from a public health standpoint, the most common cause of learning disorders and other developmental disabilities is probably multifactorial. That is, a combination of a limited genetic potential, poor infant nutrition and stimulation, and/or a poor environment. Although no specific diagnosis is found for most cases of borderline-to-mild retardation, nevertheless, a thorough genetic evaluation should be undertaken both in the affected children and, if appropriate, in parents with borderline intelligence or congenital abnormalities. In particular, detailed chromosome and metabolic studies should be pursued. This is an important category of developmental disability to recognize because, perhaps more so than in the other diagnostic categories, the child with multifactorially determined developmental delay may have substantial untapped learning potential and may benefit significantly from measures taken to counteract the effects of an educationally and environmentally impoverished home environment.

BIBLIOGRAPHY

Cronk CE: Growth of children with Down's syndrome: birth to age 3 years. *Pediatrics* 1978; 61:564–568.

Hagerman RJ: Fragile-X syndrome. *Curr Probl Pediatr* 1987; 17:623–674.

McKusick VA: *Mendelian Inheritance in Man*, ed 8. Baltimore, Johns Hopkins, 1988.

Smith DW: *Recognizable Patterns of Human Malformation*. ed 4. Philadelphia, WB Saunders Co, 1988.

Warkany J: *Congenital Malformations*. Chicago, Year Book Medical Publishers, 1971.

71 MENTAL RETARDATION

Maureen A. Fee, M.D.

Mental retardation is one of the most common of the major developmental disabilities. Six million Americans of all ages experience mental retardation. One in ten individuals in this country has a family member with mental retardation. Defined by the American Association on Mental Deficiency (AAMD), mental retardation is "significantly subaverage general intellectual functioning existing concurrently with deficits in adaptive behavior, and manifested during the developmental period." The primary care physician holds an important role in early identification, etiologic evaluation, and coordination of treatment for children with mental retardation. Familiarity with their classification and management issues is essential for fulfilling this role and responsibility.

CLASSIFICATION

Classification for mental retardation is based on intelligence quotient (IQ; mental age/chronological age × 100) that is two standard deviations or more below the mean (represented by 100) based on standardized psychological tests (Fig 71–1). The educational and functional characteristics largely follow the IQ distribution so that individuals with retardation fall into one of four categories: mild, moderate, severe, or profound. Those children with IQ scores in the 70 to 80 range are said to be borderline and are not labeled mentally retarded. They are considered "slow learners," and are usually academically at the lower end in a regular classroom within the school district. Outside of the edu-

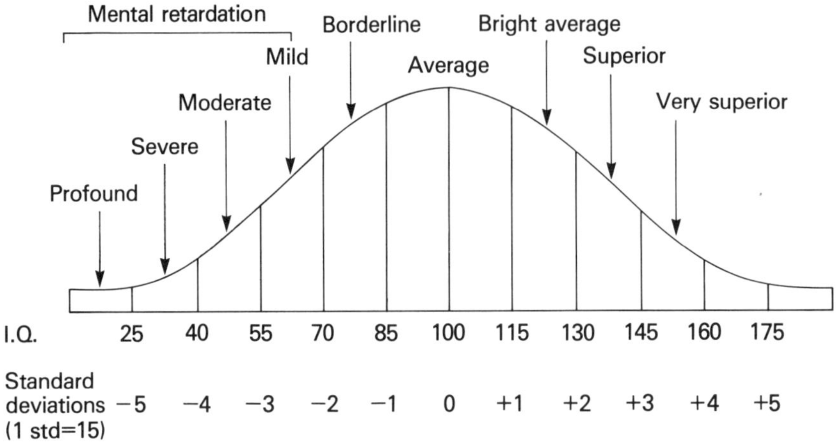

FIG 71–1
Classification of intelligence.

cational milieu they show social and vocational independence. The mildly retarded group constitutes the largest subgroup, accounting for 85% to 90% of those individuals labeled mentally retarded (Fig 71–2). Within the educational sphere they may attend EMR (educable mentally retarded) classrooms where they are able to achieve a fair degree of literacy (reading at the third- to fifth-grade level) in addition to vocational training. Such individuals can maintain gainful employment and possibly live independently and marry. Five percent to 10% of those categorized as mentally retarded are in the moderately retarded group and may attend TMR (trainable mentally retarded) classrooms. Here they can learn basic self-help skills that will allow them to live in a community-based home with ample supervision. From a vocational standpoint they are prepared for employment in a sheltered workshop. The remaining

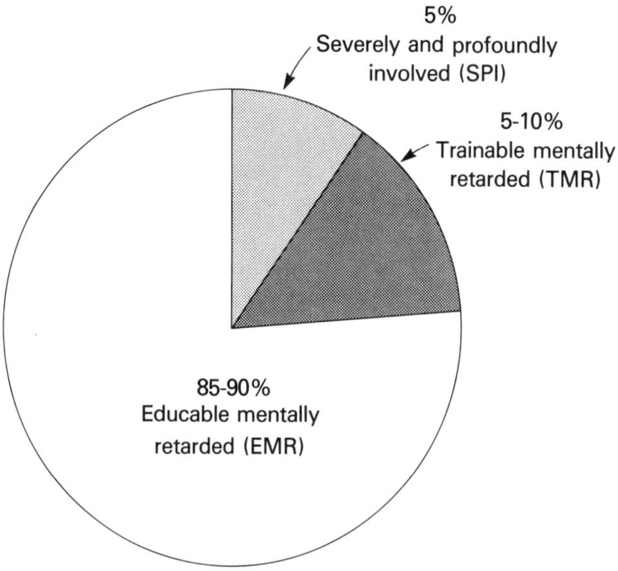

FIG 71–2
Subgrouping of mental retardation showing that 85% to 90% are mildly retarded.

TABLE 71–1
Functional/Educational Profile of Mental Retardation

IQ	RETARDATION CLASSIFICATION	EDUCATIONAL SETTING	FUNCTIONAL/ADAPTIVE OUTCOME
55–69	Mild	EMR	Identification late preschool, early school years May achieve degree of literacy (read at 3rd-5th grade level) Employed in unskilled or semiskilled capacities May be able to live independently with little supervision
40–54	Moderate	TMR	Identified during preschool years May achieve some basic academic skills Employed in sheltered workshops Independent in self-care and can live in community based home
25–39	Severe	SPI	Identified in infancy
<25	Profound		Total dependence, although some very basic self-help skills may be achieved

5% fall into the severely and profoundly retarded groups. Their educational needs are very similar and therefore allow them to be grouped together in a SPI (severely and profoundly impaired) classroom. Extensive supervision is required and minimal self-care skills can sometimes be achieved. Limited conversational skills may be seen in the severely retarded, whereas language development in the profoundly impaired is minimal indeed. Table 71–1 illustrates the educational and functional correlates of the various classifications.

PREVALENCE

Overall prevalence is 3% although prevalence figures vary with age. Because the mildly retarded are often not identified until school-age years, the prevalence of retardation in the preschool years is 0.5%. As the demands increase in the educational setting the prevalence peaks in the 6- to 16-year-old age group and may be as high as 10% in some urban settings. When individuals leave the educational environment the more mildly impaired are assimilated into the general population and the rate in the adult years is approximately 1%. Thus, the prevalence varies with age, based on whether the adaptive behavior is considered deficient. This depends on the setting and consequent expectations rather than on the subaverage intellectual functioning, which is constant. An additional factor in the decreased incidence with age is the increased death rate in the more severely affected. A preponderance of men are affected (55:45), primarily due to the sex-linked disorders (i.e., fragile-X syndrome, Menkes syndrome, adrenoleukodystrophy, mucopolysaccharidosis type II).

DIAGNOSIS

Age at diagnosis varies with severity of the disability and with associated clinical findings. Thus, the primary care physician is in a key position for early diagnosis of mental retardation. The diagnosis may be entertained because of a previously known medical diagnosis (e.g., chromosomal abnormalities, intrauterine infections, neurocutaneous disorder) or as a result of the patient being in a high-risk category based on past medical history, or family history. The more mildly involved youngsters may be devoid of physical stigmata and may only be identified by thorough developmental screening examination in the office. Once a child is suspected of having a developmental lag based on a screening tool such as the Denver Developmental Screening Test, a more definitive evaluation (e.g., Bayley Infant Scale of Mental Development) may be performed by a developmental psychologist as part of an interdisciplinary developmental assessment.

ETIOLOGY

Once the diagnosis of mental retardation is established, the physician begins the second role, of establishing a cause. The pursuit of a cause is important for identifying the medically treatable causes of mental retardation as well as those that are inheritable. As with any diagnostic problem in medicine, a thorough history is essential, including an in-depth family history as well as prenatal, perinatal, and postnatal history for the affected child. After completion of a thorough history the physician may be able to categorize the mental retardation as being either prenatal, perinatal, or postnatal in onset (Table 71–2). Further delineation of the cause is sought through the physical examination and the growth parameters, especially the serial head circumference measurements. Special attention should be given to any physical stigmata that may prove helpful in establishing a chromosomal, or teratogenic cause or a specific syndrome diagnosis. In addition, a thorough ophthalmologic evaluation will aid in the diagnosis of the neurocutaneous syndromes, intrauterine infections, various syndromes, and degenerative disorders manifested by retinal changes.

TABLE 71–2
Causes of Mental Retardation

Prenatal
- Cranial/cerebral malformations (lissencephaly, holoprosencephaly, congenital hydrocephalus, craniostenosis)
- Chromosomal abnormalities (Down syndrome)
- Intrauterine infections (toxoplasmosis, rubella, cytomegalovirus, herpes, syphilis [TORCH])
- Teratogens (phenytoin, alcohol, irradiation, trimethadione)
- Neurocutaneous disorders (Sturge-Weber syndrome, tuberous sclerosis, neurofibromatosis, linear nevus sebaceous of Jadassohn)
- Placental dysfunction
- Metabolic disorders
  - Aminoacidurias (phenylketonuria, homocysteinuria, maple syrup urine disease, prolinemia, nonketotic hyperglycinemia, citrullinemia)
  - Mucopolysaccharidoses (e.g., Hunter syndrome, Hurler syndrome)
  - Carbohydrate disorders (e.g., galactosemia)
  - Leukodystrophies (e.g., adrenoleukodystrophy, metachromatic leukodystrophy)
  - Purine disorders (Lesch-Nyhan syndrome)
- Hormonal (hypothyroidism, hypoparathyroidism)

Perinatal
- Asphyxia/anoxia
- Infections (sepsis, meningitis)
- Hemorrhage (intraventricular, subarachnoid, fetal-maternal)
- Metabolic (e.g., hyperbilirubinemia, hypoglycemia)

Postnatal
- CNS trauma
- CNS infections (viral, bacterial)
- CNS toxins (e.g., lead)
- Anoxic episodes (e.g., aborted sudden infant death, near drowning)

LABORATORY ASSESSMENT

The laboratory investigation of mental retardation should be based on the history and physical examination and directed toward the identification of the inheritable and treatable causes of mental retardation. It has been shown that routine laboratory tests (i.e., those that were not indicated by specific history or physical findings) are not usually helpful in eliciting the cause of the child's mental retardation. Also, it is important to realize that 65% to 75% of the retarded population will not have one identifiable biologic or organic cause. The children falling into the mildly retarded range have the lowest yield in terms of an identifiable organic cause. Those in the lower functioning groups will have an increased yield and are more likely to show chromosomal, metabolic, or structural cerebral abnormalities.

Computed tomography (CT) or magnetic resonance (MR) imaging may be useful when based on an indication by history or physical examination that is consistent with a progressively enlarging head, a diagnosis of a disorder such as tuberous sclerosis, focal seizures, a focal neurologic examination, or microcephaly in a child. In children with a nonfocal examination and nonspecific mental retardation, the CT scan may be nonspecific and show only cerebral atrophy. A metabolic workup including urine for metabolic screening (amino acids, organic acids, and mucopolysaccharide metabolites) is important in the children functioning below the mildly retarded range; especially in those with poor growth and/or seizure activity. In addition, thyroid screening is often helpful in children with a clinical picture suggestive of hypothyroidism. It is important to consider this diagnosis in children with previously identified causes of mental retardation, such as children with Down syndrome who have an increased incidence of thyroid disease. Chromosome analysis should be performed in children who have three or more congenital abnormalities. Also, this is an important investigation in those children who have a family history consistent with numerous spontaneous abortions. In addition to the routine karyotype analysis with banding, the fragile-X analysis should be performed in boys with an unexplained cause for mental retardation (especially those who display the phenotypic appearance of fragile-X syndrome or have features of pervasive developmental disorder (i.e., autism) and girls with mental retardation and a strong family history of retardation in men in the family.

In those children suspected of having a neurodegenerative disorder, a more comprehensive evaluation will need to be undertaken; therefore, referral to a consulting pediatric neurologist is often necessary.

MANAGEMENT

In many ways the diagnosis of mental retardation is a psychological and educational diagnosis. Very few disorders of mental retardation are treatable in the traditional medical model. Although the approach is largely an educational one (special school placement in EMR, TMR, or SPI classes), the primary care physician plays a vital role in terms of management. The group of children with mental retardation as a whole has more medical complications (seizure disorders, cerebral palsy, feeding disorders, increased incidence of congenital heart disease and chromosomal abnormalities) than the average population. The physician is often in the position of being an advocate for the child and family. In order to do this the primary care physician must have a fund of knowledge and resources that will be beneficial to the handicapped individual. A familiarity with Public Law 94–142, ensuring the legal right of education up to the age of 21 years for the handicapped, is essential. Being involved with and understanding the educational process is important for assisting parents in obtaining the optimal educational experience for their children. Knowledge of community services such as respite care, the association for retarded citizens (ARC), and residential facilities will enable the physician to direct the parents to these resources when needed.

Since Public Law 99–457 (Education of the Handicapped Amendments of 1986) was passed, the primary care physician will have an even more active role in the area of early identification and referral. The law expands services to 3- to 5-year olds and provides a mechanism of addressing the needs of infants and toddlers (birth through age 3 years) who are experiencing developmental delays or "at risk of having developmental delays if early intervention services are not provided."

Early identification, prior to the school years, will enable the physician to refer to an infant stimulation program with the triple goal of optimizing the infant's development potential, providing parental support, and identifying the child early so that transition into the public school setting is facilitated.

Involvement with the family of a mentally retarded child or adult is an ongoing process. The term "chronic sorrow" (see Chapter 79) has often been used to describe a feeling within the families of the mentally retarded. Each life milestone for the retarded individual (entry into school, expected time of graduation, sexual maturation, and entry into the work force) may provide further confirmation of the child's deficits. Also, a mentally retarded child places increased stresses on the family structure and on siblings. The primary care physician may be instrumental in exploring these aspects or may need to know resources for referral for the needed support. Thus, the role of the physician only begins with the diagnosis, and continues throughout the child's life. During this extended time, the responsibility is not restricted to the child alone, but must also encompass the family unit as well.

BIBLIOGRAPHY

Chudley AE, Hagerman RJ: Fragile X syndrome. *J Pediatr* 1987; 110:821–831.

Denhoff E: Status of infant stimulation or enrichment programs for children with developmental disabilities. *Pediatrics* 1981; 67:32.

Education of the Handicapped Act Amendments of 1986. Pub L No 99–457, 20 USC §1400, et seq.

Grossman HJ: *Classification in Mental Retardation.*

Washington, DC, American Association on Mental Deficiency, 1983.

Miller LG: Toward a greater understanding of the parents of the mentally retarded child. *J Pediatr* 1968; 73:699–705.

President's Committee on Mental Retardation 1987: *Guide for State Planning for the Prevention of Mental Retardation and Related Disabilities.* Rockville, Md, US Department of Health and Human Services, DHHS Publication No 87–21034.

Smith DW: *Recognizable Patterns of Human Malformation.* Philadelphia, WB Saunders Co, 1982.

Smith DW, Simons FER: Rational diagnostic evaluation of the child with mental deficiency. *Am J Dis Child* 1975; 129:1285–1290.

72 SPEECH AND LANGUAGE DISORDERS

Ellen R. Schwartz, M.A.

Communication problems are commonly associated with many of the developmental disabilities. During the first 5 years of life, the normal child develops communication skills without specific instruction. Any child who displays delays in acquisition of these skills, therefore, may be signaling some interference in a basic, innately human characteristic. The adage that a child will "outgrow" his speech problems is no longer acceptable. Early identification of communication delays can lead to early intervention, which may mitigate the emotional, social, and cognitive deficits of such a disability. Recognition of these delays by the primary care physician is dependent on familiarity with both normal and abnormal development of the speech and language skills utilized in communication.

Speech is the motor act of communication by articulating verbal expression whereas *language* is the knowledge of a symbol system (i.e., auditory, manual, or written) used for interpersonal communication. When considering auditory-verbal communication, receptive language includes skills in understanding what is heard, while expressive language includes the skills of putting ideas into words. Table 72–1 lists a number of major communicative milestones in both receptive and expressive language including speech articulation. Table 72–2 contains an alternative way of evaluating a child's communicative competency by citing the uppermost age at which a child should have attained certain speech and language milestones. These two lists should assist the physician in recognition and/or identification of the child with problems in communication.

LANGUAGE DEVELOPMENT

Language development, influenced by auditory, intellectual, and environmental determinants, incorporates receptive competence and expressive skills in vocabulary (semantics), grammar, syntax, and social usage (pragmatics).

DETERMINANTS

Auditory

Intact hearing is vital to the acquisition of receptive language on which expression is founded, as well as to academic learning and social adjustment. Hearing loss may be due to sensorineural impairment or to transient, recurring, conductive impairment secondary to persistent middle ear effusion. If the sensorineural loss is congenital and severe or the conductive loss recurs frequently before age 3 years, a

TABLE 72–1
Major Communicative Milestones

AGE	RECEPTIVE LANGUAGE	EXPRESSIVE LANGUAGE AND SPEECH
0–3 mo	Startles or cries at loud noises	Gurgles or coos in response to voice
3 mo	Searches for sound with eyes	Chuckles and vocalizes feelings of pleasure
5–6 mo	Reacts to music by cooing or stops crying	Uses vocalizations to get attention and express demands
7–8 mo	Localizes sound source specifically	Babbles with inflection similar to adult speech
9–10 mo	Activity stops when told "no-no" or his name	Says "mama" or "dada," not in relation to specific person
11–12 mo	Responds to simple requests ("Come here.")	Says 1st true words
13–15 mo	May identify objects, pictures, or body parts when named	4–7 true words in addition to jargon, <20%*
16–18 mo	Identifies pictures of familiar objects	10 words; some echolalia and extensive jargon, 20%–25%*
19–21 mo	Understands simple questions ("Do you want juice?")	20 words including names; spontaneous combination of 2 words (Daddy bye-bye, baby shoe, allgone milk)
21–24 mo	Recognizes new words daily	25–250 words; jargon drops out, 60%–70%*
2–2½ yr	Listens to stories, understands reasoning ("When we get to the store, I'll buy you candy.")	400–500 words; 75%*; 2–3 words per sentence; pronouns, diminishing echolalia
2½–3 yr	Follows directions incorporating 2–5 prepositions	Over 900 words; plurals and past tense, 80%–90%*, 3–5 words per sentence
3–4 yr	Classifies and compares pictures	3–6 words per sentence, asks questions, relates experiences, converses
4–5 yr	Interest in words, letters, puns, rhymes, and silly language	Defines in terms of use or class, complex syntax, 6–8 words per sentence

*Percentage of time speech is intelligible.

child's receptive and expressive language may not become fully developed (see Chapter 73). Mild to moderate hearing loss is far less easy to differentiate, since the effects on speech-language development may be subtle. Because *hearing loss should be the first factor to be determined when speech-language development is delayed*, a good audiologic assessment should be the physician's first recommendation.

Intellectual

Mental retardation is clearly the most common cause for delayed speech-language development. Most children with even mildly delayed cognitive skills demonstrate some delays in language acquisition and articulation. Severely retarded individuals may eventually develop some degree of verbal communication but with limited acquisition of symbolic-abstract vocabulary, grammatical rules and syntactic complexity, pragmatic intent, and articulatory clarity.

Mild central nervous system (CNS) impairment may be manifested in delayed speech-language development and is often one of the earliest diagnostic symptoms of learning disabilities. Children with mild, frequently subtle, specific language learning disorders may acquire language late and then become "stuck" at a particular level that is immature for their chronological expectations. Thus, some 5-year-old learning-disabled children may speak in full

TABLE 72–2
Danger Signals of Speech-Language Problems in Preschool Children

By 3 mo	No response or inconsistent response to sound or voice
By 9 mo	No response to his or her name
By 12 mo	Stopped babbling or did not babble yet
By 15 mo	Does not understand and respond to "no" and "bye-bye"
By 18 mo	No words other than mama and dada
By 2 yr	No two-word phrases
After 2 yr	Still jargons or echoes excessively
By 2½ yr	No simple sentences
By 3 yr	Speech that is not intelligible to family
By 3½ yr	Speech that is not intelligible to strangers
By 4 yr	Consistent articulation errors (besides r, s, l, th)
By 5 yr	Sentence structure is awkward
After 5 yr	Noticeable, persistent dysfluency (stuttering)
By 6 yr	Unusual confusions, reversals, or word-finding problems in connected speech
After 7 yr	Any speech sound errors
Any age	Any persistent hypernasality or hyponasality, monotone pitch, or hoarseness of voice

sentences, but still confuse pronouns me/I, him/he, etc., and may not differentiate verb tenses.

Environmental

Children typically acquire and use language if they have the potential. Environmental stresses must be extreme to interfere with language development. It is rare that parental anxiety, not "needing" to talk, sibling rivalry, or lack of playmates, have significant roles in the child who is truly delayed in language, although these are commonly the focus of blame. However, parental reaction to normal developmental dysfluencies may be partly responsible for the development of stuttering.

A bilingual home environment may cause a temporary delay in the onset of both languages, but a normal child will be proficient in both languages before age 5 years. In contrast, a child with any basic cognitive/linguistic problem is predisposed to having difficulty in mastering two competing language systems.

DISORDERS

Vocabulary Deficits

Deficits may occur in both comprehension of spoken words and in usage. Typically, a child who is delayed in comprehension will have a small expressive vocabulary. Developmentally delayed, hearing impaired, or learning-disabled children may have particular difficulty with acquisition of abstract vocabulary (denoting temporal, spatial, sequential information) or may use vocabulary without clear referents. Overuse of some word classes (i.e., nouns) may occur. Learning-disabled children, in particular, are unable to recall from auditory storage and use a word that has been, at other times, part of their vocabulary system.

Grammatic and Syntactic Deficits

These deficits are noted in difficulty with using word endings or organizing words into sentences. In many children, their syntax may remain "telegraphic," with articles, prepositions, conjunctions, and auxiliary verbs omitted and the overall utterance length reduced. Word order may be confused, particularly in production of questions and in using verb forms "do," "have," and "be." The "s" for plurals, tenses, and possession words may be omitted. Children 4 and 5 years old may seem to be fixated at the language level usually associated with 2½ -year-old children.

Pragmatic Deficits

These deficits reflect a child's difficulty with initiating or maintaining a conversation, adapting to communication roles (speaker, questioner, persuader, etc.), providing and asking for feedback, and recognizing knowledge shared in the communication interaction. Generally, pragmatic disorders accompany and compound other linguistic defects.

SPEECH DEVELOPMENT

Speech development, influenced by neuromuscular and structural determinants, incorporates skills in articulation, fluency and rate, and voice quality.

DETERMINANTS

Neuromuscular

Neuromuscular control enables the child to coordinate respiration with precise and rapidly executed movements of the articulators (lips, tongue, teeth, pharyngeal walls, and vocal cords). In an infant, dysfunction of the oral-motor mechanism (as reflected in difficulty with sucking, swallowing, and feeding skills) may signal a critical involvement of neurologic coordination related to speech. Children with neurological disabilities, such as cerebral palsy, are nearly always delayed in language acquisition and speech development.

Structural

The structural features of the oral mechanism must be intact for speech production. For example, a child with cleft lip or palate (see Chapter 74) is vulnerable to speech-language problems and is also susceptible to conductive hearing loss, which further compounds his communication problem.

Although it is a popular notion among parents that structural impairment of the tongue, specifically, "tongue-tie" of the frenulum, is a common cause of delayed speech, this is rarely true. Typically, a child with normal intelligence develops articulatory compensations for minimal tongue-tie. Only in the most severe (and rare) cases is a frenectomy required to free the tongue tip for range of motion. In many instances, a parent is incorrectly focusing on the alleged tongue-tie as the reason for child's delay, when actually the child is primarily delayed in language, not in speech.

Severe malocclusion, tongue posture (perhaps as a compensation for an obstructed airway), and tongue thrusting habits may also impede articulation. The relationship between occlusion, tongue thrusting, and articulation is complex; a dental consultation may be necessary prior to a speech evaluation.

DISORDERS

Articulation Defects

These defects are characterized by errors of substitution, as "thun" for "sun" and "wewow" for "yellow"; distortion, as "bud" for "bird"; omissions of consonants, usually at the end of words, such as "cu" for "cup." Normally, most vowels are acquired in infancy; consonants are acquired in a predictable pattern over the next few years. The sounds "s," "l," "r," "th" are generally the most difficult to be learned and are usually not considered to be errors in children before age 5 years unless combined with numerous other errors or if seriously disrupting speech clarity. Many children with speech unintelligible to those outside the immediate family have a small repertoire of consonants (typically t, d, w, p) that they substitute for others. Speech therapy is recommended if a child's speech is still unintelligible by age 3½ years. That such help must wait until the child is school-aged is an outdated notion and may unnecessarily prolong the period of frustration and social withdrawal that frequently accompanies such a speech disorder.

Stuttering or Developmental Dysfluency

Stuttering is a common characteristic of the speech of preschool children, as seen in their frequent syllable, word, or phrase repetitions, sound prolongations, or excessive pauses and hesitations. The vast majority of children do not persist with such stuttering after age 5 to 6 years, but two groups of preschoolers are at greater risk to do so: children with a genetic predisposition (family history of stuttering) and those with anxiety-provoking stress concerning communication. In either case, the primary care physician can guide parents in positive management of the problem by counseling, since just telling parents to "ignore" the problem may not be sufficient. The following suggestions are usually helpful to parents: (1) do not give the child directives about how to deal with his speech (i.e., "slow down" or "take a breath"); (2) provide a relaxed, slow speech model in your own manner of speaking to the child; (3) reduce the need/expectation for the child to speak to strangers, adults, or authority figures or to compete with others (i.e., siblings) to be heard; (4) listen attentively to the child with patience and without showing concern; and (5) seek professional guidance if his speech is not noticeably more fluent in 2 to 3 months.

Any child with strong secondary stuttering (in which he is aware of his dysfluencies and consciously attempts to modify them) is demonstrating a communication disorder requiring more direct intervention and should be referred to a speech-language pathologist for treatment.

Voice Disorders

These may result from anatomic abnormalities or upper respiratory infections. The most common symptom in young children is hoarseness, usually related to chronic vocal abuse, such as screaming and loud crying.

PRIMARY CARE PHYSICIAN'S ROLE IN EVALUATION AND REFERRAL

The primary care physician's major role in detecting problems is that of screening the child's communication on a regular basis. This is particularly true if parents have expressed concerns about delays in the child's communication. Screening can be done directly, through specific attempts to engage the child in language tasks and responses, or indirectly, through parent interview. Given the notoriously uncooperative nature of most preschool children, many physicians prefer the more expedient indirect approach. There are numerous screening measures (see Chapter 78) and journal articles available to the physician describing each approach and the physician is encouraged to become proficient with at least one of these.

If addressing the young child directly, it is best to elicit spontaneous speech by avoiding the common pitfall of asking yes/no questions ("Do you want to sit on mommy's lap?") and instead ask questions in a way that encourages longer responses ("Where do you want to sit?" "What did you have for lunch?"). Avoid asking merely for the name of an object (i.e., flashlight, tongue depressor) but ask the child "Tell me how this thing works."

The physician's second responsibility is referral for further assessment. *If a speech-language delay is suspected, the child should be referred for audiometry, even if hearing loss is not suspected, because subtle conductive hearing loss may be one contributing factor that can be easily identified.* Either concurrently with or following the audiologic referral (depending on the particular services of the facility), referral should be made to a speech-language pathologist. What this professional will do with your patient depends, of course, on the child's age and problem and whether or not a hearing loss has been detected.

A speech and language pathologist's evaluation generally incorporates a detailed family, medical, developmental, and social history from the parent as well as observation and direct assessment of the child. The latter is usually done in a nonthreatening manner, incorporating age-appropriate toys and pictures devised to elicit specific performance or verbal responses. Frequently, parents are present in the same room (especially with a child under 3 years) and may be asked to participate in the administration of some language tasks (i.e., "Ask her to give you the bottle."). The speech-language pathologist may not recommend immediate therapeutic intervention, but can provide a detailed baseline assessment against which to measure future progress. Moreover, guidance will be provided to parents regarding home language stimulation and management techniques. Therapy is recommended when the child's speech and/or language delay exceeds normal limits for his cognitive level. In therapy, the speech-language pathologist systematically elicits and generalizes production of target goals (specific phonemes, vocabulary, syntactic patterns, fluent speech, etc.). The ultimate goal of therapy is the transfer and maintenance of new communication skills to everyday, natural speaking interchanges.

BIBLIOGRAPHY

Aram DM, Ekelman BL, Nation JE: Preschoolers with language disorders: 10 years later. *J Speech Hear Res* 1985; 27:232–244.

Bradford LJ: Understanding and assessing communicative disorders in children. *Dev Behav Pediatr* 1980; 1:89–95.

Owens RE Jr: *Language development: An introduction.* Columbus, Ohio, Merrill Publishing Co, 1988.

Wanner E, Gleitman L (eds): *Language Acquisition: The State of the Art.* Cambridge, England, Cambridge University Press, 1982.

Whitman RL, Schwartz ES: The pediatrician's approach to the preschool child with language delay. *Clin Pediatr* 1985; 24:26–31.

73 PRELINGUAL HEARING LOSS

Dan F. Konkle, Ph.D.

Hearing loss prior to the third year of life, either congenitial or acquired, conductive or sensorineural, represents a severe deterrent to the acquisition of linguistic skills necesary for subsequent psychosocial, educational, and vocational development. Failure of the hearing impaired to develop adequate speech and language is recognized by most authorities as the primary reason why more than half of those with moderate-to-profound hearing loss fail to graduate from high school, while less than one third ever obtain an eighth-grade education. The average annual income of such children, over a working lifetime, will be 30% to 40% below that of the general population. Conversely, children who acquire hearing loss after the acquisition of linguistic skills fare considerably better. These children seldom suffer the same magnitude of psychosocial, educational, and vocational handicaps as do their counterparts with either congenital or prelinguistic auditory impairments.

From a developmental standpoint, therefore, it is important to minimize the detrimental influence of hearing loss on language acquisition, especially during the first 3 years of life. This goal can be achieved if there is early identification of the impairment, prompt intervention, and follow-up that combines the use of appropriate amplification or hearing aids in conjunction with an intensive program of language stimulation.

This chapter emphasizes the major concept of how early identification and intervention can minimize the developmental deficits associated with hearing loss prior to the acquisition of adequate language skills. Since language skills form the basis for subsequent communicative development and achievement, it is important to consider first several salient features of language development and auditory behavior.

LANGUAGE DEVELOPMENT

Perhaps the most widely accepted theory of language acquisition is that children, including those with hearing loss, have an innate, maturationally controlled propensity for developing language. This potential does not require formalized teaching, yet the potential is realized through an orderly learning process of perception, recognition, assessment, and analysis. Specifically, the child with normal hearing forms hypotheses about the meaning and structure of language as a consequence of exposure to oral/auditory communication (e.g., speech signals), tests these hypotheses by making efforts at oral communication, analyzes the results, and makes adjustments that are evaluated through subsequent attempts at communication.

Average children with normal hearing produce their first words at about 1 year of age, and by age 3 years have acquired a complex set of grammatical rules that represent the basis of adult language structure (see Chapter 72). This fund of language experience can be used by the child to predict correctly the meaning of distorted messages, usually received when listening under adverse conditions. Most common listening environments (e.g., home, nursery school) are characterized by a variety of acoustic signals that compete with the primary message and thus result in an adverse listening condition. In most adverse listening conditions, however, the listener can rely on other aspects of language, such as context to fill in the gaps that occur when the message is not completely received or understood.

This normal process of learning language, of course, depends on the ability to hear various components of important speech messages. If auditory input is impaired because of hearing loss, the child receives only distorted information and thus becomes either alinguistic or, at best, language delayed. The hearing loss not only restricts the normal flow of oral/auditory communication, but also distorts those portions of the message that are audible. Hence, children with hearing impairment often fail to develop adequate language skills and are forced to function with a set of incomplete auditory language experiences. Lack of auditory language skills exacts a severe penalty, since reduced language competency, necessary to predict the content of partially understood messages, forces an additional dependence on the already impaired auditory channel.

Without a solid language base, children with hearing impairment often are unable to understand spoken messages in backgrounds of noise common to most listening conditions; they are not able to fill in the gaps. The typical result is a child with hearing impairment who demonstrates confusion, frustration, and eventually, inattentiveness to auditory communications.

EARLY IDENTIFICATION OF HEARING LOSS

Early identification of hearing loss in infants and young children is a vital prerequisite to successful rehabilitation. Congenital hearing loss often can be detected within a few days after birth, and hearing sensitivity levels can be quantified in most infants by 6 months of age. Since the late 1970s, several audiometric procedures have been standardized that make it possible to identify confidently the majority of infants and young children who suffer hearing loss prior to 1 year of age. The use of surface electrodes and microcomputers to record neuroelectric activity in response to acoustic stimulation (e.g., Brain Stem Response Audiometry, BSRA) have increased dramatically the audiologist's ability to quantify hearing impairment, even in children who suffer multiple developmental disorders. Children with suspected hearing loss, therefore, regardless of age or associated problems, should be referred to an audiologist competent in the assessment of infants and children.

In the newborn or neonate population, perhaps the most efficient method to identify those with potential hearing loss is by use of an "at risk" register. The United States Joint Committee on Infant Hearing, composed of professional representatives from the American Academy of Pediatrics, Academy of Otolaryngology/Head and Neck Surgery, American Nurses Association, and American Speech-Language-Hearing Association, has published the following guidelines for identification of infants "at risk" for hearing loss:

1. A family history of childhood hearing impairment.
2. Congenital perinatal infection (e.g., cytomegalovirus, rubella, herpes, toxoplasmosis, syphilis).
3. Anatomic malformation involving the head or neck (e.g., dysmorphic appearance including syndromal and nonsyndromal abnormalities, overt or submucous cleft patate, morphologic abnormalities of the pinna).
4. Birth weight less than 1,500 g.
5. Hyperbilirubinemia at level exceeding indications for exchange transfusion.
6. Bacterial meningitis, especially *Hemophilus influenzae*.
7. Severe asphyxia, which may include infants with Apgar scores of 0 to 3 or those who fail to institute spontaneous respiration by 10 minutes and those with hypotonia persisting to 2 hours of age.

Findings from investigations that used these or similar criteria have consistently shown the incidence of moderate-to-profound hearing loss in the at risk population between 2.5% and 5%, or about 40 to 75 times greater than in infants who are not at risk for auditory impairment. This relatively high incidence of impairment, coupled with the importance of early intervention with rehabilitative strategies that minimize subsequent language-based educational and psychosocial developmental problems, clearly justifies the routine referral of at risk infants for audiologic screening with BSRA procedures. Infants who fail the screening, of course, should receive complete audiologic assessment.

Despite the advantages of screening infants at

risk for early identification of hearing loss, it remains that approximately 50% of those youngsters who suffer either congenital or early acquired hearing loss will not demonstrate a known risk factor. The responsibility for the early identification and referral of these cases rests with the primary care physician. Perhaps the most sensitive indicator of potential hearing loss in this population is the expressed concern of parents or other family members. Parents are often alerted to a potential hearing problem by their child's inconsistent attention to noises and/or delay in developing meaningful speech. Unfortunately, the physician often may fail to recognize the importance of such information. Survey data indicate that the majority of pediatricians use the case history as a routine screening tool for hearing loss, yet less than 10% will actually question the child's parents concerning the infant's hearing status. Equally important, rather than making a recommendation for an audiologic assessment when parents raise the possibility of hearing loss, the physician may inform the parent to wait until the infant is more mature to see if the problem persists. While it may be true that some delays in speech and language spontaneously resolve with time or maturation, others represent actual hearing loss, and the delay in identifying such problems only compounds the developmental sequela. *Any indication expressed by parents related to the possibility of hearing loss should therefore be investigated with a complete audiologic assessment.*

The initiation of successful rehabilitation logically depends on early identification of the auditory impairment. Most hearing impairments can be quantified via audiologic assessment by the time the child is 6 months old. Primary care physicians usually represnt the initial contact by parents concerned over their child's hearing. It follows, therefore, that these professionals must take the responsibility to initiate prompt audiologic evaluation.

EARLY INTERVENTION

When hearing loss connot be corrected surgically or medically, successful treatment depends on the early and effective use of hearing aids. Hearing aids represent the single most important rehabilitative tool available for individuals with hearing impairment. The use of hearing aids as means of amplification for the child with prelanguage hearing loss is critical for two major reasons.

First, acoustic stimulation provided by hearing aids minimizes the threat of auditory sensory deprivation, thus reducing the potential for detrimental morphologic and physiologic alterations to the auditory system. Although our understanding of auditory deprivation phenomena in humans is limited, available information from other sensory systems, findings from animal research on auditory deprivation, and a growing fund of data from various studies on children with histories of early persistent middle ear effusion lend strong support to the contention that without acoustic stimulation during some critical period following birth, the auditory system undergoes morphologic and physiologic changes that forever restrict its ability to process acoustic information.

Second, providing hearing aids early can stimulate the infant or young child with sufficient acoustic cues whereby the auditory channel can assume its normal role in language development. This premise is based on the widely accepted theory that children, including those with hearing loss prior to the acquistion of language skills, have an innate, maturationally controlled propensity for developing language. This innate capacity for language development is greatest during the first 3 years of life. The span from birth to 3 years of age must, therefore, be exploited by the effective use of amplified speech if children with hearing impairment are to develop optimal language skills.

Although audiologic management through the use of early and appropriate hearing aids is vital if the child with hearing impairment is to make maximum use of residual hearing, it is equally important that the child be exposed to a rich language environment. The child must be exposed to language experiences that are consistent with perceptual and cognitive maturation. Language stimulation should be structured in such a way that it is consistent with normal developmental experiences, especially those that relate to auditory-based concepts. This approach to language stimulation is most effective when used in conjunction with appropriate amplification, educational setting, and support services for family members.

SUMMARY

The primary concern associated with hearing loss in children prior to 3 years of age is development of language skills. To permit children with hearing impairment to fulfill their intellectual and psychosocial potential, it is necessary to identify the auditory impairment early and to provide prompt intervention in the form of amplification and language stimulation.

BIBLIOGRAPHY

Davis JM: Habilitation of language of children with mild to moderate hearing loss, in Perkins WH (ed): *Current Therapy of Communication Disorders: Hearing Disorders*. New York, Thieme-Stratton Inc, 1984, pp 75–84.

Gerkin KP, Amochaev A (guest eds): Hearing in infants: Proceedings from the national symposium, in Northern JL, Perkins WH (eds): *Seminars in Hearing*. New York, Thieme Medical Publishers Inc, 1977, pp 77–187.

Matkin ND: Re-evaluating our approach to evaluation: Demographics are changing—are we?, in Bess FH (ed): *Hearing Impairment in Children*. Maryland, York Press Inc, 1988, pp 101–111.

Ross M, Seewald MC: Hearing aid selection and evaluation with young children, in Bess FH (ed): *Hearing Impairment in Children*. Maryland, York Press Inc, 1988, pp 190–213.

74 CLEFT LIP AND PALATE

Don LaRossa, M.D.

In the early weeks of pregnancy, when many women are not certain they are pregnant, the human face and palatal structures are developing. During this time, a cleft of the lip and/or palate will occur in one of 750 to one of 1,000 gestations.

During the third to seventh week, the nasofrontal and lateral maxillary processes normally coalesce to form the nose, upper lip, and alveolar structures anterior to the incisive foramen. Failure of normal fusion will result in a cleft of the lip and alveolus (pre-palatal structures). The extent of failed fusion determines the severity of the cleft. The cleft may extend completely into the nasal cavity with a gap in the upper arch and a markedly distorted nose (complete cleft). Various degrees of "healing in utero" may occur reducing the severity of the cleft (incomplete cleft). The closure may be almost complete leaving only a minimal notch in the vermilion-cutaneous border of the lip and slight widening and retrodisplacement of the ala nasi on the cleft side. All variations of complete or incomplete clefts may occur unilaterally or bilaterally.

During the seventh to eleventh weeks of gestation, the true palate (posterior to the incisive foramen) forms. The head unflexes, mandibular growth occurs, and the tongue moves out from between the two vertically oriented palatal shelves. This allows the two hemi-palates to move downward into a horizontal position. They fuse from the incisive foramen posteriorly. Failure of the head to unflex inhibits mandibular growth, prevents the tongue from dropping out from between the palatal shelves, and prevents palatal closure. This is thought to be the etiology for Robin syndrome (Pierre Robin syndrome), with micrognathia, glossoptosis, and airway obstruction, often associated with cleft palate. In this anomaly, the cleft is often wide and horseshoe-shaped.

Failure of complete closure of the palate may leave a bifid uvula, an incidental finding seen in approximately 2% of the population. Mucosal fusion without muscular fusion results in a submucosal cleft of the palate seen in approximately one of 10,000 children. A true cleft of the palate occurs when there is a lack of closure or fusion of all layers of the palate and may be associated with a cleft of the lip and pre-palatal structures.

Clefts of only the palate are more common in girls while cleft lip is more often seen in boys. A complete, left unilateral cleft of the lip and palate is the most common variant seen. Ethnic variations are noted as well, with Asiatics affected more often than Caucasians, who are affected more frequently than Blacks. Cleft lip can sometimes be seen on uterine ultrasound (US) at 16 weeks gestation, though cleft palate cannot.

Although heredity can account for a cleft (Table 74–1), most instances are sporadic. Likewise, most clefts are not part of syndromes although a large number of associated malformations have been described. One of the most commonly seen associated malformations is Stickler syndrome with which the Robin sequence seems to be more prevalent. Van der Woude, Binders, Apert, Crouzon, and Treacher Collins syndromes are commonly seen.

Drug ingestion has been implicated as causative in mothers taking phenytoin (Dilantin) while cortisone can produce clefts in certain strains of laboratory mice. Few commonly used drugs are known to cause the defect. Folic acid deficiency has been implicated, though there is a lack of conclusive evidence in man for this and other metabolic or vitamin deficiencies causing clefts.

TABLE 74–1
Frequency of Cleft Lip and Palate or Cleft Palate Occurring in Family Members*

AFFECTED RELATIVES	PREDICTED RECURRENCE (%) CLEFT LIP/PALATE	CLEFT PALATE
One sibling	4.4	2.5
One parent	3.2	6.8
One sibling, one parent	15.8	14.9

*From Ross RB, Johnston MC: *Cleft Lip and Palate.* Baltimore, Williams & Wilkins, 1972. Used by permission.

The term cleft lip and palate inadequately describes the potential complexity of the deformity. The nose, lip, alveolus, and palate can all be involved. As a consequence, appearance, dentition, dental occlusion, facial growth, speech, and hearing can all be affected. Perhaps more far-reaching are the psychosocial implications for the affected individual.

The birth of an infant with a cleft has a profound effect on the family and presents a challenge to the primary care physician. Because of the complexity of the deformity and the long-term nature of the treatment, a multidisciplinary team approach has been used widely in the United States and worldwide, wherever sophisticated medical care is available. The specialists essential to the team are: the plastic surgeon, speech pathologist, orthodontist, pediatrician, and otolaryngologist. In an ideal situation, a psychologist, geneticist, anthropologist, pedodontist, prosthodontist, opthalmologist, and nurse are team members. A team coordinator/educator oversees the teams' functioning and its' interaction with patients. The evaluation team collaborates to plan treatment strategies, which also serve as a forum for continuing education of the team members by an exchange of knowledge from each specialty area.

GENERAL AND SPECIAL AREAS OF CARE OF THE PATIENT WITH CLEFT LIP OR PALATE

CARE IN THE NEWBORN PERIOD

The newborn period presents the greatest challenge to the physician, family, and team. Not uncommonly, those who initally provide care for the infant with a cleft are unprepared, despite the relative frequency of clefting. Intervention by someone familiar with the problem should be prompt so as to provide consolation and education to the parents. Outreach by the team nurse, coordinator or parent of a cleft patient, trained at providing support, is critical at this time. Parents need information about what has happened and where to go for help. Hospital personnel may need advice about feeding and community resources as well.

A general evaluation looking for other anomalies is undertaken. In particular, airway obstruction related to Robin syndrome must be assessed. In this anomaly, the dyad of cleft palate size and mandible size interact with each other. The degree of airway obstruction varies directly with jaw size and inversely with cleft size. That is, a wide cleft can help compensate for a small mandible (the tongue size being constant). Hence a child with a small mandible and narrow cleft may quickly get into serious respiratory difficulty, while one with a wide cleft may be adequately compensated.

FEEDING INFANTS WITH CLEFT LIP OR PALATE

Since clefts of only the lip do not interfere with normal feeding, breast-feeding is often possible. Feeding problems occur in a child with a cleft of the palate who does not suck normally because of his inability to create a seal. The nipple on the bottle must be modified to allow milk to flow easily. A preemie nipple should be crosscut with scissors or a no. 11 scalpel so that milk drips from the bottle when it is held upside-down. Too much flow will flood the infants mouth; too little will cause fatigue and malnutrition. The child should be fed in the upright or football position and burped frequently, since excess air will be ingested. The infant should sleep in an infant seat or on his side. These maneuvers are particularly important in the child with Robin syndrome, where the tongue may fall back into the oropharynx or become lodged above the cleft completely obstructing the airway. Such an infant may have to be fed in an upright position or even tipped forward to get the tongue out of the way to permit feeding. Nasogastric feeding tubes should be used only as a last resort. If one becomes necessary, it is imperative to sham feed the infant with a pacifier during nasogastric feeding lest they forget how to suck.

Children with Robin syndrome should be placed on an apnea monitor and have pulse-oximetry done during feeding to assess the degree of oxygenation. Pneumography and thermistor studies are indicated to fully assess other causes for apnea. If hypoxic episodes occur, the infant may be a candidate for a tongue-lip adhesion procedure or perhaps even a tracheostomy if the obstruction is severe enough. Most children will outgrow their respiratory difficulties (by about 3 months of age) as the mandible grows.

As a general rule, infants with cleft palate can eat and grow normally. Failure to thrive usually indicates a problem with feeding technique rather than from the mere presence of the cleft. Education and patience can overcome these difficulties. Diet can be advanced normally in these children.

OTOLOGIC PROBLEMS

Infants with palatal clefts are more prone to develop otitis media. This is thought to result from the muscle derangement within the cleft in concert with the drying effects on the eustachian tube orifice exposed to the oral cavity. The tensor palati muscle, which controls the eustachian tube orifice, is more flaccid in the unrepaired cleft interfering with normal closure. Serous otitis media is the rule, creating a milieu for repeated bouts of acute otitis media and reduced hearing. Long-term hearing loss can result from recurrent episodes of acute and chronic otitis media. Virtually all children require myringotomy with tube placement until they have completely healed following palate repair. Some have persistent difficulty, and all require close monitoring by the primary care physician, otolaryngologist, and audiologist.

DENTAL PROBLEMS

Dental development is usually delayed in children with cleft palate. Teeth bordering the alveolar cleft may be missing or rotated or may appear within the cleft, depending on the severity of the alveolar cleft. Good dental care is particularly important since many of these children will eventually need fixed bridges or prosthetic teeth to replace those missing from the clefting process. Parents must be cautioned about the milk bottle caries syndrome and directed to good dental care.

Children with clefts of the soft palate do not experience serious orthodontic problems related to the cleft itself. Posterior crossbites may be seen. However, when the cleft involves the alveolus, various degrees of maxillary arch collapse occurs as a consequence of the missing alveolar bone. This results in anterior crossbites and a lack of facial projection or even a concave appearance of the mid-face. This can be compounded by surgical scarring, which may inhibit normal facial growth. When children enter the age of mixed dentition (8 to 12 years), the upper dental arches can be orthodontically expanded and the teeth realigned and leveled. Position is then maintained with a prosthetic appliance attached to the teeth (fixed bridge) often with attached prosthetic teeth to replace those that are missing. Alternatively, bone grafts from the iliac crest, rib, or cranium can replace the missing alveolar bone. The graft stabilizes the arch, provides for the ingrowth of unstable teeth, and restores the gingival contour. Following this latter approach, missing teeth can be restored via a removable bridge or by bonding them to adjacent teeth (Maryland bridge).

SPEECH PROBLEMS

Children with cleft lip only are not expected to have speech problems related to palatal dysfunction. However, since there is an increased incidence of submucosal clefting of the palate in children with only cleft lip, the stigmata of this problem (bifid uvula, notching of the posterior edge of the hard palate and zona pellucida of the soft palate) should be sought. Most children with submucosal clefting of the palate will not have speech difficulties. However, approximately 20% will exhibit velopharyngeal incompetence producing the typical hypernasal speech associated with poor palatal function. If hypernasal speech becomes evident, surgical repair may be necessary.

Children in whom clefts of the palate have been repaired are evaluated at about 2½ years of age by the speech pathologist. The rate of speech development and any evolving problems with velopharyngeal function are particularly noted. Hypernasality and nasal escape are evidence of velopharyngeal incompetence. Lateral static radiographs of the palate obtained with the patient saying the phonemes "M," "D," "S," and "E" will confirm the clinical findings. Where the diagnosis is unclear, videoradiography of the soft palate using the Towne, base, and anterior views with contrast material and nasopharyngoscopy may demonstrate the problems. Mild degrees of velopharyngeal incompetence may be treated with speech therapy. More significant velopharyngeal incompetence may require a pharyngoplasty (posterior pharyngeal flap or Orticochea pharyngoplasty) to augment velopharyngeal closure.

PSYCHOSOCIAL PROBLEMS

In general, one may anticipate psychosocial problems proportional to the severity of clefting of the lip structures. Interesting, serious problems are not often seen. Perhaps because of the extra attention lavished on these children and their ability to successfully use their mental mechanisms to cope with the difficulties of growing up with a dentofacial deformity or speech impediment, they probably do represent a slightly higher risk group and deserve attention in this sphere. Although the physician or cleft palate team members can manage the psychologic problem, often psychiatric intervention is needed.

The plastic surgeon often oversees the entire treatment of the child, making decisions regarding primary and secondary surgery with input from the team. He or she becomes involved early in the care of the child, meeting with the parents as soon as possible after birth to evaluate the infant and to outline the short- and long-term goals. Education regarding clefting is provided to supplement that given by the outreach person. The first phase of genetic counseling is offered at this time to aid in family planning.

CLEFT SURGERY

In an otherwise healthy infant, surgery is guided by the basic tenets of pediatric surgery, which are 10 weeks of age, 10 lbs. of weight, and 10 g of hemoglobin. Hence, lip repairs are usually done at about 3 months of age in the uncomplicated cleft. General anesthesia and an overnight hospitalization are usual. Infants can be bottle or breast fed immediately after surgery without fear of disrupting the repair.

Palatal clefts should be surgically closed by 18 months of age to minimize any deleterious effects on speech. Closure before 12 months of age may improve speech. Preliminary data demonstrate better results from even earlier closure (3 to 6 months). The precise timing is dependent on the infant's overall condition and the width of the cleft (Figs 74–1, 74–2). Clefts of the soft palate only are usually closed earlier

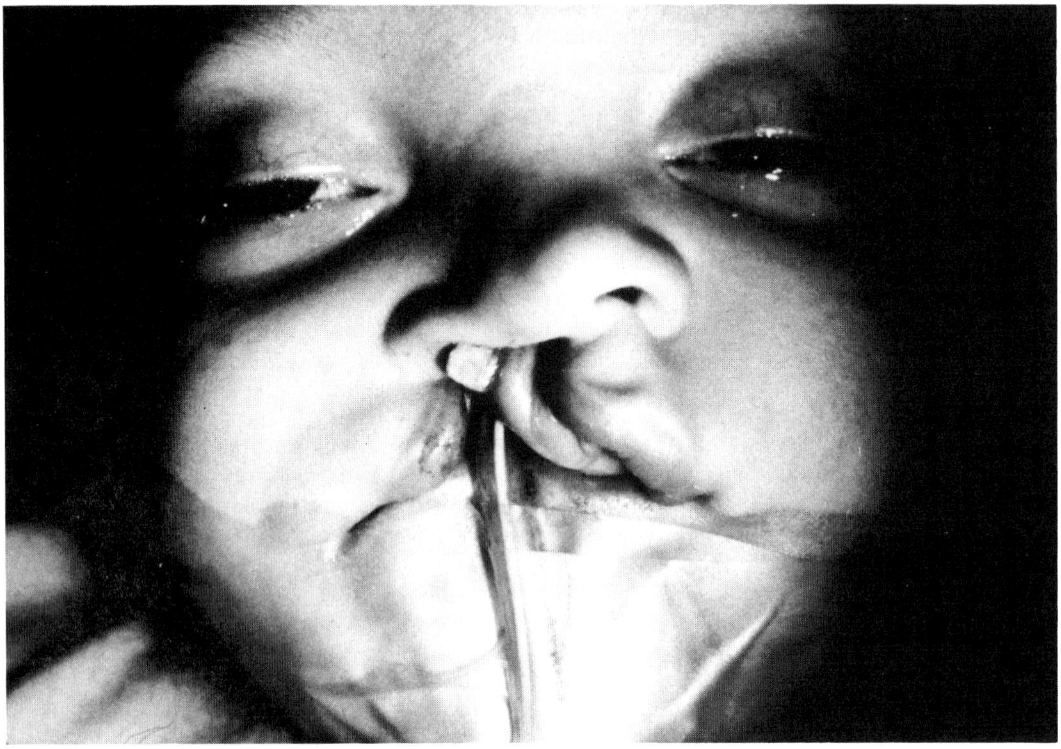

FIG 74–1
Three-month-old girl with complete cleft of the lip and palate at surgery. Note the rudimentary tooth in the cleft adjacent to the nostril rim and the effects on the nose.

(age 3 to 9 months), whereas closure of complete clefts is delayed (age 6 to 9 months). Surgery in children with Robin syndrome may have to be postponed for as long as 24 months to allow for sufficient mandibular growth and overall increase in the dimensions of the airway. Their palates are rarely closed before 12 months. A longer hospitalization is needed following cleft palate repair (1 to 3 days) to permit resumption of oral intake. Feeding is done with a spoon, cup, or Breck feeder (syringe with a rubber tube tip to permit controlled introduction of liquids into the oral cavity). Bottles and pacifiers are not permitted for 2½ to 3 weeks to prevent pressure on the repair from sucking and to reduce the risk of disruption. The cleft across the alveolus is often left unrepaired to reduce scarring in this area which could impede facial growth. It is closed later, often when bone grafting of the alveolus is done (age 8 to 12 years).

LONG-TERM CARE

Following these initial procedures, the child is followed up by the team on a yearly basis, evaluating growth, speech, dentition, hearing, and psychosocial development. Revisional operations on the lip, premaxillary bone, and nose or to improve speech (posterior pharyngeal flaps or pharyngoplasties) are recommended depending on the team's evaluation and the patient and family's desires.

As a child enters adolescence, the final phases of treatment are planned. Orthodontics and prosthodontics are completed. When severe derangements of occlusion and the facial skeleton exist, orthognathic surgery may be warranted. This is usually delayed until full facial growth has been achieved (16 years for women, 17 to 18 for men). Final revisions are made on the lip and nose, frequently including a rhinoplasty. It is at this time when the second phase of genetic counseling should be offered to the patient. They should be given access to the data they will need to make an informed

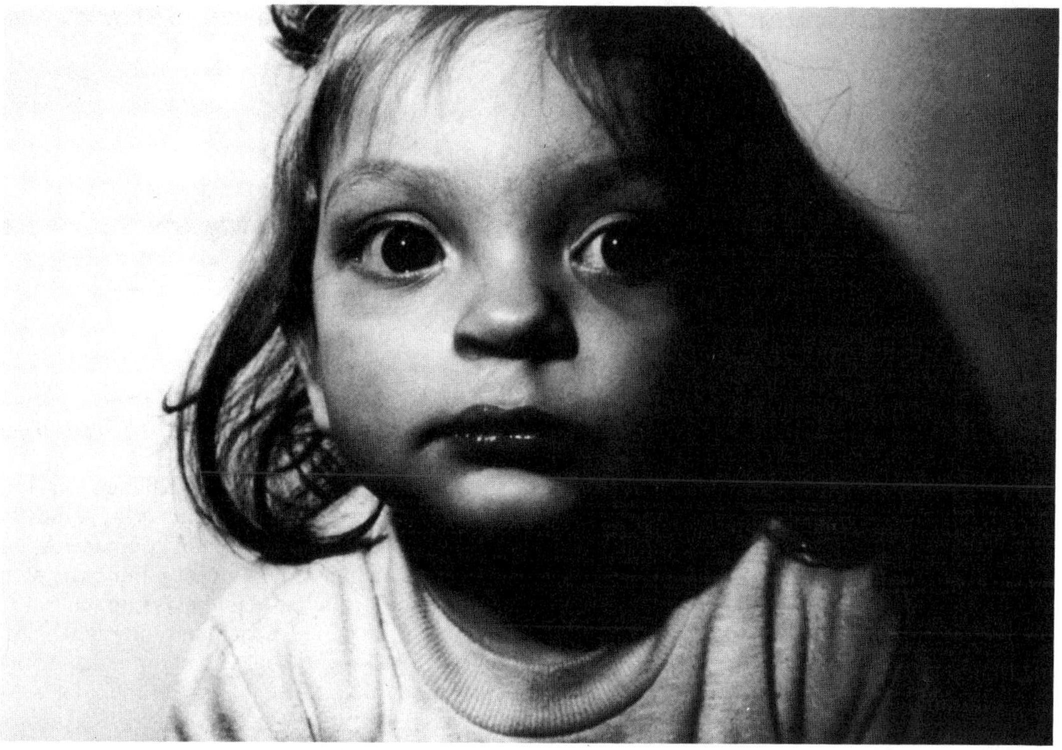

FIG 74–2
Same child at 2 years of age after repair of the lip and palate.

decision about their risk of having a child with a cleft.

Thus the treatment is complete. The team members have focused on a unique set of anatomic derangements. Appropriate interventions have hopefully been made to equip the young man or woman with the best possible appearance, speech, and confidence to enter the adult community.

BIBLIOGRAPHY

Cohen MM Jr: Syndromes with cleft lip and cleft palate. *Cleft Palate J* 1978; 15:306.

Converse: *Reconstructive Plastic Surgery,* vol 4: *Cleft Lip and Palate, Craniofacial Deformities.* Phildelphia, WB Saunders Co, 1977.

Fraser FC: The genetics of cleft lip and palate. *Am J Hum Genet* 1970; 22:336.

Grabb WC, Rosenstein SW, Bzoch KR (eds): *Cleft Lip and Palate.* Boston, Little, Brown & Co, 1971.

McWilliams BJ, Morris HL, Shelton RL (eds): *Cleft Palate Speech.* Philadelphia, BC Decker, 1984.

Millard DR: *Cleft Craft,* vols I, II, III. Boston, Little, Brown & Co, 1976, 1977, 1980.

Ross RB, Johnston MC: *Cleft Lip and Palate.* Baltimore, Williams & Wilkins Co, 1972.

Stark RB: The pathogenesis of harelip and cleft palate. *Plast Reconstr Surg* 1954; 13:20.

75 AUTISM

Maxine Field, Ph.D.

DEFINITION AND ETIOLOGY

Infantile autism, a behaviorally defined developmental disorder evident early in life (before 30 months), has three primary characteristics: social indifference or failure to develop normal social responses (autistic aloneness); absent or abnormal speech and language development; and restricted, stereotyped, or bizarre responses to objects and other aspects of the environment (insistence on sameness, perceptual inconstancy). The syndrome is heterogeneous so that these central three characteristics vary considerably in severity, and take on different appearances depending on age, intelligence, treatment, other personality attributes, and family management. Although most autistic children are also intellectually retarded, about 20% have IQs of 70 or above. The special abilities of some—precocious reading, arithmetic, drawing, musical skills, calendar calculating, or memory for intricate transportation routes—are, however, splinter skills and do not of themselves indicate greater intellectual potential or broader understanding. Autism is found in all races and social classes, is seen three to four times more often in males, and may have some genetic basis, with the families of autistics having higher than expected occurrences of autism and language disorders. The incidence of autism and autistic-like disorders varies according to definitional criteria, but ranges from four to 15 per 10,000 population.

The early hypotheses that autism resulted from parental coldness, rejection, or mishandling has been almost unanimously discarded. The current belief, that it arises from dysfunction of the central nervous system, is supported by reports of associated abnormal biochemical and neuroanatomic findings and seizures in some autistic persons. However, no specific and universal biologic marker has yet been identified.

There is controversy about whether the underlying psychological deficit is specifically one of disordered language and communication or one involving perception of more basic sensory stimuli. The first hypothesis implicates the higher brain centers, specifically the left hemisphere. The second suggests disturbance of the subcortical area, particularly the reticular activating system, which acts to prevent necessary sensory information from reaching the cortex, thus impeding the formation of normal neuronal connections. It is most likely that the behavioral abnormalities clustered together in autism do not represent a single disease, but a common outcome of a variety of pathologic processes.

DIAGNOSIS

With no consistent physical findings or definitive laboratory tests, autism is diagnosed by a pattern of abnormal behavior. Table 75–1 lists some of the specific behaviors that may fulfill criteria. It has been usual for autism to be identified at about the age of 3 years or later. The presenting complaints typically are failure to acquire speech together with temper tantrums arising from the child's communicative failure or in reaction to changes in routines. The diagnosis can and should be entertained sooner to offer the child the best opportunity for improvement and his parents guidance in optimum management. Even the most competent parents, puzzled and frustrated by a child who does not respond to them in the usual ways,

TABLE 75–1
Common Behaviors of Young Autistic Children

Mental or Chronological Age (yr)	Social Unrelatedness	Impaired/Deviant Language	Insistance of Sameness; Stereotype Behavior	Disturbed Sensory and Motor Responses	Unusual Abilities
0–1	Avoids eye contact; does not posturally anticipate being lifted; indifference or aversion to physical contact; doesn't play baby games or imitate gestures; doesn't show specific attachments	Little vocalization; decreased interest in human voice; seems deaf	Resists new foods or feeding procedures; sleep difficulties	Slow or irregular acquisition of motor milestones	
1–2	Relates to part of person, using mother's hand or lap or body without relating to whole person; does not come for comfort when hurt; requires intrusive social games, roughhouse play for any social response; most contented when left alone; aloof and avoidant	A few words may appear, but are lost, and vocabulary doesn't expand; little speech; sounds limited and atypical; listens and attends poorly or erratically	Panics and tantrums with new people/environmental changes; spends long periods of time in repetitive activities; nonfunctional use of objects: spins, dangles, stares, lines up, fascinated with movement; attachment to odd objects; rituals; little or no pretend play	Interest in small visual details or patterns; hyporeactive or hyperreactive to sound; tunes out or holds ears; indifferent to pain; smells or mouths objects; motor abnormalities: toe walking, finger or body posturing, rocking, spinning, grimacing	Interest in music; repeats melodies; looks at books for long periods; skill with puzzles, blocks, or construction toys
2–5	May develop attachment to parents, but no cooperative peer play	Speech develops in unusual patterns and is out of line with nonverbal skills; echolalia, immediate or delayed; repeats questions, TV commercials, songs out of context; difficulty using speech for communication; can't ask or answer questions; reverses pronouns; unusual pitch, volume, or intonation; short sentences; immature grammar			Letter and number recognition; early reading; good memory for routes

have little sense of how to handle the difficult behavior of an autistic child.

Early symptoms seem to arise both from the autism and the mental retardation. In a low-functioning child, there may be delayed or irregular motor development. More commonly, motor milestones are normal or even early. The autistic infant in the first year may be too content—happy to remain in his crib for long periods, not babbling or crying for food, so unreactive that parents wonder if he is deaf, showing little interest in the usual games, and failing to develop preferential attachment to his parents. Or, in a different pattern, he may be excessively irritable—a poor sleeper, a picky eater, content only when clinging to one person. At the same time he may show some unusual behaviors including interest in small visual details that would normally escape notice such as light, shadows, motes of dust, small patterns, or lines or cracks in the wall. The child may have particular difficulty with change and react violently to small alterations in routines, introduction of new food, new food textures, or methods of feeding. Some children seem to develop normally in the first year and acquire a few words, which are then lost at about 12 to 18 months as they become remote and spend increasingly long periods of time spinning objects, rocking, or banging.

Because autism is a developmental disorder, its manifestations shift over time. The minimal progress of the severely impaired child may mean that the intelligence quotient (IQ) declines as he fails to acquire new skills; some children may deteriorate or lose skills as a result of seizures. However, many children, particularly the more mildly affected who receive adequate environmental support, will show improved functioning and become more affectionate and socially responsive. The changes in the clinical picture, resulting in a child who is not so much withdrawn as odd or socially immature, may be confusing. It is, therefore, important that observations of current behavior be integrated with relevant historical data.

The child's primary care physician, who has the most regular contact with the infant and young child, is in a unique position to act effectively in the early identification of the autistic child. Yet there are difficulties. The low incidence means that individual practitioners will have limited experience with autism, and the autistic child will usually look normal and have an unremarkable physical examination. It is only by attending to and eliciting parental reports of behavioral disturbances or developmental lags that the physician may come to suspect problems that warrant further observation and questioning.

ADDITIONAL EVALUATION

The child with suspected autism should be referred for a thorough evaluation at a developmental center staffed with clinicians experienced in the range of developmental disorders of early childhood. Parents should be adequately involved in the process, which should include: physical/neurologic examinations, careful social and developmental history, audiologic testing, review of birth records, behavioral observations, and psychological testing. Because autism can occur concomitantly with blindness, hearing impairment, mental retardation, seizure disorder, and other neurologic diseases, these conditions should also be identified. Syndromes that may produce some similar symptoms must be ruled out, such as deprivation, developmental language disorders, parental mismanagement, or parental overanxiety. Depending on results of the physical examination and level of functioning, further diagnostic tests such as electroencephalography, computed tomography, chromosome studies (including fragile X), and urine metabolic screening to address the cause or concurrent medical conditions may be done. Standardized psychological tests must be appropriate to the child's mental age and assess nonverbal skills. A number of observational measure and rating scales specifically developed for autistic children are helpful in delineating strengths and weaknesses and differentiating mildly affected from more severely affected children.

The purpose of a comprehensive assessment by medical and behavioral specialists is not only to make a diagnosis, but to communicate carefully and clearly the findings to parents, begin plans for treatment, and provide for periodic reassessment. The much-criticized approach of a diagnosis given without a plan of intervention or hope for improvement is as much to be deplored as an overly enthusiastic treatment effort that proceeds without adequate study and seems to promise a miracle cure.

TREATMENT

Current treatments are educational and behavioral and consist in the most general sense of strategies to eliminate or minimize abnormal behaviors so that skills to foster the child's development can be taught. Treatment philosophies vary with the practitioner, the nature and severity of the symptoms, and the developmental age of the child, but all embody some common practices and sequences. Initial efforts with the withdrawn child must be directed to establishing awareness of and responsiveness to people, so that learning from others can begin. To achieve this, one-to-one work that is intense, intrusive, highly structured, and carried out over many hours of the day has been most effective. Parents, siblings, and volunteers have been engaged as cotherapists in such programs to decrease the amount of time the child is left to his own devices and his old routines. If and when the child becomes more related, his cognitive and language deficits become salient, and structured special education programs designed to teach specific skills and behaviors are needed. Language therapy and sign language have been used with children with severe language deficits or muteness. Supportive psychotherapy may be helpful to the older, more mildly affected child or adult.

A comprehensive plan for the autistic child should include an educational program, guidance for home management and treatment, and attention to associated medical problems. Facilities for the preschool child are just beginning to become available so that the young autistic child will usually be served in a general program for handicapped children that may or may not be equipped to handle his special problems. Public school districts have responsibility for the education of autistic children until the age of 21 years. In some areas, classes are organized statewide but in others they are still sporadic. The Autism Society of America (ASA), an organization of parents and professionals with national offices in Washington, D.C., and local chapters, disseminates information, operates a hot line, sponsors scientific conferences, and publicizes the needs of the autistic population to the general public, educational establishment, and governmental agencies.

PROGNOSIS

Prognosis is most often directly related to the severity of the child's mental retardation, which can usually be reliably assessed by the age of 4 or 5 years. Individuals with IQs less than 50 are likely never to talk and to require institutionalization. The outcome for the mildly affected is more variable and seems to depend on the level of language development and the severity of behavior problems. Autistic children as a rule do not develop the thought disorders, delusions, or hallucinations of schizophrenia; rather, they are likely to present as simple, unsophisticated adults who may have continuing difficulties with language and have trouble understanding the subtleties of normal social interactions. Some hold jobs that may utilize their special skills with numbers, music, or drawing, but most are employed at lesser levels than IQ alone might predict. Their social peculiarities and obsessive interests may interfere with job performance and social relationships. Follow-up data indicate good outcome in terms of normal or near-normal social and work function in about 10% of autistic persons, but the accepted wisdom is that autism is a lifelong condition with behavioral abnormalities continuing even in those who function best. Whether current treatment programs begun early and directed at improving behavior and socialization will alter social adjustment and functional outcome has still to be determined.

CONCLUSION

Infantile autism is a syndrome of deviant development of social, linguistic, and cognitive skills, which affects a child's relation to people, objects, and environmental events. It is present from early in life, is caused by unknown, but probably diverse, neurologic dysfunction, and is manifest in varying degrees of severity. Research into cause and treatment is in a very early stage; work in both areas is hampered by a lack of agreement on definition and insufficient differentiation of homogeneous subgroups. It is important to identify autistic children at the earliest possible time so that attempts to alter maladaptive behaviors through intensive behavioral treatment can be most effective.

BIBLIOGRAPHY

American Psychiatric Association: *Diagnostic and Statistical Manual of Mental Disorders* ed 3, revised. Washington, DC, The Association, 1987; pp 33–39.

Cohen DJ, Donnellan AM: *Handbook of Autism and Pervasive Developmental Disorders*. New York, John Wiley & Sons, 1987.

Coleman M, Gillberg C: *The Biology of the Autistic Syndromes*. New York, Praeger, 1985.

DeMyer MK: *Parents and Children in Autism*. Washington, DC, VH Winston & Sons, 1979.

Journal of Autism and Developmental Disorders. New York, Plenum.

Lovaas OI: Behavioral treatment and normal educational and intellectual functioning in young autistic children. *J Consult Clin Psychol* 1987; 55:3–9.

Park CC: *The Siege*. Boston, Little, Brown & Co, 1982.

Rutter M, Schopler E (eds): *Autism: A Reappraisal of Concepts and Treatment*. New York, Plenum Press, 1978.

Wing L: *Early Childhood Autism*, ed 3. Oxford, England, Pergamon Press, 1984.

76 LEARNING DISABILITY

William G. Sharrar, M.D.

The fundamental requirement placed on a child between the ages of 5 to at least 16 years is school attendance. For many reasons, not all children do well in school. Some reasons for poor school performance are (1) learning disability, (2) mental retardation, (3) attention deficit disorder, (4) poor health, (5) behavioral or emotional disturbances, and (6) environmental disadvantage.

A specific learning disability is but one reason and, by definition, describes the child who has at least normal intelligence and yet has difficulty learning in the traditional way in which most students are taught. The term does not apply to children who have learning problems that are primarily the result of visual, hearing, or motor handicaps; mental retardation; emotional disturbance; or cultural or economic disadvantage. Children with a specific learning disability have difficulty with the perception, organization, storage, and retrieval of information that constitutes learning. The primary distinction is the discrepancy between basic intelligence and achievement levels in such subjects as reading, writing, and arithmetic. This implies that children with learning disabilities, when taught in a different manner, have the ability to learn.

Children with learning disabilities in the past were often referred to as being either hyperactive children or as having minimal cerebral dysfunction. Children who are hyperactive because of attention deficit disorder often do quite well in a regular classroom setting after receiving proper medication whereas many learning disabled children are withdrawn or quiet in a classroom setting and do not appear hyperactive. Minimal cerebral dysfunction on the other hand, is a vague concept implying pathologic function of the central nervous system (CNS) and has little practical meaning to either educators or parents.

Learning disabilities are now called Specific Developmental Disorders in the *Diagnostic and*

Statistical Manual of Mental Disorders (DMS-III-R), and are subdivided into Academic Skills Disorders, Language and Speech Disorders, and Motor Skills Disorders. Academic Skills Disorders primarily involve difficulties with arithmetic, expressive writing, and reading. Language and Speech Disorders primarily involve difficulties with articulation, expressive language, and receptive language. Motor Skills Disorders involve coordination so poor that it interferes with academic performance. For this discussion the general term learning disability is used.

INITIAL IDENTIFICATION AND ASSESSMENT

The primary care physician is often the first person to whom the parents turn when they discover that their child is having difficulty in school. Having the advantage of knowing the child and the family over an extended period of time, the physician often has a knowledge of the child's overall developmental strengths and weakness. Evaluation of the present school problem should begin with a detailed school history that includes the following questions: At what age did the child first attend school? What were the parental reasons for sending the child to school at that time and what was the child's reaction to the initial separation from home? How did the child interact with his peers and what were the parents told by the teacher at the end of the year? When did the teacher first become concerned about behavioral or learning problems? When did the parents first become concerned, and were they surprised by their child's difficulties in school? Are the parents keeping in touch with the school regarding the child's performance? Are they in agreement with the teacher's observations, assessments, and recommendations? Has the school done any testing, or do they intend to? What specific testing or intervention strategies have been tried and what is the parental understanding of these procedures?

These questions can help place in perspective whether the child's difficulties are mainly in school or whether there are also problems elsewhere. Children with primary learning problems often begin school with no difficulty. As the learning demands increase, the child experiences failure and behavior changes. The child can become withdrawn or disruptive in class, and may even refuse to go to school.

The family history should identify the following: Have other family members had school problems? What and how are they doing now? What has been the educational experience of both parents and other siblings? What are parental expectations and hopes for this child? What kind of occupations have the parents pursued? These questions will provide information on how the family views education in general and how much pressure is on the child to perform. There is often a familial pattern of learning problems.

A social history should try to identify stresses at home that may be affecting the child's ability to concentrate. Marital discord or illness in other family members can preoccupy a child's thoughts. If such problems are uncovered, referral for psychiatric evaluation and treatment is necessary.

The medical history should be detailed and address several issues, including the possibility of a neurologic insult that might suggest a neurologic dysfunction as the basis for a learning disability. Were there any difficulties during labor and delivery that necessitated resuscitation and/or oxygen therapy? Was the neonatal course benign without a history of infection, hyperbilirubinemia, or feeding difficulties? Has there been any history of head trauma, seizure disorder, or CNS infection? A detailed developmental history with special reference to language development should be taken. Many children with speech delays are later diagnosed as being learning disabled.

The general medical examination in children with learning disabilities is often essentially normal. An assessment should be made of the child's ability to interact with the examiner. Can the child follow directions, or does he need to be told them several times? Are his speech and language patterns age-appropriate? Does he have spontaneous speech, or is he quiet and sullen? Will the child answer questions, or do the parents speak for him? Vision and hearing should be carefully checked. The presence of "soft" neurologic signs such as poor fine-motor coordination, finger agnosia, and right-left disorientation may represent either neurologic dysfunction or normal variation in neurologic maturation. There are many children with poor coordination who do well in school and, conversely, children who have difficulty in learning who excel in competitive sports.

ADDITIONAL EVALUATIONS

The primary care physician, after a careful history and physical examination, is often left without a clear-cut diagnosis for the cause of a child's poor school performance. Electroencephalograms, computed tomography scans, and blood chemistry analyses are not usually helpful, and formal neurologic consultation may often not be required. A multidisciplinary team evaluation, however, is necessary to pinpoint specifically the cause of the child's learning difficulty and to make recommendations for future educational planning. The composition of this team will vary depending on the community and may include an educational psychologist, speech and language pathologist, and social worker. The team's observations and recommendations are often used in developing the individual educational plans (IEP) for each child. The primary care physician can be vital in providing information to the team about the child's overall health status and can assist in counseling the parents.

It must be emphasized that the diagnosis of a learning disability can only be made after a battery of standardized and individually administered tests are performed that measure both the development of the impaired skills and the person's intellectual capacity. Discrepancies between verbal and performance scores, as well as "scattering" among the various subtests, are often found in children with learning disabilities. Most notable, however, is that the achievement testing of these children lags behind what one would expect based on their full intelligence quotient score. A learning-disabled child will have normal intelligence but may be two years behind other children his age with respect to reading, writing, or arithmetic ability.

Psychologists and/or learning disability specialists are also trained to evaluate the strengths and weaknesses in a child's ability to learn. Areas of evaluation include the child's perceptual motor skills and perceptual skills with respect to hearing and vision. Formal audiometric evaluation may be necessary to determine the child's level of hearing and his ability to process sound. Children with auditory discrimination problems have difficulty distinguishing words that sound alike. Children with auditory-sequential memory problems have difficulty remembering the order of verbal information presented to them. Those children with auditory processing problems learn better by visual means, whereas children with visual-spatial orientation problems or visual tracking problems learn better by listening. Speech and language pathologists may evaluate the child's communication skills in both written and spoken language, for children with reading difficulties often have associated problems in this area.

MANAGEMENT

The primary care physician needs to be knowledgeable about interpreting the test results to the parents and what special educational services are available in the community. The options may range from small, specialized classes to regular classes with time out for resource room help. In general, the major form of management for a learning disability is special education. For children with attention-deficit disorders, psychostimulants may be indicated (see Chapter 77). Antihistamines and megavitamins have been tried without any demonstrated effect. Although visual motor exercises have been recommended by some optometrists for learning problems, no known scientific evidence supports the benefit of visual training exercises. The American Academy of Pediatrics comments that "such training may result in a false sense of security, which may delay or prevent proper instruction or remediation . . . the expense of such procedures is unwarranted."

When to "mainstream" a child in a regular class, promote a child, or retain a child are often difficult situations that need careful exploration by all parties. As a general rule, repeating kindergarten or first grade is easier on a child than having to repeat a grade at a higher level. The child needs to hear from his parents that this is a good thing to do, and will help him to perform better in school.

It is important to realize that the educational environment is highly structured, with specific demands on the child. Many children with learning difficulties in school do quite well in later life. They ultimately choose professions or disciplines that accentuate their strengths and minimize their deficits. The child with difficulty in reading may work where manual skills and verbal directions are used. Children with difficulties in spatial relations may do quite well in a working position that requires verbal skills.

Finally, it is important for the primary care physician and the parents to note consistently the strengths of the child. In this manner the child will develop a good self-esteem and will be encouraged to explore the areas in which he has talent. This diversity among people is actually the strength on which society is based.

SUMMARY

Approximately 10% of children have difficulty learning in school. Some of these children have learning disabilities and require specialized instruction. This can best be determined by a multidisciplinary team of which the primary care physician is only one member. Evaluation must be done in conjunction with the school district. The parents must recognize the strengths and weaknesses of their child. Specialized educational programs should be the major form of management.

BIBLIOGRAPHY

American Psychiatric Association: *Diagnostic and Statistical Manual of Mental Disorders*, ed 3, revised. Washington, DC, The Association, 1987, p 39.

Boder EL: School failure: Evaluation and treatment. *Pediatrics* 1976; 58:395.

Block RW, Miller EK: The maladroit adolescent: Learning disorders and attention deficits. *Adv Pediatr* 1986; 33:303–330.

Committee on Children With Disabilities: Learning disabilities, dyslexia, and vision. *Pediatrics* 1984; 74:150–151.

Hartzell HE, Compton C: Learning disability: 10 year follow-up. *Pediatrics* 1984; 74:1058–1064.

Gottlieb MI, Zinkus PW, Bradford LJ: *Current Issues in Developmental Pediatrics—The Learning Disabled Child*. New York, Grune & Stratton, Inc, 1979.

Levine D, Brooks R, Shonkoff JP: *A Pediatric Approach to Learning Disorders*. New York, John Wiley & Sons Inc., 1980.

Shaywitz S, Grossman JH, Shaywitz B (eds): Learning disorders. *Pediatr Clin North Am* 1984; 31:2.

Silver LV: Acceptable and controversial approaches to treating the child with learning disabilities. *Pediatrics* 1975; 55:406–415.

77 ATTENTION DEFICIT–HYPERACTIVITY DISORDER

Marianne Mercugliano, M.D.

Hyperactivity and short attention span are childhood symptoms that parents often first discuss with their primary care physician. Many children who manifest these symptoms will ultimately fit the diagnostic criteria for attention deficit–hyperactivity disorder (ADHD). These symptoms, however, are often nonspecific and therefore, the primary care physician has a critical role in considering other causes for similar behaviors that may require different treatments. This chapter should assist the physician caring for these children and their families in developing a strategy for evaluating the severity of symptoms, establishing a differential diagnosis, and initiating a comprehensive and coordinated treatment plan.

DEFINITION AND HISTORY

ADHD may be considered a syndrome in that it has a characteristic clinical picture, yet the etiology is poorly understood, associated features are nonspecific, and the predictive value of specific components is limited. Prevalence estimates range from 2% to 20%, depending on the population selected. The most pressing reason to strive to understand and treat ADHD is that it causes significant morbidity for a large number of children. It is estimated that 25% to 50% of children with ADHD will have an associated learning disability. Diagnostic criteria from the *Diagnostic and Statistical Manual of Mental Disorders* (DSM-III-R) include a disturbance of at least 6 months duration with at least eight of the following features present considerably more often than in most children of the same mental age:

1. Fidgets (or has subjective feelings of restlessness in adolescence).
2. Has difficulty remaining seated when required.
3. Is easily distracted.
4. Has difficulty awaiting his or her turn in group situations.
5. Blurts out answers before questions are completed.
6. Has difficulty following instructions or completing tasks.
7. Has difficulty sustaining attention.
8. Shifts from one uncompleted activity to another.
9. Has difficulty playing quietly.
10. Talks excessively.
11. Interrupts or intrudes on others.
12. Does not seem to listen to what is being said to him or her.
13. Loses things.
14. Engages in dangerous activities without considering consequences.

Other requirements include onset before the age of 7 years and absence of pervasive developmental disorder. ADHD can be diagnosed in the presence of mental retardation if the behaviors are out of proportion to those expected for the child's mental age.

In 1902 George Still described a group of children with hyperactivity, attention and learning problems, and conduct disorders. He speculated that a combination of organic and environmental factors lead to this type of behavior. Kahn and Cohen in 1934 noted that children who contracted encephalitis were left with a behavior disorder characterized by hyperactivity. Although this clearly had an organic cause, colleagues noted that environmental manipulations could affect the behavior. Strauss, who studied children with a wide variety and severity of brain insults, theorized that if known brain damage resulted in the syndrome, then perhaps those children manifesting the syndrome in the absence of a known neurologic insult had subtle neurologic deficits not detectable by examination. For several decades the terms minimal cerebral damage or dysfunction and minimal brain damage or dysfunction were used to describe children with hyperactivity with or without learning disabilities and soft neurologic signs. Studies that showed nonspecifically abnormal electroencephalograms (EEGs) as well as studies which retrospectively noted a higher frequency of perinatal complications in behavior-disordered children seemed to support this concept. Ultimately these diagnoses were thought to apply to too heterogeneous a population and the label of hyperkinetic reaction of childhood was adopted in the DSM-III in 1968. It was revised in the 1980 edition to attention deficit disorder with or without hyperactivity. Attention deficit disorder, residual state, was used to refer to persistent attentional difficulties in adolescents who met full criteria at a younger age. In the DSM-III-R (1987), attention deficit disorder with or without hyperactivity has been renamed ADHD and there is no longer a residual state category. The changes in nomenclature reflect increasing recognition that attention and concentration are germinal deficits and that the same disorder has different manifestations at different developmental stages.

EVALUATION

Parental concern about hyperactivity should first be defined more specifically. Symptoms that often cluster with hyperactivity include inattention, poor concentration, impulsivity, distractibility, fidgetiness, low frustration tolerance, difficulty with compliance, and poor social interaction. Age of onset of the problem behaviors and situations in which they exist (situational vs. pervasive hyperactivity) provide further definition. An assessment of whether the behavioral characteristics are indeed abnormal for the child's cognitive level is also crucial. Several questionnaires are available to assist in gathering this type of information. These include the Conners Parent and Teacher Questionnaires, the Achenbach Child Behavior Profile, the ADHD Comprehensive Teacher Rating Scales (ACTRS), and the Yale Children's Personal Data Inventory/Yale Teacher's Behavior Rating Scale. It is important that questionnaires be completed by multiple observers, usually parent(s) and teacher(s). If the child's behavior is not thought to be outside the normal range, it may be useful to explore the possibility that other family stresses are making it more difficult to cope with normal childhood activity and inquisitiveness. Not infrequently a child with a manageable degree of ADHD symptoms presents when family issues or academic factors overstress his or her limited ability to cope and lead to an exacerbation of difficult behaviors.

DIFFERENTIAL DIAGNOSIS

If information provided by both parents and teachers reveals that activity level or attention span are not age appropriate, the primary care physician must then investigate other possible causes for these behaviors. ADHD is one cause, but there are others with the same symptoms and that require different treatment, and these should be sought first. These non-ADHD symptoms may be medical/neurologic, educational/cognitive, or social/emotional.

Medical/neurologic causes include medications (e.g., anticonvulsants, antihistamines and "mixed" cold preparations, theophylline), visual or hearing impairment, untreated absence or partial complex seizures, lead poisoning, anemia, hyperthyroidism, poor sleep patterns as in obstructive sleep apnea, and neurodegenerative diseases (particularly the leukodystrophies, Wilson's disease, and Sanfilippo-type mucopolysaccharidosis). Other neurologic conditions such as mass lesions of the brain and neurocutaneous syndromes may present with cognitive or behavioral symptoms, but usually there are additional signs and symptoms. Other syndromes that frequently have ADHD as a component include fetal alcohol syndrome, Dubowitz syndrome, and Tourette's syndrome.

Educational/cognitive causes refer to undiagnosed learning disabilities, communication disorder, mental retardation, or pervasive developmental disorder (autism) in a child who is therefore educationally misplaced. Behavioral symptoms can arise when a child faces expectations from parents and teachers that are consistently beyond his or her capabilities. Social/emotional causes include chaotic family environment; physical, sexual, or emotional abuse; and psychiatric conditions, particularly mood and anxiety disorders.

The primary care physician's objective is to rule out other treatable conditions with a thorough history, general physical examination, and neurologic examination. Referral to a pediatric neurologist is recommended if specific concerns (focal examination findings, seizures, or a degenerative course) are raised by the initial history and examination. Routine EEGs and computed tomography scans are not indicated. For social/emotional concerns, a social worker, psychologist, or professional with similar training should evaluate the child and family interaction and individual functioning. Referral to a child psychiatrist is recommended if concerns about psychopathologic conditions are raised. For educational concerns, a thorough developmental assessment must be performed. For the preschooler, an assessment focusing on cognitive skills (receptive and expressive language and visual-motor problem-solving) by a psychologist or developmental pediatrician is appropriate. If language problems are suspected, an evaluation by a speech and language pathologist should be done to assist with diagnosis and treatment planning. For the school-aged child, both cognitive (intelligence quotient) and academic achievement testing by a psychologist and perhaps a special educator are required to distinguish mild global cognitive delay (mild mental retardation) and learning disabilities.

Clearly, the chief complaint of short attention span or hyperactivity requires a complex assessment before ADHD, which is a diagnosis of exclusion, can be made. Further complicating the diagnostic process is the fact that many children with ADHD have learning or psychosocial problems as well. The primary care physician may prefer to be the central coordinator of the evaluation using individual consultants as needed and subsequently providing a synthesis of the results and recommendations for the family. Alternatively, the family may be referred to an interdisciplinary team that specializes in the evaluation of school, behavioral, and developmental problems. Such teams may be found in the child development or child psychiatry divisions of pediatric medical centers or through the school system. The team usually consists of one or more physicians (developmental pediatrician, child psychiatrist, pediatric neurologist), a social worker, and a psychologist with expertise in testing and behavior management. Other consultants such as the special educator, speech and language pathologist, audiologist, and occupational therapist are available to the team. The advantage of the team approach is that the evaluators discuss their results together, directly resulting in a better overall understanding of the child and family. Since the evaluations of different professionals may overlap in some areas, the opportunity to have findings corroborated by others as well as the necessity to explain discrepant results may lead to a more in-depth assessment. The need for stepwise intervention and reevaluation may be met more easily by a team as this can be a time and labor-intensive condition to treat. The pediatrician may retain primary responsibility for treatment and follow-up if desired, with guidance from the team, if needed. It should be noted that a comprehensive, multidisciplinary baseline assessment is becoming the standard of care for children with possible ADHD, particularly when medication is being considered.

TREATMENT

Treatment of ADHD consists of educational, behavioral, and medication intervention. Educational intervention consists of providing the necessary additional help required for the child to master academic skills. It also includes implementing strategies for reducing distractibility in the classroom such as having the child sit at the front of the class near the teacher, providing a carrel for use during independent work, and allowing frequent short breaks or changes in type of activity.

Counseling for the child and family is an important part of treatment and must be presented as such. The main type of counseling used is behavior modification therapy. Parents work with a trained professional (usually, but not always, a psychologist) to learn how to modify the antecedents and consequences of specific behaviors such that positive behaviors are encouraged and negative ones discouraged. This is a labor-intensive undertaking because parents must first learn to become systematic objective observers of the child's behavior, and then must be extremely consistent in applying the techniques they have developed with the psychologist. Parents may become discouraged because changes do not occur as quickly as they would like, but behavior modification has been shown to be effective in improving behavior and academic productivity. Other types of counseling can be helpful in selected cases. The older, insightful child may benefit from individual, cognitively oriented therapy to work on "self-modifying" certain behaviors, as well as self-esteem and social skills. Family therapy can be helpful in resolving specific family issues that may create tension and contribute to increased negative behavior. In addition, family therapy can be helpful in ameliorating the stress experienced by most families raising a child with ADHD. Parents need support since they are often made to think that poor parenting skills are the source of their child's difficulty. When parents do not perceive their child in the same way, or have the same views about discipline, marital discord may result, with the child sensing that he or she is to blame. Finally, the therapist can help a family find ways to ensure that all members' needs are met in a supportive, consistent way, creating the optimal home environment for the child with ADHD.

Methylphenidate (Ritalin), dextroamphetamine (Dexedrine), and magnesium pemoline (Cylert) are the stimulant medications most commonly used to treat ADHD. It has been proposed that children with ADHD have deficient mesocortical dopaminergic transmission, affecting circuits between the frontal lobes and basal ganglia. A modulating loop between the frontal lobes and brain stem reticular activating system may also be involved. Methylphenidate and dextroamphetamine facilitate synthesis and release of norepinephrine and dopamine and inhibit the catabolic enzyme, monoamine oxidase. Methylphenidate also blocks monoamine reuptake. Pemoline is an indirect dopamine agonist with fewer sympathomimetic effects.

Stimulants have been shown to improve several aspects of functioning from attention and impulsivity to social and fine motor skills. Improvements in scholastic achievement are controversial and despite substantial improvements in day-to-day functioning, improved long-term outcome has not been clearly documented. This may be a reflection of the importance of other factors, such as educational intervention, family support, and individual characteristics. Certainly pharmacologic management will accomplish little by itself.

Medication is recommended when educational and behavioral intervention are insufficient. The primary care physician must have a plan for evaluating efficacy and side effects. There isn't a single correct way to manage medication for ADHD, but some general principles are important. The family history should be reviewed relative to tics, movement disorders, and neurodegenerative disease. The child's current review of systems should be noted as well as other medications frequently used. Baseline vital signs, including blood pressure, and growth parameters should be obtained. Several parent and teacher rating scales should be completed before medication is started. It is important to speak with the child directly, in age-appropriate terms, about the nature of his or her difficulty and the purpose of medication. In particular, fears of being "bad," "stupid," or "sick" must be addressed. The child should be encouraged to discuss the effects of the medication with parents.

Generally, a dose of 0.3 mg/kg of methylphenidate or dextroamphetamine is given before school and response is monitored by several parent and teacher rating scales. The dose may be increased by approximately 0.1 mg/kg weekly until no further benefit is seen or side effects emerge. It is important to assess more than just activity-related items as the optimal dose for improving attention may be smaller than that required for a substantial decrease in physical activity. The lowest dose that results in significant improvement should be used to reduce the risk of side effects. A second dose is often required at lunch-time as the behavioral effects usually last about 3 to 4 hours. Older children may benefit from an after-school dose to assist with homework or structured after-school activities. While some children who receive a dose late in the day will experience insomnia, others who are restless at night may actually sleep better. Many children experience "rebound" as the medication wears off (worsening of baseline symptoms). This may be managed by using progressively smaller doses throughout the day, or for some children, by switching to slow-release capsules. The slow-release, long-acting forms of methylphenidate and dextroamphetamine may allow some children to take medication only once a day, but variable absorption and lack of longer effect can be problems.

Pemoline is given as a single daily dose of 37.5 mg before school and may take 3 to 4 weeks to begin to take effect. The dose may then be increased by 18.75 mg weekly as needed for optimal effect. Approximately 2.25 mg/kg is usually required. Hypersensitivity reactions involving the liver have occurred, making this a second-line choice and necessitating baseline and periodic liver function tests.

The *Physicians' Desk Reference* (Medical Economics Co., Oradell, N.J.) contains an extensive list of reported side effects of stimulants. Those that occur with sufficient regularity to warrant specific anticipatory guidance include insomnia, decreased appetite, dysphoria, irritability, stomachache, headache, weight loss, and small increases in heart rate or blood pressure. Long-term side effects, which are less common but of greater concern, include precipitation of tics and decreased growth. Stimulants are reported to decrease the seizure threshold so careful attention should be paid to maintaining therapeutic anticonvulsant levels in children who require both types of medication.

When properly prescribed and carefully monitored, stimulants appear to be quite safe. There is currently no evidence to suggest that adverse neurobehavioral outcomes are related to medication use in childhood. Appropriate monitoring cannot be overstressed, particularly since most children who benefit from stimulants will need to take them for several years. First, it is imperative that parents have the opportunity to see their child on and off medication during the therapeutic trial so that they may take an active role in assessing its effect. This may be accomplished by having the child take medication on one of the weekend days initially, or by having parents observe their child in a structured activity such as school, sports, or religious instruction with and without medication. Second, several parent and teacher rating scales are required at each dose to obtain the most accurate assessment of effect. Third, during dose adjustment, phone contact every 1 to 2 weeks to discuss side effects is important. Frequent checks of heart rate, blood pressure, and weight are done initially. Once a stable dose is reached, examinations can be done at 3- to 6-month intervals. Fourth, every child deserves an annual trial off medication during the school year so that efficacy can be reassessed.

Parents will frequently raise questions about controversial causes and therapies for ADHD. Immunologic mechanisms and the role of dietary substances are currently under investigation. Large well-controlled studies of additive-free or low-sugar diets have not supported these as causes for the dysfunction. It is certainly possible, however, that selected groups of children have different metabolic characteristics which would be obscured by unselected population studies. If parents elect to try controversial therapies, the primary care physician's responsibility is the same: to help them objectively monitor efficacy and to avoid possible negative consequences.

SUMMARY

ADHD is a common, clinically reproducible disorder. Although in some respects little is known about specific organic cause, enough evidence exists to conclude that there is an organic basis for this type of dysfunction. Psychosocial and environmental factors are likely to play a significant role in associated symptoms and perhaps outcome. Treatment may include educational intervention, behavior modification, other types of counseling, and medication. The role of the primary care physician is to rule out other causes of similar symptoms with the aid of consultants, to educate the family about the disorder and available community resources, to provide anticipatory guidance about the particular issues that impact on the child and family at different developmental stages, and to monitor the efficacy and side effects of treatment.

BIBLIOGRAPHY

American Psychiatric Association: *Diagnostic and Statistical Manual of Mental Disorders*, ed 3, revised. Washington, DC, American Psychiatric Association, 1987, pp 50–53.

Barkley RA: *Hyperactive Children: A Handbook for Diagnosis and Treatment*. New York, Guilford Press, 1981.

Kandt RS: Neurologic examination of children with learning disorders. *Pediatr Clin North Am* 1984; 31:297–315.

Shaywitz SE, Shaywitz BA: Diagnosis and management of ADD: A pediatric perspective. *Pediatr Clin North Am* 1984; 31:429–445.

Sleater EK, Pelham WE, Carey WB: Attention Deficit Disorder, in Cornfeld D, Silverman BK (eds): *Dialogues in Pediatric Management Series*, vol 1, no 3. Norwalk, Conn, Appleton-Century-Crofts, 1986.

Weiss G, Hechtman LT: *Hyperactive Children Grown Up: Empirical Findings and Theoretical Considerations*. New York, Guilford Press, 1986.

78 OFFICE DEVELOPMENTAL SCREENING

Susan E. Levy, M.D.

Routine developmental screening of infants and children by primary care physicians is an effective tool for early identification of developmental disabilities that cause school-related and other problems. The range of developmental disabilities includes motor impairment (e.g., cerebral palsy), cognitive impairment (e.g., mental retardation), or communication disorders (e.g., learning disabilities). During the first 18 months of life, it is easiest to measure motor progress; however, the most common symptom of developmental disability in childhood is delayed development of speech and language, affecting 5% to 10% of all children. Language is the best predictor of future intellectual development, and should be the basis of cognitive assessment in the infant and young child.

Early identification of the child with developmental disability allows for referral to appropriate diagnostic and treatment programs. These resources often assist in improving the functional status of the child and family, while providing appropriate educational opportunities and specific intervention services to mitigate the disability.

Office developmental screening should be a three-part process that must include history, physical examination, and developmental screening tests. A thorough medical, family, and developmental history is necessary. A number of medical historical risk factors of the mother's pregnancy and at the time of delivery may alert the primary care physician of increased likelihood of developmental disability (Table 78–1). In addition, a family history of

TABLE 78–1
Medical Historical Risk Factors for Developmental Disabilities

Prenatal
Maternal illness
Maternal infection
Maternal malnutrition
Exposure to toxins
Exposure to teratogens
Abnormal fetal movement
Low birth weight
Perinatal
Asphyxia
Abnormal presentation
Trauma
Placental dysfunction
Postnatal
Infection
Complications of prematurity
Asphyxia or anoxia
Seizures
Presence of congenital defects or syndrome
Hyperbilirubinemia
Poor nutrition or feeding difficulties
Abnormal sleep patterns
Central nervous system trauma
Dysmorphic features

mental retardation, delayed speech, communication disorder, or other developmental disabilities should raise the clinician's index of suspicion for a genetic-based developmental disorder. Several clinical features (neurodevelopmental markers) of the child should alert the primary care physician to the increased risk of developmental disability (Table 78–2). Parental estimate of the level of developmental functioning is helpful and has been found to be an accurate predictor of developmental status. Parents may be aided in recall of developmental milestones by bringing their child's baby book to the visit. Review of attainment of developmental milestones helps to establish the rate of development and consistency across different developmental streams when compared to norms described by Illingworth and others (Table 78–3). Slowed rates of development in cognitive and communication streams may be

TABLE 78–2
Neurodevelopmental Markers for Developmental Disabilities*

Parental concerns about delayed development
Suspected mental retardation
Lack of language development (in absence of deafness)
Patient acts as if deaf or blind
Behavioral disturbance
Excessive irritability or lethargy in infancy
Feeding dysfunction or poor sucking
Microcephaly
Dysmorphic physical features
Delay in disappearance of primitive reflexes
Hyperactive or hypoactive fetus
Abnormal fetal presentation
Excessive irritability or lethargy in infancy

*These risk factors may be obtained by parental interview or by direct observation and are listed in descending order of importance.

TABLE 78–3
Developmental Milestones*

Gross motor	**Fine motor/adaptive**
Chin up (1 mo)	Unfisting (3 mo)
Head up (wrists) (4 mo)	Reach and grasp (5 mo)
Roll (prone to supine) (4 mo)	Transfer (6 mo)
Roll (supine to prone) (5 mo)	Handedness (24 mo)
Sit alone (8 mo)	**Feeding**
Pull to stand (9 mo)	Fingers (10 mo)
Cruise (10 mo)	Spoon (15 mo)
Walk alone (13 mo)	Fork (21 mo)
Stairs (mark time; 20 mo)	Independent feed (36 mo)
Stairs (alternate feet; 30 mo)	**Dressing/self-help**
Tricycle (36 mo)	Cooperate (12 mo)
Two-wheeler (36 mo)	Pull off socks (15 mo)
	Unbutton (30 mo)
	Button (48 mo)
	Shoe tying (60 mo)
Receptive language	**Expressive Language**
Social smile (6–8 wk)	Coo (3 mo)
Recognize mother (3 mo)	Babble (6 mo)
Laugh (4 mo)	Da-da (inappropriate) (8 mo)
Gesture games (9 mo)	Da/ma (appropriate) (10 mo)
Understand "no" (9 mo)	First word (11 mo)
One-step command (12 mo)	Second word (12 mo)
Two-step command (24 mo)	Two to 6 words (15 mo)
	Two-word phrases (21 mo)
	Two-word sentences (24 mo)
	Three-word sentences (36 mo)
	Echolalia (9–30 mo)
	Four colors (48 mo)

*Adapted from: Illingworth RS: *The Development of the Infant and Young Child: Normal and Abnormal.* New York, Churchill Livingstone, 1987.

indicative of mental retardation, while a slowed rate in the motor sphere alone may be indicative of cerebral palsy. The rate of developmental progress may be assessed over time, at 3- to 6-month intervals, to determine if the delay is consistent. Significant delays in developmental progress should result in referral for more complete diagnostic assessment.

During the physical examination, particular attention should be directed to identifying abnormalities in growth (especially head circumference), dysmorphic facial or musculoskeletal features, dermal lesions (which may be characteristic of specific neurocutaneous syndromes), and neurologic abnormalities (i.e., hypotonia, hypertonia, asymmetric movements, or persistence of primitive reflexes).

A number of standardized developmental screening tests are available for use by the primary care practitioner. They differ in the scope of abilities examined: some assess language development (Peabody Picture Vocabulary Test—Revised [PPVT-R]), others test fine motor and conceptual development (Goodenough Draw-a-Person Test) or examine a broader range of functions (Denver Developmental Screening Test). The amount of time for administration (range 2 to 3 minutes to 45 minutes) and training required for administration also differ. The ideal screening test is quick, simple, inexpensive, reliable, and accurate. No single developmental screening tool meets these requirements. The primary care practitioner should be adept at administering several of the screening tests (e.g., a general and language based tool) in a standardized fashion to facilitate accuracy and promote identification of children at high risk for developmental disability.

DEVELOPMENTAL SCREENING TESTS (TABLE 78–4)

DENVER DEVELOPMENTAL SCREENING TEST

The Denver Developmental Screening Test (DDST) is administered to children aged 1 month to 5 years and measures a child's performance in four areas of function against that of a standardization sample. It was devised by the selection of 105 items from other developmental preschool intelligence scales. Periodic screening should occur at 3 to 6, 9 to 12, and 18 to 24 months and at 3, 4, and 5 years of age.

The tasks are arranged in four major sectors of function: personal/social, fine motor-adaptive, language, and gross motor. A vertical line placed at the child's chronologic age determines which tasks the child should perform. As the child passes or fails an item, a "P" or "F" is placed on each task. For scoring, inability to perform any item to the left of the vertical age line is a delay (Fig 78–1). The number and location of delays in each sector determines a total test result, categorized as either abnormal, questionable, or normal (Table 78–5).

Administration of the full test takes 15 to 20 minutes. Children with abnormal, questionable, or untestable results should be rescreened after 2 weeks. If results are consistent, referral should be made for further diagnosis and possible intervention services. A shortened version of the DDST takes 5 to 10 minutes and identifies those children who are likely to have abnormal or questionable results when given a full DDST. The short form of the DDST uses only 12 items, with three items in each sector to the left of each bar administered. If there are no failures or refusals, the test is considered nonsuspect, and no further testing is necessary until the next age for periodic testing.

Many studies have examined the validity of this screening tool. Weaknesses include assessment of language abilities, (especially after 3 years of age), and screening in high-risk populations. The standardization population had few minorities represented, and the test may be culturally biased.

DRAW-A-PERSON TEST

The draw-a-person (DAP; Goodenough-Harris drawing test) is a widely used screening test for fine motor and conceptual development. The child aged 3 years and older is asked to draw a person, which can be scored, based on the child's accuracy of observations and conceptual development, approximating a mental age. Points are assigned for each feature of the drawing (Table 78–6). This test does not provide information about the child's language or gross motor development.

TABLE 78–4
Developmental Screening Tests

	AGE	FUNCTION TESTED	RESULTS	COMMENTS	TIME (MIN)	ADMINISTRATION	SOURCE
General							
Denver Developmental Screening Test (DDST)	1–60 mo	Sectors of function: personal/social fine motor/adaptive language gross motor	Normal Abnormal or questionable Rescreen in 2 wk Refer if persists	Weaknesses in assessing language abilities and standardization sample	15–20 Short form 5–10	Parental interview Observation Direct testing	LADOCA Pub Foundation, E 51st Ave & Lincoln St, Denver, CO 80216
Goodenough Draw-A-Person Test	3–8 yr	Fine motor/conceptual	Mental age	No information on language or gross motor development	5	Child performs	The Psychological Corp, 1732 Peachtree St NE, Atlanta, GA 30309
Pediatric Examination of Educational Readiness (PEER)	3–5 yr	Neurodevelopmental examination; observe behavior and coping skills, and strategies during performance of age-appropriate tasks	Qualitative assessments of strengths and weaknesses	Duration of administration	30–45	Interview Test administration (training)	Educators Publishing Service, Cambridge, MA
Language							
Peabody Picture Vocabulary Test—Revised (PPVT-R), forms L and M	26 mo–18 yr	Single word	Vocabulary age and standard	Difficulty generalizing conclusion of overall language and cognitive abilities; cultural bias	10–15	Test administration	American Guidance Service, Publishers Bldg, Circle Pines, MN 55014
Bzoch-League Receptive-Expressive Emergent Language Scale (REEL)	1 mo–3 yr	Receptive and expressive language skills	Receptive, expressive, and combined language age and language quotients	Primarily parent interview; standardized sample small	10–15	Parental interview Observation	University Park Press, 233 E Redwood St, Baltimore, MD 21202
Clinical Linguistic Auditory Milestone Scale (CLAMS)	0–2 yr	Receptive (language comprehension) and expressive (language production)	DQs computed: <60, refer ≤80 twice, refer	In process of standardizing samples in normal population	5–10	Observation Parental interview	*Dev Med Child Neurol* 1986; 28:762–771
Early Language Milestone Scale (ELM)	0–3 yr	Sectors: auditory expressive, auditory receptive, visual	Pass or fail		1–3	Interview, observation, test administration	Modern Education Corp, PO Box 721, Tulsa, OK 74101

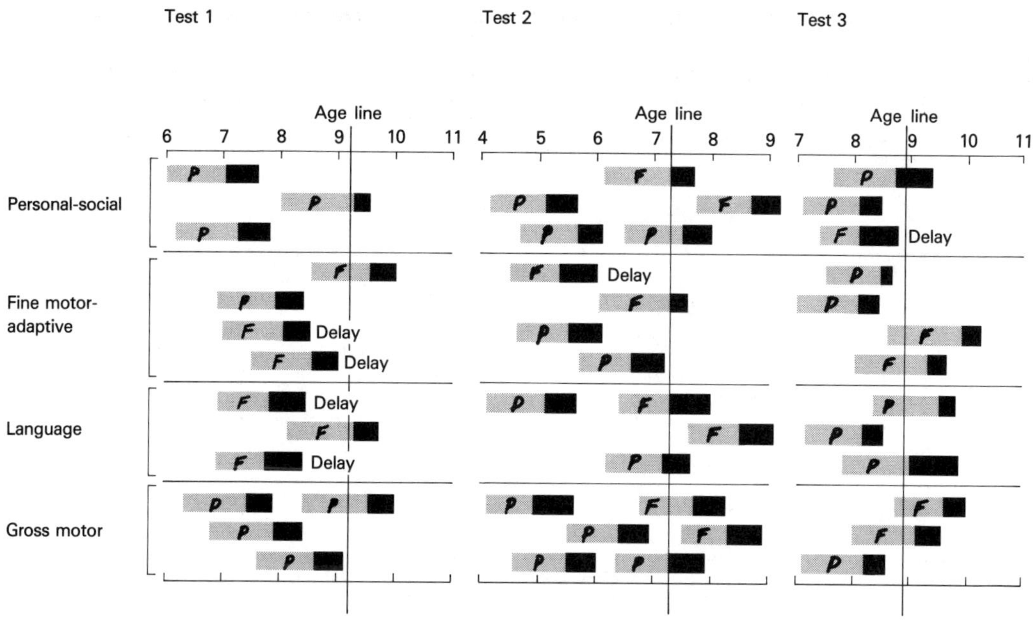

FIG 78–1

Denver Developmental Screening Test. Age is given in months. **Test 1,** *abnormal: two major sectors with two delays.* **Test 2,** *questionable: one delay and age line does not go through a passed item in the same sector.* **Test 3,** *normal: one delay but age line goes through a passed item.*

THE PEDIATRIC EXAMINATION OF EDUCATIONAL READINESS (PEER)

The PEER is a standardized observation system designed to predict school performance in the earliest grades and to uncover the need for special services or further evaluations. It includes a physical examination, sensory assessment, and a comprehensive medical and developmental historical review. The multilevel observation of function provides information about the child's developmental attainment, processing efficiency, and neurologic maturation. Simultaneously there is an assessment of the child's behavioral adaptation to the examination, with observations of adaptability, general responsiveness, cooperativeness, and reinforceability. The report provides a profile of strengths and weaknesses, with observations of behavior and attention, resulting in a composite picture of "educational readiness." The neurodevelopmental section of the PEER requires 20 to 30 minutes to complete, with 10 to 15 minutes for the physical and sensory examinations. This may be too lengthy for a routine health supervision visit.

TABLE 78–5
Denver Developmental Screening Test Categories of Scoring

Abnormal	Two sectors having ≥2 delays; one sector with ≥2 delays and one or more sectors with one delay and in that same sector no passes intersecting the age line
Questionable	Two or more delays in one sector; one or more sectors having one delay without the chronologic line intersecting a passed item
Normal	Neither abnormal nor questionable
Untestable	Refusals occur in numbers large enough to cause the test result to be questionable or abnormal if they were scored as failures

TABLE 78–6
Goodenough-Harris Draw-a-Person Test Scoring System

ONE POINT ASSIGNED PER FEATURE:	
Head present	Opposition of thumb shown (must include fingers)
Neck present	Hands present
Neck, two dimensions	Arms present
Eyes present	Arms at side or engaged in activity
Eye detail: brows or lashes	Feet: any indication
Nose present	Attachment of arms to legs I (to trunk anywhere)
Nose, two dimensions (not round ball)	Attachment of arms and legs II (at correct point on trunk)
Mouth present	Trunk present
Lips, two dimensions	Trunk in proportion, two dimensions (length greater than breadth)
Both nose and lips in two dimensions	Clothing I (anything)
Both chin and forehead shown	Clothing II (two articles of clothing)
Bridge of nose (straight to eyes; narrower than base)	
Hair I (any scribble)	
Hair II (more detail)	
Ears present	
Fingers present	
Correct number of fingers shown	

MENTAL AGE (YR)	POINTS SCORED BY BOYS	POINTS SCORED BY GIRLS
3	4	5
4	7	7
5	11	11
6	13	14
7	16	17
8	18	20

LANGUAGE-BASED SCREENING TOOLS

PEABODY PICTURE VOCABULARY TEST—REVISED

The Peabody Picture Vocabulary Test—Revised (PPVT-R) assesses single-word receptive language skills in children 2 to 18 years of age. The child is shown a series of plates with four pictures and given a stimulus word that must be matched with one of the pictures. Scoring results in a single word receptive vocabulary age and a standard score. Some drawbacks of this test are its unrepresentative standardization sample, cultural bias with some pictures, and difficulty with generalizing conclusions as to overall language and cognitive abilities based on single-word receptive vocabulary.

BZOCH-LEAGUE RECEPTIVE-EXPRESSIVE EMERGENT LANGUAGE SCALE FOR MEASUREMENT OF LANGUAGE SKILLS IN INFANCY

This Receptive-Expressive Emergent Language Scale (REEL) screens the level of receptive and expressive language skills in children aged 1 month to 3 years. It is administered by parental interview, with attempts to confirm questionable items by direct observation of the child. Items of receptive and expressive language skills are grouped in various intervals over 36 months. For example, for the age interval 1 to 2 months, receptive language items include "Frequently gives direct attention to other voices; appears to listen to speaker; often looks at speaker and responds by smiling;" expressive language items include, "Has a special cry for hunger; sometimes repeats the same syllable while cooing or babbling; develops vocal signs of pleasure." The items in each interval are scored as plus, minus, or plus-minus. The infant obtains credit for an age interval when he scores a plus in at least two of the three items. Results are scored as a receptive, expressive, and combined language age and language quotients may be computed for the highest age interval obtained. Drawbacks of this test include that it is primarily parent interview and the standardization sample is unrepresentative and small.

CLINICAL LINGUISTIC AND AUDITORY MILESTONE SCALE

The Clinical Linguistic and Auditory Milestone Scale (CLAMS) is a new tool that assesses language skills in children 0 to 24 months old, using a series of questions to determine the age of attainment of linguistic and auditory milestones. Both receptive (language comprehension) and expressive (language production) milestones are included. Ages of attainment are recorded to the nearest month and compared with norms described. Ages of attainment of receptive and expressive milestones may then be plotted on a graph demonstrating the normal data (Figs 78–2, 78–3). Infants whose attainment of milestones is consistently later than the tenth percentile are at risk of language and cognitive delay.

EARLY LANGUAGE MILESTONE SCALE

The Early Language Milestone (ELM) Scale assesses language development in children age 0 to 3 years. It is administered with the ELM

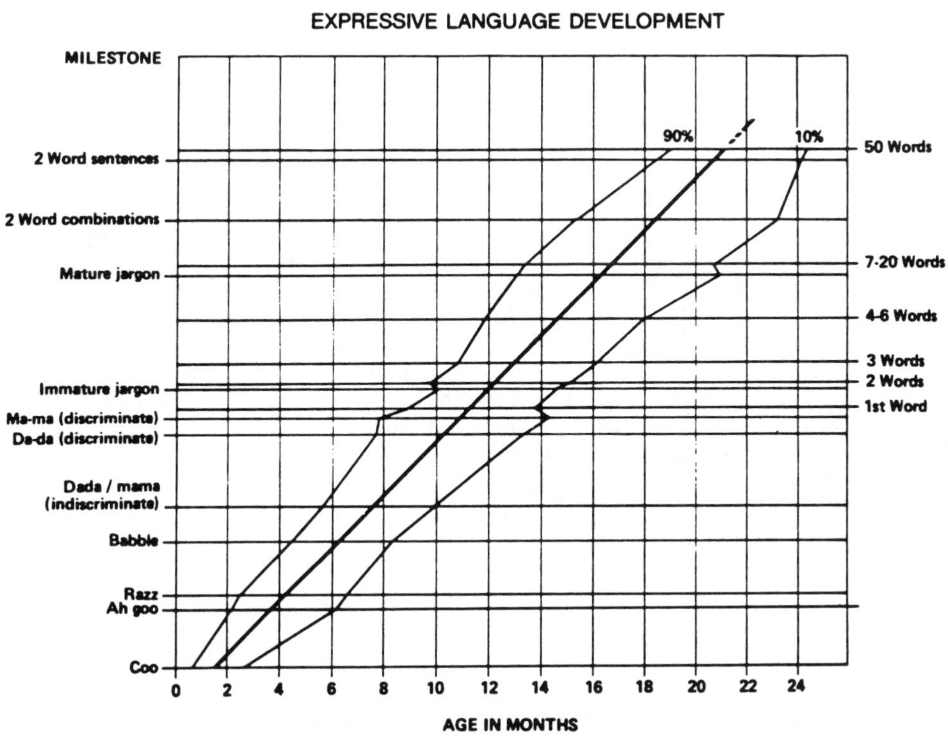

FIG 78–2

Expressive language milestones; 90th and 10th percentiles for normal population. Infants whose attainment of milestones is consistently later than 10th percentile are at risk for language and cognitive delay. Slope of line through median of each milestone is 1.0 and corresponds to developmental quotient of 100. Milestone attainment can be plotted to depict rate of development as well as plateau or degeneration patterns. (From Capute AJ, Palmer FB, Shapiro BK, et al: *Dev Med Child Neurol* 1986; 28:762–771. Used by permission.)

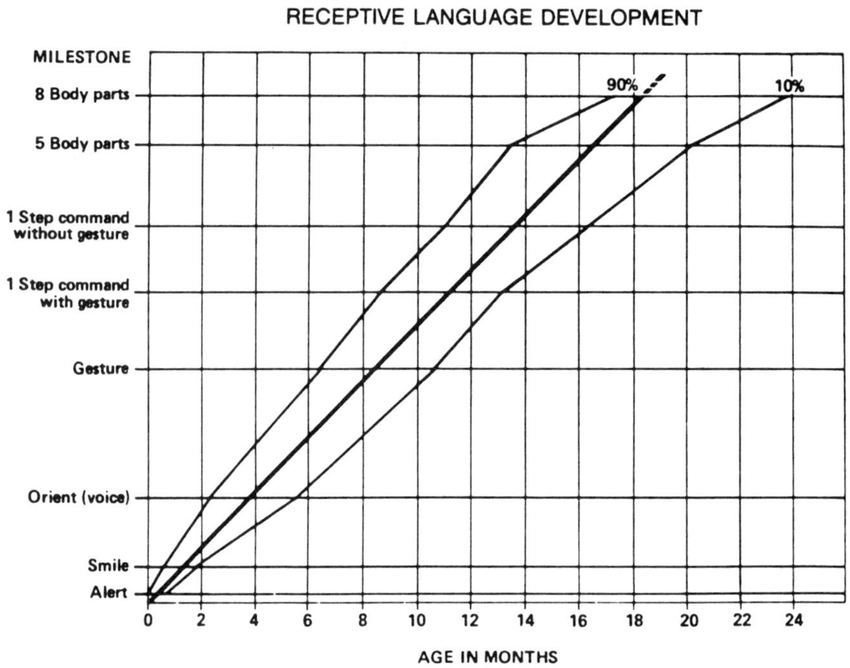

FIG 78–3

Receptive language milestones; 90th and 10th percentiles for normal population (see legend for Fig 78–2). (From Capute AJ, Palmer FB, Shapiro BK, et al: *Dev Med Child Neurol* 1986; 28:762–771. Used by permission.)

Scale recording sheet, drinking cup, spoon, crayon, 3-inch rubber ball, and one 1-inch wooden cube, in 1 to 3 minutes. The 41 items of the scale are divided into three sections: auditory expressive (AE), auditory receptive (AR), and visual (V). The ELM Scale is passed only if each division of the scale (AE, AR, V) is passed.

A vertical line is placed at the child's chronologic age. A base score is attained by proceeding backward until three consecutive items in each division are passed (Fig 78–4). A passing score is obtained if a child achieves the base score without failing any items already attained by more than 90% of children. If one or more items that have already been attained by more than 90% of children are failed, then work forward from the chronologic age until three consecutive items in that division are failed. The 50% value of the highest item passed in each division is the ceiling level. If the ceiling level is greater than or equal to chronologic age, then ELM Scale is passed. If the ceiling level is less than chronologic age, then ELM Scale is failed.

REFERRAL

Children suspected of having developmental delay and/or a specific developmental disability should be referred to a team of developmental specialists for further medical and developmental diagnostic assessment. This team may include developmental pediatricians, child neurologists, pediatric geneticists, child psychologists, special education teachers, occupational therapists, physical therapists, and/or speech/language pathologists. Further evaluation should include formal psychological test-

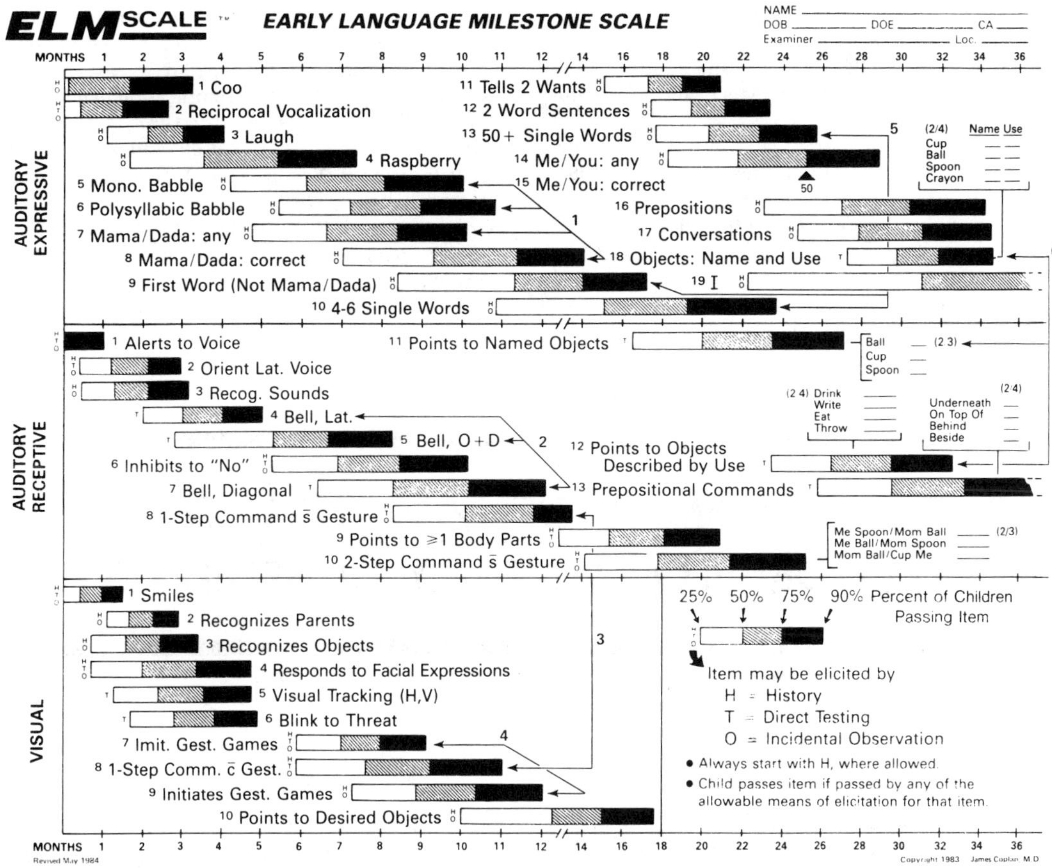

FIG 78–4

Early Language Milestone (ELM) Scale sheet. (From Coplan J: *The Early Language Milestone Scale [ELM Scale]*. Tulsa, Modern Education Corp, 1987. Used by permission.)

ing with such infant tests as the Bayley Scales of Infant Development, the Gesell Developmental Schedules, or the Catell Infant Intelligence Scale. In older children, other tests such as the Stanford-Binet Intelligence Scale, Wechsler Preschool and Primary Scale of Intelligence (WPPSI), Wechsler Intelligence Scale for Children—Revised (WISC-R), and others may be used to determine the level of cognitive or intellectual function.

SUMMARY

Developmental screening in an office setting can be effective when a comprehensive history, physical examination, and selected standardized developmental screening tests are used. A sense of the range of the child's developmental abilities can be determined when tools assessing general and language abilities are used in conjunction.

The primary care physician, therefore, has the first opportunity for early identification of a developmental disability and prevention of secondary complications. Although additional diagnostic and management recommendations may be provided by a consultant team of developmental specialists, the primary care physician maintains the active role as a case manager, and provides ongoing support for the child and family while monitoring medical status and developmental progress in the child.

BIBLIOGRAPHY

Capute AJ, Palmer FB, Shapiro BK, et al: Clinical Linguistic and Auditory Milestone Scale: Prediction

of cognition in infancy. *Dev Med Child Neurol* 1986; 28:762–771.
Capute AJ, Accardo PJ: Linguistic and auditory milestones during the first two years of life. *Clin Pediatr* 1978; 13:847–853.
Cohen HJ, Biehl R, Crain LS, et al: Screening for developmental disabilities. *Pediatrics* 1986; 78:526–528.
Coplan J: Parental estimate of child's developmental level in a high-risk population. *Am J Dis Child* 1982; 136:101–104.
Frankenburg WK, Thornton SM, Cohrs ME (eds): *Pediatric Developmental Diagnosis.* New York, Thieme-Stratton, 1981.
Illingworth RS: *The Development of the Infant and Young Child: Normal and Abnormal,* ed 9. New York, Churchill Livingstone, 1987.
Kaminer R, Jedrysek E: Early identification of developmental disabilities. *Pediatr Ann* 1982; 11:420–437.
Knobloch H, Pasmanick B: *Gesell and Amatruda's Developmental Diagnosis,* ed 3. Hagerstown, Md, Harper & Row, 1974.
Levine MD, Carey WB, Crocker AC, et al: *Developmental-Behavioral Pediatrics.* Philadelphia, WB Saunders Co, 1983.

79 DYNAMICS OF FAMILIES WITH A DEVELOPMENTALLY DISABLED CHILD

David N. Swank, M.S.W.

Under normal circumstances, the conception and birth of a child into a family presents a process of adaptation for every member of that family. With the birth of a child with a developmental disability, there are potential challenges and crises that may have a profound and long-term effect on every family member. The primary care physician needs to be familiar with the impact of the disability on the parents, siblings, and affected child. This chapter will explore some of the pertinent concepts that relate to families with a developmentally disabled child and will draw some implications that should facilitate the physician's relationship with these families.

PARENTS

When a developmental disability is diagnosed in a child, the parents are presented with a crisis that has stressful consequences. There are several affective states of parental reaction to the diagnosis. Within the first state—shock—there are frequently feelings of grief and depression. The second state may be denial of the child's problem. This defense temporarily shields the parents from the force of the crisis. The third state of the reaction, which many times is coupled with denial, consists of sadness, anger, and anxiety. The fourth state is one of adaptation and/or equilibrium, in which the previous intense feelings begin to subside. The last state of initial reaction is reorganization or adjustment. Here, parents begin to sort out their feelings and begin to deal with their responsibilities toward their child. Throughout all stages, there is often a parental mourning process for the "normal" child that they had or wanted to have. Parents often progress at different rates through these stages and there may be delayed reactions to the stress.

As a child with a disability develops, the family may experience a chronic sorrow that is not time-bound but rather is accentuated when each anticipated developmental milestone is not achieved on time. This chronic sorrow will be an enduring aspect of family life, since some children continue to be dependent on their families.

The marital bond of parents can be significantly weakened by a disabled child. If there was significant marital dysfunction present before the birth of a disabled child, the marriage may be at a significant increased risk for a separation and divorce. The blaming of one parent for the child's problem is a common response, as are feelings of anger, hostility, and depression. The need for counseling regarding the issues of sexuality and genetic concerns is something to anticipate in working with these couples. Although the negative aspects of parents' situations are anticipated, there are many parents whose marriages are strong and have been strengthened even through this type of ordeal.

Another area to watch for is a role change where one parent, particularly the mother, assumes the primary caretaking function for the disabled child. This may arise out of a mother's need to be protective while isolating fathers to the periphery of family activities.

SIBLINGS

Children with a developmental disability can significantly impact the feelings and functioning of their siblings. Birth order does not seem to matter. If the affected child is the oldest, the siblings may show regression and attention-seeking behavior because of the excessive attention that the older child receives from his or her parents. If the affected child is the youngest or one of the younger children, then the older sibling becomes a surrogate parent and may become overprotective of the child. This overinvolvement in sibling care can compromise development of normal peer relationships. The child who has assumed the role of surrogate parent can also become dysfunctional when the parents' authority and decision-making are challenged by this child. Often, siblings will worry and show anxiety for their parents as they see the pressure that their parents must experience while carrying out numerous responsibilities. This concern can contribute to somatic complaints such as abdominal pain or other school-avoidance behavior. Siblings are particularly affected if a disabled child has multiple hospitalizations. Sometimes a normal sibling (older or younger) can become a scapegoat for a family. This may indicate emotional problems on the sibling's part but also may indicate marital problems between the parents.

DISABLED CHILD

Because these children are special in terms of their developmental problems, they have an increased risk for being a "vulnerable child." This term is applicable to a wide variety of children, particularly to those children who are mentally retarded and/or physically disabled. A child may be placed in a vulnerable position with excessive overprotectiveness because of the circumstances of the birth and/or because of his or her developmental problem. These experiences linger and have an ongoing effect on how the children are viewed as individuals and how they are treated by family members. Maladaptive development can be seen in discipline problems, separation problems from parents, and phobic reactions in regard to school. When assessing a child's development, it is important to evaluate whether or not there has been achievement of trust, autonomy, initiative, and self-identity. Each of these stages represents a developmental task that if not mastered may have a profound negative effect on the child.

When a child has a poor adjustment to his disability, the adjustment pattern may fall into one of three groups. One group is marked by overdependence, fearfulness, and lack of outside contacts and interests. While such children are described by their parents as dependent, the parents themselves are viewed by health care professionals as overanxious and overprotective. The second group contains the overly independent and daring child. The child may tend to use denial of his or her problem to cover his or her own inadequacies. The third group of behavior patterns is often seen in older individuals with a chronic disability. Frequently these persons are hostile, lonely, and shy. They are hidden by their families and generally have a poor self-concept. They tend to have doubts about their health, physical condition, and sexual normalcy.

FINANCIAL STRESS

The financial stress that families of disabled children often experience has significant impact on all family members. Repeated hospitalizations for a child with a chronic illness can be an overwhelming experience. Although some families have excellent hospital insurance coverage there may be a limit to the amount the insurance company will pay. There are clinic fees, x-rays, and fees for other tests that may not be covered by their insurance. With federal monetary cutbacks in program services, parents may be required to pay fees for services such as therapy (i.e., speech and language, occupational, and physical therapy) and transportation. Bracing is often expensive and some parents may need to renovate their homes for their child to make it accessible for wheelchairs. Some families need to move to an area in an apartment complex that is on the first floor and accessible for entry and transportation. Because of financial stress, many families remain isolated from their extended families and friends. When the parents do not have enough resources, overall isolation affects parents and children.

PRINCIPLES FOR IMPROVED FAMILY COPING

Several principles of family functioning can be significant in improving a family's ability to cope with the stress of having a child with a developmental disability:

1. A firm, close marital relationship. Communication is very important in this family situation. Mutual support is vital. This means that fathers need to be involved in the child's care.
2. These families need access to supportive and understanding friends. This will decrease the isolation that a family may feel. These friends can be helpful in learning about the child's problem and provide some relief to the parents at stressful times.
3. There should be opportunities for parents to have recreation with and without family members. The ability to get away for a while is an important aspect of coping. As a child gets older, a good camp experience may be beneficial for child and parent.
4. Parents can hopefully plan ahead and prepare household management matters, instead of acting on a crisis basis.
5. Families can cope better if transportation (public or private) is close by. If families are close to shopping stores, for example, it makes for more effective use of their time.
6. Parents cope better when they have an opportunity to reach out to other parents and families in similar situations. This can be done through specialized preschool and infant programs in which there is a parents' group or through a parents' group developed around the particular disability, such as the Spina Bifida Association. Professionals can empathize, but parents in the same situation can provide immeasurable support and friendship.

SUMMARY

Families with children who have a developmental disability can experience significant stress. The concepts of mourning, chronic sorrow, and the "vulnerable child" as ramifications of the stress have relevance in the assessment of these families. These families face tremendous assaults emotionally, which are felt at birth or time of diagnosis of the problem and continue throughout the child's life. Primary care doctors need a greater sensitivity to these families and ability to assess their problem from a developmental viewpoint. Understanding that chronic disabilities have a profound impact on parents, siblings, and child is an important step toward helping these families. The help that is given must be viewed in the context of an alliance, in which medical and supportive services are available and given as the family system accepts them. The primary care physician's knowledge of the disability and sensitivity to parental and child emotional needs can often facilitate an outcome whereby a family may appropriately adapt and cope in their day-to-day life.

BIBLIOGRAPHY

Battle CU: Chronic physical disease, behavioral aspect. *Pediatr Clin North Am* 1973; 22:525–531.

Bruhn JG: Effects of chronic illness on the family. *J Fam Pract* 1977; 4:1057–1060.

Gabel H, McDowell J, Cerreto MC: Family adaptation to the handicapped infant, in Garwood S, Gray, Fewell RR: *Educating Handicapped Infants: Issues in Development and Intervention.* Rockville, Md, London Aspen Systems Corp, 1983; pp 455—493.

Goldson E: Parents' reactions to the birth of a sick infant. *Child Today* 1979; 8:13–17.

Green M, Solnit AJ: Reactions to the threatened loss of a child: A vulnerable child syndrome. *Pediatrics* 1964; 34:58–66.

Keith Barr C: Impact on the family of a chronically ill child, in Hobbs N, Perrin JM (eds): *Issues in the Care of Children with Chronic Illness.* San Francisco-London, Jossey-Bass Publishers, 1985; pp 24–40.

Moses KL: The impact of initial diagnosis: Mobilising family resources, in Mulick J, Pueschel S: *Parent-Professional Partnerships in Developmental Disability Services.* Cambridge, Mass, The Ware Press, 1983; pp 11–34.

Powell TH, Ogle P: *Brothers and Sisters: A Special Part of Exceptional Families.* Baltimore-London, Paul H. Brookes Publishing Co, 1985.

Solnit AJ, Stork MH: Mourning and the birth of a defective child. *Psychoanal Study Child* 1961; 16:523.

Travis G: *Chronic Illness in Children: Its Impact on Child and Family.* Stanford, Calif, Stanford University Press, 1976; chaps 1–3.

80 RIGHTS OF CHILDREN WITH DEVELOPMENTAL DISABILITIES

Symme W. Trachtenberg, M.S.W., ACSW

Children with special needs have the right to attain their own potential for participation in activities within the family and society at large. Therefore, no matter how handicapped a child is, he or she should be referred to an educational program. The Education for All Handicapped Children Act of 1975 (Public Law 94-142) states that free appropriate public education is provided to all children. PL 94-142 was expanded with the Education of the Handicapped Act Amendments of 1986, PL 99-457. It provides that all states receiving funds under PL 94-142 must provide a free appropriate public education for children from age 3 to 21 years by the 1990 to 1991 school year. The law also allocates additional funds for states agreeing to provide early intervention programs for infants and toddlers from birth to 3 years of age. Some states are responsible for educating children with disabilities from birth. The local public school districts in each community are responsible for the testing and educational recommendations for those children with handicaps for whom education must be provided. Early intervention programs are available throughout the United States for developmentally delayed children from birth up to the time when the public school system assumes responsibility for providing the education.

SERVICES

In addition to specialized educational settings, various other programs throughout the United States provide services to children with disabilities and their families. Federal funding for such programs is distributed to individual states, which in turn determine how to spend the allocated monies for these services. Each state, city, and county, therefore, offers different programs that may change periodically due to funding allocations. The educational programs are moving toward a mandate for an Individualized Family Service Plan (IFSP). This is an effort to strengthen family involvement, develop an interdisciplinary effort, and make the Individualized Educational Plan (IEP) more meaningful. In addition, there are programs that provide parents with assistance in finding ways to cope with their child's special needs. They often have supportive counseling for parents and families who may be seen individually, as a family unit, or as part of a professionally run or self-help support group. This supportive experience can mean the difference between a family that is functional and one that is not. Over time and with guidance, parents can learn to understand their child's disability and learn how to help him or her to reach full potential while becoming an integrated part of the family. Thus the parents will be contributing to their child's goal of reaching maximum potential.

Families should also be made aware of services that provide concrete help in the day-to-day management of their child. These services fall within two major categories: those that directly contribute to the child's psychosocial growth and development (e.g., special needs preschool and daycare; Head Start; specialized day and overnight camps; after-school, recreational, and socialization activities for the child with a handicap; vocational training, sheltered employment, transportation) and those that offer relief and assistance to the entire family (e.g., respite care, where the child can be cared for overnight; homemaker services if the parent is unable to provide care temporarily; and protective services for the child abused by a parent who is unable to cope with the stress that the child's presence has created).

Judicial, legislative, and program trends, including research findings, clearly show that institutional care is rapidly becoming obsolete and is being replaced by community-based services. Children with disabilities are increasingly remaining with their natural families and with the added supports being provided, fewer families are forced to choose separation as a way of providing for their children with special needs. For the older child, community living arrangements or group homes are an option. Parents who are concerned about who will care for their handicapped child once they themselves are unable to provide that care may want to investigate specialized guardianship and estate planning.

Occasionally the family or the physician may decide on additional diagnostic evaluations. The child may then be referred to hospital-based diagnostic services or clinics for the specific disability. In these places, the staff is a good resource for referral information or treatment (e.g., physical, occupational, and speech therapy; psychoeducational, audiology, social work, nursing, and counseling services). Primary care physicians are often called on for supplementary medical evaluations and treatment while maintaining emotional support and overall guidance for the child and family.

FINANCIAL ASSISTANCE AND RESOURCES

Financial assistance for families of children with handicaps may be obtained through state medical assistance or Social Security Administration–funded supplemental security income (SSI) programs. The former provides financial assistance to families with costly medical bills and insufficient income or medical insurance coverage; the latter uses federal funds to provide a minimum level of income to disabled people from infancy through old age. Although some children may be found ineligible for either program on the basis of parental income, all families should be encouraged to apply through their local social security office.

It is important for the primary care physician to develop a list of reliable contacts to establish a resource network in the community. Resources with national offices cited in Appendix B should be helpful in establishing contact within or nearby the local community. Most have state or local services listed in the local telephone directory. Many county services are listed under the name of the county. Those listed provide free or low-cost educational or social service programs, while others are available for information and referral to specialized services within the community. Many national organizations have support groups and counseling. The social service agencies listed under "Family Services, Children and Youth," or by religious denomination can also provide counseling and referral information.

BIBLIOGRAPHY

Federal Assistance for Programs Serving the Handicapped, Publication No. E-9022001. Rockville, Md, US Department of Education, Office of Special Education and Rehabilitative Services, Office for Handicapped Individuals, Sept 1980.

Pocket Guide to Federal Help for the Disabled Person. Rockville, Md, US Department of Education, Office of Information and Resources for the Handicapped, Sept 1983.

Summary of Existing Legislation Relating to the Handicapped, Publication No. E80-22014. Rockville, Md, US Department of Education, Office of Special Education and Rehabilitative Services, Office for Handicapped Individuals, Aug 1980.

section V

Behavior Problems

John Sargent, Section Editor

Behavior problems account for a large percentage of office visits to the primary care physician, even though the patient may have concerns of organic illness. The physician's task consists of recognizing the problems, defining which situations are in his or her purview, and developing a system to manage those that are appropriate for his expertise or orchestrating an appropriate referral when the problems are more complex.

Since the child is a member of a family, the approaches of family therapists provide many aids for the primary care physician to use in dealing with behavior problems. This section includes an outline of the principles of family therapy as well as a discussion of some of the common problems facing children and their families as the children grow and develop. Quite often, early recognition of the problems or intervention by the physician will prevent more severe problems for the child and the family. The topics in this section were selected because of their frequency of occurrence and the applicability of the information to the interested primary care physician.

81 CHILD AND FAMILY PSYCHOSOCIAL ASSESSMENT

John Sargent, M.D.

Primary care physicians are frequently the first to be consulted concerning problems of child behavior and development. These physicians may also observe that some families need assistance in coping with acute and chronic illness, school problems, and transitions in family life. Because of their special role in the lives of the families, they are in an excellent position to provide assistance to parents concerning psychosocial problems of their children which are estimated to be the reason for 10% to 20% of primary care visits.

To diagnose and manage the child's problems, primary physicians will need a model for assessment of the child's emotional and behavioral capacity. They should also be able to analyze family functioning to define these difficulties accurately and arrange for treatment.

The family, like other living systems, is organized as a hierarchy that allows for the accomplishment of several tasks:

1. Development and maintenance of integrity of family
2. Ongoing development and function of all members
3. Expression of affection, authority, and affiliation
4. Negotiation of changes and responses to stress
5. Conflict resolution, problem solving, decision making
6. Behavior control-socialization coupled with encouragement for individual action and expression

Any individual is simultaneously an independent entity, a member of the family, and a member of smaller groupings within the family. The family encourages the development of all members toward the goal of being successful as a person and in a social setting. The family is a major area for the expression of affection and affiliation as well as for displeasure and anger for children and adults. Responses to change and stress are developed within the family, problems are solved, and conflict and disagreement are negotiated so that the family maintains its integrity at the same time as it fosters individual development and achievement. The family also establishes mechanisms for behavior control that allow for both socialization and individual expression of all family members. Successful participation in all of these family endeavors promotes the emotional and behavioral development of children.

Each of the family members and subgroups (e.g., spouses, parental figures, siblings, and individuals) has special tasks and responsibilities within the family. The members of the subgroupings must be able to work together but there needs to be enough separation among them so that each can pursue individual tasks and gain competence to achieve the goals. As two adults form a family, they develop methods of interaction that encourage the expression of mutual satisfaction, psychological needs, and confirmation of accepted behaviors. Conflicts and disagreements are negotiated. Spouses help each other succeed and support each other when stress occurs. The experience and growth that occur both within and outside the family must be incorporated into the development of the spouse relationship. At the same time, the spouses must be able to be separate enough from the children and from their own parents to maintain their relationship and resolve their disagreements. The spouse relationship also can provide the children with examples of both affection and support, as well as the resolution of conflict, which can become part of the children's values and expectations and model for successful development of intimate relationships. Components of spouse behavior are summarized below:

1. Support and encouragement
2. Intimacy, affection, sex
3. Potential for procreation
4. Creation of a new culture with continuity with families of origin
5. Resolution of disagreements, collaboration

In our society, the child's caretakers have the major responsibility for promoting growth and development. Parents must provide support and nurturance to the child to establish an emotional bond. When such attachment is present, the child will desire parental approval and will usually respond to parental authority. The parents need to provide enough socialization to set limits on the child's behavior and to be able to define the child's world in such a way that the child feels safe and protected. The parents should promote their child's efforts in age-appropriate tasks. These will include consistent school performance, school attendance, relating to peers, and assuming increasing autonomy within the family as development proceeds. Parents also will need to instill within the child a sense of competence and mastery at each developmental level, so that the child successfully integrates new knowledge and new experiences and develops an ever-increasing sense of self-worth and self-esteem. Finally, parents or parental figures will need to assist their child in coping with unexpected failures, disappointments, and losses. Parental figures will need to negotiate and decide on a course of action with respect to their children in situations in which there is no clear and obvious right answer. As the parents negotiate these issues and achieve a course of action, they can increasingly gain a sense of competence and confidence in their own ability as parents and transmit these positive feelings to their children. If there are difficulties in the spouse relationship so that conflicts are not negotiated effectively, parents may find it increasingly difficult to resolve disagreements concerning their children and the children will receive inconsistent direction.

Through *parent-child interaction,* children experience support appropriate to their developmental level and learn to expect that authority and limits can be rational and predictable. Considerations in parent-child interaction include:

1. Congruence between parental behavior and child's needs and skills is important.
2. Varying parental responses and styles of parent-child interaction are required at different stages of development (e.g., infancy, preschool, school age, adolescence, young adulthood).
3. Major components of parental behavior are:
   - Support and nurturance
   - Structure, limits, definition of the world
   - Affiliation (appreciation of the child for his or her own sake, based on accurate understanding of the child's skills).

If the parents appreciate and recognize the child's abilities and competencies, the child can learn self-esteem, which will then assist him in the development of further skills. The child's own development serves, in turn, to increase the parents' sense of their own adequacy. As the child grows and develops, parent-child interaction must change. Parents must provide the older child more opportunities to make independent decisions and solve problems while also requiring the child to take increasing responsibility for his or her actions. The parents' own actions move from control and rule-setting to supervision, monitoring, and availability.

Sibling relationships within the family allow each child to learn and experience competition and cooperation among peers, specific abilities to negotiate conflict, establish autonomy, and achieve recognition for development among siblings, which can then assist the child in similar situations outside the family. It is important for the family to encourage siblings' opportunities to interact directly with one another, both to cooperate and to resolve disagreements or conflicts.

CHILD AND FAMILY ASSESSMENT

Through history taking, observation of family interaction, and assessment of the manner in which the family relates to the physician, it is possible to assess the family's patterns of interaction, their skills, capacities, assets, and difficulties as the family members relate to the presenting problem. Methods used in family evaluation are:

1. Observing interaction, monitoring
   Leadership
   Predominant features of relationships: closeness vs. distance
   Flexibility of relationships
   Verbal-nonverbal congruence of communication
   Involvement of all family members
   Task orientation
2. Response to stress or change
   Degree of disruption
   Support generated
   Commitment to cooperation
   Problem-solving behaviors
   Appreciation of new information
3. Ability to utilize extrafamilial resources effectively

The physician will want to note what takes place in his or her office as well as what is described by the family. The physician should appreciate not only how the family relates to the problem in question, but also how the family functions on a day-to-day basis in relationship to the tasks outlined above. As the physician recognizes particular skills and assets of the given family and identifies and works with them, these skills will enable the family to be more confident and competent in dealing with their child and the presenting problem. To assess families, the physician will need to have an organized framework to guide the evaluation process. Parameters for family evaluation are:

1. Relationships
2. Leadership
3. Boundaries
4. Negotiation and conflict resolution
5. Communication and expression of emotion
6. Problem solving
7. Relationship with physician

ELEMENTS OF EVALUATION

RELATIONSHIPS

Relationships between family members should be flexible so that each member can work together for support and growth and can maintain distance when limits and discipline are important. Parental figures should be able to establish relationships with the children appropriate to the situation and the children's needs. The physician should be concerned when either excessive closeness or excessive distance characterizes the relationship between parent and child. An overly close affiliation between parent and child may interfere with the parent's ability to establish important rules. The parent may hold back, either because of inability to get angry at the child or fear of upsetting the child by taking a firm stand. Such relationships may be revealed when the child and overinvolved parent are sitting close to each other, the parent answers for the child or describes how the child feels rather than encouraging the child to speak for himself, or when the parent uses the pronoun "we" to describe difficulties pertaining to the child. Very often in problematic families, one parent establishes and maintains an overly close relationship with the child in question, while the other parent is overly distant. Parents often argue with one another about appropriate responses to the child and frequently each responds independently, counterbalancing the other and confusing the child.

Excessively distant relationships may occur in disorganized families in which the parents are so involved with their own problems that the needs of the child are neglected. In such families, the child is given more autonomy than is age-appropriate and rules are either nonexistent or enforced inconsistently. Such families may be unable to focus on the child's problem and the parents may be primarily concerned about the effect of the child's problem on their lives and less concerned about the child's distress. The child may also be blamed or made a scapegoat by the parents as the source of all parental difficulties. Excessively distant or underinvolved parents may appear apathetic and unresponsive to the child's distress, leaving the child to either increasingly withdraw, persist in disturbed behavior, or try to mask his sadness.

LEADERSHIP

All families require leadership to set direction, accomplish tasks, solve problems, and satisfy the needs of the children as determined by the children's developmental status and skills. Parents are expected to set rules, enforce behavior, and respond with support, encouragement, and reinforcement for positive outcomes. Within the family, rules should be agreed on by the parental figures to minimize undermining and subversion. The physician needs to learn from each family who the leadership group is and to be sure that members of that group recognize their participation and agree on who takes part in making decisions. In general, in a nuclear family, parents take on that role, with grandparents and relatives having secondary or subordinate roles. In some families, however, grandparents maintain a leadership position, especially in single-parent families. In families with problems, there exists confusion and disagreement about the identity of the family leaders and a lack of collaboration between parental figures. The primary care physician will need to note this, especially as it relates to problem behavior or emotional responses on the part of the children. The children may be allowed to voice complaints with the understanding that the parents are the final arbiters of decisions.

BOUNDARIES

The physician should note whether family subgroupings exist and function independently. In observing the family interactions, the physician should try to decide if parents and children can act independently and as a family unit depending on the situation. The physician should pay attention to whether the spouses can protect and develop their relationship without excessive interference by the children or extended family. The physician will also want to note whether the siblings can cooperate and work together to support one another, and whether the parents can make decisions and implement them without significant intrusion from outside the family. It should be noted whether the boundary around the family allows for family participation in the extrafamilial world, at the same time as it identifies the family as a separate entity reinforcing a sense of belonging and participation. An exclusive, overly close parent-child relationship in a family in which discipline is inadequate and marital strife apparent, is indicative of an ineffective boundary between the parents and the children. Such overinvolvement with the child may occur in a family with a special child, such as one with a physical handicap or chronic physical illness. Parents in such families may be overprotective of the child, while assuming functions for him and speaking for him. The child may also avoid speaking for himself out of a limited sense of self-esteem, assertiveness, and autonomy. In such situations, the child's development of independence and maturity is often significantly delayed.

NEGOTIATION AND CONFLICT RESOLUTION

All families have disagreements among their members. In some families, some conflicts are acknowledged and confronted directly, while in others potential conflict is consistently avoided. Some families disagree openly, but are unable to reach a constructive resolution of the problem at hand. The physician should assess the capacity of the family for conflict resolution because unresolved disagreements typically lead to chronic hostility, undermining, and ineffective parenting. Families that tolerate and resolve disagreement are usually more open in their discussion of family problems and more able to use external resources and the guidance of the physician in addressing behavioral and developmental difficulties. As history is given, the physician can observe discussion and the resolution of disagreements as they occur spontaneously or as negotiation is directed through his intervention. If conflict is apparent but denied, the family tension may increase as problems of the children are discussed. Families that are unable to resolve conflict directly usually have significant marital problems that are denied but cause one parent to become overinvolved with one of the children. The child may become caught in the marital struggle of the parents and more involved in the family, further reinforcing behavior difficulties and emotional immaturity.

COMMUNICATION AND EXPRESSION OF EMOTION

The primary care physician, while assessing the family, will note whether communication is clear and whether nonverbal and verbal communication between family members is consistent and congruent. He or she will pay attention to whether family members listen to and respond to one another or act as though they haven't heard the other's statement. Confusion of verbal and nonverbal messages is especially common in the face of emotional or behavioral problems of the children or in response to significant psychosomatic symptoms.

The physician will also note whether emotional upset on the part of any family member is recognized and supported by other family members. He or she should also observe whether emotional expression interferes with important family functions, so that rules are not enforced for family members who are perceived as being particularly upset or stressed. The child's emotional upset then affects family members in a way that disrupts the family's ability to respond to his difficulties and to support his development of improved self-esteem and increased self-reliance.

CAPACITY FOR PROBLEM SOLVING

Families vary in their ability to assess situations, gather information, decide among possible alternatives, and implement strategies to resolve problems. Components of effective problem-solving are:

1. Gaining knowledge: background understanding
2. Information gathering, in specific situations
3. Information processing: assessing specific situations
4. Decision making: choosing among alternative strategies
5. Implementation: carrying out strategies
6. Assessing results and modifying strategies

Within a family, these steps are shared, negotiated, and carried out collaboratively. Some families readily address themselves to the difficulties and are effective in marshaling their resources to resolve them. Through effective problem-solving, these families gain increased confidence and competence and are more adequately prepared to resolve future difficulties. Other families, because of tenuous or difficult family relationships and an inability to resolve disagreements, fail to gather information effectively and fail to implement strategies to resolve problems. These families are likely to attempt the same solutions over and over again and to perceive other remedies as inaccessible or impossible. Their repertoire of behaviors becomes extremely limited and their responses to problems are stereotyped, rigid, and ineffective.

To resolve problems successfully, disagreeing parents must find a way to put aside their differences in the interest of the child and family. They must develop a mutually acceptable plan for responding to their child's difficulties, and, therefore, soften rigid and polarized positions. Through his assessment of the family, the physician will want to pay particular attention to the ways in which parents end up in mutually opposing positions, and, therefore, are unable to address themselves to problem situations.

RELATIONSHIP WITH THE PHYSICIAN

The physician should assess the family's ability to relate to him or her and respond to the interventions. If the family approaches the physician in an open, interested, and friendly fashion, the physician should feel more comfortable in responding to the problem and expecting parental collaboration and cooperation. The physician should also expect to experience a different, but effective relationship with each family member as he or she meets with the family. Families in which members are guarded or inaccessible are more likely to have serious difficulties. The physician also should expect that the observed family behavior will be indicative of the family's responsiveness to other extrafamilial resources, which may need to be utilized in order to solve the presenting problem. Teachers, therapists, and social agencies may either be welcomed by a family or resisted.

These characteristics of family functioning are interdependent and mutually reinforcing, so that a family with several positive characteristics is likely to have others. These competencies lead to further success in a circular fashion. Taken together, the presence of the qualities listed above describes a family that is flexible and capable of change over time as well as a family that will be able to resolve difficulties with appropriate input from the physician.

ASSESSMENT OF THE CHILD'S BEHAVIORAL CAPACITIES

Evaluation of the child's emotional and behavioral status will take place at the same time as the physician is evaluating the family. Parameters of child assessment are:

1. Physical functioning: neurologic, sensory
2. Integration ability: visual-motor, auditory-motor
3. Communication ability: understanding and expression
4. Mood and emotional tone
5. Affect: variety, expression, appropriateness, regulation and control
6. Relationships: capacity for attachment, friendship, and intimacy
7. Competence and mastery, problem-solving ability
8. Self-esteem
9. Content and style of thought
10. Temperament: behavioral style
11. Impulse control
12. Appropriateness based on developmental stage and intrinsic capacities (e.g., intelligence, physical integrity, well-being)

The physician should have the framework for appreciating the child's abilities in relationship to the age and developmental level. The physician should observe the child's *behavioral style,* ability to approach new stimuli, and curiosity. The doctor should note whether the behavior is goal-directed and modulated, rapid and diffuse, or slow and withdrawn. The physician should note the child's ability to control his or her behavior in response to the demands of the examining room situation and in response to the requests of the physician and parents. In estimating the child's degree of *impulse control,* the doctor can differentiate times when children have difficulties responding to consistent directions from situations in which the child is generally responsive but the directives are inconsistent and inappropriately given. The physician should notice the child's ability to speak directly and coherently and the overall content and manner of the child's *thinking.* Such elements as spontaneity, coherence, and articulation of *speech* are important, as well as the overall coherence and goal-directedness of the child's thinking and verbal communication. The physician may want to ask for the child's wishes, fantasies, and views of the future as a reflection of the child's self-esteem and self-concept. The doctor should also evaluate the overall *mood* or emotional tone of the child during his assessment as well as the child's ability to express and experience a variety of *affects.* The affect should reflect the content of the issue under discussion and the child should be able to respond to and mirror the physician's affect as he interacts with the child.

The physician should observe the child's ability to *relate* to him or her during the assessment process. If the child is unusually withdrawn or shy, or unusually responsive and open, these cues will indicate potential difficulties to the physician. The degree of eye contact and spontaneous speech, the degree of trust the child demonstrates in the physician, and the extent to which the child desires the physician's approval and warmth should be noted. The final component of the assessment of the child for the physician is a clear appreciation of the child's strengths in relationship to any particular difficulties that may be present. This is especially important in situations in which the child's difficulty is associated with developmental delay, physical handicap, or chronic illness. It will be through these strengths that the physician will enable the family to encourage the child in the development of appropriate self-esteem, competence, and mastery and in the achievement of maximum psychosocial adaptation.

SYNTHESIS AND CONCLUSIONS

The assessment of both family and child will take place for the physician throughout history taking, observations of family interaction, physical examination, and review and assessment of the visit. This assessment will lead the physician to a recognition of the family's strengths and capacities and their accomplishments with respect to child-rearing. It will also help the physician determine the areas of difficulty or weakness within the family corresponding to the problems the family has identified. The physician should be able to feel comfortable with the assessment and to expect that the impressions of the child and of the family make sense. A successful family in which child-rearing has proceeded without significant difficulties may be having specific problems at a point of developmental stress at which previously mastered parenting skills are no longer effective. A family in which the child demonstrates significant behavior problems may have marked unresolved conflicts between the parents, with significant overinvolvement on the part of one parent with the child so that the rules and directives of parenting are ineffective. In a family in which a psychosomatic symptom is present, there may be significant parental concern for either the meaning of the symptom or for the vulnerability of the child in question. As the physician recognizes increasingly the consistency between family assessment and child assessment, he/she will be able to intervene effectively with the family to promote their successful achievement of the tasks of child rearing and also to be able to utilize external resources or refer a family for additional assistance when the presenting problem and family difficulties require such intervention.

BIBLIOGRAPHY

Carter B, Mc Goldrick M (eds): *The Changing Family Life Cycle*, ed 2. New York, Gardner Press, 1988.

Falicov C (ed): *Family Transitions: Continuity and Change Over the Life Cycle*. New York, Guilford Press, 1988.

Greenspan SI: *The Clinical Interview of the Child*. New York, McGraw-Hill Book Co, 1981.

Hodas GR, Sargent J: Psychiatric emergencies, in Fleisher G, Ludwig S (eds): *Textbook of Pediatric Emergency Medicine*, ed 2. Baltimore, Williams & Wilkins Co, 1988.

Minuchin S: *Families and Family Therapy*. Cambridge, Mass, Harvard University Press, 1974.

Minuchin S, Minuchin PL: The child in context: A systems approach to growth and treatment, in Talbot NB (ed): *Raising Children in Modern America*. Boston, Little Brown & Co, 1976.

Sargent J: The family: A pediatric assessment. *J Pediatr* 1983; 102:973–976.

Simons J: *Psychiatric Examination of Children*, ed 2. Philadelphia, Lea & Febiger, 1974.

Walsh F (ed): *Normal Family Process*. New York, Guilford Press, 1982.

82 FAMILY TREATMENT OF CHILDHOOD BEHAVIOR PROBLEMS

John Sargent, M.D.

Family therapy has attracted the attention of many practitioners, since it deals not only with the individual who presents with a problem but also with the family who lives with the patient. This chapter describes some of the principles of family therapy and strategies used by family therapists in treating children and their families.

The primary care physician's role in working with children with behavioral problems is to make an accurate diagnosis of the child's problem and of the family's functioning and to intervene in family operations directly or to refer the family for family-oriented psychotherapy. It is important for the physician to recognize that when dealing with a child's emotional or behavioral problem, the family must also be considered. In order for the interventions to have the most beneficial effect, the assessment of the family should be complete and should reflect an appreciation of the role of the family in relationship to the child's symptom. The physician, then, will require a model of how family interaction influences the child's problem.

Family therapy is a method to change family interactions so that their functioning is effective in relationship to the child's development, adaptation, and socialization. The goal of family therapy is to assist the family to solve its own problems, to manage and direct the development of the children, and to appreciate the unique needs, skills, and abilities of each child. To effectively intervene in family interaction, the physician should have in mind a model of effective family organization and functioning and an appreciation of the influence of the family in the development and maintenance of their children's symptomatic behavior. This is not to suggest that all behavior problems are a result of faulty family interaction. Some, such as attention-deficit disorder, psychosis, and mood disorders may reflect an underlying physiologic difference on the part of the affected child. The physician has a responsibility to help the family adapt to and cope with each of their children's individual capabilities and needs, allowing maximal psychosocial functioning and adaptation on the part of each child.

Family therapy is based on the concept that symptomatic behavior in a family member arises within a family context and is an attempt to adapt to that situation.

VIEWPOINT OF FAMILY THERAPY

1. Symptomatic behavior arises within the family and is adaptive to the family.
2. Symptoms are maintained by family interaction and play a role in maintaining the stability of the family.
3. The symptom affects the entire family; the entire family affects the symptom.
4. Symptoms tend to arise in families at points of change or transition.
5. Interactions of families with symptoms are constricted. More skills and possibilities exist within the family than are utilized currently.
6. Most families can successfully respond to symptoms, foster their children's development, and accomplish other family goals.

Families with a symptomatic member are dysfunctional, that is, not capable of effectively meeting the needs for all members at the time of problem expression. The symptom is not limited to the member with a problem, but embedded in patterns of family interaction and continued by those family transactions. The problem also maintains family stability in a circular fashion. The entire family affects the symptomatic member, whose behavior, in turn, affects the entire family. Symptoms tend to arise within families at times of change or stress, especially at transitions in the family life cycle. At these times, previously adaptive patterns of family interaction are no longer satisfactory for family members. New responses are not available or are perceived as threatening because interactions among family members are inappropriately rigid. Because limited aspects of any individual's capacities are utilized by the family, family problem-solving is deficient and the symptom remains or may worsen.

The basic assumption of family therapy is that families with symptoms possess unused capabilities and unapplied strengths. Encouraging those interactions that utilize family strengths more effectively can enable the family to resolve the symptoms or adapt to underlying differences in their children. These new interactions can be integrated into the family responses, ultimately altering the family system and achieving more effective family functioning.

Dysfunctional families have inadequate leadership that occurs when there is disagreement or conflict between the parents or between a single parent and another important caretaker. Unresolved disagreement between parenting figures leads to inconsistent direction and may result in undermining decisions. As long as the caretakers have problems with their own interaction, the symptoms in the children will persist. Each parent encourages the child to side with him or her in the persistent disagreements, therefore encouraging further participation of the child in family matters, leaving the child less available to peer group and less able to develop self-control and effective self-esteem.

Problems occur when there is a blurring of the boundary between parent and child. A secret coalition of one parent and the child may develop, with the two of them acting against the other parent. These alliances may shift, with the child alternatively aligned with each parent. The physician should recognize that the child is an active participant but may not have the insight nor autonomy necessary to refuse to take sides with one parent. The child may not recognize the parents' vulnerability or may not be aware that they are rewarded with increased attention for participation in the parents' disagreement. The child's problem diminishes the stress of unresolved parental conflict and distracts the family, as a whole, from other unaddressed and important stresses. Communication among family members is likely to be confused and incomplete, with nonverbal and verbal communications contradicting each other. Within the family, there is also likely to be a chronic state of tension and stress. As each family member plays a role in the perpetuation of the child's problem, it becomes evident that the difficulty is actually a problem of the family rather than just the child.

Relationships among family members become excessively rigid and stereotyped and attempts to resolve the problem by one parent or by the child individually become part of the system that maintains or worsens the problem. At that point, advice that does not alter the rules of family organization and habitual family interaction also further maintains the problem. Interventions that directly change family organization and the actions that maintain the problem are required so that the parents, together, can collaborate to assist the child to grow, appropriate to his developmental stage and age. Treatment will require change on the part of all family members. The parents will need to work together more effectively, the child will need to be supported when in trouble and yet limited when out-of-control, and the siblings will need to be able to cooperate more effectively. As the parents collaborate to resolve the difficulty or appreciate the special needs of their child, they then can be encouraged to resolve their marital difficulties at the same time as the child is encouraged to learn skills and develop maturity. Indications for family therapy are listed below.

INDICATIONS FOR FAMILY THERAPY

1. Poor compliance with medical treatment.
2. Poor control of chronic illness and repeated hospitalizations.
3. Less than expected physical function despite adequate medical treatment, or psychosomatic symptoms.
4. Social withdrawal, depression, emotional immaturity in a child.
5. Poor school performance with adequate learning skills.
6. Aggressive, reckless, out-of-control behavior.
7. Family strife in raising children.
8. Family concern about child's ability to mature into adolescence or adulthood.
9. Psychosis, suicidal behavior.
10. Nonorganic failure to thrive, parent-child attachment disorders.
11. Substance abuse.
12. Child abuse or neglect with appropriate legal supervision.

Several distinct models of family-oriented treatment for childhood behavior problems have been developed. Each model responds to the symptomatic behavior of children by assisting the family to resolve the child's symptoms and proceed with family life successfully. One clearly articulated model of family treatment has been developed and described by Minuchin. Derived from a consistent model of effective family functioning, it has been utilized in response to a variety of emotional and behavioral problems of children. Outcome studies have shown Minuchin's structural family therapy to be effective for serious psychosocial and psychophysiologic disorders in children including psychosomatic disorders and adolescent drug abuse and habituation. It is particularly relevant for physicians caring for children because of its focus on change and development throughout family life and its normative expectations of parental and child behavior, especially in response to problems or stress. The treating person assists the family in responding to crises and transitions and then expects the family to reestablish control over its behavior and functioning as soon as the problem is resolved. The treating person remains available to the family for assistance in future crises. This therapist, then, has a role with the family analogous to that of primary care physician for illnesses. Primary care physicians can learn the techniques of family therapy and can, with interest, training, and experience, treat a variety of uncomplicated behavioral, emotional, and psychosomatic problems of children. The following discussion reflects this and identifies the physician as a treating person. The approach to treatment and the techniques of treatment will be similar if the primary care physician chooses to refer the family and patient to a family-oriented therapist.

STRUCTURAL FAMILY THERAPY

1. Therapy is aimed at changing family relationships and family behavior in the present.
2. Therapy highlights family strengths and assists the family in developing confidence and ability to manage the child's care and development.
3. Therapy is geared toward action.
4. A clear understanding of the child's physical and intellectual capacities must be developed and agreed on by the parents.
5. Therapy uses family concern about the disabled or ill child to change family relationships.
6. The parents must work together.
7. The parents can then enhance treatment and require maturity of the child.
8. As the child's symptoms become manageable for the family, the focus of therapy can shift to other issues troubling the family: the marriage, difficulties of the siblings, etc.

The primary goal of structural family therapy is to alter inappropriate patterns of family interaction by reestablishing and restructuring family relationships. The physician, then, can create and support more effective family activity, at the same time as the parents encourage and support the child's development and maturity. Treatment supports effective functioning of all family members and requires that the family actively solve problems in the presence of the physician. Changes in family relationships induce changes in behavior of all members—first the child and subsequently the parents—and these changes can be reinforced, first by the physician and ultimately by family members in their lives at home.

INITIAL EVALUATION

The initial treatment stage is one in which the physician completes an assessment of the child's physiologic, emotional, and behavioral functioning and integrates that assessment into his appreciation of the family system's operation. The physician can note whether the parents collaborate effectively, whether both parents appreciate the child's difficulties in the same way, which pattern of family interaction interferes with successful approaches to the presenting problems, and which areas of family difficulty are reflected in the parents' inability to deal effectively with the child's behavior problem. The first step in successful treatment is for the physician to work with the family developing a relationship with each family member and appreciating each individual point of view without blaming anyone. The physician also learns and respects the culture, idiosyncrasies, and style of the family, and notices and highlights strengths and competencies of each family member in the family as a whole. The physician also should maintain an attitude of impartiality, which will convey the belief that each family member is presenting only that individual's perspective of the family reality.

During the evaluation phase, the physician will identify predominant family relationships and preferred patterns of interaction, noting who talks to whom, what the tone of the conversation is, what the predominant features of the relationships between both parents and the identified patient are, and how family members address the problem. A hypothesis is developed about the family structure and the difficulties in family organization that are impeding resolution of the symptoms. During this assessment, the physician may note significant overprotectiveness on the part of one parent, marked rigidity that leaves one parent overly close to the child with the problem while the other parent is excessively distant and critical, and significant difficulty in negotiation and conflict resolution between the parents. The physician should also develop an appreciation of the role of the child's symptoms in the family. Are there stresses on family members that the symptoms are masking or diverting attention from? Does the symptom play a role in maintaining contact between the child and a distant or undervalued parent? Is there a particular reason why the parents are having difficulties with this child with this set of problems?

It is important for the physician to remember at this time that it is not the child's particular temperament or behavioral style that is important in any family, but rather the fit between that child's style and the family's expectations and abilities to respond effectively to that child. As the physician gathers history concerning the presenting problem, attention should be paid to methods that each family member has used to try to resolve the problem and what other family members have done when a particular member was attempting to apply his preferred solution. Does the father provide support and encouragement to the child as the child misbehaves for the mother, or does the father rather support and encourage the mother's disciplinary efforts? Is the mother overly close or protective of the child while the father is harsh and disciplinary? When the child becomes symptomatic, does the mother or father become anxious, confused, and therefore unable to respond? The physician, gaining experience in observing family interactions, will note the same patterns occurring over and over again in any particular family and will observe the ways in which parents interfere with each other's efforts, leaving the child unsupported and without consistent direction. As history is obtained concerning recent family circumstances, the physician may also note other unresolved difficulties that the family has and incompetencies that the family has recognized, but is not able to address. Examples of this may be recent death, concern about the child's overall well-being, economic stress, or interference of extended kin.

INTERVENTION IN FAMILY OPERATION

The physician's first goal in working with the family is to establish a spirit of teamwork and collaboration with the parents, with the expectation that all three adults will gain the same appreciation of the child's needs and work together to come up with effective solutions to the child's problems. At this point, the physician should be clear about the definition of the child's problems and gradually and directly help the parents to share this assessment. Often, however, a direct statement of the child's capabilities and problems by the physician may only lead to increased family resistance and denial of the child's problems. It is important for the physician to develop ways of asking parents to note and recognize the child's behavior in response to parental directives. As the parents become increasingly adept at observing and identifying their child's skills, and negotiating between themselves a consistent appreciation of the child, they will then be able to develop ways of acting to limit problematic behaviors and support effective behaviors of the child. This may include the parents' noticing that the child has difficulty following inconsistent directions, therefore becoming able to address more consistent rules and expectations to the child. It may also include the parents' reinforcing impulse control, expecting performance of homework, or expecting continued functioning despite moderate interfering functional physical symptoms. As the parents monitor their child's behavior and negotiate actively between themselves a response that they can both carry through and feel comfortable with, they will increasingly become competent at limiting the child's behavior and supporting the child's need for nurturance and attention.

The physician will generally ignore ineffective family operations, encourage a task-orientation on the part of the parents, and demonstrate optimism and support of the family's success. At the same time as he or she encourages the parents to be more competent and successful with the child, the physician will want to support the child's self-esteem and encourage the child to achieve appropriate developmental and behavioral goals. The physician will need to encourage the family to express sadness and disagreement and provide support and congratulations when interventions are successful. The physician should monitor the family's success in dealing with the child and intermittently encourage the parents to collaborate more effectively with each other on other issues of their lives, especially with regard to particular family stresses. Specific techniques for treatment for the child, including relaxation training so that the child can deal effectively with painful or fearful experiences, drug treatment (e.g., using stimulants for attention-deficit disorder), and consistent responses to problematic behaviors through the use of behavior modification techniques may be useful and integrated into the therapy. As treatment progresses, the physician may want to meet independently with the parents to identify with them any particular stresses in their marriage that will need to be addressed either by the physician or through referral to a therapist. The physician may also want to meet independently with the child, especially for older children and adolescents, to be sure that the child's self-esteem is improving and interest in the world of peers is increasing. The techniques of family therapy are summarized below:

1. The therapist should be aware of the child's physical condition and intellectual capacity.

2. The therapist develops and conveys respect for family problems and possibilities.
3. The therapist collaborates with medical and educational specialists working with the child and family.
4. Family members resolve problems and interact during therapy.
5. The therapist maintains focus of the session upon issues of his choice.
6. The therapist highlights the responsibility of the family to solve problems.
7. The therapist builds disagreements among family members during the sessions so that motivation is developed to resolve conflict and develop plans that all are committed to following.
8. The therapist regulates participation in the sessions, allowing for the creation of new family relationships and the most effective methods of family operation.
9. The therapist monitors family performance supporting new relationships and skills.
10. The therapist can shift to sessions for marital therapy with the parents and individual sessions for the child as indicated.

These interventions are directed at changing boundaries within the family, the family's beliefs about their relationships and their child's abilities, and the realities of family relationships. Family members become increasingly flexible and able to respond to the child's problem and other stresses. As increasing capacity and competency on the part of the family as a whole is noted, the physician can decrease the involvement and return to a primary care approach, remaining available to the family to provide assistance in future stressful or crisis situations. For many behavior problems and emotional problems, the physician can carry through the interventions described here independently. The parents can achieve an experience of success that reinforces their effectiveness in raising the children. In some situations, such as those described in this section, the child's problems may be significant. In other situations, unresolved marital difficulties and severe communication problems among family members may also be noted. In these situations, it is necessary to refer these families for psychotherapy.

The physician, attuned to family problems as a basis for manv of the complaints of children, will develop skills for detection and early intervention. For more details, consult the works by Minuchin listed in the bibliography.

BIBLIOGRAPHY

Allmond B, Buckman W, Goffman H: *The Family Is the Patient.* St Louis, CV Mosby Co, 1979.

Coherty W, Baird M: *Family Therapy and Family Medicine.* New York, Guilford Press, 1983.

Crouch M, Roberts I (eds): *The Family in Medical Practice.* New York, Springer-Verlag, 1987.

Haley J: Toward a theory of pathological systems, in Watzlawick J, Weakland J (eds): *The Interactional View.* New York, WW Norton, 1977.

Heneo S, Grose N (eds): *Principles of Family Systems in Family Medicine.* New York, Bruner-Mazel, 1985.

Hodas GR, Sargent J: Psychiatric emergencies, in Fleisher G, Ludwig S (eds): *Textbook of Pediatric Emergency Medicine,* ed 2. Baltimore, Williams & Wilkins Co, 1988.

Hoffman L: *Foundation of Family Therapy.* New York, Basic Books Inc, 1981.

Langsley DG, Kaplan DM: *Treatment of Families in Crisis.* New York, Grune & Stratton, 1968.

Minuchin S: *Families and Family Therapy.* Cambridge, Mass, Harvard University Press, 1974.

Minuchin S, Fishman HC: *Family Therapy Techniques.* Cambridge, Mass, Harvard University Press, 1981.

Mirkin M, Koman S (eds): *Handbook of Adolescents and Family Therapy.* New York, Gardner Press, 1985.

Pittman F: *Turning Points: Treating Families in Transition and Crisis.* New York, Norton, 1987.

Sargent J: Family therapy: A view for pediatricians. *J Pediatr* 1983; 102:977-981.

83 EFFECTIVE USE OF PSYCHIATRIC CONSULTATION

Henry Berger, M.D.

In a psychiatric consultation a psychiatrist and primary care physician work together in evaluating a child's emotional climate and well being, formulating a treatment plan, or facilitating the execution of the plan. Effective use of psychiatric consultation requires the physician to (1) have a good working relationship with the consultant; (2) learn to recognize and respond to emotional "red flags" in his patients and families; (3) recognize what issues are beyond his or her own expertise and time limitations; and (4) know how to enable the child and family to overcome their fears and reluctance in obtaining necessary help. Part of the job of a consulting psychiatrist is to help the practitioner to fulfill these requirements. This section describes each of these in detail.

WORKING RELATIONSHIP BETWEEN CONSULTANT AND PHYSICIAN

The primary tools of a psychiatric consultant are the ability to establish rapport and sensitivity to the feelings of others, as well as the more specialized diagnostic and therapeutic skills. The physician who cannot feel comfortable in discussing problems with the psychiatrist and develop confidence in the consultant's abilities may well ask how the troubled patients might feel with the same individual. The lack of an open, cooperative working relationship may force the physician to avoid utilizing the consultant until there is a "serious problem." Finally, the practitioner may inadvertently give away a feeling of discomfort or distrust to the child or family, thus affecting their relationship with the psychiatrist. The primary care physician should also consider his or her own attitudes toward emotional issues and psychotherapy in general. On the other hand, the psychiatrist should be interested and comfortable with medical issues, while acknowledging a lack of expertise in these areas. One of the most destructive obstacles to resolving a child's and families' emotional difficulties is a conflict between the practitioner and psychiatrist. Even the most positive teamwork is often tested and stressed by the disruptive nature of certain emotional difficulties. Thus, it is particularly important to select the right psychiatric consultant and to maintain a sound working relationship.

"RED FLAGS"

The primary care physician should be alert to signs and signals that suggest a need for further exploration and perhaps immediate or eventual therapeutic intervention. While a more detailed description of the diagnostic categories and criteria can be found in the *Diagnostic and Statistical Manual of Mental Disorders* (third edition, revised) prepared by the American Psychiatric Association, a physician will want to be alert at least to signals suggesting underlying disorders or difficulties. Such warning signs range from the severe and more obvious one, suggesting psychiatric disorders, to the more common emotional problems and family dysfunction. The problems suggesting underlying disorders and certain associated diagnostic or etiologic categories are listed in Table 83–1. These categories are not meant to be all-inclusive, nor are the symptoms or signs pathognomonic.

Various studies of pediatric inpatient, outpatient, and physically disabled populations

TABLE 83–1
Underlying Disorders and Diagnostic Categories

PROFILE	DIAGNOSTIC CONSIDERATION
Preschool	
Numerous developmental and behavioral delays in language, social, and motor skills	Mental retardation
Severely withdrawn; noncommunicative; emotionally unresponsive	Childhood autism; pervasive developmental disorder
Significantly anxious or depressed; delayed development; evidence of repeated physical injury; aggressive behavior	Child abuse or neglect
Chronic sleep or eating difficulties; oppositional behavior	Inconsistent or irregular parenting; lack of nurturance
Mild complaints in apparently well-developed child, with age-appropriate behavior	Overwhelmed, emotionally unsupported, anxious parent
School Age	
Poor school performance; aggressive behavior; tantrum; overactivity	Attention-deficit disorder; learning disability
Chronic somatic complaints, with frequent school absence	School avoidance, with family dysfunction
Severe moodiness; social isolation; poor school performance	Childhood affective disorders
Poorly controlled childhood asthma or diabetes, or other "psychosomatic illness"	Stress; family dysfunction
Frequent behavior problems; stealing; fighting; oppositional behavior	Family dysfunction
Adolescence	
Severe personality changes; withdrawn or bizarre behavior; agitated behavior becoming worse; confused behavior	Schizophrenia
Severe weight loss; frequent compulsive vomiting; frequent laxative use	Anorexia nervosa, bulimia
Self-destructive behavior; continual moodiness; school failure; sleep difficulties	Affective disorder
School failure; delinquent behavior; drug abuse; promiscuity	Attention-deficit disorder; learning disability; borderline personality disorder
Poorly controlled chronic illness; asthma, diabetes, colitis	Family dysfunction
School failure, labile mood, personality change	Drug and alcohol abuse

show a high incidence of undiagnosed psychopathology. This suggests at least the need to be alert to complaints and receptive to a family's requests for help and to be willing to take the time, when necessary, to explore these complaints adequately to develop a treatment plan.

Stressful episodes and conditions that should alert the physician to the need for further exploration to determine the impact on the child and the possible need for intervention are listed below. This list is certainly not complete but is meant as a demonstration of the need for a broader perspective in considering the child's emotional environment as well as his individual symptoms and behavior.

1. Loss of family member through death or divorce.
2. Depressed or psychotic parent or guardian.
3. Chronically or severely ill child, parent, or sibling.
4. Chronic parental conflict or other type of severe family dysfunction.
5. Child with learning disability or attention-deficit disorder.
6. Physical or sexual abuse of child or other family member.

FORMULATING A SOLUTION TO THE PROBLEM

Once a decision is made that a particular behavior or situation requires further evaluation, a practitioner must decide whether to proceed alone or to call in a consultant. In either case, time needs to be set aside for a meeting for all family members to discuss the particular situation or complaint. While sometimes this can be done immediately, often it requires a return visit for all family members scheduled at a time that is convenient for both the practitioner and the family and child. The purpose of such a meeting is to gather necessary information, both by hearing from all family members as well as by observing their relationships together. During this meeting a treatment program can also be developed with the cooperation and consent of the family. This therapy can mean immediate suggestions and intervention on the part of the practitioner to alleviate problems that are more simple or the involvement at the next stage of the psychiatric consultant for further assessment and possible intervention. The meeting avoids the risk of the practitioner reassuring a family about a particular complaint without adequate data or prematurely dismissing a complaint as something the parents "might want to see a psychiatrist about." Furthermore, such a meeting increases the chances of enlisting the cooperation of all family members in pursuing a particular decision or treatment plan. In a family meeting, the physician can obtain a history while simultaneously observing family members' reactions to one another. The physician should encourage a family discussion of the problem so that interactions can be observed better. Such family sessions are also useful to discuss relative medical findings, school reports, or testing data. If a problem-solving approach is maintained in a supportive and accepting atmosphere, most families will readily accept appropriate advice. Methodical data gathering through conjoint family meetings helps the physician to avoid becoming involved in an overly complex, explosive, or time-consuming situation.

Most primary care physicians will find they have neither the training nor the time to deal with problems such as a severely dysfunctional family, significantly depressed child or adult, or the variety of problems created by some of the more serious issues mentioned above. Thus, one possible outcome of the evaluation meeting is a decision to consult a psychiatrist for further evaluation and possible treatment. To carry out this decision, it is often necessary for the practitioner to help the family overcome their resistance and anxieties concerning psychiatric involvement.

Often the primary care physician is involved in short-term counseling and in prescribing psychotropic medication. It is estimated that over 50% of emotionally ill patients are being seen by the primary care physician. In such situations, it may be particularly important for the primary care physician to maintain an ongoing relationship with a consulting psychiatrist.

FACILITATING A DIRECT MEETING BETWEEN FAMILY AND PSYCHIATRIC CONSULTANT

The value of considering the psychiatric consultation as a joint process involving the practitioner, family, and consultant makes it possible to view the psychiatrist as participating as an advisor prior to his beginning therapy with the family. In this role, the psychiatrist may help the practitioner identify the problem, gather information, and evaluate the information prior to meeting the family. Such a process naturally means that the practitioner must have a comfortable, ongoing, working relationship with the consultant and that the consultant be available (at least by phone) as needed. Often the practitioner's comfort with the psychiatric consultant will be apparent to the family and enable them to be comfortable in meeting with him. Even under these conditions, however, the most sensitive and supportive physicians may meet enormous resistance to involving a psychiatrist. At this point, the family may attempt to minimize a potentially serious problem to convince the practitioner that they can handle it themselves with a little help, stating it is really just "the teacher's problem" or "he'll grow out of it." Helping the family and child overcome this resistance can be extremely beneficial, both to obtain the necessary assistance and to help them solve problems realistically and cooperatively.

There are a few general approaches and techniques that are useful in overcoming such resistance. First, it is helpful to try to determine its cause. Is the family trying to protect the child? Does someone feel they are to blame for the problem and wish to avoid being criticized? Has there been a previous bad experience with a psychiatrist? Is the involvement of a psychiatrist viewed as an admission of failure? These and other difficulties may be at the root of such resistance and may be clues to more underlying family dysfunction. Sometimes the first visit can be set up as a consultation and a "test," just as a referral to a radiologist is a consultation to find out if anything is wrong and if further treatment is necessary. Whatever the underlying issue may be, the physician will want to maintain a clear stance concerning his or her opinion about obtaining psychiatric help, while, on the other hand, recognizing the legitimate fears of family members. The physician's strongest ally in overcoming such fears is an ongoing positive relationship with the patient and family. In certain instances, friendly understanding but firm encouragement is not enough. In acute crises, one may look for extended family members, friends, church, or school personnel as allies—both in efforts in supporting a disorganized, fragmented family and in assisting further encouragement in obtaining psychiatric help. In other instances, further private consultation between the psychiatrist and physician can be useful and possibly a decision may be reached and agreed to by the family to have a meeting with the psychiatrist in the family physician's office as a form of further evaluation.

SUMMARY

As in working with any other consultant, the primary care physician's relationship with the psychiatric consultant requires a mutual respect and rapport. A general broad focus on the part of the primary care physician is needed to recognize a wide array of problems, including psychosocial dysfunction and to respond to and adequately assess these problems. Naturally, the physician must be able to recognize personal limitations and be able to ask for help when indicated. The psychiatric consultation, however, requires special consideration because of the unique discomfort that families and individuals have in dealing with and working through psychosocial problems and in requesting the help of a psychiatric consultant.

BIBLIOGRAPHY

Beardslee WR, Benporad J, Keller MB, et al: Children of parents with major affective disorders, a review. *Am J Psychiatry* 1983; 140:825–832.

Bennett LA, Wolin SJ, Reiss D: Cognitive, behavioral and emotional problems among school-age children of alcoholic parents. *Am J Psychiatry* 1988; 145:185–190.

Borus JF: Psychiatry and the primary care physician, in Kaplan H, Sadock B (eds): *Comprehensive Textbook of Psychiatry*, vol 4. Baltimore, Williams & Wilkins, 1985.

Breslau N: Psychiatric disorders in children with physical disabilities. *J Am Acad Child Psychiatry* 1985; 24:87–94.

Cantwell DP: Prevalence of psychiatric disorders in a pediatric clinic for military dependent children. *J Pediatr* 1974; 85:711–714.

Hauts CB, et al: Cost of medical/surgical delays: Prevented by psychiatric treatment. *J Am Acad Child Psychiatry* 1985; 24:227–230.

Last CG, Hersen M, Kayden A, et al: Pschiatric illness in mothers of anxious children. *Am J Psychiatry* 1987; 144:1580–1583.

Livingston R, Taylor JL, Crawford SL: A study of somatic complaints and psychiatric diagnosis in children. *J Am Acad Child Adolesc Psychiatry* 1988; 27:185–187.

Orleans CT, George LK, Haupt JL, et al: How primary care physicians treat psychiatric disorders. A national survey of family practitioners. *Am J Psychiatry* 1985; 142:52–57.

84 FAMILY RESPONSE TO DEATH

Linda Gordon, M.D.

Bereaved families commonly will turn to their physician for expert advice and counsel during the period of a child's death. To help them, it is important to understand how the family's developmental levels and structure influence how they react to death and how they can be helped to adjust. The first part of this chapter will explore the grief response of individual family members to the death of the child and the impact on the whole family system. This will be followed by the role of the physician in assisting families through their bereavement toward the successful resolution of their grief.

THE GRIEF REACTION

Grief is an intense emotion, deeply felt in response to the personal loss caused by the death of a child. Mourning is the expression of grief that typically involves physiological disturbances, withdrawal from others, and total preoccupation with the lost love object. This process includes reviewing the experiences, meanings, and emotional significance of the relationship with the deceased individual. The length of mourning will depend on the personal value derived from the relationship with the deceased, the responsibility felt for the death, one's emotional resiliency, and the availability of emotional support (both for the grieving and for recovery). This period of mourning is usually 6 to 12 months. Kubler-Ross described a common progression through five stages of grieving, both for dying individuals and their survivors. These stages of grieving are denial and isolation, anger, bargaining, depression, and acceptance.

DENIAL AND ISOLATION

The news of a death evokes a feeling of surprise as well as sadness. Commonly disbelief or denial follow, both as a mechanism to adjust to the need and as a time delay that allows a time for processing both the fact and how it affects the remaining members of the family. Because of demands of funeral arrangements and of daily living needs, family members are forced to remain somewhat functional.

ANGER AND GUILT

When the defense of denial breaks down, parents of a child who is dying may experience anger or resentment that is displaced in all directions. They commonly experience intolerable self-reproach and guilt or attack a member of the health team for errors or decisions, real or imagined. At this time, family members are prone to accidents such as careless driving. Suicidal ideation, without intent, is often felt and sometimes expressed. As a demonstration of an outward projection of the parents' sense of guilt and failure, one parent may blame the other for the child's death. Doing this, parents may isolate themselves from one another at a critical time.

BARGAINING

Bargaining may be the parent's reaction formation against feelings of intolerable helplessness and the ultimate inability to protect the child. Bargaining usually takes place prior to death in a hope to gain more time or relieve guilt. This overcompensation may take varied behavioral expressions, as parents bargain with God for their child's life. Parents may become extremely protective of their child or focus on career achievement, both in attempts to fulfill their bargain to be better parents. They may overfunction as nurses for their own child at this stage to compensate for feelings of incompetence.

DEPRESSION

Sadness and depression, which follow this phase of increased activity, are associated with physiologic difficulties such as: loss of sleep, appetite, and libido; inability to concentrate; memory problems; distractibility; fatigue; weakness; and complaints of pain. Some parents seek relief with medication or alcohol. Parents physically identify with their dying child and experience pain as if their child were being forcibly wrenched away from them. The parent is completely preoccupied with thoughts of the child and is apathetic to everyone else.

ACCEPTANCE

Ultimately acceptance is reached at the point at which parents integrate the child's illness into the family structure and begin to plan for the future.

Generally, the family that can experience its grief before the child's death will make a smoother transition through the stages of grief. Families that undergo anticipatory grief have time to develop a strong and broad support network that includes the physician. The family may choose a home care program where there is greater opportunity for family intimacy and communication. Through this program the family participates more in decisions about their child and family and has been able to exert more control over the child's course. Even with anticipatory grieving, the acute grief reaction ensues.

ACUTE GRIEF REACTION OF PARENTS

Since the majority of childhood deaths are unpredictable and sudden, most families find themselves totally unprepared. Family members individually undergo an acute grief reaction lasting 4 to 8 weeks. This five-stage period involves a loss of self-esteem, various somatic disturbances, and decreased level of functioning. A period of psychological adjustment follows the physiologic changes. This depression stage usually remits by 12 to 15 months, followed by a readjustment period with renewed interest in the future by 24 months.

Despite the similarities, each family member suffers the loss in a personal way. Culturally determined patterns as well as the age of the child and the cause of death will provoke a different pattern of grief. Studies by Mandell and associates and Smialek point out important differences in parents' grieving patterns. Fathers often assume a controlled, manager-like role, utilizing intellectualization, and increase their career involvement outside the home. They are more reluctant to share their emotional pain, perhaps due to a sense of loss of power. Many fathers require extra encouragement and permission to cry and to express feelings of sadness. Parents often verbalize guilt at not having spent enough time with the deceased child. Mothers, usually the primary caretaker, often assign themselves the majority of blame for their child's death. They are more likely to utilize professional support. In most instances, parental guilt is an emotional reaction without any basis in reality. However, in some situations such as a child with a congenital malformation, parents may be realistically dealing with the guilt of having contributed to the child's death. In these families, mourning becomes complicated and often prolonged.

Serious marital discord after the death of a child is common. Preexisting marital problems are generally intensified by the loss. Couples who are married for a short time before the child's death or who lose their first and only child are also at risk. One short-term follow-up study by Mandell and associates of families of victims of sudden infant death syndrome reported a 20% rate of divorce.

Parents commonly react to the death of one child by desiring another "substitute child" as soon as possible. The planned conception of another child during the mourning is fraught with dangers. There is a higher rate of infertility and spontaneous abortion 1 year after a child's death (Mandell et al.). The identity of the replacement child may become fused with that of the deceased child bringing on additional behavior problems.

ACUTE GRIEF REACTION OF CHILDREN

Siblings experience similar grief reactions to their parents. They suffer the loss of their identity as brother or sister and mourn for their deceased sibling in ways appropriate for their age and understanding. An estimated 50% of children may experience emotional and behavioral adjustment disorders after a sibling's death (Mulhern et al.).

The child under 3 years of age is mainly concerned with the physical presence of the parents and the integrity of his or her body. Children of this age group do not consider the permanence of death. They see characters who die in one television program reappear in another role. Their games include dying and returning to play. Some children fear loss of body parts or physical mutilation as concomitants of death. For some children a clinical picture of acute separation anxiety may be the prominent dynamic, while other children may regress in eating and toilet training. In one study of siblings of victims of sudden infant death syndrome performed by Mandell et al., sustained sleep disturbances lasted 2 to 12 months.

Children between 3 and 5 years view death as a reversible separation. The child experiences magical thinking and lacks a concept of causality. They understand better the death of animals but do not appreciate the permanence of the death of the family member. The child may repeatedly ask where the deceased sibling is and when will he return. Their inability to differentiate between thought and deed increases the preschool child's risk of feeling responsible for his sibling's disappearance by having merely wished that the brother or sister would go away. Many children verbalize fears of dying in their sleep and talk of nightmares with monsters chasing them to go to heaven. Behavioral changes such as withdrawal, hyperactivity, and aggression toward other children were also common.

Between the ages of 5 and 10 years, death is personified as an evil person who carries others away. Using concrete operations, children may view death as murder or punishment for being bad or for crying. Sometimes children this age will perceive illness also as a punishment. Children often express their fears in nightmares. Through stories and games they attempt to master their fear of death. School problems, peer problems, sleep disturbances, and changes in their dynamics with their parents were frequently observed in this age group (Mandell et al.).

From age 10 years to early adolescence, children acquire formal operational or logical thinking. At this time, children understand death as a universal biologic process both final and inevitable. Verbalization is greatly increased, leading to better communication and greater understanding about the death of their siblings. The grieving of children of this age group follows the stages outlined above, although their expressions of the feelings are more appropriate for their age.

THE ROLE OF THE PHYSICIAN

The primary care physician due to the longstanding involvement with the family, the personal relationship with the deceased child, and the familiarity with the family dynamics is in a powerful position to support bereaved families. In dealing with the families, the physician should not only have an understanding of grief reaction and the developmental capacity for children to comprehend death, but also an awareness of his or her own emotional reactions to the death of the child. Physicians often experience a sense of inadequacy and powerlessness, not unlike that felt by the family. The physician needs to meet his or her own need for support, to work through his or her own personal grief prior to helping the family.

The physician who cares for the terminally ill child has an opportunity to monitor the family's interactions, including the degree of communication, availability of emotional supportiveness, and the appropriateness of the children's behavior. The physician may act as a facilitator for increased family communication among estranged or noncommunicative members and help the family express their emotions. The physician can be a consultant to the parents regarding the child's developmental capabilities and guide them to age-appropriate expectations.

When a terminally ill child is hospitalized, the doctor has an opportunity to help staff members share their emotional reactions in caring for the child. Families, whose grief is expressed privately or in ways unfamiliar to hospital staff, may sometimes experience a subtle loss of staff support. The physician may help the staff by sharing views about the range of normal variations in the expected grief response and highlighting the family's style of grieving as unique but not inappropriate.

At the time of the child's death, the physician has several important responsibilities that are outlined in the protocol provided by Frader and Sargent: making contact, providing support, allaying guilt, appreciation of cultural and social influences, organizing social support, seeing the patient, and follow-up.

The physician first informs the family of the child's death in a straightforward but sensitive way. Preferably, the family will be shown to a room where they will be allowed to share their acute grief privately. The apparent cause of death should be explained as simply and clearly as possible. In many cases of sudden or unexplained death, an autopsy may be required or requested (Berger). Families may be told that an autopsy may be helpful by uncovering hidden congenital malformations (information that would be useful to other family members), infectious disease that may be a public health concern, or valuable medical information to help other children in the future. Families may be allowed to specify certain restrictions or to donate organs for transplant into other children. This choice may help parents derive meaning from the death.

The physician can help the family make their separation from the child in a personally meaningful way. Family members should be given the opportunity to see and hold the child's body in a private room. Some families may want to hold their child; some may want to have the siblings with them.

Perhaps the most difficult, but the most important, part of acute supportive care of the family is supportive listening. Physicians are trained to be helpful to others by active treatment or technical procedures. At this time, listening to the family's concerns and sadness in an active and supportive way is most helpful to grieving families.

Families may seek guidance from physicians to plan for funeral and burial arrangements. In many situations, nursing services or social workers will have more experience with the actual methods of calling funeral directors to begin the arrangements. The usual problem for the physician is to help the family explain the death to the siblings and to help them make a decision about siblings' attendance at the funeral. An honest and direct explanation to the other children is the best approach, keeping in mind their developmental level and their own feelings about their imagined contribution to the death. The physician might review with the parents what they will say and might offer to be present. Parents should be told that euphemisms about death, such as "he went to sleep" or "he went away" do not address the questions children have and may be frightening. A more direct approach is to say that the sibling died because of an illness or accident and that he or she will never return to the family. When appropriate, the religious views of the family can be reinforced also. Parents should be encouraged to share feelings of sadness with their children and to reassure them that they will not be alone or forgotten. The family's routine should be as close to normal as possible. Parents need to listen closely to the surviving siblings to discover their hidden fears and worries to comfort them appropriately.

The physician, anticipating the parents' harsh self-recrimination, can discuss these feelings while explaining the medical reason for death. To disabuse the family of their misconceptions about the child's death, the physician should first elicit the family's particular concerns. Leading questions such as "Many parents in your situation feel responsible for their child's death. Do you have any feelings like that?" may be productive. If the physician feels uncomfortable using that phrase, another one that fits the physician's style should be used. Once the parents' worries are identified, the physician can then help to demystify death by clarifying the medical etiology, while reassuring the family that they were not responsible.

The physician, as a medical expert, has a major role in reassuring parents that their feelings and symptoms are expected and not signs of impending psychosis. For instance, parents frequently experience acute vision of their child alive and healthy. It is not uncommon for parents to feel that their life, not their child's, should have been taken. Acute physical changes need to be anticipated and understood. Short-term use of tranquilizers may sometimes be necessary. Caution should be used to avoid oversedation and blunting of the emotional grief response. Physicians should help keep families focused on the child to facilitate grieving. It is helpful to review the special place the child had in the family and to recall a pleasant or meaningful experience. The family may join into the discussion and mix smiles and tears. The sooner and greater the catharsis, the more likely will be its successful resolution.

The physician may inquire how the parents have dealt with other crises, asking the parents how they supported one another through that time. A high level of communication and contact between family members will help facilitate the process.

Routine follow-up visits are beneficial to grieving families. Visits may be scheduled at 1 month after the child's death. The visit gives the families another chance to ask questions and clarify any issues that were not resolved at the time of the death. At this visit, the physician can assess the functioning of the family in their resolution of their grieving. The family should have begun to return to a level of functioning at which the daily routine of living is accomplished. The family's understanding of the cause of death can be reviewed. The autopsy results, if available, can be discussed. The family will benefit from further reassurance that they were not responsible for the child's death.

The physician intervenes in the family system when there is an inability to resume an appropriate level of functioning. Psychiatric referral is indicated when family members present a danger to themselves or others by expressing persistent suicidal ideation or intent or by acting in a negligent manner with respect to their health or personal responsibilities. A parent may be dangerous to others by not appropriately attending to the health and safety needs of other family members. Parent support groups exist in some communities to help families who have experienced the death of a child.

Families may experience adjustment reactions after the death of a child. Often children express behavior problems or somatic complaints, for example, a depressed child may have abdominal pain or sleep disturbance or withdrawal from peers as an equivalent of unresolved sadness shared by one or more family members. Therefore, assessment of the symptomatic child should include assessment of all family members.

The primary care physician has an important and unique role in helping the family who experiences the death of a child. By understanding the developmental issues in regard to the remaining children (especially how they understand death), the family structure, and the family's method of functioning under stress, the physician can help the family through the adjustment period.

BIBLIOGRAPHY

Aradire C: Books for children about death. *Pediatrics* 1976; 57:372.

Berger L: Requesting the autopsy: A pediatric perspective. *Clin Pediatr* 1978; 17:445.

Brent DA: A death in the family: The pediatrician's role. *Pediatrics* 1983; 72:645.

Cain A, Cain B: On replacing a child. *J Am Acad Child Psychiatry* 1964; 3:443.

Elliott BA: Neonatal death: Reflections for parents. *Pediatrics* 1978; 62:100.

Elliott BA, Hein HA: Neonatal death: Reflections for physicians. *Pediatrics* 1978; 62(1):96.

Frader JE, Sargent J: Sudden death or catastrophic illness: Family considerations, in Fleisher GR, Ludwig S (eds): *Textbook of Pediatric Emergency Medicine*. Baltimore, Williams & Wilkins Co, 1983, chap 64.

Friedman SB, Chodoff P, Mason JW, et al: Behavioral observations on parents anticipating the death of a child. *Pediatrics* 1963; 32:610.

Kubler-Ross E: *On Death and Dying*. New York, Macmillan Publishing Co, 1970.

Mandell F, McAnulty E, Reece RM, et al: Observations of paternal response to sudden unanticipated infant death. *Pediatrics* 1980; 5:221.

Mandell F, McAnulty EH, Carlson A: Unexpected death of an infant sibling. *Pediatrics* 1983; 72:652.

Mulhern RK, Lauer ME, Hoffmann RG: Death of child at home or in the hospital: Subsequent psychological adjustment of the family. *Pediatrics* 1983; 71:743.

Sargent AJ: The family: A pediatric assessment. *J Pediatr* 1983; 102:973.

Schulman JL, Rhem JL: Assisting the bereaved. *J Pediatr* 1983; 102:992.

Smialek Z: Observations on immediate reactions of families to sudden infant death. *Pediatrics* 1978; 62:160.

Wessel MA: The primary physician and the death of a child in a specialized hospital setting. *Pediatrics* 1983; 77:443.

Wilson AL, Fenton LJ, Stevens DC, et al: The death of a newborn twin: An analysis of parental bereavement. *Pediatrics* 1982; 70:587.

85 DELINQUENCY, RUNNING AWAY, AND PROMISCUITY

Edwin F. Castillo, M.D.

Delinquency, running away, and promiscuity are significant social problems characteristic of adolescence. Mann reports in 1974 that there were reportedly 6,100,000 arrests in the United States for serious crimes, such as criminal homicide, forcible rape, robbery, aggravated assault, and arson. Of these, 1,700,000, or just over 27%, were committed by persons under 18 years of age.

Juveniles commit 10% of all murders, 32% of all robberies, 17% of all the aggravated assaults, and 58% of all the arson. Nationally, when burglary, larceny, and motor vehicle thefts are added to this list, more than half of all the serious crimes in the United States are found to be committed by youths from 10 to 17 years of age (Youth Crime Plague, 1977). Over 1 million youths have currently run away from home. Delinquent behavior occurs five times more frequently in boys than in girls, and boys are more likely to demonstrate violent behavior directed against others. These behavioral disorders are not restricted to any particular socioeconomic group, although they are most frequently seen in the lower socioeconomic strata.

Most often these problems come to the attention of the physician through an emergency caused by drug or alcohol intoxication, running away, suicide attempts, or aggressive or violent behavior. At times, these problems can be identified in the physician's office, particularly when the child and family are known to the physician and are under undue stress and call on the physician for advice. When serious behavior problems such as these occur, one person in a family is likely to seek help from the local physician.

In delinquency, the problem behavior starts before the age of 15 years, usually from earliest school years, and persists into adulthood. Delinquency represents a chronic pattern of antisocial behavior. The behavior may involve violence or aggression (e.g., vandalism, mugging, assault, and rape), or may involve behavior that is socially unacceptable, but nonaggressive (e.g., truancy, expulsion from school, academic achievement below expected level, running away, theft, lying, excessive drinking, or drug abuse).

Children who run away generally exhibit nonaggressive behavior. The runaway episode is usually short-lived, lasting from a few days to 2 weeks. Teenagers who run away frequently find solace with friends or adults that they know and trust. They often get into trouble and are caught by the police. These adolescents, from all socioeconomic groups, frequently leave home after physical or sexual abuse by parents and parental figures. Very often the child has tried in his own way to express to his parents what his needs are and what kinds of frustration or emotional difficulties he is experiencing. He may ask for more independence and have tried to negotiate for more flexibility concerning rules. When the parents respond critically or by rigidly adhering to their rules, the child can then have difficulties that result in his receiving punitive attention, rather than the support and nurturance that he needs. The child, feeling totally unsupported in the family and with the sense that there is nothing he can do to change the situation, runs away. Leaving the family can be seen as a sign of hope or a cry for help for the individual as well as for the family. When delinquency, running away, and promiscuity occur simultaneously in girls, incest is a common precipitating factor. Here, the running away is a form of communication through which the adolescent may say, "I can't deal with this anymore, so I might as well run away."

There is some confusion in our society regarding the degree of sexual experimentation that is permissible. It is important for the physician to recognize the moral values of a family and the culture they live in before making a definite judgment about this issue. Promiscuity can be defined as out-of-control and excessive sexual behavior, due to an inability on the part of the child and family to control or deal with it.

DIFFERENTIAL DIAGNOSIS

Before labeling children as delinquent, it is important to rule out other medical conditions, intoxications, and other psychiatric disorders, since aggressive, violent, and unacceptable behavior can be the result rather than the cause. Children with psychotic symptoms frequently commit serious and violent offenses. Similarly, depression and hyperkinetic syndrome during adolescence are associated with significant antisocial behavior. Somatization can also be seen in connection with behavioral problems, particularly when these youths are dealing with a tremendous amount of stress and anxiety or depression.

RECOGNITION

In some instances, recognition will be easy because these problems will be identified by the family. In other instances, parents may either conceal the problems or be indifferent to them. The problem behaviors frequently are initially manifested during the school years and early adolescence. These children show impulsive behavior, irritability, labile affect, poor frustration tolerance, and temper outbursts. They may have other problems such as school suspension, smoking, drinking, drug dependence, precocious sexual activity, pregnancy, and venereal disease. They may get in trouble with the law due to stealing, mugging, reckless driving, running away, and prostitution.

The presence of delinquency and conduct disorder represents a failure of the socialization process in which the families are unable to enforce societal rules and set limits adequately. As a result, the child is unable to learn to control his impulses. The families of these children and adolescents present a typical pattern of inadequate and inconsistent limit setting and enforcement of rules and do not hold the child accountable for his behavior. The parents frequently undermine each other in their efforts to discipline the child, which only contributes to the perpetuation of the problem. The adolescent avoids responsibility for his behavior and, as a result, comes to believe that he will be excused from any consequences of his actions. In some families, discipline may fluctuate from being mild, at times, to being overly punitive and physically abusive at other times. These families also present a variety of other problems. They are poorly organized and role expectations of different members of the family are unclear. Parental role models show poor impulse control and disregard of societal norms. Frequently parents of these children are going through separation or divorce or suffer from mental illness, or drug or alcohol abuse. Criminality and incarceration occur in some of these families.

EVALUATION

The history, to be as complete as possible, should be obtained from both parents. Everybody should be encouraged to be as open as possible. If hostility exists between the child and the parents, the child should also be interviewed alone. Special attention should be given to the child's safety and well-being. It is important to explore family relationships (past or present), peer relationships, alcohol and drug use, hobbies, enjoyed activities, emotional well-being, and self-concept. How the child views himself and how he is viewed by others is important. Is the child experiencing any painful or emotional difficulties, crying spells, sadness, depression, or anxiety? The physician should inquire about academic performance, school attendance, and relationship to teachers and authority figures. How does the child handle frustration and anxiety? Is the child prone toward irritability or temper tantrums? How do the family members relate to one another? Is there open communication between family members or is there indifference? Do both parents agree on setting limits and in disciplining the child? How are conflicts expressed? How does the child ask for what he wants and does he get it? In the case of the runaway child, what is the child running away from or running to? Is there any evidence of sexual or physical abuse? A complete physical examination should be performed to determine if there is any evidence of physical abuse, intercurrent illnesses, or signs of marijuana, alcohol, or other drug use. In cases of promiscuity, the physician should be attentive to evidence of sexually transmittable illness and pregnancy.

OFFICE COUNSELING

It is important for the physician to assess the severity of each case and determine if immediate psychiatric care is needed. The physician should determine the potential for violence, the presence of suicidal ideation and previous suicidal behavior, chronicity of the problem, and the history of any previous treatment and its outcome. In less serious situations, the physician can help the parents agree on disciplinary measures and insist on their consistency concerning limit-setting. The physician can also help the parents develop a set of expectations around chores, homework, and curfew time, determine which parent will be the enforcer of the rules, and assess if the other parent will support this plan. With early sexual acting-out or promiscuity, the physician should support and help the parents set their own rules in determining sexual behavior. The child should be helped to assist the parents to understand his or her own needs and desires concerning sexual behavior. In this way the family can resolve this issue themselves in accord with their culture and the child's developmental level. With moderately serious behavior problems, especially in the presence of emotional disturbance and significant family conflicts, the child and family should be referred for outpatient psychotherapy. For more seriously disturbed children, the presence of violent outbursts and/or suicidal behavior necessitates a referral for psychiatric hospitalization.

The physician also has the responsibility to report suspected sexual or physical abuse by contacting the local child protective services agency. Families who refuse referrals for psychotherapy or children whose behavior fails to improve in treatment may need referral to the juvenile justice system for chronic delinquent behavior.

OVERVIEW OF TREATMENT

While some adolescents with behavior disturbance are seen as psychiatrically disturbed and in need of treatment, other authorities view these *same children* as juvenile delinquents who need to be handled by the juvenile justice system. This dichotomy in approach continues to be an unresolved issue.

The treatment of the juvenile delinquent is difficult and complex. Reports from the literature of results from individual, group, and family therapy are not very promising. The families are difficult to involve in therapy. In many instances, through the use of a court order or probation, the judicial system may provide some leverage to engage families in treatment, but with only limited success. The best results are reported for adolescents who live in group homes or residential placements that provide more structure and control to prevent self-destructive and violent behavior. Individual counseling and group therapy are frequently effective tools in assisting adolescents to work through difficulties with peer relationships, relationships with authority figures, and/or a long history of abuse and neglect. Family participation and therapy is indicated at a later stage, once the staff has established trust and a cooperative relationship with the patient.

In the case of runaway behavior, family-oriented psychotherapy is the treatment of choice. One should not assume that these patients and their families cannot be treated. Typically, these youngsters are unable to ask for and get what they want and need verbally. Frequently, the parents are either indifferent or insensitive to the adolescent's needs or too rigid and inflexible to respond appropriately. The runaway behavior induces a crisis in the family that brings attention to the family problems. These families do not readily seek psychiatric treatment, so physicians should actively encourage them to do so. In cases in which the behavior is chronic, severe, and/or life-threatening, it may be necessary to hospitalize the child. This approach is particularly effective in instances in which parents deny or fail to recognize the seriousness of the problem. Once the child is hospitalized, therapy can assist family members to reconnect with one another, which is the first step in a process aimed at improving communication and ultimately strengthening family relationships.

TREATMENT OF PROMISCUITY

The physician can treat an isolated situation of sexual experimentation or acting-out by helping the family develop a set of expectations concerning the sexual behavior and assisting the child to express his or her own needs and desires so that the parents can respond appropriately. The physician should keep in mind that the child may be expressing a need for companionship, affection, and nurturance through the sexual behavior. Depressed children with low self-esteem may also use sexual behavior to gain approval and be liked by peers. In situations in which promiscuity is associated with other serious behavioral, emotional, or communication problems within the family, the physician should make referral for psychiatric therapy. In general, if this problem is approached early, before it has spread to other areas of the adolescent's life, the treatment can be quite effective.

BIBLIOGRAPHY

Aichorn A: Underlying causes of delinquency, in *Wayward Youth*. New York, Viking Press, 1935; pp 92–116.

Cantwell DP: Hyperactivity and antisocial behavior. *J Am Acad Child Psychiatry* 1978; 17(2).

Johnson AM: Sanctions for superego lacunae of adolescents, in Eissler KR (ed): *Searchlights on Delinquency*. New York, International Universities Press, 1949, pp 225–234.

Patteson GR, Dishion TJ: Contributions of families and peers to delinquency. *Criminology* 1985; 23:63–79.

Patterson GR, Stoathamer-Leober M: The correlation of family management practices and delinquency. *Child Dev* 1984; 55:1299-1300.

86 DEPRESSION

Gordon R. Hodas, M.D.

Depression during childhood and adolescence is a serious and potentially life-threatening condition that implies dysfunction at three distinct levels: individual, interpersonal, and biochemical. At the individual level, childhood and adolescent depression implies a significant disturbance in mood, most commonly persistent sadness, self-deprecation, and suicidal ideation. There are myriad presentations, varying from a full-blown depressive syndrome with physiologic concomitants to a less complete but often equally serious adjustment reaction with serious alterations of mood toward sadness and hopelessness. At the interpersonal level, childhood and adolescent depression signifies a breakdown in the process of care-taking and support on the part of the parents as well as an interference in the capacity of parents and child to acknowledge and talk about the problem. The biochemical level becomes relevant in the more severe cases of childhood and adolescent depression in which disturbances in mood and self-concept are accompanied by physiologic and other associated impairments in functioning. In such instances there is often a family history of depression. The office-based physician should appreciate that effective treatment of childhood and adolescent depression need not involve pharmacotherapy, even when a biochemical imbalance is present.

Although some children and adolescents have been depressed for a prolonged period, depression usually implies a recognizable change from an earlier more adaptive mode of functioning. The office-based physician should recognize that depression in childhood and adolescence may present directly, in the form of overt sadness, or indirectly, in the form of persistent somatic complaints, frequent office visits, and school avoidance patterns. Similarly, depression may be readily acknowledged by some children and adolescents and their parents and strongly denied by others. Since some parents may be unaware of depression when it exists, the office-based physician can often serve a crucial role in relinking parents and child while also making a referral when indicated.

PRESENTATION

The common presentations of depression in childhood and adolescence are summarized below:

1. Sad, hopeless mood
2. Suicide attempts
3. Recurrent "accidents"
4. Recurrent somatic complaints
5. School avoidance
6. Exacerbation of medical disorder
7. Eating disorders (anorexia nervosa, bulimia)
8. Alcohol and drug abuse
9. Conduct disorder
10. Academic problems
11. Attention deficit disorder

The findings may occur singly or in combinations. The child or adolescent may describe directly his sad, hopeless feeling, or the mood state may be so evident that the physician recognizes it readily and the patient confirms it. When the patient shows a capacity to acknowledge his depression and discuss it with the physician, there is a more favorable prognosis, even if the symptoms are severe. Any overt suicide attempt should be regarded as serious, since all suicidal behavior represents a genuine statement of distress and self-destructive urges. Repeated accidents are a frequent manifestation of depression and may take the form of unconscious recklessness or risk-taking, or deliberate life-endangering acts. It would appear that many accidents, especially car accidents, are really unacknowledged suicide attempts.

The depressed child or adolescent may present with recurrent somatic complaints and have frequent office visits. The complaints (such as headaches, abdominal pain, nausea, and dizziness) typically have no organic basis despite repeated evaluation. Upon further questioning, the office-based physician may discover a persistent pattern of school avoidance of many months' or years' duration. Depression may also occur in children with a chronic medical disorder, who may present with an unexplained exacerbation of the condition. An underlying depression, in conjunction with less effective coping, can contribute to a worsening of the illness.

Depression can also present in other forms that superficially appear unrelated to it. For example, depression is quite frequent in two common eating disorders, anorexia nervosa and bulimia. Depression may be masked by alcohol and drug abuse when the substances are used to offer an escape from the painful, sad affect. Similarly, many children and adolescents with conduct disorders may also be masking an underlying depression.

Children who present with a rapid deterioration of school performance may have an underlying depression that has interfered with the ability to concentrate. Children with special limitations (such as a learning disability or an attention deficit disorder) encounter special problems in school and are thus vulnerable to depressive episodes.

RECOGNITION

The cardinal features that assist the office-based physician in recognizing overt or underlying depression are presented in the following lists. The diagnosis of depression is best made by seeing the child with the parent(s) and also by talking with the child or adolescent alone and observing the patient for signs of depression, while noting the relationship that unfolds. In most instances, a gently sympathetic approach on the part of the physician will make the sad affect more apparent and will enable the child to begin to discuss some of the sources of distress. The three major criteria for recognizing depression are dysphoric mood (a pervasive sense of distress and ill-being), self-deprecatory ideation, and associated impairments of functioning.

The major feature of the *dysphoric mood* of depression is a persistent sense of sadness; features of this mood are:

1. Sad affect
2. Irritability
3. Anxiety
4. Lability
5. Crying
6. Exhaustion

The other characteristics listed may occur singly or in combination. Lability refers to persistent moodiness and the tendency to be verbally abusive. The sense of exhaustion may be overwhelming and may be experienced both emotionally and physically.

Self-deprecatory ideation frequently manifests itself in terms of self-doubt and indecisiveness. The subjective expressions of self-deprecation are:

1. Self-doubt
2. Low self-esteem
3. Sense of worthlessness
4. Indecisiveness
5. Sense of guilt
6. Sense of powerlessness and helplessness
7. Sense of hopelessness
8. Suicidal ideation

Suicidal wishes are likely to occur when the child sees himself as powerless, helpless, and hopeless.

In general, *associated impairments of functioning* occur in more severe depressions and may have physical, academic, interpersonal, and behavioral manifestations. These impairments of functioning are:

1. Physical alterations
   - Sleep pattern
   - Eating pattern
   - Energy pattern
   - Somatic preoccupations
   - Exacerbated medical condition
2. Academic
   - School absence
   - Visits to school nurse
   - Drop in grades
3. Interpersonal
   - Withdrawal from peers and family
   - Increased isolation
   - Increased conflict at home
4. Behavioral
   - Suicide attempts
   - Acting out
   - Eating disorders

Physical alterations may involve changes in three physiologic patterns: sleep (excessive sleep or insomnia), eating (poor appetite and weight loss), and energy (psychomotor retardation, fatigue, and inability to concentrate). Exacerbation of both psychosomatic and chronic medical illnesses may also occur. Academic impairments may involve lower grades, poor work habits, school absence (often unreported), and visits to the school nurse.

A careful drug history is helpful in making the diagnosis. In general, exogenous substances tend to produce symptoms that mimic acute schizophrenia rather than acute depression. Amphetamine, cocaine, and hallucinogen withdrawal may produce some depression, but usually this is superficial and is often accompanied by severe agitation. Depression can be distinguished from schizophrenia because the depressed patient, however withdrawn and preoccupied, speaks in a goal-directed manner and may exhibit some warmth. Hallucinations and delusions are uncommon in adolescent depression and, when present, relate only to themes of worthlessness.

Recognition and diagnosis of depression are the office-based physician's primary tasks. It is not always easy to distinguish between significant adolescent depression and the moodiness and lability that often accompanies this developmental period. However, in view of the increasing acceptability of self-destructive behavior among adolescents, both through individual acts and suicide pacts, it is especially prudent for the office-based physician to remain alert to the possibility of depression and to take a cautious approach. Screening for signs of depression should be done with every child and adolescent and should include questions about drug and alcohol use, school performance and attendance, family relationships, future plans, suicidal thoughts, and direct self-destructive behavior.

When discussion elicits concern on the part of the physician about a sad or suicidal child or adolescent, the physician should talk further to that patient, seeking to learn sources of stress, attempts at coping, and available sources of support. The physician should ask about the child's relationship with parents, the extent to which the child has shared his or her concerns with the parents, and how the child would expect the parents to react if they were aware of his crisis. Additional questions about suicide should focus on the immediate possibility of suicide on the part of the child or adolescent and on the child's ability to make a firm non-suicide agreement, first to the physician and later to the parents. With actively suicidal patients, immediate psychiatric referral, either to the pediatric emergency room or to an immediately available private psychiatrist, should be made. The physician should make certain that both parents are present or should have them come in immediately so that the parents can deal with the crisis together.

REFERRAL

The referral process may be more difficult with a depressed but not actively suicidal patient who needs psychiatric referral, since the family's pattern of rationalization and denial may preclude follow through with the referral. The urgency created by an acutely suicidal or psychotic patient is absent in these cases. In addition, the referral recommendation is typically made by the physician only to the mother; as a result, the father may feel excluded and threatened and may block referral. To promote a successful psychiatric referral by avoiding some of these pitfalls, it is recommended that the office-based physician regularly take the following steps:

1. The physician, after talking with the child alone, should arrange for a family conference at which both parents and the child will be present. The physician should personally call the father, since this will enable the physician to explain the purpose of the conference while gaining rapport with the father.
2. The physician should privately encourage the child to share his concerns with the parents at the family conference.
3. At the family conference the physician should highlight the need for psychiatric consultation to understand the child's depression better and to learn how the family can help in promoting personal and family development. The specific name of a psychiatrist is given to the parents, who are encouraged to call that day. The office-based physician assures the family that he will actively communicate with the psychiatrist and that he will remain available to the child and family, both now and after the depression resolves.

BIBLIOGRAPHY

Carlson G, Cantwell D: Unmasking masked depression in children and adolescents. *Am J Psychiatry* 1980; 137:445–449.

Cytryn L, Mc Knew DH Jr, Bunney WE Jr, et al: Diagnosis of depression in children: A reassessment. *Am J Psychiatry* 1980; 137:22–25.

Kashani J, Husain A, Shekim WO, et al: Current perspectives on childhood depression: An overview. *Am J Psychiatry* 1981; 138:143–153.

Petti T: Depression in children: A significant disorder. *Psychosomatics* 1981; 22:444–447.

87 DRUG AND ALCOHOL ABUSE

John Sargent, M.D.

In recent years, it has been estimated that between 80% and 90% of adolescents in the United States have used a drug for nonmedical purposes. The use of these substances to alter mood, perception, and behavior has become an integral part of coming of age in our society. Many young people experiment with drugs and do not repeat the experience. Others use the drugs intermittently, or regularly, in a controlled fashion and suffer few adverse consequences. For some, however, early experimentation may progress to a pattern of abuse that becomes compulsive and repetitive and may become associated with physical and psychosocial deterioration. In addition to psychological difficulties that can arise as a result of the effects of the drug use, these substances interfere with other developmentally important behaviors and experiences during adolescence. Furthermore, irresponsible drug and alcohol use can lead to death or disability due to accidents that occur under the influence of these substances.

It is important for the primary care physician to be familiar with different categories of adolescent drug use. The majority of adolescent drug use is *experimental* and carried out for its effects on mood or behavior. Experimental drug use is controlled, limited to specific situations, and the adolescent ingests enough of the drug to alter his mood, but rarely enough to cause acute intoxication or overdose. *Intoxication* refers to significant use of a given drug on a particular occasion that will lead to a dramatic alteration in mood, behavior, and physical status that interferes with judgment, inhibition, and control of behavior and places the drug user at significant risk, especially if engaging in dangerous activities. *Overdose* refers to the excessive use of a drug that interferes with bodily functions and can lead to significant physiologic impairment or death. *Habituation* describes a pattern of repetitive drug use that is compulsive and engaged in regardless of external circumstances. *Addiction* implies physical dependency upon a drug with physiologic symptoms resulting from abrupt cessation of its use. Addiction occurs only with substances that induce *tolerance*, a decreased effect from repeated administration of the same dose of a specific drug. Habituation and addiction describe patterns of drug use over time, while intoxication and overdose refer to a response to a drug ingestion on one particular occasion.

As the physician deals with adolescent substance use, it is always important for him to bear in mind the age and developmental stage of each adolescent and the expectations and mores of that adolescent's family and culture. The primary care physician will find that drug or alcohol use may be a problem for particular teenagers or their families at different stages of use. Some families may find experimental or infrequent use of drugs to be problematic, even though it is highly intermittent and controlled by the adolescent, whereas other families may not be significantly concerned even though the adolescent's use of a drug has become repetitive and may be interfering with that adolescent's overall functioning.

Drug and alcohol use among adolescents is culturally influenced and can be supported by the teenager's peer group. An adolescent's use of a particular substance may reflect both use in the adolescent's family as well as the activities of that adolescent's peers. Studies of adolescents who use drugs repeatedly indicate that these youths, who harbor a more critical attitude toward conventional society, often place a higher value on independence and autonomy and lower values on academic achievement. The use of drugs may also be reinforced by a perceived lack of confidence and competency, lack of attention and support within the family, and a lack of overall adaptation to the academic environment.

Drug use is an age-graded behavior. It can be seen by adolescents as a developmental milestone and, therefore, is identified as a marker of enhanced maturity. There is often a hierarchy of drug use. Cigarettes and alcohol are often tried first, marijuana subsequently. A smaller proportion of adolescents may try other drugs of abuse, including opiates, hallucinogens, cocaine, or amphetamines. Drug use is a learned behavior. The adolescent experiences a sense of belonging and participation within the peer group through the use of drugs or alcohol and often drugs are used as recreation. The adolescent then associates stress reduction and social pleasure with drug use and this association continues through repetitive use. The adolescent also may gain a feeling of independence through drug use. The adolescent's view of himself begins to include substance use as well as the lack of other enjoyments without drug use. As the adolescent increasingly withdraws from other experiences and fails to continue to participate in other aspects of teenage behavior, developmental lags can occur that further reinforce repetitive drug or alcohol use. Substance abuse, then, can lead to a stance of pseudoindependence and pseudoconfidence for the adolescent who believes that he is in control of his behavior. However, he does not take responsibility for problems resulting from the drug use. At the same time, family, school, and other social systems often react in a helpless fashion, leaving the adolescent increasingly isolated and his drug use out of control.

Drug use during adulthood most closely resembles the amount and frequency of drug use in an individual's family, rather than drug use among adolescent peers. Excessive drug use is commonly a time-limited behavior, with a decrease in use often occurring after approximately 10 years. The physician should identify patterns of substance use in parents and adult relatives as he works with adolescents who have difficulties with drug use. Drug use is more worrisome when associated with other problem behaviors such as truancy, marked aggressiveness, communication problems within the family, runaway behavior, or sexual promiscuity. Drug and alcohol use is also a greater concern when the substance use interferes with school or work performance or with participation in other peer group activities that might lead to a sense of increased competency and social effectiveness. Since adolescents with mood or adjustment disorders more commonly have chronic drug use, it is important for the physician to pay attention to the potential for suicide, either through the adolescent's deliberate or inadvertent overdosage or through self-destructive behavior such as driving a car under the influence of an exogenous substance.

An adolescent who is confused about goals for his life may use drugs and alcohol more excessively. Drug use is likely to become a more significant problem when poverty or educational deficiencies are also present. This is also the case when the adolescent experiences education and other peer group activities as ritualized, uninvolving, and unsatisfying. Adolescents may use drugs in a repetitive fashion when they are experiencing significant emotional distress. In these situations, the drug or alcohol use may actually be an attempt to relieve the pain of a psychiatric disorder through self-medication. It is also important for the primary care physician to remember that adolescents may have accurate information about the effects of drugs upon their mood or behavior at the same time as they are misinformed about the effects of drugs upon their judgment or physiology. In general, the teenager's use of drugs is goal-directed, although the adolescent's lack of judgment or control in specific circumstances may affect the amount consumed.

TYPES OF DRUGS

Table 87–1 reviews commonly abused substances and describes toxic signs, treatment of intoxication, signs of overdose, and treatment of acute overdoses. References are provided in the bibliography for further information concerning the treatment of severe overdosages with these substances. Alcohol, the most commonly used substance of abuse consumed by adolescents, is used most often in social situations. Within the past ten years initiation into alcohol use has occurred at increasingly

TABLE 87–1
Common Drug Poisonings, Signs of Toxic Effects, and Treatment*

DRUG	MILD TOXIC SIGNS	SPECIMEN FOR DIAGNOSIS	TREATMENT	SEVERE OVERDOSE SIGNS	TREATMENT
Opiates					
Heroin Morphine Demerol Methadone	"Nodding" drowsiness, small pupils, urinary retention, slow and shallow breathing; skin scars and subcutaneous abscesses; duration 4–6 hr; with methadone, duration to 24 hr	Blood, urine	Naloxone (Narcan) 0.01 mg/kg IV	Coma; pinpoint pupils, slow irregular respiration or apnea, hypotension, hypothermia, pulmonary edema	Naloxone
Depressants					
Alcohol	Confusion, rousable drowsiness, delirium, ataxia, nystagmus, dysarthria, analgesia to stimuli	Blood, urine, breath	Alcohol excitement: diazepam or chlorpromazine	Stupor to coma; pupils reactive, usually constricted; oculovestibular response absent; motor tonus initially briefly hyperactive then flaccid; respiration and blood pressure depressed; hypothermia; with glutethimide, pupils moderately dilated, can be fixed; with meprobamate, withdrawal seizures common; with methaqualone, coma, occasional convulsions, tachycardia, cardiac failure, bleeding tendency	Intubate, ventilate, gavage; drainage position; antimicrobials; keep mean blood pressure above 90 mm Hg and urine output 300 ml/hr; avoid analeptics; hemodialyze for severe phenobarbital poisoning
Barbiturates		Blood	None needed for acute toxicity; withdraw drug under supervision if patient is chronic user		
Glutethimide (Doriden)		Blood			
Meprobamate (Equanil)		Blood			
Methaqualone (Quaalude, Sopor, Mandrax)	Hallucinations, agitation, motor hyperactivity, myoclonus, tonic spasms	Blood, urine			
Chlordiazepoxide (Librium)	Usually taken with another sedative if poisoning is attempted	Blood			As above; diuresis of little help
Diazepam (Valium)		Urine			

*From Wyngaarden JB, Smith LH (eds): *Cecil Textbook of Medicine,* ed 17. Philadelphia, WB Saunders Co, 1985. Used by permission.

TABLE 87–1 *(continued)*
Common Drug Poisonings, Signs of Toxic Effects, and Treatment*

DRUG	MILD TOXIC SIGNS	SPECIMEN FOR DIAGNOSIS	TREATMENT	SEVERE OVERDOSE SIGNS	TREATMENT
Stimulants					
Amphetamines Methylphenidate	Hyperactive, aggressive, sometimes paranoid, repetitive behavior; dilated pupils, tremor, hyperactive reflexes; hyperthermia, tachycardia, arrhythmia; acute torsion dystonia	Blood, urine	Reassurance if mild Diazepam or chlorpromazine if severe	Agitated, assaultive and paranoid excitement; occasionally convulsions; hypothermia; circulatory collapse	Chlorpromazine
Cocaine	Similar but less prominent than above; less paranoid, often euphoric	Blood	Reassurance Diazepam or chlorpromazine	Twitching, irregular breathing, tachycardia	Sedation
Psychedelics LSD Mescaline Psilocybin STP Phencyclidine	Confused, disoriented, perceptual distortions, distractable, withdrawn or eruptive, leading to accidents or violence; wide-eyed, dilated pupils; restless, hyperreflexic; less often, hypertension or tachycardia		Reassurance; "talk down"; do not leave alone Diazepam	Panic	Reassure; diazepam satisfactory; avoid phenothiazines Symptomatic supportive; Acidify urine with ammonium chloride
Atropine-scopolamine (Sominex)	Agitated or confused, visual hallucinations, dilated pupils, flushed and dry skin		Reassure	Toxic disoriented delirium, visual hallucination; later, amnesia, fever, dilated fixed pupils, hot flushed dry skin, urinary retention	Reassure; sedate lightly; (1) avoid phenothiazines; (2) do not leave alone
Antidepressants					
Imipramine (Tofranil) Amitriptyline (Elavil)	Restlessness, drowsiness, tachycardia, ataxia, sweating	Blood		Agitation, vomiting, hyperpyrexia, sweating, muscle dystonia, convulsions, tachycardia or arrhythmia	Symptomatic; gastric lavage
MAO inhibitors Tranylcypromine (Parnate) Phenelzine (Nardil) Pargyline (Eutonyl)	Hypertensive crises, agitation, drowsiness, ataxia	Blood	Withdrawal	Hypotension; headache; chest pain; agitation; coma, seizures and shock	Symptomatic; gastric lavage
Phenothiazines	Acute dystonia, somnolence, hypotension	Blood	Benadryl 0.50; withdrawal	Coma; convulsions (rare); arrhythmias; hypotension	Symptomatic; gastric lavage

younger ages, frequently in junior high school. The psychoactive effects of alcohol are similar to those of other depressants and tranquilizers. The degree of intoxication depends upon the amount of alcohol consumed and correlates roughly with blood alcohol levels. Mild intoxication may lead to reduction in anxiety and individuals who are mildly intoxicated may feel that they perform more readily in social situations. Alcohol use becomes a significant problem as the user becomes increasingly dependent on the alcohol for its effect in reducing anxiety and increasing ease of performance in social situations. Problem drinking may also develop as a reaction to a stressful situation, especially within the adolescent's family or peer group. Alcohol consumption then becomes increasingly frequent and may begin to occur when the adolescent is alone as he prepares for worrisome or potentially stressful situations. The acute intoxicating effects of alcohol are important causes of disability and death among young people. These acute effects may include overdosage, suicide, violent behavior, or accidents. Any physician working with adolescents will need to strongly reinforce the fact that adolescents should never drive when drinking (or after). Alcoholism is rare among adolescents but chronic alcohol use can lead to significant worsening in school performance and social adjustment.

Marijuana is the second most commonly used substance by adolescents. Half of those teenagers who use alcohol also use marijuana. It affects perception, behavior, and emotional state. It may lead to an increased sense of well-being or euphoria, accompanied by feelings of relaxation or sleepiness. Differential effects of marijuana may be seen due to differences in amount ingested of its active substance tetrahydrocannabinol (THC). With increasing ingestion, marijuana may significantly interfere with information processing, attention, and perception, as well as performance of simple motor tasks and reaction time. Thinking may become confused and disorganized and altered time perception is a frequently noticed effect. Excessive doses of marijuana can induce hallucinations and depersonalization, although most smokers can adjust the dosage to avoid severely unpleasant effects. It is important for adolescents to appreciate that marijuana use may significantly interfere with performance of motor tasks, especially driving a car.

Adolescents currently use other drugs much less frequently and often in an experimental fashion. Less than 0.5% of all adolescents use any other drug in a repetitive fashion. Phencyclidine (PCP) is a commonly used hallucinogen that may lead to bizarre behavior, an inability to integrate sensory input, changes in body image, and marked disorganization of thinking. PCP is generally used to increase sensitivity to external stimuli and to elevate mood, but it may induce hallucinations and a frightening disorientation that may persist for up to 2 to 3 days. The use of LSD and other psychedelic drugs also alters perceptions and leads to hallucinations, alteration of subjective time, and marked lability of mood. Acute and chronic use of PCP warrants complete medical evaluation and the patient may require hospitalization when acutely intoxicated for monitoring, protection, and support, while the symptoms of disorientation and panic persist.

Stimulants such as amphetamines and cocaine are used to heighten the sense of accomplishment, induce a feeling of well-being, and reduce fatigue. Amphetamines and cocaine may also lead to a feeling of euphoria, excitement, and a perception of enhanced clarity of thinking. Their use may be extremely reinforcing, leading to chronic repetitive use. Acute overdosage may lead to extreme anxiety, assaultiveness, hallucinations, and psychotic effects. Chronic overdosage with both cocaine and amphetamines can lead to visual hallucinations and paranoid delusions; chronic use of cocaine can lead to increased craving of the drug, with heightened irritability and depression and discomfort when the user is not able to obtain the substance. Massive overdose of cocaine can also lead to cardiac arrest and sudden death.

Recently there has been a significant increase in the use of cocaine. Most worrisome has been the popularity of smoking the crystalline form of cocaine, crack. This has become readily available and inexpensive and has been used regularly by disaffected adolescents involved in alcohol and drug abuse. Crack is especially dangerous because of its powerful addictive quality. Physicians who learn that an adolescent is using crack regularly will want to discuss the danger of that substance frankly with the adolescent and refer the young person for inpatient drug rehabilitation treatment.

Sedatives are less frequently used by adolescents and are generally used in association with other drugs. They induce a feeling of peace and tranquility and a reduction in anxiety and inhibition. It is possible, but unusual, to find adolescents physically dependent upon sedatives. The use of opioids, including heroin, has become more common among adolescents within the past 20 years. However, their use continues to depend on availability and patterns of substance abuse among a particular teenager's peer group. Heroin use continues to be more common in poor environments where adolescents have limited alternative opportunities for expression and accomplishment. Users of opioids often develop a pattern of addiction and physical dependence. Physical problems seen in drug addicts including phlebitis, endocarditis, and malnutrition are common complications of chronic heroin use that the physician must be prepared to identify and treat in individuals with a history of opioid ingestion.

During routine outpatient care, the primary care physician should question adolescents about drug use. The adolescent's pattern of drug use and associated psychosocial adjustment should be ascertained. It is rare that an adolescent will visit the physician specifically for difficulties with drugs or alcohol, although visits for somatic symptoms or anxiety or psychological concerns may mask worries about substance abuse. In obtaining the history, the physician should identify which drugs are used, how much is ingested at any particular time, and how frequently and under what circumstances the drug is used. It is also extremely important for the physician to determine from the adolescent the reason why he is using a particular substance and to appreciate the adolescent's knowledge about the effects and dangers of the drugs used. As has been stated above, tension, boredom, anxiety, a feeling of inadequacy, curiosity, or an attempt to alter perceptions or activity level may lead an adolescent to experiment with drugs or use them regularly. The physician may learn more about an adolescent's drug use by interviewing the teenager alone. The physician should also determine what the parents know about the teenager's drug use and their response to it. The physician should also note the parents' appreciation of the difficulties the adolescent is experiencing that may be reinforcing drug use and their attempts to help the teenager decrease these stresses.

The primary care physician should also obtain a profile of the adolescent's functioning in school and peer-group activities; identify the adolescent's interests, overall accomplishments, sense of competency, and self-esteem; and understand the adolescent's relationship within his family. In addition to obtaining a history concerning drug or alcohol use, the physician should learn the teenager's impressions of his drug use and his ability to control their use and to vary his sources of recreation. The physician should also learn if the adolescent experiences any difficulties in association with his drug use, including social isolation because of the drug use. Use of drugs and alcohol in adolescence becomes drug abuse when it is an ineffective way of coping with developmental or environmental stresses or when the drug use itself leads to further difficulties in overall psychosocial functioning. The physician will also want to obtain information from parents concerning their impressions of the adolescent's psychological well-being and social functioning. A complete examination is often helpful in identifying any physical effects of drug use and especially in identifying physical difficulties associated with repetitive use of substances such as amphetamines or sedatives.

At the close of his evaluation, the physician will have developed an impression of (1) the seriousness of the drug use itself and its potential acute and chronic ill effects; (2) the adolescent's psychosocial level of adaptation; and (3) the opinions of the adolescent's family concerning both drug use and emotional and behavioral difficulties associated with it. As a result of this evaluation, the pediatrician can determine whether an adolescent's use of drugs is experimental and controlled or if it is repetitive or habitual and indicative of severe adjustment problems.

MANAGEMENT

For the group of adolescents for whom drug use is experimental and for whom there are no significant associated difficulties in functioning, the physician should involve the family to support the adolescent's accomplishments, to encourage alternative recreational experiences, and to provide adequate supervision for the adolescent. The physician should discuss drug use during health maintenance visits and will especially want to ensure that adolescents and their families have accurate information concerning alcohol, drugs, and smoking. The physician should point out the addictive qualities of nicotine, alcohol, cocaine, and crack and help adolescents recognize the danger of street drugs and PCP.

Adequate supervision will include helping the parents set rules about drug use. These rules should be aimed at preventing irresponsible drug use. The physician should also strongly encourage communication and emotional support within the family. Consideration of the adolescent's age, the type of substance, and the circumstances of substance use are important in these decisions. The physician should avoid power struggles with adolescents and help parents recognize that they are capable of limiting their teenager's behavior and ensuring his safety. It is probable that adolescents under the legal drinking age may experiment with alcohol use and parents need to strongly reinforce and support good judgment concerning this. The parents need to feel that they can limit drinking or drug use in an uncontrolled fashion and can prevent driving when under the influence of either alcohol or marijuana. The physician's goal should be to help the family and the teenager to make responsible choices about drug and alcohol use. The physician will then help the family to ensure that the adolescent continues to develop in other areas of his life, learns varied methods of obtaining pleasure and enjoyment, learns to be able to identify and discuss stresses and anxieties that he is experiencing and to react to difficult circumstances without habitually using exogenous substances.

Adolescents with patterns of frequent or habitual drug use will require referral for mental health treatment, ideally treatment involving the entire family. Patterns of frequent drug use in association with other evidence of poor adaptation and family difficulties require outpatient psychotherapy for the entire family. Adolescents with habitual drug use, significant underlying psychopathology, and serious family problems may need inpatient care followed by regular outpatient individual and family therapy. Patients with physical dependency upon a drug will need hospitalization to supervise withdrawal from the drug. The physician and psychiatric consultant will also identify specific adolescents and families with serious drug-related problems who require the special expertise of an inpatient drug-treatment program for adolescents.

ANTICIPATORY GUIDANCE

The physician can counsel families with adolescents concerning drug and alcohol use as part of anticipatory guidance in adolescent primary care. The physician should ensure that both teenagers and their families have adequate information concerning the potentially dangerous effects of psychoactive drugs and prepare them as a family to make decisions concerning appropriate recreational use of drugs. A family will do better by discussing these issues openly. In areas where there are not organized programs for education, the physician will need to work with school personnel and the school system to heighten parents' sense of responsibility and surveillance concerning the use of these substances at parties. The physician can support strong community efforts to limit teenage driving under the influence of either alcohol or marijuana. Physicians can also help school personnel to identify adolescents with particular adjustment difficulties and associated substance abuse and then assist in referral for appropriate mental health treatment.

BIBLIOGRAPHY

Abelson HI, Fishburne PM, Cisin I: *National Survey on Drug Abuse: 1977*. National Institute on Drug Abuse, US Dept of Health, Education and Welfare, 1978.

Brecher EM, Editors of *Consumer Reports: Licit and Illicit Drugs: The Consumer's Union Report*. Mount Vernon NY, Consumer Union, 1972.

Collins M: Adolescent emergencies, in Fleischer G, Ludwig S, Henretig FW, et al: *Textbook of Pediatric Emergency Medicine*. Baltimore, Williams & Wilkins Co, 1982.

DuPont RI, Goldstein A, O'Donnell J (eds): *Handbook on Drug Abuse*. National Institute on Drug Abuse, US Dept of Health, Education and Welfare and Office of Drug Abuse Policy, 1979.

Gwinner PDV: The young alcoholic: Approaches to treatment, in Madden JS, Walker R, Kenyon WH (eds): *Alcoholism and Drug Dependence*. New York, Plenum Press, 1977, pp 263–270.

Hamburg BA, Kraemer HC, Jahnke WA: Hierarchy of drug use in adolescence: Behavioral and attitudinal correlates of substantial drug use. *Am J Psychiatry* 1975; 132:1155–1167.

Litt IF, Cohen MI: The drug-using adolescent as a pediatric patient. *J Pediatr* 1970; 77:195–202.

Litt IF (ed): *Adolescent Substance Abuse: Report of the Fourteenth Ross Roundtable on Critical Approaches to Common Pediatric Problems.* Columbus, Ohio, Ross Laboratories, 1983.

Millman RB, Botruin GJ: Substance use, abuse and dependence, in Levine MB, Carey WB, Crocker AC, et al (eds): *Developmental-Behavioral Pediatrics.* Philadelphia, WB Saunders Co, 1983.

Stanton MD, Todd T: *Family Therapy of Drug Addiction.* New York, Guilford Press, 1981.

Wells CF, Stuart I (eds): *Self-Destructive Behavior in Children and Adolescents.* New York, Guilford Press, 1981.

88 EATING DISORDERS

John Sargent, M.D.

Anorexia nervosa and bulimia, prototypes of biopsychosocial disorders, represent diagnostic and therapeutic challenges for the primary care physician who must complete physical, psychological, and familial assessments and direct the interventions necessary to have the patient recover and change the pattern of adapting to stress. Since the management of this serious and potentially fatal disease is beyond the area of primary care, the doctor must recognize early signs and symptoms and be able to refer the patient for appropriate therapy. This section will explain the dynamics of families of these patients and several therapeutic plans.

ANOREXIA NERVOSA

Anorexia nervosa is the diagnosis applied to individuals, mostly women, who demonstrate a relentless pursuit of thinness and an absolute refusal to maintain minimum body weight. Weight loss is achieved through reduction in dietary caloric intake, especially foods containing carbohydrates and fats. For some patients, weight loss is also achieved through the use of diet pills, vomiting, laxatives, or diuretics. Because of a marked disturbance in body image, the patient experiences herself as fat even when underweight, and feels strongly that she needs to diet to lose more weight. The term anorexia is, in fact, a misnomer because there is no loss of appetite, only the absolute control of appetite by the patient. In anorexia there is no known physical or psychiatric disorder to account for the weight loss. However, anorexia nervosa can occur in association with chronic underlying physical and psychiatric illness. The identification and treatment of anorexia nervosa should occur when a patient is under a minimum healthy weight for age, sex, and height, continues to diet, and strongly believes that she needs to lose more weight. The diagnosis of anorexia is a positive diagnosis that is reached through obtaining a history of relentless, intractable dieting and weight loss and an absolute refusal to begin to eat more to maintain normal weight. Ninety-five percent of cases of anorexia are in women. The onset of the disorder occurs more often in adolescence, and currently 1 in 200 adolescent girls develops the symptoms of anorexia. There is no identified specific organic etiology for anorexia nervosa. Anorexia can and often does become chronic, with the symptoms extending over years. Mortality associated with anorexia has been estimated to be 5% to 10%.

CLINICAL FEATURES

The primary physical features of anorexia nervosa occur as a result of starvation. Patients with anorexia have significant disturbances in endocrine function associated with starvation-induced hypothalamic disturbances that usually resolve with weight gain. Patients generally have low body temperature, low pulse rate, and low blood pressure. They may have significant gastrointestinal complaints, including abdominal pain, and may experience bloating when eating small amounts of food. At significantly low weight, patients have muscle-wasting, weakness, and slow movements. They may have marked thinning of their hair as well as the development of fine lanugo hair over their body. Although thyroid hormone levels are generally within normal limits, patients usually complain of being cold when others are warm; often the patients are amenorrheic. At moderate amounts of weight loss, there are generally no other significant physical disturbances and results of most laboratory studies are within normal limits. Patients may have a slight amount of leukopenia, with white blood cell (WBC) counts in the range of 4,000/mm^3, and hemoglobin level may be increased, usually on the basis of chronic dehydration and reduction in level of total body fluids. Death generally occurs because of cardiovascular collapse only after more than a 40% weight loss. Patients often think slowly and in a rigid fashion. They may identify problems in concentrating. With severe weight loss, an organic psychosis can occur. Patients who use laxatives or vomit regularly can also have alterations in electrolyte levels, with vomiting resulting in hypokalemic alkalosis and laxative abuse leading to dehydration.

Resumption of normal dietary intake and cessation of vomiting generally lead to physical recovery and normal physical signs and symptoms described above. Upon refeeding, some patients, after prolonged periods of malnutrition, may have gastrointestinal complaints, malabsorption, and diarrhea. This generally occurs only in patients whose dietary intake has been under 500 calories/day. Dramatic increases in caloric intake from 500 calories/day to 3,500 to 5,000 calories/day over a short period of time have resulted in the development of cardiac failure, which was reversed when caloric intake was reduced. Moderate caloric intake of 2,500 to 3,000 calories/day after slowly increasing caloric intake by 200 calories/day has been tolerated well by patients recovering from anorexia.

PSYCHOLOGICAL AND BEHAVIORAL FEATURES

Patients with anorexia nervosa demonstrate characteristic psychological and behavioral disturbances. They deny other problems and state that they feel fine, have no physical complaints, and only need to lose a few more pounds. They report a pervasive sense of helplessness and ineffectiveness and, when asked, generally have little respect for their previous accomplishments. An individual with anorexia may also be markedly nonassertive. She is generally perfectionistic and may describe herself as feeling out of control. Her weight loss gives her a sense of mastery and control. She generally does not disagree overtly and yet maintains a stance of intractability through resistance. The patient is usually brought to the physician's attention by someone else (most often her parents) rather than coming voluntarily. She may be very attentive to her parents' feelings and highly concerned for the well-being of her family.

Anorectic patients may have bizarre or unusual eating habits; they may eat in a compulsive fashion and often refuse to eat with others, eating only in private. They may also compulsively exercise, usually performing it in a ritualized fashion and not for fun, but rather for its continued effect on caloric consumption, inducing weight loss. Most patients continue to attend school, studying excessively for hours at a time. The patient is usually socially isolated and withdrawn from peers and group activities. Individuals with anorexia also may become highly emotional and upset when frustrated. The symptoms of anorexia may develop after a significant psychosocial stress such as loss of a boyfriend, divorce or death of a parent or may develop following an increased awareness of one's body or disappointment with one's accomplishments or attractiveness. Individuals who develop anorexia have been unhappy and dissatisfied with themselves for some time prior to the onset of dieting and weight loss. Dieting and weight loss lead to a worsening of the psychological state and increased social withdrawal, which further reinforce focus on weight and dieting behavior.

DIFFERENTIAL DIAGNOSIS

The differential diagnosis for anorexia nervosa includes other causes of weight loss and appetite restriction. It is rare, though, for significant organic illnesses to mimic the psychological and behavioral features of anorexia as well as its purposeful and relentless course. Chronic gastrointestinal disease including Crohn disease or ulcerative colitis can present with reduction in food intake and abdominal pain and frequently diarrhea, gastrointestinal bleeding, and evidence of malabsorption. Patients with cancer may have significant weight loss and reduction in appetite. However, these patients do not diet and lose weight on purpose. Central nervous system tumors and Addison disease have also, at times, been confused with anorexia. However, in the appropriate age range, history and physical examination appear to clearly differentiate anorexia from chronic organic illness.

THE FAMILY AND ANOREXIA

Minuchin and colleagues investigated the interaction of families with an anorectic member at the time the symptoms were present. Five predominant characteristics of family interaction were present in these families and detrimental to overall family functioning: *enmeshment, overprotectiveness, rigidity, lack of conflict resolution, and involvement of the sick child in unresolved parental conflict.*

Enmeshment refers to a tight web of family relationships in which family members are highly sensitive to one another. They often infer moods and needs of others and submerge individual interests for the good of the whole. Overt criticism is rare. Enmeshment characterizes appropriate relationships between spouses or parents and adolescents or young adults. *Overprotectiveness* describes a relationship in which autonomy is sacrificed and highly nurturant interactions predominate. Family members feel a strong sense of vulnerability. The anorectic patient is often as highly protective of her parents and siblings as they are of her. Within these families, the interactions of enmeshment, protectiveness, and conflict avoidance are rigidly preferred. Even at times of stress or necessary developmental change, one observes the family to utilize, repeatedly and ineffectively, a narrow range of behaviors. In dealing with the anorectic child, the family responds as they would to a much younger child. Families with anorectic members have marked difficulty allowing for and encouraging the resolution of disagreement. As these disagreements remain, a chronic state of tension and stress develops. These characteristics are mutually reinforcing creating a family organization that is fragile and unable to respond effectively to the symptoms of anorexia. The final common feature of these families is *involvement of the symptomatic child in unresolved parental conflict.* The patient helps maintain family integrity by joining the side of one parent in a stable coalition against the other parent, by providing a focus for common concern and action through her symptoms, or by being caught between her parents in a loyalty conflict. Because of the *rigidly* preferred family patterns of interaction, the parents may be more concerned with the rightness of their own actions rather than their effectiveness. They may try (one parent by pleading, the other parent by demanding) to help the patient to eat, but then when each fails, each parent recoils and leaves the anorectic patient alone and without support. Because the family members do not resolve conflict well, they do not compromise and work together.

If the family is highly overinvolved with the patient, she need not perceive her own sensations. Others may recognize them first or deny their presence. The child must also be vigilant to perceive and respond to the signs of distress from others. In a context in which everyone is vulnerable and protection is necessary, interpersonal trust does not develop. When conflict and distress are denied or not resolved, the child does not develop a sense of competence and an appropriate use of problem-solving skills.

BULIMIA

Bulimia is a syndrome in which patients eat excessively and then follow these periods of overeating with episodes of purging through vomiting, laxative abuse, or diuretic use. We reserve the term bulimia for patients who are of at least normal weight at the time of diagnosis. Most bulimic patients weigh between normal and 10% to 15% above normal. Approximately a third of anorectic patients develop episodic binging and purging as they regain and maintain normal weight. Other patients who are bulimic may never have been significantly underweight. The frequency of binges generally varies from patient to patient and may vary also in any individual patient. Some patients can go days or weeks without binging or purging; other patients may pursue this activity daily or several times daily. The exact incident of bulimia is unknown, although recent studies of eating habits of women college students indicate that some 10% to 20% of high school and college students engage in this behavior. Bulimia also occurs much more frequently in women (80% to 90% of cases). Foods consumed during binging are frequently high in carbohydrates. These periods of binging occur in addition to normal eating at regular mealtimes. However, some patients report episodes of excessive dieting or fasting, fluctuating with binges that then result in purging. Bulimic patients may also have a history of drug or alcohol abuse.

PHYSICAL FEATURES

The physical difficulties associated with bulimia in normal weight patients are caused by repetitive purging. Patients who induce vomiting may have calluses on the backs of their hands; they may also have parotid swelling. They may experience epigastric distress associated with chronic esophagitis or may have episodes of mild to moderate gastrointestinal bleeding occurring as a result of excessive repetitive vomiting. All patients with significant repetitive vomiting have some degree of tooth enamel erosion as a result of chronic irritation by gastric acid. Cardiac arrhythmias may result from hypokalemic alkalosis associated with significant chronic vomiting. Patients who use laxatives excessively may become dehydrated.

PSYCHOLOGICAL FEATURES

Bulimic patients are aware of their problem and are distressed by their symptoms. They report that the bulimic symptoms are habitual and outside of their control. Usually acting in secrecy, the patients are generally quite ashamed of their symptoms and reluctant to admit to them. Many patients describe that the binges are planned; others will describe periods of overeating that occur almost involuntarily. They also describe a point in eating at which they are sure that they have eaten too much and, therefore, will purge after finishing eating. This decision then leaves them free to continue to eat as much as they would like with the knowledge that they will be able to get rid of the food after completing the binge. Usual caloric intake in a binge often exceeds 2,500 calories. Patients describe a battle with themselves to gain control over the symptoms and prevent future binges. They continually fail to master the problem that leads to worsening of the symptoms. Increase in frequency of binging can lead to lessening of their self-esteem and increased social isolation. Many bulimic patients, however, report successful performance in work, school, or social activities. Patients describe binges occurring during periods of loneliness, boredom, anxiety, or anger so that the eating and purging can be used to dissipate disturbing emotions. The loss of food relieves the anxiety but also leads to increased self-criticism and increased frequency of the binging. The entire experience of overeating and purging also is physically and psychologically consuming and exhausting. Patients then experience a period of quiet and relaxation, distracting them from stresses in their environment. The cycle then repeats itself.

DIFFERENTIAL DIAGNOSIS

As with anorexia, the diagnosis of bulimia is made through confirmation of symptoms by history and elimination of organic causes for the vomiting by physical examination. Causes of repetitive vomiting, such as Addison disease, need to be considered; however, the self-induced nature of the purging and excessive calorie intakes in episodes of binge eating are not present in other organic diseases.

THE FAMILY WITH A BULIMIC MEMBER

Enmeshment, rigidity, and poor conflict resolution are frequent in families with patients with bulimia. The patient maintains a stance of independence and acts as if she is responsible for herself, yet she is often sad, lonely, and unsupported. While the patient frequently will state that the symptoms are secret, family members are aware and concerned about the eating disorder. The family fluctuates between attempting to stop the symptoms through injunctions or cajoling and retreating when ineffective. The family then becomes angry, blames the patient, and abandons her. This stance persists for awhile, and then the cycle occurs again. The fluctuation between overinvolvement and abandonment is characteristic of families with bulimic members. It happens concerning the symptoms of bulimia and in other areas of family life. Within these families, conflict is apparent. However, it is still not resolved. The parents may not have gotten along for many years. This fixed arrangement of argument, retreat, and reconciliation is stabilized by concern for the symptomatic child with bulimia. There may also be other overt and recognized difficulties with impulse control in families with bulimic members. One or both parents may have difficulty with their temper, often leading to explosive behavior in the house. There may be a history of substance abuse within the family, especially alcohol abuse, and concern that one or both parents may become depressed and incapacitated. There may also be a history of incest in the family, reflecting the lack of personal boundaries and poor impulse control.

OFFICE EVALUATION

The physician's evaluation of an eating disorder should include a determination of the patient's physical status, an assessment of the patient's psychosocial difficulties and developmental level, and an assessment of the family. The physician's efforts with respect to the physical symptoms and medical difficulties related to the eating disorder must be coordinated with efforts to deal with psychosocial and familial difficulties that occur simultaneously. The treatment approach must be one in which the body and mind of the patient are dealt with in concert and the patient is treated in relationship to her family. The goals of the medical evaluation of a patient with an eating disorder are (1) identification of underlying disease processes present at the time of the referral and ascertainment that no physiologic process explains the weight loss; (2) clarification of the patient's physiologic condition and the nature of any metabolic difficulties resulting from the patient's symptoms that require immediate remediation; and (3) effective preparation of the patient and family for resolution of the physical, psychosocial, and familial difficulties associated with the eating disorder.

The physician's evaluation can be performed on an outpatient basis. The presence of all parental figures is essential and underscores the need of parents and all family members to be involved in the treatment. The physician obtains history concerning the development of the symptoms, methods utilized to achieve weight reduction if this has occurred, current dietary practices, and information concerning the use of self-induced vomiting or exogenous substances. The physician should also obtain history concerning other physical symptoms including weakness, faintness, muscle cramping, loss of concentration, periods of dehydration, and difficulties with fluid retention. For women, menstrual history should be accurately established and any further medical difficulties should be noted. In particular, the physician will want to pay attention to the presence of symptoms that are not generally associated with either anorexia or bulimia, such as frequent diarrhea or bloody stools indicative of possible inflammatory bowel disease, neurologic signs or symptoms associated with central nervous system tumors, or evidence of an endocrine disorder. The patient's report that she is actively pursuing dieting or purging after eating is a positive indication of the presence of an eating disorder.

After obtaining each parent's perception of the problem, the symptoms should be discussed with the patient in the parents' presence. The physician should inform the patient that the frequency and severity of eating-related symptoms cannot be kept secret because of the seriousness of the symptoms and because all family members will be involved in the treatment of the eating disorder. The physician will also want to ask the patient directly concerning her weight goal and her feelings about her body shape. The physician should also learn from each parent how they have tried to resolve the eating-related symptoms.

The physician can also obtain information

concerning the patient's psychosocial adaptation, the family medical history, recent changes in the home, and other current family stresses. The physician should ask the patient about emotional difficulties and suicidal ideation or behavior. The patient's level of functioning should be determined, including such factors as school or work attendance and performance, peer relationships, social activity, career interests, level of self-esteem, and sense of competency. As the patient is questioned, the physician should attempt to help the parents to remain silent and to listen. Overinvolvement within the family is demonstrated when one or both parents interrupts frequently, corrects the patient, or offers alternative explanations. The physician will also want to develop an initial assessment of the family system by noting whether the parents act together and respect each other during their meeting with him. The physician's evaluation of the family will include an assessment of family leadership and the commitment of the family as a whole to effective problem resolution.

The physician will also need to carry out a thorough physical examination and appropriate laboratory studies to be certain of the medical diagnosis and the patient's physical condition. It is our strong impression that the diagnosis of the eating disorder is a positive diagnosis achieved through recognition of symptoms and history of anorexia or bulimia. Usually a complete blood cell (CBC) count, a sedimentation rate, urinalysis, and chemical profile studies, are adequate tests. In patients with significant weight loss, who may have an arrhythmia, an electrocardiogram is performed. If there is concern about the patient's neurologic condition, computed tomography of the brain may be ordered. Patients who describe significant gastrointestinal (GI) tract symptoms that would not be expected in either bulimia or anorexia should have GI radiographs, including an upper GI study and barium enema. If there is sufficient concern about the patient's endocrine status beyond that expected on the basis of the weight loss, thyroid studies and cortisol studies can be performed. However, in uncomplicated cases of anorexia nervosa or bulimia, these values are usually normal. The patient's estrogen levels in anorexia will be low, purely on the basis of starvation-induced hypothalamic dysfunction.

Most patients with mild to moderate symptoms have normal physical examination and laboratory studies. On physical examination, in underweight patients, the pulse rate and blood pressure may be significantly lower. A pulse rate of 120 beats per minute and a blood pressure of 110 to 120 over 85 to 90 mm Hg may be indicative of significant dehydration in a patient who is severely underweight and whose usual pulse rate is 50 beats per minute and usual blood pressure is 80 to 90 over 50. Worrisome findings of laboratory studies in patients with eating disorders include leukopenia, indicating potential immune compromise; hypoglycemia; and elevation in values of hemoglobin, hematocrit, and blood urea nitrogen, indicative of dehydration. The patient's electrolyte levels deserve special attention. Hypokalemic alkalosis may be seen in patients with repetitive vomiting. A disturbing sign, the absence of ketones in the urine of a patient who is acutely starving may indicate the total utilization of muscle stores for energy. Abnormalities in liver enzyme levels usually occur after significantly chronic and severe malnutrition. Any unusual findings of laboratory studies or unexplained physical signs on examination require further evaluation.

MANAGEMENT

The initial assessment includes the patient's diagnosis, physical condition, medical status, developmental level, and the family's organizational and functional status. The presence of acute medical complications (such as dehydration, electrolyte abnormalities, or impending cardiovascular collapse indicated by postural hypotension) necessitates immediate medical hospitalization and appropriate physical treatment. Psychiatric hospitalization is recommended for patients with eating disorders when the patient's weight is dangerously low and when the symptoms are sufficiently out of control to seriously compromise the patient's functioning in other areas of her life. Suicidal ideation or behavior or psychotic behavior requires hospitalization of the patient. An inpatient psychiatric program can be used to demonstrate the severity of the symptoms to the family and to augment outpatient treatment that has previously been ineffective. Medical or psychiatric hospitalization is required in 15% to 20% of patients with anorexia nervosa or bulimia, either to deal with acute complications or crises in treatment.

All patients with anorexia or bulimia and their families will require outpatient treatment that addresses both the physical and psychosocial problems of the patient and the problems in organization and interaction within the family. Treatment is a collaborative effort among family, patient, physician, and therapist. The physician will need to remain available to monitor the patient's physical condition, to reinforce the goals of treatment for the patient including goal weight and expected rate of weight gain, and to provide dietary information as necessary. Patients who purge either through vomiting or laxative abuse will require regular medical evaluation in order to be certain that the patient's physical condition is stable, to reinforce improvement, and to be certain that the patient remains safe for treatment on an outpatient basis.

Early referral and effective treatment can lead to resolution of eating disorders. The physician can follow patients with small amounts of weight loss, but the follow-up period should be brief. In situations that fail to improve with the physician's intervention or in situations for which the physician believes psychotherapeutic attention is required following his initial assessment, patients should be referred to a therapist who is experienced in treating eating disorders, capable of working successfully with adolescents and their families, and willing to collaborate with the physician concerning the medical aspects of treatment. The therapist should also be able to use the physician's information and his determinations of the patient's condition to foster improvement of the family and the patient. The physician should inform the therapist of his impressions, his availability to monitor the patient physically and his desire to collaborate in treatment. The physician's referral for psychotherapy should be made in a positive fashion, orienting the family and patient toward resolution of the eating disorder symptoms. Frequently, families with members with eating disorders either will deny the severity of the symptoms, or deny the presence of psychological difficulties. It is important for the physician to help the family appreciate that psychotherapy is necessary.

The physician should arrange a follow-up meeting with the family after making a referral for psychotherapy to discuss the family's initial impressions of psychotherapy and to ensure that the family has begun therapy. The physician can reiterate his expectation that the family continue treatment as well as encourage them to resolve any questions concerning their initial impressions of treatment with the therapist. Throughout the course of treatment, it is important that the physician and therapist communicate regularly and work actively to resolve any areas of disagreement, either concerning the impressions of the patient or family, therapeutic approach, or goals of treatment.

PHYSICIAN'S ROLE IN THE PREVENTION OF EATING DISORDERS

The physician can take an active role in the prevention and early identification of eating disorders. Media reports and advertisements suggest that anyone can be thin while eating whatever he or she would like. Especially for women, one's physical appearance is viewed as a sign of one's worth as a person. The family physician can work with families to support the development of a more moderate approach to physical appearance and dieting behavior as he provides primary care. The physician also should be particularly attuned to difficulties in the development of effective control and effective autonomy throughout adolescence and young adulthood. A complete dietary history, including questions concerning dietary behavior and the existence of binging and purging, should be part of the physician's routine evaluation of adolescent health. The physician should monitor the adolescent's sense of self-esteem, autonomy, and personal control. Finally, the physician will need to be attentive to the ability of the family to respond effectively to the adolescent's need for supervision and direction, and for autonomy and privacy. While working with families, the physician may note that there are some in which parents have significant difficulty in encouraging the young person's individuation and sense of personal responsibility. In some of these families, the symptoms of an eating disorder may occur and be reinforced through family behavior. Early diagnosis of the eating disorder and institution of effective treatment is essential.

The physician can also work with school nursing personnel to identify instances in which dieting and eating-related behavior have caused problems. Early identification of these situations can then lead to treatment and their effective resolution. The physician also can encourage early identification and treatment of eating disorders and the individual's satisfaction with his own physiology and acceptance of the limitations of his own body through working with schools and within the community. This will include advocating a more thoughtful and patient and a less impulsive and moralistic approach to food and diet. If the physician also encourages alternative means of expression, appropriate and adequate family relationships, and an increased acceptability of varieties of body shape, the incidence and the severity of eating disorders can be reduced, while symptoms can be treated in an effective and humane manner.

BIBLIOGRAPHY

Boskind-White M, White WC: *Bulimarexia: The Binge/Purge Cycle*. New York, Norton, 1983.

Bruch H: *Eating Disorders*. New York, Basic Books, 1973.

Bruch H: *The Golden Cage*. Cambridge, Mass, Harvard University Press, 1978.

Cauwels JM: *Bulimia: The Binge-Purge Compulsion*. Garden City, NJ, Doubleday, 1983.

Collins M, Hodas GR, Liebman R: Interdisciplinary model for the inpatient treatment of anorexia nervosa. *J Adolesc Health Care* 1983; 4:3–8.

Crisp AH: *Anorexia Nervosa: Let Me Be*. New York, Grune & Stratton, 1980.

Garfinkel P, Garner D: *Anorexia Nervosa: A Multidimensional Perspective*. New York, Brunner/Mazel, 1982.

Garner D, Garfinkel P (eds): *Handbook of Psychotherapy for Anorexia Nervosa and Bulimia*. New York, Guilford Press, 1984.

Halmi KA, Falk JR, Schwartz E: Binge-eating and vomiting: A survey of a college population. *Psychol Med* 1981; 11:697–706.

Harkaway J (ed): *Eating Disorders: The Family Therapy Collection*, vol 20. Rockville, Md, Aspen Publications, 1987.

Hirschmann J, Zaphiropoulos L: *Are You Hungry?* New York, Random House, 1985.

Johnson C, Connors M: *The Etiology and Treatment of Bulimia Nervosa: A Biopsychosocial Perspective*. New York, Basic Books, 1987.

Minuchin S, Rosman BL, Baker L: *Psychosomatic Families: Anorexia Nervosa in Context*. Cambridge, Mass, Harvard University Press, 1978.

Palazzoli MS: *Self-Starvation*. New York, Jason Aronson, 1978.

Pope HG Jr, Judson JL, Jonas JM, et al: Bulimia treated with imipramine: A placebo-controlled, double-blind study. *Am J Psychiatry* 1983; 140:554–558.

Sargent J, Liebman R, Silver M: Family therapy for anorexia nervosa, in Garner DM, Garfinkel PE (eds): *The Treatment of Anorexia Nervosa and Bulemia*. New York, Guilford, 1984.

Sargent J, Liebman R: The outpatient treatment of anorexia nervosa. *Psychiatr Clin North Am* 1984; 7:235–45.

Schwab AD (moderator): Anorexia nervosa. *Ann Intern Med* 1981; 94:371–381.

89 PSYCHOSIS

Gordon R. Hodas, M.D.

Psychosis is a state of severe impairment in functioning characterized by a loss of contact with reality, poor interpersonal relationships, and disturbances in thinking. Behavior may be aggressive, withdrawn, or both. Younger children express psychosis as a global withdrawal from relationships and reality in a way that may affect nearly all phases of development. Adolescents with acute onset of schizophrenia or manic episodes show a clinical picture similar to that of adults with these conditions. Psychoses of childhood and adolescence can be divided into two categories: organic and psychiatrically based psychosis. The distinction between these two is based on the presence of some identifiable physical source for organic psychosis, such as a medical or traumatic condition or an exogenous substance, whereas no such identifiable source can be ascertained for psychiatrically based psychosis.

Psychiatrically based psychosis of childhood and adolescence is divided into four major categories: (1) infantile autism (onset prior to the age of 30 months); (2) pervasive developmental disorders (onset between 30 months and 12 years); (3) schizophrenic episodes (onset in adolescence); and (4) manic-depressive illness (onset in adolescence).

ORGANIC PSYCHOSIS

Although the majority of psychoses are psychiatrically based, the primary care physician must be alert to the possibility of organic psychosis and consider possible sources. This is especially pertinent given the increasing use of nonprescription drugs by adolescents. The four major sources of an organic psychosis are medical conditions, trauma, prescribed medications, and drug intoxications.

CAUSES OF ORGANIC PSYCHOSIS

Medical conditions

- Central nervous system lesions
  - Tumor
  - Brain abscess
  - Cerebral hemorrhage
  - Meningitis or encephalitis
  - Temporal lobe epilepsy
- Cerebral hypoxia
  - Pulmonary insufficiency
  - Severe anemia
  - Cardiac failure
  - Carbon monoxide poisoning
- Metabolic and endocrine disorders
  - Electrolyte imbalance
  - Hypoglycemia
  - Hypocalcemia
  - Thyroid disease (hyperthyroidism and hypothyroidism)
  - Adrenal disease (hyperadrenocorticism and hypoadrenocorticism)
  - Uremia
  - Hepatic failure
  - Diabetes mellitus
  - Porphyria
- Rheumatic diseases
  - Systemic lupus erythematosus
  - Polyarteritis nodosa
- Infections
  - Malaria
  - Typhoid fever
  - Subacute bacterial endocarditis
- Miscellaneous conditions
  - Wilson disease
  - Reye syndrome

Trauma

- Acute
- Chronic

Prescribed medication(s)

- Side effect

Toxicity
Discontinuation

Drug intoxications (toxic psychosis)
Accidental ingestion
Proprietary medications
Drug experimentation or abuse
Alcohol abuse
Suicide attempt

Most of the medical conditions will have been previously diagnosed, but some (e.g., cerebral lupus erythematosus and Reye syndrome) may present as acute psychosis. Chronic trauma can be more easily overlooked and requires a careful history and neurologic evaluation. Prescribed medications may cause psychosis, either as a side effect when the medication is given in high doses or as an untoward effect when it is being tapered off and discontinued.

Drug or alcohol experimentation is the most common cause of organic psychosis in adolescence. The following exogenous substances may induce a toxic psychosis either singly or in combination: alcohol, barbiturates, antipsychotics (e.g., phenothiazines), amphetamines, cocaine, crack, hallucinogens (e.g., LSD, peyote, mescaline), marijuana, phencyclidine (PCP), methaqualone (Quaalude), anticholinergic compounds, heavy metals, corticosteroids, reserpine, opiates (e.g., heroin, methadone). The physician should always consider the possibility of a suicide attempt when an adolescent presents with an organic psychosis.

ACUTE ADOLESCENT SCHIZOPHRENIA

Schizophrenia, despite substantial research efforts over the past several decades, remains a mystery. Although a genetic predisposition exists, it is not entirely clear what factors produce this state of emotional disorganization and why it occurs when it does. The prognostic range is extremely wide, from individuals who experience a single psychotic break and recover completely, to persons who remain symptomatic and require either institutional or supervised living arrangements.

Schizophrenia occurs in 1% of the population. Schizophrenia, equally distributed between men and women, is more common in nonwhite populations and in lower socioeconomic groups. There is a significantly greater likelihood for schizophrenia in an individual whose parent(s) or sibling has the disorder. While the peak age for patients to have hospital admission for schizophrenia is 25 to 34 years, acute schizophrenic episodes occur commonly in middle to late adolescence and young adulthood, prior to the age of 25 years, and can begin as early as 12 years of age.

Many individuals with an acute schizophrenic episode are found to have led isolated lives prior to the psychosis. Other individuals may have achieved higher levels of functioning and may have a better prognosis. In addition, the family often fails to support the development of independence and autonomy of a schizophrenic member. Such adolescents typically fall short of convincing their parents of their capability, and parents frequently remain overinvolved out of concern that their child will fail without them. This can become chronic, entrapping both parents and adolescent, while also maintaining family stability.

The family with a schizophrenic member also often avoids direct communication and fails to achieve resolution of conflict. The family may appear disorganized, superficial, and distant. Marital problems may be evident, but denied. Some families respond poorly to the symptomatic patient, who may have been in distress for some time prior to the family requesting assistance. The disruptive effect of the illness itself on overall family functioning must also be appreciated. In addition, some families with children with schizophrenia have greater cohesiveness and the ability to acknowledge and discuss problems and conflicts.

MANIC-DEPRESSIVE ILLNESS

Manic-depressive illness usually occurs prior to the age of 30 years, and there is increasing recognition that the disorder can occur in late childhood and in adolescence. Manic-depressive illness may present in different ways: (1) as an acute manic state, with or without prior history of mania and depression; (2) as an acutely depressed state, in a patient with one or more manic attacks in the past; (3) as rapid alternation between mania and depression.

An acute manic episode may emerge suddenly in adolescence, but often there are early clues. A family history of depression or manic-depressive illness can often be obtained. The patient may have had previously untreated depressive episodes or have been regarded as "moody." The patient may identify past and present mood swings with irritability and an accompanying loss of personal control.

INFANTILE AUTISM AND PERVASIVE DEVELOPMENTAL DISORDER OF CHILDHOOD

Together, infantile autism and pervasive developmental disorder of childhood account for most cases of psychosis in children from birth to 12 years of age. Both disorders, which are three times more common in boys than girls, are extremely rare, with approximately two cases per 10,000 children. The major distinguishing feature is age at onset, with infantile autism by definition occurring prior to 30 months of age. Tasks of the primary care physician for these children are to diagnose the condition, refer the child and family for appropriate service, and work collaboratively with this treatment network.

INFANTILE AUTISM

The cardinal feature of autistic children is a generalized lack of responsiveness to people, together with a failure to develop normal attachment behavior. The manner of presentation can be quite variable and the diagnosis is usually made after the child is 12 months old. Often the mother can describe sensing a "differentness" or "strangeness" about the child going back to the first several months. The child is often described as having been aloof. Developmental milestones may be erratic or delayed. Only 30% of autistic children have an IQ above 70. Some of these children have an underlying medical condition such as maternal rubella syndrome or previous encephalitis or meningitis, but the etiology for the vast majority of autistic children is unknown. The autistic child uses toys inappropriately and in a bizarre manner. Stereotyped behaviors (such as rocking, twirling, or whirling) may occur. The single most important prognostic sign is the development or absence of language by the age of 5 years (see Chapter 72).

PERVASIVE DEVELOPMENTAL DISORDER

Children with a pervasive developmental disorder have had apparently normal development during the first 2½ years of life. Typically, the child acquires language. Developmental milestones are often variable and mental retardation, when present, is less severe than with infantile autism. The key deficiency again is in social relationships and attachment. Pervasive development disorder accounts for most cases of psychosis in children under the age of 12 years.

OFFICE EVALUATION

Table 89–1 indicates some of the differentiating features of organic and psychiatrically based psychosis. *History* often reveals an acute onset for an organic psychosis, as compared to a more gradual, insidious onset for psychiatrically based psychosis. With the latter, a history of prior psychotic episodes or a family history of psychosis may be obtained. With an organic psychosis, the panicked patient sometimes admits to an ingestion of drugs or a history of drug use is obtained from family or friends. History of the circumstances of the ingestion, including the possibility of a suicide attempt, should be obtained. On *physical examination*, alteration of vital signs may occur with organic psychosis, or there may be other findings of an underlying medical or traumatic disorder. *Mental status evaluation* points toward an organic psychosis if there is impairment in orientation, recent memory, and other cognitive functioning. In organic psychosis, *hallucinations* tend to be visual and may also be tactile, olfactory, and gustatory; in contrast, psychiatrically based psychosis is most frequently accompanied by auditory hallucinations. Finally, the immediate *response to support, reassurance,* and small doses of *medication* are frequently more dramatic with organic psychosis than with psychiatrically based psychosis.

A patient experiencing an *acute schizophrenic episode* appears strange, preoccupied, and private. Affect is flat and the patient has little interest in relating to the physician. Speech appears disconnected, lacking goal-directedness and clear transitions. There may be inappropriate smiling and/or giggling or other inappropriate comments. The patient typ-

TABLE 89–1
Differentiating Features of Organic Psychiatrically Based Psychosis

ASSESSMENT FEATURE	ORGANIC	PSYCHIATRIC
History		
Nature of onset	Acute	Insidious
History before illness	Prior illness or drug use	Prior psychiatric history (self or family)
Physical evaluation		
Level of consciousness	May be impaired	Normal
Vital signs	May be impaired	Usually normal
Pathologic autonomic signs	May be present	Normal
Laboratory studies, including urine screening	May be abnormal	Normal
Mental status evaluation		
Orientation	May be impaired	Intact
Recent memory	May be impaired	Intact
Intellectual functioning	May be impaired	Intact
Nature of hallucinations	Not auditory (e.g., visual, tactile)	Auditory
Response to support and medication	Often dramatic	Often limited

ically finds it excruciatingly difficult to make decisions, such as that of agreeing to psychiatric treatment.

The following are the most commonly found signs and symptoms of acute schizophrenic episodes: auditory hallucinations; flatness of affect; thoughts spoken aloud; and delusions of external control. Auditory hallucinations typically involve voices of persons talking negatively about the patient in the third person. At times, the voices may also direct the patient toward suicidal or homicidal acts. The patient may feel that others can read his mind or can either add to or take away the patient's ideas at will. The patient also has delusions of external control that involve the belief that the patient's mind, thoughts, behavior, spirit, and/or body are being externally controlled by some outside force or person. An acutely psychotic individual may also be depressed and may have suicidal and homicidal ideations.

An acute schizophrenic episode can be differentiated from an organic psychosis on the basis of history, which usually reveals chronic deterioration in functioning and the gradual emergence of psychotic symptoms. A positive family history of schizophrenia may be helpful. Findings of physical examination of the acutely schizophrenic patient are usually negative, except for that of possible tachycardia associated with anxiety.

The *manic patient* presents with an expansive, often grandiose, and elevated mood. The patient reports feeling extremely good and readily describes his exploits, which may include great achievements and plans, lack of sleep, and buying sprees. The patient speaks rapidly with pressured speech, and may show a "flight of ideas," rapidly shifting from one topic to the next without completing earlier thoughts. The patient may also become irritable and emotionally labile if someone disagrees with him. Extremely aggressive and combative behavior may be displayed. The patient overestimates himself and has little or no awareness of his distortion of reality. If the patient is also experiencing a significant depression, emotional lability will be even greater. Overall, the range of sudden emotional responses may include any of the following: euphoria, anxiety, irritability, combativeness, panic, and depression. There may also be a history of previous episodes of mania or depression.

The office-based physician can make the diagnosis of *infantile autism* on the basis of the history, the mother's concerns, and the findings of regular visits during the first 2½ years of life. Children with a *pervasive developmental disorder* may also be identified through history and clinical presentation. The patient may demonstrate extreme anxiety, difficulty in separation, hypersensitivity to sensory stimuli, irregular physiologic patterns, and extreme mood lability. Posturing and self-mutilation may occur. Speech may be abnormal, and affect may be inappropriate. Typically, these children appear to have a "strange" quality noted by the physician.

In encountering an acutely psychotic adolescent, the office-based physician should recognize that the patient as well as the family are often extremely anxious. The patient's mood may be extremely labile, as the world is seen as dangerous, threatening, and unpredictable. Whether agitated or withdrawn, the patient may pose a suicidal and/or violent risk, and violence can be directed at the physician and emergency room staff as well as the family and outside world.

MANAGEMENT

The management of psychosis in the acute phase includes the following goals:

1. *Differentiating Organic Psychosis from the Psychiatrically Based Psychosis.*—This distinction is made on the basis of history (individual, family, illness, and drug histories), mental status, physical examination, and laboratory studies, including toxicology screen. When in doubt, the patient should be observed for a longer period of time. This differentiation of organic from psychiatrically based psychosis will influence all subsequent management decisions.

2. *Determining Possible Suicidal Danger or Other Risk of Self-Harm.*—All acutely psychotic patients may represent an immediate suicide risk, due to impaired judgment and possible depression. In addition, the patient may harm himself unintentionally. It is essential to ascertain from patient, friends, and family whether any deliberate or accidental life-endangering events have taken place. The patient should be asked directly about suicidal thoughts. This assessment will influence significantly the decision of whether or not to hospitalize the patient.

3. *Determining the Nature of Family Resources.*—To address the emergency created by the acutely psychotic patient, the office-based physician should call in all important family members. The nature of the family response and the degree to which the family can collaborate with the physician in developing a treatment plan for the patient guide the physician in deciding upon treatment and disposition.

4. *Determining the Need for Medical Hospitalization.*—Medical hospitalization may be necessary in cases of organic psychosis due to newly diagnosed or exacerbated chronic illness or toxic psychosis to manage medical complications. With an intoxication, the patient and family often deny the significance of the acute episode after it resolves. Therefore, it is essential that the psychiatrist see the patient and family as soon as he is able to speak coherently. If medical hospitalization is employed, the patient should be placed on a floor that is experienced in the acute management of psychotic and possibly suicidal patients. A psychiatrist should be available on an emergency basis.

5. *Determining the Need for Psychiatric Hospitalization.*—Under ideal circumstances, the acute schizophrenic or manic patient is managed on an outpatient basis, with intensive psychiatric intervention beginning at the time of diagnosis. Outpatient treatment for acute psychiatrically based psychosis is indicated under the following circumstances: *(a)* the patient is not suicidal, homicidal, or at significant risk of accidental self-harm; *(b)* the patient recognizes his own impairment and is cooperative; *(c)* the family is organized and appears capable of supervising the patient; *(d)* a therapist is available at the time of the crisis to work immediately with patient and family; *(e)* the patient responds to antipsychotic medication in the emergency room.

Psychiatric hospitalization, on the other hand, is required in the following cases: *(a)* the patient is suicidal, violent, or incapable of supervised self-care; *(b)* the family is disorganized, absent, or unable to assume responsibility for the patient; and *(c)* no therapist is available to assume immediate control of the case.

6. *Using Psychotropic Medication, When Indicated.*—Antipsychotic medication may be utilized in the acute management of both organic and psychiatrically based psychosis. Many toxic psychoses resolve with support and reassurance, involvement of the family, isolation from other patients, the passage of time, and physical restraint, if needed. When these measures fail, and especially when the ingested drug is known, low doses of an antipsychotic agent may be quite helpful. When severe psy-

chiatrically based psychosis requires psychiatric hospitalization or when no therapist is available to take responsibility for the case, it is recommended that the patient *not* be given antipsychotic medication on an emergency basis, since the partial response to this medication may result in the patient's being turned away by the psychiatric hospital. In such circumstances, the intramuscular or intravenous use of diphenhydramine (Benadryl), 20 to 50 mg, and physical restraints, when necessary, are preferable. Other minor tranquilizers such as diazepam (Valium), oxazepam (Serax), and alprazolam (Xanax) may also be utilized.

Common antipsychotic medications, relative potency, and usual dosage ranges are listed in Table 89–2. It is recommended that the office-based physician select several drugs and gain familiarity with their usage in emergency situations. The physician should also be familiar with common side effects of antipsychotic medications and inform patients and parents of these. Lethargy, dizziness, and hypotension may occur with those drugs given in high doses (chlorpromazine, thioridazine), and vital signs should be monitored. Extrapyramidal side-effects are common with low dosage drugs (haloperidol, trifluoperazine, fluphenazine); these side effects include acute dystonia (abnormal muscle contractions); akathisia (abnormal motor restlessness); pseudo-Parkinsonism (rigidity, slowness, stooped posture, drooling, inexpressive facies). Tardive dyskinesia (often irreversible, with long-term use) may occur with either high or low dose antipsychotic medication.

Acute dystonic reactions are common in the adolescent and young adult age group and can be treated prophylactically with benztropine, 1 to 4 mg/day orally. Emergency treatment of dystonia involves the intramuscular or intravenous use of diphenhydramine, 25 to 50 mg. For manic-depressive illness, lithium is the mainstay of treatment but requires several days to achieve maximum beneficial effect. The administration of lithium should be the responsibility of the treating psychiatrist.

TABLE 89–2
Common Antipsychotic Medications

GENERIC NAME (BRAND NAME)	ESTIMATED EQUIVALENT DOSAGE (MG)	TOTAL DAILY DOSAGE (MG)
Phenothiazines		
Chlorpromazine (Thorazine)	100	5–1,000
Thioridazine (Mellaril)	100	50–800
Trifluoperazine (Stelazine)	5	5–30
Fluphenazine (Prolixin)	2	1–20
Butyrophenones		
Haloperidol (Haldol)	2	2–40

FOLLOW-UP

Once the acute psychotic episode has resolved, whether organic or psychiatric, the office-based physician can broaden his own relationship with the adolescent, encourage personal competence, and help the family deal with important issues, such as parental limit setting and appropriate levels of closeness, as well as independence, autonomy, and eventual separation. If the patient requires continuing medication, the physician supports this. If specialized education is required or treatment programs are needed, the physician becomes familiar with these programs and serves as an advocate for the patient, ensuring that appropriate services are being provided and that communication between institutions also occurs.

BIBLIOGRAPHY

Haley J: *Leaving Home*. New York, McGraw-Hill Book Co, 1980.

Kessler K, Waletsky JP: Clinical use of the antipsychotics. *Am J Psychiatry* 1981; 138:202.

Werry JS (ed): *Pediatric Psychopharmacology: The Use of Behavior Modifying Drugs in Children*. New York, Brunner-Mazel, 1978.

Wiener JM: *Psychopharmacology in Childhood and Adolescence*. New York, Basic Books, 1977.

90 SCHOOL REFUSAL

Gordon R. Hodas, M.D.

School refusal, also known as school phobia and school avoidance, has been called "the great imitator" because the patient frequently presents with other symptoms, often recurrent somatic complaints such as headache or abdominal pain. Although school refusal may on occasion be the presenting concern, usually this diagnosis is made by the office-based physician's considering this possible diagnosis and pursuing it in the history. School refusal implies a separation problem between child and parents, usually the mother, and a block in the development of competence and autonomy on the part of the child. Other family problems may exist as well. School refusal is distinguished from truancy because school refusal occurs with the knowledge and accommodation of the parents, while truancy usually occurs in the absence of parental awareness and consent. Even when the medical evaluation is normal, children who still refuse to attend school are typically seen by parents as too sick and too upset to return to class.

Incidence figures for school refusal are not available, but the condition is not uncommon and is probably underdiagnosed. School absence may be long and continuous, sporadic over time, or interspersed with regular attendance the majority of each week. The primary care physician should appreciate the frequent association between chronic somatic complaints, depression, and school refusal.

Overprotected children with somatic symptoms are at highest risk for school refusal and may include previously vulnerable but now healthy children, special children, and children from unstable families at risk for divorce and from families in which parents have physical symptoms and possible disability. Children with chronic medical illnesses more typically strive actively to remain in school.

OFFICE EVALUATION AND DIAGNOSIS

The triad of findings that leads to the diagnosis of school refusal includes: (1) poor school attendance, (2) vague physical symptoms, and (3) normal physical and laboratory findings. These findings often occur in association with depression and anxiety.

School attendance patterns vary from continuous to intermittent. Sporadic school absence occurs most commonly in the fall after the school year begins, and following holidays and weekends. The child may function quite well without physical complaints and anxiety when school is not in session, but symptoms develop when classes resume. This pattern may have occurred over several academic years. On the other hand, when a child has missed several consecutive weeks of school or more, this situation represents a major crisis and must be responded to immediately and decisively by the physician. The child with good grades who misses one or two days of school each week can more easily escape detection; it is here that the careful history of the office-based physician is rewarded.

The vague physical complaints and symptoms that, despite a normal medical evaluation, may accompany the school refusal pattern are as follows:

1. General
   Insomnia
   Excessive sleeping
   Fatigue
   "Fever"
2. Skin
   Pallor
3. Ear, nose, and throat (ENT)
   Recurrent sore throat
   Constant "sinus trouble"

4. Respiratory
   Hyperventilation
   Coughing tics
5. Cardiovascular
   Chest pain
   Palpitations
6. Gastrointestinal
   Abdominal pain
   Anorexia
   Nausea
   Vomiting
   Diarrhea
7. Renal
   None
8. Genital
   Dysmenorrhea
9. Skeletal
   Bone pain
   Joint pain
   Back pain
10. Neuromuscular
    Headaches
    Dizziness
    Syncope
    "Weakness"

Although the most common symptom is abdominal pain, there may be multiple complaints. Anorexia in the absence of weight loss may occur, as may diarrhea. Nausea may be present, with or without associated vomiting. Vomiting often follows stressful events. The serious complaint of vomiting should not mislead the physician into an overly extensive workup that unwittingly reinforces disability. Similar considerations apply to skeletal complaints that may occur—bone pain, joint pain, and back pain. Other possible symptoms that may mask the school refusal syndrome include chest pain, dysmenorrhea, muscle weakness, coughing, tics, and recurrent sore throats.

Certain family characteristics of the child with school refusal have been identified. Berger described four important elements: (1) An overprotective infantilizing attitude toward the patient. The child is excused from family responsibilities, and his wishes are quickly granted. (2) A belief in the physical or emotional vulnerability of the mother. This belief is fostered by the mother herself, who may express fear of emotional breakdown and complain of various physical symptoms. (3) An isolated and devalued father, frequently seen as uninterested and unreliable, perhaps even as violent. There may be accompanying marital tension. (4) Occurrence of a major change in family composition (such as the departure from home of an older sibling), which has focused new attention on the younger child.

The major responsibility of the office-based physician is the detection of school refusal. Hints in history taking include the following: (1) The child has had multiple somatic complaints or recurrent complaints involving one somatic symptom, in the absence of significant medical findings. (2) A substantial amount of missed school has occurred. (3) Child and parents are often evasive about how much school has been missed and under what circumstances. (4) The parents may agree to the child's remaining home out of frustration, to avoid further conflict, after the child cries out in distress, refuses to leave home, and the parents argue fruitlessly with the child and with each other. (5) The child may function well at home after the morning crisis has passed and may do well on the weekends also. (6) The child may have a history of limited peer relationships and of previous episodes of school refusal. (7) Some major family event—illness, depression, or a family member leaving home—often preceded the school refusal by several weeks or months.

MANAGEMENT

The office-based physician can manage many cases of uncomplicated childhood school refusal himself. The physical examination should be done in the presence of the parent(s) in a thorough manner, with the physician emphasizing the absence of physical findings. Appropriate, but not excessive laboratory work should be performed, and medication should not be prescribed. *No letters condoning further school absence should be written.*

Once the physician has established the absence of organic disease, he should set up an immediate family conference with both parents present and the child outside the office. At the family conference, while acknowledging the child's subjective pain or distress, the physician should make a firm and unequivocal statement to the parents that this child has no serious illness and needs to learn to function and attend school despite his symptoms. Eventually the symptoms will diminish but the return to normal functioning cannot await this development, lest the child become seriously disabled emotionally. The parents are then encouraged to discuss how they will inform their child that he must return to school immediately and are given a chance to develop a plan of action in the event that the child refuses. At this point, the child can enter the room. The parents should inform him of the physician's findings and of his immediate need to return to school. The child is invited to cooperate so that the entire family can work together and is informed, when necessary, that the parents will persist even if he fails to cooperate.

This approach is effective with many cases of childhood school refusal. When it fails (e.g., the parents are unable to make an agreement or to carry it out successfully) psychiatric referral is indicated. Psychiatric referral is also indicated in the following situations: long-standing continuous school refusal, recurrent episodes, severe depression, psychosis, and most cases occurring in adolescence.

When the office-based physician manages school refusal himself, it is important that he contact the school nurse to reassure her of the child's state of health, describe his proposed approach to the school refusal and obtain her support. The physician should encourage the family to maintain close telephone contact with him over the next several days until he sees the child and family again, ideally after the first day of successful return to school. When psychiatric referral is made, the physician should underline the urgency of this process and make sure that the family follows through. The family-oriented treatment of this problem addresses both the child's return to school and underlying precipitating stresses. The physician frequently needs to support the treatment actively; with the most difficult cases, the physician and psychiatrist may need to meet with the family jointly to clarify issues and underline the need for treatment. Following completion of treatment, the office-based physician should continue to encourage the child during the primary care visits, while remaining alert to the possibility of recurrence.

BIBLIOGRAPHY

Berger H: Somatic pain and school avoidance. *Clin Pediatr* 1974; 13:819–826.

Nader PR, Bullock D, Caldwell B: School phobia. *Pediatr Clin North Am* 1975; 22:605–716.

Schmitt B: School phobia: The great imitator: A pediatrician's viewpoint. *Pediatrics* 1971; 48:433–442.

91 SUICIDE ATTEMPT

Gordon R. Hodas, M.D.

The acutely suicidal patient, together with the acutely psychotic patient, represent the two most serious psychiatric emergencies that the office-based physician faces. Broadly defined, suicidal behavior involves thoughts or actions that may lead to self-inflicted serious injury or death. Suicidal ideation involves the wish or plan to die, not yet acted upon, while a suicidal attempt implies that actual behavior to take one's life has occurred. It is important for the office-based physician to regard all suicide attempts as serious and reject the notion of "suicidal gesture" for apparently less serious attempts, since many of these children may remain strongly suicidal and try again.

A suicide attempt by a child or adolescent

signifies a cry for help as well as a breakdown in the system of mutual supports in the family that guides and protects a child while also promoting his autonomy. Therefore, the physician must select the treatment that addresses the needs of child and family and not just child alone. Most suicidal children are depressed, and all share a pervasive sense of hopelessness and helplessness. Alternate solutions are viewed as absent or unrealistic, and suicide is seen as the only solution for the child's and family's problems. In addition to depression, suicide attempts occur in the context of major losses (e.g., serious illness or death in the family), major family conflict or instability (e.g., separation, divorce, and physical or emotional abuse), and psychosis.

While incidence figures for both suicide attempts and successful suicides have climbed rapidly over the past 30 years, there has been some stabilization of incidence during the 1980s. This trend is significant but should not be falsely reassuring. In contemporary American society, too often suicidal behavior is seen as an acceptable response to personal crisis and distress. At times suicide is even viewed as heroic. One consequence of these changing social values is adolescent suicide pacts, in which groups of adolescents try to kill themselves either by prior agreement or through a process of negative modeling. Such events have been common during the past decade and have created tragedies in many communities.

In addition to the recent trends described, it has been recognized for some time that suicide attempts and completed suicides are often underreported and are at times classified as accidents to avoid shame for child and family. For children under 10 years of age, suicide is not even classified as a cause of death in registries. Available data indicate that suicide attempts occur in children as young as 5 years old. In children between the ages of 10 and 14 years, the rate of completed suicide tripled from 1955 to 1975. For persons between 15 and 24 years, suicide is now the third leading cause of death, after accidents and homicides, and the rate of attempted suicide doubled in this group from 1965 to 1975. In 1983 there were an estimated 400,000 adolescent suicide attempts, 6,000 of which were successful. Furthermore, many accidents, especially car accidents, are believed to be masked suicides.

Suicidal thinking is not uncommon in childhood and adolescence and can present in many psychiatric conditions. For example, 72% of children ages 6 to 12 years who were sequentially admitted to a psychiatric inpatient unit were found to have suicidal ideation or attempts. Suicidal thinking is even more common in depressed children. In one study, over 80% of outpatient depressed children reported suicidal ideation during some point in their depression.

A suicide attempt by a boy is two times more likely to be fatal than one by a girl; on the other hand, girls attempt suicide at least three times more often than boys. Overall, approximately 80% of suicide attempts are by ingestion. More lethal methods (such as jumping, shooting, or attempted hanging) are more common with boys and often express greater suicidal intent. It would be incorrect to assume that other methods do not often reflect a genuine wish to die.

The office-based physician should suspect a possible suicide attempt with "accidental" ingestions, vehicular accidents, and other suspicious accidents. The index of suspicion is higher if the child appears sad, has made a previous suicide attempt, or comes from an unstable family environment. When younger children present with an accident or injury, the possibility of inadequate parental supervision or child abuse must be considered.

Immature conceptions of death by preadolescent children complicate the assessment of suicide attempts in that age group. Although variability exists, an appreciation of the irreversibility of death usually does not occur until the age of 9 years; even then the child may believe that, in his or her case, death will not be irreversible and will be pleasant. It is not until adolescence that the adult concept of an irreversible death is firmly in place.

OFFICE EVALUATION

Common characteristics associated with suicide attempts in children aged 6 to 12 years are:

1. Depression
2. Hopelessness
3. Low self-esteem
4. Worthlessness

5. Positive family history
6. Positive wish to die
7. Death seen as temporary

These characteristics distinguish high-risk suicidal children from other emotionally disturbed, but nonsuicidal children. The first four features, all related to significant depression, are juxtaposed with a wish to die without fully appreciating the irreversibility of death. A family history of suicide attempts increases the risk.

The sequence of events commonly associated with adolescent suicide attempts is summarized below, following the work of Teicher.

1. Continuing family instability
2. Withdrawal from parents and communication breakdown
3. Acute precipitating event, with loss of self-esteem

Typically, there is a history of family instability of many years' duration, characterized by residential and environmental changes and unexpected losses through divorce, illness, and suicide. With the onset of adolescence, a period of mutual alienation between parents and adolescent may occur, characterized by withdrawal, misunderstandings, and communication breakdown. This further loss of support, coming at a time of developmental transition, lowers the adolescent's self-esteem, rendering him vulnerable to an acute disappointment (e.g., peer rejection, broken romance, poor grades) which may precipitate a suicide attempt.

High-risk suicide situations for children and adolescents are summarized below.

1. Attempted suicide
2. Threatened or planned suicide
3. Desire for death
4. "Accidental" ingestion or other questionable accident
5. Severe depression
6. Significant interpersonal withdrawal
7. Sadness and recurrent somatic complaints
8. Violence
9. Psychosis

As can be seen, many different clinical situations may be associated with a high risk for suicide. The office-based physician should be alert to these possibilities so that further assessment and treatment can be pursued when indicated.

MANAGEMENT

With an immediate suicide attempt, the goal is to get the child and family to the pediatric emergency room as soon as possible so that proper medical treatment can be provided and further evaluation pursued. With a child who admits to serious suicidal intent without an overt attempt, either emergency room evaluation or direct psychiatric referral is indicated. When a child or adolescent admits to a recent suicide attempt that no longer requires medical evaluation or treatment, psychiatric referral is appropriate unless continuing suicidal intent necessitates emergency room evaluation and possible hospitalization.

As a general guide, the following four principles of assessment and management are offered:

1. *Routinely screen for suicide ideation.* The screening for suicidal ideation, especially with adolescents, should not be neglected even when a patient does not appear depressed or under obvious stress. The physician should raise the question of suicide in a matter-of-fact manner. (Physician: "How often do you feel down?" "When you get really down, do you sometimes wish you were dead or think of killing yourself?") With higher-risk children, questioning about suicide should be more extensive. (Physician: "When you're really sad like this, do you sometimes wish you were dead?" "Have you been feeling that way lately?" "Have you tried to kill yourself?")

2. *Consider all suspicious accidents to be possible suicide attempts.* In this way, the office-based physician may detect a seriously depressed child and prevent a completed suicide.

3. *Regard all suicide attempts as serious.* Some suicide attempts may have only limited medical consequences but that does not mean they are not serious (the child who takes ten diazepam [Valium] tablets and survives may be just as suicidal as the child who takes ten digitalis pills and dies). It is suicidal intent that matters.

4. *Determine the level of suicidal intent—the actual wish to die—with all suicide attempts.* This includes the child's direct statements about dying and is also reflected in the child's overall mental status and in the nature of the actual suicide attempt.

The systematic assessment of a suicidal child or adolescent involves an appreciation of the child's current medical status and his or her wish to die and context of support. Critical information is gained through assessment of medical lethality, suicidal intent, and strengths of the child, the family, and social context.

Medical lethality refers to the severity of the medical consequences of a suicide attempt.

ASSESSING MEDICAL LETHALITY

1. Need for emergency room treatment
2. Vital signs
3. Loss of consciousness
4. Evidence of drug/alcohol intoxication (e.g., pupils, smell on breath)
5. Need for emesis, lavage, and catharsis
6. Acute medical complications: cardiac complications, respiratory arrest, convulsions
7. Indications for medical hospitalization
8. Indications for intensive care treatment
9. Residual abnormalities

The physician assesses such factors as the necessity for emergency room treatment, alteration of vital signs, loss of consciousness, signs of drug or alcohol intoxication, and development of acute complications such as cardiac complications, or respiratory arrest and seizures. The physician should also evaluate the requirement of medical or intensive care hospitalization and possible residual effects of the attempt.

Suicidal intent is inferred by the physician following a suicide attempt based on the circumstances of the attempt, the patient's self-report of the seriousness of his intent at the time of the attempt, and an assessment of the child's mental status.

ASSESSING SUICIDAL INTENT—WISH TO DIE

Circumstances of suicide attempt (from child and family)
- Use of violent means (hanging, shooting, jumping, deliberate car accident)
- All available pills ingested
- Use of multiple pills and alcohol
- Hidden suicide note
- Child found unexpectedly
- Previous suicide attempts

Child's self-report
- Premeditation of attempt
- Irreversible concept of death
- Nature of precipitating stresses
- Anticipation of death
- Desire for death, then and now
- Attempt to conceal suicide attempt

Child's mental status
- Orientation and possible psychosis
- Unwillingness to relate to or cooperate with physician
- Unwillingness to accept family support
- Negative orientation toward future
- Continuing suicidal impulses

It is important to determine how serious the suicide intent was and the extent of continuing suicide risk. It is strongly recommended that the physician rely not only on the data regarding circumstances and self-report, but also on his overall impression of the child as revealed in the physician-patient relationship. A child who relates warmly to the physician and expresses remorse is usually a better risk than one who verbalizes the risk to die or continues to deny the attempt.

Finally, the physician should evaluate the *strengths of child, family, and social context.*

ASSESSING STRENGTHS AND SUPPORTS

Strengths and assets of child
- Ability to relate to physician
- Ability to utilize parents
- Ability to acknowledge problem
- Positive orientation toward future

Strengths and assets of family
- Commitment to child
- Ability to unite during current crisis
- Ability to unite during past crises
- Problem-solving abilities
- Capacity to supervise child
- Ability to utilize external supports

Nature of external supports
- Family physician, pediatrician, psychiatrist
- Extended family
- Neighbors, other significant adults
- Religious community

Since a suicide attempt represents a fundamental crisis in child development and parenting, it is essential that the physician seek out all possible strengths and supports. As listed above, these include strengths of the family and child and the strengths offered by external supports. It is only by appreciating these strengths that a safe and realistic plan can be undertaken.

Every suicide attempt, regardless of its ap-

parent seriousness, requires psychiatric consultation for that patient, and many patients will require psychiatric hospitalization. The degree of the psychiatric involvement will depend on the circumstances of the suicide attempt. The alert child can be interviewed alone and with his parents in the emergency room, while the obtunded child may need to be seen the next morning on the medical floor on which he is hospitalized. When psychiatric hospitalization is deemed necessary, it should be effected as soon as the child has been cleared medically. Psychiatric hospitalization becomes substantially easier when the office-based physician prepares child and parents for the possibility and then supports the decision once made. On occasion, the emergency psychiatrist may need to initiate an involuntary commitment for psychiatric hospitalization.

The primary physician should arrange for immediate psychiatric referral for those patients who do not require psychiatric hospitalization. This is best achieved by addressing both parents, either alone or in the presence of the child. The physician should contact the family shortly after this to be sure that his recommendations for psychiatric care were followed. In like manner, when the physician learns about a suicide attempt made weeks or months earlier, it is imperative that he not be lured into the denial pattern that the patient may be demonstrating. *All suicide attempts, regardless of when they are detected, should receive psychiatric consultation and referral.* Hospitalization is indicated under the following circumstances: (1) the physician has had difficulty in gaining the cooperation of the child and family; (2) the child has made a serious suicide attempt and continues to have strong suicidal intent; (3) the child has made a repeated suicide attempt; (4) the child is psychotic; (5) the family appears unable to provide necessary supervision and support to the child; and (6) there is rapid denial by child and family of the significance of a serious suicide attempt.

After psychiatric referral, the office-based physician maintains a health-oriented primary care relationship with child and family. The physician and treating psychiatrist should communicate regularly so that each is aware of and can support the other's efforts. The physician should appreciate that, with appropriate individual and family psychotherapy, suicidal children and adolescents with their families are often able to reverse the self-destructive cycle and move constructively ahead into the future.

BIBLIOGRAPHY

Duncan J: The immediate management of suicide attempts in children and adolescents: Psychological aspects. *J Fam Pract* 1977; 4:77–80.

Garfinkel BD, Golombek H: Suicide and depression in childhood and adolescence. *Can Med Assoc J* 1974; 110:1278–1281.

Hofman A: Adolescents in distress: Suicide and out of control behavior. *Med Clin North Am* 1975; 59(6):1429–1437.

McAnarney E: Suicidal behavior of children and youth. *Pediatr Clin North Am* 1975; 22:595–604.

McIntire M, Angle C, Schlicht M, et al: Suicide and self-poisoning in pediatrics. *Adv Pediatr* 1977; 24:291–309.

Pfeffer C: Suicidal behavior in latency-age children: An outpatient population. *J Child Psychol Psychiatry* 1981; 18:679–692.

Teicher J: Children and adolescents who attempt suicide. *Pediatr Clin North Am* 1970; 17:687–697.

section vi

The Primary Care Physician and the Subspecialist

When the primary care physician shares the management of certain patients with subspecialist colleagues, communication and decision-making responsibility help determine the success of a clear definition of management. In this section, certain conditions are described for which the subspecialists offer expertise and management decisions while the primary care physician helps implement the treatments and manages the patient's other health problems. Although the topics include conditions that are not typically within the realm of primary care, it is important for the physician to know about them and understand some of the specialists' thoughts that help formulate the decisions. The separation of chapters into Section III and this section are based on this concept as well as on local practice patterns. Just as it is difficult to define primary care, the description of its contents and limitations lacks universal agreement. The organization of this section is done without any intention to limit the scope of practice of the primary physicians.

The specialists who contributed to this section have described what they do to assess and manage patients referred to them. The primary care physician can then better understand the complexities and limitations of a referral as well as define his or her role in the care of such patients.

92 CARDIOLOGY

Anthony C. Chang, M.D.
Bernard J. Clark III, M.D.

CARDIOLOGY AND THE PRIMARY CARE PHYSICIAN

The primary care physician is often the first medical person to identify a cardiac problem and after referral is responsible for following up the patient in conjunction with the cardiologist. The purpose of this chapter is to present some important, common problems in pediatric cardiology, which will aid the physician in (1) recognizing problems; (2) heightening the awareness of potential problems; and (3) answering some routine office practice questions that come up when dealing with the pediatric patient with heart disease. The following topics are covered: congestive heart failure; surgical treatments of congenital heart disease; and issues surrounding the handling of fever and preventing bacterial endocarditis, Kawasaki disease, acute rheumatic fever, mitral valve prolapse, hyperlipidemias, and irregular rhythms.

CONGESTIVE HEART FAILURE

Heart failure in infancy and childhood represents a clinical syndrome that reflects the inability of the myocardium to meet the metabolic requirements of the body. Most commonly, failure results from excessive volume overload associated with left-to-right shunts, valvular insufficiency, and iatrogenic causes. Excessive pressure overload (as seen in valvular stenosis, coarctation or interruption of the aorta, systemic hypertension, and pulmonary hypertension) is the next most common cause. Following these are: primary myocardial dysfunction from myocarditis, cardiomyopathies, or metabolic and endocrine abnormalities (hypoxemia, sepsis, anemia, hypoglycemia, and electrolyte abnormalities). Finally, rhythm abnormalities from either tachyarrhythmias (supraventricular or ventricular) or severe complete heart block may cause heart failure.

Excessive volume and pressure-loading situations predominate in the infant as causes of CHF. After 1 year of age, rheumatic heart disease, bacterial endocarditis, endomyocardial disease, myocarditis, and severe cardiac arrhythmias as well as complications from surgical repair of heart malformations are frequent causes of CHF.

The earliest onset of CHF occurs in the hypoplastic left-heart syndrome, interrupted aortic arch or severe coarctation of the aorta, or severe myocardial disease. Most infants with septal defects or patent ductus arteriosus, endocardial cushion defects, unobstructed anomalous pulmonary venous connections, and less severe coarctation of the aorta usually do not develop CHF until the second week of life or later. Except for newborns with transient myocardial ischemia from perinatal stress causing CHF, patients with anatomic heart disease generally improve only slightly and should be referred immediately for complete evaluation.

Clinical Manifestations of Congestive Heart Failure

Growth failure may be a sign of CHF in the infant and young child. Feeding difficulties combined with respiratory distress often preclude attainment of adequate nutritional balance. A history of easy fatigability, dyspnea on exertion, or failure to keep up with siblings or peers suggests the presence of CHF. Recurrent pulmonary infections may be a result of overperfused lungs from large left-to-right shunting defects.

On initial examination, the general state of health or illness can usually be readily determined. A baby with reduced oxygen delivery to the tissues, whether from cyanotic heart disease or CHF, will show little spontaneous movement. Dysmorphism of face or body may suggest one of many syndromes associated with congenital heart disease such as Down syndrome (endocardial cushion defect or ventricular septal defect), Turner syndrome (coarctation of the aorta, bicuspid aortic valve), Noonan syndrome (pulmonic valve stenosis), and fetal alcohol syndrome (septal defects and tetralogy of Fallot).

Blood pressure measurements should be obtained in all four extremities for every infant and child being evaluated for congenital heart disease to rule in or out the presence of a coarctation of the aorta or other arch abnormality. A heart rate of more than 160 beats per minute in an infant or 100 beats per minute in an older child at rest is suggestive of increased adrenergic tone in response to diminished cardiac output. Tachypnea typically is a part of the clinical picture of CHF. Rapid, shallow respirations with flaring of the alae nasi and retractions with wheezes are characteristic of pulmonary overcirculation. Rales, a late finding in the infant, can be heard in the older child who may also have dyspnea on exertion, orthopnea, and a chronic cough. Hepatomegaly, jugular venous distention, and peripheral edema are all signs of elevated central venous pressure and accompanying CHF.

Examination of the cardiovascular system may reveal specific abnormalities. Palpation of the pulses in upper and lower extremities, an essential part of the examination, can be diagnostic of coarctation of the aorta or one of the various interruption complexes, as well as generalized low-output states in which all pulses are diminished. The heart may be enlarged to palpation or percussion, which will be confirmed with chest radiography (Fig 92–1). A third heart sound may be present indicating decreased ventricular compliance. Murmurs may suggest an etiology but definitive diagnosis will be made in conjunction with a cardiologist. Auscultation of the rhythm may suggest an arrhythmia, which can be documented with an electrocardiogram (ECG).

The infant or child with the spectrum of abnormalities described above requires immediate attention. Such a patient is in a tenuous position and his condition may rapidly deteriorate. Therefore, when the diagnosis of possible

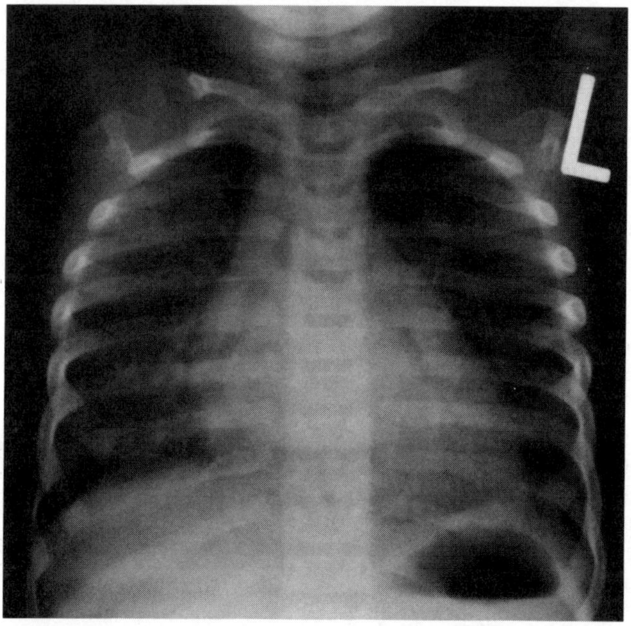

FIG 92–1
Chest roentgenogram in a patient with heart failure shows enlarged heart and increased pulmonary vascular.

congenital heart disease with CHF is entertained, the patient is best served by referral to a pediatric cardiologist.

Management of Congestive Heart Failure

Treatment of heart failure includes supplemental oxygen and placement of an intravenous line to aid in drug administration. The patient should be positioned with the head and shoulders elevated to decrease pulmonary blood volume by increasing peripheral pooling. An arterial blood gas analysis should be performed to evaluate acid/base status. If severe metabolic acidosis (pH less than 7.2) is found, bicarbonate therapy should be instituted. Additionally, if respiratory insufficiency or failure is confirmed, positive-pressure mechanical ventilation, which may improve both respiratory and cardiovascular function, should be instituted. It may be difficult in the infant or young child to separate sepsis or pulmonary infection from CHF, and in these circumstances antibiotics may be administered after appropriate cultures have been performed.

In most CHF, regardless of the underlying cause, initial pharmacologic therapy will include digoxin and diuretic therapy. Diuretics decrease blood volume and intrapulmonary fluid. Furosemide, 1 mg/kg intravenously, can be administered in the first 24 hours with a dramatic improvement in respiratory status. Because of the kaliuretic effects of the diuretics, serum potassium levels should be monitored during initial therapy and supplemental potassium administered as necessary.

The mainstay of long-term medical management of CHF remains the use of digitalis to improve myocardial function. The digitalization schedule is outlined in Table 92–1. If the patient is in mild or moderate heart failure, the digitalis may be given intramuscularly. In cases of severe CHF, where absorption of medication from the tissues would be variable and possibly incomplete, the digitalis doses are given intravenously with a 25% reduction in the calculated intramuscular dose. A lower total dose is used in the presence of myocarditis or cardiomyopathy due to an increased predisposition to arrhythmias. A total digitalis dose is given over 24 hours: half initially, one quarter in 8 hours, and the final one quarter in another 8 hours. The patient is monitored for changes in heart rate and rhythm during this period. The daily maintenance dose is one quarter the total digitalis dose divided every 12 hours. The parenteral form of the drug contains 100 μg/mL while the oral preparation contains 50 μg/mL.

The oral bioavailability of digoxin is less than 100% (usually 70%) because it is incompletely absorbed from the gastrointestinal (GI) tract. Disease states or drugs that are characterized by hypermotility may decrease digoxin absorption, while drugs that retard gastrointestinal motility tend to increase absorption. Taking digoxin with meals does not affect the total amount of digoxin absorbed; however, it does retard the rate of absorption. After the administration of digoxin tablets, peak serum levels are reached in 1 to 1½ hours, whereas with intravenous injections, peak levels are obtained almost immediately. After approximately eight hours, the distribution phase of the drug is completed and the central and peripheral compartments are in equilibrium.

Digitalis Toxicity

A relatively high incidence of toxic manifestations has accompanied the widespread use of digoxin. Intoxication has been reported to be as high as 20% in patients receiving the glycosides. Although the most common and earliest side effects are related to the GI tract (anorexia, nausea, vomiting, abdominal discomfort), disorders of cardiac rhythm are the first manifestation in one third of patients and can be seen in up to 80% of patients with other toxic effects.

Certain ECG abnormalities occur more fre-

TABLE 92–1
Digitalization Schedule for Pediatric Patients (Intramuscular or Oral)*

AGE	WEIGHT (G)	TOTAL DOSE OF DIGITALIS† (μG/KG)
Premature infants	500–1,000	20
	1,000–1,500	25
	1,500–2,000	30
	2,000–2,500	30–40
Term to 1 mo	. . .	60
1 mo to 2 yr	. . .	60–80
2 yr to 10–12 yr	. . .	40–60

*The intravenous dose is 75% of oral or intramuscular.
†No dose greater than 1.5 mg.

quently than others though none are pathognomonic of digoxin toxicity. The most common abnormalities include bigeminy, multifocal premature ventricular beats, and paroxysmal atrial tachycardia with block. A prolonged PR interval is not a sign of digoxin toxic effect, but it is a sign of digoxin effect. Toxic response may be precipitated by several factors. These include (1) potassium losses (diuretics, adrenocorticosteroids, cathartics), (2) hypercalcemia (usually only with very high serum levels), (3) hypoxemia (accounts for high incidence of toxic effects in patients with cor pulmonale), and (4) renal insufficiency, as digoxin is excreted primarily by this route. A patient with signs or symptoms that can be ascribed to digoxin toxic effects should be referred to a cardiologist.

Although most studies demonstrate elevated digoxin levels (more than 2.0 ng/mL) in patients with digoxin toxic effects, a number of patients with apparent toxic effects have levels in the therapeutic range (1.0 to 2.0 ng/mL). Though the likelihood of toxic effects increases with increasing concentration, there is no precise value that clearly separates toxic from nontoxic levels. Therefore, the serum digoxin level is not, in itself, sufficient for a diagnosis of digoxin toxic response. However, levels may be of value (1) as an adjunct in the diagnosis of toxic effects, (2) in the evaluation of an accidental ingestion, (3) in the assessment of the adequacy of digitalization, and (4) in the management of digitalization of patients with renal insufficiency.

SURGICAL TREATMENT OF CONGENITAL HEART DISEASE

The terms "definitive operation," "corrective surgery," and "total repair" are misleading; a definitive repair may be accomplished but residual defects may persist and sequelae or late complications may develop that may jeopardize the well-being of the patient. Therefore lifelong cardiac follow-up should be provided by an experienced cardiologist. Since the events leading to cardiac surgery begin with the primary care physician and since the patient is generally returned to his or her care, it is important for the physician not only to have an understanding of the preoperative anatomy of the defect and knowledge of the types of surgical procedures (Table 92–2), but also of the presence, extent, and likelihood of development of postoperative residua, sequelae, or complications (Table 92–3).

Curative procedures are ones in which no residua or sequelae exist. Today these are confined to division of a patent ductus arteriosus in a patient without pulmonary hypertension and closure of a secundum atrial septal defect (though this may be associated with conduction and rhythm disturbances).

Palliative procedures include shunt operations for tetralogy of Fallot and other lesions associated with inadequate pulmonary blood flow. Valvulotomy for valve stenosis can only be considered palliative surgery, as residual or recurrent stenosis, valvular regurgitation and continued predisposition for endocarditis remain. Furthermore, prosthetic valves do not grow, and if inserted in children will require another operation (possibly more than once) before the patient attains adult size. Both synthetic and tissue valves are at risk for thrombus formation and endocarditis, while tissue valves (porcine and pericardial) are associated with calcifications and early degeneration when inserted in children.

Anatomic corrections include closure of ventricular septal defects, correction of endocardial cushion defects, intracardiac repair of tetralogy of Fallot, and arterial switch procedures for complete transposition of the great arteries. Physiologic correction (diversion of blood flow as opposed to anatomic correction) is best represented by the Mustard and Senning procedures (atrial repairs) for complete transposition of the great arteries.

Despite an initial postoperative success, important residua, sequelae, and late complications have been reported in many of these lesions. The most common of these are presented in Table 92–3. Children, after undergoing repair of coarctation of the aorta, have risks of systemic hypertension as well as of recoarctation. From a recent study of 87 patients seen 5 to 15 years after repair, 14% had recoarctation and 23% had systemic hypertension. In addition to these risks are stenosis and regurgitation of an accompanying bicuspid aortic valve and cerebral complications due to aneurysms of the circle of Willis. Right ventriculotomy used in the repair of several malformations may result in right ventricular dysfunction or conduction

TABLE 92–2
Surgical Procedures for Congenital Heart Defects

LESION	PROCEDURE
Aortic stenosis	Valvulotomy, prosthetic valve insertion (tissue or mechanical)
Pulmonary stenosis	Valvulotomy
Coarctation of aorta	Resection and end-to-end anastomosis, patch angioplasty, subclavian flap angioplasty
Ventricular septal defect (VSD)	Patch closure through right atrium or ventricle
Atrial septal defect (ASD)	Patch or suture closure through right atrium
Endocardial cushion defect	Patch closure of ASD and VSD, division of common AV valve and construction of mitral and tricuspid valves
Tetralogy of Fallot	Various shunt procedures for palliation; patch closure of VSD, relief of right ventricular outflow, obstruction with valvulotomy and outflow patch, with or without resection of infundibular muscle
Transposition of great arteries	Mustard or Senning repairs (atrial baffle and venous return diversion); arterial switch with transplantation of coronary arteries
Tricuspid atresia	Fontan procedure (anastomosis of right atrium to pulmonary artery either directly or via valved or nonvalved conduits)
Pulmonary atresia with associated lesions	Various shunt procedures for palliation; Rastelli procedure (valved or nonvalved conduit from right ventricular outflow tract to pulmonary artery

disturbances. The conduction defects are the result of peripheral scarring, which may also become a focus of ventricular irritability. Ventricular septal defect closure may result in injury to the proximal conduction system with a late risk of heart block, which may be sudden and life-threatening. Intraatrial repair of transposition of the great arteries, atrial septal defects, and endocardial cushion defects may be associated with sinus node and atrioventricular node dysfunction as well as atrial arrhythmias such as supraventricular tachycardia, atrial flutter, and fibrillation.

Long-Term Postoperative Perspective

Long-term postoperative outlook for children and young adults with congenital heart disease varies. Three groups of patients must be considered: (1) patients who have undergone a definitive operation with no residual disease and no expectation of late complication or future surgery; (2) patients who have had successfully repaired cardiac lesions but in whom significant complications occur with some frequency and in whom further surgery might eventually be necessary; and (3) patients who have had either palliative or limited corrective operations, but who have severe residual disease for which no further palliative or definitive surgical therapy is possible.

TABLE 92–3
Postoperative Residua, Sequelae or Late Complications

LESION	RESIDUA, SEQUELAE, COMPLICATIONS
Aortic stenosis	Residual or recurrent stenosis, aortic insufficiency; prosthetic valve dysfunction or stenosis; thrombosis; life-long anticoagulation
Ventricular septal defect (VSD)	Residual VSD with congestive heart failure; poor ventricular function; AV block; pulmonary vascular disease
Endocardial cushion defect	Mitral, tricuspid regurgitation/ stenosis; pulmonary vascular disease; AV block; atrial arrhythmias; residual left-to-right shunt
Tetralogy of Fallot	Residual VSD or pulmonary stenosis; ventricular arrhythmias, AV block; pulmonary, tricuspid insufficiency; ventricular dysfunction
Transposition of great arteries	Atrial repair: atrial arrhythmias and conduction disturbances, ventricular dysfunction, caval and/or pulmonary venous obstruction, pulmonary stenosis, tricuspid regurgitation; arterial switch: semilunar valve insufficiency, coronary artery ostia, narrow great vessel stenosis at anastomosis site
Rastelli repair	Conduit stenosis; valve stenosis or insufficiency
Fontan repair	Elevated right atrial pressures at rest and with exercise; abnormal cardiac response to exercise

Patients in the first group have had lesions such as atrial septal defect (ASD) of the secundum type, ventricular septal defect (VSD), patent ductus arteriosus, coarctation of the aorta, and total correction of tetralogy of Fallot repaired successfully without residua or sequelae. These patients may have normal exercise tolerance, physical examination, ECG, and chest radiographs. Little ambulatory management is required beyond an occasional checkup. No restriction need be placed on regular daily activity, including sports. Prophylaxis for bacterial endocarditis is obligatory in all of these patients except those who have had a patent ductus arteriosus closed. Patients with ASD or VSD closure should be treated prophylactically for 6 months to a year after complete closure to allow for patch endothelialization. Patients who have had a coarctation repair continue to require prophylaxis because of the high incidence (about 80%) of an associated bicuspid aortic valve. The low additional risks of having offspring with congenital heart disease as compared with the general population (2 to 4 per 100 vs. approximately 1 per 1,000, respectively) is the general problem. Though patients with uncomplicated complete repair of tetralogy of Fallot have done well 10 to 15 years after surgery, the long-term status of right and left ventricular function in patients undergoing repair in infancy in unknown.

The patients in the second group have had cardiac malformations corrected but have residua or complications as listed in Table 92–3.

Patients with aortic stenosis treated with valvulotomy may develop restenosis or severe aortic insufficiency and require another operation (in as high as 50% of the cases). Some patients with repaired coarctation of the aorta will have systemic hypertension and a number of these will have evidence of recoarctation. Previously competent or minimally regurgitant atrioventricular valves may show progressive insufficiency and require replacement. Although Mustard and Senning repairs of transposition of the great arteries yield physiologic correction, the right ventricle continues to support the systemic circulation and may show progressive dysfunction. The arterial switch procedure theoretically avoids this risk. The operation involves transsecting the great vessels above the semilunar valves and "switching" the arteries so that the pulmonary artery is now anterior, attached to the right ventricle while the aorta is posterior and attached to the left ventricle. The coronary arteries must also be "switched" to the new aorta. However, this procedure is associated with occasional semilunar valve insufficiency and coronary artery ostia narrowing. In patients with conduits, stenosis from pseudointima formation ("peel") or from patient growth requires replacement. Any residua or anomaly may be the site of endocarditis regardless of its functional severity. Periodic evaluation for potential rhythm disturbances, residual lesions, prosthetic valve dysfunction, hypertension, and myocardial dysfunction must be carried out at intervals commensurate with the patient's clinical status and medical or surgical therapy instituted when necessary. Prophylaxis for endocarditis is obligatory in all these patients. These patients may participate in sports activities as long as it is not in a competitive (organized sports) role.

The final group of patients are those with severe residual disease, usually with complex intracardiac anatomy and inadequate pulmonary blood flow. These patients may have had one or more "shunt" procedures for palliation, which may indeed be the only procedures possible. Other patients may have residual pulmonary vascular obstructive disease from previous large systemic-pulmonary anastomoses or despite correction of the basic cardiac defect, such as a large VSD, endocardial cushion defect, or transposition of the great arteries with a VSD. Still others may have chronic progressive myocardial disease and CHF; in such patients no anatomic problem remains that can be corrected surgically. Shunts may be revised or a different anastomosis utilized. A corrective procedure may now be available for certain children previously receiving palliation. If no further surgical procedures are possible or warranted, medical management must be carefully monitored. This includes appropriate treatment of CHF and rhythm disturbances, prophylaxis against bacterial endocarditis, and observation and therapy for progressive polycythemia from persistent hypoxemia (the hematocrit should be measured frequently by venipuncture method and if found to be in excess of 65%, exchange transfusion should be performed).

FEVER

Children with congenital heart disease and fever pose challenging problems for the primary physician. In addition to the common viral and bacterial infections that afflict all children, some children with congenital heart disease, particularly those with congestive failure or the small group of patients with heterotaxia syndrome and splenic dysfunction, are at increased risk for serious and even life-threatening bacterial infections. Thus the evaluation of such patients with fever must include an understanding of the underlying heart disease, a willingness to search for a specific cause of the fever, and avoidance of the indiscriminate use of oral antibiotics, which can often confuse and delay diagnosis.

When possible, the treatment of the common respiratory and GI tract infections of childhood should be managed with the same approach taken with children without congenital heart disease: administration of antipyretics and fluids, and observation. In small children and infants a search for the specific bacterial source for the fever should be performed. This evaluation should include a chest radiograph if there is tachypnea or abnormal findings on examination of the chest. Often it is difficult to separate evidence of congestive failure from an infectious infiltrate with radiography. In these situations, it is often necessary to admit the patient to the hospital for observation and, if the suspicion of infection is high, for intravenous administration of antibiotics.

If a patient is sick enough to require antibiotic therapy, a blood culture drawn prior to the commencement of antibiotics can be helpful in confirming the presence of a bacterial vs. viral infection and can act as a guide to appropriate antibiotic choice. Since the incidence of endocarditis in young children and infants with congenital heart disease is small, the presence of a positive blood culture should not be taken as evidence of endocarditis. The duration of antibiotics can be limited to treatment of the specific infection. If there is a suspicion of endocarditis, the decision for extended treatment should be made in consultation with the patient's cardiologist.

SUBACUTE BACTERIAL ENDOCARDITIS

Bacterial endocarditis must be ruled out in persistently febrile older children or in patients of any age who have undergone cardiac operations. Often older children will present with only a history of malaise or mild anorexia and weight loss and not have the physical stigmata classically described, such as systemic signs of embolization in the form of splinter hemorrhages or abnormal findings on funduscopic examination. Changes in the character of cardiac murmurs or the appearance of a new murmur should raise suspicion. Laboratory evidence will include an elevated sedimentation rate and, often, evidence of mild anemia and hematuria secondary to an immune complex nephritis. The sine qua non of subacute bacterial endocarditis (SBE) is a positive result of blood culture.

Various regimens have been described to properly gather sufficient blood cultures to rule out SBE. Some guidelines suggest that at least 1% of the patient's blood volume should be cultured over 48 hours, while others think that three properly obtained blood cultures will be sufficient to pick up 97% of cases of SBE. It is now clear that blood cultures can be obtained at any time, since the bacteremia of SBE is continuous.

Sterile surgical gloves should be worn when obtaining blood cultures to rule out SBE and the skin carefully cleansed, because a blood culture result often suggests there was contamination by skin flora. Generally, it is desirable to wait for the identification of an organism prior to commencing antibiotic treatment. In the ill patient, however, therapy with anti-staphylococcal penicillin and an aminoglycoside can be started. Echocardiography has been very helpful in identifying vegetations and should be routinely done in any patient with positive results of blood culture and a suspicion of endocarditis. Once an organism is identified and appropriate antibiotics chosen, the patient should be followed up closely for any sign of embolic phenomena from the breakup of a valvular vegetation.

Duration of treatment is 6 weeks of intravenous antibiotics. Most treatment schedules suggest that an aminoglycoside be added for the first 2 weeks of therapy. The only exception to 6 weeks of antibiotics would be the treatment of *Streptococcus viridans* endocarditis, which has been shown to be adequately treated with 4 weeks of penicillin.

Because the complications of SBE are often not predictable and can occur at any point in the treatment period, most patients should be monitored carefully in concert with a cardiologist skilled in pediatrics or should be referred to a major center for the duration of the antibiotic treatment.

Subacute Bacterial Endocarditis Prophylaxis

Table 92–4 outlines the indications for SBE prophylaxis and type and dose of antibiotic. In general these guidelines are based on the assumption that a surgical procedure that interrupts the epithelial or mucosal surface of an area normally contaminated by microorganisms should be preceded by a sufficiently large dose of antibiotic to provide a level adequate to prevent significant bacteremia. For this reason the antibiotic is guided by the predominant organism in the area to be operated on. The most common situation in which this is used is prior to any dental procedure, including routine cleaning and scaling.

Patients who are receiving daily penicillin for either splenic dysfunction or rheumatic fever prophylaxis require a change in antibiotics to erythromycin for dental procedures because of the development of penicillin-resistant oral flora.

KAWASAKI SYNDROME

Kawasaki syndrome, first described by Tomisaku Kawasaki, M.D., of Japan in 1967, is a vasculitis syndrome that involves the medium and

TABLE 92–4
AHA Recommendations for Prophylaxis Against Infective Endocarditis*

FOR DENTAL PROCEDURES AND SURGERY OF THE UPPER RESPIRATORY TRACT		FOR GASTROINTESTINAL AND GENITOURINARY TRACT SURGERY AND INSTRUMENTATION	
Oral penicillin for most patients	Children less than 60 lb: 1 g of penicillin V 1 hr before procedure and then 500 mg 6 hr after initial dose.	Ampicillin plus gentamicin for most patients	Timing of doses is same as for adults. Doses are ampicillin 50 mg/kg and gentamicin 2 mg/kg. Given 30 min before procedure; may repeat once 8 hr later.
Erythromycin for those allergic to penicillin (may also be selected for those receiving oral penicillin as continuous rheumatic fever prophylaxis)	20 mg/kg orally 1 hr before procedure and then 10 mg/kg 6 hr after initial dose.	Vancomycin plus gentamicin for patients allergic to penicillin	Timing of doses is same as for adults. Doses are vancomycin 20 mg/kg and gentamicin 2 mg/kg.
Ampicillin plus gentamicin for those patients at higher risk of infective endocarditis (especially those with prosthetic heart valves) who are not allergic to penicillin	Doses are ampicillin 50 mg/kg, gentamicin 2 mg/kg, and penicillin V 500 mg (for children under 60 lb). Given 30 min before procedure, then penicillin V orally 6 hr after initial dose.	Amoxicillin (oral regimen) for minor or repetitive procedures in low-risk patients	50 mg/kg 1 hr before procedure and then 25 mg/kg 6 hr after initial dose.
Vancomycin for higher-risk patients (especially those with prosthetic heart valves) who are allergic to penicillin	Vancomycin 20 mg/kg IV over 60 min, begun 60 min before procedure; no repeat dose is necessary.		

*Adapted from Committee on Rheumatic Fever and Infective Endocarditis. Reprinted with permission of the American Heart Association.
Note: In patients with compromised renal function, it may be necessary to modify or omit the second dose of antibiotics. Intramuscular injections may be contraindicated in patients receiving anticoagulants. Children's doses should not exceed adult doses.

large arteries. It is an acute illness characterized by fever for 5 days and at least four of the five following criteria set by the CDC (Rauch): nonexudative, bilateral *conjunctivitis;* nonvesicular, polymorphous *rash; oral mucosal inflammation*—fissuring of lips, pharyngeal erythema, and "strawberry" tongue; *extremity changes*—erythema of palms and soles, desquamation of digits, induration of hands and feet, and transverse nail grooves ("Bow's lines"); and *cervical adenopathy*—usually unilateral and nonsuppurative (at least 1.5 cm or greater in diameter).

Kawasaki syndrome has stirred interest recently because of the potential life-threatening sequelae of coronary artery ectasia, aneurysm formation, and thrombotic occlusion. Coronary aneurysms occur in 15% to 25% of all patients with Kawasaki syndrome with a 1% fatality rate. Risk factors for the development of coronary aneurysms include: age less than 1 year, male sex, fever for more than 16 days, erythrocyte sedimentation rate (ESR) greater than 100, elevated ESR more than 30 days, hemoglobin level less than 10 g/dL, white blood cell (WBC) count greater than 30,000, arrhythmia, cardiomegaly, and abnormal ECG (Asai).

Although epidemiologic data and clinical course seem to support an infectious cause, the exact cause of this disease is still not known. The annual incidence is 0.59 per 100,000 children less than 5 years of age (Bell), but there seems to be a seasonal peak in the spring and winter. Although 80% of cases occur in children less than 5 years of age, the peak incidence occurs in children between 12 and 24 months of age. Cases have been reported in patients as young as 2 months of age. In addition, asians and blacks have higher incidence rates than whites.

Cardiovascular manifestations are not limited to coronary arteritis, and may include myocarditis, pericarditis, pericardial effusion, mitral regurgitation, AV conduction, inflammation, and aneurysm of peripheral arteries (most frequently involving the axillary, iliac, and renal arteries).

Noncardiovascular involvement includes myositis and myalgia, arthritis and arthralgia, urethritis and pyuria, aseptic meningitis, hydrops of the gallbladder, pancreatits, hepatitis, diarrhea, and pneumonitis.

DIAGNOSIS

Laboratory abnormalities include elevated ESR, elevated WBC count, mild anemia, rise in platelet count (usually in the second week); presence of C-reactive protein (CRP), elevated liver function tests, proteinuria, and cerebrospinal fluid (CSF) pleocytosis. Changes on chest radiographs include cardiomegaly. Changes on ECG include prolonged PR interval, reduced QRS voltages, ST segment changes, and flattened T waves. Findings on echocardiography include pericardial effusion, decreased shortening fraction, and coronary aneurysms.

The differential diagnosis includes Stevens-Johnson syndrome, juvenile rheumatoid arthritis, streptococcal infection, toxic shock syndrome, and other infections (including Epstein-Barr virus, measles, leptospirosis, and Rocky Mountain spotted fever).

The process of the illness starts with an acute phase, which lasts for 1 to 2 weeks, characterized by fever, rash, lethargy, and oral mucosal inflammation. This is followed by a subacute phase lasting 3 to 8 weeks. It is during this period that most of the coronary aneurysms occur. The convalescent phase lasts for the next 4 months.

THERAPY

Aspirin, the mainstay of therapy, may not stop aneurysmal formation but may prevent thrombosis of these lesions. The dose is 80 to 100 mg/kg/day during the acute stage of the illness, and can be reduced to 3–5 mg/kg/day in the convalescent period. Patients with evidence of coronary aneurysms should continue to receive low-dose aspirin therapy.

Intravenous gamma-globulin is now readily available and initial reports of its efficacy have been encouraging (Furosho and Newburger). The dose presently recommended is 400 mg/kg/day for 4 days.

After the initial period of illness, patients should be followed up with serial echocardiography and ECGs. Cardiac catheterization is used to study the coronary anatomy in detail in selected patients with clinical manifestations of myocardial infarction, ischemic changes on ECG, or echocardiographic evidence of decreased left ventricular function.

The natural course of the coronary aneurysms in Kawasaki syndrome is such that there can be a regression of these lesions in 1 to 2 years. Patients who are at high risk for coronary aneurysms that persist include those who have: fever for more than 21 days, age of onset more than 2 years, aneurysm diameter of more than 8 mm, and aneurysm shape of the saccular type.

The major cause of death appears to be cardiogenic shock due to acute myocardial infarction. Other causes of death include congestive heart failure, rupture of coronary aneurysm, myocarditis, and arrhythmia.

The characteristic signs and symptoms of Kawasaki syndrome have prompted early recognition and therapeutic intervention by physicians. Atypical and recurrent cases do occur, however, and may confuse even the most astute of clinicians.

Children who have had Kawasaki syndrome may be at risk for coronary artery disease in the future as mural thickening occurs even in the absence of aneurysmal formation. It is important therefore to remember Kawasaki syndrome as a coronary risk factor.

An aggressive approach to Kawasaki syndrome with early diagnosis and treatment is crucial to successful management of this serious illness.

ACUTE RHEUMATIC FEVER

As recently as the 1920s, rheumatic fever was the leading cause of death in the pediatric population. Furthermore, sequelae from rheumatic fever often resulted in crippling heart disease. By the 1970s, however, rheumatic fever had become extremely rare in the industrialized world, with an incidence of less than 1 per 100,000 per year.

The recent resurgence of rheumatic fever has the younger physicians eager to learn an unfamiliar disease. Outbreaks have occurred in several areas in the United States including Columbus and Akron, Ohio, Pittsburgh, and Salt Lake City (Kaplan). The reason for this recent comeback of rheumatic fever is not certain. Epidemiologic evidence suggests rheumatic fever to be a disease of poverty, as it is more commonly found in overcrowded urban areas and in underdeveloped countries.

It has been known since 1930 that rheumatic fever is caused by an antecedent group A streptococcal upper respiratory tract infection. Although there was a decline in the incidence of rheumatic fever concomitant with the introduction of antibiotics, many authorities do not support the notion that antibiotics were responsible for the disappearance of rheumatic fever.

A set of clinical and laboratory criteria was originally described by T. Duckett Jones in the 1940s and is now revised by the American Heart Association. The diagnosis of rheumatic fever is made if two major criteria *or* one major and two minor criteria *plus* evidence of a preceding group A streptococcal infection (e.g., scarlet fever, positive results of culture, elevated or rising streptococcal antibody titer such as ASO or anti-DNAse B) are present.

MAJOR MANIFESTATIONS

Carditis (40% to 50%)
Polyarthritis (60% to 85%): migratory, usually involving large joints
Sydenham chorea (15%): purposeless, jerking movements occurring in convalescence
Erythema marginatum (10%): evanescent, nonpruritic rash
Subcutaneous nodules (2% to 10%): small nontender nodules along tendon sheaths

MINOR MANIFESTATIONS

Clinical findings: arthralgia, fever, previous rheumatic fever or rheumatic heart disease
Laboratory data: prolonged PR interval, positive acute phase reactants (ESR, CRP)

Carditis is the most important sequela of rheumatic fever. It can be manifested by a pathologic murmur, pericarditis, or congestive heart failure. Rheumatic heart disease involves the mitral valve in three fourths of the cases and involves the aortic valve in the remaining cases.

The differential diagnosis for rheumatic fever includes systemic lupus erythematosis, juvenile rheumatoid arthritis, infective endocarditis, collagen vascular diseases, infectious arthritis, serum sickness, or viral myopericarditis.

The treatment of acute rheumatic fever involves both eradicating the group A streptococcal infection and reducing the inflammation of arthritis and carditis. The recommendation for *primary eradication* from the Committee on Prevention of Rheumatic Fever of the American Heart Association is intramuscular benzathine penicillin G or oral penicillin V or erythromycin for 10 days. *Secondary prophylaxis*, or prevention of recurrence of disease in a patient who already had rheumatic fever, consists of daily penicillin or sulfadiazine orally or monthly benzathine penicillin G by injection. Children who have rheumatic heart disease and who need *SBE prophylaxis* should receive either erythromycin or vancomycin.

Bed rest and salicylates were and still are the mainstay of therapy for arthritis and carditis in rheumatic fever. Salicylates should not be started, however, until the diagnosis of rheumatic fever is certain. The use of steroids is controversial at present. Some authorities advocate the use of steroids for a short course only in the presence of severe carditis.

The implications of making a diagnosis of rheumatic fever in a patient are not insignificant. Prolonged antibiotic prophylaxis and extended bed rest are more than mere inconveniences. It is vital, however, for primary care physicians to recognize the resurgence of this disease that "licks the joints and bites the heart" (Bland).

MITRAL VALVE PROLAPSE

In 1963 Barlow described a constellation of cardiac findings that have come to be known as mitral valve prolapse (MVP). The hallmarks of MVP on examination include a midsystolic to late systolic click and a systolic murmur. This is thought to be caused by redundant mitral valve tissue, which prolapses into the left atrial cavity during ventricular contraction. A great deal of interest has been focused on this problem because of associated symptoms in adults identified with MVP.

Mitral valve prolapse has been found in 1% to 6% of children of all ages. There is a 2:1 female-male ratio. A subset of patients show a familial incidence with approximately 45% of the children of an affected first-degree relative having MVP. The most common auscultatory abnormality in MVP is a midsystolic click and a late systolic murmur. These findings may vary from day to day. In children the murmur may be a honking musical sound, which is loudest just off the left midsternal border. A holosystolic murmur is less common. The diagnosis is confirmed by two-dimensional or M-mode echocardiography. The risk is highest in women in the third and fourth decade of life with a previous syncope or a positive family history of MVP and sudden death. Many of these patients have previous ECGs that show premature ventricular contractions, ventricular fibrillation, or ventricular tachycardia.

Although most children with MVP are asymptomatic, it is very disturbing for parents to find that their child has MVP, especially when they read of the small but significant incidence of lethal arrhythmias in adults with prolapse.

Evaluation of a child suspected of having MVP should include chest radiography, ECG, and echocardiography. In patients with a history of syncope, palpitations or other symptoms suggesting an arrhythmia, a 24-hour Holter ECG and exercise stress testing may be done. Because of the small risk of SBE, only the patient with a systolic murmur should receive prophylactic antibiotics at the time of surgical procedures.

HYPERLIPIDEMIA IN CHILDHOOD

Since coronary artery disease is the leading cause of death in the western world, many physicians have become increasingly aware of coronary risk factors in the pediatric population. These risk factors are hypertension, diabetes, cigarette smoking, and increased plasma lipids. It is the last of these risk factors that is now most often discussed.

Cholesterol and triglycerides are the two major lipids that are responsible for the genesis of atherosclerosis. These lipids are carried by the four classes of lipoproteins: *chylomicrons* carry fat as triglycerides, *very-low-density lipoproteins (VLDL)* carry triglycerides, *low-density lipoproteins (LDL)* carry cholesterol to the body tissues, and *high-density lipoproteins (HDL)* carry cholesterol back to the liver for removal in the bile.

The Framingham study has shown that increased plasma cholesterol is clearly related to increased risk for developing coronary artery disease (Dawber). Recent surveys have shown that 5% to 25% of children and teenagers in the United States have serum cholesterol levels above 200 mg/dL. Because of the high percentage of the pediatric population with elevated cholesterol levels, there is a recent emphasis on change in dietary habits as well as on monitoring of plasma cholesterol.

The diagnosis of hyperlipidemia can be made as early as the first or second year of life (Freedman). A plasma lipid profile, which includes plasma cholesterol, plasma triglycerides, and HDL cholesterol, should be obtained only in those pediatric patients who are at high risk, that is, those children from families with hyperlipidemia, sudden death, xanthomas, hypertension, or premature (less than 60 years of age) myocardial infarction, angina, cerebrovascular accident, or peripheral vascular disease.

There are three familial hyperlipidemias that lead to premature atherosclerosis: familial hypercholesterolemia, familial combined hyperlipidemia, and familial hypertriglyceridemia. These genetic disorders affect about 0.5% to 1% of the general population. Causes of secondary hyperlipidemia include diabetes, hypothyroidism, obstructive liver disease, nephrotic syndrome, excessive dietary intake, and the use of steroids, oral contraceptives, and alcohol (Lavie).

Therapy for hyperlipidemia includes dietary modification, weight control, aerobic exercise, and pharmacologic agents. The American Heart Association has recommended that children older than 2 years of age should have decreased amounts of cholesterol and fat in their diets (with cholesterol limited to 100 mg/1,000 kcal and with total fat restricted to 30% of caloric intake). This low-fat diet, which restricts total cholesterol and limits saturated fats in the diet, includes five simple modifications: restrict egg intake to three per week, drink low-fat milk, use polyunsaturated fat containing margarine instead of butter, use corn oil in cooking, and limit meat intake and increase intake of fish and fowl (Breslow). Patients with diagnosed hyperlipidemia should have further restrictions of cholesterol and fat in their diets. In addition, a weight reduction program and an exercise regimen is usually instituted.

Some children may require the use of pharmacologic agents to reduce plasma cholesterol. The drug of choice is a bile acid sequestrant resin such as cholestyramine or colestipol. The main side effects of these agents are constipation, diarrhea, and bloating.

The association of hyperlipidemia and atherosclerotic heart disease is well known in the adult population. Since the process of atherosclerosis probably starts in childhood and adolescence, primary prevention needs to be emphasized by the primary care physician.

PEDIATRIC DYSRHYTHMIAS

With the recent further development of sophisticated noninvasive and invasive diagnostic tools such as Holter monitoring, transtelephonic monitoring, electrophysiologic study, esophageal stimulation and exercise testing, the area of pediatric cardiac dysrhythmias has broadened in scope in the past decade. Dysrhythmias in the younger pediatric patient are often difficult to diagnose. In the newborn infant symptoms of dysrhythmias include such nonspecific findings such as fussiness or poor feeding, while preschool children may complain of poorly localized pain or a "funny" feeling in the chest. Syncope can pose an especially difficult differential diagnosis. It is common in school-aged children, has several causes, and the actual incidence of cardiac syncope is small. A complete family history for dysrhythmias, syncope, and sudden death coupled with an ECG to specifically evaluate the corrected QT interval should be part of every evaluation of syncope unless the episode can clearly be ascribed to a noncardiac cause such as a vasovagal attack.

An irregular rhythm is occasionally heard during a routine physical examination. There are several common mechanisms for an irregular rhythm: 1) *Sinus arrhythmia* is an irregular sinus rhythm due to the respiratory cycle (Fig 92–2). It is benign in children. 2) *Premature atrial contractions (PAC)* are manifested by premature and abnormal P waves. These premature contractions are often seen in the neonate and often disappear in the first few days of life. In infants, although occasional PACs are common, frequent PACs can be associated with supraventricular tachycardia and may require therapy. Although usually benign in children, PACs also occur the setting of heart diseases such as myocarditis, hyperthyroidism, indwelling lines, or medications. 3) *Premature ventricular contraction (PVC)* (Fig 92–2) is manifested by a premature widened QRS complex. These premature beats can also be benign, especially if single and uniform and abated with exercise.

Initial workup of PVCs should include: EGG (to rule out prolonged QT syndrome), Holter monitoring, and chest radiography or echocardiography if indicated. Often an exercise stress

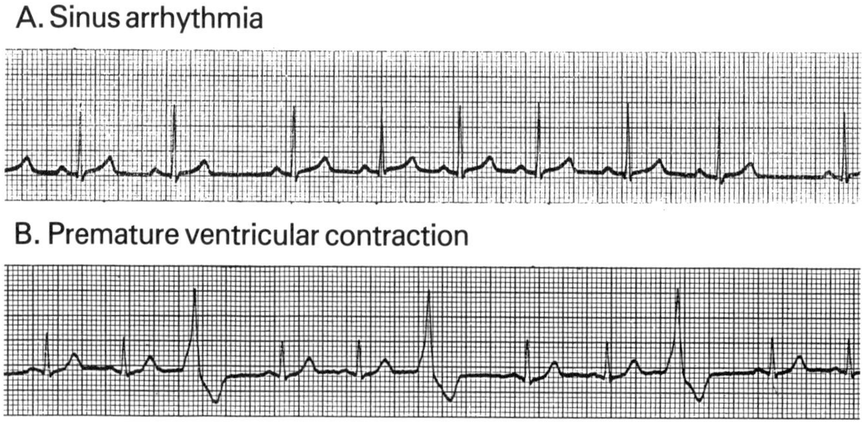

FIG 92–2
A, electrocardiogram of sinus arrhythmia. Note irregular distance between QRS complexes. **B,** premature ventricular contractions.

test is helpful to evaluate PVCs. Predisposing conditions for PVCs include electrolyte abnormalities, drugs, congestive heart failure, cardiomyopathy, and after cardiac surgery.

Supraventricular tachycardia (SVT) is the most common symptomatic dysrhythmia in children (Garson). An infant with supraventricular tachycardia usually presents with poor feeding or lethargy, and has a heart rate above 200 beats per minute. The most common cause of SVT in infants less than 4 months old is idiopathic. Older children with SVT, however, are much less likely to present with congestive heart failure because the heart rate is much slower and also because they are capable of verbalizing their symptoms. The older child with SVT is more likely to have a predisposing factor such as congenital heart disease (preoperative or postoperative), myocarditis, cardiomyopathy, pre-excitation syndrome, drugs, or other causes such as hyperthyroidism and usually will undergo an electrophysiologic study as part of their evaluation. Immediate management of SVT includes evaluation of the hemodynamic state. If the patient is unstable, then cardioversion is indicated. If the patient is hemodynamically stable, as are most children who present with SVT, then diagnostic evaluation including a full ECG and the use of vagal maneuvers in children or placing a ice pack over the face of an infant can be tried. Maintenance therapy usually includes digoxin and other drugs, such as propranolol and procainamide as well as newer agents such as flecainide and mexiletene.

BIBLIOGRAPHY

Asai T: Evaluation method for the degree of seriousness in Kawasaki disease. *Acta Paediatr Jpn* 1983; 25:170.

Beerman LB, Neches WH, Patnode RE, et al: Coarctation of the aorta in children: Late results after surgery. *Am J Dis Child* 1980; 134:464.

Bell DM, Morens DH, Holman RC, et al: Kawasaki syndrome in the United States 1976 to 1980. *Am J Dis Child* 1983; 137:211–214.

Bergman AB, Stamm SJ: The morbidity of cardiac nondisease in school children. *N Engl J Med* 1967; 276:1008.

Bland E: Rheumatic fever: The way it was. *Circulation* 1987; 76:1190–1195.

Breslow J: Pediatric aspects of hyperlipidemia. *Pediatrics* 1978; 62:510–520.

Carr RP: Psychological adaption to cardiac surgery, in Kidd BSL, Rowe RD (eds): *The Child With Congenital Heart Disease After Surgery*. Mount Kisco, NY, Futura Publishing Co, Inc, 1976.

Dawber T, Kannel W, McNamara P: The prediction of coronary artery disease. *Trans Assoc Life Insur Med Dir Am* 1971; 47:70.

Freedman D, Sriniwasan SR, Cresanta JL, et al: Serum lipids and lipoproteins. *Pediatrics* 1987; 80:789–796.

Furosho K, Kamiya T, Nakano H, et al: High dose intravenous gamma globulin therapy for Kawasaki disease. *Lancet* 1984; 2:1055–1058.

Garson A, Gillette P, McNamara D: Supraventricular tachycardia in children: Clinical features, response to treatment, and long-term follow-up in 217 patients. *Pediatrics* 1981; 98:875–882.

Gilette P: Cardiac dysrhythmias in children. *Pediatr Rev* 1981; 3:190–198.

Kaplan E: The startling comeback of rheumatic fever. *Contemp Pediatr* 1987; 4:20–34.

Kawasaki T: Acute febrile mucocutaneous syndrome with lymphoid involvement with specific desquamation of the fingers and toes in children: Clinical observations of 50 cases (in Japanese). *Jpn J Allergol* 1967; 16:178–222.

Lavie C, et al: Management of lipids in primary and secondary prevention of cardiovascular diseases. *Mayo Clin Proc* 1988; 63:605–621.

McGoon DC: Long term effects of prosthetic materials. *Am J Cardiol* 1982; 50:621.

Newburger JW, Takahashi M, Burns JC, et al: The treatment of Kawasaki syndrome with intravenous gamma globulin. *N Engl J Med* 1986; 315: 341–347.

Perloff JK: Adults with surgically treated congenital heart disease: Sequelae and residua. *JAMA* 1983; 250:2033.

Rauch A, Hurwitz E: Centers for Disease Control (CDC) case definition for Kawasaki syndrome. *Pediatr Infect Dis* 1985; 4:702–703.

Rowland TW: The pediatrician and congenital heart disease—1979. *Pediatrics* 1979; 64:180.

Talner NS: Heart failure, in Adams FH, Emmanouilides GC (eds): *Moss' Heart Disease in Infants, Children and Adolescents*. Baltimore: Williams & Wilkins Co, 1983.

Vetter VL, Horowitz LN: Electrophysiologic residua and sequelae of surgery for congenital heart defects. *Am J Cardiol* 1982; 50–588.

93 ENDOCRINOLOGY

Mary M. Lee, M.D.
Jose F. Cara, M.D.
Thomas Moshang, Jr., M.D.

Endocrinology involves diagnosis and treatment of chronic endocrine disease as well as differentiation of pathologic patterns of growth and development from variations of normal. The diagnosis of an endocrine disorder often rests on the primary physician's ability to discern subtle abnormalities of growth and development, to recognize clinical manifestations suggestive of disturbances in hormone regulation, and to evaluate commonly available endocrine laboratory tests.

This chapter discusses both the management of some common endocrine problems and the appropriate initial evaluation and subsequent referral of children with more complex endocrine disorders by the primary care physician.

DISORDERS OF GROWTH

Growth is a dynamic process that reflects genetic potential, nutritional status, and physical and emotional health. Consequently, height and weight measurements are a fundamental and necessary component of all medical examinations. Although clinically useful information can sometimes be derived from isolated heights and weights, normal and abnormal growth patterns can only be recognized through accurate plotting of sequential, consistent measurements on a growth chart. Both the growth rate and the absolute height need to be considered when making a determination of growth failure.

An abnormal growth rate can be defined as a rate of increase in linear height that is consistently below the mean growth velocity for age (Fig 93–1).

The average full-term newborn measures approximately 20 inches, grows 10 inches within the first year of life, 5 in the second, 3 in the third, and 2 inches a year thereafter until the pubertal growth spurt. A slower than normal growth rate often results in a flattening of the growth curve or a decrease in percentiles on the growth chart. Growth failure is present when the growth rate is subnormal even though the height for age is still normal. The term "short stature" implies a height for age below the 3rd percentile, independent of growth rate. Not all children with short stature have abnormal growth. In variants of normal growth such as familial short stature and constitutional delay of growth and development the absolute height may be below the 3rd percentile, but the growth rate is normal for age.

A patient with an abnormal growth rate signifying growth failure requires further study. The history and physical findings are of major importance in the evaluation. The laboratory evaluation should be directed at confirming the diagnosis suspected by the clinical findings. Screening studies include a complete blood cell (CBC) count, a sedimentation rate, a biochemical profile, a urinalysis, thyroid studies, and a bone age determination. A delayed bone age is compatible with constitutional delay, growth hormone deficiency, or any severe systemic illness, and is suggestive of a correctable cause of the growth failure. Since short stature may be the only phenotypic expression of Turner syndrome, a karyotype analysis is a critical screening test in girls (Fig 93–2).

In some centers, somatomedin C levels are useful in confirming the clinical impression of lack of illness or may help in recognizing patients with growth hormone deficiency. How-

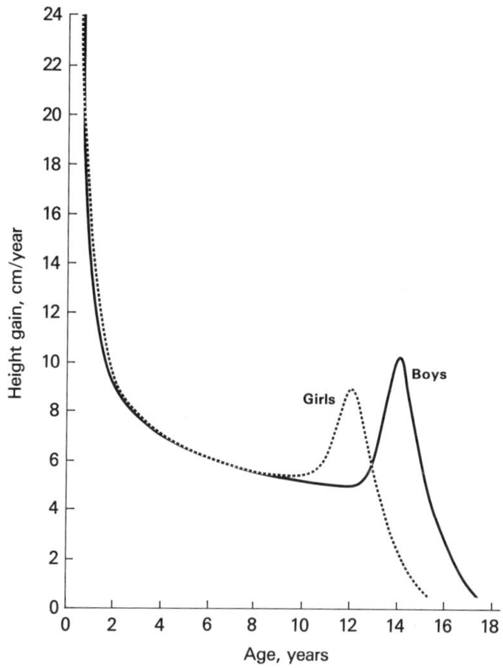

FIG 93–1
Growth velocity chart for children indicates yearly increments of change.

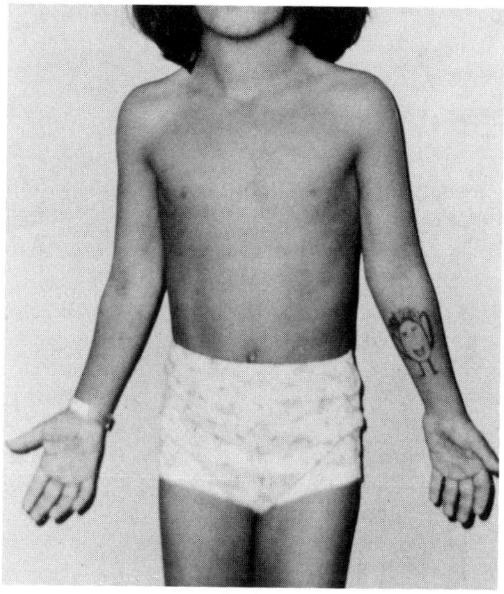

FIG 93–2
Patient with Turner syndrome demonstrates increased carrying angle of elbows.

ever, low somatomedin C levels are found in normal children in whom physiologic maturation is less than 4 years (as might be found in a 5- or 6-year old child with a delayed bone age) and systemic illnesses other than growth hormone deficiency. If an intracranial pathologic lesion is suspected, computed tomography (CT) or magnetic resonance (MR) imaging of the head is indicated. In general, the more common nonendocrine causes of growth failure must be excluded before growth hormone deficiency or other less common disorders are considered.

CONSTITUTIONAL DELAY AND FAMILIAL SHORT STATURE

Constitutional delay of growth and development and familial short stature are two of the most frequently encountered causes of short stature. The hallmark of both constitutional delay and familial short stature is a normal rate of growth and a prominent family history. In constitutional delay, a slowing of the growth rate generally occurs between 1 and 3 years of age with a correspondent delay in physical maturation and bone age. Subsequently, growth is normal, and physical development and bone age progress at a normal rate, although generally 2 or 3 years behind chronologic age. Adolescent development begins 2 to 3 years later than average in these patients and the ultimate adult height attained is usually within the normal range. Because of the excellent prognosis, an explanation of the disorder and reassurance is the most effective therapy. However, if psychosocial difficulties arise in boys because of their pubertal delay, short-term low-dose testosterone therapy may initiate sexual development in these patients and improve their psychosocial outlook. Testosterone therapy for boys with constitutional delay probably has no effect on ultimate height.

Familial short stature is characterized by short stature, normal rate of growth, normal bone age, and a strong family history of short stature. Therapy is limited to reassurance and general counseling. Growth hormone (GH) treatment is not indicated in children with constitutional delay or familial short stature. The use of growth hormone in otherwise normal children may result in abusive use of this potent hormone and related serious side effects may occur (e.g., abnormal glucose tolerance, diabetes, tumorigenesis). A questionable increase in the incidence of leukemia has been associated with GH treatment.

GROWTH HORMONE DEFICIENCY

The child with abnormal growth rate can be screened for growth hormone deficiency with measurement of the somatomedin C level. Since serum somatomedin C concentrations are low in many chronic diseases as well as in growth hormone deficiency, a low value may not be diagnostic of growth hormone deficiency, but a normal value would exclude this diagnosis. Somatomedin C levels correlate with bone age and vary with age, being lowest during infancy. Consequently, serum levels must be interpreted in light of the patient's bone age and physiologic maturation.

The possible diagnosis of GH deficiency suggested by low somatomedin C levels needs to be confirmed with GH provocative tests. Because growth hormone secretion is pulsatile in nature and basal levels are often low, random GH levels are not diagnostic of GH deficiency. Several tests that stimulate GH secretion are available for the diagnosis of GH deficiency, as shown in Table 93–1. These provocative tests are not free of side effects and their use is restricted to inpatient or closely monitored outpatient services. It is generally accepted that at least two provocative tests must show subnormal GH response to be diagnostic of GH deficiency.

Human GH is usually given intramuscularly or subcutaneously three times a week. Although hypersensitivity reactions to GH are rare, an occasional patient will complain of minor skin rashes. These will often disappear spontaneously or with small doses of antihistamines. The reconstituted GH is fairly stable and can be conserved for four to six weeks under refrigeration. Patients should be cautioned that should a precipitate develop on reconstitution, the vial of GH should be discarded.

DISORDERS OF THE THYROID

THYROID FUNCTION TESTS

The most common tests utilized to evaluate thyroid function at present include the measurement of total thyroxine (T_4), triiodothyronine resin uptake (T_3RU), and thyroid-stimulating hormone (TSH). Serum T_4 measurement, the most useful indicator of thyroid function, usually correlates well with the clinical disorders. However, the serum T_4 concentra-

TABLE 93–1
Tests of GH Secretory Capacity

TESTS	CONDITIONS	OBSERVATIONS
Physiologic tests		
Exercise	15 min of moderate exercise followed by 5 min of vigorous exercise	Frequent findings of low response in normal subjects
Sleep	Deep sleep (EEG stages 3–4); 60%–70% of normal children will have a response of at least 7 ng/mL of GH during deep sleep	Best utilized in association with sleep EEG
Provocative tests		
Insulin	Regular insulin, 0.05-0.1 U/kg, IV	Severe hypoglycemia
Arginine	0.5 g/kg, IV, over 30 min	Local irritation, numbness, nausea, vomiting, hypoglycemia
Levodopa	0.5 g/m^2, orally	Cardiac and BP changes, nausea and vomiting
Glucagon	0.03 mg/kg, IM, up to 0.5 mg, IM	Nausea and vomiting
Propranolol	1.0 mg/kg up to 40 mg orally; can be used to augment responses to primary stimuli (glucagon, exercise, levodopa or arginine)	Changes in heart rate or BP, hypoglycemia

tion must be interpreted with the knowledge of those factors that may alter the serum T_4 concentration but are not related to alteration of thyroid function. Chronic illness, such as starvation (malnutrition) or hypoxia, may lower serum T_4. Since the determination of serum T_4 measures total hormone, protein bound as well as free (or unbound) hormone, an alteration of the concentration of circulating T_4-binding proteins will result in altered concentrations of serum T_4. Only free T_4 is metabolically active. T_4 binding globulin (TBG), the main binding protein, varies with age, illness, and serum estrogen concentration.

T_3RU is an indirect measurement of TBG and other thyroid hormone binding proteins. T_4 and T_3RU levels are elevated in hyperthyroidism and low in hypothyroidism. When the T_3RU and the serum T_4 levels are discordant, alterations of thyroid hormone binding protein concentrations rather than abnormalities of thyroid function should be suspected. The calculated "free T_4 index" (the product of T_3RU and T_4) provides an estimation of free T_4 and correlates closely with measured free T_4. Free T_4 and TBG assays are also available, although more expensive.

Since the thyroid gland is under negative feedback control by the pituitary gland, TSH determinations represent a sensitive in vivo measure of the adequacy of thyroid function. Thyroid failure results in elevated TSH levels. With the recent development of a more sensitive TSH assay, the suppressed low levels of TSH seen in hyperthyroidism can now be distinguished from the low basal values seen in the normal euthyroid state.

A number of less common disorders may result in unexpected low TSH findings when the clinical findings suggest hypothyroidism. Low T_4 and low TSH values are found in secondary (pituitary) hypothyroidism, tertiary (hypothalamic) hypothyroidism, and in chronic illnesses ("euthyroid sick syndrome"). The rare syndrome of peripheral resistance to T_4 is biochemically characterized by high T_4 values, a normal or slightly elevated level of TSH, and a normal TSH surge in response to thyrotropin releasing hormone (TRH) stimulation.

In general, T_4 concentration and T_3 resin uptake are the most useful tests in confirming the clinical suspicion of hypothyroidism or hyperthyroidism. The measurement of total T_3 should be reserved for the rare occasion when clinical findings indicate hyperthyroidism but the serum T_4 and T_3RU levels are not confirmatory (the syndrome of T_3 thyrotoxicosis). A TSH level should be obtained once hypothyroidism has been established or in the clinical presence of a goiter.

Other useful tests that the endocrinologist might order for delineating the unusual conditions include the TRH stimulation test, radioiodine uptake and scan, ultrasonography, and fine-needle or open biopsies of the thyroid gland.

CONGENITAL HYPOTHYROIDISM

Congenital hypothyroidism can be difficult to diagnose clinically. In addition, irreparable neurologic impairment and mental retardation often are established before the clinical findings of hypothyroidism become manifest. Consequently, newborn screening programs have been developed and are now required by law in most states to allow the prompt diagnosis and treatment of hypothyroid infants. With the institution of these programs, the incidence of congenital hypothyroidism has been determined to be approximately 1 in 4,000 newborns (Fig 93–3).

Thyroid screening tests are designed to identify newborns with T_4 concentrations in the lower 3% of the general population. Most screening programs include determinations of TSH concentrations in patients with low T_4 concentrations. An elevated TSH level in association with a low T_4 concentration is highly suggestive of congenital hypothyroidism. A normal or low TSH level in association with a low T_4 is compatible with congenital TBG deficiency, the "euthyroid sick syndrome" in small or sick newborns or secondary (pituitary) or tertiary (hypothalamic) hypothyroidism. If the screening tests are abnormal, further evaluation with serum concentrations of T_4, TSH, and TBG is necessary for diagnostic confirmation. Radioactive iodine studies, ultrasonography, or serum thyroglobulin determinations may be useful in determining those infants with ectopic thyroid tissue or a hormone synthesis defect.

Treatment is 6 to 8 μg/kg/day of levothyroxine, given as a single daily dose. Serum T_4 and TSH concentrations should be repeated 6 to 8

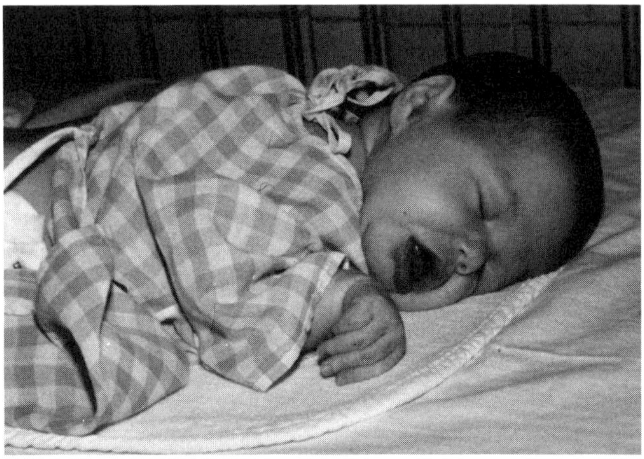

FIG 93–3
Patient with congenital hypothyroidism. Note large tongue and puffy eyelids.

weeks after treatment is started and every 3 months thereafter to assess the adequacy of therapy. Serum T_4 concentrations are maintained in the upper range of normal. In infants less than 1 year of age, TSH concentrations are very difficult to suppress to normal levels on the usual replacement doses. Consequently, if the T_4 and free T_4 concentration (as evaluated by the T_3RU or TBG level) are appropriate, slightly elevated TSH levels are acceptable. Using higher than usual doses of levothyroxine in order to suppress the TSH to normal levels in these children may result in complications often associated with hyperthyroidism, such as premature closure of the cranial sutures. The prognosis is usually good if therapy is begun early; however, even appropriately treated infants may have a slight decrease in intelligence when compared with their siblings.

ACQUIRED HYPOTHYROIDISM

The causes of acquired hypothyroidism can be classified as primary (thyroid gland dysfunction), secondary (pituitary insufficiency), and tertiary (hypothalamic disease). The most frequent is primary hypothyroidism, often due to chronic lymphocytic thyroiditis (Hashimoto thyroiditis). Other less frequent forms of acquired hypothyroidism include thyroid ectopy, dyshormonogenesis, and pituitary tumors or trauma.

Hypothyroidism will usually present clinically with the slow onset of growth failure, dull, placid expression, myxedema, cold intolerance, constipation, bradycardia, hypotension, brittle hair, and dry, pale skin. Occasionally, the only presenting sign is poor growth and, therefore, a high index of suspicion for thyroid dysfunction is warranted to make the diagnosis. In females, primary or secondary amenorrhea can be the presenting complaint. An unusual presentation is that of hypothyroidism associated with pseudoprecocious puberty and galactorrhea. The sexual precocity is occasionally complete with breast development, pubic hair, galactorrhea, and vaginal spotting in girls and testicular enlargement in boys. These changes often regress with adequate thyroid replacement. Finally, hypothyroidism can be subclinical or "compensated" when the gland begins to fail but continues secreting adequate amounts of hormone due to increased TSH stimulation.

The diagnosis of hypothyroidism can be easily confirmed by measuring TSH, T_4, and T_3 resin uptake. An elevated TSH level indicates primary gland failure. A low TSH level in the presence of a low T_4 level and low T_3RU is compatible with the diagnosis of pituitary or hypothalamic hypothyroidism or euthyroid hypothyroxinemia secondary to illness.

Once diagnosed, therapy with levothyroxine should be initiated. The usual dose is 3 to 4 μg/kg/day taken as a single oral dose (usually 0.1 to 0.15 mg/day). Adequacy of thyroid hormone replacement should be evaluated clinically and by T_4 and TSH determinations 6 to 8 weeks after starting therapy and every 6 to 12 months thereafter.

Parents should be cautioned that once their child begins thyroid hormone replacement the child will appear livelier and less docile. The child's school work will occasionally deteriorate because of relative hyperactivity and decreased attention span. Most patients will lose their excess myxedematous water weight and their coarse, dry hair will be lost and slowly replaced by hair of normal texture. Stomach ache (due to increased peristalsis) and headache are occasionally encountered. These complaints are generally transient and do not require specific therapy.

Once the child is euthyroid on levothyroxine therapy, there is no contraindication to full physical activity. There is no increased risk for surgical procedures. In addition, there are no problems with the use of other medications, including those drugs containing iodides.

The prognosis in acquired hypothyroidism is excellent. Normal physical and neurological development and function can be expected if the patient is receiving adequate replacement therapy. In addition, treatment is easy, inexpensive, and well-tolerated.

HYPERTHYROIDISM

Graves disease, the most common cause of thyrotoxicosis in children, is an autoimmune disorder characterized by the presence of antithyroid immunoglobulins that bind to the TSH receptor of the thyroid gland and stimulate excessive thyroid hormone secretion. In the presence of these thyroid-stimulating immunoglobulins (TSI), the gland, independent of pituitary control, hypertrophies and secretes large amounts of hormone. The older patient often has gradual onset of goiter and complains of nervousness, palpitations, heat intolerance, increased appetite, and amenorrhea. Younger children often exhibit hyperactivity and behavior problems.

The measurement of serum T_4 and T_3RU level will usually confirm the clinical diagnosis. The syndrome of T_3 thyrotoxicosis is unusual in childhood except during treatment with thionamide drugs. Determinations of serum T_3 levels are generally not necessary until after the initiation of medical therapy.

At the Children's Hospital of Philadelphia, the thionamide drugs are the treatment of choice for juvenile thyrotoxicosis. These drugs block the organification of iodide by the thyroid gland and thus decrease the amount of thyroid hormone synthesized. Propylthiouracil and methimazole are the most often used thionamides. The dose of propylthiouracil is 8 mg/kg/day, given three times a day. The dose of methimazole is one tenth that of propylthiouracil. Clinical improvement occurs in several weeks with the thionamides alone. If the patient is very symptomatic or the cardiovascular findings of hyperthyroidism very pronounced, propranolol can be used in conjunction with the thionamides. The dose of propranolol is 1 to 2 mg/kg/day. The dose of the thionamides should be adjusted to maintain the T_4 and T_3 levels within the normal range.

Methimazole and propylthiouracil are both associated with side effects that can complicate medical therapy. Minor side effects include vomiting, stomach upset, leukopenia, arthralgia, arthritis, and urticarial rashes. In general, these are not an indication for discontinuing therapy unless they are very severe. The major complication of thionamide therapy is agranulocytosis. Although rare, it can be life-threatening and must be recognized early. Routine blood cell counts are ineffective in predicting this complication since agranulocytosis can appear in a previously healthy patient. However, blood cell counts should be obtained if a patient receiving thionamides develops fever. If agranulocytosis is present, blood cultures should be obtained and antibiotic therapy started immediately. The thionamides should be discontinued and alternate forms of therapy used.

Hyperthyroid patients should be evaluated clinically and with thyroid function tests every 4 to 6 months. At The Children's Hospital of Philadelphia, therapy is discontinued once the patient has been euthyroid for at least 2 years. The patient must be followed up closely, and if hyperthyroidism recurs, therapy reinstituted.

Failure of medical therapy is due to lack of drug compliance, complications of drug therapy, and unresponsiveness to thionamide drugs. In these cases, thyroid ablation through radioiodine or surgical therapy is indicated. Although the advantages of one form of therapy over the other are a matter of great debate, both are effective forms of therapy. In general, the choice depends on the availability of an experienced surgeon and the patient's personal inclinations.

THYROID GOITERS AND NODULES

Thyroid goiters are a common occurrence in childhood and can be accompanied by signs of hypothyroidism, hyperthyroidism, or euthyroidism (Fig 93–4). The most common cause of thyroid gland enlargement in children is chronic lymphocytic thyroiditis, which accounts for 40% to 60% of simple, nontoxic goiters. Chronic lymphocytic thyroiditis is a pathological diagnosis characterized by interfollicular lymphocytic infiltration of the thyroid gland with formation of germinal follicles and destruction of functioning thyroid tissue. Antimicrosomal or antithyroglobulin antibodies are present in 80% to 85% of patients. Other causes of simple goiters include inborn errors of T_4 synthesis, adolescence in females, and drugs.

Drug-induced goiters occur more commonly than expected. Drugs implicated in thyroid gland enlargement include iodine (and other halogens), lithium, paraamino salicylic acid, phenylbutazone, thionamides, and the white turnip plants. Breast milk from mothers receiving antithyroid therapy may induce thyroid gland enlargement in their newborn infants.

Thyroid nodules are not uncommon in childhood. Thyroid nodules in children are more often malignant than nodules in adults. The malignant nodule is often "stony hard" and associated with lymphadenopathy. The child with a thyroid nodule should be referred for evaluation and therapy. The evaluation will include radioactive scanning as well as ultrasonography (Fig 93–5). A nodule that does not take up the radioiodine, i.e., a "cold" nodule, should be surgically removed if ultrasound shows a mixed solid/cystic lesion. A needle biopsy can be performed on a completely cystic lesion before deciding further therapy.

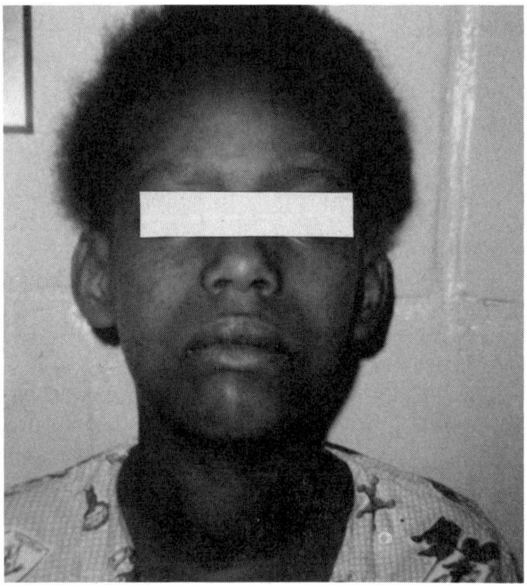

FIG 93–4
Patient with hyperthyroidism with goiter.

DISORDERS OF THE ADRENAL GLANDS

ADRENAL INSUFFICIENCY

Adrenal insufficiency may be due to primary failure of the adrenal gland or may be secondary to pituitary or hypothalamic disorders. In childhood, primary adrenal failure due to autoimmune processes, infectious disorders such as tuberculosis or histoplasmosis, and malignancies is relatively uncommon. Primary acute adrenal insufficiency during childhood is more likely to be due to congenital adrenal hyperplasia or meningococcal infections with resulting acute adrenal crisis. Chronic adrenal insufficiency during childhood is more likely to be secondary to either pituitary or hypothalamic disease.

The clinical findings of chronic adrenal failure include weakness, lethargy, exercise intolerance, poor weight gain, anorexia, nausea, vomiting, headaches, salt craving, polyuria, and dehydration. In primary gland failure, hyperpigmentation may be present and is best noted in the areolae, mucous membranes, extensor surfaces of joints (knees, elbows, and fingers), and surgical scars. Routine laboratory tests may reveal hyponatremia, hyperkalemia, acidosis, and eosinophilia. A morning cortisol level may be low but a normal level does not rule out the possibility of adrenal insufficiency.

The diagnosis of adrenal insufficiency requires adrenocorticotropic hormone (ACTH) stimulation testing and demonstration of the lack of response in primary adrenal failure or inadequate response of the adrenal in secondary adrenal failure. Once adrenal insufficiency has been diagnosed, appropriate tests should

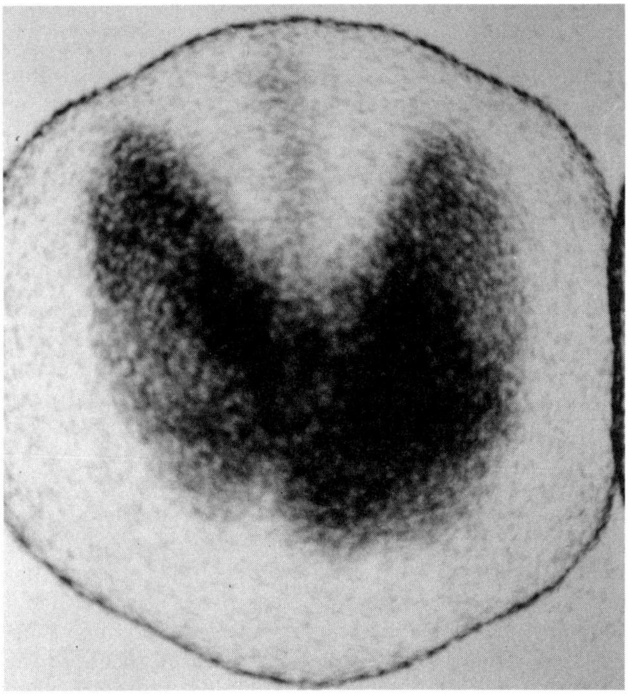

FIG 93–5
^{123}I uptake scan shows goiter and nodule.

be performed in an effort to elucidate the cause.

Adrenal insufficiency requires chronic replacement therapy with glucocorticoids and, usually, mineralocorticoids. Although a number of glucocorticoids can be prescribed, hydrocortisone is the most frequently used corticosteroid because it is the naturally occurring hormone. Physiological replacement is achieved with 15 to 25 mg/m^2/day of hydrocortisone taken orally in three divided doses. Mineralocorticoid deficiency requires replacement with a steroid such as fludrocortisone (Florinef) in doses of 0.05 to 0.1 mg once a day.

Patients on corticosteroid replacement will require an increase in their steroid dose during times of severe illness, trauma, or stress. Under these circumstances, patients can be instructed to increase their usual daily dose threefold. They should receive at least 75 mg/m^2/day of hydrocortisone. If vomiting should occur, the oral dose should be repeated in 10 to 15 minutes. If vomiting persists, intramuscular cortisone acetate, at three or four times the usual daily dose, is indicated. This dose can be repeated every 24 hours if necessary for several days. If severe vomiting, prostration, or acute adrenal failure develop, intravenous fluid therapy is required immediately. All patients should be instructed to continue the increased dose of steroids during the acute phase of the illness and to then return to their maintenance dosages within several days.

Patients with secondary (pituitary) adrenal insufficiency are very sensitive to steroid therapy and may not need maintenance treatment or may require only one-third to one-half the usual physiologic replacement dose. Most of these patients, however, will require increased or pharmacologic doses (75 mg/m^2/day of hydrocortisone) during times of illness or stress. Mineralocorticoid production in these patients is usually normal and replacement with salt-retaining steroids is not indicated.

Careful follow-up of children on glucocorticoid therapy is essential to ensure that they do not develop signs of steroid excess. Determinations of height and weight are helpful since poor growth and excessive weight gain are often the first signs of corticosteroid excess. Weight loss, nausea, and hypotension may be indicative of insufficient glucocorticoid treatment.

ACUTE ADRENAL INSUFFICIENCY (ADRENAL CRISIS)

Acute adrenal failure is a life-threatening condition that must be treated early and aggressively to ensure survival. Adrenal crisis may be the first manifestation of Addison disease (chronic adrenal insufficiency) or of congenital adrenal hyperplasia. Adrenal crisis may also occur with acute decompensation in a patient known to have these disorders. The patient in adrenal crisis may present in an acutely dehydrated state, and be moribund and cachectic. Routine laboratory studies may demonstrate hyponatremia, hyperkalemia, and, occasionally, hypoglycemia.

The most important facet of therapy of adrenal crisis is aggressive fluid and electrolyte management. Most patients present with severe water and salt loss. Cardiovascular collapse is the principal cause of death. To treat hypotension, normal saline containing 5% dextrose should be given as a 20 to 30 ml/kg bolus over 10 to 20 minutes or faster, if necessary. Blood pressure should be monitored closely and normal saline should be continued until a normal blood pressure is attained. After acute resuscitation, normal saline containing 5% dextrose is infused at a rate to provide maintenance requirements and correct any fluid and electrolyte deficits. If hyponatremia becomes symptomatic (usually less than 120 mEq/dL), it should be corrected immediately and vigorously with 3% saline solution. The dose (in milliliters) of 3% saline solution to be infused over 15 minutes can be calculated by the formula

$$[120 - \text{Na level (mEq/L)}] \times 0.6 \times \text{weight (kg)} \times 2$$

While the resuscitative phase is under way, hydrocortisone in the hemisuccinate form should be given initially as an intravenous bolus in a dose of 2 to 4 mg/kg followed by 200 to 400 mg by constant intravenous infusion over the next 24 hours. If available, desoxycorticosterone acetate at a dose of 2 to 3 mg (intramuscularly) should be given to provide mineralocorticoid activity. Glucocorticoids can be subsequently supplied by giving cortisone acetate in a dose of 50 to 100 mg intramuscularly every 24 hours. Desoxycorticosterone acetate and cortisone acetate should be continued intramuscularly until the patient is well enough to return to his usual therapeutic regimen.

TAPERING OF GLUCOCORTICOID ADMINISTRATION

Chronic, large-dose steroid therapy is often necessary in children with certain diseases, for example, bronchial asthma, nephrosis, nephritis, leukemia. Consequently, steroid withdrawal often becomes a problem that must be handled with extreme caution. Acute, life-threatening adrenal insufficiency may occur when the adrenal-pituitary axis has not had time to recover following suppressive corticoid therapy. If the patient has not previously received steroid therapy and has received acute, intensive therapy for less than 3 days, it is not necessary to taper the medication and the steroids can be suspended abruptly. If therapy has persisted for 3 to 10 days, the dose can be tapered quickly, changed to a single morning dose, then to an alternate-day dose, and finally discontinued. If chronic, high-dose therapy has been used, gradual tapering of glucocorticoid dosage is necessary to avoid the possible exacerbation of the primary disease process or the precipitation of acute adrenal failure. Several protocols have been developed for this purpose. In general, if the primary disease permits, the steroid dose can be decreased by 50% each week until maintenance levels are reached. Subsequently, the dose may be decreased by 20% every three days until the glucocorticoids are finally discontinued. It is advisable that steroids be given at three times the maintenance doses if the patient is stressed either medically or surgically up to 1 year after cessation of therapy. If signs of adrenal insufficiency develop while corticosteroids are being tapered, the dose should be increased again to previous levels. Symptoms of impending adrenal failure include anorexia, nausea, vomiting, lethargy, headache, and hypotension.

DISORDERS OF THE REPRODUCTIVE SYSTEM

HIRSUTISM

Hirsutism refers to the increase in short, thick, terminal hair that is usually associated with signs of masculinization. An increase in terminal hair over the upper lips, beard area, upper back, and chest in females is consistent with hirsutism, especially if accompanied by other signs of virilization, such as clitoromegaly or amenorrhea.

The most common cause of hirsutism is excessive androgen production in late-onset congenital adrenal hyperplasia or in polycystic ovary syndrome. The differential diagnosis of hyperandrogenism must include ovarian and adrenal tumors. Hirsutism can also be familial, a side effect of diazoxide or diphenytoin use, or secondary to hypothyroidism, malnutrition, or central nervous system injury.

In evaluating a patient complaining of hirsutism, it is important to determine if there has been a change in the amount or location of the body hair and if it has been accompanied by a change in weight, voice pitch, or menstrual irregularities. A history of drug intake and a family history of hirsutism should be sought. On physical examination, the location of the body hair, the presence of acanthosis nigricans, and signs of virilization (change in body fat or muscle, clitoral enlargement) should be noted. Patients with true hirsutism, menstrual irregularities, or signs of virilization should be formally evaluated.

The laboratory studies include serum levels of testosterone, free testosterone, dihydroepiandrosterone (DHEA), 17-hydroxyprogesterone, androstenedione, follicle-stimulating hormone (FSH), luteinizing hormone (LH), and prolactin. A karyotype analysis might be necessary. In women, serum testosterone concentrations greater than 200 ng/dL that are not suppressible by dexamethasone suggest the possibility of an adrenal or ovarian tumor. The patient should undergo further evaluation, which would include ultrasound and CT of the abdomen and pelvis.

A mild increase in the serum androgen levels suggests the possibility of an androgen excess syndrome. The serum androgen most often elevated is free (unbound) testosterone. The androgen excess syndromes include late-onset congenital adrenal hyperplasia, polycystic ovary syndrome, and mixed gonadal dysgenesis. To differentiate the various androgen disorders, ACTH stimulation and dexamethasone suppression tests are necessary. The measurement of various steroidal precursors along the cortisol biosynthetic pathway, including 17-hydroxypregnenolone, 17-hydroxyprogesterone, and 11-deoxycortisol, should be determined during ACTH testing. The patient with elevated androgen levels should be referred to an endocrinologist, because the interpretation of the results of the various stimulation or suppression tests is often difficult.

Therapy is to be directed at the underlying pathologic disorder. Surgery is indicated for adrenal or ovarian tumors, while glucocorticoids are used for congenital adrenal hyperplasia. Birth control pills containing progesterone have been found to be effective in the polycystic ovary syndrome since they interrupt the constant estrous cycle and lead to normal ovarian function. Since glucocorticoids have been shown to decrease ovarian steroid production, they have also been used as therapy for polycystic ovary syndrome with mixed success. Other medications that have been beneficial include clomiphene citrate, cyproterone acetate, and spironolactone. Cosmetic improvement can be occasionally obtained with electrolysis, although some degree of facial hair usually remains.

PRECOCIOUS PUBERTY

Sexual precocity is the appearance of secondary sexual characteristics before 8 years of age in girls and 9 years of age in boys. True precocious puberty refers to sexual precocity produced by an elevation of FSH or LH levels. Pseudoprecocious puberty refers to sexual precocity induced by an increase in sex steroids that occurs independently of gonadotropin stimulation. True precocious puberty is generally complete, with a normal rate of progression of the secondary sexual characteristics. Pseudoprecocious puberty is usually incomplete; not all of the secondary sexual characteristics appear.

The most common problems of premature sexual development in children are premature thelarche and premature pubarche (adrenarche). Both conditions are benign but require separation from true sexual precocity or pseudosexual precocity. Premature thelarche often presents in the young female infant. The breast development may be present from birth or appear several months after birth and progress slowly from several months to years. The bone age may be slightly advanced and the vaginal smear may reveal some more mature cells. The general neurologic examination is normal. Levels of LH, FSH, and estradiol are normal. Most often, the breast development progresses very slowly for several months and then stabilizes. Breast tissue in a significant percentage of patients will decrease in size in several years, although a smaller number will persist or continue to increase in size.

Premature pubarche occurs both in boys and girls. There is often a strong family history of premature pubarche. The development of hair in this condition may be as early as 4 years of age, although the most common age for premature pubarche is 6 and 7 years. The bone age is normal to slightly advanced in premature pubarche. Unfortunately, mild forms of the adrenogenital syndrome may also present with premature hair development without attendant bone age advancement. A rapidly developing tumor with marked elevations of androgens might cause pubic hair development with only a slight advancement in bone age. When appropriate, the possibility of androgen excess should be evaluated by determination of serum concentrations of testosterone and androstenedione.

In girls, over 80% of cases of true precocious puberty are idiopathic, whereas in boys over 80% have an organic basis. Sexual precocity can be produced by disorders of the hypothalamic-pituitary axis, excessive steroid production by the adrenal gland or gonads, increased sensitivity of the peripheral tissues to circulating sex steroids, and exogenous hormone. Idiopathic precocious puberty is relatively common in girls. In boys, most cases are produced by organic lesions of the central nervous system. Adrenal or gonadal causes and idiopathic sexual precocity is much less common in males. The aim of the clinical and laboratory evaluation is to separate those boys and girls with an organic cause of precocious puberty from those with idiopathic true precocity. Other than premature thelarche or pubarche, the child with precocious puberty should be referred for evaluation of possible organic causes of sexual precocity and for appropriate treatment.

Therapy is directed at the underlying pathologic disorder. Glucocorticoids are indicated for congenital adrenal hyperplasia and surgery, if possible, for tumors of the adrenal, ovary, or central nervous system. In idiopathic precocious puberty, treatment is directed at suppressing gonadotropin secretion to prevent premature epiphyseal fusion and consequent short stature. The treatment of idiopathic sexual precocity has been unsatisfactory in the past. The drugs utilized included medroxyprogesterone, cyproterone acetate, and bromocriptine. Although medroxyprogesterone decreased breast size and caused cessation of menses, bone age advancement often progressed, resulting in short stature.

Recently, an analogue of gonadotropin-releasing hormone (GnRH) with the property of sustained duration of action has been used with great success to suppress FSH and LH secretion by the pituitary. This GnRH analogue is now available for clinical use and is given as a daily subcutaneous injection. At adequate doses, sexual maturation is halted and may even regress. The increased growth rate and rapid advancement in bone age will also improve. On discontinuation of therapy, pubertal changes will resume and can progress rapidly.

SEXUAL INFANTILISM

Sexual infantilism is defined as the lack of secondary sexual characteristics by 13 years of age in girls and 14 years of age in boys. In addition, an age-appropriate onset of puberty but a lack of progression of secondary sexual maturation may also indicate a sexual infantilizing organic disorder. Sexual infantilism can be due to lack of hypothalamic or pituitary stimulation of gonadal maturation (hypogonadotropic hypogonadism), or primary gonadal failure (hypergonadotropic hypogonadism).

Often, the most difficult differential diagnosis is to separate the child with constitutional delay of growth and development from the child with sexual infantilism, especially if secondary to hypogonadotropic hypogonadism. The findings in constitutional delay of growth and development have been discussed earlier. A bone age and serum concentrations of LH, FSH, and testosterone or estradiol should be obtained. Since Klinefelter syndrome occurs in 1 of every 600 boys and Turner syndrome in one of every 2,000 girls, a karyotype analysis should be performed if the gonadotropin levels are elevated or clinical phenotypic findings of these syndromes are present. If the gonadotropins are low, and sexual infantilism is suspected, further evaluation including a complete pituitary evaluation is necessary.

Therapy of sexual infantilism consists of replacement of sex steroids. Treatment is generally begun when the bone age is 13 or 14 years, or when the patient has reached an appropriate height. In boys, Depo-Testosterone (enanthate or cypionate) is the treatment of choice. For development of secondary sexual characteristics, the usual starting dose is 50 mg intramuscularly once a month. This dose is progressively increased over the next 2 to 3 years until a final adult replacement dose of 300 mg every 3 weeks is attained. The patient must also be referred to a urologist for testicular prosthetic implants, when appropriate.

While receiving testosterone therapy, boys will often complain of breast tenderness, increase in body hair, spontaneous erections, increased libido, and the pain of intramuscular injections. If these symptoms are exceptionally bothersome, a smaller dose of testosterone may be tried until "tolerance" develops. Most patients will be pleased at the secondary sexual development and tolerate the intramuscular injections without major objections.

In girls, estrogens are used to induce pubertal development. Oral ethinyl estradiol in a daily dose of 5 to 10 μg is the preferred therapy. Once secondary sexual characteristics have progressed to a Tanner stage III or IV level, ethinyl estradiol is only administered on the first 21 days of the month. When menstrual bleeding occurs regularly, medroxyprogesterone acetate is given with the estradiol on days 15 to 21 of the month. A monthly cycle is thus established, simulating normal menstrual cycles. If breakthrough bleeding occurs before an appropriate level of sexual and mental maturity is obtained, a smaller dose of ethinyl estradiol should be used. On the other hand, if poor sexual development is observed on 5 to 10 μg of ethinyl estradiol, the dose should be increased to 10 to 20 μg per day.

AMBIGUOUS GENITALIA

A newborn infant with genital ambiguity requires urgent attention and expedient referral to a tertiary center for thorough examination. The decision on gender assignment needs to be postponed until results of the initial diagnostic studies are available, and should be a joint decision involving the patient's primary care physician, an endocrinologist, a pediatric urologist or surgeon, and a psychologist who is conversant with the parents' concerns. Gender assignment is based primarily on the patient's potential for normal sexual functioning. Future fertility and the feasibility of reconstructive surgery are secondary issues. The chromosomal sex is not critical to the decision.

Vital aspects of the physical examination include the absence or presence of palpable gonads, the location of the urethral meatus, the length and width of the phallus, and the presence of other anomalies. Karyotype analysis is helpful diagnostically in distinguishing an undervirilized boy from a virilized girl, or an infant with chromosome mosaicism. Other useful tests include baseline serum 17-hydroxyprogesterone, testosterone, and gonadotropin concentrations, pelvic ultrasound, and genitourethrography. hCG and cosyntropin (Cortrosyn) stimulation tests, and fibroblast studies for 5_{α}-reductase activity and androgen receptor disorders may help establish the diagnosis.

Treatment of the patient depends on the cause of the disorder and on the gender assignment, and often includes reconstructive surgery and parental counseling.

BIBLIOGRAPHY

Burke CW: Adrenocortical insufficiency. *Clin Endocrinol Metab* 1985; 14:947.

Fisher DA: Hypothyroidism in childhood. *Pediatr Rev* 1980; 2:67.

Foster CM, Kelch RP: New hope for youngsters with precocious puberty. *Contemp Pediatr* 1986; 105.

Frasier SD: Short stature in children. *Pediatr Rev* 1981; 3:171.

Glorieux J, Desjardins M, Letarte J, et al: Useful parameters to predict the eventual mental outcome of hypothyroid children. *Pediatr Res* 1988; 24:6.

Lippe BM, Landaw EM, Kaplan SA: Hyperthyroidism in children treated with long term medical therapy; Twenty-five percent remission every two years. *Pediatr Res* 1987; 64:1241.

Miller WL, Levine LS: Molecular and clinical advances in congenital adrenal hyperplasia. *J Pediatr* 1987; 111:1.

Milner RDG: Which children should have growth hormone therapy? *Lancet* 1986; 483.

New M, Temeck J, Grimm R, et al: An overview of disorders of sexual differentiation. *Res Staff Phys* 1985; 31:21.

Rimoin DL, Horton WA: Short stature. *J Pediatr* 1978; 92:523.

Rimoin DL, Horton WA: Short stature. *J Pediatr* 1978; 92:697.

Root AW: Endocrinology of puberty. II: Aberrations of sexual maturation. *J Pediatr* 1973; 83:187.

Rosenfield RL: Androgen disorders in children: Too much, too early, too little, or too late. *Pediatr Rev* 1983; 5:141

Saxena KM, Crawford JD, Talbot NB: Childhood thyrotoxicosis: A long-term perspective. *Br Med J* 1964; 2:1153.

White PC, New MI, Dupont B: Congenital adrenal hyperplasia (first of two parts). *N Engl J Med* 1987; 316:1519.

White PC, New MI, Dupont B: Congenital adrenal hyperplasia (second of two parts). *N Engl J Med* 1987; 316:1580.

94 NEPHROLOGY

John W. Foreman, M.D.

Although chronic renal failure occurs in only eight children per million, the primary care physician may be called to see such children for acute illnesses and general pediatric care. Because of this, it is helpful for the general pediatrician to understand certain aspects of this problem, although major renal decisions lie in the realm of the nephrologist. This chapter will describe the major problems associated with chronic renal failure, aspects of chronic dialysis, and general indications for a renal biopsy.

PROBLEMS OF CHRONIC RENAL FAILURE

Biochemical abnormalities are often not evident until the glomerular filtration rate is reduced to less than 30% of normal. Symptoms suggestive of renal failure, such as fatigue, poor school performance, anorexia, nausea and vomiting, and edema, are usually not noticed until the glomerular filtration rate falls below 25% of normal and often not until it falls to 15% of normal. Because of the marked redundancy of renal function, patients with renal insufficiency are able to survive without dialysis until the glomerular filtration rate falls below 10% and often 5% of normal. However, with specific disease processes, certain manifestations and symptoms may be evident with only minimal reductions in glomerular function.

Specific problems associated with chronic renal failure are seen in the following list:

PROBLEMS OF CHRONIC RENAL FAILURE

- Growth retardation
- Renal osteodystrophy
- Hypocalcemia
- Hyperphosphatemia
- Acidosis
- Hyperkalemia
- Hypertension
- Edema
- Anemia
- Uremia

Growth impairment, one of the earliest signs of chronic renal failure, is evident when the glomerular filtration rate is reduced to only 50% of normal. The etiology of the growth failure in renal insufficiency is multifactorial, including acidosis, disturbances in vitamin D metabolism, and problems with calcium and phosphate regulation. Activation of vitamin D by the kidney is impaired with renal failure. Activated vitamin D, 1,25-cholecalciferol, has many functions including absorbing calcium and phosphorus from the intestine, aiding the mineralization of growing bone, and, possibly, reabsorbing calcium in the kidney. Impairment of this activation step leads to rickets. Prolonged and severe depression of this activation of vitamin D produces hypocalcemia and tetany.

With moderate reductions in glomerular filtration rate, it becomes more and more difficult for the kidney to excrete the normal dietary load of phosphate, leading to a small rise in blood phosphate levels, but inducing a clear increase in parathyroid hormone (PTH) secretion. This increase in PTH facilitates phosphate excretion by the kidney, maintaining a nearly normal blood phosphate concentration. However, the rise in PTH also acts to demineralize bone. Therefore, the bone disease in renal insufficiency, renal osteodystrophy, is a mixture of the effects of activated vitamin D deficiency and increased PTH on growing bone. Both of these influences lead to demineralization of the bone with bowing, flaring, and, eventually, fracturing of the long bones.

With reduction of the glomerular filtration rate to less than 30% of normal, the kidney is no longer able to excrete the normal dietary load of phosphate, which results in a clearly elevated blood phosphate concentration. This rise in blood phosphate level, in concert with poor gut absorption of calcium, causes a further depression of serum calcium concentration, which is a typical feature of marked renal impairment. However, tetany is an unusual symptom in spite of the hypocalcemia because of the concomitant acidosis associated with renal failure.

Acidosis is also a common feature of chronic renal failure, especially when the glomerular filtration rate falls below a third to a quarter of normal. It may be evident earlier if the renal disease predominantly involves the tubules, such as in cystinosis. Acidosis occurs because there are not enough nephrons to excrete the normal dietary load of acid, although individual nephrons excrete supranormal amounts of acid. In the forms of renal failure characterized by tubular disease, acidosis is enhanced by bicarbonate loss from the kidney. In spite of the acidosis, the blood pH rarely falls below 7.2 because the acid that is not secreted by the kidney is buffered by bone. However, the price paid for this buffering is further demineralization and osteomalacia.

Because the acid production of the average child is 2 to 4 mEq/kg of body weight per day, the acidosis of chronic renal failure typically requires a similar amount of alkali given as either sodium bicarbonate or as the sodium or potassium salt of citrate. Citrate is metabolized by the liver to bicarbonate and is easily given to children. When correcting acidosis in renal failure, especially in severe renal failure, hypocalcemia must be corrected concomitantly to prevent tetany.

The renal handling of sodium and potassium is also often disturbed in chronic renal failure. Sodium problems range from an absolute need for sodium seen in some children with marked tubular or interstitial disease to children who require very restricted intakes of sodium, especially those children with glomerulonephritis. All children with renal failure tolerate extremes of sodium intake poorly.

Potassium also needs to be followed carefully. Most children with renal insufficiency do not have hyperkalemia until their renal failure is quite advanced; however, hyperkalemia is a common cause of death in such patients. When hyperkalemia is evident, dietary potassium should be restricted. If this is not sufficient, then resins such as sodium polystyrene sulfonate, which bind potassium secreted into the gut, can be employed. Failure of these agents to control the serum potassium level necessitates the institution of dialysis. Some children with renal insufficiency require supplemental potassium, especially those with tubular disorders such as renal tubular acidosis or the Fanconi syndrome.

Hypertension is a very common problem in chronic renal failure, especially that secondary to glomerulonephritis. Hypertension in glomerulonephritis often is evident before there is any impairment of the glomerular filtration rate. Increased blood pressure arises for a number of reasons, including impaired sodium and water excretion leading to volume expansion, and the liberation of vasoactive hormones, especially those of the renin-angiotensin system. (For treatment of this problem, see the section on Hypertension.)

Edema, another problem of renal failure, is usually present early in glomerulonephritis, but appears, if at all, late in tubular or interstitial diseases. Edema is present either because of impaired sodium and water excretion leading to expansion of the intravascular space, or because of proteinuria with the development of the nephrotic syndrome. In both situations, sodium restriction and often diuretics are helpful in controlling the edema. With severe impairment of renal function, fluid intake may also need to be limited, since the kidney is unable to excrete a normal intake.

Anemia is a major and predictable consequence of chronic renal failure. It may even be the presenting sign, especially in medullary cystic disease. The anemia, characterized by normal indices and a low reticulocyte count, is caused primarily by decreased production of erythropoietin by the diseased kidney. Treatment consists mainly of blood transfusions, although androgens have been used in adolescents. Recently, recombinant human erythropoietin has been given to adult patients with renal failure with dramatic results. Although not used in children, recombinant erthropoietin holds great promise for treating the anemia of chronic renal failure and obviating blood transfusions.

The diet is very important in children with renal failure. Typically, it must be high in calcium and low in phosphorus, with attention to the amount of sodium. As mentioned before, some children tolerate a normal amount of sodium or even require extra sodium, whereas others need sodium restriction. Another important consideration in the diet of these children, as in normal children, is the caloric content. As renal failure progresses, these children often become anorectic and uninterested in food, resulting in undernourishment. It is, therefore, important to make sure that they take in an adequate number of calories. This is often a challenge for all concerned: the mother, the dietician, and the pediatrician. Protein intake should be restricted when the blood urea nitrogen (BUN) level rises over 50 to 70 mg/dL. In infants, protein requirements can be met by 2 g/kg of body weight per day and in older children by 1.5 g/kg of body weight per day. The protein offered should be of high biologic value, such as egg protein. Obviously, trying to design a restricted diet that is both palatable and nutritious is quite difficult.

Uremic symptoms usually begin to appear when the BUN level rises above 75 mg/dL and especially when it rises above 150 mg/dL. Early symptoms of uremia are lethargy, increased fatigability, shortened attention span, and poor school performance. Later, persistent nausea and vomiting occur. More serious signs and symptoms of uremia are coma, seizures, pericarditis, and bleeding, especially gastrointestinal, from a platelet dysfunction.

Another important consideration to bear in mind when treating children with renal failure is the adjustment of medication dosages. The kidney is an important excretory organ for many drugs, e.g., gentamicin. With renal insufficiency, dangerous levels can develop if adjustments are not made. Recommendations for specific medications are beyond the scope of this chapter and such questions should be referred to a pediatric nephrologist or nephrology text.

DIALYSIS

Since there are no precise indications for when to institute chronic dialysis, this decision must be individualized for each child. Usually, chronic dialysis is begun when the serum creatinine rises to 8–10 mg/dL or glomerular filtration rate falls to less than 5–10 mL/min per 1.73 m^2. In younger children and infants, chronic dialysis may need to be undertaken with much lower levels of serum creatinine reflecting the smaller muscle mass and creatinine production by such individuals. Irrespective of the serum creatinine, dialysis should be considered if other biochemical abnormalities, such as acidosis, hyperkalemia, hyponatremia, hypocalcemia, hyperphosphatemia, and marked azotemia cannot be managed with more conservative means. However, more important than biochemical criteria in making this decision is the presence of progressive fatigue, weakness, lassitude, anorexia, nausea, and vomiting. Furthermore, clinical problems related to volume overload, that are unresponsive to sodium restriction, fluid restriction, and diuretics, such as anasarca, hypertension, and congestive heart failure will require dialysis, again irrespective of the biochemical status of the patient.

Having made the decision to put a child on chronic dialysis, the next question to answer is which mode of dialysis is best suited to the patient and his family. The choices available are hemodialysis, continuous cycled peritoneal dialysis, and continuous ambulatory peritoneal dialysis (CAPD). Each method has advantages and disadvantages, and it is not known which method is most effective in terms of the long-term goals of growth and survival. Therefore, the decision of which modality to use is based on a number of factors including availability of facilities, educability of the family and patient, and the interest and time the family and patient have in performing home dialysis.

The traditional mode of chronic dialysis is hemodialysis. Hemodialysis is accomplished by passing arterial blood along one side of a semipermeable membrane while a balanced salt solution, called the *bath*, is pumped along the other. Because the bath solution does not contain urea, creatinine, or other nitrogenous waste products, these compounds diffuse from the blood into the bath and are removed. Since the blood is pumped along this membrane under pressure, a filtrate of the plasma, composed of water, salts, and waste products, is also forced into the bath, further cleansing the blood and allowing the removal of excess sodium and water.

Vascular access that allows a large blood flow volume (100–300 mL/min) is required for hemodialysis. Such access can be achieved by connecting an artery to a vein either directly or via synthetic graft. In small children, proximal vessel grafts, such as the bronchial artery to cephalic vein or femoral artery to saphenous vein, are necessary. The synthetic graft may be used more quickly after surgery than a natural arteriovenous fistula but carries a greater risk of infection or aneurysm formation.

A major problem common to both modes of vascular access is thrombosis. This can often be recognized by the loss of the palpable thrill associated with a well-functioning shunt. If detected early enough, it is sometimes possible to remove the clot without changing the access site.

Because of the expense and family disruption that hemodialysis causes, new interest has been raised in chronic home peritoneal dialysis. A peritoneal dialysis catheter designed by Tenckhoff and his colleagues has made this possible by reducing the incidence of infection through the use of a long subcutaneous tunnel prior to the catheter's entry into the peritoneum. In spite of this tunnel, infection remains the major problem associated with chronic peritoneal dialysis. However, it affords the most normal lifestyle for a child with end-stage renal failure.

The two major methods of performing home peritoneal dialysis are CAPD and cycled continuous peritoneal dialysis (CCPD).

In CAPD, dialysate is allowed to remain in the abdomen for 4 to 6 hours and then replaced with fresh dialysate approximately four to six times a day. Extra fluid is removed by this technique by using a concentrated glucose solution in the dialysate. This has been a very effective method of dialysis, but does require that either the child or a caretaker constantly change the dialysis solution. With CCPD, the dialysate exchanges are done every other hour for 8 to 12 hours a night, 5 to 7 days a week. A simple machine can perform this while the child is asleep, minimizing the disruption that chronic renal failure can wreak on family life. With both modes of peritoneal dialysis, meticulous care of the catheter is necessary to prevent infection of either the subcutaneous tunnel or the peritoneum. Diagnosis and treatment should be undertaken at the first sign of infection. Unfortunately, tunnel infections often require removal of the catheter to eradicate the infection. Also in both forms of peritoneal dialysis, there are constant protein losses into the dialysate, necessitating a more liberal intake of protein than is usually possible with hemodialysis.

TRANSPLANTATION

Because chronic dialysis imposes significant dietary and social restrictions on children, the ultimate goal of most pediatric end-stage renal programs has been successful renal transplantation. Over the last 15 years, renal transplantation in children has become an established procedure. The two potential sources of kidneys that are available to patients with end-stage renal disease are from compatible, healthy, immediate relatives (live related donor) or from a brain-dead but otherwise healthy patient (cadaveric donor).

Transplants from living relatives have longer graft survival and can be performed more quickly once the disease reaches end stage. For these reasons, these transplants are the choice of many pediatric centers.

Lifelong immunosuppression is necessary in these patients to prevent rejection, except in transplants between identical twins. The traditional immunosuppressive agents are prednisone and azathioprine. Cyclosporine has dramatically improved graft survival, especially in cadaveric transplants. However, cyclosporine can be nephrotoxic, making its use problematic at times. Another class of immunosuppressive agents coming into use are antibodies directed at the T-lymphocyte. These agents hold great promise for more selective immunosuppression, avoiding some of the infectious risks of current immunosuppressive agents.

Three major problems continue to plague renal transplantation. First, in spite of immunosuppression, a significant percentage of renal grafts are rejected and for this reason continual monitoring of renal function is necessary. Secondly, because of the immunosuppression, infection remains a constant threat. These patients need to be evaluated promptly for any symptom suggestive of an infection, a task that the primary care physician is often asked to perform in consultation with the transplant center. Finally, hypertension is quite common in transplant patients for a variety of reasons and the management is similar to that in other patients.

RENAL BIOPSY INDICATIONS

There are few absolute indications for a renal biopsy, therefore the reasons for biopsy vary between nephrologists. A renal biopsy can provide information on both diagnosis and prognosis and occasionally on therapy. Complications arising from the procedure, mainly related to bleeding, are quite low when done by individuals experienced in performing it in children. Recent studies have shown that it need not be performed in prepubertal children in the initial presentation of nephrosis who respond to steroids, since the overwhelming majority have minimal disease change. Because adolescents presenting with nephrosis have less than a 50% response rate to steroids, a renal biopsy is a useful procedure for guiding therapy in these patients. A renal biopsy is not necessary in a healthy child with microscopic hematuria in the absence of proteinuria, urinary casts, and hypertension. Persistent proteinuria, after excluding orthostatic proteinuria, is an indication for a biopsy since there is a high probability for significant renal disease.

BIBLIOGRAPHY

Chesney RW, Mehls O, Anast C, et al: Renal osteodystrophy in children: The role of vitamin D, phosphorus, and parathyroid hormone. *Am J Kidney Dis* 1986; 7:275–284.

Eschbach JW, Egrie JC, Downing MR, et al: Correction of the anemia of end-stage renal disease with recombinant human erythropoietin. *N Engl J Med* 1987; 316:73–78.

Fine RN: Peritoneal dialysis update. *J Pediatr* 1982; 100:1–7.

Foreman JW, Chan JCM: Chronic renal failure in children. *J Pediatr* 1988; 113:793–800.

Offner G, Aschendorff C, Hoyer PF, et al: End-stage renal failure: 14 years' experience of dialysis and renal transplantation. *Arch Dis Child* 1988; 63:120–126.

95 ONCOLOGY

Beverly Lange, M.D.

This chapter provides background information and practical guidelines for the primary care practitioner participating in the care of a child with cancer. The classification, presentation, and differential diagnosis of pediatric neoplasms are discussed in Chapter 63, and some aspects of supportive care are given in Chapter 105.

PRINCIPLES AND COMPLICATIONS OF CANCER THERAPY

Over the past two decades combinations of surgery, chemotherapy, and radiation therapy, as well as intensive supportive care, have brought long-term survival and possibly cure to over half the children with cancer (Fig 95–1). Surgery is used to remove bulky tumors, but it fails to cure most tumors even when the tumor is removed completely. Irradiation is usually given to the tumor bed and sometimes to areas of local extension. Chemotherapy is intended to treat all sites of disease. More recently, extraordinarily high doses of radiation therapy and chemotherapy followed by bone marrow transplantation have successfully controlled some childhood leukemias or solid tumors refractory to standard therapy. Most children with malignant tumors are treated according to institutional or national collaborative protocol studies that are designed to provide the therapy currently most effective while avoiding life-threatening toxic reactions.

Virtually all malignancies are treated with more than one chemotherapeutic agent because multiple-agent therapy discourages emergence and growth of resistant populations of cells that eventually manifest themselves as metastases or recurrences. In many instances chemotherapy or even radiation therapy is used in a prophylactic or "adjuvant" way: that is, the chemotherapy for solid tumors is given before the pulmonary metastases are large enough to be seen on a chest radiograph. In leukemia, intrathecal medications and cranial irradiation are given before leukemic meningitis occurs. Controlled clinical trials have shown that adjuvant therapy prevents metastases in many pediatric solid tumors and overt central nervous system disease in acute lymphoblastic leukemia.

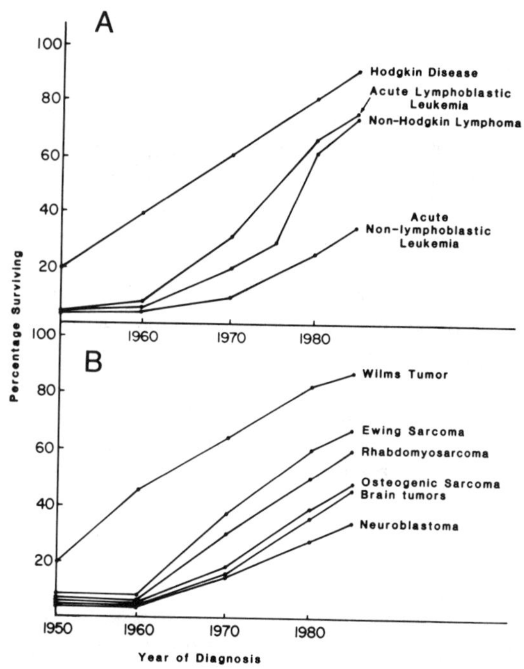

FIG 95–1
Approximate 5-year survival rates in pediatric leukemias and lymphomas (A) and solid tumors (B) by year of diagnosis from 1950 to 1985.

Most cancer chemotherapy acts on the DNA, the RNA, or protein synthesis of proliferating cells, both normal and malignant and results in injury, death, or mutation of the cells. The effects of chemotherapy on cells of the hematopoietic system and gastrointestinal tract, respectively, cause anemia, thrombocytopenia, leukopenia, and severe mucositis. Toxic effects that involve the leukocytes, causing functional or absolute neutropenia or lymphopenia, lead to opportunistic infection. Furthermore, many of the diseases are themselves immunosuppressive. Thus, infection is the most common cause of death in children with cancer.

INFECTION IN THE COMPROMISED HOST

Three infectious conditions occur that are not usually encountered in the normal host: (1) fever and neutropenia; (2) interstitial pneumonitis; and (3) serious viral illness from viruses generally not considered dangerous. Most other infections are not so life-threatening, and one can manage them as in an otherwise healthy child.

FEVER AND NEUTROPENIA

Neutropenia is defined as an absolute neutrophil count of less than 500 or less than 1,000/μL and falling. Fever is defined as three temperature readings above 38° C in 24 hours or a single temperature over 38.5° C. Fever, a highly reliable sign of infection, may often be the only sign. However, in patients who have received steroid therapy for months even fever may be suppressed and metastatic foci of infection and clinical deterioration may be the only signs of sepsis. Only 25% of febrile neutropenic patients have microbiologically documented infection. Most bacterial infections are caused by endogenous flora, *Escherichia coli*, *Staphylococcus aureus*, or *Pseudomonas* species, which have become invasive because of altered host defenses. Although it is recommended that blood, urine, and throat cultures be obtained, routine lumbar punctures are not indicated unless the child has clinical symptoms of meningitis. The child should be treated promptly with broad-spectrum antibiotics, which cover all possibilities. Combinations of an antistaphylococcal penicillin or cephalosporin plus an aminoglycoside plus an anti-*Pseudomonas* penicillin are recommended. Specific agents are best discussed with the subspecialist. Shock must be corrected promptly. Many children receive oral trimethoprim-sulfamethoxazole to prevent bacterial infection.

Fungal disease is also a cause of fever in neutropenic patients. Candidial esophagitis occurs in some patients receiving steroids and presents as dysphagia and substernal pain. Other invasive fungal diseases occur such as aspergillosis in hospitalized patients receiving antibacterial antibiotics and having prolonged neutropenia. The treatment of invasive fungal disease in most cases is amphotericin B. Many oncologists now add amphotericin B empirically to treat persistent or recurrent fever in the neutropenic patient. Simple thrush can be treated with nystatin, clotrimazole, or ketoconazole.

INTERSTITIAL PNEUMONITIS

Ten years ago, *Pneumocystis carinii* pneumonitis was the leading cause of death in children with lymphoblastic leukemia in remission. Now most children who are at risk for this pneumonia receive prophylactic therapy with oral trimethoprim-sulfamethoxazole. Nonetheless, children not receiving or not complying with prophylaxis are still at risk: *Pneumocystis* pneumonia presents as cough, fever, progressive tachypnea, and cyanosis. Chest radiographs show interstitial pneumonitis with prominent hilar infiltrates. The necessity of prompt tissue diagnosis with aspirate or biopsy is controversial. In many places, susceptible children are admitted, given trimethoprim-sulfamethoxazole, observed, and reevaluated. Other causes of interstitial pneumonia include: cytomegalovirus, common respiratory viruses, *Mycoplasma* pneumonia, and, rarely, legionnaires' disease or fungal disease, as well as radiation- or chemotherapy-induced pneumonitis.

VARICELLA AND RUBEOLA

Although varicella and rubeola do not usually cause life-threatening infections in healthy children, they can be fatal in children with leukemia or lymphoma or in children who have had extensive irradiation and immunosuppressive therapy with agents such as steroids or cyclophosphamide. Varicella can cause pneumonitis, encephalitis, hepatitis, and a hemorrhagic diathesis with disseminated intravascular coagulation. Varicella should be treated promptly with acyclovir. All chemotherapy, except long-term steroid administration, should be stopped.

More important, fatal varicella can be prevented. Protection and prevention are achieved by the parents advising the child's school and friends about the risk of varicella and asking them to acknowledge exposures promptly. Administration of varicella-immune globulin (VZIG) or zoster-immune plasma (ZIP) within 72 hours of exposure will attenuate or abort the disease. These are available at American Red Cross regional centers. The child's oncologist should be contacted, and, in most cases, chemotherapy should be discontinued and administration of steroids tapered to maintenance levels. Children should receive ZIP or VZIG if they have a household contact or if they have been playing closely with a child who develops varicella. The disease is contagious 24 hours before the rash and until all lesions have become scabs. Varicella vaccine is currently under investigation for prophylaxis of varicella in the compromised host.

Zoster, or shingles, is common in children with Hodgkin's disease or leukemia or in marrow transplant recipients. Zoster should be treated with acyclovir.

Children who have received adequate immunization with measles, mumps, and rubella (MMR) vaccine should be immune to rubeola. Those inadequately or unimmunized should receive 0.05 mL/kg of immune serum globulin immediately on exposure and, usually, chemotherapy should be stopped.

COMMON CHILDHOOD ILLNESSES

If a child does not have neutropenia, is not seriously ill, is not receiving prolonged steroid therapy, is not at risk for *Pneumocystis* pneumonia, and does not have varicella or rubeola, then it is likely that most illnesses can be treated according to the principles of good pediatric practice. Chemotherapy is usually stopped when the child is febrile. Otitis, mild bronchopneumonia, streptococcal pharyngitis, and urinary tract infection can be treated with specific appropriate antibiotics. Bactericidal antibiotics rather than bacteriostatic antibiotics should be used. Rubella, mumps, infectious mononucleosis, enteroviruses, and influenza do not require special care or precautions. Hepatitis B infection is becoming less common because of screening of blood products, but children with leukemia who are hepatitis B surface antigen (HBsAg)-positive shed extraordinarily high quantities of virus in saliva and stool.

NONINFECTIOUS SIDE EFFECTS OF CANCER AND CANCER THERAPY

In addition to predisposing to leukopenia and opportunistic infection, cancer therapy also causes anemia and thrombocytopenia. Anemia is well tolerated, but packed red blood cell transfusions are used to maintain a hemoglobin level of about 10 g/dL in patients who are unlikely to be able to make their own erythrocytes and who are ill or symptomatic. Spontaneous bruising and bleeding occur with platelet counts of under 20,000/μL. Platelets are not given routinely for prophylaxis because they increase the risk of platelet resistance. However 0.2 U/kg are given for bleeding or in patients with falling platelet counts who repeatedly bleed at counts under 20,000/μL. Children with thrombocytopenia should avoid contact sports and should receive platelets for trauma. If possible, blood products should be irradiated to avoid graft-vs.-host disease and, if possible, cytomegalovirus-negative blood products should be used in children who are expected to receive a marrow transplant.

Like the marrow, the intestinal tract is susceptible to transient damage from therapy. This most often manifests itself as mouth ulcers and denuded mucosa. Local and systemic analgesics, good oral hygiene (brushing with a soft toothbrush), a diet with cool bland foods, and, sometimes antibiotics are helpful. Potential dental problems should be treated as soon as possible to avoid abscesses as sources of infection.

Specific drugs have some unusual side effects that should be recognized. These are in Table 95–1. It should be noted that temporary hair loss, nausea and vomiting, and hematopoietic toxic effects are almost universal.

TABLE 95–1
Acute and Delayed Toxic Effects of Commonly Used Chemotherapeutic Agents

DRUG	ACUTE TOXIC EFFECTS*	DELAYED TOXIC EFFECTS*
Bleomycin	2,7,8	E†
Cisplatin	1,2,3,6,13,15	D†,F†
Corticosteroids	See chapter 93	
Cyclophosphamide	1,2,3,4,6,14,15	A†,E†,I†
Cytarabine	1,2,3,4,6,7,12	
Dacarbazine	1,2,3,7	
Dactinomycin	1,2,3,5,6,12	B,E†
Daunorubicin	1,2,3,5,6,8	B,C†,E†
Doxorubicin	1,2,3,5,6,8	B,C†,E†
L-Asparaginase	7,8,9,10,12	
Melphalan	1,2,3,4,5,6,7	A,I†
Mercaptopurine	3,4,6,10	
Methotrexate	1,2,3,4,6,7,10,12	E†,H
Nitrogen mustard	1,2,3,4,6	A†,I†
Nitrosoureas (lomustine, carmustine)	1,2,3,4,6,7,13	A,D,E,I
Procarbazine	1,3,4,12	I
Thioguanine	3,4,6,10,12	H
Vincristine	2,5,7,11,13,15	
Vinblastine	2,3,5,11	
VM-26 (teniposide), VP-16 (etoposide)	1,2,3,11,8	

*Explanation of codes: 1 indicates nausea and vomiting; 2, alopecia; 3, myelosuppression; 4, immunosuppression; 5, tissue necrosis with extravasation; 6, mucosal ulceration; 7, fever; 8, urticaria; 9, pancreatitis; 10, chemical hepatitis; 11, neuromuscular pain; 12, rash; 13, renal tubular damage; 14, hemorrhagic cystitis; and 15, syndrome of inappropriate antidiuretic hormone (SIADH). A indicates sterility; B, radiation recall; C, cardiac failure; D, renal failure; E, pulmonary fibrosis; F, hearing loss; H, hepatic fibrosis; and I, secondary leukemia.
†Effect enhanced by radiation therapy.

IMMUNIZATIONS

Children may receive diphtheria-pertussis-tetanus (DPT) and influenza immunizations but vaccinations should be given in collaboration with the subspecialists, as there may be times when the child is unlikely to respond well. Inactivated (Salk) polio vaccine and influenza vaccine may be given. Live polio vaccine should not be given to children receiving chemotherapy and siblings should not receive this vaccine if the patient is not immune. Inactivated vaccine can be given to siblings or the child. If a sibling receives live polio vaccine, the children should be separated. Current recommendations are for 4 to 6 weeks of separation, but these recommendations apply more to recent marrow transplant recipients or for children with severe combined immune deficiency. In children with leukemia it is practical for siblings to avoid any form of fecal-oral contact so that dishes, clothing, towels, etc., should be kept separate and physical contact and close play avoided. Likewise measles, mumps, and rubella vaccine should not be given, as measles vaccine may lead to fatal rubeola. γ-Globulin is indicated for protection after exposure to measles or hepatitis A. *Hemophilus influenzae* B vaccine has been recommended for compromised hosts, and there are data to show that children receiving chemotherapy can respond to *H. influenzae*-diphtheria conjugate vaccine.

GROWTH AND DEVELOPMENT

Growth is retarded during chemotherapy and radiation therapy. At the time of cessation of therapy, there is usually substantial catch-up growth although ultimately there may be a reduction in predicted stature. If high doses (>3,000 rad) and large-field irradiation have been used, major growth disturbances occur; skeletal and soft tissue abnormalities appear months and years later. Late-onset damage to heart and lung are also of great concern. Radiation therapists who specialize in the care of children attempt to minimize these sequelae.

Children and pubertal or postpubertal patients who have received alkylating agents (cyclophosphamide, melphalan, nitrogen mustard, lomustine, carmustine, busulfan, chlorambucil) or irradiation to the gonads are likely to suffer gonadal failure. This may present as failure to develop secondary sex characteristics or infertility. Boys seem more susceptible than girls. These problems should have been or should be discussed by the subspecialist who has obtained informed consent for therapy. Thyroid function and pituitary function may be damaged by irradiation to these glands.

Most children are able to resume normal activities and to return to school within weeks or months of diagnosis. However, some therapies may interfere with mental development. High doses of irradiation to the brains of infants and young children with primary brain tumors may cause major learning disabilities. In the young child with leukemia, the combinations of moderate doses of irradiation and methotrexate and overt central nervous system (CNS) leukemia may cause learning disabilities. Children should be tested and placed in appropriate classes if learning disabilities occur. More importantly, there is much ongoing research about how to avoid these problems.

NUTRITION

Parents have many questions regarding nutrition and receive spurious unsolicited advice about nourishing their children. Few guidelines exist and cancer and some cancer therapy cause wasting and malnutrition. There is no firm evidence that maintenance of an absolutely normal nutritional status favorably or unfavorably influences the outcome of disease. Parenteral hyperalimentation is used for malnourished children without a properly functioning intestine; nighttime nasogastric feeding may be used in the anorectic wasted child who has a normal intestinal tract. General dietary recommendations are the same as for a healthy child, except that when mucosal ulceration is severe, bland cold foods are soothing. If a child is neutropenic, uncooked vegetables should be avoided as they have a high content of gram-negative bacteria. Megadose vitamins are contraindicated. Children may take vitamin supplements that provide the minimal daily requirements of essential vitamins; however, folinic acid should not be given routinely to children receiving methotrexate; large quantities of folate should not be prescribed. Supplemental iron is usually not necessary as the anemia of cancer comes from arrested production of erythrocytes or low-grade hemolysis, and not from iron deficiency.

DISEASE RECURRENCE OR SECOND TUMORS

Most recurrences occur within the first 2 years after diagnosis. Brain tumors tend to recur with symptoms of increased pressure or cranial nerve abnormalities; rarely, they metastasize to the spinal cord or outside the CNS to bone or marrow. Other solid tumors metastasize most commonly to lung; frequently, metastasis is detected on routine surveillance radiographs. The tumors occasionally recur at their original site. Leukemia may recur in marrow and often shows itself by reproducing the symptoms that occurred originally. In about 10% of patients, leukemia recurs in the nervous system as sterile meningitis. This may be silent or may cause meningeal signs and symptoms. In boys, leukemia may appear in the testis as painless, hard testicular enlargement.

In most cancers recurrence is a sinister event in that it often means that cure is unlikely. However, in some tumors, such as Wilms tumor, Hodgkin disease, and, rarely, in osteosarcoma and acute leukemia, major changes in treatment strategy appear to be allowing increasing numbers of patients who have had a relapse to achieve long-term survival and possible cure. Furthermore, for acute leukemia and solid tumors such as neuroblastoma, Ewing tumor, and non-Hodgkin lymphoma, investigative therapies may be available at a few specialized centers in the country and all the physicians responsible for the child may need to investigate these possibilities.

EMERGENCIES

Few tumors present medical emergencies. However, there are certain situations that require either immediate attention or immediate referral. These emergencies occur because of the mass effects of the tumor compressing or obstructing a vital organ, the metabolic effects of cancer treatment or the cancer itself, and the hematologic consequences of leukemias or cancer therapy. Common oncologic emergencies are listed below. It should be noted that severe intractable pain is common to all forms of malignancy. Cancer pain is best controlled by specific anticancer therapy, but when that is not possible, narcotic analgesics are often required.

ONCOLOGIC EMERGENCIES

Mass effects of cancer
Superior vena cava syndrome
Superior mediastinal syndrome
Spinal cord compression
Increased intracranial pressure
Bowel obstruction
Bladder obstruction
Severe intractable pain
Metabolic effects of cancer
Tumor lysis syndrome, renal failure
Hypercalcemia
Hypertension
Syndromes of inappropriate antidiuretic hormone
Hematologic effects of cancer of its treatment
Hyperleukocytosis (WBC $>200,000/\mu L^3$)
Fever and neutropenia
Severe anemia (Hgb <3 g/dL)
Disseminated intravascular coagulation
Septic shock

COMMUNICATION

Because of the complexity and cost of care of children with cancer, it is necessary for most families to have access to a number of physicians. Currently, many primary care physicians are helping in care of these children by administering chemotherapy or blood products as prescribed by the subspecialist or center, monitoring blood counts, evaluating and treating intercurrent infections, coordinating activities with the school and other organizations, and caring for the handicapped or dying child. The participation of the community physician is essential to help relieve the financial and emotional strain that cancer brings on a family. For the physician the work is gratifying and challenging. However, for shared care to be a help rather than a hindrance, mutual trust and written and verbal communication between the community physician and the cancer center are essential.

Finally, the Leukemia Society, the American Cancer Society, and the Gandlelighters (a national organization that provides an accurate, incisive newsletter for parents and physicians), and many local charitable and paramedical organizations are invaluable resources in the care of the child with cancer. Local hospice organizations may provide assistance to the family of a child dying at home.

BIBLIOGRAPHY

Allegreta GJ, Weisman SJ, Altman AJ: Metabolic and space occupying consequences of cancer and cancer treatment. *Pediatr Clin North Am* 1985; 32:601–611.

American Cancer Society: *Cancer in Childhood*. New York, Professional Educational Publication, 1985.

Fledman S, Lott L: Varicella in children with cancer: Impact of antiviral therapy and prophylaxis. *Pediatrics* 1987; 80:465–472.

Hughes WT, Kuhn S, Chaud HS, et al: Successful chemoprophylaxis for pneumocystis carinii pneumonitis. *N Engl J Med* 1977; 297:1419–1426.

Pizzo P, Robichaud KJ, Wesley R, et al: Fever in the pediatric and young adult patient with cancer: A prospective study of 1001 episodes. *Medicine* 1982; 61:153–165.

96 OPHTHALMOLOGY

Gary R. Diamond, M.D.

The primary care physician is an important member of the team concerned with the care of a child's vision. The initial contact and referral, as well as periodic follow-up of the postoperative patient, are usually the role of the primary care physician or pediatrician. This chapter is intended to help the nonophthalmologist to better understand the reasons for and timing of ophthalmologic referrals and postoperative problems of their patients.

In this chapter, the following problems will be discussed: strabismus, cloudy cornea, hemangioma, ptosis, tearing, conjunctivitis and corneal abrasion, cataracts, glaucoma, retinoblastoma, and rhabdomyosarcoma.

STRABISMUS

Any child with a turned eye or poor vision in one eye should be referred to an ophthalmologist as soon as it is noted (see Chapter 53). Assuming that strabismus surgery is indicated, it is usually performed on an outpatient basis. Postoperatively, eye patches are generally unnecessary and combination antibiotic eyedrops or ointment can be administered for the week following surgery. Normally, the patient is seen 1 to 3 weeks after surgery, then about every 4 to 6 months, if stable. Common postoperative restrictions include prohibiting sandbox play, showers, and swimming for a week until the incision heals. In our experience, the child usually is able to return to school the next day. It should be noted that subconjunctival hemorrhage and edema may last up to 2 weeks. Reoperation is necessary in about 35% of cases.

CONGENITAL CLOUDY CORNEA

If abnormalities of the cornea are detected, the physician should refer the patient to the ophthalmologist for examination, given the possibility that a corneal transplant will be indicated. Common causes of corneal cloudiness are:

- Glaucoma
- Corneal dystrophies
  - Congenital hereditary endothelial dystrophy
  - Posterior polymorphous dystrophy
- Sclerocornea
- Mucopolysaccharidoses
  - Hurler syndrome
- Infection
  - Syphilis
  - Herpes simplex
- Mesodermal dysgeneses
  - Peter anomaly
- Dermoid cyst
- Birth trauma

In addition, certain instances of cloudy cornea are associated with heritable disorders of metabolism, such as mucopolysaccharidoses, and may represent the first clue to the diagnosis of a systemic disorder.

HEMANGIOMA AND PTOSIS

Any demonstrable structural abnormality of the eye or adnexal tissue warrants prompt referral to an ophthalmologist for diagnosis and parental reassurance. A lesion covering the visual axis such as hemangioma (a benign tumor composed of newly formed blood vessels) or ptosis (prolapse of the upper eyelid) should be referred at once, since the problem of amblyopia (decreased vision of nonuse) with structural abnormalities is significant in a very young child. Often definitive treatment of the underlying condition can wait, but the reversal or prevention of amblyopia is of prime consideration.

TEARING

The primary care physician should refer a child with tearing at age 3 months since the condition may represent a blocked nasolacrimal system or increased intraocular pressure. The age for referral requires communication with the ophthalmologist since opinions vary. Occasionally, tearing is indicative of structural eyelid abnormalities that cause the lashes to encroach on the cornea. A mass at the medial canthus should prompt immediate referral because it may represent dacryocystitis secondary to obstruction of the nasolacrimal system, or, more rarely, a malignancy.

CONGENITAL CATARACT

The mainstay of modern therapy for congenital cataract is early diagnosis and surgery (Fig 96–1). If the cataracts are bilateral and complete, it is essential that surgery be performed on both eyes before 3 to 6 months of age. If the cataract is unilateral and the decision is made to operate, the surgery should be performed before 6 to 8 weeks of age, the earlier the better.

The current practice involves outpatient surgery if the child is over 3 months of age, or an overnight stay the day of surgery if the child is younger. Using a microscope for visualization, with the patient under general anesthesia, a small incision is made in the eye to remove the lens by a mechanized vitreous cutting device. Some ophthalmologists leave the posterior capsule of the lens and perform a discussion of this capsule at the time of surgery or shortly thereafter; other surgeons remove the posterior capsule and perform an anterior vitrectomy. After discharge, the patient is fitted with an eye patch and plastic shield. Therapy with topical cycloplegic eyedrops, steroid eyedrops, and broad-spectrum antibiotics follows. The patient should have daily outpatient examinations for one week and, when possible, be fitted with a contact lens 1 or 2 weeks postoperatively. The ophthalmologist will perform visual acuity examinations and refraction every week or two, depending on the age of the child.

In considering a diagnosis of congenital cataract, the primary care physician should be alerted to the following possible associations:

- Inherited mendelian disorder
  - Autosomal dominant
  - Autosomal recessive (rare)
  - X-borne recessive (rare)
- Associated with chromosomal abnormalities
  - Trisomy 21
  - Turner syndrome (XO)
  - Trisomy 13
  - Trisomy 18
- Associated with head and face abnormalities
  - Oxycephaly
  - Crouzon disease
  - Apert syndrome
  - Hallermann-Streiff syndrome
  - Pierre Robin syndrome
- Associated with skeletal disease
  - Conradi syndrome
  - Stippled epiphyses
- Associated with central nervous system syndromes
  - Sjögren-Larsson syndrome
  - Marinesco-Sjögren syndrome

(cont.)

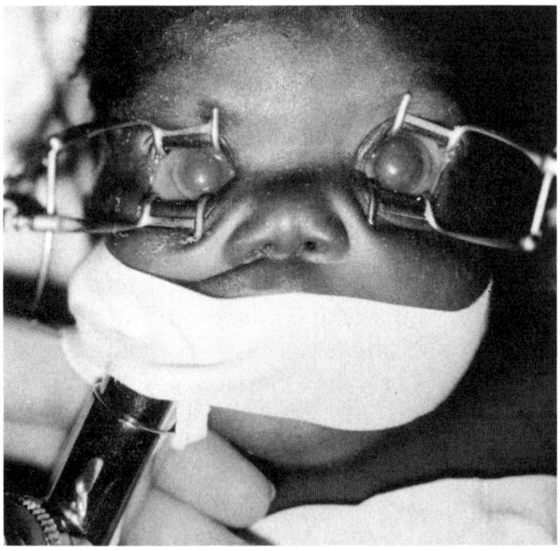

FIG 96–1
Patient with congenital glaucoma prior to surgery. (Courtesy of David Schaffer, M.D.)

Associated with renal disease
- Lowe syndrome
- Renal insufficiency and renal dialysis
- Congenital hemolytic icterus

Associated with metabolic disturbances
- Galactosemia
- Galactokinase deficiency
- Hypocalcemia
- Hypoglycemia
- Diabetes mellitus
- Wilson disease
- Fabry disease
- Refsum syndrome
- Mannosidosis

Associated with muscular disease
- Myotonic dystrophy

Associated with embryopathies
- Rubella
- TORCH association (toxoplasmosis, rubella, cytomegalovirus, herpes virus, and syphilis)

Associated with drug therapy
- Corticosteroid

The primary care physician is in an ideal position to work with the ophthalmologist in the workup of systemic associations of cataracts such as galactosemia, Lowe syndrome, TORCH association, and others. In addition, the primary care practitioner provides valuable support for parents through the period of patching and contact lens manipulation, recognizing that this is a very difficult time for many parents who expected to be bonding with their child in an entirely different manner.

Upon discharge from the hospital, the physician should be alert for a cloudy cornea (which may indicate a secondary glaucoma), hemorrhage in the eye, or red eye with a discharge. If any of these conditions is noted, the operating ophthalmologist should be contacted immediately.

CONGENITAL GLAUCOMA

The primary care physician should suspect congenital glaucoma in a child with photophobia, tearing and enlarged corneas, a red eye, a cloudy cornea, breaks in the cornea (Haab striae) (Fig 96–2), and with a positive family history.

As with congenital cataract, the mainstay of therapy demands early diagnosis and early therapy. Present surgical techniques involve creating a channel between the anterior chamber and Schlemm canal by incision of the trabecular meshwork. It is uncertain whether children with congenital glaucoma have an imper-

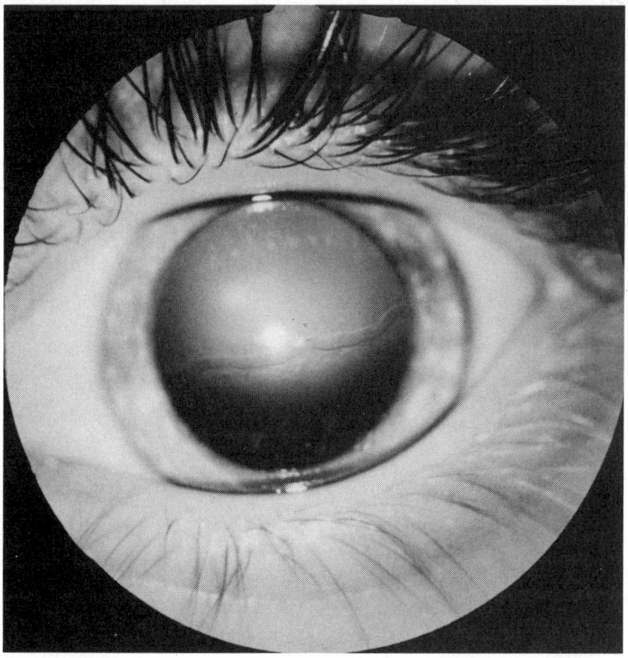

FIG 96–2
Haab striae (breaks in cornea) in patient with congenital glaucoma. (Courtesy of David Schaffer, M.D.)

forate membrane blocking aqueous outflow or whether faulty attachments of the muscle of the ciliary body are to blame.

Surgery precedes an overnight stay in the hospital if the child is younger than 3 months of age. If the patient is older, the procedure usually is performed on an outpatient basis. A patch and shield are placed on the eye postoperatively; often, a topical steroid and antibiotic eyedrops are prescribed. The ophthalmologist usually examines the child each day for a week following surgery, then approximately every three months thereafter. Examination under anesthesia will be performed until evaluation of the optic nerve and intraocular pressure can be accurately ascertained with the child awake. It should be noted that in approximately 50% of cases of congenital glaucoma, it is necessary to repeat the surgery.

Since the management of congenital glaucoma in a child is lifelong (a significant percentage of these children will develop secondary glaucoma as teenagers or young adults), the primary care physician's role is crucial in participating with the ophthalmologist in the care of the patient and providing support to the family. In addition, preoperative control of pressure with osmotic agents or acetazolamide (Diamox) may be necessary. As in the case of congenital cataract, the primary care practitioner is in a position to collaborate on the workup of systemic associations of glaucoma, such as Lowe syndrome, aniridia, Sturge-Weber syndrome, and neurofibromatosis.

The primary care physician should examine the postoperative patient for red eye with discharge, return of presenting signs and symptoms of congenital glaucoma, and increased irritability in the child. If any of these conditions appears, the ophthalmologist should be consulted without delay.

RETINOBLASTOMA AND RHABDOMYOSARCOMA

The two ophthalmic conditions presenting to the primary care practitioner that have potentially life-threatening consequences are retinoblastoma and rhabdomyosarcoma. A patient with a retinoblastoma often presents with leukokoria (white pupil) and should be referred for ophthalmologic examination. Other causes of leukokoria are as follows: congenital cataract, choroidal coloboma, retinoblastoma, persistent hypertrophic primary vitreous (PHPV), Norrie syndrome, Coats disease, *Toxocara*, cloudy cornea, retinopathy of prematurity, and toxoplasmosis.

Any child with a poor red reflex or in whom fundus details cannot be examined should be considered to have a retinoblastoma until proved otherwise. The majority of patients present at 5 years of age or less, although there are cases that have been described at later age. Retinoblastoma can present as strabismus in a young child if the visual axis is compromised by tumor.

Rhabdomyosarcoma is an orbital tumor that presents in an older child, commonly between the ages of 6 and 10 years. It is often a rapidly progressive lesion causing proptosis and signals immediate referral. With increasingly effective radiation therapy and chemotherapy available, the prognosis for saving of life is much improved, so timely referral may have a significant effect on outcome.

BIBLIOGRAPHY

Beller R, Hoyt CS, Marg E et al: Good visual function after neonatal surgery for congenital monocular cataract. *Am J Ophthalmol* 1981; 91:559.

de Luise V, Anderson D: Congenital glaucoma. *Surv Ophthalmol* 1983; 28:1.

Hiles DA, Carter BJ: Classification of cataracts in children. *Int Ophthalmol Clin* 1977; 17:15.

Parks MM: *Ocular Motility and Strabismus*. Harper and Row, New York, 1975.

97 ORTHODONTICS

James L. Ackerman, D.D.S.

The several million children receiving orthodontic care in the United States today represent only about 15% of patients who could benefit from this therapy. The purpose of this chapter is to help the primary care practitioner recognize orthodontic problems, make the necessary referral to an orthodontist, and have a basic understanding of the rationale of orthodontic treatment. More specifically, this chapter will discuss how the patient's medical history impacts on orthodontic treatment and how orthodontics can affect the patient's overall health.

MALOCCLUSIONS

In the transition from the edentulous state of the neonate to the complete primary dentition at approximately 3 years of age to the complete permanent dentition (with the exception of the permanent third molars) at age 12 years, environmental influences on the development of the dentition and heritable factors lead to a variety of abnormalities that require orthodontic consultation. In the normal anteroposterior relationship of the gum pads in the neonate, the mandible is somewhat posterior to the maxilla. Parents rarely recognize this anteroposterior disproportion between the maxilla and the mandible since it causes no symptoms, unless it is severe as in the case of the Pierre Robin syndrome. Occasionally, when the maxillary and mandibular primary incisors have fully erupted by age 1 year, the parent might note that when the child closes the jaws the mandibular incisors bite in front of the maxillary incisors (anterior crossbite or underbite) (Fig 97–1). Although in an older child an anterior crossbite is justification for seeking an orthodontic consultation, at this early phase it is often merely a habit or imitative of a parent. It is wise to ask the parents if anyone in the family, including older siblings, has an anterior crossbite. This often offers a clue as to whether this trait is an early manifestation of mandibular prognathism or maxillary hypoplasia that will require orthodontic or even surgical correction at a later date. Abnormal bite relationships in the primary dentition do not occur with great frequency so it is unusual to have to seek an orthodontic consultation for a child under 3 years of age unless there is a severe craniofacial abnormality.

Crowding of the permanent teeth is the most common form of malocclusion (Fig 97–2). When the primary teeth emerge, spacing between the primary teeth is normal. If interdental spacing does not exist, the permanent teeth, which are much larger, will emerge in a crowded and overlapped position. The primary care physician should be wary of the patient whose primary dentition looks "too perfect," whose mother admiringly notes that her child has "beautiful baby teeth." Perfectly aligned and nonspaced primary teeth are often a clue that there will be crowding problems later in the development of the permanent dentition. Other factors involved in attaining good alignment of the permanent teeth include the comparison between the widths of the primary teeth (Fig 97–3) and their permanent successors as well as jaw growth. There is little increase in the transverse dimension of the dental arches once the permanent first molars erupt at approximately age 6 years. The greatest dimensional arch changes that take place are when the accessional teeth erupt (permanent teeth without primary tooth counterparts, i.e., the permanent first and second molars) adding arch

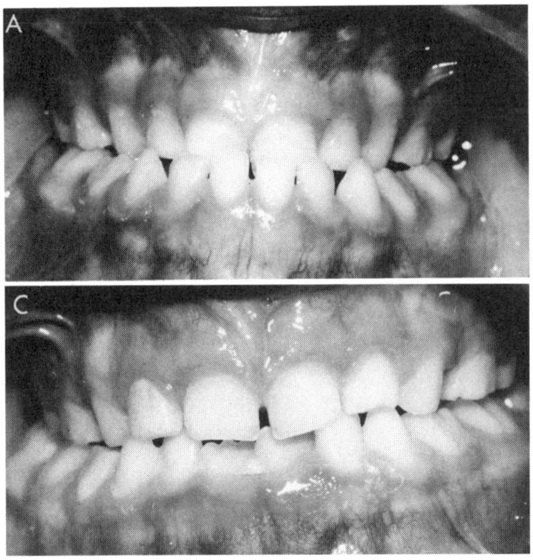

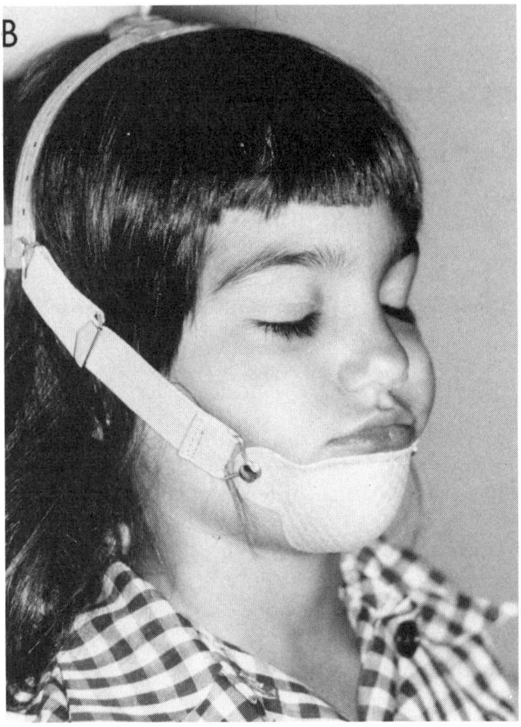

FIG 97–1
A, anterior crossbite in the primary dentition. Note that the mandibular primary incisors are anterior to the maxillary primary incisors. **B,** in some cases a chin cup is effective in treating anterior crossbite in the primary dentition. **C,** same patient as in **A,** 1 year after chin-cup wear. Note that mandibular permanent central incisors have erupted. Chin cups are used when mild mandibular prognathism is the cause of the anterior crossbite.

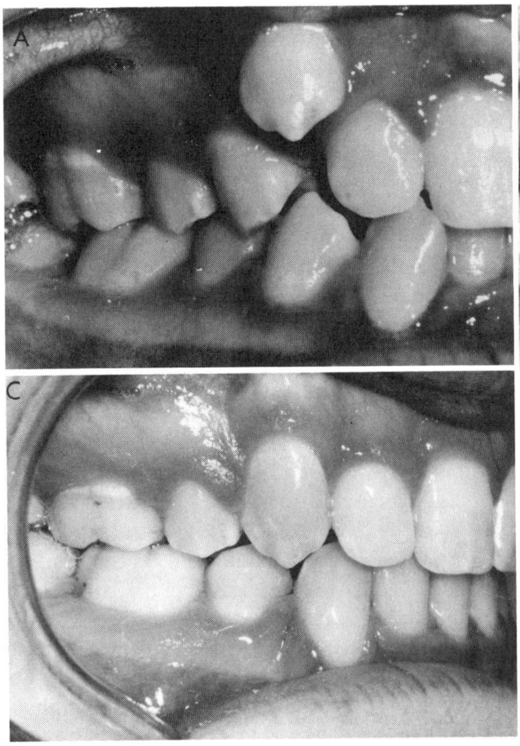

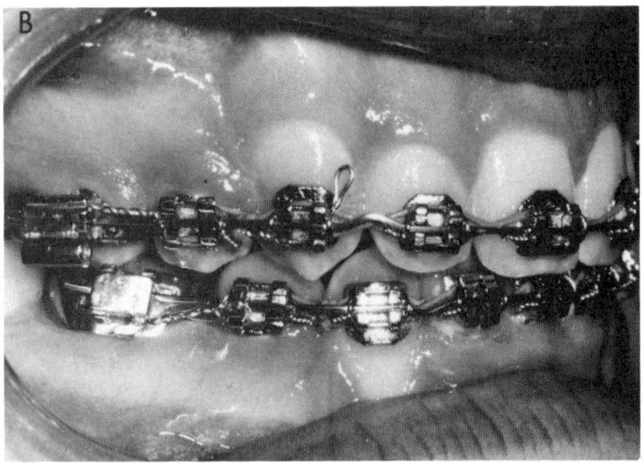

FIG 97–2
A, crowding occurs when there is insufficient arch perimeter available in the dental arch to accommodate all of the permanent teeth. In this example of a common problem, the maxillary permanent canine is completely "blocked out" of the dental arch and has erupted ectopically. **B,** in this patient, first premolar teeth were extracted to relieve the crowding. Permanent canine teeth, no matter how badly malaligned, are rarely extracted for orthodontic purposes. **C,** alignment of teeth after the orthodontic appliances were removed. Treatment time was approximately 2 years.

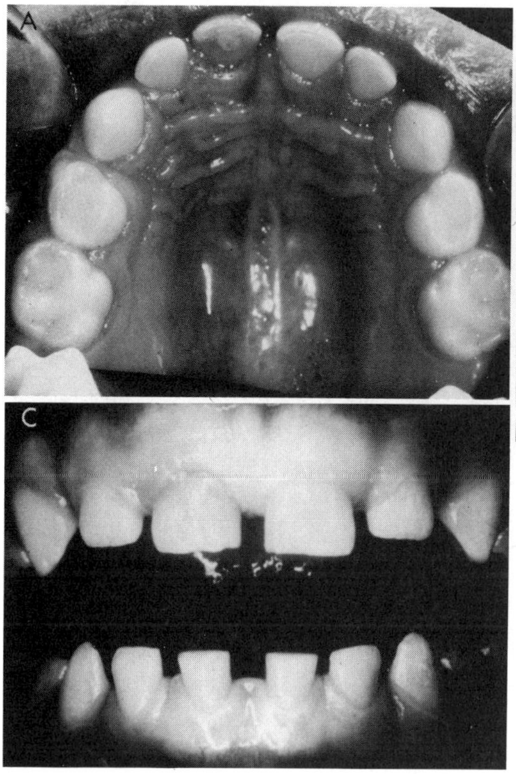

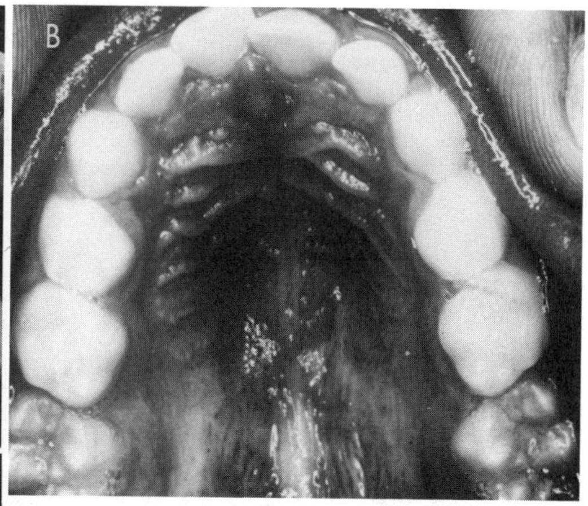

FIG 97–3

A, interdental spacing of maxillary primary anterior teeth is prerequisite for well-aligned successional permanent incisor teeth. **B,** patient with no interdental spacing of the maxillary primary anterior teeth. One can predict with some assurance that this patient will have crowding of the permanent incisor teeth when they emerge. **C,** patient with excessive interdental spacing of the primary teeth. Depending on the size of the succedaneous permanent incisors, this patient may also have spacing in the permanent dentition.

length at the posterior portion of the dentition. Since bone does not grow interstitially, there is no increase in the length of the anterior portion of the dental arches due to growth once the primary molar teeth emerge.

Crossbite problems (either anterior or posterior) in the primary dentition should be referred to an orthodontist, since early correction of these problems is sometimes quite simple and can prevent the development of more serious problems at a later date (Fig 97–4). It is unlikely that the primary care physician would have much need to consult an orthodontist about a patient until the patient is approximately 6 or 7 years of age. A question often asked of the primary care physician relates to the eruption of the mandibular permanent incisors, which normally develop lingually to the mandibular primary incisors and often erupt in this position prior to exfoliation of the primary incisors. Commonly, the primary care physician or dentist receives a call from a mother who has discovered that her child has "a double row of teeth." Often in this circumstance, it is necessary to extract the overretained primary teeth. If there is sufficient space, normal tongue pressure alone usually guides the lingually displaced permanent teeth into their positions in the dental arch (Fig 97–5). If there is sufficient space for the erupting permanent incisors, additional primary teeth may have to be removed, more or less "robbing Peter to pay Paul." This procedure should only be done after careful evaluation by an orthodontist, since this procedure of "serial extraction" often leads to the necessity of extracting permanent teeth at a later date to establish the desired esthetic and functional goals of the orthodontic treatment (Fig 97–6).

During the ages of approximately 7 to 9 years, the primary care physician might be queried most by the mothers about developing orthodontic problems, since it is at this point that malocclusion is first easily recognized by the parent. When maxillary permanent lateral incisors erupt, the crowns of these teeth may appear displaced because the developing unerupted maxillary permanent canines normally press on the lateral portion of the roots of the erupted permanent lateral incisors, causing the teeth to tip. This stage of dental development, the "ugly duckling" phase, often corrects

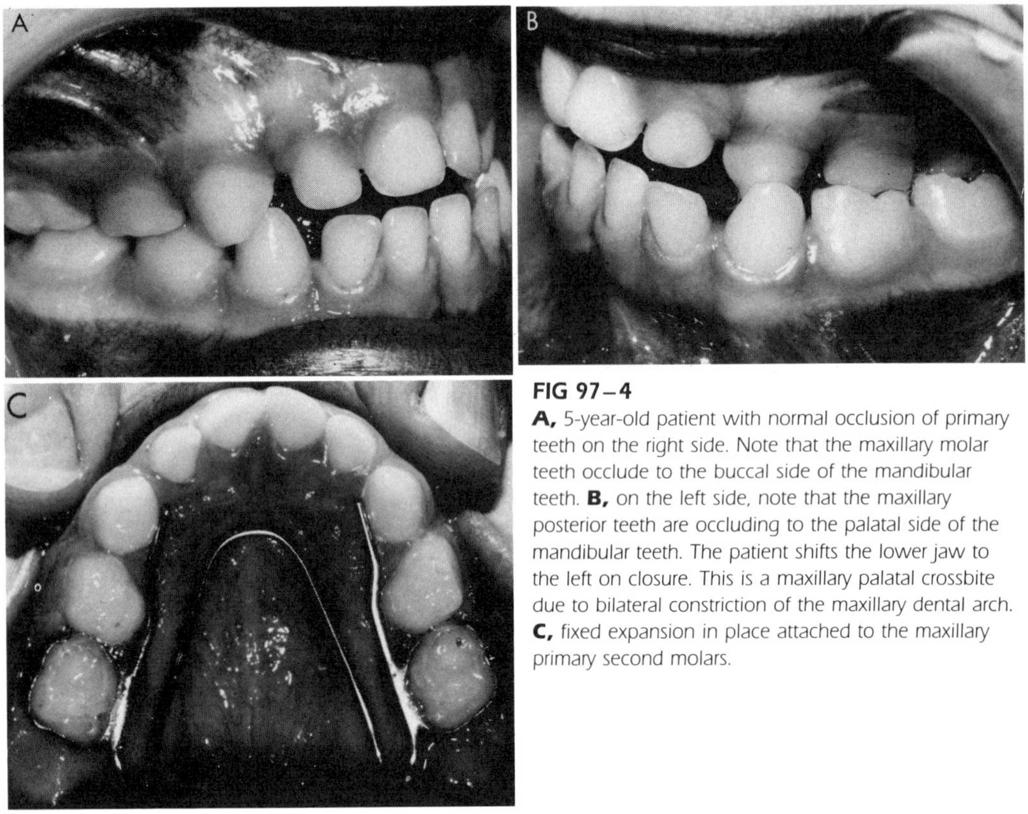

FIG 97–4

A, 5-year-old patient with normal occlusion of primary teeth on the right side. Note that the maxillary molar teeth occlude to the buccal side of the mandibular teeth. **B,** on the left side, note that the maxillary posterior teeth are occluding to the palatal side of the mandibular teeth. The patient shifts the lower jaw to the left on closure. This is a maxillary palatal crossbite due to bilateral constriction of the maxillary dental arch. **C,** fixed expansion in place attached to the maxillary primary second molars.

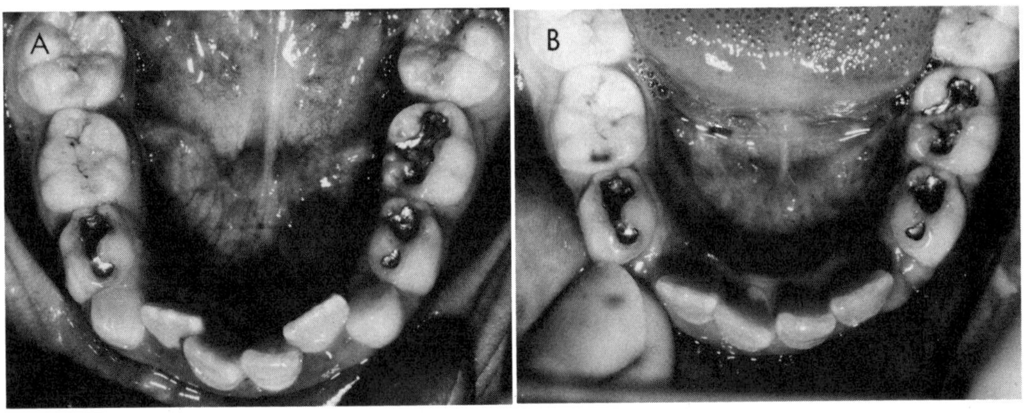

FIG 97–5

A, anterior arch perimeter deficiency in the early transitional dentition. When there is insufficient space, mandibular permanent lateral incisors erupt ectopically to the lingûal side. **B,** mandibular primary canine teeth have been removed and autoalignment of these teeth has occurred due to the molding effect of tongue and lip pressure. This approach amounts to "robbing Peter to pay Paul," since ultimately there will probably be insufficient space for the mandibular permanent canines.

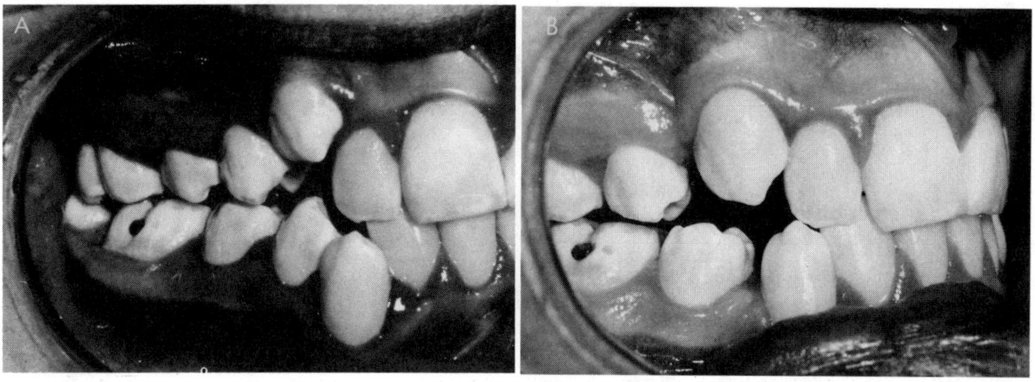

FIG 97–6
A, example of serial extraction shows that if the first premolar teeth are extracted at the propitious time, the ectopically erupting canines often spontaneously drift into the correct position. **B,** note the absence of the first premolars and the nearly complete extraction space closure from the result of serial extractions without orthodontic appliance therapy. The vast majority of serial extraction cases do require fixed orthodontic appliance therapy to achieve optimal tooth positions.

itself as the rest of the permanent teeth emerge. Maxillary permanent canines sometimes become impacted and simply do not emerge at age 12 or 13 years when they are due to erupt. These teeth can become impacted in the palate or can also be impacted on the facial side of the alveolar ridge. Permanent canine teeth are important teeth, from an esthetic as well as functional point of view. As a result, orthodontists generally recommend that these teeth be surgically exposed and an orthodontic attachment be bonded to the tooth (Fig 97–7). With orthodontic traction, the tooth can gradually be brought into its normal position in the dental arch.

Another common concern among parents of children in the transitional or mixed-dentition stage (some primary and some permanent teeth) relates to the space, or diastema, which occurs normally between the newly emerged maxillary permanent central incisors. Unless there is an exceptionally thick band of tissue (frenum) that is preventing the natural mesial drift of the permanent incisor teeth (Fig 97–8), or unless the maxillary permanent incisors are unusually small, this space will close naturally, particularly when the maxillary permanent canines emerge at approximately age 11½ years in girls and 12½ years in boys.

There is a wide range of variation in terms of the timing of tooth eruption. In general, girls are somewhat more advanced than boys in terms of their dental age. Dental age may vary by as much as a year or two when compared with the chronologic age, giving a very low correlation between dental age and skeletal age.

In general, if the child's orthodontic problem relates to a disproportion in the size or position of the jaws, the referral to an orthodontist should be made on the basis of skeletal age, since part of the treatment may involve an attempt to achieve facial growth modification. On the other hand, if the orthodontic problem is one relating to tooth position and either intra-arch spacing or crowding, the orthodontic referral perhaps should be made on the basis of the dental age.

Just as the maxillary posterior teeth can be occluding palatally in relationship to the mandibular molar teeth, the opposite condition, whereby the mandibular molars are occluding too far lingually in relationship to the maxillary molars, can also occur. Thus, there are a number of different types of crossbites that can occur unilaterally or bilaterally and can occur between individual antagonist teeth or can include entire segments of the dental arch. Long-term crossbites cause abnormal loading forces on the teeth, which can ultimately cause stresses within the supporting structures of the teeth leading to periodontal problems. Crossbites can also cause deflection of the mandible while biting, which can cause stress on the temporomandibular joints. This problem can ultimately lead to pain and dysfunction in the jaw joints. Many individuals maintain excel-

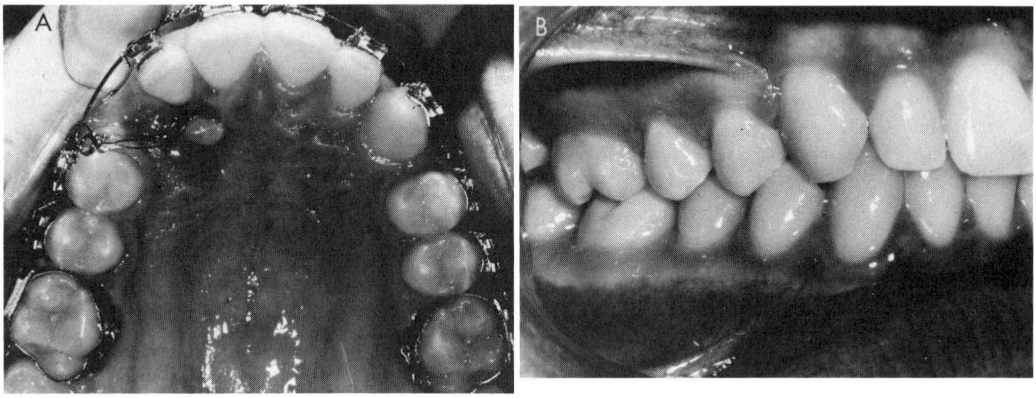

FIG 97–7
A, palatally inpacted permanent canine surgically exposed and orthodontic appliances applying traction to the tooth to bring it into the dental arch. **B,** orthodontic appliances are removed when the permanent canine has achieved a good esthetic and functional position.

lent oral health throughout life with severe crossbites, and the judgment of whether these problems should be corrected requires careful analysis of the problem. The common, easily recognizable orthodontic problems are those that relate to the anteroposterior dimension or the sagittal plane (Fig 97–9).

The vertical dimension must be considered when defining malocclusion. The major categories of bite problems in the vertical dimension are anterior open bite (Fig 97–10), in which there is insufficient vertical overlap of the anterior teeth, and anterior deep bite, in which the mandibular incisors are biting too deeply toward the palate, often impinging on the palatal mucosa (Fig 97–11). It is also possible to have a posterior open bite, in which the maxillary and mandibular teeth are not in contact. Problems in the vertical dimension can be caused by skeletal disproportion or merely insufficient dental compensation for an underlying skeletal dysplasia.

There is an enormous range of variations for jaw positions and some patients who are at the outer limits of the normal range of jaw disproportion often have quite normal dentition based on natural dental compensation that can occur from the positions and inclinations of the teeth. On the other hand, some patients whose jaw proportions are seemingly more harmonious and proportional can have severe malocclusion based on the malpositions of the teeth themselves in all three planes of space. From an epidemiological point of view, only a small segment of the population has ideal occlusion. Thus, in many respects, malocclusion must be

FIG 97–8
In this patient a hypertrophied maxillary labial frenum has prevented the natural closure of a midline diastema. When the maxillary permanent canines erupt they usually exert a mesial force, which closes this space. Frenectomies are rarely performed for hypertrophied maxillary labial frenum unless it is in conjunction with orthodontic treatment.

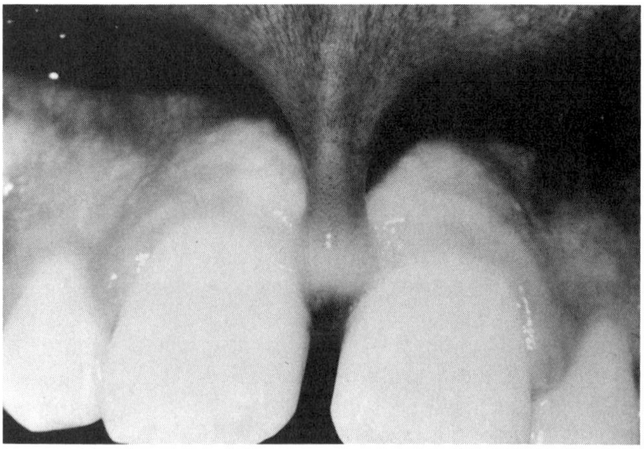

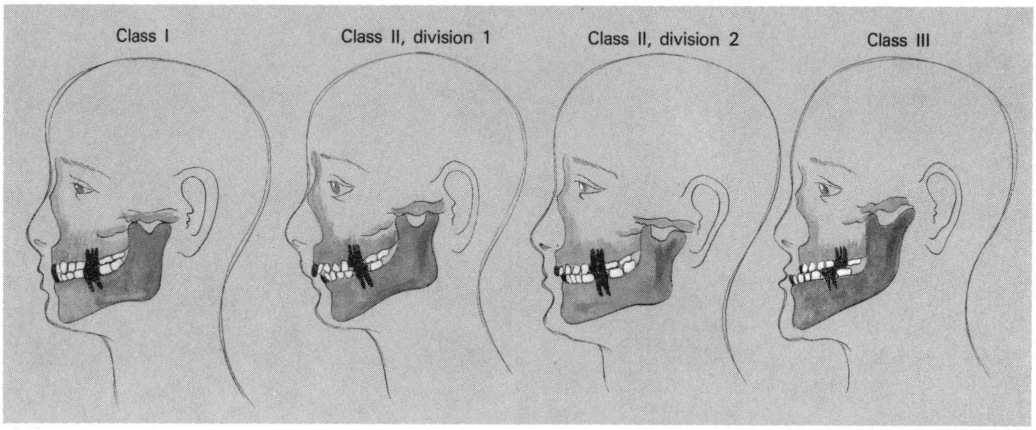

FIG 97–9
Malocclusion is classified according to the anteroposterior relationships of the teeth (i.e., the relationship of the permanent first molars). Angle (1898) described three major types of malocclusion: class I, normal occlusion but crowding of teeth; class II, upper teeth forward; class III, lower teeth forward. (Courtesy of T.M. Graber.)

considered as the usual rather than the unusual finding in a pediatric population and the decision as to whether orthodontic treatment is indicated is based on dentofacial esthetics, psychosocial factors, and functional considerations.

TREATMENT

There are three basic modalities for treating malocclusion and dentofacial deformity. The first of these is orthodontic tooth movement alone, the second is redirecting the growth of the jaws as well as regulating the positions of

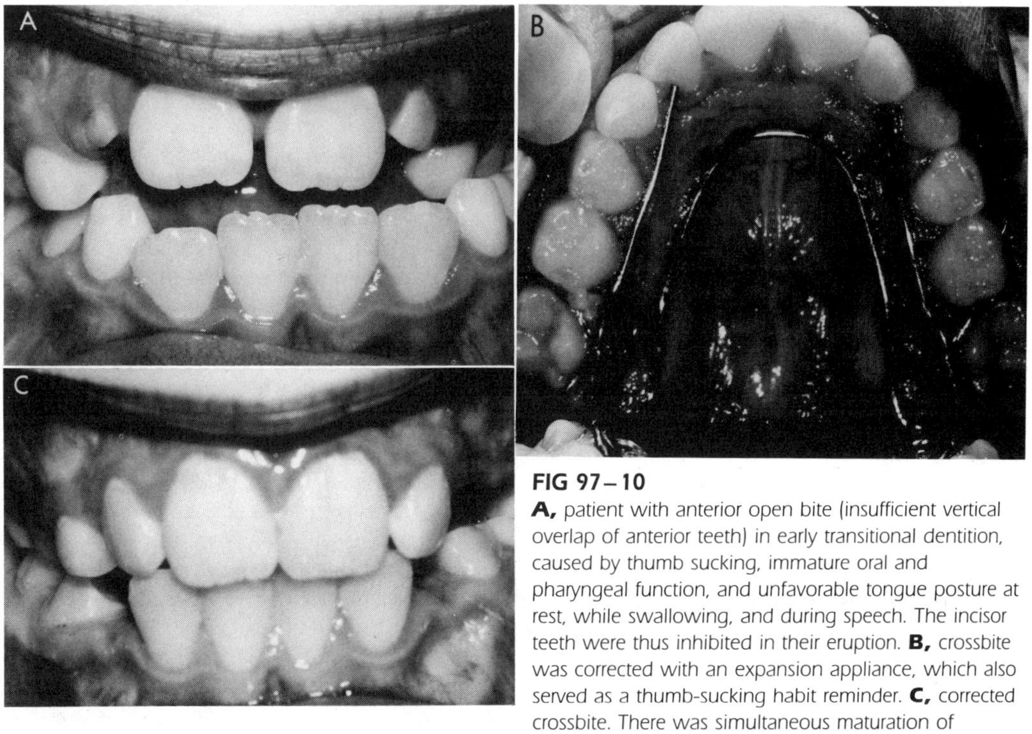

FIG 97–10
A, patient with anterior open bite (insufficient vertical overlap of anterior teeth) in early transitional dentition, caused by thumb sucking, immature oral and pharyngeal function, and unfavorable tongue posture at rest, while swallowing, and during speech. The incisor teeth were thus inhibited in their eruption. **B,** crossbite was corrected with an expansion appliance, which also served as a thumb-sucking habit reminder. **C,** corrected crossbite. There was simultaneous maturation of oral-pharyngeal function.

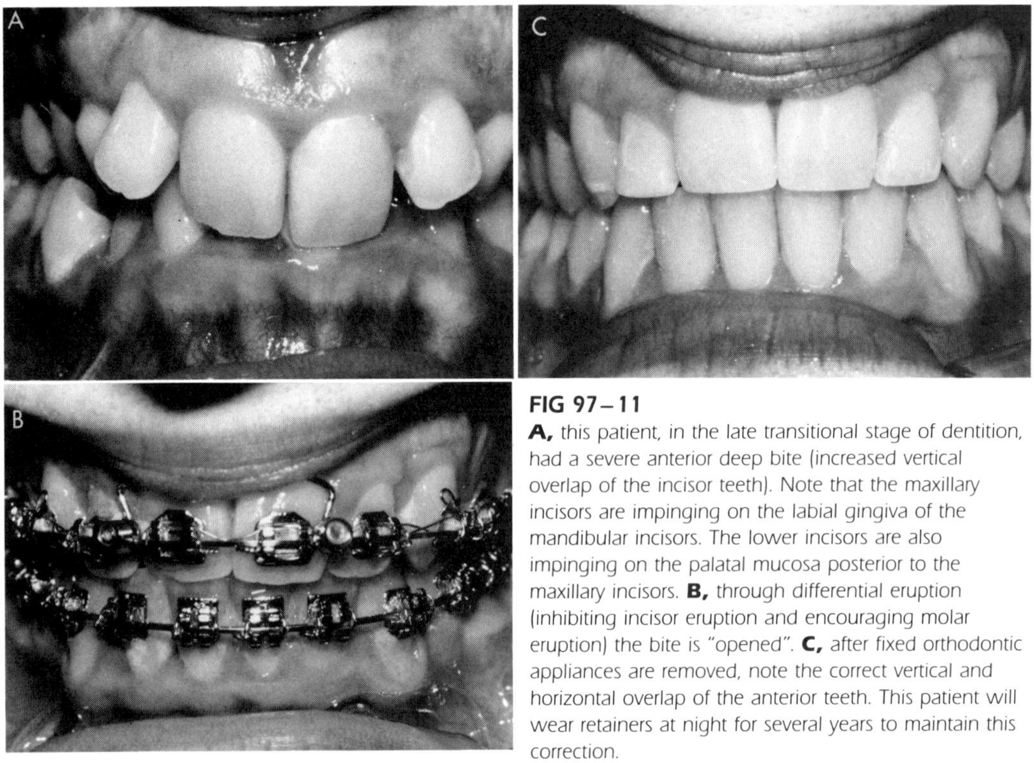

FIG 97–11
A, this patient, in the late transitional stage of dentition, had a severe anterior deep bite (increased vertical overlap of the incisor teeth). Note that the maxillary incisors are impinging on the labial gingiva of the mandibular incisors. The lower incisors are also impinging on the palatal mucosa posterior to the maxillary incisors. **B,** through differential eruption (inhibiting incisor eruption and encouraging molar eruption) the bite is "opened". **C,** after fixed orthodontic appliances are removed, note the correct vertical and horizontal overlap of the anterior teeth. This patient will wear retainers at night for several years to maintain this correction.

the teeth, and the third is the utilization of surgical techniques for repositioning the jaws in conjunction with orthodontic tooth movement. The nature and degree of the deformity and the age of the patient (growth potential) help determine which mode of treatment is selected.

The simplest type of treatment, preventive and interceptive orthodontics, is utilized when there is some event or insult to the developing dentition that, if not modified, will certainly lead to a malocclusion. A good example of such an event is the early loss of a primary molar tooth, which would allow the mesial drift of the posterior teeth, leaving insufficient space for eruption of the successional tooth. If indicated, an appliance called a *space maintainer* can be placed on the adjacent teeth to hold the space where the primary tooth was lost. On the other hand, if a primary tooth has been lost prematurely and some of these unfavorable sequelae have already occurred, a simple appliance can sometimes be utilized to regain the space. This mode of treatment is called interceptive orthodontics. Once the early treatment is performed, no further therapy will be required on the remaining permanent teeth. Thus, preventive and interceptive orthodontic treatment is usually performed in the primary and transitional dentitions, and its goal is to achieve a substantial result with minimal effort.

Orthodontic tooth movement is based on the principle that the force applied to the crown of a tooth is transmitted to the periodontal ligament, which is interposed between the root surface (cementum) and the lamina dura of the dentoalveolus. Since all these tissues are cellular, the resulting differential apposition and resorption that takes place within the tooth socket is mediated by cellular responses. The periodontal ligament consists of fluid plus fibers that connect the root of the tooth to the alveolar bone. Thus, the periodontal ligament acts as a type of "shock absorber," which is both suspensory and hydraulic in nature. The periodontal ligament and the suspensory apparatus of the tooth seems particularly well-designed to resist the normal type of forces that are applied to the teeth, which is along their long axis during mastication. The forces of mastication are usually quite strong but are of an intermittent nature. If, on the other hand, a

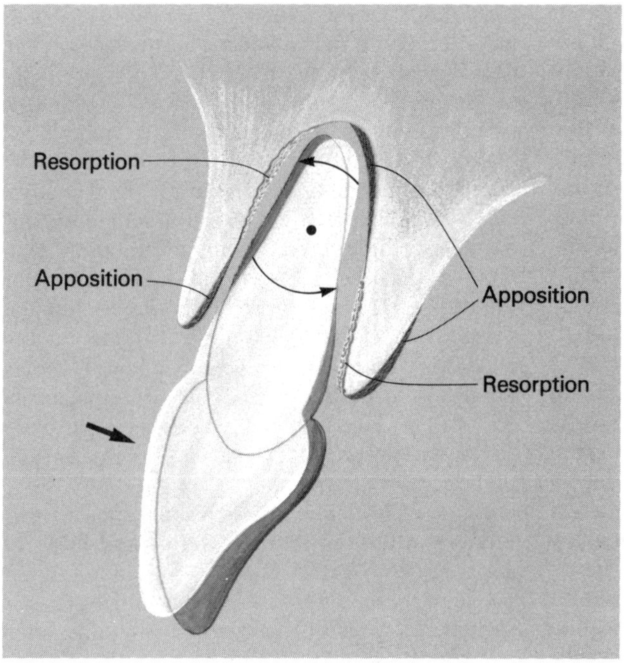

FIG 97–12
Diagram of the tissue reaction to orthodontic tooth movement, where differential apposition and resorption at the tension and pressure sites causes the tooth socket to "drift" slowly along with the movement of the tooth. (Courtesy of T.M. Graber.)

light continuous force is applied to the tooth, particularly if it is in an eccentric direction, adaptive changes take place within the alveolar bone and the tooth drifts along with the tooth socket (Fig 97–12). Cells in the cementum of the root cause resorption of the tooth root, but the cellular activity on the alveolar bone surface is much more labile and the osteoclastic and osteoblastic activity at the alveolar bone level operates at a more rapid rate than does the resorption of the root. If the opposite were true, it is obvious that orthodontic tooth movement would not be a possibility. In the most simple type of orthodontic tooth movement, which is the tipping of a tooth, there is a center of resistance; along the alveolar wall on the compression side of a periodontal ligament there is osteoclastic activity, and on the tension side there is osteoblastic activity. This is the mechanism whereby the suspensory mechanism of the tooth in the alveolar bone remains intact during orthodontic tooth movement. The most biologic manner for orthodontically moving a tooth results from the application of light, continuous force. These pressures can be applied to the teeth through either removable appliances or fixed appliances. The removable appliances are constructed of acrylic and wire and can incorporate a variety of springs and levers to apply the light, continuous forces to the teeth. Since the forces of removable appliances can only be applied to a single point on each tooth, one is only able to tip the teeth. With this method, there is only a minimal amount of control of individual tooth movement.

Since the patient must be willing to wear the appliance on a full-time basis, patient compliance is a major consideration with this treatment. Fixed appliances, the major type of orthodontic treatment, consist of bands usually constructed of stainless steel that are fitted and adapted to the tooth and cemented with a luting medium such as zinc phosphate cement. These bands have welded attachments consisting of tubes or brackets in which wires can be engaged for applying more controlled force to the tooth. The other method of attaching brackets to teeth is direct bonding, in which an adhesive is used to directly adhere the bracket to the tooth. With fixed appliances, arch wires of stainless steel or titanium alloys are used to apply controlled forces to the teeth. It is the relative strength, stiffness, and range of these wire elements that allow the orthodontist to control the magnitude, direction, and distance over which these forces operate.

COMPLICATIONS

These mechanical devices can be quite physically irritating to the oral mucosa. If a patient has a predilection for aphthous ulcers he can have considerable discomfort during the firs week to 10 days that he is wearing orthodontic appliances. Palliative treatment such as warm saline rinses, the use of benzocaine in Orabase, and the use of soft wax over any element of the appliance that is particularly sharp can minimize the discomfort to the oral soft tissues Within several weeks, almost all patients adapt to even the most complex types of orthodontic appliances. When the appliances are placed, particularly when small elastomeric units called separators are placed in between the teeth to gain room for applying the orthodontic bands, and when the bands themselves are fit, there is a transient bacteremia that occurs due to the trauma to the teeth. If a patient has a health history of rheumatic fever or congenital heart disease, which places him at risk to this type of transient bacteremia, prophylactic antibiotics should be prescribed.

Root resorption is another hazard of orthodontic treatment. Almost all patients who have had orthodontic tooth movement do demonstrate minor signs of root resorption on radiographs. In some cases, as much as a quarter to a third of the root can be lost through root resorption. Appliances make maintenance of good oral hygiene difficult. Decalcification of the enamel adjacent to the orthodontic band or bracket may occur if the plaque and debris are not removed thoroughly at least once a day. Many orthodontists prescribe a fluoride mouth rinse that is utilized daily for 1 minute after the patient has brushed his teeth to further prevent decalcification of the enamel. If this decalcification proceeds sufficiently, there can actually be cavitation of the enamel surface, which requires restoration of the tooth after the orthodontic appliances are removed. The gingiva can become hypertrophied and inflamed during treatment (Fig 97–13). Although this particular sequela usually resolves spontaneously once the orthodontic appliances are removed, under some circumstances, the gingival inflammation can cause increased resorption of the alveolar bone and can, under unusual circumstances, lead to periodontal defects. Patients at puberty, particularly girls, seem more prone to this type of gingival hypertrophy.

When orthodontic appliances are placed and forces applied to the teeth, the patient initially experiences a great deal of tooth tenderness, particularly on palpation (such as during mastication). As a result, for the first few days after orthodontic appliances are placed, the patient should eat a soft diet and take acetaminophen or aspirin.

Forces applied to the teeth are also transmitted through the jaws to growth sites considerably removed from the teeth themselves and, as a result, orthodontic force systems can have an effect on facial sutures, synchondroses, the mandibular condyle, and other growth sites. When an orthodontist is attempting to accomplish this type of growth redirection, usually stronger forces are used, and often the anchors for such forces are extraoral (such as headgear, facial masks, and chin cups). If the maxilla is

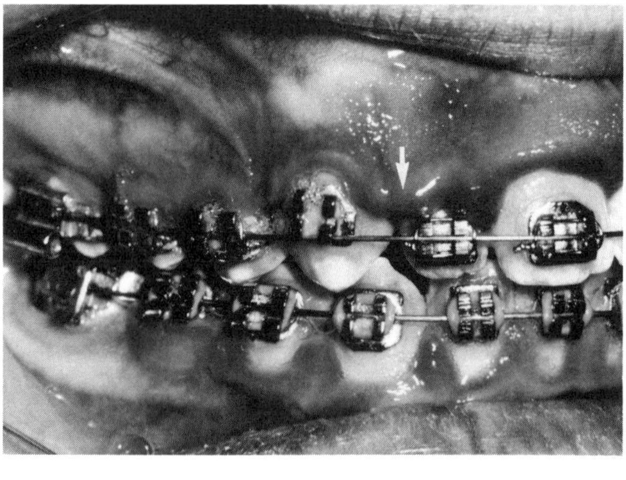

FIG 97–13
Gingivitis, partly attributable to mouth breathing. The additional gingival irritation from the appliance and space closure compressing the gingiva leads to further inflammation and hypertrophy of the tissues.

extremely constricted, under some circumstances an orthodontist might use a fixed appliance with a screw in the midline of the palate, which causes rapid separation of the two halves of the maxilla. Over a period of several weeks after this rapid separation, bone fills in the midpalatine suture. This type of orthopedic device often sounds quite radical to parents, and frequently they will consult with their primary care physician about the wisdom and efficacy of such an appliance.

In a late adolescent sometimes there is a skeletal disproportion and facial imbalance that is sufficiently great to warrant surgical repositioning of one or both jaws to improve both facial esthetics and oral function.

MYOFUNCTIONAL THERAPY AND ORTHODONTICS

Since form and function in the oral-pharyngeal area is important in the development of the dentition and the overall growth of the craniofacial complex, it is not surprising that the issue of swallowing and speech has received considerable attention as it relates to oral architecture. It is currently thought that the infantile pattern of swallowing and speech in which the tongue is placed in a forward position, interposed between the anterior teeth and in approximation with the lip, is an early maturational feature. At some point, the child goes through a transition in which a more adult pattern of tongue posture both at rest and in swallowing and speech is adopted. The adult pattern is thought to be with the tongue tip posterior and superior to the maxillary anterior teeth, without the tongue protruding or thrusting in between incisor teeth during speech or swallowing. The more immature pattern has been called "tongue thrusting," and speech therapists and orthodontists over the past two decades have developed an approach that attempts to correct this immature oral-pharyngeal function. The method is called myofunctional therapy and consists of a series of exercises that the child practices to overcome this "habit." Both the American Speech and Hearing Association and the American Association of Orthodontists have taken the position that there is little evidence that myofunctional therapy is efficacious, and that more research is required before this method can be embraced as a clinical tool that should be widely used. Surely, there are patients for whom myofunctional therapy is useful, and those patients are usually ones whose speech problems are also the result of immature oral and pharyngeal function. At the present time, the view of the orthodontist is that the best approach to these patients is to change the architecture of the mouth so that the improved function will follow the new form. Since there has been greater utilization of surgical correction of jaw position in severe malocclusions, the clinical results have led orthodontists to the expectation that, in many patients, function can follow form of the jaw.

On the other hand, American orthodontists have begun to use removable orthodontic appliances, which have been popular in Europe for nearly 50 years and are called *functional appliances*. The purpose of these appliances is to alter oral function in an attempt to redirect the growth of the jaws. Unlike the heavy forces used with orthopedic devices to inhibit growth, these appliances attempt to alter muscle activity and jaw posture in such a way as to stimulate and redirect jaw growth. Since most of these appliances are toothborne, they also, obviously, cause considerable orthodontic tooth movement; over the years there has been considerable debate as to whether their greatest effect is as tooth-moving devices or in redirecting growth of the jaws. There is some evidence that over a short time interval, such as a year or two, there can be changes in skeletal proportions created by these appliances. Whether these changes are permanent and what the implication is for the ultimate configuration of the craniofacial complex in these children is yet to be determined. Nonetheless, these appliances have become popular in the United States and, unfortunately, there are more extravagant claims being made about the efficacy of these appliances than the evidence would support.

When patients are utilizing removable orthodontic appliances, these appliances should not be worn during active play and sports. As well, if fixed appliances are being worn, a special mouth guard to protect the lips from trauma should be utilized while playing active sports.

When orthodontic appliances are removed, there is a tendency for physiologic rebound or recovery (relapse) to occur, and the teeth have a tendency to move in the direction of their original positions. As a result, retaining devices (which are made of acrylic and wire) are worn either full-time or just at night for some period of time after the fixed orthodontic appliances are removed. These devices hold the teeth in their corrected positions and serve as a template to ascertain whether the teeth are shifting. Very little relapse is required before a retainer becomes tight and, as a result, the patient has an early warning signal that his teeth are not maintaining their original corrections. In some instances, fixed retainers are utilized rather than removable retainers (Fig 97–14).

THE VISIT

When a patient is referred to an orthodontist, the first visit usually consists of an initial evaluation in which the orthodontist performs an oral examination and thoroughly reviews the medical/dental history. Based on these initial findings, the orthodontist usually recommends that orthodontic records be taken, which consist of impressions of the teeth to make plaster models that carefully reproduce the anatomy of the oral structures, facial and intraoral photographs, intraoral roentgenograms, and a cephalometric roentgenogram. The cephalometric roentgenogram is taken in norma lateralis at a fixed anode-to-target distance and can be used for ascertaining the nature of the orthodontic problem based on skeletal proportions. These roentgenograms can be taken at intervals and the patient's craniofacial growth and development can be studied by superimposing tracings of the roentgenograms. The results of treatment and growth can also be ascertained using the same clinical tool.

With increasing concern of the public regarding diagnostic roentgenograms, the orthodontist is being asked more frequently whether it is necessary to take roentgenograms as part of the diagnostic regimen. Because of the complex nature of the developing dentition and the fact that many patients can profit from early treatment, there is no alternative at the present time other than to take a survey series of dental roentgenograms to establish a proper orthodontic diagnosis and treatment plan. Issues such as congenital absence of teeth, supernumerary teeth, impacted teeth, cysts, and other pathologic conditions, as well as just the normal sequence, position, and timing of eruption of teeth, are factors that cannot be ascertained in any other way other than with roentgenograms.

In all of the health sciences, the risks of treatment must be weighed against the benefits. Orthodontics is no exception. When orthodontic treatment is elective, it may be decided that it is inadvisable due to one or more aspects of the patient's health history. For some patients orthodontics is mandatory, such as those with craniofacial and dentofacial anomalies as well as those with other handicapping orthodontic conditions. For these patients, especially those

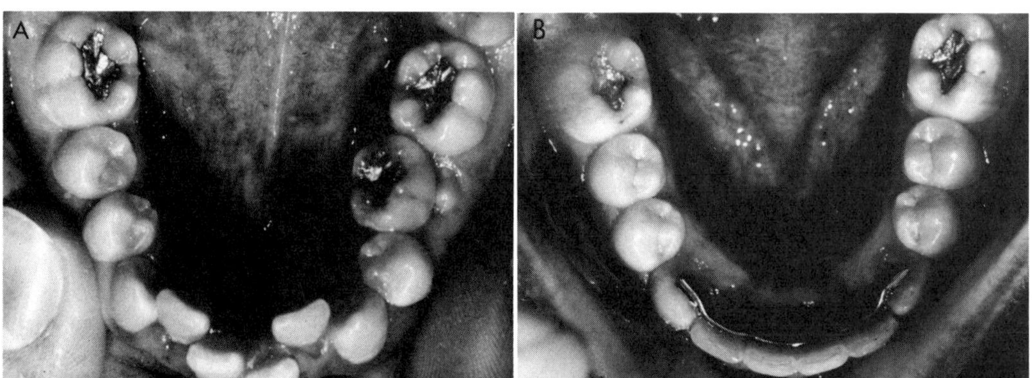

FIG 97–14
A, malaligned mandibular incisors. **B,** after orthodontic correction, it is not uncommon for the patient to wear a bonded mandibular canine-to-canine fixed retainer. There is a greater tendency for mandibular incisor teeth to become crowded, and these fixed retainers are sometimes left in place until the fate of the mandibular third molars (wisdom teeth) is determined, which usually occurs during college years.

with other health problems, close cooperation between the primary care physician and various specialists can reduce the complications of orthodontic treatment.

BIBLIOGRAPHY

Epker BN, Fish LC: *Dentofacial Deformities: Integrated Orthodontic and Surgical Correction*. St Louis, CV Mosby Co, 1986.

Forrester DJ, Wagner ML, Fleming J: *Pediatric Dental Medicine*. Philadelphia, Lea & Febiger, 1981.

Graber TM, Swain BF: *Orthodontics: Current Principles and Techniques*. St Louis, CV Mosby Co, 1986.

Proffit WR: *Contemporary Orthodontics*. St Louis, CV Mosby Co, 1986.

98 OTOLARYNGOLOGY

Ralph F. Wetmore, M.D.

Frequently, primary care physicians share responsibility for their patient's care with an otolaryngologist. The primary care physician with a better understanding of the management of an otolaryngologic problem is better able to coordinate the patient's overall treatment and communicate more effectively with the patient and his family. In this section, the following topics will be discussed: (1) diagnostic evaluation of hearing loss, (2) management of ear ventilation tubes, (3) current indications for tonsillectomy and adenoidectomy, (4) management of a foreign body of the upper aerodigestive tract, and (5) management of a chronic tracheostomy.

DIAGNOSTIC EVALUATION OF THE CHILD WITH HEARING LOSS

The three major categories of hearing loss include (1) conductive, (2) sensorineural, and (3) mixed. An accurate determination of the type of hearing loss has important implications for prognosis and management.

A conductive hearing loss can result when sound is impeded at any point from the external auditory meatus to the footplate of the stapes. This may include a cerumen impaction of the external canal, a perforation of the tympanic membrane, or a disruption of the ossicular chain. Conductive hearing losses are often reversible by medical or surgical therapy.

Damage to the cochlea, the cochlear nerve, or the brain stem may result in sensorineural hearing loss. This type of loss may be secondary to infection, metabolic abnormality, or genetic transmission. With rare exceptions, most cases of sensorineural hearing loss are not reversible. A mixed hearing loss has both conductive and sensorineural components. Each component can be evaluated and treated separately.

An audiogram, including both pure-tone and speech thresholds, remains the keystone in the evaluation of hearing loss (Fig 98–1). In children, the skill of the audiologist and the age and cooperation of the subject determine the accuracy of the test. Hearing loss greater than 20 dB is abnormal and should be referred to an otologist for further evaluation.

The evaluation of a child with conductive hearing loss begins with a detailed history, including its duration, previous occurrence, and presence of a recent ear or upper respiratory

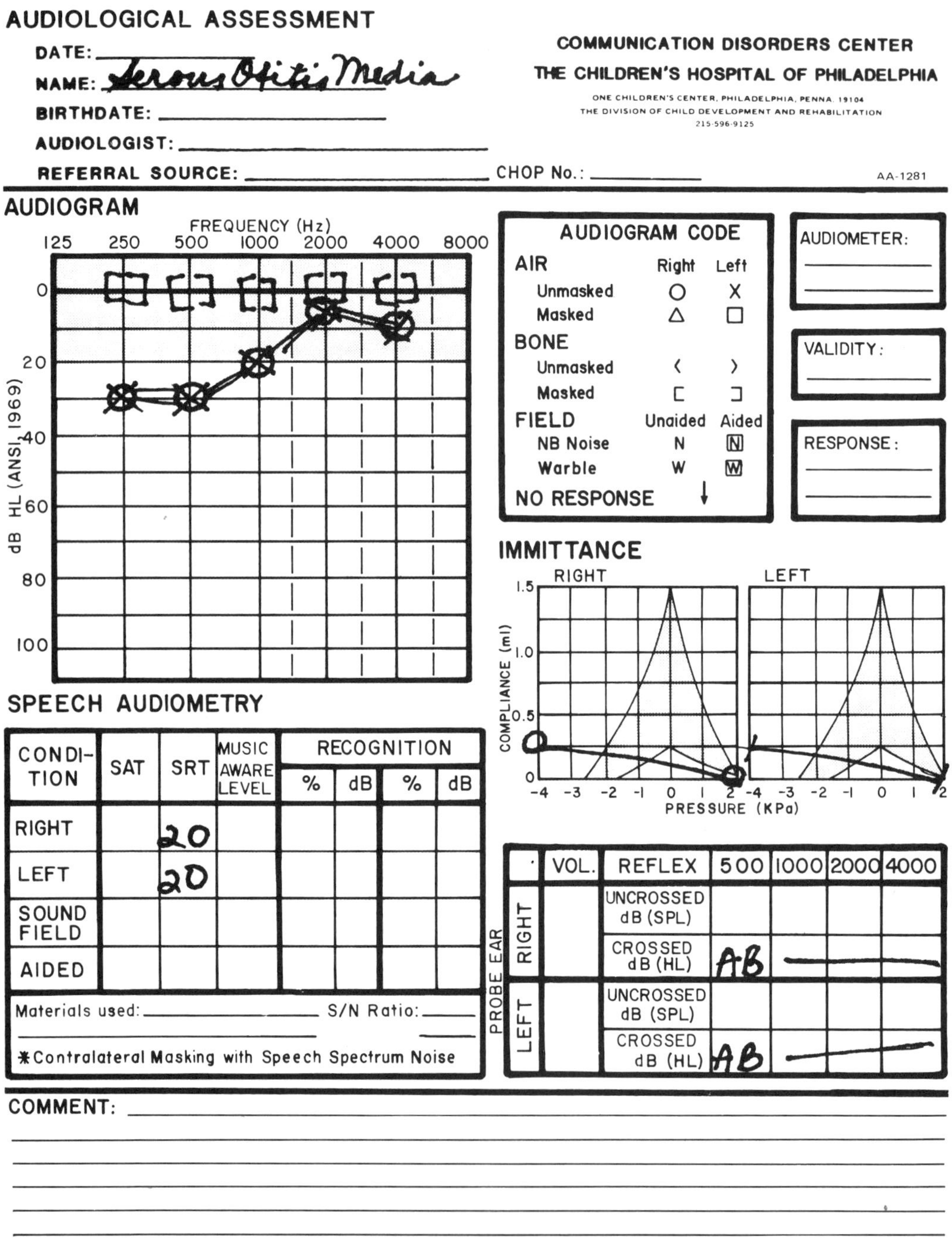

FIG 98–1

Hearing test. Decreased air conduction in 250 to 1,500 Hz range. Tympanogram on both sides shows a flat curve, indicating minimal tympanic membrane motility.

tract infection. Physical examination of both ears should be made with attention to possible occlusion of the external canal with either cerumen or a foreign body. A tympanic membrane perforation or evidence of infection such as purulent drainage may also result in a conductive hearing loss. Assessment of tympanic membrane mobility by pneumatic otoscopy is crucial in the evaluation of a conductive hearing loss. Tuning-fork testing (Weber and Rinne) can be used to confirm a unilateral conductive hearing loss. In the Weber test, the sound produced by the tuning fork will lateralize to the ear with the conductive hearing loss. By demonstrating that bone conduction is louder than air conduction in the Rinne test, one can verify a conductive, as opposed to a sensorineural, hearing loss.

In addition to an audiogram, which should confirm the amount of the conductive hearing loss, additional information can be obtained by impedance audiometry (tympanometry), an additional method of quantitating tympanic membrane mobility (Fig 98–2). Normal mobility is indicated by a type A curve, with the peak at O. An A_D curve has an extremely high peak, characteristic of hypermobility of the tympanic membrane. This finding may occur in the presence of an ossicular discontinuity or with a very atrophic tympanic membrane. An A_S curve has a shallow peak, indicative of stiffness of the tympanic membrane. This may be seen in conditions such as otosclerosis or tympanosclerosis. B (or flat) curves demonstrate little or no tympanic membrane mobility, such as seen in otitis media with effusion. C curves peak in the negative-pressure range, indicating varying degrees of eustachian tube dysfunction.

Occasionally, additional confirmation of conductive hearing loss in a young or difficult-to-test child may require brain-stem evoked response audiometry. Brain stem audiometry does not require subjective responses from a patient to determine the level of auditory acuity. Objective data obtained by this procedure can support routine audiometry.

Evaluation of sensorineural hearing loss also includes a complete medical history with special attention to episodes of meningitis, major neurologic insults, or family history of hearing loss. Otologic examination in most cases of sensorineural hearing loss is normal. Routine audiometry confirms and quantitates the degree of

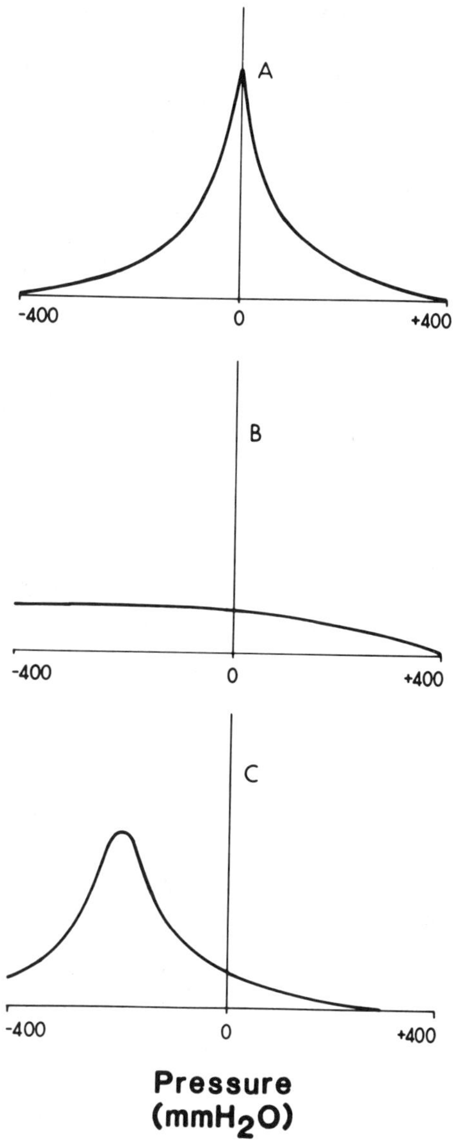

FIG 98–2

Tympanogram types: *1*, normal curve; *2*, B curve (seen with middle ear effusion); *3*, C curve (seen with eustachian tube dysfunction).

hearing loss. In infants, brain-stem audiometry can supplement behavioral testing. Brain stem audiometry is also useful in the difficult-to-test or malingering patient. Tympanometry is usually normal in a purely sensorineural hearing loss although the stapedial reflex may be absent if a substantial loss is present.

Sensorineural hearing losses follow one of

several audiometric patterns. With flat losses, all frequencies are affected equally. A sloping high-frequency loss consists of a progressive increase in hearing loss with an increase in testing frequency. The development of high-powered audio and stereo equipment has increased the susceptibility of adolescents to noise-induced hearing loss. Depending on the intensity and duration of exposure, this type of loss may be temporary or permanent. Noise-induced hearing loss produces a characteristic sloping pattern, with the greatest loss at 6,000 Hz.

In most children with a sensorineural hearing loss, the etiology cannot be determined. Metabolic abnormalities affecting hearing may be discovered by a series of tests including: complete blood cell (CBC) count, urinalysis, serologic analysis, serum lipids determination, thyroid function studies, and serum glucose determination. A mastoid radiologic series may pinpoint genetic abnormalities of the cochlea.

MANAGEMENT OF THE CHILD WITH EAR VENTILATION TUBES

The child with tympanostomy tubes need not have any restrictions of activity other than avoidance of water in the ears. Because tympanostomy tubes provide ventilation of the middle ear cavity, children with functioning tubes should have no difficulty adjusting to changes in pressure, such as that experienced on airplane flights.

Because cerumen tends to collect lateral to the tympanic membrane, it rarely blocks the tympanostomy tube. Blockage of tubes occurs when attempts at cleaning may force cerumen deeper into the canal and obstruct the tube. Superficial amounts of cerumen may be carefully debrided in most children with a cerumen curet. The pinna can be pulled in a posterior-superior direction, exposing the external meatus. The lateral portion of the canal may then be inspected and cleaned. With large or deep impactions, use of eardrops, such as those normally used for infection in the patient with tubes (e.g., Cortisporin Otic Suspension, a polymixin B-neomycin-hydrocortisone suspension), may prove helpful. *Use of hydrogen peroxide drops or irrigation with water should be avoided.*

The participation of children with ventilation tubes in water activities remains controversial. Some otologists recommend complete avoidance of such exposure to water, although most tend to allow such participation if care is taken to prevent infection of the tubes. The use of earplugs or molds provides an excellent method of excluding water from the ear canal. The other option is to place an antibiotic eardrop in the ear canal after exposure to water.

The management of ear drainage in the child with tubes usually includes either oral antibiotics, antibiotic eardrops, or both. Strict avoidance of water exposure should be practiced until the drainage has stopped. Failure of the ear to clear within 2 weeks on such a regimen should signal the need for an otologic referral. On occasion, a tympanostomy tube will become blocked with dried secretions. Antibiotic eardrops may prove useful in such situations to restore patency of the tube.

CURRENT INDICATIONS FOR TONSILLECTOMY AND ADENOIDECTOMY

While tonsillectomy and adenoidectomy have been widely practiced for over a century, no definite criteria have ever been established as absolute indications for surgery. Recurrent infection remains one of the major indications for tonsillectomy and adenoidectomy. This includes recurrent episodes of either tonsillitis, adenoiditis, or adenotonsillitis. Because it may be difficult to obtain cultures prior to beginning antibiotic therapy, documentation of recurrent bacterial infections with positive throat cultures is often lacking. In some patients, cultures remain negative even in the presence of a bacterial infection. Infection deep within the tonsillar crypts is often difficult to culture and completely eradicate with antibiotics. This failure to clear the infection may account for complaints of chronic sore throats in the absence of clinical signs of infection.

Prior to the development of ear ventilation tubes, adenoidectomy or tonsillectomy and adenoidectomy were widely practiced in the treatment of recurrent acute otitis media and otitis media with effusion. While tympanostomy tubes remain the standard surgical treatment for otitis media, one recent study has demonstrated the efficacy of adenoidectomy in the management of chronic otitis media with effusion.

Chronic upper airway obstruction provides another major indication for tonsillectomy and adenoidectomy. Obstruction may be due to adenoid, tonsillar, or adenotonsillar hypertrophy. Symptoms of upper airway obstruction are often more prominent during sleep. Loud snoring is indicative of partial obstruction, while complete obstruction may result in apnea. Sleep disturbances including abnormal positions and enuresis are not uncommon. Chronic mouth-breathing, hypersomnolence, complaints of dysphagia, and failure to thrive are the major daytime symptoms of chronic airway obstruction. Since many children have minor obstructive problems with large tonsils and adenoids, the point at which these problems become serious enough for surgery is subjective and judgmental. Most patients with severe obstruction have relief after surgery; the majority of patients with mild-to-moderate symptoms improve with no treatment.

Formerly, tonsillectomy was recommended in all patients with peritonsillar abscess, several weeks after the infection cleared. This recommendation was based on a presumed significant recurrence of abscess formation. More recent studies have shown this recurrence rate to be lower than suspected. Tonsillectomy should be considered when peritonsillar abscess fails to respond to aggressive antibiotic therapy or if the patient has a history of recurrent tonsillitis.

In rare situations, significant tonsillar asymmetry or other symptoms suggestive of a tumor within a tonsil are also indications for tonsillectomy. Although some tonsillar asymmetry may be present as a result of infection, sudden enlargement of one tonsil in the absence of infection is highly suggestive of neoplasm. In children, the occurrence of tonsillar neoplasm is rare.

Occasionally, a child may have large tonsils without symptoms of chronic upper airway obstruction or recurrent infection. In these cases, tonsillectomy is usually not indicated, because the lymphoid tissue will decrease as the child ages.

MANAGEMENT OF FOREIGN BODY IN THE UPPER AERODIGESTIVE TRACT

The child who has aspirated a foreign body that has lodged in the larynx or upper trachea, producing partial airway obstruction, typically presents with dyspnea and stridor. There may or may not be a witness to the aspiration or a history consistent with such an event, e.g., choking, gagging, or acute paroxysms of coughing. No attempts to dislodge the foreign body should be made, as this may result in complete obstruction of the airway. If the situation permits, a radiologic evaluation, including lateral neck and chest radiographs, may prove helpful; however, the child should be accompanied by a physician at all times during these studies. At the same time, a referral should be made to a physician skilled in airway management.

If a partial obstruction is converted to a complete obstruction, a potentially fatal situation develops. Management of complete obstruction remains controversial at the present; some favor a Heimlich maneuver, while others suggest the use of a physical slap to the midportion of the back. During such a critical event, both should probably be used to try to convert a complete obstruction to a partial one.

The child with a foreign body of the lower trachea or bronchus will also have a history of choking, gagging, or coughing. Nuts, raw vegetables, and popcorn are commonly aspirated materials. Physical examination of the chest frequently reveals diminished breath sounds and wheezing over the affected lung areas. A chest radiograph may demonstrate a radiopaque object. The presence of a radiolucent foreign body may be more difficult to confirm. A hyperlucent lung field distal to a radiolucent foreign body may be demonstrated by fluoroscopy, comparison of inspiratory and expiratory radiographs, or failure of the mediastinum to shift on a decubitus film. A child with a suspected upper respiratory tract foreign body should be referred to an endoscopist skilled in its removal.

The child with a foreign body lodged in the esophagus may also present with a history of gagging and choking. There may also be an inability to swallow secretions. An object located high in the esophagus may press on the larynx from a posterior position, causing stridor. Some children may point to the area of the neck in which they feel the sensation of the foreign body; however, this is not a valid indication of where the foreign body is located.

The initial evaluation should include lateral neck and chest radiographs. These may confirm the presence of a radiopaque object. Air in the upper esophagus may provide a clue to a radiolucent foreign body in that region. A barium swallow may also help to pinpoint radiolucent objects, but a negative study does not always exclude a foreign body. As with foreign bodies of the airway, suspicion of an ingested foreign body can only be excluded definitely by an endoscopic evaluation of the esophagus.

MANAGEMENT OF THE CHILD WITH A CHRONIC TRACHEOSTOMY

Although many parents and even some physicians fear caring for the child with a tracheostomy, anxiety may be reduced by good training and adherence to a few basic principles of chronic care.

While plastic tracheostomy tubes have replaced those made of metal, there are still physicians who favor tubes made of stainless steel or silver. Metal tubes have the advantage of possessing an inner cannula, which can be removed periodically for cleaning without replacing the entire tube. Today, most pediatric tracheostomy tubes in use are made of plastic, which can either be disposed of when soiled or cleaned and resterilized (Fig 98–3). To prevent stomal infection, tracheitis, or occlusion with secretions, tracheostomy tubes should be changed on a regular basis.

Cloth tapes with foam rubber lining are the best material for securing the tracheostomy tube. In small children who are prone to decannulation, a harness can be fashioned with cloth tapes under the axillae to secure the tube more adequately.

Routine tracheostomy care usually consists of daily cleaning of the tracheostomy stoma with either water or half-strength hydrogen peroxide. Soiled tracheostomy strings can be changed as necessary. Suctioning need not be done at regular time intervals, but rather as needed if the patient is having difficulty clearing secretions. Because the tracheostomy bypasses the nose and pharynx, which normally warm and humidify the inspired air, use of a

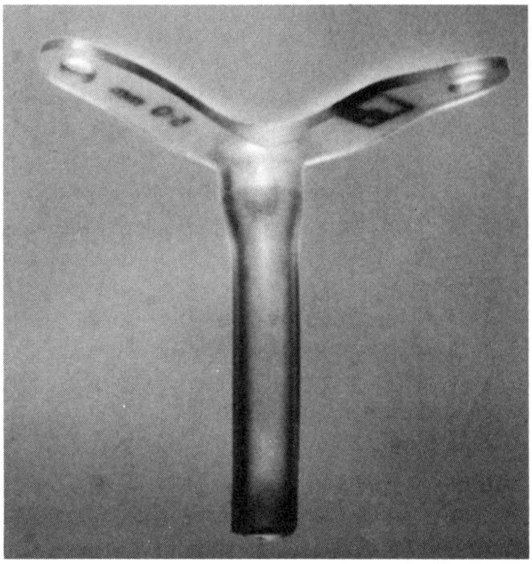

FIG 98–3
Plastic tracheotomy tube.

humidifier is recommended to help thin secretions and prevent excessive drying of the tracheal mucosa (Fig 98–4).

The major problems with a chronic tracheostomy include maintaining the patency of the

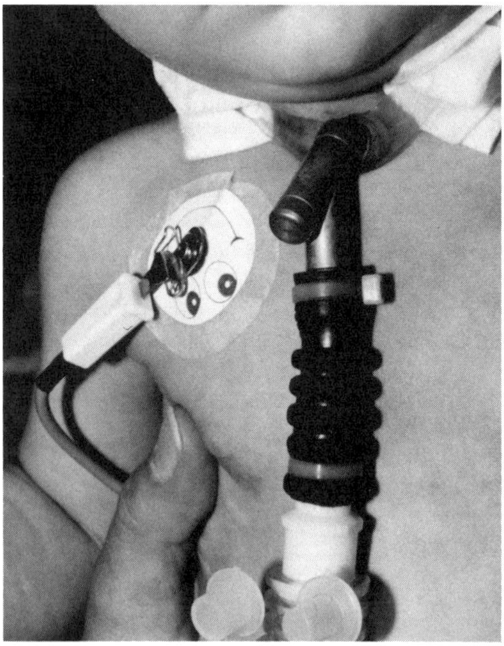

FIG 98–4
Swivel atachment connects tracheotomy tube to humidifier.

airway and managing infection. Accidental decannulation and plugging of the tracheostomy tube with secretions are the usual causes of airway occlusion and tracheostomy-related mortality. Most problems with accidental decannulation occur soon after the tracheostomy has been performed, before the stoma has matured. Even in a child with a mature tracheostomy site, decannulation of the tube may result in severe hypoxia or death. To avoid such a calamity, a family member or friend skilled in tracheostomy care, including tube replacement, should always be near a child who has a chronic tracheostomy. Use of a pulse oximeter or cardiorespiratory monitor at night or when the child cannot be closely observed may provide an early warning of airway problems.

Plugging of the tracheostomy tube may occur if secretions are allowed to collect and crust within the tube. Dyspnea and noisy breathing are early signs of occlusion and indicate a need for tube replacement. Routine tracheostomy care, including humidification, suctioning, and periodic changing of the tube, and treatment of infection tend to prevent acute plugging.

Infection of the tracheostomy stoma is usually indicated by erythema and crusting of purulent secretions around the tube. Mild infections can be treated with antibiotic ointment, while more serious involvement requires a systemic antibiotic. Since the pathogen is frequently *Staphylococcus aureus*, antibiotic therapy should include coverage for this organism. Skin lacerations caused by the tracheostomy tapes can be managed best with a dressing, to prevent further irritation and to keep the area dry.

Tracheitis, an acute bacterial infection of the trachea, occurs in patients with a chronic tracheostomy. Diagnosis is made by the development of purulent tracheal secretions. Fever and radiographic evidence of infection may or may not be present. A Gram stain of secretions will show the presence of both bacteria and polymorphonuclear leukocytes. A culture of secretions will often indicate a predominant organism. Humidification and appropriate systemic antibiotics are the keystones of management.

BIBLIOGRAPHY

Gates GA, Avery CA, Prihoda TJ, et al: Effectiveness of adenoidectomy and tympanostomy tubes in the treatment of chronic otitis media with effusion. *N Engl J Med* 1987; 317:1444–1451.

Gates GA, Avery C, Prihoda TJ, et al: Delayed onset post-tympanotomy otorrhea. *Otolaryngol Head Neck Surg* 1988; 98:111–115.

Jackson C: Foreign bodies in the air and food passages. *Otolaryngology* 1983; 5:1–94.

Kennedy AH, Johnson WG, Studevant EW: An educational program for families of children with tracheostomies. *Maternal-Child Nurs* 1982; 7:42–49.

Laks Y, Barzilay Z: Foreign body aspiration in childhood. *Pediatr Emerg Care* 1988; 4:102–106.

Line WS, Hawkins DB, Kahlstrom EJ, et al: Tracheostomy in infants and young children: The changing perspective 1970–1985. *Laryngoscope* 1986; 96:510–515.

Luxford WM, Sheehy JL: Myringotomy and ventilation tubes: A report of 1,568 ears. *Laryngoscope* 1982; 92:1293–1297.

Meyerhoff WL: Symposium on hearing loss—The otolaryngologist's responsibility. Medical management of hearing loss. *Laryngoscope* 1978; 88:960–973.

Paradise JL: Tonsillectomy and adenoidectomy, in Bluestone CD, Stool SE (eds): *Pediatric Otolaryngology*. Philadelphia, WB Saunders Co, 1983, pp 992–1006.

99 UROLOGY

William Tarry, M.D.
Howard Snyder, M.D.

Management of urologic problems changes as concepts are modified and evaluations are undertaken. The purpose of this chapter is to discuss the present understanding of common urologic problems that are encountered in a primary care physician's practice. These include ureteral reflux, use of the cystoscope, circumcision, cyptorchidism, meatal stenosis, and dysfunctional voiding. These topics are presented so that the physician will be aware of the potential treatments and have a better understanding of the approach taken by the urologist when caring for these patients.

VESICOURETERAL REFLUX

Urinary tract infection (UTI) is one of the most common bacterial infections of childhood. The treatment of UTI in children is discussed in Chapter 60. Every child with a UTI should undergo voiding cystourethrography (VCU) and intravenous pyelography or renal ultrasound (US) after the urine has been sterilized.

Because of the frequency of vesicoureteral reflux, many urologists and nephrologists recommend a VCU after the first infection. The initial VCU assesses the status of the bladder and urethra, ruling out obstructing lesions such as posterior urethral valves, diaphragms, and strictures. It documents the presence and severity of vesicoureteral reflux (VUR), and demonstrates trabeculation and diverticula that suggest outlet obstruction. To ensure the most accurate assessment of the degree of reflux, the cystogram should be obtained with the child awake and the radiographs should be taken at the time of peak flow of the voiding phase. The cystogram may not give reliable information about bladder size or postvoid residual urine. Many children do not empty completely on each voiding, and many will experience a reflex bladder contraction prior to reaching full capacity.

IVP or renal US will be diagnostic in most cases of obstructing lesions of the upper urinary tract that can occasionally present with infection. IVP also provides useful information about renal scarring, renal size, and interval growth in patients who have reflux demonstrated on the cystogram. Ureteral duplications and other upper tract abnormalities coexisting with VUR represent complex cases, which are managed on an individual basis by a urologist.

Reflux is the most common abnormality discovered in the radiographic evaluation of a child with an infection, and is one of the most significant congenital anomalies in children in terms of morbidity and long-term disability. In the first year of life, 50% of infants with a UTI will have VUR. Between ages 1 and 16 years, reflux occurs in 15% to 35% of children presenting with a UTI. The remainder of this section will consider VUR and infection in the absence of other anatomic or neurologic lesions.

Vesicoureteral reflux occurs secondary to an abnormality of the ureterovesical junction. The more severe the abnormality, the greater the degree of reflux. As the ureterovesical junction does change with growth of the child until the age of puberty, children may "grow out" of reflux.

Grading the severity of reflux helps to predict the likelihood of spontaneous resolution. The international grading system for reflux and the rates of spontaneous resolution by grade are given in Figure 99-1 and below:

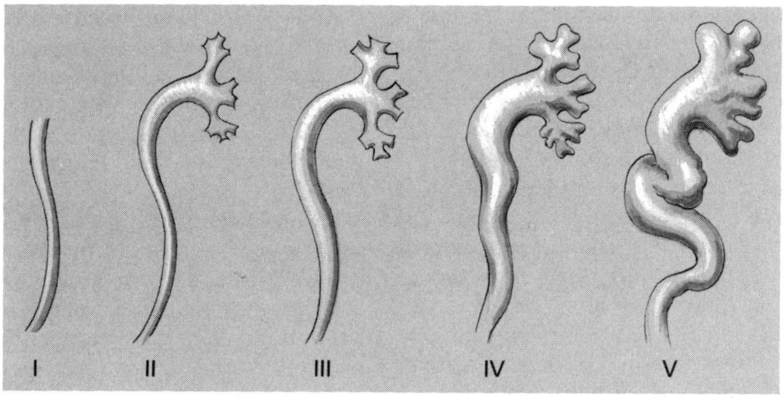

FIG 99–1

International classification of vesicoureteral reflux. Grade I, ureter only. Grade II, ureter, pelvis, and calyces; no dilatation, normal calyceal fornices. Grade III, mild or moderate dilatation or tortuosity of ureter and mild or moderate dilatation of renal pelvis; no or slight blunting of the fornices. Grade IV, moderate dilatation or tortuosity of ureter and moderate dilatation of renal pelvis and calyces; complete obliteration of sharp angle of fornices. Grade V, gross dilatation and tortuosity of ureter; gross dilatation of renal pelvis and calyces; papillary impressions no longer visible in majority of calyces.

GRADE OF REFLUX	RATE OF SPONTANEOUS RESOLUTION (%)
I	85
II	63
III	53
IV	34
V	0

The grading system reflects a combination of aspects of two older systems derived by Perlmutter and Parkkulainen. The system helps the clinician predict the natural history of reflux in a general way; the spontaneous resolution rates observed enable one to pursue the conservative or medical management of reflux with some confidence.

The factors influencing the decision of whether to employ medical or surgical therapy include: grade of reflux, extent of renal scarring, renal growth, compliance, relative cost, family preference, breakthrough infections, and age of patient. If the grade of reflux is III or less, the child has a better than 50% chance of growing out of this problem. As long as the urine can be maintained free from infection, there is little likelihood that reflux will produce renal damage. Medical management of reflux consists of (1) prevention of infection by constant antibiotic prophylaxis; (2) surveillance by quarterly urine culture; and (3) evaluation of progress by periodic radiologic imaging. Prophylactic treatment consists of bedtime administration of one fourth to half of the therapeutic dose of nitrofurantoin or trimethoprim-sulfamethoxazole. Cephalexin, 2-4 mg/kg/day, can also be used. These regimens usually do not alter gastrointestinal (GI) tract flora or lead to monilial infections. Quarterly cultures are necessary because occasional asymptomatic or minimally symptomatic infections may occur. Additional cultures at any time the child exhibits unexplained fever, abdominal pain, or voiding symptoms should be carried out. Fortunately, "breakthrough" infections in children on antibiotic suppression occur in less than 10% of children. The addition of anticholinergic drugs such as oxybutinin (Ditropan) to the regimen in children with reflux and "wetting" problems or other symptoms of an unstable bladder may enhance spontaneous resolution of reflux.

Resolution or progression of reflux may be documented by yearly conventional cystography or nuclear voiding cystography, which, although more costly, has the advantage of providing less radiation exposure. Renal growth and progression of scarring may be monitored by IVP, renal scanning or US. Nuclear and US studies reduce the radiation dose but may be more subject to errors of interpretation unless carried out by radiologists familiar with such studies in children.

The surgical alternative is ureteral reimplantation (Fig 99–2). The advancement techniques (Cohen reimplant) used in most centers today produce excellent success in correcting reflux with minimal complications. IVP and VCU are usually done 3 months after surgery and if the findings appear satisfactory, administration of the suppressive antibiotics is stopped. Although in most cases the 3-month studies will demonstrate a good result, reflux will occasionally persist for up to 1 year after surgery, probably secondary to edema of the trigone area. By 1 year, the success rate should be greater than 95%. Obstruction is exceedingly rare with ureteral advancement techniques; persistent reflux may occur in 2% to 4% of cases but may be corrected by a second reimplantation reimplant. The patient with normal upper tracts probably needs no radiologic follow-up beyond a year after surgery. Those with scars or poor renal growth should be followed up into puberty for changes in size and function, and into adulthood for possible development of hypertension secondary to renal scarring. With unilateral renal scarring, the long-term risk of hypertension is 10%; with bilateral scarring, the risk is 20%. A few infants with poor general health and massive reflux may be managed initially by vesicostomy. The reimplantation and vesicostomy closure may be done safely when continence becomes a concern for them (age 2 to 3 years).

Several factors influence the choice of surgical therapy. In general, increasing grade, progressive scarring, poor growth or compliance, and breakthrough infections lead one toward surgery either at the onset or after a trial of medical treatment. The relative cost of an operation vs. several years of roentgenograms and medications must be considered, as well as the preference of the family and their level of understanding and reliability. Reimplantation is preferable to loss of renal function due to the patient's being lost to follow-up. The question of the prepubertal girl with persistent reflux remains unresolved. Most urologists think that a girl with persistent reflux and a history of infections should undergo reimplantation before child-bearing age, especially if renal scarring is present. This may reduce the risk of pyelone-

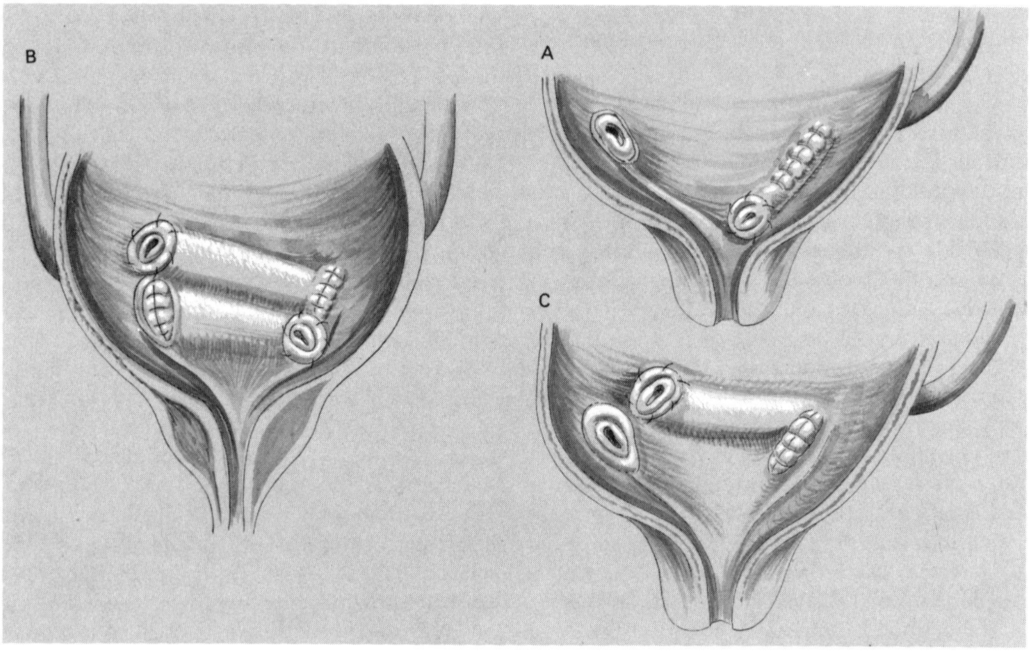

FIG 99–2

Reimplantation procedures. ***A,*** Anderson advancement: Left ureter is moved distally to prevent reflux. ***B,*** Cohen procedure: Bilateral transverse tunnel created by moving left ureter through mucosa to right side and right ureter to left. ***C,*** Cohen procedure: Unilateral reimplantation.

phritis during pregnancy with possible harmful effects on both the mother and fetus.

ROLE OF CYSTOSCOPY IN CHILDREN

The role of cystoscopy in the evaluation of pediatric patients has been steadily declining in recent years. It has traditionally been employed to evaluate hematuria, obstructing lesions, infection, reflux and voiding dysfunctions. With the improvement in radiographic techniques and the advent of new techniques such as US and renal scanning, cystoscopy, along with retrograde pyelography, has lost its place in the workup of many of these entities.

In the past, one of the most common indications for cystoscopy was urinary tract infection, with or without vesicoureteral reflux. At present, vesicoureteral reflux can be diagnosed and graded with careful VCU, and a reliable prediction can be made on that basis as to the likelihood of spontaneous resolution of the reflux. The endoscopic observation of the bladder and ureteric orifices rarely adds any useful information. Data from the Mayo Clinic and Children's Hospital of Philadelphia indicate that in intermediate grades of reflux, the endoscopic judgment of position and shape of the orifice and ureteral tunnel length was only 50% accurate in predicting resolution of reflux. Associated findings such as cystitis cystica, trigonitis, and urethritis do not alter the management in these cases. Urethral stenosis in women is no longer thought to be a cause of infection or reflux, *so that cystoscopy in combination with urethral dilation for recurrent UTI is no longer warranted.*

Cystoscopic evaluation of patients with voiding dysfunctions is unnecessary. The symptoms in this group include enuresis, daytime wetting, frequency, urgency, and dysuria. Positive radiographic findings tend to be confirmed, while patients with normal radiographs have normal cystoscopic examinations. Neither patients with dysfunctional voiding or true neurogenic bladders resulting from myelomeningocele or other spinal cord disorders benefit by cystoscopic evaluation, since adequate information can be obtained from standard radiography and selective urodynamic testing.

Endoscopy is not helpful in evaluating most hematuria. Episodic asymptomatic hematuria occurs most commonly secondary to benign urethritis (urethrorrhagia) or a lacuna magna (congenital diverticulum of the fossa navicularis), hypercalcemia or medical renal disease. These are diagnosed by other tests and procedures (Chapter 33).

At present, cystoscopy is useful primarily to confirm a diagnosis made on the basis of a radiograph at the same time that intervention is applied, particularly in cases where the intervention can be carried out by endoscopic means. Lesions requiring cystoscopy after radiographic diagnosis are urethral valves, strictures, diaphragms, ureteroceles, bladder tumors, fibroepithelial polyps, and intersex states. Cystoscopy also is useful in completing the evaluation of various intersex states and imperforate anus or cloacas. It is sometimes used postoperatively to evaluate a reconstructed urethra or bladder neck. Retrograde pyelography is no longer often required, as the ureter can be evaluated both anatomically and functionally by means of careful application of IVP, antegrade pyelography, US, and renal scanning techniques.

CIRCUMCISION

Routine neonatal circumcision began in this country in the 1870s and was practiced on both boys and girls for the ensuing two decades. It has persisted as a routine operation for 75% to 85% of newborn boys at present. The medical rationale has been questioned and the pediatric urologic community and the American Academy of Pediatrics are now in agreement that there is no medical indication for routine circumcision in this country. The only well-substantiated argument in favor of routine circumcision is that 10% of uncircumcised males will eventually require surgery for balanitis, phimosis, or dyspareunia. Most often, the need for surgery will arise in the adult at a time when it can be carried out under local anesthesia on an outpatient basis. Other putative benefits of neonatal circumcision include a decreased incidence of urinary tract infection, penile carcinoma, and cervical carcinoma in sex partners of circumcised men, and herpetic infection. None of these has been substantiated in comparative studies of populations in which circumcision is not routinely done.

The estimated 1% to 3% incidence of complications after newborn circumcision covers only the immediate postoperative period prior to the infants' discharge from the hospital. The reported risks are hemorrhage in 1%, infection—occasionally leading to sepsis—in 0.5%, meatitis and meatal stenosis, urethrocutaneous fistula, adhesions between the glans and remaining prepuce, secondary phimosis, and cosmetically unsatisfactory results. The rate of subsequent repeat surgery to correct adhesions of the glans, meatal stenosis, fistula, and phimosis with buried penis is unknown, but our practice at Children's Hospital of Philadelphia includes about two such cases per month. While this is not a large percentage of the total number of circumcisions performed, it is a significant number of children undergoing surgery for complications of this operation. (At 1.25 million newborn circumcisions per year, the 0.5% infection rate translates to 6,250 cases per year, and the 4% overall rate of complications requiring treatment represents some 50,000 patients experiencing avoidable morbidity.)

Recent epidemiologic studies in the pediatric literature have supported the contention that the presence of the foreskin promotes pyelonephritis in male infants. Statistical and methodologic problems with these studies preclude their acceptance as definitive. Even if their conclusions are correct, a positive impact on the cost-benefit ratio for prophylactic circumcision remains to be demonstrated. Furthermore, no justification exists for the assertion that circumcision in any way alters the likelihood of contracting acquired immune deficiency syndrome (AIDS) or other sexually transmitted diseases. One obvious caveat is that the collection of urine specimens for culture, always difficult in the infant, must be by suprapubic aspirate in the uncircumcised infant or toddler; catheter specimens are often contaminated unless the foreskin can be retracted to expose the meatus.

As a general rule, it seems wise to counsel expectant parents that no medical indications exist for routine neonatal circumcision, and that few if any benefits result from the procedure. On the other hand, it is unreasonable to be so dogmatic as to refuse to perform the procedure.

No special care is required by the uncircumcised boy during the first years of life. The normal foreskin is adherent to the glans and gradually separates during the first years of life. The foreskin is nonretractable in 80% of boys at 6 months of age, 50% at 1 year, 20% at 2 years, and 10% at 3 years. In some normal boys, it is not retractable until school age. Forcibly retracting the foreskin is painful to the child and may lead to a true phimosis from traumatic rupture of glans-foreskin adhesions. There are no harmful effects from failure to clean under the foreskin in childhood. By the time a child is old enough to bathe himself, the adhesions usually will have spontaneously separated and he can be taught normal penile hygiene.

UNDESCENDED TESTIS

The primary care physician's task is to differentiate a retractile testis, which requires no surgical correction, from a truly undescended testis. Retractile testis occurs secondary to the pull of the cremaster muscle on the small prepubertal gonad. Occasionally this distinction is difficult and in some cases, it can only be made with the patient under general anesthesia. If the testis can be manipulated into a dependent portion of the scrotum without tension on the spermatic cord, it is a retractile testis even though it spends most of its time in the inguinal canal. No harm comes to the gonad. Such testes will eventually reside in the scrotum as the child grows older. Gentle pressure by the fingers on the inguinal region will usually push the testis low enough that it can be grasped by the fingers of the opposite hand and gently drawn into the scrotum. This maneuver requires a relaxed patient and careful manipulation on the part of the examiner. Examining an obese boy in a squatting or "catcher's" position may push the testis down to where it may be grasped and drawn into the scrotum. If it reaches no farther than the pubic bone or upper scrotum or if it cannot be palpated at all, surgical exploration is warranted. If it reaches the scrotum but pops up into the canal as soon as it is released, the testis is undescended and surgery is required.

The cause of testicular maldescent remains unclear. One plausible theory is that decreased local testosterone production produces failure of descent. Mechanical factors have been implicated as well, and the role of the gubernaculum remains to be defined. Maldescent can occur as part of several syndromes including chromosomal anomalies, endocrine deficiencies and midline cranial developmental defects. Although undescended gonads are frequent in intersex states, most of these children come to medical attention because of their ambiguous genitalia. One should be aware that a child who appears to be a normal boy but who has no palpable gonads must be assumed to be a girl until proved otherwise, as the adrenogenital syndrome can rarely produce this degree of virilization. A karyotype analysis will clarify this issue. As about one fourth of boys with hypospadias and an undescended testis are found to have an abnormal chromosomal analysis, a karyotype is indicated. Most frequently, a genetic mosaicism is found, requiring only hypospadias repair and orchiopexy. These patients are likely to be sterile.

Treatment of undescended testes by administration of human chorionic gonadotropin (HCG) has been popular in Europe, but American urologists have found it unrewarding. Recently, intranasally administered gonadotropin-releasing hormone (GnRH), not yet available in the United States, has achieved better results. When GnRH is followed by a course of HCG, an overall success rate of 74% has been reported. Such a success rate suggests that this form of therapy is most promising and may enable a large number of patients to avoid surgery in the future.

Surgical orchidopexy is still the standard treatment for cryptorchidism. Currently, urologists feel that orchidopexy should be carried out by age 2 years as pediatric anesthesia is now quite safe and the results seem to be improved. Histologic changes can be seen as early as 1 to 2 years of age, and are progressive. Fertility is poor in the patient subjected to orchidopexy late in childhood. Logic dictates earlier orchidopexy to improve fertility, although no large group has yet been followed up sufficiently long to prove this hypothesis. Orchidopexy can be done on an outpatient basis even when accompanied by intraperitonel exploration. If both gonads are intra-abdominal, it is wise to stage the procedures.

About 85% of undescended testes will be found in the inguinal canal and are easily placed in the scrotum by one of several standard procedures. Fewer than 5% of testes will be absent; the remainder will be found within the abdomen along the course of normal descent, usually adjacent to the internal inguinal ring. These may require mobilization on a vasperitoneal pedicle with ligation of the spermatic vessels (Fowler-Stephens orchidopexy). After Fowler-Stephens orchidopexy, gonadal survival is about 70%.

The major considerations in terms of surgical results are fertility and malignant potential. Oligospermia occurs in 20% to 65% of patients after orchidopexy. The best sperm counts are seen in patients whose orchidopexy was performed prior to age 4 years. No improvement in fertility can be shown to result from orchidopexy at or beyond puberty so that the pubertal undescended testis is usually removed unless it is solitary.

The risk of gonadal malignancy in a cryptorchid testis is 20 to 40 times that for a normally descended testis. Malignant potential is greater in the abdominal testis than in the canalicular or ectopic one. Tumors rarely have developed in testes brought down early (under age 4 years), while orchidopexy at puberty does not decrease the risk of malignancy, highlighting another reason that undescended testes after puberty should be removed, and earlier orchidopexy emphasized. Even at age 10 years, germ cell hyperplasia or carcinoma in situ may be present in 8% of undescended testes.

Most surgeons will follow up the patient for some months postoperatively to assure that the testis remains in good position without atrophy. Beyond that, it becomes the burden of primary care physicians to be alert for the development of malignancy. Ten percent of germ cell tumors occur in undescended testes. Regular examination of the testis should be carried out after puberty and can be taught to the patient much as self-examination of the breasts is taught to adult women. Any increase in size or change in consistency after completion of pubertal growth warrants referral to a urologist.

MEATAL STENOSIS

Meatal stenosis is a term that is often applied to any urethral meatus that appears to be narrow or pinhole in nature. Such an appearance seems to result from ammoniacal and/or mechanical irritation of the exposed meatus in many circumcised boys. The lesion is almost unknown in the uncircumcised patient. An appearance suggesting significant meatal stenosis can often be misleading, as the meatus may in fact be quite pliable and can be shown by calibration to be normal. In such cases, the voided stream is completely normal and the meatal appearance has no functional significance. In boys with functionally significant meatal stenosis, the urinary stream will be seen to spray or to be deflected, usually dorsally. Such voiding symptoms as frequency and enuresis should not be blamed on meatal stenosis, which should not be regarded as significant obstructive uropathy. Those patients who have a sprayed or deflected stream require a meatotomy, which can usually be carried out as an office procedure under local anesthesia. A distinction should be made between this lesion and the meatal stenosis occurring after urethral surgery, which, although it is called by the same name, is a result of scarring and can indeed produce significant bladder outlet obstruction.

DYSFUNCTIONAL VOIDING (HINMAN SYNDROME)

The spectrum of voiding disorders that includes enuresis, urinary frequency, and diurnal urge incontinence are all related pathophysiologically. At the worst end of the spectrum are a few patients whose disorder includes urinary tract infection and upper urinary tract damage. These patients' conditions can progress to end-stage renal disease if not recognized early and managed aggressively. Because bladder dysfunction occurs as a spectrum of disorders, the distinction between true dysfunctional voiding or Hinman syndrome and the more common pediatric uninhibited bladder may initially be difficult.

In infancy, voiding occurs by reflex; as the detrusor contracts, the striated external sphincter relaxes automatically. Voiding to completion is usual. At the age of toilet training, the child becomes aware of bladder filling and emptying and initially attempts to gain control over a bladder contraction by "holding on" with the striated external sphincter. Tightening the sphincter during a bladder contraction raises intravesical pressure, but eventually most children gain the ability to inhibit detrusor contractions by a poorly understood central mechanism that is largely subconscious in nature. During the transition to central control over the bladder, uninhibited detrusor contractions can lead to wetting either during the day or the night. Attempts to control this by contracting the external sphincter engender the squatting or cross-legged stance that such children exhibit, as well as the sensation of urgency that leads some children to run to the bathroom many times in succession while producing only small amounts of urine. Once central control of the detrusor develops, coordinated relaxation of the sphincter during voiding ensues in most cases. In that event, the enuresis or urge incontinence resolves without sequelae. Most of these children do not exhibit abnormalities on roentgenograms or have significant problems with urinary tract infection.

In some instances, for reasons that remain unclear, a transitional pattern persists, and the child fails to relax the external sphincter during voiding. Elevated intravesical pressure during voiding and incomplete bladder emptying results, leading to infection, incontinence, and, in severe cases, hydroureteronephrosis. None of these children have any underlying neurologic or muscular disease, and careful electromyography will demonstrate normal action potentials and conduction velocities in the involved musculature. The role of urodynamic investigation in the care of children with dysfunctional voiding is therefore unclear. The information provided by such investigations does not usually alter the management. The diagnosis may be suspected on the basis of the following historical, physical, and radiographic findings: older child (>7 years); wetting and infection; chronic constipation, encopresis; infrequent voiding, intermittent stream; elevated residual urine volume; increase in anal sphincter tone; trabeculated bladder; and hydronephrosis and reflux. Only the progress of the condition over time will establish the severity of this disorder.

Children with radiographically normal upper urinary tracts may be managed as follows: an anticholinergic, with or without antibiotics; timed voiding; focus on relaxation and sustained stream; relief of chronic constipation; and careful follow-up. Many such patients will ultimately be shown to have simple, uninhibited bladder or persistent transition-phase voiding. These measures can be applied to patients falling all along the spectrum of voiding dysfunctions up to the point at which upper tract dilation has occurred. Constipation often accompanies these voiding dysfunctions and can usually be resolved with dietary maneuvers that provide more bulk. Follow-up includes urine cultures, and US or radiographic assessment of bladder emptying and upper urinary tract drainage in patients in whom infections develop or whose conditions fail to improve with this regimen. Any change in the upper tracts dictates referral to a urologist for further treatment. In our experience, clean intermittent self-catheterization has been most successful in such cases.

BIBLIOGRAPHY

Bartholomew TH: Neurogenic voiding: function and dysfunction. *Urol Clin North Am* 1985; 12:67–74.

Duckett JW: Vesicoureteral reflux: A 'conservative' analysis. *Am J Kidney Dis* 1983; 111:2.

Gairdner D: The fate of the foreskins. *Br Med J* 1949; 2:1433–1437.

Johnston JH (ed): *Management of Vesicoureteric Reflux*, vol 10, *International Perspectives in Urology*. Baltimore, Williams & Wilkins, 1984.

Kaplan GW: Complications of circumcision. *Urol Clin North Am* 1983; 10:543.

Metcalf TJ, Osborn LM, Mariani EM: Circumcision: A study of current practices. *Clin Pediatr* 1983; 22:575.

Rajfer J (ed): Symposium on cryptorchidism. *Urol Clin North Am* 1982; 9:3.

Snyder HM, Duckett JW: Endoscopic evaluation problems in refluxing orifices. *Dialogues Pediatr Urol* 1983; 6:12.

Wallerstein E: Circumcision: The uniquely American medical enigma. *Urol Clin North Am* 1985; 12:123–132.

Walther PC, Kaplan GW: Cystoscopy in children: Indications for its use in common urologic problems. *J Urol* 1979; 122:717.

Wiswell TE, Roscelli JD: Corroborative evidence for the decreased incidence of urinary tract infections in circumcised male infants. *Pediatrics* 1986; 78:96.

Wiswell TE, Cohen ML, Ozere L, et al: Corroborative evidence for the decreased incidence of urinary tract infections in circumcised male infants (letters to the editor). *Pediatrics* 1986; 78:951, 1986; 79:649, 1987; 80:303, 763.

100 PAIN

Barbara S. Shapiro, M.D.

In children, pain is usually thought of as a diagnostic clue to an underlying disorder, which once identified can be appropriately treated. Until recent years, there has been little discussion of pain as a concurrent or separate problem. A complete approach to the care of children includes the assessment and management of pain, both as a symptom and as a problem in its own right.

PATHOPHYSIOLOGY

Pain is the perception of unwelcome bodily hurt or injury; this may or may not involve clinically detectable changes or pathologic conditions. Neurologically, pain is a complex phenomenon. Stimulation of peripheral pain receptors produces an impulse that is filtered through connections in the spinal cord, reticular formation, hypothalamus, thalamus, limbic system, and other areas of the cerebral cortex on the way to the somatosensory centers. Within this complex network are multiple ascending and descending inhibitory and excitatory inputs. Because areas of the cerebral cortex involving memory, cognition, and emotion are recruited, the character of the pain is affected by context, developmental stage, and emotional factors. For example, a sensation signaling the presence of a disease such as cancer may be experienced as more severe than an equivalent stimulus resulting from strenuous but pleasant physical activity. Therefore, because of the neurophysiology, the perceived sensation may differ from the intensity of the impulse.

Pain originates from somatic, visceral, and neural structures. Neuropathic pain affects the central nervous system (CNS), the peripheral nervous system, and the autonomic nervous system, and includes such syndromes as phantom limb pain, sciatica, causalgia, and reflex sympathetic dystrophy.

TYPES OF PAIN

Understanding the type of pain facilitates institution of appropriate therapy. Pain can be defined as acute or chronic, by quality, and by cause.

ACUTE AND CHRONIC PAIN

Acute pain and chronic pain are very different in character and treatment (Table 100–1). Acute pain, such as postoperative pain or pain from fractures or infection, may serve as a warning of injury and tissue destruction. The pain does not cause major and persistent changes in lifestyle and relationships. Behaviors from the discomfort do not become a part of the child's repertoire. In contrast, chronic pain does not have a predictable resolution, may be expected to recur, and often produces substantial alterations in activities and relationships. Chronic pain may be recurrent or steady. Recurrent pain, such as recurrent abdominal pain and headache, is the most common form of chronic pain in children. The recurrences may be predictable or unpredictable; unpredictable pain, especially if severe, can lead to more difficulty in coping.

ORGANIC, NONPATHOLOGIC, AND PSYCHOGENIC PAIN

Traditionally, pain has been defined as either organic or emotional (also called functional or psychogenic). However, this dichotomy can result in unnecessarily aggressive diagnostic workups, erosion of trust between the physician and the family and patient, inadequate treatment of the psychologic effects of organically based pain, unnecessary referral for psychotherapy, and lack of acceptance by the patient and the family of the behavioral and emotional components of all pain.

It is more accurate and useful to regard pain as a variable mixture of many factors (Fig 100–1). Depending on the relative balance of these factors, three overlapping categories can be distinguished. The pain may result from (1) a defined emotional disorder, (2) a disease process or tissue injury, or (3) a physiologic pro-

TABLE 100–1
Comparison of Acute and Chronic Pain

ACUTE PAIN	CHRONIC PAIN
Warning symptom of tissue damage	Pain serves no physiologic function
Escape behavior	Withdrawal, decreased mobility
Anxiety	Depression
Crying, irritability	Apathy, irritability
Vital sign changes	No vital sign changes
Time limited	Unknown or long duration
Unlikely to return, or is infrequent or mild	Likely to return, frequent or severe
No major changes in lifestyle	Lifestyle alterations
No or little effect on family	Major impact on family
No learning of pain behavior	Pain behaviors incorporated
Ideal treatment simple and rapid	Ideal treatment complex and multidisciplinary

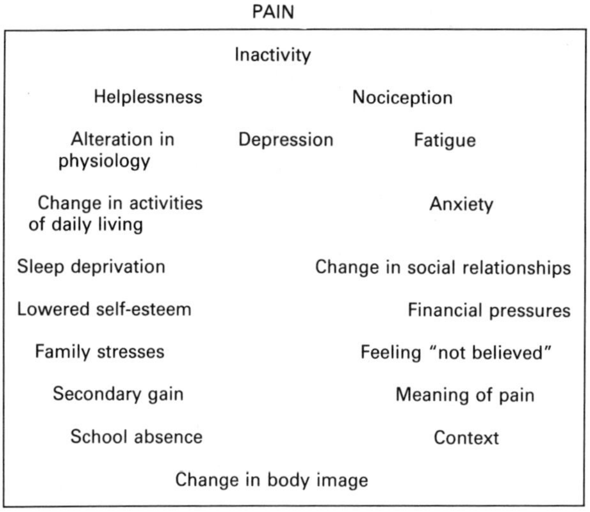

FIG 100–1
Interplay of factors in pain.

cess or alteration that does not cause actual pathologic alterations or disease. Most recurrent pain disorders in children fall into the third category, as the child has no clear organic or psychologic disorder. Thus, unless there are clues in the history or physical examination that a disease process is present, an extensive diagnostic workup is not necessary in the majority of patients.

Nonpathologic pain resulting from physiologic processes may have a known or unknown organic basis and may or may not result in dysfunction in daily activities, such as school and relationships with family and friends. Factors influencing the degree of dysfunction are listed in Figure 100–2. An example is migraine headache. The pain is not secondary to a disease or tissue destruction; rather, the headache results from alterations in the vascular and biochemical physiologic milieu. The majority of patients with migraine headache do not have an emotional disorder that causes the headache. However, the headache can be precipitated or aggravated by environmental or intrapsychic stressors, which affect neurohumoral vascular control and erode coping skills. As in all pain syndromes, the presence of secondary gain can cause amplification of the pain perception and behavior. Recurrent or chronic pain syndromes are nonpathologic in most cases, but are not benign, as the pain itself can cause significant dysfunction and distress. Although emotional stressors may precipitate nonpathologic pain, the pain is not

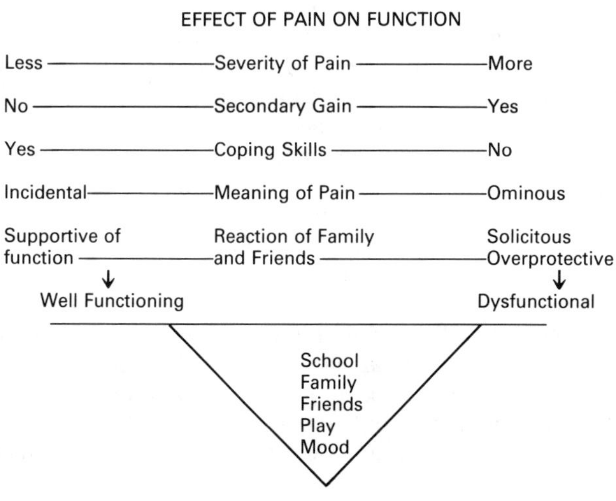

FIG 100–2
Factors influencing degree of dysfunction with pain.

solely psychogenic but results from an interaction between physiology, emotion, perception, and environment.

The diagnosis of psychogenic pain is made by establishing the definitive presence of an emotional disorder or stressor causally related to the pain, and not by the lack of documented organic disease. An example is abdominal pain in a child who is being sexually abused, which disappears with appropriate situational intervention. The child with emotionally based pain often does not have a serious psychologic disorder, and the pain may not affect function. Children (and adults) frequently experience abdominal pain before a stressful event such as a public performance; this does not necessarily interfere with the activity. Children with a mild injury may respond to an oversolicitous and worried parent with amplification of the sensation. Emotional pathologic conditions may or may not be etiologic; persistent severe pain, whether disease related or nonpathologic, can produce depression, school absence, and troublesome family relationships. A child with cancer and severe family dysfunction may indeed have organically based pain, but the perception of the pain and the extent to which the child can cope may be mediated by stress within the dysfunctional family. Consequently, in any chronic pain problem the psychosocial function of the child should be assessed; problems warrant intervention whether or not a causative relationship can be established.

Secondary gain from pain can amplify pain perception or behavior. The child with abdominal pain who is allowed to stay home from school and watch television, while the parents express great concern and stay home from work, may readily go back to school after learning that he or she now has to stay in bed all day, with a parent in another part of the house and with no television or toys. If the secondary gain is removed and the pain disappears, then the secondary gain may be viewed as a causative factor. The presence of secondary gain does not in and of itself indicate a psychogenic cause for the pain, as secondary gain can occur with all pain syndromes. In fact, parents of children with disease-related pain syndromes benefit from being taught how to avoid amplification of pain behaviors because of secondary gain.

ASSESSMENT

Pain is complex and multifaceted. However, within a chief complaint it tends to be communicated in global and vague terms, such as "bad," "better," or "worse." The nebulous complaint of pain takes on form and color as the physician explores the patient's perceptions. Parameters of pain perception are listed in Table 100–2. The severity or intensity of the pain, as well as provocative and palliative factors, can be documented. The quality of the pain (throbbing, tight, shooting, burning) can be important in delineating cause and therapy. Region and radiation (with and without movement) of the pain, as well as temporal factors (hourly, daily, weekly, on all days or just school days) must be assessed. When determining the part of the body affected, the presence of referred pain should be considered. For example, hip disease may produce knee pain, and sinusitis may produce toothache. The effect of the pain on activities of daily living, friends, family, school, mood, and overall well-being (energy level, fatigue, and sleep patterns) is important in chronic pain problems. Assessment of the meaning of the pain to the patient and to the family, as well as psychologic factors such as anxiety, helplessness, and depression, are necessary to understand a complex pain problem.

The extent of assessment will vary with the problem. For a child with cellulitis or a fracture, a simple assessment of pain intensity will guide the choice of analgesic agent. In contrast, a patient with persistent headaches that are significantly interfering with daily activities, with no symptoms or signs of a space-occupying or infectious lesion, needs a careful evaluation of all aspects of the pain, psychosocial status, and coping mechanisms.

Developmentally appropriate tools for assessing pain intensity are available (Table 100–3). These methods are clinically useful, and have been shown to be reliable and valid. The child over the age of 6 or 7 years who understands the concepts of rank and order can easily be taught a simple numerical scale. The child is asked how much hurt he or she has on a scale of 0 to 10 (or 0 to 100), where 0 represents no pain at all and 10 means the worst pain imaginable. Alternatively, a visual analogue scale may

TABLE 100–2
Parameters of Pain Perception

PAIN DESCRIPTORS	RHEUMATOID ARTHRITIS	REFLEX SYMPATHETIC DYSTROPHY	RECURRENT ABDOMINAL PAIN	EMOTIONAL
Severity	Mild to severe	Moderate to severe	Mild to severe	Varies, described diffusely
Provocative factors	Inactivity	Light touch, movement	Eating, stress	Usually difficult to elicit
Palliative factors	Mild activity, aspirin	Splinting, transcutaneous electrical nerve stimulation	Heat, curling up	Often none or avoidance of activity
Quality	Aching, pressing	Burning, pins and needles	Diffuse, crampy	Usually poorly described
Region	Joints	Distal extremity, not dermatomal	Abdomen	Diffuse or very circumscribed
Radiation	None	Occasional stabbing, proximal extremity	None	Variable
Temporal	Worse in morning	Worse in afternoon or evening	Intermittent, unpredictable	Usually nonspecific or associated with secondary gain
Meaning	Presence of chronic illness	Usually unknown, frightening to patient	Variable	

be used. The visual analogue scale is a straight line, usually horizontal and 10 cm long, anchored on one end with "no pain," and on the other end with the "worst pain." The child is asked to place a vertical mark on the line corresponding to the amount of pain or hurt. A measurement of the distance of the mark from the left end can then be made by the physician to produce a numerical value. Children who do not understand numbers may be able to use a visual analogue scale. If consecutive pain reports are being obtained over time, the patient may remember and be influenced by the past numbers used on a numerical scale, but may be less likely to remember the exact placement of the line on the visual analogue scale. However, numerical scales may be easier to use in a busy clinical setting, especially if the child is in the hospital. Both the numerical and visual analogue scales can be used to help the child and the physician separate out the factors of pain per se and fear or sadness.

Perhaps even more important than the pain intensity is the extent to which the pain actually bothers the child. Certainly the two are related. However, depending on context, meaning, and coping skills, pain that is moderately intense may not bother some children. Children over the age of 7 years can usually understand this concept and can rate the "bother" on a numerical or analogue scale. If the intensity and the bother are rated at different levels, therapy should be directed at the latter.

For the child from 3 to 7 years of age, other

TABLE 100–3
Age-Appropriate Methods of Assessing Pain Intensity*

- Age 6–7 years and older
  - Numerical scale: 0 to 10 or 0 to 100
  - Visual analogue scale: ⟵⟶ No pain — Worst pain
  - Body map
- Age 3–7 years
  - Cartoon faces scale
  - Pieces of hurt
  - Body map
- Age 18–36 months
  - Behavioral observation
  - Simple verbal statements ("Does it hurt?")
- Age less than 18 months or nonverbal child
  - Behavioral observation

*Adjust for developmental age.

assessment tools have been developed. A cartoon faces scale is easy to use in the office setting. The child is shown the series of faces, and is told that the smiling face is of a child with no hurt at all, the next one has a little hurt, and so on to the last face which has the most hurt ever. The child picks the face corresponding to his or her current state. Other scales available include Hester's poker chip scale, in which the child is shown four poker chips or similar objects and is told to show the interviewer how many pieces of hurt he or she has now.

The assessment of pain intensity in babies and toddlers is much more difficult. Acute pain in these children can be categoried as none, mild, moderate, and severe by assessing cry intensity and quality, active resistance, body tension, irritability (especially to movement), guarding or lack of movement of the affected body part, responsivity to favorite toys and food, and sleep. For example, a baby with mild teething pain may be more cranky than usual but is easily distracted with parental comforting, whereas a baby with severe pain of any cause is unlikely to respond for any length of time to parental comforting. Chronic pain is more difficult to assess, and may be manifested by general irritability and crankiness, diminished interest in feeding and playing, decreased activity, withdrawal or apparent depression, and apathy. The toddler may be able to verbalize pain in a simple fashion, such as "yes" or "no" or "a little" or "a lot" as long as the pain is not too severe. At times, however, it is difficult to know whether behaviors observed in a baby or toddler represent pain. If the child has an organic process that can cause pain, a therapeutic trial of analgesia may be given. A positive response to such a trial confirms the presence of pain.

For children over the age of 3 or 4 years, body maps may be useful to discern the region as well as intensity of the pain. This can be useful in a disease like polyarticular juvenile rheumatoid arthritis, in which the pain occurs in variable intensity in multiple regions. A dorsal and ventral body outline is presented. The child is given crayons or markers and told to pick the colors representing no pain, a little pain, more pain, and the most pain. The body outline is then colored according to the current severity and region of the pain.

Children over the age of 5 or 6 years, are usually able to define the quality of the pain if given words and descriptions appropriate to development. The pain of reflex sympathetic dystrophy and other neuropathies is often characterized as burning (or like sunburn), stinging, or pins and needles. Deafferentation or nerve compression pain is described as shooting, like electric shocks, or like a needle. Myofascial or somatic pain is throbbing or drumlike, aching, tight, or heavy; and visceral pain is crampy, intermittent, sharp, and often poorly defined (although it may be referred to myofascial structures and described as such).

Temporal factors may help define cause and effect on daily activities. Exacerbation after inactivity or sleep may be a clue to rheumatoid arthritis. Stomachaches may occur on school mornings only (although this must be distinguished from other factors that can vary on school days, such as diet). Migraine headaches may occur on weekends or vacations, concurrent with altered sleep or food intake patterns. Pelvic pain from endometriosis often follows a cyclic pattern. Headaches that occur daily are far more significant as far as cause and impact than headaches that occur for a few hours every few weeks.

The distinction among disease-related, nonpathologic, and psychologic causes is more difficult. The history and physical examination usually provide clues to organic pathologic conditions; these clues include well-defined and described pain and other symptoms and signs of illness. Similarly, psychopathology such as psychosis, sexual abuse, or school phobia may be evident on assessment. In most cases, however, psychosocial factors, such as depression or family stress, could easily result from rather than cause the pain.

Pain that has a large emotional overlay typically is described in nebulous and diffuse terms, even after the physician has taught the child developmentally appropriate methods for communicating intensity, quality, and region. The child may seem actively or passively resistant to answering questions despite a nonthreatening, supportive atmosphere with clear assurance that the physician needs to understand the pain to help.

When assessing chronic pain, the physician should be aware that memory of pain is often inaccurate and may reflect the current state of the pain rather than the actual history. The child with migraine headaches who is brought to the physician's office because of an increase in frequency and severity over the past few days may, along with his or her parents, overestimate the number of headaches over the preceding few months.

The diary system helps circumvent the problems of memory. The child or parent is asked to keep a daily record of pain occurrence, intensity, preceding events, action taken, and results. The format for recording this information should be easy to understand and complete. In addition to aiding in diagnosis and therapy, the diary enables the child to become part of the team by taking an active role in assessment and treatment. The pain is communicated in a positive and controlled manner rather than through global pain complaints and acting out. The complaint of pain is given credence, but at the same time, decisions about diagnostic and therapeutic intervention are postponed until a more complete picture is gained. Finally, the patient and the family may realize when reviewing the record that the amount of time spent in pain is not that significant.

Overall, the assessment of pain may range from a quick determination of intensity and region to a complex and ongoing assessment of multiple factors. The assessment should be tailored to the individual situation, and performed in a developmentally appropriate manner, with an understanding of the physiologically determined subjectivity of the pain experience. Assessment, if done in this manner, is in itself therapeutic because it validates the pain experience without obviating the importance of clinical judgment on the part of the physician, teaches the child to communicate rather than act out the pain, and sets the stage for an ongoing productive relationship between the physician, the patient, and the parent(s). It is impossible to decide for the patient how much pain he or she has. There is no right answer. Rather, the task of the caretaker is to assess the pain and its overall impact on the patient's functioning and then to take steps to enhance the overall function and well-being, both now and in the future. If the patient's perception of pain is not believed, the physician's efforts to help the child return to a more functional state may be resisted actively or passively.

TREATMENT

The type and intensity of the pain, effect on activities of daily living and relationships, expected time course, and cause determine the treatment. Intervention can be divided into two basic categories: therapy that decreases the pain or the perception of pain, and enhancement of the ability to cope with the pain. Treatment must be accompanied by an ongoing assessment to determine efficacy.

TREATMENT OF PAIN

Pharmacologic
Nonnarcotic: acetaminophen, aspirin
Narcotic: morphine, codeine
Adjuvant: tricyclic antidepressants, stimulants (Ritalin, amphetamine), anticonvulsants (carbamazepine)

Behavioral
Hypnosis
Relaxation
Biofeedback
Desensitization
Psychotherapy
Distraction
Music/art/play therapy

Rehabilitative
Physical therapy
Orthopedic: braces, splints
Exercise

Neurologic
Transcutaneous electrical nerve stimulation
Acupuncture

Cognitive
Preparative education
Symptom diary

Supportive
Physician availability
Financial
Religious
Social

Developmental
Occupational therapy
Stimulating environment

Anesthetic
Local
Regional blocks
Epidural/intrathecal blocks
Sympathetic blocks

Neurosurgical
Ablative
Stimulatory

If the cause of the pain is not clear and there are no worrisome symptoms, signs, or laboratory abnormalities, the physician can focus intervention on disruption and dysfunction in the child's daily activities. Such a therapeutic plan is important for all patients and can be implemented without establishing the relationship of the pain to organic and psychosocial factors. If significant organic or psychopathologic conditions exist but have been missed on initial assessment, clues to these issues will surface if close follow-up and ongoing assessment are maintained. This approach buys time for the physician to establish a trusting relationship with the patient and the family, validates the experience of pain while avoiding unnecessary testing and referral, and provides for immediate and ongoing therapeutic intervention.

Although pharmacologic agents are often considered first, they may not be appropriate or necessary or may be more efficacious when used with other interventions. Cognitive and behavioral approaches such as education, distraction, relaxation, and self-hypnosis can be very helpful, especially for chronic pain. Most children can easily learn the techniques of relaxation, self-hypnosis, and imagery. Music, art, and play therapy can be used. Psychotherapy or family therapy are indicated for specific difficulties.

Since the emphasis in treating most chronic pain is on enhancing function, rehabilitative approaches are important. Exercise and physical activity within a developmentally appropriate framework may help to counteract the mutually interactive effects of pain, inactivity, depression, and fatigue. When prescribed by the physician, physical activity or physical therapy serve dual purposes of showing the physician's concern about the pain and increasing function, without the side effects found in pharmacologic therapy. Depending on the complexity and severity of the pain, simple rehabilitative measures can be taught by the physician or referral can be made to a physical therapist or other specialist. For example, the child with reflex sympathetic dystrophy of short duration following mild trauma can be given a simple set of exercises to be practiced at home. If the condition has not improved on follow-up in a few days, referral to a physical therapist is indicated.

Cognitive therapy includes education, demystification of the cause of the pain, supportive counseling, and the keeping of a symptom diary. Since young children often view pain as a punishment, education may be used to counteract this impression. Pain is perceived by humans and animals as a signal of injury that must be avoided to avert further injury or destruction. Children with nonpathologic pain can benefit from an explanation of the fact that their pain is different than the pain of a fracture, represents hurt only and not harm, and does not signal the need to stop an activity to avoid further injury. Children and parents easily understand the concept that focusing on pain makes the pain worse because of the lack of other stimuli, and this can be presented as a reason to continue daily activities as much as possible. Counseling includes identifying financial, supportive, and religious resources within the community that can decrease the stresses that augment the *perception* of pain.

The objective of pain management, especially for chronic pain, is not to make the patient free of pain but to make the pain tolerable to the patient and to maximize functioning. Attempts to make the child pain free can lead to frustration on the part of the patient and the physician.

REFERRAL

The majority of children with acute and recurrent pain can be treated by the primary physician (Fig 100–3), who can use pharmacologic therapies, such as acetaminophen, aspirin, and other nonsteroidal anti-inflammatory agents (NSAIAs; peripherally acting analgesics), and opioids (narcotics); education, diaries, and demystification; simple exercises and physical therapy; and referral to community resources. The physician can intervene in the family and environmental factors that may be reinforcing or augmenting the pain and are not associated with significant psychopathologic problems. Secondary gain can be removed with instructions to the parent and the child. To be effective, this must be done in a positive manner that allows the child to "save face." The primary physician can teach relaxation and self-hypnosis if he or she has received training in this area. Close follow-up is necessary in chronic pain problems.

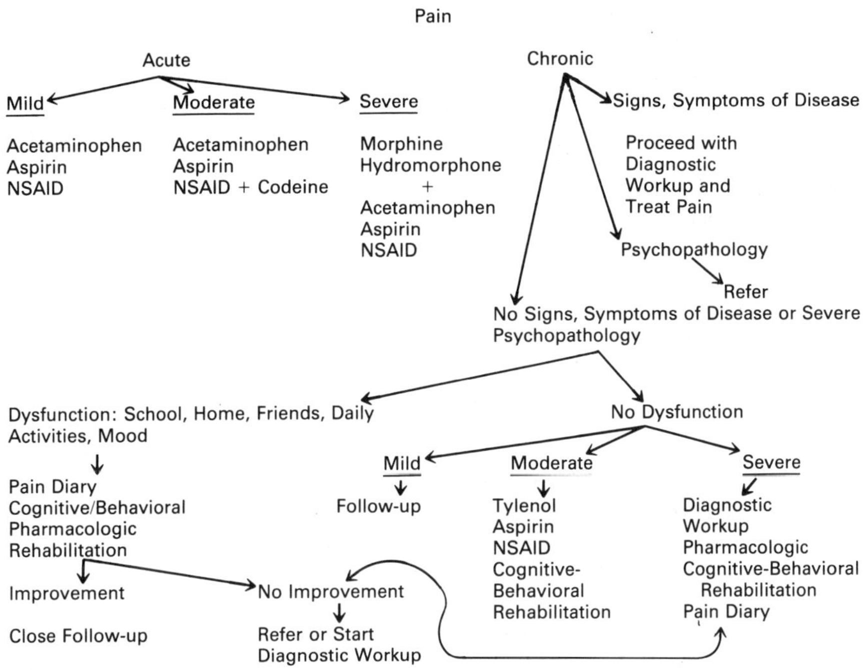

FIG 100–3

Flow chart shows management of acute and chronic pain.

Referral is necessary if a patient continues to have pain that significantly interferes with function or mood despite intervention or if the pain is associated with a disease that is best treated by consultation with a specialist. Careful assessment of the problem is necessary to decide when and to whom to refer. Involvement of a mental health worker, such as a psychologist, psychiatrist, or a psyciatric social worker, is indicated for significant psychosocial disorders, for adjustment problems that do not respond easily to the physician's efforts, or for the child who may benefit from learning behavioral techniques of pain control that the physician is not trained to teach. Similarly, the physician may refer to a physical therapist for a vigorous rehabilitative program and transcutaneous electrical nerve stimulation. After making such referrals, the physician should continue to see and assess the patient regularly so that the family and the patient perceive all members of the team as working together under the supervision of the primary care physician.

The manner in which referral to a mental health professional is made can be instrumental in determining the success of the intervention. Groundwork for such referral is laid when the primary physician validates the pain experience and does not reinforce the common perception of pain as being either organic or emotional if an organic cause is not found. The family and patient should be educated initially about the interplay of emotion, context, and meaning with the perception of and ability to cope with all pain, and the effect of pain on psychosocial status. A workup that initially focuses on ruling out all diseases, and only then proceeds to evaluate psychosocial factors relegates psychosocial intervention to a lesser status. The patient and the family are often distressed and angry if the psychosocial workup is presented as a separate entity, and may insist on more and more tests to definitively eliminate a pathologic process.

PHARMACOLOGIC TREATMENT

Pharmacologic agents available for the treatment of pain include the peripherally acting analgesics, such as acetaminophen and aspirin, opioids (narcotics), and other agents that can be beneficial in certain pain syndromes, such as the tricyclic antidepressants, some anticonvulsants, and stimulants.

Placebos have no place in the assessment or management of pain and should not be given to demonstrate an emotional overlay to the pain. Under conditions of mild pain or anxiety, 30% of all patients will have a placebo response. The percentage of placebo responders increases under conditions of severe pain and anxiety. The person who responds to a placebo is likely to have severe organic pain without any secondary gain. Secondary gain tends to interfere with placebo response.

By the same token, however, the principle of placebo response can be used to enhance response to therapy. After the physician has assessed the pain and chosen a therapy or combination of therapies, the treatment plan should be presented with authority, confidence, and optimism for the patient's good response.

The choice of medication depends on the severity of the pain. Mild pain is best managed with a peripherally acting agent. For moderate pain, a weak opioid (such as codeine) can be added to the regimen. Severe pain calls for the use of strong opioids, again usually in conjunction with a peripherally acting agent if the child can take medication by mouth.

PERIPHERALLY ACTING ANALGESICS

Acetaminophen, aspirin, and other NSAIDs are the most commonly used and prescribed analgesics. A pharmacologic dose of acetaminophen or aspirin is approximately equal in analgesic potential to a pharmacologic dose of codeine. Furthermore, the analgesia from the peripherally acting agents is additive to the analgesia from an opioid; 10 mg/kg of acetaminophen plus 0.5 mg/kg of codeine offers twice the analgesia of either agent separately. There is no reason to prescribe codeine or other opioids without also using a peripherally acting analgesic unless there is a specific contraindication to all peripherally acting agents.

There is no difference between aspirin and acetaminophen as far as analgesic efficacy, and no extra analgesia is achieved by using both agents at the same time. However, most clinicians would use acetaminophen in preference to aspirin for analgesia in children because of concerns about Reye syndrome. Aspirin and other NSAIDs offer advantages when an anti-inflammatory action is desired.

OPIOID ANALGESICS

In using opioids, the appropriate agent, dose, schedule, and route must be used. One must ask, "For which patient? In which situation? With what disease? Can the pain be well managed using other approaches?" (See Table 100–4 for dosing information.)

In the patient who can take medications by mouth, moderate pain can be managed with codeine and a peripherally acting agent. More severe pain can be managed with a peripherally acting analgesic supplemented by oral hydromorphone, oxycodone, or morphine.

Of the parenteral analgesics, morphine is the drug of choice. If a patient develops side effects from morphine that are not easily controlled, hydromorphone can be substituted. Methadone and levorphanol are difficult to correctly titrate and should be used only by a physician familiar with dosing principles.

Although meperidine is a commonly used agent for pain control, there are disadvantages to its use. It is absorbed poorly when given by mouth. Intravenous administration results in very high initial serum levels, with a short duration of action. Intramuscular administration should not be used with children, as they would often rather have pain than a shot and will hide or deny their pain. In adults, the use of meperidine for more than 24 hours has been shown to be associated with significant dysphoria, which may compound and exacerbate the pain. Normeperidine, a metabolite of meperidine, has a half-life much longer than meperidine and can cause agitation and seizures.

The principle of equianalgesia is important in determining the dose of opioids. In analgesic potency, 7.5 mg of oral hydromorphone is equal to 10 mg of intravenous morphine. Morphine is effective by mouth, but must be used in at least three times the amount given intravenously to produce the same analgesia. Therefore the decision as to route (intravenous or oral) rests on the ability of the patient to take medicine by mouth and the desired length of time to peak effect. Because intravenous opioid reaches peak effect sooner than oral, and is thus easier to titrate, this route is preferable in the immediate treatment of severe pain.

When possible, pain should be controlled with oral medications. Intramuscular injections should be avoided, because they produce extreme anxiety in most children. If enteral and intravenous routes are not available and if the

TABLE 100–4
Dosing Information

DRUG	EQUIANALGESIC DOSE (MG)	RECOMMENDED STARTING DOSE (MG/KG)	AVERAGE T(HR)	RECOMMENDED STARTING DOSING INTERVAL (HR)	ONSET (MIN)
Morphine					
Parenteral	10	0.1	2–4	3	15
Oral	30	0.3	2–4	4	30–60
Hydromorphone					
Parenteral	1.5	0.015	2–3	2–3	<15
Oral	7.5	0.08	2–3	3–4	30–60
Meperidine					
Parenteral	75	0.8–1.0	3–4	3	<15
Oral	300	Not recommended			
Codeine					
Oral	200	0.5–1.0	3	4	30

patient is not dehydrated, subcutaneous injection or continuous infusion of morphine or hydromorphone can be used.

When using an opioid in a patient who has not recently taken such medications, the physician should start with the recommended initial doses. However, many patients require much higher doses, especially those with very severe pain or those who have received opioids for any length of time in the immediate past. The dose can be increased as long as analgesia, sedation, and respiratory depression are monitored. For acute pain, a higher dose may be necessary to attain control of the pain. After control is achieved, less medication may be required to keep the pain away, because of the decrease in attendant anxiety.

The analgesic requirement must be determined for each individual patient by assessing analgesia and sedation at the time of peak effect and again before the next dose. If the initial dose provides inadequate analgesia, the next dose can be increased by 20%. Further increases of this amount can be made with each dose. If a constant infusion is being used, the dose can be increased by about 20% to 25% every 8 to 12 hours, with a loading bolus equal to the hourly increase.

For severe pain, assessment of pain, sedation, and respiratory depression should take place 30 minutes to 1 hour after the initial dose of a parenteral opioid. If there is no analgesia and no sedation or respiratory depression, 50% of the initial dose can be repeated at that time. If there is some decrease in pain and minimal sedation, 25% of the initial dose can be given. This should be done under close observation. It is possible to titrate the dose to the patient's requirement much faster and more aggressively than described here; however, this should only be done by a physician experienced in the use of opioids.

The schedule of medication depends on the specific pain syndrome, the intensity of the pain, and the expected time of resolution. In any pain syndrome in which pain can be expected to last for more than a few hours, medication "as needed" should be avoided. Such a schedule necessitates the return or increase of pain before it is treated and puts the patient in a position of having to ask for medication and endure delay.

Preventing the return of pain by giving medication around the clock provides better pain relief, and usually a lower total amount of analgesic is required. The as-needed schedule reinforces pain behaviors such as whining, begging, or crying. The patient who does not exhibit this behavior may not receive the medication. The delay and uncertainty of pain relief increases anxiety, which in turn reduces the patient's ability to utilize such coping methods as relaxation and distraction. Children are at a particular disadvantage on a medication as needed schedule, as they may be unable to articulate their pain or gain the attention of the nurses.

The dosing interval should prevent an increase in pain intensity before the next dose. Many patients do well on conventional schedules of every 3 or every 4 hours around the clock. However, because of the physiologic variation in opioid requirement, some patients need doses at closer intervals. For example, 0.1 mg/kg of morphine may provide good analgesia with minimal sedation for 2 hours, followed by an increase in pain intensity at 2½ hours. In this case a dosing schedule of every 3 hours is inadequate and should be decreased to every 2 hours with no change in dose. If the dose of 0.1 mg/kg provides inadequate analgesia even at the time of peak effect, the dose should be increased until adequate analgesia is achieved and then the schedule adjusted to prevent the recurrence of pain. Similarly, if 0.1 mg/kg of morphine every 3 hours produces moderate sedation with good analgesia lasting 2½ hours, both the dose and the interval should be decreased.

When the pain is variable in intensity or is resolving, doses given around the clock do not provide flexibility in decreasing or weaning the medication. A flexible dosing or reverse as-needed schedule may be used to circumvent this problem. In the reverse as-needed schedule, the physician writes an order stating that the patient must be asked at regular intervals whether he or she wishes to have pain medication. For flexible dosing, the medication is given around the clock, but the patient is given a choice of a higher or lower dose. If the patient is too young to use this approach (less than 7 or 8 years old) and if a parent is present most of the time, he or she can be educated in pain assessment and can participate in the flexible dosing. Obviously, flexible dosing can cause some of the same problems as the as-needed schedule; especially for a child, the way in which the choice is presented can influence the decision.

Opioids can be administered by bolus injection or by infusion. Boluses are useful in titrating the dose of analgesic to the patient's requirements. However, once a dose is determined, if the pain is going to last for more than 1 day and if the dose of boluses is greater than 0.05 mg/kg/hr of morphine equivalents or if boluses are required more often than every 2 hours, an infusion can give better control. The dose of the infusion is determined by calculating the milligrams of analgesic required over time for adequate analgesia and dividing this total dose into milligrams per hour.

Opioids can be used in babies under 3 months of age, but the dosing must be approached with caution. Pharmacokinetics of opioids in the neonate are different than in the older child, and there is a risk of apnea in the unventilated infant because of altered metabolism and prolonged excretion. The starting dose should be no more than 30% to 50% of the usual recommended starting dose, and the interval should be determined by observing the time required for the recurrence of pain. A cardiorespiratory monitor and pulse oximetry should be used, along with close observation.

Constipation, the most frequent side effect of opioids, is preventable with proper bowel regimens. Respiratory depression is the most feared problem and is almost always avoidable with proper attention to individual dosing and close monitoring. Sedation is frequent within the first days of therapy and must be distinguished from sleep deprivation resulting from pain. The patient in whom sedation is secondary to opioids is usually easily arousable with stimulation, but on the cessation of stimulation lapses into sleep. Pruritis, urinary retention, and nausea and vomiting are common within the first days of therapy. Frequently these problems are self-limiting. Pruritis often responds to hydroxyzine, and nausea and vomiting to low doses of antiemetics. If the problem continues and is not controlled with adjuvants, another opioid may have fewer side effects.

The fear of addiction keeps many physicians from prescribing opioid analgesics. However, the risk of addiction with the use of opioids for the treatment of pain is very low. Addiction and psychological dependence must be distinguished from tolerance and physical dependence. Tolerance is a poorly understood phenomenon, involving a receptor interaction in which the patient requires higher doses of analgesic to achieve the same amount of analgesia with no change in the underlying process. The first sign of tolerance is a decreased duration of action of the agent. Physical dependence is common after receiving opioid analgesics for more than 7 days. On abrupt discontinuation of the agent, one observes symptoms of withdrawal, which include abdominal pain, diarrhea, lacrimation, salivation, diaphoresis, and jitteriness. This is easily avoided by tapering the medication more slowly. Tolerance and physiological dependence do not indicate the presence or risk of psychological dependence or addiction. The patient who is psychologically dependent uses the medication for other than its pain relieving potential, perhaps to assuage anxiety or depression. Psychological dependence must be carefully distinguished from the normal and adaptive behavior of seeking the medication for the relief of pain, which itself can produce anxiety and depression. Unrelieved pain causes drug-seeking behavior; however, the therapy is treatment of the pain rather than focusing on medication use. Addiction is a pattern of behavior in which the patient is psychologically dependent on the medication and actively procures its supply.

ADJUVANTS

Benzodiazepines and phenothiazines provide little or no analgesia; rather, they alter behavior, so that the patient complains about the pain less and has fewer behavioral manifestations of pain without altering the experience of pain. Thus they should generally not be used in the treatment of pain. Benzodiazepines can be useful in the treatment of anxiety. In most situations involving pain, however, the anxiety is secondary to untreated pain, and the treatment is analgesia. When pain relief is provided, the anxiety resolves.

Tricyclic antidepressants (TCAs) can be useful in the treatment of severe chronic pain syndromes, especially when the pain is neuropathic. The analgesic effect of TCAs is exerted at approximately one-third to one-half the dose required for the treatment of depression. Usually 1 to 2 weeks of TCA therapy is required to see full analgesic effect; therefore these agents are not recommended for acute or temporary pain. When given at bedtime, TCAs in low doses also have a soporific effect that is seen immediately. This can help combat the sleep disturbance associated with severe pain. TCAs can be used alone in neuropathic pain or for migraine prophylaxis or as adjuvants to opioid analgesics. Amitriptyline is the most commonly used agent. The starting dose in children is 0.2 to 0.3 mg/kg, given as a single bedtime dose, with increments every 2 or 3 days to a usual maximum of 1 to 1.5 mg/kg/day in one dose. The rate of increase is based on tolerance of side effects, such as dry mouth, orthostatic hypotension, and morning sedation.

PROCEDURAL PAIN

For procedural pain, patients can be premedicated with a combination of an opioid and a benzodiazepine. In this combination the benzodiazepine assuages anticipatory anxiety and the opioid provides analgesia for the actual procedure. Chloral hydrate produces sedation without effect on anxiety or pain. Its use for procedural pain typically results in a child crying throughout the procedure and sleeping afterward. The combination of meperidine, phenergan, and thorazine often does not work well for procedural pain and has been associated with untoward side effects. Any child given premedication for procedural pain should be closely observed.

ACKNOWLEDGMENT

The review and substantive evaluation on which this article is based was supported in part by National Institute of Mental Health Grants MH-19156 and MH-44193 and in part by a grant from the Institute for Experimental Psychiatry Research Foundation.

BIBLIOGRAPHY

Anand KJS, Hickey PR: Pain and its effects in the human neonate and fetus. *N Engl J Med* 1987; 317:1321–1329.

Beaver WT: Combination analgesics. *Am J Med* 1984; 10:38–53.

Berde CB, Warfield CA: Pediatric pain management. *Hosp Pract* 1988; 30:83–101.

Foley K: Current controversies in opioid therapy, in Foley K, Inturrisi C (eds): *Opioid Analgesics in the Management of Clinical Pain.* New York, Raven Press, 1986; pp 3–11.

McGrath PJ, Unruth AM: *Pain in Children and Adolescents.* Amsterdam, Elsevier, 1987.

Newburger PE, Sallan SE: Chronic pain: Principles of management. *J Pediatr* 1981; 98:180–189.

Ross DM, Ross SA: *Childhood Pain: Current Issues, Research, and Management.* Baltimore, Urban & Schwarzenberg, 1988.

Schechter NL: *Pain and Pain Control in Children. Current Problems in Pediatrics.* Chicago, Year Book Medical Publishers, 1985; pp 1–87.

Schechter NL (ed): Symposium on recurrent pain in children. *Pediatr Clin North Am* 1984; 31.

Yaster M, Deshpande JK: Management of pediatric pain with opioid analgesics. *J Pediatr* 1988; 113:421–429.

101 RHEUMATOLOGY

Balu Athreya, M.D.

Primary care physicians are likely to be called on to manage the following problems related to arthritis: (1) diagnosis of arthritis in a child, (2) follow-up of children with juvenile rheumatoid arthritis (JRA) in collaboration with specialists, (3) dealing with toxic effects of drugs used in the management of rheumatic diseases, and (4) working with local school systems and outpatient physical therapy centers in treatment of children with arthritis and rheumatic diseases.

DIAGNOSIS OF ARTHRITIS

The primary care physician is the one most likely to see children in the initial phases of arthritis. Initial tasks include the establishment of the diagnosis and a search for the cause of the arthritis. The following criteria must be fulfilled for a diagnosis of arthritis: (1) swelling or effusion of a joint *or* (2) two or more of the following: limitation of range of motion, tenderness or pain on motion, increased heat.

Swelling of the joint, due to synovial thickening, is felt as a soft, velvety cushioning between the skin and the bone landmarks. Soft, gentle palpation is required to appreciate this finding. Effusion can be elicited by displacement of the fluid in the joint. Even if fluid can be demonstrated inside the joint, it is clinically impossible to say whether it is blood, inflammatory fluid, or noninflammatory fluid without looking at the fluid directly. Therefore, joint fluid aspiration and analysis are essential, particularly in single-joint disease (monarticular arthritis).

Patients with isolated joint pain or stiffness do not have arthritis. In the absence of swollen joints, two or more of the additional criteria mentioned above must be present.

Figure 101–1 summarizes an algorithm developed at the Children's Hospital of Philadelphia as a guideline in the differential diagnosis of arthritis in children. This approach helps the physician to separate acute arthritis from chronic arthritis. Acute arthritis, particularly of a single joint and associated with fever or rash, needs immediate attention. Chronic arthritis, on the other hand, is most often associated with one of the rheumatic disorders.

CAUSES OF ACUTE ARTHRITIS IN CHILDREN

Monarticular (single joint)
- Trauma
  - Stress fracture
  - Child abuse
  - Foreign body synovitis
  - Acute chondrolysis of the hip
- Sickle cell disease
- Hemophilia
- Infectious agent (septic) arthritis (e.g., *Staphylococcus, H. influenzae, Gonococcus*)

Polyarticular (many joints)
- Infectious agent arthritis
  - Rubella arthritis
  - Gonococcal dermatitis-arthritis syndrome
  - Enteric pathogens
- Rheumatic disorders
  - Acute rheumatic fever
  - Henoch-Schönlein purpura
  - Serum sickness
  - Kawasaki disease
  - Juvenile rheumatoid arthritis
- Hematologic
  - Sickle cell arthropathy
  - Leukemia

CAUSES OF CHRONIC ARTHRITIS IN CHILDREN

Monarticular
- Congenital lesions (e.g., discoid meniscus in the knee)

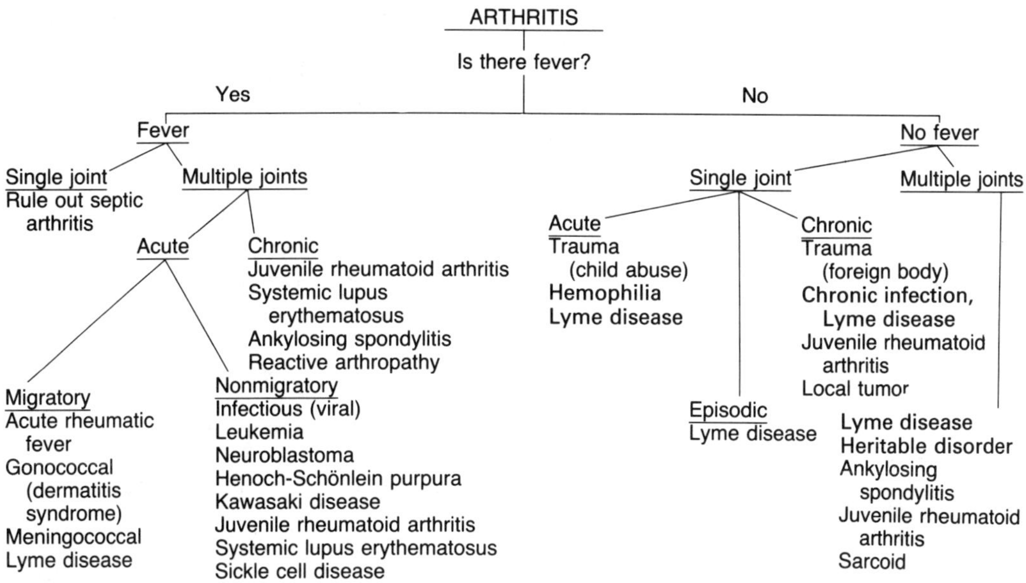

FIG 101–1
Algorithm developed at Children's Hospital of Philadelphia as a guide in the differential diagnosis of arthritis in children.

Foreign body arthritis (e.g., plant thorn synovitis)
Infectious agent arthritis (e.g., tuberculosis, fungus, Lyme arthritis)
Juvenile rheumatoid arthritis
Local tumors: Hemangioma
Other: Hemophilia, joint hypermobility with recurrent effusions

Polyarticular

Rheumatic disorders (e.g., juvenile rheumatoid arthritis, systemic lupus erythematosus, ankylosing spondylitis)
Chronic inflammation: Sarcoidosis, Lyme arthritis
Other: Heritable disorders of connective tissue, hypertrophic osteoarthropathy (e.g., cystic fibrosis)

Common errors in the diagnosis of arthritis are (1) mistaking conditions involving periarticular structures for arthritis, (2) mistaking true arthritis for other conditions, (3) mistaking aches and pains for true arthritis, leading to overdiagnosis of rheumatic disorders, and (4) excessive reliance on laboratory tests, such as rheumatoid factor (RF), antinuclear antibody (ANA), and HLA-B27.

MISTAKING CONDITIONS INVOLVING PERIARTICULAR STRUCTURES FOR ARTHRITIS

Conditions such as urticaria, cellulitis, tenosynovitis, and osteomyelitis may mimic arthritis. Careful history taking, clinical examination, and proper application of criteria for arthritis mentioned earlier should help differentiate among these conditions.

It is relatively easy to recognize urticaria from the history, characteristic physical appearance of the lesion, and the observation that there is no swelling of the joint all around. There is thickening of the skin over only portions of the skin around the joint. The joint also will have full range of movement.

Cellulitis can produce swelling all around the joint. The skin is tender and hot, making it difficult to decide whether there is an associated arthritis. Usually, the child can move the joint through a full range of motion by himself, though he may not allow others to do so. Laboratory studies may not be helpful in differentiating cellulitis from septic arthritis, since high white blood cell count, elevated sedimentation rate, and positive blood cultures may be seen in both conditions. Plain roentgenograms of the area and technetium or gallium scans may be necessary to rule out underlying osteomyelitis or arthritis. Caution should be exercised in aspirating the joint or bone, since passing a needle through an area of cellulitis may carry the infection to deeper structures.

Swelling of the tendons around the joint due to tenosynovitis may also present with pain, swelling, and limitation of motion. The swelling of tenosynovitis is diffuse, extending proximally and distally to the joint, in contrast to localized swelling of the joint. Tenderness along the tendons and inability to extend the fingers are clues to tenosynovitis of the flexor tendons of the hand. In addition to complete blood cell count, sedimentation rate, and blood cultures done as routine investigations, aspirations of tendon sheaths for culture may be needed.

Leukemia may present with joint pain and swelling. In children with leukemia, the bone pain is more prominent and the severity of pain is often out of proportion to the swelling of the joint. A blood cell count should often give clues to the actual diagnosis, though there are reports of children with a prolonged history of arthritis (up to six months) without evidence of leukemia in the peripheral smear. Bone marrow aspiration should be done when the index of suspicion is high. Roentgenograms may show the characteristic "leukemic" lines. Neuroblastoma may also present with joint pain and swelling.

MISTAKING JOINT PAINS (ARTHRALGIA) FOR TRUE ARTHRITIS

Confusing arthralgia (joint pains) with true arthritis leads to overdiagnosis of specific rheumatic disorders such as acute rheumatic fever, JRA, and systemic lupus erythematosus (SLE). This in turn leads to unnecessary referrals, laboratory tests, and treatments. The anxiety generated is often disabling.

Of the 110 children referred with a diagnosis of acute rheumatic fever, JRA, or SLE to our pediatric rheumatology center during one year, only 60 had a true rheumatic disorder. Criteria for the diagnosis of these common rheumatic disorders have been developed by the American Rheumatism Association and are available in standard textbooks of rheumatology. Strict application of criteria, wise use of laboratory data, and the use of consultants should help to rule out these diagnoses. The following are some of the common reasons for the overdiagnosis of these conditions.

COMMON CAUSES OF OVERDIAGNOSIS OF RHEUMATIC DISORDERS

- Overdiagnosis of acute rheumatic fever
  - Interpretation of arthralgia as arthritis
  - Interpretation of innocent murmurs or murmurs of congenital valvular lesions as murmurs of acute rheumatic fever in a patient with arthralgia
  - Overinterpretation of laboratory results, such as elevated ESR and antistreptococcal antibody titers
- Overdiagnosis of JRA
  - Mistaking bone pain and musculoskeletal pain for arthritis
  - Diagnosis too early in the course of the disease
  - Diagnosis before exclusion of other conditions
  - Overreliance on laboratory results, such as rheumatoid factor (RF) and antinuclear antibody (ANA)
- Overdiagnosis of SLE
  - Loose application of criteria
  - Diagnosis before exclusion of other conditions
  - Overreliance on laboratory tests, such as ANA
  - Mistaking hyperactive vascular response for Raynaud disease

OVERRELIANCE ON LABORATORY TESTS

Rheumatic disorders are difficult to diagnose, because they are chronic and except for acute rheumatic fever evolve over time. There are no specific laboratory tests, except in the case of SLE, and diagnosis is made on the basis of clinical findings and exclusion of other diseases.

Rheumatoid factor (RF) is *not* a diagnostic test for JRA. The sensitivity of this test at the Children's Hospital of Philadelphia is less than 5%. Since the prevalence of the disease is less common in the community than at a tertiary center, this test is useless as a screening test for JRA in office practice. However, once a child is known to have JRA (by using standard criteria), an RF test will be of help in defining the subset of JRA and as an aid to prognosis.

Antinuclear antibody (ANA) is *not* a diagnostic test for JRA. Once a diagnosis of JRA is made, the presence of ANA may help define the subset of JRA (pauciarticular arthritis in young girls, and with high risk for iridocyclitis), or may also suggest that the child's disorder may evolve into SLE or scleroderma. In the diagnosis of SLE, however, the ANA is an excellent screening test.

FOLLOW-UP OF CHILDREN WITH JRA

Rheumatic disorders are chronic disorders with varying courses, indefinite prognosis, exacerbations, and remissions. Management of rheumatic disorders requires the expertise of various specialists, including pediatric rheumatologists, orthopedic surgeons, nephrologists, dermatologists, ophthalmologists, and allied health personnel such as nurses, physical therapists, occupational therapists, social workers, and child guidance specialists. Therefore, a team leader who can coordinate the activities of these specialists and therapists and who can tailor the therapy to the needs of the child and the family is a necessity. The primary care physician is an ideal candidate for this leadership position. This is fully discussed in Chapter 106.

The main goal of therapy in the management of children with JRA is to keep the children active and allow them to lead as normal a life as possible. Therefore, in addition to helping with the treatment of JRA and other acute medical problems, the primary care physicians should take care of the routine medical and developmental needs of these children. Routine immunizations, including rubella vaccination, should be completed *except in those children on steroids and on immunosuppressive drugs,* who should not receive live virus vaccines. Developmental assessments and counseling should be continued as for normal children.

Some of the specific problems associated with arthritis that may come to the attention of the primary care physician are (1) generalized growth retardation, (2) localized growth abnormalities, (3) eye problems, (4) fever, (5) morning stiffness, (6) anemia, and (7) toxic effects of drugs. In addition, the primary care physician may be called on to answer questions by the physical and occupational therapists.

Growth Retardation.—Growth retardation is common in children with systemic and polyarticular-type JRA who are often the shortest in their class. The exact cause is not known, though it is probably related to chronic inflammatory disease. In some children, growth retardation is related to steroid therapy with or without vertebral collapse.

General attention to good nutrition is essential, as in any chronic disease, but there is no proved benefit to any of the popular diet therapies. In patients with growth retardation due to steroid therapy, every effort should be made to withdraw the medication. Localized growth disturbances such as leg-length discrepancy and small feet are also common in JRA

Eye Problems.—Iridocyclitis, a major cause of disability in children with JRA, is a particular problem for children with pauciarticular arthritis, who also exhibit ANA in their serum. The onset is insidious and may be asymptomatic. Therefore, all children with JRA should have an initial comprehensive eye evaluation. The following routine is suggested for periodic slit-lamp examination: every 3 to 4 months for pauciarticular arthritis with positive ANA; every 6 months for pauciarticular JRA without ANA, systemic-type JRA, and RF-negative polyarticular JRA; and every year for RF-positive polyarticular JRA and children receiving steroid therapy.

Once the disease enters remission, the slit-lamp examination should be repeated every year for at least three or four years as iridocyclitis can occur even after arthritis has cleared.

Fever.—Elevated temperature, a common sign in children, presents a problem to the physician to decide whether the fever is related to JRA or is due to some other cause. Statistical probability favors the diagnosis of an intercurrent respiratory or urinary tract infection as the most likely explanation for fever. However, there are some specific problems to consider in children with JRA.

First, these children are on aspirin or one of the other nonsteroidal anti-inflammatory drugs. Therefore, when fever occurs, one of the questions is whether to add another drug. Generally, it is not necessary. An occasional dose of acetaminophen (one or two doses per day) should not cause any harm.

Some of the nonsteroidal drugs, specifically indomethacin, may mask localized evidence of inflammation. Therefore, one should perform a thorough physical examination and appropriate laboratory tests to rule out common infections, such as otitis media and urinary tract infection.

Children with systemic JRA who have recurrence of fever always present a diagnostic dilemma. The fever may represent recurrence of JRA or an intercurrent infection. Absence of localizing signs of infection, a fever pattern resembling the earlier course associated with the characteristic rash should suggest exacerbation of the disease. Since leukocytosis may be seen as part of systemic JRA, a WBC count may not help in differentiating fever of JRA from that of an infection. Urinalysis and cultures of other body fluids need to be obtained as indicated.

In any child with JRA and fever, there is always a concern that septic arthritis has been added onto the rheumatoid process. The usual findings are increased pain in the affected joint, warmth and limitation of range of movement. Pain on moving the joint is very intense and the child usually does not allow even minimal degrees of motion. Joint fluid aspiration for cell count and culture is absolutely necessary if septic arthritis is suspected.

Morning Stiffness.—This can be disabling for some children with JRA. Two of the measures that can ameliorate this symptom are (1) a warm tub bath for 10 to 20 minutes in the morning, and (2) sleeping in a sleeping bag at night.

Anemia.—Anemia seen in association with JRA may be due to the chronic inflammatory process, iron deficiency, or both. The anemia is usually of the normocytic normochromic type, but associated iron deficiency may give a microcytic hypochromic picture. Serum iron concentration is low, as in iron deficiency anemia, but iron-binding capacity is normal in anemia of chronic disease. Oral iron therapy may be tried, but is not always successful. The anemia corrects itself when the disease enters remission.

Other causes of anemia in JRA are blood loss through the gastrointestinal tract, hemolysis (either related to the disease or to drugs), and drug-related bone marrow depression.

PHYSICAL THERAPY

The goals of physical therapy measures are: (1) relief of pain, (2) maintenance or improvement of range of motion, (3) improvement of muscle strength, and (4) improvement of activities of daily living.

Splinting of an acutely inflamed joint is the best method of achieving pain relief. It is easy to make splints for the knee and the wrist using plaster of paris. The splint should be removed twice daily and the child allowed to move the joint actively. If this is not possible, the child should be taught to do muscle-setting exercises.

Various types of exercises are used to maintain the range of movement of joints and of muscle strength. They vary from passive (therapist moves the limb) to active range (child voluntarily moves the limb), active assistive (child contracts the muscle with help from the therapist), and active resistive (child contracts the muscle against resistance supplied by the therapist).

In children, therapy measures should take into account the child's developmental status and the need for motivation. Play activities that are age-appropriate and that include principles of physical therapy are more likely to be acceptable to children than are drab daily routines. For example, swimming is an excellent exercise for children with arthritis. A tricycle can be used to improve the range of movement of the knee joint. With the seat adjusted high, pedaling will force the child to extend the knee and is ideal for children with knee flexion contractures. On the other hand, for a child who cannot bend the knee fully, gradually lowering the seat on the tricycle will demand increasing flexion.

ANTIRHEUMATIC DRUGS AND TOXICITY

Most of the drugs used in the management of rheumatic disease have major side effects. Table 101–1 summarizes the drugs used in the management of JRA and their usual side effects.

Aspirin, still the most commonly used drug in the treatment of JRA, requires a higher dose than that used for the treatment of fever. Antirheumatic activity is seen only at serum sali-

TABLE 101–1
Drugs Commonly Used in the Treatment of Rheumatic Diseases and Their Side Effects

DRUG	USUAL DOSAGE	SIDE EFFECTS
Acetylsalicylic acid (aspirin)	80–100 mg/kg/day (in young children); older, larger children and adolescents, start with about 6–8 tablets of 375 mg each in divided doses	Rapid breathing, easy bruising, GI tract irritation, tinnitus, temporary hearing loss, allergy, hepatotoxic effects (elevated SGOT, SGPT); rarely, Reye syndrome
Tolmetin sodium (Tolectin)	15–30 mg/kg/day; maximum, 1,800 mg/day	GI tract irritation, hematuria, proteinuria, hepatotoxic effects, drop in the hematocrit reading (due to hemodilution)
Indomethacin (Indocin)	1.5–3.0 mg/kg/day; maximum, 100 mg/day	Headache, dizziness, GI tract irritation and bleeding, dermatitis, masking of infections
Ibuprofen (Motrin)	Approximately 20–35 mg/kg/day	GI tract irritation, tinnitus, hepatotoxic effects, aseptic meningitis syndrome, allergy
Naproxen (Naprosyn)	10–20 mg/kg/day in 2 divided doses; maximum, 750 mg/day	GI tract irritation, GI tract ulcer, headache, tinnitus, hepatotoxic effects, allergy
Hydroxychloroquine (Plaquenil)	5–7 mg/kg/day maximum; 400 mg/day	Dermatitis, keratopathy, retinopathy, GI tract irritation, bone marrow depression, change of color of hair
Parenteral gold preparations (Myochrysine or Solganal)	Weekly injections gradual increase in dose; maximum dose of 1 mg/kg for once-weekly injection	Rash, bone marrow depression, renal toxic effects, aphthous ulcers
Oral gold (Ridaura)	0.15–0.2 mg/kg/day in one dose at bedtime; maximum 6–9 mg/day	Diarrhea, rash
D-Penicillamine	5–10 mg/kg/day	Same as for gold, plus myasthenia, dermatomyositis, and lupus-like syndrome
Corticosteroids	Varies with preparation, e.g., prednisone 0.5–2.0 mg/kg/day	Growth retardation, cushingoid facies, hirsutism, elevated blood pressure, osteoporosis, fractures, aseptic necrosis, collapse of vertebrae, GI tract irritation, peptic ulcer, cataracts, psychosis, myopathy, opportunistic infections, masked infections

cylate levels of 20 to 30 mg/dL. The usual starting dose is 80 mg/kg/day given in four divided doses during the child's waking hours. It is *unnecessary* to give aspirin at 6-hour intervals, which interferes with a good night's rest for both the child and the parents. Serum salicylate levels can be measured (after 5 to 7 days of therapy) and the dose readjusted to reach therapeutic levels. Once the correct dose has been established, there is no reason to recheck salicylate levels too often. Since aspirin can cause hepatotoxic effects, serum glutamic oxaloacetic transaminase (SGOT) and serum glutamic pyruvic transaminase (SGPT) levels should be checked frequently during the first 2 to 3 months of therapy. If a child receiving aspirin therapy develops chickenpox, it is wise to discontinue therapy, as there is some evidence that children with JRA receiving chronic aspirin therapy also may have a higher risk of developing Reye syndrome. Children receiving aspirin therapy who develop nausea and vomiting need to have their SGOT and SGPT levels checked. If these values are high, it is best to stop therapy and follow them closely until liver function abnormalities normalize.

Two to 6 weeks of treatment are usually required with therapeutic doses of aspirin before any effect on the course of arthritis can be seen. If fever, rash, and arthritis are brought under control, the treatment is continued and the child followed up at two- to three-month intervals. If there is no response to therapy with aspirin, it is reasonable to try one of the new nonsteroidal anti-inflammatory drugs listed in Table 101–1. Among these, the most accepted is tolmetin sodium (Tolectin). Naprosyn may also be used, particularly in older children who find the twice-daily dosage more acceptable. Indomethacin is not to be used routinely in the treatment of JRA, but should be reserved for children with uncontrollable fever and those with pericarditis.

If after an adequate trial with one or more of the nonsteroidal anti-inflammatory drugs for 3 to 6 months the disease is not under control, or if it is rapidly progressive, one of the slow-acting antirheumatic drugs (injectable gold, D-penicillamine, hydroxychloroquine, oral gold) is then added to the treatment program. Frequent monitoring of the patient is essential to watch for serious side effects on the bone marrow and the kidneys.

Steroids are used only in the presence of fever that is uncontrollable by other drugs, severe pericarditis, rapidly progressive arthritis with severe pain and limitation, and eye disease. Topical steroids are used for the treatment of iridocyclitis.

Combinations of drugs are often used in the treatment of rheumatic diseases. Many of these drugs are associated with serious side effects, and some are potentially lethal (e.g., bone marrow depression due to gold administration). These potentially dangerous drugs should be used by physicians with experience, and it is imperative that there is communication between the specialists who initiate treatment with these drugs and the primary care physician.

WORKING WITH LOCAL REHABILITATION CENTERS AND SCHOOL SYSTEMS

Juvenile rheumatoid arthritis is characterized by morning stiffness and arthritis in all cases. Fever, rash, and eye disease are seen in certain subtypes of JRA only. All children with JRA take daily medications and a dose may have to be administered at school. Though the general philosophy in the management of these children is to keep them active and leading as normal a life as possible, there are times when some restrictions are needed. During a flare, a child may not be able to take part in regular physical education activities. All of these disease features create some problems in relation to school attendance and activities.

In the presence of morning stiffness, the child may not be able to arrive in time for the first class period or may be stiff and unable to move rapidly from one classroom to another. Therefore, he or she may have to start earlier than the others at the end of each class. These children may need two sets of books, one for home and one for school, to spare them having to carry heavy books. The physical education teacher may need a note from the physician to excuse the child completely, or to arrange a special program for the child. (The latter is ideal, so that the child does not become totally excluded.) If the hands are severely involved, these children may be allowed to do their homework and reports with a tape recorder, rather than have to write.

In the presence of fever and rash, schoolteachers and school nurses often feel nervous and send the child home. This may be appropriate before the diagnosis is made, but unnecessary once the diagnosis is certain and the child is receiving treatment. Children with eye problems may need special seating arrangements.

To aid in the management of all these problems, and many more, the schoolteacher and the school nurse require resources and support. Many specialty clinics in academic centers have special programs to work with the school systems. There are monographs and books that may be of use to the school nurses. However, as a person living in the community who knows its resources, as a leader in the community, and as one who knows the family and the school system, the family practitioner is the ideal resource person for the school system.

ACKNOWLEDGMENT

My thanks to David B. Rosenberg, M.D., of Vineland, N.J., who helped formulate the ideas expressed in this chapter.

BIBLIOGRAPHY

Athreya BH: Differential diagnosis of arthritis in children. *Pediatr Digest* 1976; 18:12–14.

Athreya BH, Yancey C, Eichenfeld AE: Rheumatologic emergencies, in Fleisher G, Ludwig S (eds): *Textbook of Pediatric Emergency Medicine*, ed 2. Baltimore, Williams & Wilkins, 1988.

Brewer EJ, Giannini EH, Person DA: *Juvenile Rheumatoid Arthritis*, vol 6, *Major Problems in Pediatrics*. Philadelphia, WB Saunders Co, 1982.

Cassidy JT (ed): *Textbook of Rheumatology*. New York, John Wiley & Sons, 1982.

Eichenfield AH: Goldsmith DP, Benach JL, et al: Childhood Lyme arthritis: Experience in an endemic area. *J Pediatr* 1986; 109:753–758.

Fithian J (ed): *Understanding the Child with a Chronic Illness in the Classroom*. Phoenix, Oryx Press, 1984.

Jacobs JC: *Pediatric Rheumatology for the Practitioner*. New York, Springer-Verlag, 1982.

section vii

Talking With Parents

Effective communication is an important task for the primary care physician who needs to interact well with his patients and families, using interpersonal skills to increase awareness of health, improve compliance, and promote well-being. The topics in this section include one person's method of conveying a diagnosis and plans to parents of children with medical problems. The authors offer interesting approaches to communication of sensitive information.

102 INNOCENT MURMUR

Sidney Friedman, M.D.

Approximately 90% of children referred to a cardiologist for evaluation are referred because of the presence of a cardiac murmur. The two common types of heart disease in childhood, congenital and rheumatic heart disease, usually present with a cardiac murmur. Skill in cardiac auscultation is important in pediatrics, since approximately 40% of normal children between the ages of 2 and 12 years have so-called functional or innocent murmurs. Thus, physicians are beset with the problem of determining in every second or third patient examined whether a murmur is a significant one, indicating the presence of heart disease, or an innocent one, indicating the absence of heart disease.

A label of functional or innocent murmur has the following implications: (1) no pathologic changes are present in the heart or great vessels; (2) the cardiac murmur does not affect the future health or prognosis of the patient; (3) no further diagnostic investigation or long-term follow-up systematic observation is necessary; (4) no prophylaxis against bacterial endocarditis is necessary; (5) no antistreptococcal prophylaxis is needed in order to prevent a recurrence of rheumatic fever.

There is abundant evidence in the literature and from the personal experience of pediatric cardiologists that functional or innocent murmurs can be identified accurately by simple auscultation. A recent study by Newberger and associates supported the concept that a qualified pediatric cardiologist can identify accurately the categories of "no heart disease" or "definite heart disease" without the use of simple or complex diagnostic testing. The close correlation of the separate clinical examinations of Friedman and Wells in a survey of approximately 5,000 schoolchildren in Philadelphia also supports this concept. There is ample evidence that innocent murmurs are truly benign with regard to future cardiac health. A 20-year follow-up study by Marienfeld and associates, published in 1962, demonstrated that the incidence of real heart disease in a group of adults identified as having an innocent murmur 20 years earlier was the same as in a group of controlled patients without a cardiac murmur in childhood.

In a survey of over 20,000 schoolchildren, Bergman and Stamm pointed out the high incidence of the false diagnosis of heart disease resulting from the misinterpretation of innocent murmurs and suggested the term "cardiac nondisease." The inaccuracy in diagnosis often resulted in unnecessary restriction and anxiety about heart disease in children and parents. The authors pointed out the frequency of confusion in the lay person's understanding of heart disease in children—specifically, fear of heart attacks from overexertion, a concept derived from the symptoms of adult degenerative heart disease. They concluded that the amount of disability from cardiac nondisease was greater than that due to actual heart disease in children. Failure of adequate communication between physicians and parents and the false diagnosis of heart disease resulting from the misinterpretation of innocent murmurs were the main sources of the cardiac nondisease.

Since many children are examined in routine school physical examinations or in presports or precamp examinations by physicians other than their family physician, and since many children are followed in group practices in which examinations are carried out by a number of different doctors, it is wise to mention the presence of a cardiac murmur to parents and to enter this information into the written records.

The skill and subjective confidence of physicians in deciding whether a cardiac murmur is innocent or significant vary widely. Nevertheless, an effective policy of management of children with cardiac murmurs can be established. If the presence of the murmur is reported to the family, the primary care physician must first decide whether he or she is certain or uncertain about the identification of the cardiac murmur. If the murmur is an innocent one, then the physician can proceed with the verbal type of communication outlined below. The physician may decide to observe the cardiac murmur on several occasions and come to a final conclusion at a later date. This scheme should be carried out without involving the parents in one's own indecision. If the diagnosis is uncertain, or if the parents are aware of the presence of the murmur, the physician must take further steps promptly to clarify the situation by appropriate consultation and study. It is unwise and unfair to permit parents with an unsettled question about the presence or absence of heart disease in their offspring to suffer this indecision for any significant length of time. When logistically possible, the use of such basic studies as an electrocardiogram (ECG) or chest radiograph is expected as a further confirmation and should be ordered to enhance the attitude of certainty. However, these studies are not a substitute for a skillful physical examination.

The following dialogue is an example of an appropriate approach to the discussion of the diagnosis of innocent murmurs with parents.

> I can hear a heart murmur in my examination of John, but I do not think it is of any importance. It falls in the category of heart murmurs that are called functional or innocent. Are you familiar with these terms? (The answer is usually "no.")
>
> There are a large number of children who have heart murmurs that we know from experience are not related to heart disease or a heart defect. These murmurs are called functional or innocent murmurs, because they have no relationship to any defect of the structure of the heart but rather are related to the function or working of the heart. These murmurs are due to a vibration of the heart muscle itself rather than to the turbulence of blood flow related to a defect such as a hole between two of the chambers or an abnormality of one of the valves in the heart.
>
> There is a considerable and lengthy experience in following patients with functional or innocent murmurs. It has been shown by long-term follow-up studies that patients with functional or innocent murmurs do not have any higher incidence of heart disease than patients without such murmurs, even after they are observed for 20 or 30 years. Therefore, you can be certain that this murmur will not turn into something else in the future. It is not the beginning of some other condition that will be a problem later on.
>
> I think it would be a good idea to do a routine survey of your child's heart to gain even more reassurance that the murmur is of no importance. I think that we should do an electrocardiogram and a chest radiograph in order to get further information indicating that the heart is normal. If results of these studies are normal, then I do not think there is any need to pursue this matter further. If results of these studies are normal, which I expect they will be, the accuracy of the diagnosis is extremely high, approaching 100% in the presence of a murmur of this character.

At this point, it is appropriate to answer any questions that arise and to send the family off to have the studies done. This provides parents with some time to think over what has been said and to identify any questions they want answered. When they return, I look at the radiograph and ECG. If results of these are normal, then I have a further conversation with the parents along the following lines:

> Both of the tests, the radiograph and the ECG, are entirely normal so everything seems to fit together, the physical examination and the studies. There are a few things I want to be sure you understand about functional or innocent murmurs. First and foremost, there is nothing anatomically wrong with your child's heart. He can be on the football team. This murmur does not mean that he has any struc-

tural defect or disease of his heart. The second point I want to make is this: While it is true that about 90% of these murmurs disappear when the child is around 10 or 14 years of age, not 100% of them disappear. However, it makes no difference whether the murmur disappears or does not disappear, as far as the future cardiac health of your child is concerned. For this reason, it is not necessary to have any follow-up examinations in children with functional or innocent murmurs. It is important to identify the murmur, but there is no need to continue to examine this child until the murmur is no longer audible. That will not contribute anything to the future health care of your child. The identification of the murmur is what we are doing today, and it is clear that the murmur is a functional or innocent one.

The third point I want to make is that you may, indeed, hear about this murmur again. These functional or innocent murmurs are variable in how loud they sound on different occasions. They are made to sound louder by any condition that increases the work of the heart. Thus, if a child has a fever or is anemic, or perhaps is apprehensive about something, these functional or innocent murmurs will sound very loud to the listener. Sometimes, when the murmurs are quite loud, they are interpreted by the person who is examining the child to be more important and significant than they really are. In this way, you may hear about the presence of a loud murmur again, particularly at a time when the heart is working hard. The clinical setting in which this sequence may occur is a school physical examination, or during a family trip when the child develops an illness with fever. A physician who does not know the child from previous examinations may mention to you, under these circumstances, that a loud heart murmur is present, and advise further evaluation. You must remember not to push the panic button under these circumstances, because the murmur will almost certainly be the same murmur present today, but will have been accentuated by fever or apprehension.

The goal of this presentation is to transmit a sense of certainty to both parents and child about the absence of heart disease. Contributing to this are (1) firmness of expression by the physician. This is largely an expression of the confidence he or she has in his or her own cardiac auscultation skills. Expressions such as "he can be on the football team" offer more reassurance to parents than the expression, "no restrictions are necessary" or "don't worry about it"; (2) the lack of need for follow-up is a strong point of reassurance for parents and should be stressed and the rationale repeated; and (3) some form of diagnostic testing should be employed to support the clinical diagnosis. This may not be essential on a statistical analysis for an experienced pediatric cardiologist, but testing provides a great deal of additional psychological support for parents and referring physicians.

Above all, be definite!

BIBLIOGRAPHY

Bergman AB, Stamm SJ: The morbidity of cardiac nondisease in school children. *N Engl J Med* 1967; 276:1008–1013.

Friedman S, Robie WA, Harris TN: Occurrence of innocent adventitious cardiac sounds in childhood. *Pediatrics* 1949; 3:782–789.

Friedman S, Wells CR: Experience in secondary screening of cardiac suspects of school age. *J Pediatr* 1956; 49:410–416.

Marienfeld CJ, Telles N, Silvera J, et al: A 20-year follow-up study of "innocent" murmurs. *Pediatrics* 1962; 30:42–48.

Newberger JW, Rosenthal A, Williams RG, et al: Noninvasive tests in the initial evaluation of heart murmurs in children. *N Engl J Med* 1983; 308:61–64.

SUGGESTED READING

Friedman S: The innocent (functional) cardiac murmurs of childhood. *Clin Pediatr* 1965; 4:77–81.

Friedman S: Some thoughts about functional or innocent murmurs. *Clin Pediatr* 1973; 12:678–679.

Caceres CA, Perry LW (eds): *The Innocent Murmur—A Problem in Clinical Practice.* Boston, Little, Brown & Co, 1967.

103 MENTAL RETARDATION

Thomas Curry, M.D.

During the course of monitoring a child's development, the primary care physician will be able to detect children who fail to progress through established normal ranges of development. Using a developmental screening test such as the Denver Developmental Screening Test, the physician can identify the children in need of more extensive evaluation, which usually involves other members of the medical team: geneticists, neurologists, and psychologists. This panel of physicians permits a refined approach to the multitude of problems. Unfortunately, the diversity of styles and methods of individual team members can often be a source of uncertainty to the family. Either as the coordinator of the evaluation or as the translator of the recommendations from the diagnostic team, the primary care physician is frequently the one who must tell the parents that their child is retarded.

Discussion with the parents of a mentally retarded child requires sensitivity and forethought. The pressure of time can severely impair the physician's ability to appropriately explain a diagnosis, interpret an evaluation, and react to parental concerns. Prior to a parent conference, the physician must prepare for the meeting. A few seconds to review documents immediately prior to talking with the parents is insufficient and can frequently lead to a most unsatisfactory outcome. The physician should understand the details of the evaluation that has taken place, the nature of the testing that was performed, and the specific results of the testing.

A short list of goals to be accomplished during the meeting is helpful in focusing the discussion and developing a general format for the meeting.

THE CONFERENCE

Although working parents frequently find it difficult to arrange a time that both may be present, efforts should be made to avoid delivering the news to one person. The absent parent will frequently demand explanations and ask questions that the parent who was present finds difficult or impossible to answer. It is helpful to determine in advance of the conference if the parents wish other members of the extended family to attend the meeting. This conference may require several sessions. The amount of time spent at the meeting is dependent upon the ability of the parent to comprehend and absorb all the facts and attitudes that are presented.

Structuring the parent conference is important. A typical outline is presented below.

STRUCTURE OF PARENT CONFERENCE

The diagnosis
Interpretation of diagnosis
Review of tests
Emphasis on normal features
Planning
Effect on child
Effect on family
Closing
Need for second opinion
Definite follow-up

Giving the conclusions at the beginning of the conference rather than at the end permits the parents to react to the diagnosis throughout the interview. For some, the shock of the diagnosis may cease any further meaningful dialogue. Since many parents have some idea that their child is retarded, the risk of stating the diagnosis early is limited. The diagnosis can be expressed in a variety of terms, such as below-normal intelligence or below-average potential. It is important, however, for the parents to hear the term "retardation" from the physician. If retardation is not mentioned, parents may leave the meeting feeling their child is just slow or delayed but not retarded. Occasionally, a physician will spend considerable time enumerating in great detail the results of testing prior to giving a final diagnosis. This technique only heightens the parents' tension and anxiety as they wait for the conclusion.

After presenting the diagnosis, the physician can interpret the diagnosis for the family. This discussion should include review of the tests performed. The physician's demonstration of a working knowledge of the tests employed will understandably enhance the parents' acceptance of the diagnosis. Clarification of the results of psychological testing or other evaluations from the subspecialists should be done prior to the meeting so that the physician's poor understanding of the tests does not give the parents an excuse to doubt the diagnosis.

During the conference, the parents need to hear positive statements about their child. A special effort should be made to emphasize those aspects of the child's evaluations that are normal. If appropriate, this is the time to state that the child will walk or speak but at a slower rate than peers. While parents may focus on the areas of delay, the positive features such as ability to attend school or participation in sports should be mentioned.

Even though the diagnosis is mentioned at the outset of the conference, the problem needs to be put in the perspective of the child and the family. Parents will want to know the effect all this information will have on their child. What are the recommendations for the short term as to the special educational placement, schooling, and therapy? The child should be given an opportunity to use all of his or her capabilities. Overprotection is not helpful for the child; optimal training is. Specific opportunities for schooling such as Association for Retarded Children or public school can be mentioned. Achieving full potential, however limited, is the goal that must be reinforced several times in the discussion.

The physician should attempt to deal with the potential effect of the diagnosis on the family. Usually the parents worry about the possibility of this occurring in another child. They may try affixing blame on themselves or others for this problem. This concern about genetic implications should have been anticipated in the evaluation. If appropriate, metabolic screening or genetic considerations are helpful in detecting an inherited disorder. Parents want to know if they are responsible for their child's retardation. Mothers have questions about events in their pregnancies that may have caused the problem. The parents may need help in explaining the diagnosis to their other children. This explanation should be brief and appropriate to the level of understanding of the child. Obviously, sensitivity is needed in dealing with this issue. The family may also appreciate help in how to explain the diagnosis with its difficult implications to nonfamily members.

Finally, a complete parent conference deals with the parents' need to doubt the diagnosis. The parents can be told that it is normal to have doubts about the diagnosis and they may need to have a second opinion. The mention of another opinion should be followed by a list of facilities or personnel who can provide this service, rather than allowing the parents to seek out persons who provide advice that either is unhelpful or delays acceptance or training. A file of Academy of Pediatric Committee Reports can be offered to the family to help them understand problems of vitamin therapy or exercise in treating retardation. Not all families will require another opinion, reflecting either their own personality and experience or the adequacy of the evaluation and conference. Rather than interpret the need for a second opinion as a threat to intelligence or skill, the physician should be a facilitator to make this second opinion a learning experience and an ability for the family to build confidence in their physician. During the conference it is appropriate to pause and permit periods of silence to aid the family in adjusting to the information and to allow an opportunity to formulate questions on sensitive topics.

At the conclusion of the conference, a specific follow-up appointment should be made. This second meeting serves to continue the dialogue about the problem as well as to indicate to the parents that they are not being abandoned by their physician who will be part of their support system.

PROBLEMS AND PITFALLS

Some parents have anticipated the diagnosis of mental retardation. By comparing their child with peers or siblings, they are aware that development is delayed. Others may be upset and alarmed. Their response is similar to the grief response popularized by Kubler-Ross—denial, rage, depression, acceptance, and adjustment. Some parents may have to symbolically bury their expectations for an ideal child before they can begin to deal with their child. On occasion, the initial reaction of the parents to the specific diagnosis or the specific test results is so overwhelming that the remainder of the material anticipated for the conference must be postponed. The physician needs to be willing to reschedule a conference under these circumstances. To plow through the remaining agenda with parents who are unable to focus or participate in the conference is inappropriate.

More commonly, the parents demonstrate resistance to the diagnosis. The physician should appreciate at least some degree of denial. It is understandable that the parents hope that the information is inaccurate or incorrect. Expressing an understanding that the family may wish that these facts were not true permits alignment with the family at a crucial time. The physician needs to remain firm, however, in the presentation of the conclusion.

Infrequently, anger is directed toward the person conducting the parent conference. Hostility by the physician does not aid the parents in the acceptance of the news. Quietly pointing out their anger and asking them to explain their feelings are of greater value.

During the discussion highly technical aspects should be avoided. Parents cannot always appreciate the intricate detail of testing or of laboratory evaluations. It is important to explain the test results with a language that is appropriate for the parent. Pausing frequently and asking if they wish an explanation repeated or restated is helpful.

Making very specific long-term predictions of outcome is inappropriate. Repeatedly, parents relate anecdotes of physicians who told parents that their child would never respond to treatment, only to prove the physician wrong. Physicians' expectations of eventual outcome have been shown at times to be too pessimistic compared with those of other health professionals. The long-term outcome needs to be addressed, but an attempt at the initial conference with the parents to make specific predictions is hazardous.

CONCLUSION

Mental retardation is often suspected by the primary care physician, who will also be the individual responsible for presenting the diagnosis to the family. To be effective, the physician must have familiarity with the tests, present the diagnosis in a firm but gentle manner, and then be prepared to support the family as they accept the diagnosis and make plans for the future.

BIBLIOGRAPHY

Kaminer RK, Cohen HJ: How do you say, "Your child is retarded"? *Contemp Pediatr* 1988; 5:36–49.

Korsch BM: What do patients and parents want to know? What do they need to know? *Pediatrics* 1984; 74:917–919.

McInerny T: The role of the general pediatrician in coordinating the care of children with chronic illness. *Pediatr Clin North Am* 1984; 31:199–209.

Myers BA: The informing interview: Enabling parents to "hear" and cope with bad news. *Am J Dis Child* 1983; 137:572.

Olson J, Edwards M, Hunter JA: The physician's role in delivering sensitive information to families with handicapped infants. *Clin Pediatr* 1987; 26:231–234.

Schulman JL: Coping with major disease: Child, family, pediatrician. *J Pediatr* 1983; 102:988–991.

Wolraich ML, Superstein GN, O'Keefe P: Pediatricians' perceptions of mentally retarded individuals. *Pediatrics* 1987; 80:643–649.

Zwerling I: Initial counseling of parents with mentally retarded children. *J Pediatr* 1954; 44:469.

104 DOWN SYNDROME

Deborah L. Eunpu, M.S.
Elaine H. Zackai, M.D.

Down syndrome, the most common cause of mental retardation, occurs in approximately one in 600 live births. Because of the high incidence, most pediatricians will be confronted at some time with the necessity of informing parents that their child has this condition. How the physician informs the parents about the diagnosis can be a critical determinant of how well the parents accept this unexpected event and adjust to its implications.

CONFIRMING THE DIAGNOSIS

As soon as the diagnosis is suspected, the physician should arrange the confirming chromosome analysis so that parents can be told the diagnosis at the earliest time. Results of the study can usually be obtained 72 hours after culture initiation if prior arrangements are made with the referral laboratory. When asked their preference, the vast majority of parents of children with Down syndrome express a desire to be informed of the diagnosis as soon as possible. Many parents are aware that a problem exists before the physician has mentioned the suspicion, and a delay in providing the diagnostic information can result in parents being informed inappropriately by another source. Early informing will also allow the parents to consider all options for the care of the child with Down syndrome. Delaying the disclosure can also reduce the parents' trust of the primary care physician.

When an infant has associated problems requiring immediate medical attention (e.g., a congenital heart defect or duodenal atresia), it is equally important that the parents be apprised of the diagnosis of Down syndrome as soon as possible. This will help them to view the infant's problem(s) in the context of the overall diagnosis and not to focus on isolated aspects of the child's condition.

Although most often the mother is first informed alone, most parents prefer to be told together. Telling both parents together allows them to support each other and permits each one to obtain answers to his or her questions. Other parent preferences include being told in a private setting and if possible having the baby present during the discussion. Parents have found it beneficial if there is another professional present who can be available to them for questions and discussion after the initial informing session. The physician must also consider the specific family constellation in deciding how to proceed with informing the parents.

INFORMATION FOR PARENTS

The information relayed to the parents should include an explanation of the chromosomal basis of the diagnosis, the risk of recurrence, the availability of prenatal diagnosis in a future pregnancy, a description of the associated physical features and medical problems, and a discussion of the developmental expectations for children with Down syndrome. The discussion should be in language and terms that the parents can understand. Telling parents their child will be mentally retarded can have very different meanings to different parents. Some associate retardation with violent behavior; others have a concept that retardation implies no development. Thus, it is most important to use descriptive examples to provide a frame of reference that parents can comprehend meaningfully. Parents need to know that although acquisition of milestones is expected to be delayed, the child with Down syndrome is expected to sit, walk, talk, and be able to manage self-care tasks such as dressing, going to the toilet, and feeding. The physician must also describe the expected limits. Since individuals with Down syndrome continue to learn by rote rather than by progressing to higher cognitive levels of integrative learning, they will not be able to attain full independence as adults. Again, the physician should give specific, concrete examples that are more helpful than simply giving an expected IQ level (mean, 50 to 60) or telling parents the child will probably function in the trainable range of retardation. Overall, one should present a balanced view of the significance of the diagnosis of Down syndrome. Expected limitations, potential medical problems, and positive characteristics all merit discussion.

Every parent deserves to know the possible alternatives for caring for their child with Down syndrome. While most parents will want to raise the infant in their family, it is important that parents at least know that foster care (temporary or leading to adoption) can be arranged. Residential placement may not be an option in the newborn period, because many residential facilities will not accept infants for admission. In addition, it is agreed that children with Down syndrome do best in a one-to-one care setting. Temporary foster care can serve as a valuable alternative if the parents are ambivalent about their plans for the child. Foster care leading to adoption is a very feasible option if the parents decide not to rear their child with Down syndrome. Since infants with Down syndrome are regarded as being very adoptable, local social service agencies can usually provide ready access to adoption agencies and resources. In presenting such information, the physician should encourage the parents to consider these possible options and help them see that the choice they make should be determined by what best suits their specific family situation. Parents should not be told which choice to select nor should they be urged to make permanent decisions without adequate consideration.

Parents who will raise their child with Down syndrome in their home should be apprised of locally available infant stimulation programs, the local Association for Retarded Citizens (ARC), parent support groups, and other supportive services (financial, social, and psychological).

Follow-up discussions will frequently be required to cover all information. Many parents, on hearing the diagnosis, cannot absorb additional information. These couples will require time to adjust to the shock of the unexpected news and to grieve for the lost normal child that they anticipated. One must tailor the length and content of the discussion to the parents' needs and abilities.

Even if the parents are ready to hear all of the information, follow-up is still important. New questions will arise and parents will need clarification of information that was heard only partially or incorrectly. One study of parental adjustment found that parents typically experience a second wave of grief that is initiated by delayed acquisition of a social smile and poorer eye contact than expected for the infant's age. At later times, follow-up visits can also prove beneficial by providing parents an opportunity to discuss their child's progress and their own adjustment, questions, or concern. At times of transition (e.g., first school placement and completion of formal education), intervention in the form of anticipatory guidance can be particularly helpful to parents. In fact, such follow-up is desired by most parents.

Parents who have other children often ask how to tell the older siblings and whether the child with Down syndrome will have an adverse effect on them. One should urge parents to answer the other children's questions at their level of understanding since older siblings usually detect the parents' sadness and preoccupation and are, therefore, aware that a problem exists. Although siblings may show some sadness at learning of the problem and experience some initial awkwardness in talking about the problem, siblings (and their friends) are typically understanding of the child's limitations, will include him or her in activities, and usually assume a protective role toward the child.

Throughout all dealings with parents who are trying to understand the significance of the diagnosis of Down syndrome in their child, the primary care physician should use sensitivity in the disclosure and maintain a stance of openness and acceptance. Such an approach will assist the parents in exploring their fears, hopes, and feelings to allow the healthiest adjustment to their experience.

BIBLIOGRAPHY

Carr J: Effect on the family of a child with Down syndrome. *Physiotherapy* 1976; 62(1):20–24.

Cunningham CC, Morgan PA, McGucken RB: Down's syndrome: Is dissatisfaction with disclosure of diagnosis inevitable? *Dev Med Child Neurol* 1984; 26:33–39.

Emde RN, Brown C: Adaptation to the birth of a Down's syndrome infant: Grieving and maternal attachment. *J Am Acad Child Psychiatry* 1978; 17:299–323.

Gallagher UM: The adoption of mentally retarded children. *Children* 1968; 15(1):17–21.

Gath A: Parental reactions to loss and disappointment: the diagnosis of Down's syndrome. *Dev Med Child Neurol* 1985; 27:392–400.

Gayton W, Walker L: Down syndrome: Informing the parents. *Am J Dis Child* 1974; 127:510–512.

Golden DA, David JG: Counseling parents after the birth of an infant with Down syndrome. *Children Today* 1974; 3:7–11.

Hockey A: Evaluation of adoption of the intellectually handicapped: A retrospective analysis of 137 cases. *J Ment Defic Res* 1980; 24:187–202.

Murphy A, Duffy T, Brady E, et al: Meeting with brothers and sisters of children with Down's syndrome. *Child Today* 1976; 5:20–23.

Pueschel S, Murphy A: Assessment of counseling practices at the birth of a child with Down syndrome. *Am J Ment Defic* 1976; 81:325–330.

Pueschel SM: Changes of counseling practice at the birth of a child with Down syndrome. *Appl Res Ment Retard* 1985; 6:99–108.

Pueschel SM, Tingey C, Rynders JE, et al (eds): *New Perspectives on Down Syndrome.* Baltimore, Paul H. Brookes Publishing Co, 1987.

Solnit AJ, Stark MH: Mourning and the birth of a defective child. *Psychoanal Study Child* 1961; 16:523–537.

Stone H: The birth of a child with Down syndrome: A medico-social study of thirty-one children and their families. *Scott Med J* 1973; 18:182–187.

105 POTENTIALLY FATAL DISEASE

R. Beverly Raney, Jr., M.D.,
Nancy L. Kashlak, R.N., P.N.P./O.,
Karen Bringelsen, M.D.

Discussing death is one of the most difficult tasks for the primary care team. This chapter offers an approach to help communicate the serious nature of the child's disease to the parents. There are three stages in the course of a life-threatening illness at which the possibility of death must be faced. The first occurs at the time of diagnosis of a potentially lethal disease. The second stage takes place at the time of relapse, after some period of active treatment, or when the disease fails to respond to initial therapy. The third stage is that period during which further medical intervention, with the goal of cure, is no longer feasible. At that time palliative measures may be used, but eventual death has become a certainty and life expectancy is limited to days or weeks.

DIAGNOSIS

How should the primary care physician describe to the parents the diagnosis and management of a possibly lethal disorder? The physician should outline the symptoms and signs of the child's illness and then discuss the diagnosis, attempting to keep the conversation simple and limited to practical issues such as the need for hospitalization, the types of treatment available, and the expected outcome of therapy. Ideally, both parents should be present in a quiet, private room, separate from the child so they can feel free to react emotionally and to ask questions without frightening the child. The parents are told calmly and sympathetically that the child has a life-threatening and potentially fatal disease. In many cases, treatment can alleviate the symptoms, perhaps permanently. The probability of control of the disease should be stressed, as should curability if that is possible.

The diagnosis of acute lymphoblastic leukemia is used here as an example. Once the diagnosis is confirmed by examination of the bone marrow, we inform the parents by saying "Your child has acute leukemia. That is why the child is pale and feels tired and sometimes has fever. The bone marrow is producing the wrong kind of blood cells. We can nearly always eradicate leukemia for a period of time by giving the child several drugs. If the disease goes away and does not reappear within 3 years, your child may eventually be cured."

Parents also need to know at this point whether hospitalization is advisable. We believe that the shock of the diagnosis of cancer, for example, is such that outpatient management is psychologically very difficult for the parents and may be inadvisable for the child. Also, the parents need time to learn about the disease and to become familiar with medical terms and procedures. The parents should also be told whether imminent death is likely. In addition, they need to know whether the child can lead a virtually normal life, both during and after the period of treatment. The time required for this discussion should ideally not exceed 30 minutes, because parents are generally incapable of absorbing and retaining overly detailed information when under stress. The physician should close by emphasizing that he or she will be available to talk with them again and will answer their ongoing questions as much as possible. It may be helpful at this point to schedule a regular time to talk with one or both parents each day. We then say, "If you think of a question when we are not around, write it down and we can discuss it at our next meeting." It is important to warn them that neighbors and friends will give opinions and anecdotes about similar cases. These stories, which may confuse the parents, should be brought to the conference for discussion.

After the methods of management have been instituted, further instruction of the parents can take place.[1] The parents may need assistance or encouragement in informing their child with words and explanations that are not frightening. The child needs to know that he or she has a serious disease that requires treatment. The child should be reassured that the medicine will help make him well again. We inform the parents and the child about the benefits and side effects of treatment, citing primarily the major and most noticeable types of toxic effects. For example, we say, "Your child with acute lymphoblastic leukemia will need injections, blood cell counts, bone marrow tests, and occasionally spinal taps to eliminate the leukemia cells and determine when they have disappeared. The drugs will probably cause increased appetite (glucocorticosteroids) and hair loss (vincristine); sometimes vomiting or constipation occurs. We can help minimize the stomach and bowel problems with other medicines, but your child may want to wear a hat at school or when outside the home."

Other caregivers such as nurses,[2] social workers, and psychiatrists[3,4] specially trained to work with families of seriously ill children are part of the management team and provide additional counseling and information. Educational material should be distributed and discussed. As parents see their child's health becoming restored they become more capable of asking cogent questions about the disease, the treatment, their child's outlook for survival, and the quality of life. We emphasize that the attainment of remission is the first and most important goal, because children who cannot be rendered free of detectable disease are not likely to survive. Often parents' anxieties begin to dissipate after remission is documented. The parents need to be encouraged to treat the child as normally as possible during the period of remission, because cure is possible and perhaps likely.[5]

RELAPSE

Relapse, or recurrence of the disease, is as difficult and frustrating for the patient, parents, and physician as is the diagnosis. In fact, the period of relapse is often perceived as worse, since it is known that relapse nearly always signifies death from the disease. Thus there is actually less hope for long-term survival after recrudescence of the illness than there was before. Nonetheless, it is realistic and honest to emphasize that some children do recover after relapse. To provide the child another opportunity to overcome the disorder, further therapy should be undertaken, even if the likelihood of a successful outcome is low. At this stage parents need to understand the various options for further management and the problems that may arise as the therapeutic choices become more limited. Both parents should be present for support and to minimize misunderstanding. During this and subsequent interviews the primary physician can reevaluate the emotional state of the parents and determine how well they are able to cope with distressing events. The parents may need help explaining to the patient that the previous treatment is no longer working and that new medicine and possibly other measures are needed to regain control of the disease. The primary physician can also begin to prepare for the likelihood that the child will die in a relatively finite period of time. As an example, the physician may say, "The tests show that the medicines are no longer effective, because the malignant cells have returned. That is bad, because we give our best drugs at the beginning, and the disease has clearly become resistant to them. Still, there are some different medicines that have helped other children in this situation, and we would like to use them to try once more to eradicate the disease. Although permanent cure is now much less likely, it is not necessarily impossible."

IMPENDING DEATH

Once it becomes clear that active medical management can no longer control the disease, the physician is faced with having to tell the parents that death is a certainty. At this time the physician must be compassionate but honest. As an example, the physician may say, "We have now tried all the reasonable forms of treatment and yet the disease continues to come back. We really have nothing left to fight the disease, except some new experimental drugs that may well make your child even sicker. We can try one of them, if you want, but you know as well as we do that miracles don't usually happen when you need one."

The dying child will often have some psychological distress, such as fear of separation from the parents or fear of intractable pain.[6, 7] The child will also experience increasing loss of control and of stamina. The child's difficulties are intensified if a vital organ such as the liver, lungs, or brain is involved, adding physical distress to the emotional trauma. During this period the physician should strive to alleviate symptoms whenever possible, being liberal about the use of narcotics for pain control and sedatives to help the patient sleep at night. The physician should encourage the family and patient to live for each day. The physician should also avoid the temptation to appear definite about the duration of a child's survival. We believe that it is preferable to give parents some guide, such as the statement that the child probably has several weeks to a few months to live, rather than a finite time. If the child is of school age, home tutoring and visits by friends and classmates should be arranged. Often a trip to a favorite vacation spot or to a child's playground or amusement park can help the family realize a worthwhile goal that the patient would enjoy and that the survivors will later recall with pleasure. The physician can also help by suggesting that the parents should not become completely antidisciplinarian; goals still need to be set and accomplished within the limits of the child's diminishing capabilities. The more normal each day can be, the better. Referral to a hospice association for support during this phase can be very helpful.

There is always discussion about how much to tell the child who is about to die. This area is complex and varies with each person's particular situation. We believe that most children already know when they are dying, but they generally avoid seeking a point-blank confirmation, because all hope is thereby removed. However, honesty and trust must be maintained. It is not usual in our experience for a child to ask either the physician or a parent, "Am I going to die?" If the child does ask, one may begin by responding, "Do you feel that bad? Does the thought of dying scare you? Let's talk about that now." Then the child can express feelings openly. If he or she asks "Am I dying now?", one may answer, "Yes, it is possible, and some children do die from the disease you have. But we will do everything we can to prevent it, and we will be here with you, even if things become worse."

The primary physician should also advise the parents that the sick child's siblings may, like the parents, have considerable feelings of stress, including depression and guilt. The parents need help to understand that the surviving children must not be shunted aside as the sick child is dying. The siblings also need to comprehend the gravity of the illness and know that their brother or sister may die within a short time. We suggest that the parents gather the whole family and outline the fact that the affected child's condition is not improving, that he or she may need more sleep and be less capable than formerly. The parents can say, "It is not anyone's fault, but your brother (sister) is really not getting better just now, and we all need to think about just how we can help. Maybe there is something we can all do together as a family, soon, in case he (she) becomes sicker as time goes by."

Ideally, in advance of the child's death the parents should discuss with the physician how to begin to make funeral arrangements. This area is difficult and sometimes painful to address, but the actual shock of a child's demise intensifies the parents' distress and renders them less capable of making decisions afterward. At this point the physician may say, "I wonder if you have any questions about what is going on. Sometimes families request an autopsy to learn more about their child's disorder and possibly to help the physicians learn more to benefit other children later. Would you like me to explain what is involved?"

The primary physician can and should strive to be available when the patient dies. That physician who has known the child through many years is the medical person best qualified to be with the family at or just after the moment of death, to pronounce the patient dead, and to assist the family by providing a limited amount of sedatives if requested. In this way the grieving parents will not be forced to take the child's body to an emergency room for pronouncement of death. The physician should help the parents tell the siblings that the child has stopped breathing and is no longer alive on earth. The clergy, especially if previously involved, should be notified right away.

Even after the child has died, the physician can help the parents by recalling with them the good times of the child's life, by being thankful that the struggle is over for that child, and by emphasizing that everything reasonable was done before death supervened. Any lingering questions should be answered, and contact by letter, telephone, or personal visit should be maintained with the family after the child has died.[6, 8, 9] Even after the death, families may need reassurance from the physician that a new treatment described in the newspaper would not have saved the child's life and that everyone involved did everything possible to prolong the child's period of useful life.

BIBLIOGRAPHY

1. Conatser C: Preparing the family for their responsibilities during treatment. *Cancer* 1986; 58:508–511.
2. Coody D: High expectations: Nurses who work with children who might die. *Nurs Clin North Am* 1985; 20:131–142.
3. Koocher GP: Psychosocial issues during the acute treatment of pediatric cancer. *Cancer* 1986; 58:468–472.
4. Adams-Greenly M: Psychological staging of pediatric cancer patients and their families. *Cancer* 1986; 58:449–453.
5. Spinetta JJ, Deasy-Spinetta P: The patient's socialization in the community and school during therapy. *Cancer* 1986; 58:512–515.
6. Siegel BS: Helping children cope with death. *Am Fam Physician* 1985; 31:175–180.
7. Speece MW, Brent SB: Children's understanding of death: A review of three components of a death concept. *Child Dev* 1984; 55:1671–1686.
8. Newton RW, Bergin B, Knowles D: Parents interviewed after their child's death. *Arch Dis Child* 1986; 61:711–715.
9. Pollock GH: Childhood sibling loss: A family tragedy. *Pediatr Ann* 1986; 15:851–855.

SUGGESTED READING

Koocher GP, Berman SJ: Life threatening and terminal illness in childhood, in Levine MD, Carey WB, Crocker AC, et al: *Developmental-Behavioral Pediatrics*. Philadelphia, WB Saunders Co, 1983; pp 488–501.

Spinetta JJ, Deasy-Spinetta P: *Living with Childhood Cancer*. St Louis, CV Mosby Co, 1981.

106 CHRONIC ILLNESS

Balu Athreya, M.D.

The primary care physician is in an ideal position to help children with chronic illness and their families since he or she knows the family background, the strengths and weaknesses of the family members, and establishes lasting relationships with them. Unfortunately, there is reluctance on the part of some physicians to handle children with chronic disease in their practice. The reasons for this reluctance are many—some real, some not so real! The major differences between the management of patients with acute illness and of those with chronic illness are that there is often hope of "cure" in acute illness, whereas the main theme in chronic illness is "care," and in acute illness, the physician is in full control of the management, whereas in chronic illness, the physician is only one member of a multidisciplinary team. This shift from "cure" to "care" and the need to share decision-making powers may be difficult for some physicians. Others are afraid that they may not be able to handle the psychosocial problems of the child with chronic illness. Caring for these children requires time, and time is what busy physicians lack. Also, there is no financial reward for the enormous amount of time needed to coordinate the care and to talk with the families of these children.

However, considering the magnitude and importance of the problem and the unique position the family physician occupies, it makes good sense for family physicians to be the team leaders in giving coordinated long-term care to children with chronic illness and handicapping conditions.

TALKING WITH PARENTS

In managing serious and chronic disease, information must be gathered before advice is given. Therefore, it is important to determine what the family wants to know and hear about before presenting to the family an elaborate discussion on the etiology, pathogenesis, and treatment of the disease in question. Effective, sympathetic, and sensitive listening is the first step.

SETTING

It is important to have a proper setting in terms of time, place, and emotional climate in order to have worthwhile discussions with these families. Busy offices with multiple interruptions from telephone calls and office staff or bustling hospital corridors are not good settings. Ideally, the physician should be prepared to set aside a period of approximately 45 to 60 minutes for discussion.

For the initial discussion, it is essential that both parents be present. An emotionally relaxed atmosphere is essential as well. The parents should realize by the physician's posture, the way he prompts them, and the way he answers their questions that he is interested in their problems and that he is listening.

COLLECTING INFORMATION

The educational and intellectual level of the parents, their socioeconomic conditions, anxiety levels, support systems, and coping abilities should be determined before the physician can answer their questions. The physician has to look for clues by observing these families and by listening to them carefully.

One has to know the strengths and weaknesses of these families. Strengths may be apparent or potential. Similarly, weaknesses may be real or hidden. It is important to build on the strengths. The strength may be a schoolteacher who is especially interested in this child or a social worker in an agency who knows the family well and speaks their language. It is also essential not to stress their weaknesses and vulnerabilities.

Families of children with chronic illness who cope well and lead a reasonably "normal" life have the following characteristics:

1. Parents who have a good marital relationship before the onset of the chronic illness
2. Parents who mutually agree on issues after some reasonable discussion
3. An extended family support system
4. Religious faith
5. Faith in their physician

These personal observations were confirmed by Schulman in his study of families of children with leukemia. It is, therefore, useful to find out how many of these characteristics are present or absent in any particular family. If many of these characteristics are absent, it may be wise to concentrate on preventative counseling.

The usual concerns and questions of the family are:

1. What is the diagnosis? How sure are you about the diagnosis?
2. What is the cause? Could we have prevented it? Is it my fault?
3. What can you do about it? How can I help?
4. Why me? Why us?
5. What are the tests? Why are they done? At what cost?
6. What is the future likely to be?
7. Will it go away?
8. Can he/she get married and have children?
9. What are the vocational possibilities and problems?

PROVIDING ANSWERS

It is not necessary to answer all the questions at one meeting. It may be better to give only as much information as the family can handle at one time. The first task is to answer questions that are of major concern. Both the physician and the family have to learn that answers to some questions come only with time.

It is easy, given the mystique of being a physician, to come up with definite answers for all questions. The physician, having been trained to be certain and to know everything, finds it difficult to say "I don't know," but the physician should be bold enough and secure enough to say "I don't know" if that is a truthful statement. Most parents will accept and appreciate honesty. But for certain technical questions, an appropriate answer may be, "I don't know, but I will find out." If the physician says this, he should make sure he finds the answer as soon as possible.

Simple words should be used to describe the diagnosis. If there are doubts about the diagnosis, or if there is a possibility that the diagnosis will have to be added to or changed, this should be indicated at the initial conference. A good booklet with a diagram of the organ involved (or a clay or plastic model of that organ) may help the families understand the explanation better. The physician can suggest that the family return with their questions during the next visit.

There are a number of patient education booklists that are available. Physicians may be able to obtain more information from voluntary social service agencies or the local chapter of the foundation dealing with the disease in question (e.g., Arthritis Foundation).

In addition, the physician may also wish to refer the families to a parent support group or to a parent of a patient with a similar problem. This establishes the fact that there are other children with similar problems and lessens the family's feelings of having been singled out for bad luck. Parents are also more likely to ask other parents, rather than the physician, about their personal concerns. Parents who have similar problems can be extremely supportive. If the physician is not aware of any such parent support group, information such as this can be obtained from a nearby academic medical facility.

The explanation the physician gives on the disease may have to be repeated many times before the message is fully understood. Soon after the diagnosis is made, parents are often in a state of shock, grief, and denial and are not prepared to hear all the physician may have to say. They may not comprehend and may deny much of what the physician has told them. It is necessary for the physician to be patient, not to defend himself, but to repeat his explanations often.

Another idea, used by many physicians, is to audiotape the discussion with the family's permission and give the tape to them. They can listen to this at their leisure. This tape will also provide other family members with the same information.

When parents inquire about the cause of the disease, they are not asking just for medical explanations. They also want to know if they did something wrong—by omission or by commission. This feeling of "guilt," a universal phenomenon, should be addressed with sensitivity and honesty.

Questions such as "Why did it happen to me?" or "Why did it happen to my child?" are personal, philosophical questions. Some parents tend to dwell indefinitely on these questions and are immobilized because of their preoccupation with this unanswerable question. This occurs less commonly in people with deep religious faith. In fact, some families turn to religion after a chronic illness is diagnosed in a child. Some families with deep problems regarding this question tend to become depressed and socially isolated and may require special help.

Another major area of concern for the children and their families is the use of laboratory tests. Most families want to know what tests are being done, when they are being done, and at what cost. They also wish to know why some tests are repeated and whether they have to be repeated so often. Special efforts must be made to explain the tests being ordered, and how these tests will help in the management of the child's disease. Risks and benefits should be explained, whenever necessary, depending on the physician's relationship with the family and the invasiveness of the procedure. Some children and adults need sufficient notice to enable them to get prepared. Others want to be told just prior to the test. Truthfulness is necessary, but not at the expense of frightening families.

After the test results are known, it takes only a few minutes to call the families and inform them of the results. Most families appreciate this courtesy and thoughtfulness, and such a call coming from a physician breaks down barriers and allows for improved patient-physician relationships. If the physician is too busy, a nurse should provide the information.

Questions on prognosis are difficult to answer, particularly for a disease with indefinite course, such as juvenile rheumatoid arthritis and systemic lupus erythematosus. It is hard to live with uncertainty. Families cope better when they know what to expect. But, unfortunately, the physician cannot be definite in giving a prognosis for certain diseases. Therefore, it becomes a fine balancing act for the physician to be truthful and realistic, without being too optimistic or pessimistic.

Physicians need to understand themselves and their strengths and weaknesses before answering questions on prognosis. Some cannot give bad news and tend to soften the news that may then be interpreted as good news by families. Others tend to be overly pessimistic, even with mild disease. Both these extremes are to be avoided.

It is possible to convey bad news without shocking the parents to numbness, and it is unnecessary to constantly crush their hopes. Families need hope to sustain them. As long as parents are planning for and dealing with the current situation appropriately, do not be concerned if they periodically express their hopes that the disease will miraculously go away. It does not matter what they say. It is what they do that the physician should observe. If what they do suggests that they are coping well, leave things alone, encourage them, "cruise along." If what they do suggests poor coping, get involved quickly.

When parents inquire about prognosis, they have three other hidden concerns: (1) The first concern is related to the genetic nature of the disease and whether it can occur in a sibling or future offspring. (2) The second question relates to the chances of the affected child being able to grow up, marry, and have children. They are asking whether the affected child may pass the disease on to his or her offspring. (3) The third concern centers around physical activity and independence. The parents want to know if their child can go through the educational program and be able to earn a living.

When discussing treatment, simple explanations should be given. Written instructions should be helpful. Also, instructions should not be unrealistic or strain the family's resources. Compliance decreases as the treatment plan becomes more and more complicated.

The family should know that they are the principal members of the treatment team. Each family has its own special problems and special solutions. It is important to listen to them, and allow enough room in the plans for them to manage their problems in their own way. Plans should be made to suit the needs of each family and support structures should be built to make sure the plan is carried out. For example, it is unwise to give an elaborate morning care plan to the mother of a child with myelomeningocele if she also has other school-aged children. Contacts with the school principal, local social service agency, or child guidance clinic may have to be arranged to help these families. At times, it is better for the physician not to be too specific with his recommendations. Most chronic diseases have an unpredictable course, unique in each child, that requires flexibility in planning on the part of the parent and the physician.

CONCLUSION

Taking care of patients with chronic illness is a difficult task. Yet it is an area that brings into focus everything grouped under the term of "Art of Medicine." It helps the physician grow and mature. It is exciting and rewarding in its own way.

Physicians are all in the medical profession to help people with disease, people in pain, people with handicaps. Ambroise Paré said that "we seek to cure sometimes, relieve often and comfort always." That is the essence of taking care of patients with chronic illness. Primary care should become more interesting and rewarding by including a few children with chronic illness.

BIBLIOGRAPHY

Batshaw ML, Perret YM: *Children with Handicaps. A Medical Primer*, ed 2. Baltimore, Paul H. Brooks Publishing Co, 1986.

Community checklist for care of children with special needs. Publication of Association for the Care of Children's Health. Washington, DC, 1987.

Forman MA, Hetznecker W: The physician and the handicapped child: Dilemmas of care (commentary). *JAMA* 1982; 247:3325–3326.

Grant WW: What parents of a chronically ill or dysfunctioning child want to know, but may be afraid to ask. *Clin Pediatr* 1978; 17:915–917.

Green M: Coming of age in general pediatrics. *Pediatrics* 1983; 72:275–282.

Hobbs N, Perrin JM: *Issues in the Care of Children with Chronic Illness*. San Francisco, Jossey Bass Publishers, 1985.

Hobbs N, Perrin JM, Ireys HT: *Chronically Ill Children and Their Families*. San Francisco, Jossey Bass Publishers, 1985.

Martin EW: Pediatricians' role in the care of disabled children. *Pediatr Rev* 1985; 6:275–282.

McCollum AT: *The Chronically Ill Child: A Guide for Parents and Professionals*, ed 2. New Haven, Yale University Press, 1981.

McInerny T: The role of the general pediatrician in coordinating the care of children with chronic illness. Symposium on chronic disease in children. *Pediatr Clin North Am* 1984; 31:199–209.

Pless IB, Roghmann KJ: Chronic illness and its consequences: observations based on three epidemiological surveys. *J Pediatr* 1971; 79:351–359.

107 CHILD ABUSE AND NEGLECT

Toni Seidl, A.C.S.W., L.S.W.

In child abuse cases, good communication is crucial. We are for the most part dealing with psychologically fragile adults whose children have been and will continue to be dependent on them at least until the mandatory agencies or the courts intervene. Physicians and nurses find it difficult to accept the concept that these children need and want the parents who have caused them pain. In child abuse cases there are in effect two patients: at least one adult and one child. Thus the practitioner needs to promote parental involvement within the bounds of safety for the child and to encourage healing of both parent and child. To accomplish this task, a bond of trust has to be created between the practitioner and the parents. This relationship need not compromise the care of the child or prevent practitioners from contacting those systems they are mandated to report to. Practitioners must be aware of the presentations and dynamics of child abuse or neglect, skillful at obtaining factual histories, and capable of treating and providing care in a neutral and nonthreatening setting. Child abuse is an unacceptable phenomenon but an all too often predictable event when the parent is childlike, frustrated, isolated, emotionally impoverished, poor, unemployed, and has minimal parenting skills. In addition the practitioner should not view the reporting process as a loss of rapport with the family or the automatic creation of an adversarial situation but as a legal duty essential to the treatment process. An understanding of ourselves and of the child's parents is the only way the practitioner can position himself or herself to communicate effectively and subsequently help the child and family.

Alternatively, one could suspect child abuse and consider intervention as someone else's responsibility. Although this distancing does provide the practitioner with a temporary absence of conflict, it does not affect change in the family nor provide safety for the abused child and his or her siblings, or facilitate a working relationship between the practitioner and the family. The subject of violence toward children and the more insidious but equally devastating neglect have historically been avoided by our culture and the helping professions. The language and appropriate style required to cope with this problem are alien to most professionals.

A pivotal constraint to productive communication is the common and deeply held myth that those individuals who abuse and neglect their children have essentially different goals for their children than other caregivers do. This is inaccurate; most parents want their children to thrive and become productive human beings. It must be emphasized that the creation of an understanding between parties will require that practitioner to search beyond surface presentations. Another myth is that child abusers are alcoholic, psychotic, or both. This perception can serve to hamper communication profoundly unless dispelled. In fact, psychosis occurs in less than 5% of abusers, and the prevalence of alcoholism is similar in abusive and nonabusive parents.

Providers need to take responsibility for learning how to interpret parental hostility and resistance as potent symptoms of fear and inadequacy. They also should acknowledge that, given the same set of variables, they might very well be capable of abusing or neglecting a child. Individuals who act out assaultively with children are likely to be passive to a fault when dealing with authority figures whom they perceive to be powerful and in control. Fear of retribution is a common anxiety that impedes physicians functioning as parent counselors. However, when a reality-based relationship develops between the parents and health workers, retribution rarely occurs.

THE CONFERENCE

In talking to parents in the hospital or in the office, the physician must be in charge in every sense of the word. Arrange the conference site so it is private, quiet, and relatively free from interruptions. An unhurried appearance on the part of the practitioner and single-minded purpose is essential. Positioning of the conference participants is especially important when the subject for discussion is child abuse. Threatened individuals need us to firmly establish that we are comfortable and that we are in control of ourselves and of them. To do this, we must convey a sense of calm, a sense of direction, and a sense of eagerness for involvement with the parents.

The following points reflect a helpful style of managing the conference. Sit close and lean forward to demonstrate attentiveness to the parents as individuals. Do not be intimidated by their predictable passivity, hostility, or hyperactivity. The articulation of the role of reporter of suspected child abuse and caregiver rather than apportioner of blame or investigator needs to be threaded throughout the contacts with the family. By maintaining a child-focused stance, parental anxiety and anger can be successfully avoided.

It is preferable to begin the parent conference with a positive or approving comment such as, "I am glad that you brought Lilly to the hospital today; it was the right thing to do. She is a very pretty infant." After such an opening, the parents' conversation, body language, and posture will usually become less defensive and more open in response to our approval, which they will translate as a degree of acceptance.

The next step is the sharing of the medical facts without establishing etiologic conclusions. This needs to be done clearly and concretely, with explanations of medical terminology and concepts in a nonpatronizing manner. Individuals who abuse and neglect their children constantly struggle with feelings of incompetence. Try to avoid the possibility of this negative attitude, which creates a fertile atmosphere for the escalation of hostility and other aberrant behaviors. The following is the type of dialogue often used: "We are glad that Lilly is breathing by herself now, but we are still worried about the blood under the covering of her brain." These same parents will need generous amounts of reassurance and a sense of a plan. "We are doing more tests to find out just how serious the injury is so that we can treat your daughter in the best way possible." By doing this, the practitioner's expertise is established and the stage is set with the deliberate use of the word "injury" for the discussion of nonaccidental trauma or child abuse. Then, to demonstrate again a nonrejecting atmosphere and to validate the parent-child relationship, a comment such as: "We will let you see your daughter as soon as we can, because we know how much she needs you." This avoids the abusive and neglectful parent's compulsion to prove to us that they love their child when, of course, the issue for us is not one of love but of behaving in a caring and protective manner.

Next obtain a history of the events leading up to the presentation of symptoms. This is an extraordinarily important step, both diagnostically and in terms of separating accidental from nonaccidental injury or neglect and to become prepared psychologically and factually. To proceed in relative comfort and with credibility, one needs to be secure in the suspicion of abuse or neglect. Only when the information is gathered personally and meshed with the physical findings can the suspicion be presented to the parents in a clear and unwavering manner. After the parents have presented their version of the events they can be gently confronted with the reality that their presentation of the history does not fit their child's physical findings. "Mr. and Mrs. Jones, what you are telling me is puzzling in that we see hundreds of children each year who fall off beds and they do not have the type and severity of injury Lilly has. Is there anything else you can think of that might have injured her?" Here reality is supportively threaded into the conversation while giving the parents an opportunity to acknowledge the abuse. If the answer is no, move on to further explain the configuration and mechanism of injury in as concrete a way as possible. This should be supplemented with radiographs, a computed tomography scan, any other aids available, and an explanation of the syndrome of child abuse.

It is productive to preface this portion of the discussion with the comment, "I have something to tell you that is going to be upsetting for you to hear and difficult for me to say." By doing this, we are reinforcing a partnership in treatment. An effective follow-up comment can be "We see children every day who are abused and neglected by parents and caretakers, and because of my training, knowledge, and judgment, I believe Lilly's injury is the result of child abuse." By doing this, we are carefully avoiding the apportionment of blame while reemphasizing our expertise and being straightforward with concern. The use of the powerful words "child abuse" also serves to decrease the potential for denial and misinterpretation later.

Requirements to report child abuse, as stated in the specific civil and criminal statutes of the particular community, plus information regarding the process and implications of reporting and protective services investigation must be explained to the parents. Most practitioners feel compelled to do this in a rather formal style, realizing that families are not necessarily able to internalize all that is said. This serves not only to cause the family to appreciate how firmly the suspicion of child abuse or neglect is held but also to appreciate the commitment to reporting child abuse. Middle- and upper-class educated families who may very well try to derail the reporting process can be effectively managed with this approach. "When I have a suspicion of child abuse, the law clearly states that I must report it to children's protective services, and that is what I have done." In addition, messages of caring and mutuality need to be transmitted. "This does not mean that I will be less involved with you or that your daughter's care will be compromised. The staff and I are here to help you and Lilly." Assurances of confidentiality within the parameters of legal mandates need to be reiterated. Parents also deserve information regarding the implications and process of the protective services and criminal investigations.

All of this is best accomplished with a multidisciplinary approach, as the needs of abusive or neglectful families are overwhelming and complex, requiring varied expertise and monumental energy. This, coupled with the requisite involvement with the criminal and civil systems, is more than any individual or discipline can master and manage alone.

The medical and psychosocial management of child abuse or neglect offers an extraordinary challenge to us as practitioners, not only in terms of rescuing children but in terms of restoring a significant group of adults to their functional role as parents.

BIBLIOGRAPHY

Brahams D: Child abuse and the doctor's duty of care. *Lancet* 1987; 2:51–52.

Finkelhor D, Gelles RJ, Hotaling GT, et al: *The Dark Side of Families: Current Family Violence Research*. Beverly Hills, Calif, Sage Publications, 1983.

Golan N: *Treatment in Crisis Situations*. New York, Free Press, 1978.

Goldberg G: Breaking the communication barrier: The initial interview with an abusing parent. *Child Welfare* 1985; 54:4.

Hartman C, Reynolds D: Resistant clients: Confrontations, interpretation, and alliance. *Social Casework*, April 1987.

Helfer E: Children Today. May/June 1975.

Ludwig S: A multidisciplinary approach to child abuse. *Nurse Clin North Am* 1981; 16:161.

108 EXPLAINING EPILEPSY

Robert Ryan Clancy, M.D.

Epilepsy, a common chronic neurologic disorder, affects millions of persons worldwide. After the physician has concluded that the diagnosis of epilepsy is warranted, the patient and family usually have many questions and concerns regarding the nature and significance of this condition. The physician should anticipate these healthy questions and be prepared to respond in a clear and timely manner. The purpose of this chapter is to review common questions raised by individuals with epilepsy and their families and to illustrate one approach to answering these questions. The physician's response constitutes a vehicle to patient self-education and participation in the comprehensive management of the disorder.

What is "epilepsy"?

The term epilepsy refers to an individual's tendency to experience repeated seizures. Each seizure is the individual attack of altered brain function that arises from temporary abnormal electrical patterns in the brain. Some individuals with epilepsy may have only two seizures in their lifetime; others have more frequent attacks.

Is there a difference between "epilepsy," "seizure disorder," and "convulsions"?

The terms epilepsy and seizure disorder are synonymous. Because of the stigma attached to the term epilepsy by some members of society, there has been an increased emphasis on the diagnostic label seizure disorder rather than epilepsy; however, they are the same condition. Medically speaking, the term convulsion is not strictly identical to epilepsy or seizure disorder, even though the diagnosis convulsive disorder is encountered occasionally. For example, after some individuals faint they may display a brief *nonepileptic* convulsion.[1] The convulsion appears as jerks or twitches of the muscles of the face or limbs, due to the brief period of low blood pressure during the fainting episode. However, convulsion does not indicate excessive brain electrical activity from a tendency for recurrent seizures. On the other hand, seizures in some people with epilepsy are properly described as convulsive if they display forceful, repeated contractions or movements of the musculature.

Who gets epilepsy?

Anyone can have epilepsy. It is estimated that about 1% of the population is prone to recurrent seizures and thus warrants the diagnosis. When all types of seizures are collectively considered (including febrile seizures, single seizures, and epilepsy), the incidence of affected individuals increases to 10%. Seizures can arise at any age, from newborn infants to the elderly. Epilepsy occurs with equal frequency in all parts of the world and in all races.

What happens to the brain during each individual seizure?

Let's start with a more familiar experience. Most individuals have had an opportunity to undergo electrocardiography (ECG). You may recall that electrodes were attached to your arms, legs, and chest. The electrical signals that control the heart are detected and monitored with each heartbeat. The brain also runs on electrical impulses. Normal electrical signals are very orderly and tightly controlled by the brain. During an individual epileptic seizure, excessive amounts of electricity temporarily take over the normal function of part or all of the brain. This results in the seizure and the temporary interruption of normal brain function.

How many kinds of seizures are there?

Because the brain is a complicated and specialized organ, it has many ways to express seizures.[2] Historically, epileptic seizures were broadly characterized as big seizures (grand mal epilepsy) and little seizures (petit mal epilepsy). Today we recognize numerous types of epileptic seizures. It is for this reason that you must provide your physician with a careful description of the seizures. It is on the basis of this careful description of the components of the attack that the physician can best diagnose the specific type of seizure.

Most individuals with epilepsy experience only one or a few different types of seizures. Slight differences in the duration or intensity of a typical seizure do not warrant the diagnosis of a new type of seizure. Rather, this is reserved for seizures that are distinctively different in their quality.

What causes the tendency for seizures?

Anything that is potentially harmful to the brain may be a cause for seizures. A serious head injury, encephalitis, meningitis, chemical imbalances, drugs, stroke, or even a brain tumor can disrupt the normal functioning of the brain and give rise to the excessive electrical activity that is the basis for the individual seizure. It is for this reason that the doctor conducts a careful history and physical examination of the patient with newly diagnosed seizures. In some cases, additional blood testing or a computed tomography (CT) scan of the brain or magnetic resonance (MR) imaging may be suggested. Still, in many individuals, no specific cause for the recurring seizures is discovered. The cause of the seizures may then be described as idiopathic. This reflects our incomplete knowledge of the cause(s) of seizures in many individuals. Sometimes the seizures arise from genetic (inherited) influences, but in most cases medical science has simply failed to uncover the fundamental cause of the seizures.

Is epilepsy contagious?

Absolutely not! There is no way you can catch epilepsy by observing a seizure or associating with an affected individual. However, inheritance may play an important role in some cases of epilepsy. In others, inheritance seems to play little or no role. According to some medical authorities[3, 4] the risk for seizures occurring in close relatives of those with epilepsy varies from 2% to 50% depending on the specific type of seizures. When one parent has epilepsy, the risk of epilepsy in their children is about 6%; if both parents have epilepsy, the risk of epilepsy in their children increases to about 10%.

What is the difference between epilepsy, cerebral palsy, and mental retardation?

These three conditions are entirely different. Epilepsy refers only to the tendency for recurring seizures. Cerebral palsy represents a physical handicap in which the individual has faulty muscle control due to a neurologic disturbance. This may result in abnormal walking, impaired use of the hands, or speech difficulties. Mental retardation reflects an impairment of intellectual skills (subnormal intelligence), visible as slow mental development and a reduced ability to learn. It is true that some individuals with multifaceted neurologic problems can have *combinations* of these three separate problems. For example, some individuals with cerebral palsy may also be mentally retarded and experience recurring seizures (epilepsy).

Who is qualified to treat epilepsy?

Any knowledgeable general practitioner, family physician, internist, pediatrician, general neurologist, or epileptologist may successfully diagnose and treat seizure disorders. In addition to individual practitioners who care for patients with epilepsy, there are a variety of comprehensive epilepsy clinics available throughout the United States and Canada. The Epilepsy Foundation of America (EFA) can provide the names and locations of physicians who are especially knowledgeable in the diagnosis and treatment of seizure disorders.

What is the purpose of treating epilepsy?

The physician usually recommends medication to prevent the individual seizures of the epilepsy. Such medications are called antiepileptic drugs or anticonvulsants. The physician selects the drug most likely to be effective from a wide choice of available medications. The purpose of medication is to help protect the patient from future seizures. Drug treatment does not necessarily erase or remove the underlying tendency for the seizures but rather provides protection against the individual attacks. Because most individuals cannot predict when a seizure will occur, it is necessary to faithfully consume antiepileptic drugs on a daily basis to prevent recurrence. This is a difficult chore for most individuals, because few are accustomed to taking medications on a regular basis. However, the price of poor compliance is high: seizures may recur during play, school, driving, or work.

How successful is treatment with antiepileptic drugs?

About 80% of individuals with epilepsy are successfully treated with medications. They enjoy a total or substantial reduction of their seizures. As long as they faithfully use their medications as prescribed, they can reasonably expect good seizure control. Unfortunately, about 20% of people do not adequately respond to the medications currently available. For some of these patients, neurosurgery may be necessary.

Can one stop worrying about seizures once started on medications?

No. The faithful consumption of medication is not a 100% guarantee against the possibility of future seizures. It would be more reasonable to consider the medication as a safety net rather than as total ironclad protection. One should always be aware of the possibility of an unexpected seizure arising even if previously well controlled. For this reason, individuals with seizures should maintain constant vigilance for their personal health and safety.

How long will antiepileptic drugs be continued?

For many types of epilepsy, medications can be withdrawn 2 to 5 years after total seizure control. This is especially true for some of the so-called benign epilepsy syndromes of childhood. Those are considered benign because the majority of affected people are entirely healthy aside from the seizures and eventually outgrow their tendency for seizures. For a few types of seizures, the outlook is less optimistic and withdrawal of treatment may result in a relapse of the seizures. Consequently, although the goal of withdrawing medications several years after establishing total seizure control is desirable, it is not attainable in all individuals.

When the time does come to discontinue medication, the reduction is always conducted gradually. In this clinical setting, anticonvulsants are never abruptly withdrawn. Precipitous discontinuation of antiepileptic drugs can cause serious consequences including the appearance of repeated or prolonged seizures.

Do antiepileptic drugs have side effects?

The person who consumes medication must remain alert to the possibility of side effects: just as individuals are different so may be their reaction to medications. Each antiepileptic medication has its own individual spectrum of side effects. The physician should discuss the possible side effects of each drug you may be consuming. This serves to inform you of possible adverse effects and help minimize their occurrence.

Don't be overly concerned about the initial side effects of antiepileptic drugs. It takes a little while for most people to adjust to their temporary initial reactions. Some medications have more lasting side effects than others. Ask your doctor about choosing the anticonvulsant that is least likely to interfere with your lifestyle.

In general, there are two broad types of side effects: physical and mental. Examples of physical side effects include swollen gums, increased hair growth, weight gain or loss, facial cosmetic changes, or alterations of internal organs such as the liver. Examples of mental side effects include sleepiness, irritability, poor attention or concentration, or slurred speech.

What side effects should be reported to the doctor?

Drowsiness or trouble concentrating are common after starting some antiepileptic drugs and need not be reported unless severe or persistent. Swollen glands, rash, hives, or ulcers in the mucous membranes may indicate an allergic reaction and should be reported. Unusual nosebleeding, easy bruisability, or blood in the urine or stool should be promptly reported.

Can one become addicted to antiepileptic medications?

Usually not. Most antiepileptic medications are not physically addicting. For example, there is no physical dependency created from the long-term consumption of phenytoin, carbamazepine, or valproate. Physical dependency can result from the long-term consumption of benzodiazepam drugs (including diazepam, Valium; clorazepate dipotassium, Tranxene; and clonazepam, Klonopin) and barbiturates (including phenobarbital; mephobarbital, Mebaral; and primidone, Mysoline). When the time comes to taper these medications, they are slowly withdrawn over an extended period to minimize any possible physical signs of withdrawal. Because phenobarbital normally leaves the body very slowly, it automatically provides its own slow method of tapering.

Psychologic addiction to anticonvulsants can occur in some individuals who enjoy the comforting thought of safety from seizures symbolized by the drug. They understandably react adversely when advised to discontinue their medications. Individuals can become psychologically dependent on medications even though there is no physical addiction. This depends as much on their personality as on the nature of the drug.

Do antiepileptic drugs cause mental retardation?

Antiepileptic drugs do not lower the intelligence quotient (IQ) or cause mental retardation. However, they do affect the workings of the nervous system as they achieve their desired effects (seizure control) and in the process introduce unwanted neurologic side effects. These can be expressed as disturbances of behavior, mood, sleeping, attention span, or concentration. For some individuals, these side effects may be trivial; for others they materially impair the speed and accuracy of some mental processes. In that circumstance, it is sometimes necessary to reduce the dose or switch to a different antiepileptic drug.

Can antiepileptic drugs be taken with other medications?

In general, yes. Most medications can be safely administered with antiepileptic drugs without any untoward side effects. However, there are some important drug interactions that your physician knows about. It is wisest to check with your doctor or pharmacist before taking drugs together. For example, some women who consume antiepileptic medications are at risk for failure of oral birth control pills. Because some seizure medications increase the rate of drug elimination by the liver, birth control pills may be metabolized too rapidly. This may result in conception or breakthrough bleeding. Even vitamins can be removed from the body too quickly while consuming seizure medications. Therefore, many doctors recommend taking a daily multivitamin supplement.

What is the purpose of the blood test recommended by the doctor?

The dosage of individual antiepileptic drugs is usually given on a per pound basis; lighter individuals receive smaller doses than heavier individuals. The completeness of absorption from the intestinal tract and the rate of drug breakdown in the body also differ between individuals. In the final analysis, what is most important is how much medication appears in the bloodstream available for delivery to the tissues of the brain. Adequate seizure control often depends on maintaining a specific concentration of medication in the bloodstream. Your doctor may request that a drug level be obtained to measure the exact concentration of medication in your body. This allows more rational dose manipulation to achieve optimal seizure control. A low blood level may indicate a marginal protection against seizures. A high blood level may indicate impending signs of overmedication.

For some medications it is also advised that periodic blood tests be obtained to monitor the health of some internal body organs such as the liver, kidneys, pancreas, or the blood-forming organs. Your doctor will use these tests to evaluate how your body reacts to the drugs.

What about generic antiepileptic drugs?

Many physicians prefer that their patients do not consume some generic anticonvulsants. Generic phenobarbital is the rule rather than the exception. However, manufacturers' formulations of phenytoin (Dilantin), carbamazepine (Tegretol), and valproate (Depakene, Depakote) may differ sufficiently to cause a change in blood levels that could result in the reappearance of seizures (if the levels fall too low) or intoxication (if the levels rise too high).

For some families, the expense of purchasing antiepileptic medications is a major burden. Do not be afraid to shop around to find the least expensive supplier of medication. If possible, buy in bulk rather than in small 1-month amounts, which are generally more expensive. The EFA offers a mail order pharmacy that may be less expensive than your local retailers.

What can I do to help the doctor manage the seizure disorder?

The patient and family are the eyes and ears of the doctor. It is rare for the physician to personally witness the patient's seizures. Therefore it is most helpful for a clear description of all the events before, during, and after the seizure to provide the physician with accurate information to make the most precise diagnosis. Many physicians recommend that their patients maintain a seizure calendar or log. This provides a written record of the time, duration, description, and circumstances of the seizures.

The patient with epilepsy and the family must become informed partners with the doctor for successful health care. It is recommended that they be as knowledgeable as possible about seizures, take the time to read about the condition, and keep the doctor informed of the patient's status.

Patients should also be familiar with the name(s) and dose(s) of prescribed medication and with expected common drug side effects. Pill organizers can be purchased at the pharmacy to help you keep the medication schedules straight.

How can I help reduce the risk of seizures?

By maintaining a seizure calendar, it is occasionally possible to identify factors in the environment that trigger the attacks. By keeping an accurate seizure calendar, you and the physician may identify and avoid such precipitating factors. The second major job of the individual is to be totally compliant with prescribed medications. This is easier said than done, but the medication cannot help while safely stored in the medicine cabinet! Any physical illness such as the flu or fever can lower the resistance to seizures and possibly precipitate an attack. Similarly, extreme sleep deprivation or the immoderate consumption of alcohol and some illicit drugs can substantially increase the risk of seizures. Unnatural degrees of emotional distress may precipitate seizures. However, the normal healthy stresses that are encountered in everyday life do not aggravate seizures. It is not recommended to keep the patients perpetually calm. All patients with epilepsy should shoulder their fair share of life's excitement, challenges, stresses, and disappointments. Indeed, it seems that some people are more prone to seizures while they are idle. In general, the advice "keep busy" is healthy.

Are seizures painful?

Seizures are almost never painful. In fact, most persons have no recollection of the event at all.

What do you do at the scene of a seizure?

When most people first witness a seizure, their immediate reaction is: "He or she is dying." This is not true. The seizure will pass and the individual will be safe and sound in only a few minutes, so keep calm. There is nothing you can do to stop the seizure sooner; it will run its course. Most seizures last only a few minutes. Remove glasses or dentures if possible and place something soft under the person's head so they do not bump it on the ground. Do not attempt to restrain the movements. Tight clothing may be loosened. Some people will have erratic breathing during the seizure, but this is a natural part of the attack. Roll the person on their side so they do not choke on vomit or their saliva. Do not attempt to insert anything into the mouth. Although some can bite their tongue, you cannot stop this. It is a myth that someone can swallow their tongue during a seizure. In the rarest of circumstances, individuals may not resume breathing after a seizure and so cardiopulmonary resuscitation (CPR) should be started. Some families make it a point to learn CPR through qualified instructors at the American Red Cross.

It is also recommended that persons with epilepsy possess a "medical alert" bracelet, neck chain, or wallet card that describes their condition and provides relevant phone numbers.*

What happens after a seizure?

After a grand mal seizure, most individuals will awaken but seem confused or groggy and may fall asleep soon afterward. Headache, muscle soreness, or bloody saliva (if the tongue was bitten) may be noted. The person's color improves quickly even if he or she was pale, gray, or bluish (cyanotic) during the seizure. A deep state of relaxation immediately follows the attack, during which the person remains still and offers no resistance to movement. Even the muscle sphincters of the bladder and rectum can relax and lead to incontinence of urine and stool.

Some people bounce back immediately after a seizure, others require more time to recuperate. If consciousness is not regained promptly, medical attention should be sought. Do not offer the individual anything to eat or drink until they are awake and able to swallow safely.

Are seizures harmful to the brain?

Although they are dramatic and may be frightening to the onlooker, individual seizures do not produce brain damage or result in a lower IQ.

---

*Medical alert items are available from: Medic Alert Foundation International, Box 1009, Turlock, CA 95381 (1-800-ID-Alert); Emergency Information, American Medical Association, 535 N. Dearborn St., Chicago, IL, 60610; National Identification Co, Inc, 3955 Oneida Street, Denver, CO 80207.

Do you automatically take the child to a hospital after a seizure?

It is not obligatory to take a child to the doctor or hospital after each and every seizure. It would be best to clarify with your doctor when to go. If any injury occurred during the seizure (such as a laceration from falling), the patient should obviously be examined. Similarly, if the episode is unusually long, different from previous seizures, or recovery incomplete after the attack is over, the individual should be evaluated by a physician.

Can seizures occur during sleep?

Yes. Nocturnal epilepsy refers to some individuals' tendency to have seizures during sleep. Indeed, some people have their attacks only while asleep. Unfortunately, this sometimes means that seizures are unrecognized or poorly described. Parents find this unsettling since many desire to be with their child during the seizure. There is no perfect solution to this dilemma. An inexpensive auditory home intercom (usually intended to monitor a baby's crying) can allow the parents to hear the child's activities in their own room during the night.

What is "status seizures"?

Although the vast majority of seizures occur as brief individual attacks, long uninterrupted seizures may rarely occur and are potentially harmful. Prolonged seizures lasting hours can result in brain damage or death. This of course can be totally avoided by prompt medical attention. If a single seizure lasts 15 minutes or more, many physicians recommend that the family bring the patient for medical evaluation. It would be best to have a specific plan of action prepared in advance in the case of such an emergency.

In what circumstance could a seizure be harmful?

As already discussed, individual seizures themselves are not harmful to the brain. However, harm can occur if the seizure occurs in a circumstance that would produce an injury. For example, a person who has a seizure while swimming could drown unless there was immediate help from a partner or supervising adult. Bicycling amidst traffic could produce harm if the child lost control and swerved into the path of a vehicle. A seizure at great heights (e.g., rock climbing) could produce a serious fall. Similarly, seizures while operating heavy machinery or driving could result in personal injury.

What restrictions or limitations apply to the epileptic child?

All parents and guardians should exercise a healthy degree of authority and discipline over their children, including those with epilepsy. Most physicians recommend that they receive no special treatment or sheltering lest they stigmatize themselves as incapable or different. They should not be removed from challenges, excused from their transgressions, or spared the normal disappointments that constitute formative experiences of childhood.

Driving restrictions are enforced for most individuals, but all states permit driving once complete seizure control has been established for 6 months to 2 years. Unfortunately, some employers do restrict epileptics from filling some types of jobs.

What about school?

It is generally recommended that school personnel be informed of the presence of a seizure disorder. The teacher can be a valuable asset since they have ample opportunity to directly observe the child for seizures and potential drug side effects. The teacher will be best prepared to help the student during a seizure with foreknowledge of what to expect and instructions about what to do. The teacher can also be encouraged to read and learn more about seizure disorders.[5]

It is known that learning disabilities and attention deficit disorders are overrepresented in epileptic school-aged children. If the teacher observes these in your child, be prepared to deal realistically with the problems since specific treatment may be available that may materially improve school performance.

What about employment?

Children with epilepsy should plan their education with realistic career goals. For example, children with uncontrolled seizures will not be issued licenses to drive commercial vehicles or pilot airplanes. Naturally, they should be advised against pursuing such careers. Vocational counselors in school may be helpful in determining the individual's strengths, weaknesses, and aptitude for a host of appropriate careers.

Are there any limitations on participation in sports?

There is generally no restriction in participation in athletics, including contact sports such as football. However, participation in any athletic competition inherently conveys some risk, and the individual contemplating such athletics should be physically well and capable of participation. Ideally, this includes good seizure control.

What about planning for a family?

It is strongly suggested that women who desire to raise a family should confer with their doctor long before conceiving. Some medications may be harmful to the developing fetus and should be withdrawn before conception. Seizure control can deteriorate during pregnancy so the physician may wish to follow up the patient or monitor drug levels more frequently until delivery.

Is it difficult to obtain life insurance with epilepsy?

Life insurance is obtainable through many companies. Some companies have overpriced their premiums to discourage people with epilepsy from seeking a policy. However, other companies offer reasonably priced insurance. A listing is available through the EFA.

What other sources of services are available to me?

Individuals seeking specific services may direct inquiries to their Public Health Department or Public Health Nurse. Most states also provide vocational rehabilitation and disability counsels. The State Department of Social Services or Mental Health Services may also provide assistance in some circumstances.

Where can I find more information about epilepsy?

A series of well-written and informative brochures is available on request from the EFA.* Several books about epilepsy are also available for patients and families.[6, 7]

REFERENCES

1. Lin JT-Y, Ziegler DK, Lai C-W, et al: Convulsive syncope in blood donors. *Ann Neurol* 1982; 11:525–528.
2. Commission on Classification and Terminology of the International League Against Epilepsy: Proposal for classification of epilepsies and epileptic syndromes. *Epilepsia* 1985; 26:268–278.
3. Jennings T, Bird TO: Genetic influences in the epilepsies. *Am J Dis Child* 1981; 135:450–455.
4. Newmark ME, Penry JK: Genetic aspects of the epilepsies: A review. New York, Raven Press, 1981.
5. Chee C, Clancy R: Children with epilepsy, in Fithian J (ed): *Understanding the Child with Chronic Illness at School.* Phoenix, Oryx Press, 1984, pp 57–79.
6. Reisner H (ed): *Children With Epilepsy: A Parents Guide.* Kensington, Md, Woodbine House, 1988.
7. Jan JE, Ziegler RG, Erba G: Does your child have epilepsy? Baltimore, University Park Press, 1983.

---

*The Epilepsy Foundation of America, 4351 Garden City Drive, Landover, MD, 20785 (301-459-3700).

109 CONGENITAL ANOMALIES

Richard Polin, M.D.

Few events are more emotionally devastating for new parents than to be told their newborn child is not properly formed. Most frequently, either the pediatrician or family practitioner is the physician with whom parents speak first and, therefore, these individuals must have an organized approach to such meetings. The purpose of this chapter is to provide practical guidelines for speaking with families about children with congenital anomalies or malformations.

Before meeting the parents of a child with a congenital anomaly, it is vitally important to perform a careful physical examination. Parents need and seek an accurate diagnosis and detailed description of abnormalities—not a general impression that their child is not properly formed. Nothing is more frustrating for families than to have multiple meetings with their physician, each meeting describing an additional problem. Frequently, small cleft palates are overlooked, and so it is important to examine this area carefully. The overall pattern of both major and minor malformations must be considered. Even minor malformations can be significant when found in association with other anomalies. In general, a child with a single defect should not be considered to have a specific syndrome. When two or more malformations are present, however, the risk of detecting a major malformation rises to 90%. Attention should be directed to describing and categorizing the anomalies and, if possible, determining which of the defects occurred earliest in morphogenesis. This information can help determine the timing of the embryonic insult. Funduscopic examination by an experienced ophthalmologist may be especially informative, as many eye abnormalities are unique and suggest a specific diagnosis. Laboratory tests (e.g., cytogenetic studies, radiographs) should be obtained to evaluate abnormalities in specific organ systems, rather than used as a "fishing expedition" that can be both costly to parents and not very fruitful.

The first meeting with the parents following the child's birth is often the most important in the counseling process. Whenever possible, both parents should be present at all conferences. Because of cultural teachings, however, some husbands will attempt to exclude their wives from meeting any physician and insist that all communications occur through them. The husbands assume this attitude because they fundamentally believe their wives are not capable of accepting unpleasant news. Contrary to these beliefs, women often accept the truth better than their husbands and frequently are more communicative. Other family members (e.g., grandparents) can be included in these meetings; however, they should be passive participants, allowing the parents of the child to formulate their own questions and reach their own conclusions. Parents need to know that they alone will best be able to support each other emotionally.

The initial meeting with the parents of a child with congenital anomalies generally follows a common format whether the child has a single abnormality or multiple-malformation sydrome. The purpose of this meeting is threefold: (1) to state and describe the problem; (2) to obtain pertinent historical information; and (3) to answer parental questions.

EXPLAINING THE PROBLEM

A description of the anomalies should be given in the simplest possible terms. It is inadvisable to give parents a list of all possible diagnoses and the outcome for each disorder. Too much information given to families is likely to overwhelm and confuse them. An exception to this rule exists when the physician is talking with the parents of a child with a suspected chromosome abnormality. In retrospect, most of these families wished to know the diagnosis as soon as it was suspected by a physician. It is appropriate in these situations to inform parents that the overall pattern of malformations suggests a chromosome disorder and to briefly describe the significance of such an abnormality. The parents should be encouraged not to focus on any one single anomaly but should be told that the presence of many abnormal features indicates the chromosome problem.

The prognosis for single or multiple malformations should be realistically communicated. When a single malformation such as cleft lip is present, the correctable nature of this defect should be emphasized. Discussions with parents concerning nonlethal malformations ideally should take place with the infant in the room. The physician should demonstrate that their child is normal, with the exception of a single anomaly. The discussion concerning the child with multiple congenital anomalies should be approached in a similar fashion. Even when the prognosis for survival or normalcy is poor, parents should be encouraged to interact with and touch their child.

Some parents may find themselves unable to make an emotional commitment to a child with congenital anomalies. This refusal to bond to these children may be an attempt by these families to protect themselves from further emotional suffering. Occasionally, families will try to abandon a child with only a cosmetic problem. In these situations the stimulus for continuing parental involvement should come from other family members, physicians, nurses, and social service personnel. No attempt should be made to discuss withdrawal of life support systems at the first meeting. Parents must first understand the seriousness and extent of the anomalies before they are able to reach a decision concerning ongoing intensive care.

HISTORY

A second goal of the parent conference should be to obtain historical information that will help make a diagnosis. The age, sex, and past and present health of parents, siblings, and other closely related family members should be determined. The ethnic background of the infant's family and the geographic area from which they originated may also be important. Specifically, a history of maternal diabetes, polyhydramnios, or epilepsy should be sought. A detailed description of drug exposure and viral illness during the pregnancy should be obtained; however, it is important to emphasize to both parents that neither maternal drug use nor an upper respiratory tract infection in the first trimester of pregnancy is likely to be related to congenital malformations in the infant.

ANSWERING QUESTIONS

The four most common parental questions are: (1) What caused the malformations? (2) Will my child be mentally retarded? (3) Will my child survive? (4) Have we done something that caused the malformations? Although a detailed discussion of the causes of malformations might be left for a genetic counselor when there is one available, there are certain fundamental concepts that can be transmitted by the family physician. The simplest response to the first question regarding cause is that until a specific diagnosis is determined, there can be no definite answer. Parents can be told that there are four general etiologic categories for malformations: mendelian disorders (e.g., achondroplasia), multifactorial disorders (e.g., cleft lip), environmental disorders (e.g., thalidomide-induced phocomelia), and chromosome disorders (e.g., Down syndrome); however, it must be emphasized that their child's anomaly is most probably unrelated to something the parents did or neglected to do at the time of conception or during the pregnancy.

The question of handicap should also be dealt with in general terms. If the malformation is a single structural anomaly such as club foot, the remedial nature of this malformation should be stressed, as well as what is normal with the rest of the body. The prognosis for multiple malformation syndromes will vary with etiology. Trisomy chromosome disorders are uniformly associated with moderate to severe mental retardation. Other malformation syndromes (such as the VATER association: *v*ertebral, *a*nal anomaly, *t*racheo*e*sophageal, *r*adial upper limb, hypoplasia, and renal defects) have a normal mental outlook despite the severity of malformations.

Most parents assume their children will survive, regardless of the extent of their anomalies. Survival will ultimately depend on the severity of cardiac and central nervous system malformations. If the infant requires assisted ventilation, the parents should be told the life support will continue until they have had sufficient time to evaluate the appropriateness of continued care. The question of discontinuation of ventilation should be raised by the physician once it is clear that the neurologic outlook for the infant is extremely poor or if the child has malformations that are incompatible with an existence outside the hospital and are not correctable. The life-support issue is generally broached by the practitioner once the family has been given a definitive statement regarding prognosis. At that meeting, the parents should be told they will be permitted as much time as needed to reach a decision; however, the date of future meetings with the family should not be left open-ended and a new time should be set. Many families find the involvement of a clergyman welcome support at this stage. When discontinuing support is considered, the hospital ethics committee will also help define the issues and offer an opinion.

If the decision is made to remove an infant from the ventilator, some families request that they be allowed to hold their infant while the lines and tubes are removed. *All families should be encouraged to hold their infants.* This may be their only opportunity to truly function like a parent with their son or daughter. The child should be wrapped in a blanket and given to the family in a quiet area where they can be left alone to grieve. After the child has died, it is important to have the family schedule a return visit to the office for post-death counseling and discussion of autopsy findings.

The majority of infants with malformations can be cared for in smaller hospitals without immediate referral to a tertiary center. Chromosome studies as well as standard radiologic procedures and biochemical tests can be obtained in most community hospitals. It is advisable, however, to consult a geneticist before discharging the infant from the hospital, so that the family can meet the individual who will provide the majority of counseling. Infants with life-threatening anomalies involving the central nervous system, heart, or lungs should be cared for in a hospital with an intensive care nursery and surgical subspecialists. The pediatric geneticist should be consulted as quickly as possible in such cases to facilitate the diagnostic process.

SUMMARY

The initial meeting with the family should be considered the first step in the process of genetic counseling and emotional support. Further meetings should be attended by a geneticist, but not at the exclusion of the generalist. The tenor set by these initial meetings will determine parental attitude and ability to cope with their child.

BIBLIOGRAPHY

Graham JM: *Smith's Recognizable Patterns of Human Deformation*, ed 2. Philadelphia, WB Saunders Co, 1988.

Jones KL: *Smith's Recognizable Patterns of Human Malformation*, ed 4. Philadelphia, WB Saunders Co, 1988.

Miller LG: Towards a greater understanding of the parents of the mentally retarded child. *J Pediatr* 1968; 73:699.

A NUTRITION AND DIET

Donna Gruskay, M.S., R.D.
Mary Beth Zitarelli, B.S., R.D.

NUTRITION

This Appendix provides the private practitioner with an office reference to which he or she can refer for nutritional instruction material. The information provided is intended to assist the physician in routine counseling and to provide parents with concrete lists, guidelines, and reference material. We ask the community to recognize those specific instances in which referral to a trained, registered dietitian for comprehensive nutritional assessment, diet teaching, and follow-up is necessary.

INFANT FORMULAS AND TUBE FEEDINGS

The following formulary is comprised of infant formulas and tube feedings that have been most widely utilized at The Children's Hospital of Philadelphia. This is not an inclusive list of all the commercial products available but a compilation of representative formulas with which our institution has experienced the greatest success. It is of primary importance that the constituents of these formulas be carefully selected to coincide with the alterations in gastrointestinal (GI) tract function that may occur in specific disease states. A careful workup may be necessary to assess GI function. Intolerances will often exist because of inappropriate administration rather than the composition of a feeding.

The physician's cross-reference may be especially useful to practitioners in the community in selecting an appropriate infant formula.

INDICATIONS FOR COMMERCIAL INFANT FORMULAS (FOR INFANTS YOUNGER THAN 1 YEAR)

Formulas Appropriate for the Full-Term Infant

Products listed in the following sections are suitable for the full-term infant when a cow's milk formula of normal dilution or a calorically concentrated formula is desired. Nutrient distribution is essentially the same as that of human milk, and there is little difference in composition among these products.

Physician's Cross-Reference for Infant Formulas

DISORDER	FORMULA
Allergy: severe cow's milk protein allergy or multiple food allergies	Nutramigen, goat's milk
Biliary atresia	Portagen, Pregestimil
Congestive heart failure or other cardiac anomalies	Similac, PM 60/40
Cow's milk allergy	Isomil, Prosobee
Corn allergy	Nursoy, Soyalac-i
Cystic fibrosis	Pregestimil, Portagen
Elimination diet testing	Nutramigen
Galactosemia	Isomil, Prosobee, Nutramigen
Gluten sensitivity	Prosobee
Glycogen storage disease	RCF
Intractable diarrhea	Pregestimil

Continued.

Physician's Cross-Reference for Infant Formulas—cont'd

DISORDER	FORMULA
Lactose intolerance	Isomil, Prosobee
Leucine-sensitive hypoglycemia	S-14
Maple syrup urine disease	MSUD
Pancreatic insufficiency	Portagen
Prematurity	Similac Special Care, Premature Enfamil, S-M-A Preemie, initially Similac PM 60/40
PKU	Lofenalac
Short bowel syndrome	Pregestimil, Portagen
Steatorrhea	Portagen, Pregestimil
Sucrase-deficiency	Prosobee, Isomil SF

Physician's Cross-Reference for Tube Feedings

DISORDER	TUBE FEEDING
Bile acid deficiency	Portagen
Bowel rest	Vital HN
Inflammatory bowel disease	Precision
Lactose intolerance	Isocal, Osmolite, Complete B Modified, Ensure, Precision, Portagen, Magnacal
Lymphatic anomalies	Portagen
Pancreatic insufficiency	
Mild	Portagen
Severe	Vital HN
Radiation therapy to bowel	Vital HN
Short bowel syndrome	Vital HN, Portagen
Steatorrhea	Portagen, Vital HN
Tube feedings	
Standard	Isocal, Osmolite Complete B Modified
Long-term	

Normal dilution (20 kcal/oz)

Available as ready-to-feed (R-to-F), concentrate, or powder. (1) Similac 20 with or without iron; (2) Similac with whey, iron fortified only; (3) Enfamil, new whey-predominant formulation with or without iron; (4) S-M-A Formula.

Concentrated caloric density

24 kcal/oz Similac and Enfamil are available with or without iron; Similac with whey only comes iron fortified

27 kcal/oz Similac is available without iron; all dilutions can be prepared using liquid concentrate or powder form (including 30 kcal/oz), because they are not commercially available as R-to-F preparations. Mixing directions are available from the manufacturer.

Formulas Appropriate for the Premature Infant

Formulas designed for the premature infant necessitate manipulation of all three major nutrients. Lactose is found in human milk and may therefore have special significance; however, the low birth weight (LBW) infant's lactase activity does not reach that of the full-term infant until the ninth month of gestation. Therefore in these formulas only 40% to 50% of the carbohydrate is available as lactose. This mixture of carbohydrates facilitates utilization because multiple digestive and absorptive pathways are involved. The whey-casein ratio (60:40) of human milk is incorporated in these formulas because (1) whey forms smaller, more digestible curds, avoiding lactobezoar formation, and (2) whey offers a more appropriate amino acid composition that is higher in cystine (may be essential to the LBW infant) and lower in tyrosine, an amino acid that an LBW infant may not have the metabolic pathways to handle. LBW infants frequently are unable to digest long-chain saturated fats that form insoluble calcium–fatty acid complexes, resulting in impaired absorption of fats, calcium, and other minerals. This poor digestion is thought to be related to low bile acid pools or to poor resorption of the bile acids; thus medium-chain triglyceride (MCT) oil has been used. None of these formulas is fortified with iron, nor is any available outside the hospital. The feeding of the LBW infant still requires supplementation with a multivitamin preparation when these products are used.

Formulas Specially Designed for Premature Infants With an Immature GI Tract

FORMULA	COMMENT
Similac Special Care, 20 kcal/oz	Requires approximately 8–10 oz/day to meet calcium needs
Similac Special Care, 24 kcal/oz	Requires approximately 8–10 oz/day to meet calcium needs
Premature Enfamil, 20 kcal/oz	Requires approximately 12–14 oz/day to meet calcium needs
Premature Enfamil, 24 kcal/oz	Requires approximately 12–14 oz/day to meet calcium needs
S-M-A Preemie	Requires approximately 16–18 oz/day to meet calcium needs

Composition of Special Premature Infant Formulas

	KCAL/OZ	CARBOHYDRATE	PROTEIN	FAT	mOsm/100 mL H_2O
Similac Special Care	20	42% (50% lactose, 50% corn syrup solids)	11% (60% lactalbumin, lactoglobulin; 40% casein)	47% (50% medium-chain triglyceride (MCT) oil, 30% corn oil, 20% coconut oil)	220
Similac Special Care	24	42% (50% lactose, 50% corn syrup solids)	11% (60% lactalbumin, lactoglobulin; 40% casein)	47% (50% MCT oil, 30% corn oil, 20% coconut oil)	300
Premature Enfamil	20	44% (60% corn syrup solids, 40% lactose)	12% (60% lactalbumin, 40% casein)	44% (40% MCT oil, 40% corn oil, 20% coconut oil)	244
Premature Enfamil	24	44% (60% Corn syrup solids 40% lactose)	12% (60% lactalbumin, 40% casein)	44% (40% MCT oil, 40% corn oil, 20% coconut oil)	300
S-M-A Preemie	24	43% (50% lactose, 50% maltodextrins)	10% (60% lactalbumin, 40% casein)	47% (13% MCT oil)	268

Formulations With Low Renal Solute Load

FORMULA	COMMENT
S-M-A, 20 kcal/oz, with iron; S-M-A, 24 kcal/oz, with iron; S-M-A, 27 kcal/oz, with iron	Available in R-to-F, concentrate liquid, and powder form; can be easily diluted to formulas with 20, 24, 27, and 30 kcal/oz
PM 60/40, 20 kcal/oz	Not iron fortified; only 20 kcal/oz available as R-to-F; other dilutions can be easily mixed from concentrate liquid or powder form

Formulas With Manipulations of Carbohydrate Source Secondary to Allergy or Disaccharidase Deficiency

All formulas are designed for the full-term infant and are iron fortified.

FORMULA	COMMENT
Soy-protein base and lactose free Isomil, 20 kcal/oz	Hypoallergenic soy protein isolate is to be used when cow's milk allergy is diagnosed. Lactose free for the management of lactose intolerance due to diarrhea, primary lactose intolerance, and galactosemia. The formula with 20 kcal/oz dilution is available as R-to-F; concentrate liquid and powder form can be easily mixed to increase kcal concentration. Will be substituted for Soyalac. Use in the premature infant can induce phosphorus deficiency rickets.
Soy-protein base, lactose and sucrose free Prosobee, 20 kcal/oz	Same as for Isomil. In addition, it is appropriate when chronic or transient diarrhea also causes sucrase deficiency. Can also be used in gluten sensitivity. Available in R-to-F and liquid concentrate that can be diluted to 20, 24, 27, and 30 kcal/oz.
Soy-protein base, lactose and corn free Nursoy, 20 kcal/oz	For use when corn allergy is diagnosed; available in R-to-F and liquid concentrate. Soyalac-i can be substituted for Nursoy.

Formulas for Infants Who Require a Low-Sodium Intake

These formulas are often used when the infant's status requires a low-sodium intake because they contain approximately half the sodium of other infant formulas. Both formulas have often been used with the premature infant because of their whey-to-casein ratio (60:40) and have been well tolerated. However, less than optimal features for the premature infant include (1) carbohydrate content as 100% lactose and (2) inadequate levels of folic acid, calcium, and vitamin E.

Formula for Infants With Carbohydrate-Induced Diarrhea

FORMULA	COMMENT
RCF, 20 kcal/oz	For dietary management in infants or children unable to tolerate disaccharides or other carbohydrates found in commercial formulas. Specific indications include intractable diarrhea and glycogen storage disease. The concentrate does not provide a completely balanced formula unless diluted with table sugar, dextrose, polycose (glucose polymers), or corn syrup. Allows the physician to prescribe type and amount of carbohydrate that can be tolerated. Also contains soy protein to avoid symptoms of cow's milk allergy or sensitivity. Available only as 24 kcal/oz concentrate. Iron fortified.

Fat Source Modified for Use in Significant Steatorrhea

FORMULA	COMMENT
Portagen, 20 kcal/oz	Should be used when significant steatorrhea occurs in cystic fibrosis, intestinal resection, pancreatic insufficiency, lymphatic anomalies (e.g., intestinal lymphangiectasia), celiac disease, or biliary atresia. Available only in powder form. Iron fortified. Contains 86% of fat kcal as medium-chain triglyceride (MCT) oil.

Hypoallergenic Protein Hydrolysate for Easy Protein Digestion

FORMULA	COMMENT
Nutramigen, 20 kcal/oz	Indicated primarily for infants with cow's milk allergy or other protein allergic sensitivity, severe or multiple food allergies, severe or persistent diarrhea, or other GI disturbances; also used as maintenance diet during elimination diet testing and in galactosemia. Iron fortified. Available R-to-F and as powder that can easily be calorically concentrated.
Pregestimil, 20 kcal/oz	Appropriate for use in infants with idiopathic defects in digestion or absorption, intestinal resection, intractable diarrhea, cystic fibrosis, steatorrhea, or food allergies. Contains 40% of fat kcal as medium-chain triglyceride (MCT) oil. Iron fortified. Available R-to-F and as powder form that can easily be calorically concentrated.

Formula for Infants With Phenylketonuria

FORMULA	COMMENT
Lofenalac	Contains 11 mg phenylalanine dl, which is not adequate to meet the total daily requirement of the growing infant. Sufficient phenylalanine from other sources such as infant formula, breast milk, or cow's milk must be added to Lofenalac to meet the patient's minimum requirements for growth and development.

INDICATIONS FOR COMMERCIAL TUBE FEEDINGS AND SUPPLEMENTS (FOR CHILDREN OLDER THAN 1 YEAR)

Complete Diets Without Lactose

Appropriate for patients with normal gut function or slight dysfunction of the GI tract, these diets contain normal nutrient distribution, with an optimal nonprotein kcal-nitrogen ratio of 150–200:1 and are available in a ready-to-use form. They can be used for patients with hypermetabolic states, head and neck injuries (i.e., radiation to these areas or wired jaws), coma, burns, protein-calorie malnutrition, inflammatory bowel disease, celiac disease, or mild pancreatic insufficiency. These formulas contain intact nutrients that require normal digestion, and are not suitable in the presence of severe pancreatic insufficiency, short or damaged intestine, or when the patient needs bowel rest (e.g., during treatment of intestinal fistulas). All require additional free water secondary to solute load. Unless otherwise indicated, all products are unpalatable when taken orally; contain no lactose, gluten, or oxalate; and are very low in purine, cholesterol, and residue content. Most provide 1 kcal/ml. Certain formulas indicate nasojejunal or jejunal administration as an acceptable, well-tolerated route of administration and should usually be given as continuous infusions.

Tube Feedings Without Lactose

FORMULA	ADMINISTRATION	INDICATIONS AND COMMENTS
Complete B modified	NG, G, bolus	To be used when a home-blenderized diet is anticipated. Contains moderate amounts of fruit and plant fiber. Lactose-containing version is still available (with dry skim milk) and may be beneficial when a higher residue diet is needed. Contains purines.
Isocal	NG, G, NJ, or J bolus	Contains intact sources of nutrients (protein isolates) with exception of fat: of 37% fat content, 30% is soy oil, 7% MCT oil. Has been successfully used as an NJ or J feeding. Can be used as a home-blenderized diet and is isotonic.

G = gastric; NG = nasogastric; J = jejunal; NJ = nasojejunal.

Continued.

Tube Feedings Without Lactose—cont'd

FORMULA	ADMINISTRATION	INDICATIONS AND COMMENTS
Osmolite	NG, G, NJ, or J bolus	Is very similar in composition to Isocal, except a greater percentage (16%) of kcals come from MCT oil and therefore may be helpful in the management of fat malabsorption. Also isotonic.
Portagen	NG, G, NJ, or	Unique in that 34% of total kcal come from MCT oil. Should be used when fat absorption is impaired, such as may occur in pancreatic insufficiency, bile acid deficiency, some intestinal resections, and lymphatic anomalies. Needs to be ordered as 1 kcal/ml, because it is also available as an infant formula; requires mixing.

G = gastric; NG = nasogastric; J = jejunal; NJ = nasojejunal.

Tube Feedings and Oral Supplements Without Lactose

FORMULA	ADMINISTRATION	INDICATIONS AND COMMENTS
Precision	Oral, NG, G, bolus	Slightly lower fat content at 28%. This oral supplement has been well tolerated, particularly in patients with inflammatory bowel disease. Orange and vanilla flavors available. Isotonic; requires mixing.
Ensure	Oral, NG, G bolus	Because it is slightly hypertonic, should be sipped slowly to avoid diarrhea, and is not suggested as a transpyloric feeding. Vanilla, chocolate, and strawberry flavors; all but chocolate are purine free.
Ensure Plus, 1.5 kcal/ml	Oral, continuous NG or G	Contains less than optimal nonprotein calorie-nitrogen ratio but is actually more palatable than Ensure 1 kcal/ml. It is particularly important that the formula be sipped slowly (600 mOsm/H_2O), and it is not recommended as a transpyloric feeding. Vanilla, chocolate, and strawberry flavors.
Magnacal, 2 kcal/ml	Oral, continuous NG or G	Particularly useful in fluid restriction or when patient is unable to ingest adequate volumes of food (e.g., patients with cancer). Transpyloric feedings not recommended. Available in bland vanilla so a variety of flavors can be added. Product is a concentrated source of nutrients, and fluid balance must be closely monitored.

G = gastric; NG = nasogastric.

DIET

WEIGHT CONTROL DIET

Diet Structure

1. Each patient's goals need to be individualized and realistically attainable.

2. A guideline for meeting energy expenditure needs is Standard Basal Calories. From 0% to 50% increments are added for activity levels.

Basal Metabolic Rate

This Table (Standard Basal Calories) is very comparable to other calculations used to determine basal metabolic rate that utilize age and body surface area. Many variables (e.g., age, sex, diet history, activity) can make precise calculations of energy expenditure difficult. For the best results, knowledge of diet history, basal metabolic rate, and recommended daily allowance (RDA) of calories for age can be used

Standard Basal Calories*

WEIGHT (KG)	CAL/24 HR† MALE	MALE AND FEMALE	FEMALE
3		140	
5		270	
7		400	
9		500	
11		600	
13		650	
15		710	
17		780	
19		830	
21		880	
25	1,020		960
29	1,120		1,040
33	1,210		1,120
37	1,300		1,190
41	1,350		1,260
45	1,410		1,320
49	1,470		1,380
53	1,530		1,440
57	1,590		1,500
61	1,640		1,560

*From Nelson WE, et al (eds): *Nelson's Textbook of Pediatrics,* ed 12. Philadelphia, WB Saunders Co, 1983. Used with permission.

†*Increments or decrements:* Add or subtract 12% of above for each degree C (8% for each degree F) above or below rectal temperature of 37.8° C (100° F).

for this determination. It is important for growth and development to also continue during this period.

Adherence to a "prudent" diet of approximately 12% protein calories, 30% fat calories, and 58% carbohydrate calories is recommended. Weight changes should be monitored so that alterations can be made as necessary in dietary regimen. Massively obese (180%) children and adolescents may require more intense medical or dietary intervention.

Weight Reduction Programs

The tables in this section offer guidelines for initiating a weight-reduction program. An obese child benefits most by participation in a structured, multidisciplinary approach to weight loss.

Guidelines for Controlling Caloric Intake

The following steps to weight control can be implemented by the patient as an initial step. When a child is overweight, the goal is to develop a new approach to eating habits so that changes are made for a lifetime. An important key is an awareness of the ingredients of the foods that are eaten by careful attention to product labels. The following general guidelines will assist in controlling caloric intake.

Food Preparation.—

- Bake, broil, or boil foods instead of deep-fat or pan frying.
- Do *not* add extra butter, margarine, oil, mayonnaise, cream, or salad dressing to foods. *Avoid* creamed dishes.
- Serve meat well trimmed of fat. Use a rack when broiling, roasting, or baking so the fat can drain off. To keep meat moist, pour bouillon or tomato juice over it.
- When a recipe calls for browning meat, try browning it under a broiler instead of pan frying.
- When serving gravy, make it fat free. Make gravy for meat or poultry after the fat has hardened and has been skimmed off the top.
- Remove skin from poultry.
- Cooking with Pam will result in considerable calorie reduction.
- Herbs and spices offer a tasty alternative to sauces of any kind as well as salt.
- Measuring and weighing foods may help some individuals meet their caloric goals.

Food Purchasing.—

- Look for lean cuts of meat.
- Buy foods without cream fillings or rich frostings. THE PLAINER THE FOOD, THE FEWER THE CALORIES.
- Do *not* buy all special dietetic foods. The idea is to eat the right amount of food for your body and learn good eating habits.
- Buy skim milk or 2% milk instead of whole milk.
- Buy canned or fresh fruit for dessert instead of pies, cakes, and pastries.
- Choose water-packed over oil-packed tuna.
- Excessive consumption of salt-containing foods can cause fluid retention. These foods and additional salt should be used in moderation.

Activity.—

- Increase activity by encouraging participation in active sports (e.g., swimming, skating, tennis, bicycling, playing ball, brisk walking).

Approach.—

- A casual positive approach is the *best* way to help a child lose weight. A child will need encouragement, not nagging, to be able to assume the responsibility for food intake.
- A real desire on the child's part to lose weight is an essential factor for a successful outcome.

Low-Calorie Substitutions.—

- Artificial sweeteners can be used on cereals, in beverages or desserts, etc.
- Diet sodas are a smart alternative.
- Salads are a healthy change and should be encouraged in any weight-reduction diet, but use a low-calorie dressing.
- Remember, low-calorie mayonnaise is also available.
- *Non*-presweetened cereals should be encouraged.
- Popcorn with butter salt is a delicious low-calorie snack.

Additional Guidelines.—

- To maintain good growth and development while losing weight, a child's diet should include choices from each of the basic four food groups.
- With any weight-reduction diet, a multivitamin supplement is recommended.
- In general, foods labeled as having no preservatives and health or natural foods are not necessarily lower in calories.

SODIUM-CONTROLLED DIET

The low-sodium diet is designed to lower the dietary intake of sodium to a prescribed level to restore normal sodium balance to the body. Sodium-controlled diets are used as adjunctive therapy in the treatment of liver, renal, and cardiac disease when associated edema or hypertension is present or in hypertension and adrenocortical therapy.

Mean Height and Weight and Recommended Energy Intake*

		WEIGHT		HEIGHT		ENERGY NEEDS		
	AGE (YR)	(KG)	(LB)	(CM)	(IN.)	(KCAL)	RANGE	(MJ)
Infants	0.0–0.5	6	13	60	24	kg × 115	95–145	kg × 0.48
	0.5–1.0	9	20	71	28	kg × 105	80–135	kg × 0.44
Children	1–3	13	29	90	35	1,300	900–1,800	5.5
	4–6	20	44	112	44	1,700	1,300–2,300	7.1
	7–10	28	62	132	52	2,400	1,650–3,300	10.1
Males	11–14	15	99	157	62	2,700	2,000–3,700	11.3
	15–18	66	145	176	69	2,800	2,100–3,900	11.8
	19–22	70	154	177	70	2,900	2,500–3,300	12.2
	23–50	70	154	178	70	2,700	2,300–3,100	11.3
	51–75	70	154	178	70	2,400	2,000–2,800	10.1
	76+	70	154	178	70	2,050	1,650–2,450	8.6
Females	11–14	46	101	157	62	2,200	1,500–3,000	9.2
	15–18	55	120	163	64	2,100	1,200–3,000	8.8
	19–22	55	120	163	64	2,100	1,700–2,500	8.8
	23–50	55	120	163	64	2,000	1,600–2,400	8.4
	51–75	55	120	163	64	1,800	1,400–2,200	7.6
	76+	55	120	163	64	1,600	1,200–2,000	6.7
Pregnancy						+300		
Lactation						+500		

*From *Recommended Daily Allowances*, ed 9. Washington, DC, National Academy Press, 1980. Used with permission.

Calorie-Controlled Diet: Nutritional and Exchange Values for Fast Foods*

	NUTRITIONAL VALUES				EXCHANGE SYSTEM		
	TOTAL CALORIES	CARBOHYDRATE (GM)	PROTEIN (GM)	FAT (GM)	BREAD	MEAT	FAT
Kentucky Fried Chicken (fried chicken, mashed potatoes, gravy, coleslaw, roll)							
3-piece dinner							
Original	830	61	50	43	4	6	2½
Crispy	1,070	74	54	62	5	6	6½
2-piece dinner							
Original (wing and side breast)	604	48	30	32	3½	3½	3½
Crispy (wing and side breast)	755	60	33	43	4	3½	4½
Long John Silver's (fish, chips, coleslaw)							
3-piece dinner	1,190	100	55	63	7	6	7
2-piece dinner	955	89	38	50	6	4	6
McDonald's							
Hamburger	255	30	14	12	2	1½	1
Double hamburger (make your own)	350	34	20	15	2	2	1
Quarter Pounder	424	37	25	24	2	3	1½
Big Mac	563	44	21	34	2½	3	4
French fries	220	20	3	10	2	—	2
Chocolate shake	383	53	9	8	3½	—	1½
Pizza Hut (cheese pizza)							
Individual: Thick crust	1,030	143	71	19	9½	7½	—
Thin crust	1,005	128	61	28	8½	6	—
½ of 13-inch: Thick crust	900	113	65	21	7½	7	—
Thin crust	850	103	50	26	7	5	—
½ of 15-inch: Thick crust	1,200	148	83	31	10	9	—
Thin crust	1,150	144	66	35	9½	7	—
Burger Chef							
Hamburger	250	23	12	12	1½	1	1½
Double hamburger	325	28	20	15	2	2½	1
Super Chef	530	36	30	29	2½	3½	2
Big Chef	535	41	25	30	3	3	3
French fries	240	30	3	12	2	—	2
Chocolate shake	310	48	9	9	3	½	1
Burger King							
Hamburger	290	29	15	13	2	1½	1
Double hamburger	325	24	24	15	2	3	1
Whopper	630	50	26	36	3½	3	4
Whopper, Jr	370	31	15	20	2	1½	2
French fries	210	25	3	11	1½	—	2
Chocolate shake	340	57	8	10	4	—	2

*From *Pediatrics Diet Manual*. Saga Corp, 1985. Used with permission.

Sodium-controlled diets range in restriction from 250 mg/day to 2,000 to 3,000 mg/day. Because extremely restrictive sodium-controlled diets are generally not prescribed by the private practitioner, only moderate restriction (2,000 mg) and mild restriction (2,000 to 3,000 mg/day; also called no-added-salt diet) diets are included here.

1,000-Calorie Diet With 55 gm Protein*

Breakfast
- ½ cup fruit or unsweetened juice
- 1 cup skim milk
- 1 slice bread OR ¾ cup unsweetened cereal
- 1 tsp butter or margarine

Lunch
- 1 oz meat, fish, poultry, or cheese OR 1½ tbsp peanut butter OR ¼ cup cottage cheese
- 1 slice bread
- 1 small piece of fresh fruit OR ½ cup unsweetened fruit
- 1 tsp butter or margarine or mayonnaise
- raw vegetables as desired
- 1 cup skim milk

Dinner
- 2 oz lean meat, poultry, or fish
- 1 slice bread OR ½ cup rice, pasta, potatoes
- 1 cup cooked vegetable
- 1 tsp butter or margarine
- 1 small piece of fresh fruit OR ½ cup unsweetened fruit
- 1 cup skim milk

*Supplemental multivitamin with iron recommended.

1,200-Calorie Diet With 64 gm Protein

Breakfast
- ½ cup fruit or unsweetened juice
- ¾ cup unsweetened cereal OR ½ cup cooked cereal OR 1 egg
- 1 slice toast
- 1 tsp butter or margarine OR 1 strip bacon
- 1 cup skim milk

Lunch
- 2 oz lean meat, poultry, cheese, fish OR ½ cup cottage cheese OR 1 tbsp peanut butter and diet jelly OR ½ cup cottage cheese
- 2 slices bread OR 1 cup potato, pasta, or rice OR 1 slice bread plus ½ cup potato, rice, or pasta
- 1 tsp butter, margarine, or mayonnaise
- ½ cup fruit OR 1 small piece of fruit
- 1 cup skim milk

Dinner
- 2 oz lean meat, poultry, or cheese
- 1 slice bread OR ½ cup pasta, rice, or potato
- 1 cup plain vegetables
- 1 tsp butter or margarine
- ½ cup fruit OR 1 small piece of fruit
- 1 cup skim milk

1,500-Calorie Diet With 80 gm Protein

Breakfast
- 1 cup fruit or unsweetened juice OR 1 small piece of fruit
- 1 egg (any style except fried); limit to 3 times per week
- 2 slices toast OR 1 slice toast plus ¾ cup unsweetened dry cereal
- 1 tsp butter or margarine
- 1 cup skim milk

Lunch
- 2 oz lean meat, fish, poultry, or cheese OR 1 tbsp peanut butter OR ½ cup cottage cheese
- 2 slices bread OR 1 slice of bread plus ½ cup pasta, rice, or potato
- 1 tsp butter, margarine, or mayonnaise
- ½ cup of fruit OR 1 small piece of fruit
- raw vegetables as desired
- 1 cup skim milk

Dinner
- 3 oz lean meat, fish, or poultry
- 2 slices bread OR 1 cup potato, rice, or noodles OR 1 slice bread plus ½ cup potato, rice, or noodles
- 1 cup plain vegetables
- 2 tsb butter or margarine
- ½ cup of fruit OR 1 small piece of fruit
- 1 cup skim milk

NO ADDED SALT DIET (2,000 TO 3, 000 MG)

In this diet sodium (Na) and salt (NaCl) are very mildly restricted. It allows the use of a SMALL amount of salt for cooking, but NONE added at the table. This includes use of celery, garlic, and onion salts.

Regular fresh meats, all vegetables (especially frozen vegetables), and all fruits are allowed. Regular breads, butter, margarine, and desserts are also allowed.

The intake of very salty foods must be eliminated or modified; this includes:

- Salted and smoked meats: bacon, hot dogs, ham, salt pork, sausage, bologna, cold cuts, luncheon meats, chipped or corned beef, kosher meats, tuna fish (oil-packed)

Recommended and Actual Intake of Sodium by Age

AGE (YR)	ESTIMATED SAFE AND ADEQUATE DAILY INTAKE OF SODIUM (MG)	AVERAGE SODIUM CONTENT OF US DIET (1977–1980) (MG)
0–0.5	115–350	706–887 (age 6 mo)
0.5–1	250–750	1,605–1,805 (age 2 yr)
1–3	329–975	
4–6	450–1,350	
7–10	600–1,800	
11+	900–2,700	6,692–6,851 (male aged 15–20 yr)

- Salted and smoked fish: salted cod, herring, sardines, salmons, anchovies, caviar, clams, oysters, and other saltwater fish
- Cheeses: especially processed cheeses, cheese spreads, cheese sauces, and other cheese products (e.g., pizza)
- Commercial soups, bouillon, gravies, and canned stews
- Foods with salt toppings: crackers, potato chips, popcorn, pretzels, nuts, corn chips, and other salted snack foods

2,000 mg Sodium (Na) Diet

FOOD GROUP	FOODS ALLOWED	FOODS RESTRICTED
Milk 120 mg Na/8 oz (2–3 servings/day)	Whole, low-fat, skim; evaporated (½ cup), powdered (3 tbsp reconstituted), yogurt, cocoa powder	Buttermilk, instant cocoa mix, processed Dutch cocoa, other commercial instant milk beverages, malted milk
Vegetable *Group A:* 9 mg Na/½ cup (as desired)	Fresh or dietetic canned vegetables, frozen vegetables not in group B, unsalted canned vegetable juices	Sauerkraut or other vegetables prepared in brine, regular mixed vegetable juices, regular tomato juice
Group B: 100 mg Na/½ cup	Frozen lima beans and peas	Same as group A
Group C: 230 mg Na/½ cup (limit to 1 serving day)	Regular canned vegetables and those with salt added during cooking.	Same as group A
Bread/starch *Group A:* Regular 120 mg Na/serving (limit to 5 servings/ day)	Regular bread (1 slice), dry cereal (¾ cup), melba toast (4), graham crackers (2), bagel, English muffin, frankfurter bun, hamburger roll (½), yeast donut; seasoned pasta, rice, potatoes; lentils, parsnips, split peas (½ cup)	Breads, crackers, and rolls with salted tops; corn chips, potato chips, pretzels; instant cooked cereals; salted popcorn
Group B: 5 mg Na/serving	Low-sodium bread (1 slice), unsalted regular cooked cereal (½ cup), Puffed Rice, Puffed Wheat, Shredded Wheat (1 cup), unsalted popcorn (1 cup), unsalted crackers (6-in. squares), matzo (1, 6-in square), Uneeda biscuits (4); all-purpose flour (2½ tbsp); unsalted pasta, rice, potatoes, dried lentils, parsnips, split peas (½ c), low-sodium potato chips, or unsalted pretzels (1 oz)	All others, self-rising flour
Fruit 2 mg Na/serving (3 servings/day)	Any fresh, frozen, or canned fruit or fruit juice; avocado	All crystallized and glazed fruit, maraschino cherries, fruit dried with sodium sulfite, olives
Meat 3–5 servings/day *Group A:* 69 mg Na/oz	Fresh or frozen meat; poultry, or fish seasoned as in recipe; shellfish cooked with no added salt	Regular canned or smoked meat, poultry, or fish; bacon, luncheon meats, ham, chipped or corned beef, frankfurters, salt pork, sausage, meats koshered by salting
Group B: 25 mg Na/oz	Unsalted cottage cheese (¼ cup); low-sodium peanut butter (2 tbsp); unsalted fresh meat, fish, poultry; dietetic canned meat, fish, poultry; low-sodium cheese	Regular cheese, regular peanut butter
Eggs 60 mg Na (maximum of 1/day)	Fresh or whole	Frozen with salt, egg substitutes

Continued.

2,000 mg Sodium (Na) Diet—cont'd

FOOD GROUP	FOODS ALLOWED	FOODS RESTRICTED
Fat 50 mg Na/serving (limit to 3 servings/day)	Butter or margarine (1 tsp); cream, half & half, mayonnaise (2 tsp); cream cheese (1½ tbsp) Use freely: unsalted butter or margarine, cooking oil or fat, unsalted nuts, low-sodium salad dressings	Bacon, bacon fat, salt pork, salted nuts, party spreads and dips, regular salad dressings
Beverage (as desired, in moderation)	Coffee, tea, coffee substitutes, carbonated beverages, canned or frozen fruit drinks	Limit use of carbonated beverages to that amount equal to 50 mg Na (see conversion table)
Dessert (as desired, in moderation)	Low-sodium pudding and gelatin, fruit ices, popsicles, low-sodium baked products	All others
Group A: Negligible amount of Na (as desired, in moderation)		
Group B: 50 mg Na/serving (in moderation)	Brownie (1 small); cookies: brown-edge wafer (3), butter cookie (2), chocolate chip cookie (1¾-in. diameter, 2), fig bar (1), gingersnap (1), ladyfinger (6), marcaroon (7), oatmeal-raisin cookie (2), chocolate or vanilla sandwich cookie (1), shortbread cookie (10), sugar cookie (2), vanilla wafers (5); ice cream, sherbet, flavored gelatin (½ cup); pound cake (1 slice);	All others
Group C: 150 mg Na/serving (limit to not more than 1 serving/day)	Angel food cake; plain cake with frosting; custard or pudding (½ cup); pie (1.5-in. arc); Boston cream pie (2.5 in. arc)	Pastries, any desserts containing salted nuts or regular peanut butter
Soup 40 mg Na/cup (1 serving/day)	Homemade cream or meat broth soups made without salt (for cream soup, count sodium value of milk used in recipe); low-sodium canned soups; use only those vegetables listed in group A	Regular canned soup, stews, or bouillon (cubes, liquid, or powder); dehydrated soup mixes
Miscellaneous (as desired, in moderation)	Unflavored gelatin, lemon, lime, vinegar, cream of tartar, yeast, pure cocoa, nonsalt herbs and spices	Catsup, chile sauce, cooking wine, cerery salt, garlic salt, onion salt, pickles, relishes, prepared mustard, soy sauce, meat sauces, meat tenderizers, monosodium glutamate, barbecue sauce, Worcestershire sauce
Sweets	Candy corn, gumdrops, jam, jelly, jelly beans, hard candy, chocolate, syrup	Processed Dutch cocoa

Sample Meal Plan in a 2,000-mg Sodium Diet for Children 4 to 6 Years Old*

BREAKFAST	LUNCH	DINNER
4 oz orange juice 1 hard-boiled egg ½ cup regular farina 1 tsp regular margarine 1 tsp sugar 8 oz lowfat milk	Chicken sandwich: 2 oz regular chicken, 2 slices regular bread, 1 tsp regular mayonnaise, lettuce leaf ½ cup low-sodium green beans with 1 tsp regular margarine ½ medium banana 4 oz lowfat milk	2 oz regular roast beef ½ cup regular rice with 1 tsp low-sodium margarine ½ cup low-sodium diced carrots with 1 tsp low-sodium margarine 2 chocolate chip cookies 4 oz lowfat milk
	SNACK	SNACK
	2 graham crackers 4 oz lowfat milk	1 tbsp low-sodium peanut butter 4 low-sodium crackers 4 oz lowfat milk

*From *Pediatrics Diet Manual.* Saga Corporation, 1985. Used with permission.

- Sauerkraut, pickles, olives, and other foods prepared in brine or heavily salted
- Highly salted sauces: limited amounts of catsup, mustard, chili sauce, Worcestershire sauce, barbecue and steak sauces, meat tenderizer, soy sauce, mayonnaise, salad dressings
- Salt substitutes and medications should not be used without permission from a physician

SUGGESTIONS FOR ADDING FLAVOR AND VARIETY TO LOW-SODIUM DIETS

General Recommendations

1. Add lemon juice or vinegar *after* vegetables have been cooked; otherwise, cooking time will be lengthened.
2. To obtain a delicate flavor, spices should be used sparingly and to taste.
3. Sprinkle seasonings on vegetables or blend them with unsalted fat.
4. Rub herbs or spices on surface of meat before roasting or add them to flour before browning meat in unsalted fat.

SODIUM IN FAST FOODS

Many foods available in fast-food restaurants are similar in sodium content. The values given on p. 930 are averages of comparable items purchased at Arthur Treacher's, Burger Chef, Burger King, Jack-in-the-Box, Kentucky Fried Chicken, Long John Silver's, McDonald's, and Taco Bell. There may be some 10% to 15% variation in sodium content between similar products from various establishments.

FLAVORING AIDS THAT MAY BE USED

Allspice
Almond extract
Anise seed
Basil
Bay leaf
Caraway seed
Cardamom
Chili powder
Chives
Cinnamon
Cloves
Cumin
Curry
Cyclamate, calcium (sugar substitute)
Dill
Fennel
Garlic, garlic juice, or garlic powder
Ginger
Horseradish root or horseradish prepared without salt
Juniper
Lemon juice or extract
Mace
Maple extract
Marjoram
Mint
Mustard: dry or mustard seed

Continued.

FLAVORING AIDS THAT MAY BE USED—CONT'D

Nutmeg
Onion, onion juice, or onion powder
Orange extract
Oregano
Paprika
Parsley or parsley flakes
Pepper: fresh green or red
Pepper: black, red, or white
Peppermint extract
Pimiento peppers for garnish
Poppy seed
Poultry seasoning
Purslane
Rosemary
Saccharin
Saffron
Sage
Savory
Sesame seeds
Sorrel
Sugar
Tarragon
Thyme
Tumeric
Vanilla extract
Vinegar
Wine
Walnut extract

LACTOSE-RESTRICTED DIET

The lactose-restricted diet is used when the body is unable to tolerate large amounts of lactose-containing foods due to lactase deficiency secondary to congenital lactase deficiency, acute or chronic diarrhea, or acquired lactase deficiency with certain disease states. Gastrointestinal symptoms among individuals vary but usually become apparent after the consumption of one or two glasses of milk. It is therefore essential that the diet be designed with flexibility. Most individuals are able to

Sodium Values of Foods in Fast-Food Restaurants*

FOOD	PORTION	SODIUM (MG)
Breakfast Foods		
Egg sandwich	1 oz cheese, 1 egg, 1 bun	960
Scrambled eggs	2–3 eggs	205
Omelette	2–3 eggs	1,000
Pancakes	3 pancakes, syrup, butter	1,400
Hash browns	½ cup	450
Juice	8 oz fruit juice	0
Lunch/Dinner Foods		
Hamburger	1½ oz meat on bun	530
Cheeseburger	1 oz meat, 1 oz cheese on bun	690
Deluxe burger	3–3½ oz meat on bun	950
Deluxe with cheese	3 oz meat, 1 oz cheese on bun	1,120
Fish sandwich	1½–2 oz fish on bun	630
Chicken sandwich	2½–3 oz chicken on bun	710
Roast beef sandwich	2½–3 oz meat on bun	900
Chicken nuggets	3 oz chicken meat	525
Sauce		
Sweet and sour	1 oz	186
Honey	½ oz	2
Hot mustard	1 oz	259
Barbecue	1 oz	309
Fried chicken	3½–4 oz chicken (2 pieces)	495
Fried fish	2–3 oz fish (2 pieces)	270
Taco	1–2 oz meat	715
Burrito	2 oz meat	925
French fries	5 oz	210
Onion rings	1 serving	385
Soft drinks	10 oz	25
Milkshakes	10 oz	260

*From *Pediatrics Diet Manual.* Saga Corporation, 1985. Used with permission.

tolerate small quantities of milk and milk products such as cheese, yogurt, cultured buttermilk, and butter and margarine in cooked products. The fermented dairy products (yogurt and cultured buttermilk) are better tolerated because the bacteria will again exert lactase activity in the intestinal tract. If symptoms persist, a more ridid regimen should be followed. Some guidelines for the varying lactose content of selected foods are as follows:

- Small amounts of lactose
  - Prepared mixes: cookie, cake, biscuit, muffin
  - Noncream fillings
  - Instant cereal
  - Sweet rolls
  - Canned cream soup made with water
  - Instant potatoes
- Medium amounts of lactose
  - Half and Half, 1 tbsp
  - Camembert cheese, 1 oz
  - Cream cheese, 1 oz
  - Cottage cheese, 2 tbsp
  - Ricotta cheese, 2 tbsp
  - Hard cheese
    - Swiss, 1 oz
    - Cheddar, 1 oz
    - Parmesan, 2 tbsp
    - Bleu, 1 oz
    - Brick, 1 oz
    - American (pasteurized processed), 1 oz
  - Milk chocolate, ½ oz
  - Sherbet, ½ cup
- Large amounts of lactose
  - Cheese food, 2 tbsp
  - Yogurt, ½ cup
  - Ice milk, ½ cup
  - Ice cream, ½ cup
  - Condensed milk, 2 tbsp
  - Evaporated milk, 2 tbsp
  - Cheese spread, 2 tbsp
  - Dry milk powder, 2 tbsp
  - Skim milk, ½ cup
  - Eggnog, ½ cup
  - 2% Milk, ½ cup
  - Buttermilk, ½ cup
  - Whole milk, ½ cup
  - Whipping cream, ½ cup

A lactose-hydrolyzed milk or lactose-free dietary supplement (e.g., soy milk, Isomil) may be an alternative. Lact-Aid enzyme can be added to whole milk, 2% milk, nonfat milk, half-and-half, whipping cream (prior to whipping), sweet acidophilus milk, eggnog, goat's milk, instant cocoa mix, and Carnation Instant Breakfast Drink. By following the package directions, the lactose can be hydrolyzed from 70% to 100%. Lact-Aid cannot be used in some milk products, such as buttermilk, cheese, cottage cheese, sour cream, ice cream, sherbet, and yogurt. Information on where this product is available as well as recipes can be obtained from: SugarLo Co, 600 Fire Rd, PO Box 1100, Pleasantville, NJ 08232.

Remember that ingestion of ¼ to ½ cup of milk four times a day, when permitted, is preferable to 1 cup or more of milk at one time. Milk may be better absorbed if taken with other foods.

Additional products to be avoided are those that have as ingredients butter, buttermilk, cheeses, condensed milk, cow's milk, curds, custards and puddings, evaporated milk, frozen custard, half-and-half, ice cream, lactalbumin, lactoglobulin, 1% milk, 2% milk, milk solids, nonfat dry milk, skim milk, sodium caseinate, sour cream, sour half-and-half, whey, or yogurt.

Special Products Guide for Lactose-Free Commercial Products

The following list* excludes those products containing lactose. This list does not include all commercial products that could be used; many more could be added. Check the label for

*From *Pediatrics Diet Manual*, Saga Corporation, 1985. Reprinted with permission.

Diet Structure—Lactose-Restricted Diet

FOOD GROUP	FOODS ALLOWED	FOODS RESTRICTED
Milk (2 or more)	Yogurt and buttermilk in small amounts, if tolerated	All milk and milk drinks, cocoa, cocoa malt, Olvaltine, condensed or evaporated milk
Milk substitutes	Soy milk products (e.g., Isomil, Prosobee, Nursoy, Mocha-Mix, Lidalas, Ensure, Ensure Plus, Citrotein, Nutramigen, Pregestimil, Precision, Soyalac-i Soyalac)	
Vegetable (2 or more)	All except those "restricted"	Any canned or frozen vegetables prepared with milk or milk solids or seasoned with butter, margarine (if not tolerated), cream or cheese sauces, breaded vegetables, corn curls
Bread/starch Bread, cereal, starchy vegetables (8 or more)	Water breads, hard rolls, bread and rolls made without milk (e.g., Italian bread, soda crackers), prepared and cooked cereals that contain milk solids (read labels), rice, all pastas, potatoes prepared without milk or milk solids	Bread made with milk or milk solids, crackers made with butter or margarine (if not tolerated), French toast made with milk, muffins, biscuits, waffle, cereals containing milk, milk solids, or lactose (i.e., instant Cream of Rice/Wheat, Special K, Fortified Oat Flakes, Cocoa Krispies, Total), commercial french fries, creamed or instant potatoes, Zweiback, frozen french fries processed with lactose
Fruit (2 or more)	All fruits and juices unless listed as "restricted"	Orange Julius
Meat (5 or more)	All except those listed as "restricted"	Cold cuts or frankfurters containing milk solids; creamed or breaded meats; fish, poultry, or sausage; cheese; if not tolerated, omelettes and souffles containing milk
Eggs	All	
Fat (in moderation)	Milk-free margarine (Kosher); gravies; mayonnaise oil; if tolerated, butter, margarine; bacon; Rich's whipped topping; some nondairy creamers; nuts.	If not tolerated, butter, margarine, and dressings made with milk; cream; cream cheese; peanut butter with milk-solid fillers; sour cream
OTHER FOOD CATEGORIES		
Beverage (in moderation)	Coffee, tea, carbonated drinks, instant coffee and cereal, beverages (read labels), freeze-dried coffee	Instant coffee or cereal beverages containing milk solids; powdered soft drinks with lactose curds
Dessert (in moderation)	Gelatin, angel food cake, homemade cake made with vegetable oils and no milk solids, water and fruit ices, puddings made with milk	Cake mixes or other baked product mixes containing milk solids, any product made with milk or milk solids (e.g., ice cream, sherbert, custard, gelatin made with carregeenan), pie crust made with butter or margarine
Seasoning (in moderation)	Pure seasonings and spices	MSG with lactose added
Soup (in moderation)	Cream soups made with mocha mix or nondairy creamers, meat- and vegetable-based soups, clear soups	Cream soups and all soups made with milk
Sweets (in moderation)	Sugar, jams, jellies, and candies made without milk or milk solids; corn syrup and honey	Any sweets made with milk (e.g., chocolate, peppermints, butterscotch, toffee, dietetic preparations)
Miscellaneous	Popcorn without butter, nut butters, soy sauce, carob powder, olives, corn syrup, Baker's cocoa, pickles, molasses	Caramel, chewing gum, milk gravies, ascorbic acid tablets (in moderation), certain vitamin and mineral preparations (check with your druggist), Equal, Sweet n' Low, Wee-Cal

Sample Meal Plan—Lactose-Restricted Diet

BREAKFAST	LUNCH	DINNER
4 oz orange juice 1 poached egg 1 slice French bread toast 1 tsp milk-free margarine 1 cup milk substitute	1 oz turkey 1 slice French bread ½ cup carrots 1 tsp milk-free margarine 1 medium apple 1 cup milk substitute	2 oz roast beef ½ cup rice ½ cup green beans 2 tsp milk-free margarine 1 cup milk substitute
	SNACK	SNACK
	1 tbsp peanut butter 1 slice French bread 1 tsp milk-free margarine ½ cup milk substitute	½ cup Rice Krispies banana ½ cup milk substitute

ingredients when purchasing any processed foods, because ingredients may change from time to time.

Beverages

Coffee
- General foods
  - Regular and instant coffees (Maxwell House, Yuban, and Sanka brands)
- Maxim freeze-dried coffee

Fruit-flavored drinks
- General Foods
  - Birds Eye Awake frozen concentrate for imitation orange juice
  - Birds Eye Orange Plus frozen concentrate for orange juice drink
  - Instant Postum beverages
  - Kook Aid, regular or presweetened soft drink mixes
  - Kool Aid Pop bars
  - Start instant breakfast drink
  - Tang instant breakfast drink
  - Twist imitation lemonade, grapeade, orangeade, and punch mixes

Breads, cereals, crackers, flour

Breads
- Most Italian breads (read label)
- Most French breads (read label)

Cereal
- General Foods
  - Post brand cereals (except Fortified Oat Flakes)
- General Mills
  - All cereals except crackers
- Kellogg's
  - Cornflakes
  - Frosted Flakes
  - Product 19
  - 40% Bran Flakes
  - Raisin Bran
  - Rice Krispies

Crackers
- Premium saltines
- Ritz crackers
- Zesta saltines
- General Mills Bows, Bugles

Flour
- General Mills Gold Medal flour (regular, Softasilk cake flour, Wondra)
- Swans Down cake flour
- Swans Down self-rising cake flour

Other
- General Foods Birds Eye potato products
- General Foods Minute Rice
- General Foods Minute rice mixes (Drumstick and Rib Roast only)
- General Foods Calumet baking powder

Desserts

Duncan Hines angel food cake mix

General Foods
- Baker's chocolate (unsweetened, semisweet, German sweet)
- Baker's semisweet chocolate chips (not glazed chips)
- Baker's Redi-Blend chocolate products for baking
- Baker's cocoa
- Baker's coconut (all varieties)
- Certo fruit pectin
- D'Zerta gelatin desserts
- D'Zerta pudding (chocolate only)
- Jell-O gelatin desserts
- Jell-O lemon chiffon pie filling
- Jell-O pudding and pie fillings (except milk chocolate flavor)
- Jell-O tapicoa pudding
- Minute tapicoa

- Sure-Jell fruit pectin
- Swans Downs angel food cake mix

General Mills
- All angel food cake mixes
- All chiffon cake mixes
- All fluffy frosting mixes
- Chocolate Chip Fudge Brownie Mix
- Chocolate Fudge Brownie Mix
- Graham cracker pie crust
- Ready-to-serve lemon pudding
- Walnut Brownie Mix
- Royal Puddings and Pie Filling (except milk chocolate)

Fruit

General Foods
- Birds Eye frozen fruits
- Birds Eye frozen concentrated fruit juices

Margarines

Mother's Brand
Diet Mazola
Willow Run soybean margarine
Nucoa

Meat products

Roessler's all-beef frankfurters
Armour frankfurters
Kosher all-beef cocktail franks
Nepco frankfurters
Oscar Mayer frankfurters
Swift's Premium frankfurters
Swift's Premium Brown 'N Serve sausage (fully cooked)

Salad dressings

General Foods
- Good Seasons dressing mixes (Creamy French, Garlic, Italian, Low-Calorie Italian, Old-Fashioned French, Onion)
- Good Seasons Open Pit barbeque sauces (Original, Hickory Smoke, and Mild Garlic)
- Good Seasons Thick 'N Creamy salad dressing mixes (Coleslaw, French, Thousand Island)

Soups

Campbell's
- New England Clam Chowder
- Chili Beef
- Noodles and Ground Beef
- Turkey Vegetable
- Chicken Gumbo
- Manhattan Clam Chowder
- Chicken Noodle
- Vegetarian Vegetable
- Old-fashioned Vegetable
- Chicken with Rice
- Chunky Turkey

Habitant
- Chicken Noodle
- Chicken Rice

Lipton's
- Country Vegetable Soup
- Noodle mixed with chicken broth
- Onion

Pepperridge Farm
- Petite Marmite Beef and Vegetable Soup

Sweet Life
- Vegetable Beef

Vegetables

General Foods
- Birds Eye vegetables without sauce or butter

Miscellaneous

General Mills Bacos
General Foods Log Cabin syrup (except Log Cabin buttered syrup)
Cream substitutes
- Borden Cremora
- Carnation Coffeemate

Peanut butter
- Jiff
- Peter Pan
- Planter's
- Sweet Life

FOOD INTOLERANCE

Diets from which a food or family of foods have been eliminated should be evaluated carefully and frequently to ensure that all essential nutrients are included in the diet. Calorie and protein requirements are the same as those for other children of the same age.

Diet Structure—Milk Free

See "Lactose-restricted Diet."

Diet Structure—Wheat-Free*†

FOOD GROUP	FOODS ALLOWED	FOODS RESTRICTED
Milk (2–3 servings)	Whole, lowfat, skim milk; evaporated milk; dry milk powder; buttermilk; cocoa; yogurt	None
Vegetable (2–3 servings)	All plain vegetables; any prepared with allowed flours	Any breaded, creamed, or prepared with wheat flour
Bread/starch (3–4 servings)	Breads made from allowed flours (corn, rice, potato, barley, oat, rye, arrowroot)	Breads, bread products, and crackers made from whole wheat, white, bread, all-purpose, cake, pastry, self-rising, wheat, graham, gluten, durum flours
	Any cereal not made from wheat, to which no wheat has been added in manufacture	
	White potatoes, sweet potatoes, rice	Wheat germ, wheat bran, farina, semolina, cracker meal, bread crumbs, malt
		Commercial pancake, waffle, biscuit, rolls, cake, bread mixes; rye bread or cornbread containing wheat flour
		Wheat cereals or pastas
Fruit (2 servings, 1 citrus)	All prepared and served products without wheat	None unless prepared or served with wheat products
Meat/meat alternates (4–6 oz)	Plain meats, prepared without wheat; peanut butter; eggs; dried peas, beans; cheese; all-meat hot dogs, bologna, lunch meats	Any creamed, breaded, or with wheat flour gravy; meats containing wheat fillers (hot dogs, bologna, lunch meats, meat loaf)
Fats (in moderation)	Butter, margarine, oils, shortening, pure mayonnaise, cream	Commercial salad dressings; gravy made with wheat flour
Beverages (in moderation)	Water, fruit juices, fruit drinks, carbonated beverages	Postum
Desserts (in moderation)	Homemade ice cream and sherbert; cornstarch, rice, and tapioca puddings; baked products made with allowed flours; custard; gelatin dessert; Bavarian cremes; mousse	Cakes, cookies, pastries, pie, ice cream cones, commercial frozen desserts, commercial frosting, mixes, puddings prepared with wheat flour
Soups (in moderation)	Any homemade soup with allowed ingredients	Soups thickened with wheat flour or containing noodles, alphabet noodles, or dumplings
Sweets (in moderation)	Sugar, honey, jelly, jam, corn syrup, maple syrup; candies made without wheat products; hard candy	Commercial candies, such as those with cream centers
Miscellaneous (in moderation)	Popcorn, pickles, olives, vinegar, cornstarch, catsup, mustard, herbs, spices, salt, pepper	Pretzels, some yeast MSG, some brands of soy sauce

*Products should be avoided if the following ingredients appear on the label: bran, buckwheat, buckwheat groats, farina, graham flour, malt, MSG (monosodium glutamate; not all MSG comes from wheat, but wheat is a common source), wheat flour, wheat germ, wheat gluten, wheat starch, white enriched flour, and whole-wheat flour.

†From *Pediatrics Diet Manual*, Saga Corporation, 1985. Used with permission.

Diet Structure—Egg-Free*†

FOOD GROUP	FOODS ALLOWED	FOODS RESTRICTED
Milk (2–3 servings)	All milk and milk drinks, cocoa, Ovaltine, yogurt	Malted cocoa drinks, any containing eggs or egg protein
Vegetable (2 servings)	All except those "restricted"	Any prepared vegetable combined with egg (e.g., souffle or with Hollandaise sauce)
Bread/starch (3–4 servings)	Homemade breads or bread products made without eggs; any breakfast cereal prepared without egg; plain dumplings, macaroni, spaghetti, noodles made without egg	Any commercial product or mix unless label shows no egg, egg powder, or albumin. Any bread or rolls with egg as an ingredient or brushed on top, pancakes, waffles, muffins, French toast, donuts unless made without egg
Fruit (2 servings, 1 citrus)	All fruits and juices prepared without egg	None
Meat/meal alternates (4–6 oz)	Any prepared without egg	Eggs, egg substitutes, meat loaf, sausages, loaves or croquettes with egg as a binding agent
Fats (in moderation)	Butter, margarine, vegetable fats and oils; salad dressings made without egg	Tartar sauce, Thousand Island dressing, mayonnaise, commercial salad dressings made with egg
Beverages (in moderation)	Coffee, tea, carbonated drinks, instant coffee	Any prepared with egg, root beer in which egg has been used as a foaming agent
Desserts (in moderation)	Homemade products prepared without egg, gelatin fruit and water ices	Custard, angel and sponge cake, macaroons, meringues, pie filling containing egg, ice creams, puddings, cakes and cookies made with egg
Soups	Any prepared with allowed ingredients	Alphabet and egg noodle soups, any soup cleared with egg (consommé, bouillon)
Sweets (in moderation)	Sugars, jams, jellies, candies made without egg	Marshmallows, divinities, chocolate candies brushed with egg for luster
Miscellaneous (in moderation)	Popcorn, nuts, olives, pickles, spices	Pretzels; any made with egg

*Products should be avoided if the following ingredients appear on the label: dried eggs, egg albumin (ovalbumin), egg white solids, egg whites, egg yolk solids, powdered eggs, and whole eggs.
†From *Pediatrics Diet Manual.* Saga Corporation, 1985. Used with permission.

B NATIONAL ORGANIZATIONS THAT AID CHILDREN WITH DEVELOPMENTAL DISABILITIES

Administration of Developmental Disabilities
330 Independence Ave. S.W.
Washington, DC 20201
(202) 245-7719

Association for Children with Learning Disabilities
4156 Library Rd.
Pittsburgh, PA 15234
(412) 341-1515

Council for Exceptional Children
1920 Association Dr.
Reston, VA 22091
(703) 620-3660

Epilepsy Foundation of America
4351 Garden City Dr.
Landover, MD 20785
(301) 459-3700

Hellen Keller National Center—Deaf/Blind
111 Middle Neck Rd.
Sands Point, NY 11050
(516) 944-8900 (voice or TTY)

March of Dimes
1275 Mamaroneck Ave.
White Plains, NY 10605
(914) 428-7100

Muscular Dystrophy Association Inc.
810 Seventh Ave.
New York, NY 10019
(212) 586-0808

National Association of Protection and Advocacy Systems
220 I St. N.E., Suite 150
Washington, DC 20001
(202) 546-8202
(Monitoring of architectural accessibility and equal rights)

National Association for Retarded Citizens
P.O. Box 6109
2501 Ave. J
Arlington, TX 76011
(800) 433-5255

National Easter Seal Society for Crippled Children and Adults, Inc.
70 E. Lake St.
Chicago, IL 60601
(312) 726-6200

National Information Center for Handicapped Children and Adults
7926 Jones Branch Dr., Suite 1100
McLean, VA 22102
(703) 893-6061

Spina Bifida Association of America
1700 Rockville Pike, Suite 540
Rockville, MD 20852
(301) 770-SBAA

United Cerebral Palsy Association of America
66 E. 34th St.
New York, NY 10016
(212) 481-6300

Variety Club International
1560 Broadway, Suite 1209
New York, NY 10036
(212) 704-9872
(For physically handicapped)

INDEX

F

J

K

L

M

N

Q

R

W